# Adult CNS Radiation Oncology

Eric L. Chang • Paul D. Brown • Simon S. Lo
Arjun Sahgal • John H. Suh

Editors

# Adult CNS Radiation Oncology

Principles and Practice

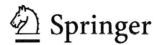 Springer

*Editors*

Eric L. Chang, MD, FASTRO
Department of Radiation Oncology
Keck School of Medicine of USC,
Norris Cancer Hospital
Los Angeles, CA
USA

Simon S. Lo, MB, ChB, FACR, FASTRO
Department of Radiation Oncology
University of Washington Medical Center
Seattle, WA
USA

John H. Suh, MD, FACR, FASTRO
Department of Radiation Oncology
Taussig Cancer Institute Cleveland Clinic
Cleveland, OH
USA

Paul D. Brown, MD
Department of Radiation Oncology
Mayo Clinic
Rochester, MN
USA

Arjun Sahgal, MD
Department of Radiation Oncology
Sunnybrook Health Sciences Centre
University of Toronto
Toronto, ON
Canada

ISBN 978-3-319-42877-2      ISBN 978-3-319-42878-9    (eBook)
https://doi.org/10.1007/978-3-319-42878-9

Library of Congress Control Number: 2018948825

Printed on acid-free paper

This Springer imprint is published by the registered company Springer International Publishing AG part of Springer Nature.
The registered company address is: Gewerbestrasse 11, 6330 Cham, Switzerland

*Adult Central Nervous System Radiation Oncology is dedicated to our parents, our families, and mentors who have greatly supported our careers.*

*We also dedicate this new textbook to countless patients who continue to motivate and inspire us. It is hoped that by disseminating and advancing knowledge through this new textbook, we will improve our collective capability to control disease, palliate patient suffering, and alleviate caregiver burden related to CNS disease.*

—Eric L. Chang, Paul D. Brown, Simon S. Lo,
Arjun Sahgal, John H. Suh, the editors

# Foreword

Thirty-one years ago, I became interested in adults patients with both benign and malignant brain tumors. I had to travel from the medical mecca of America (Boston) to do a mini-fellowship in San Francisco to work with Drs. Sheline, Liebel, Gutin, Larson, and Wilson—some of the most distinguished neuro-oncologists in the world—all in one institution (UCSF). In the first week of my time there, I saw more patients with benign and malignant brain tumors than I had in my entire residency in Boston. In San Francisco, I was exposed to research and clinical investigators, neuropathologists, and neuroradiologists who had dedicated their lives to improving the outcome for patients with these diseases. While the first comprehensive textbook on cancer had just been printed (*Cancer: Principles and Practice on Oncology*, Editors DeVita, Hellman, and Rosenberg), only a few chapters were dedicated to brain tumors. Fast-forward 31 years later and I am so excited to review this textbook completely dedicated to the role of radiation oncology in the treatment of these tumors.

Twenty years of studying the impact of treatment volume, fractionation schemes, dose, concurrent chemotherapy, and radiation sensitizers yielded little in the overall outcome for patients with malignant primary and metastatic disease. However, in the mid-1980s the introduction of MRI and internal and external stereotactic technologies allowed for better imaging definition of disease and the ability to deliver the most conformal treatments ever available. Intensity-modulated photons and protons soon followed to expand our armamentarium to increase dose and reduce late effects of radiation on normal brain tissue.

The editors and authors should be congratulated in putting together this fabulous new pedagogical addition to document where we are currently and where our dreams will take us in the future for the role of radiation in the treatment of our patients with brain tumors. I am particularly proud and humbled that I had a role in the training of two of the editors.

Boston, MA, USA                                                    Jay S. Loeffler, MD, FACR, FASTRO

# Preface

As active clinicians, educators, and researchers in the field of neuro-radiation oncology, the co-editors of this book identified a strong need to fill a gap in the medical textbook literature which until now lacked a modern comprehensive book dedicated to addressing the intersection of two important fields: radiation oncology and adult central nervous system (CNS) diseases.

The past two decades have witnessed remarkable developments and rapid advances in the field of neuro-radiation oncology, aided by image guidance, increasing sophistication of computers, software, radiation technology delivery, and ongoing development of molecular prognostic and predictive factors leading to improvements and refinement in the patient selection, and care of patients with CNS diseases.

Most recently, the World Health Organization classification of CNS tumors was updated in 2016 and now includes molecular subtypes in diagnoses as an important component. Therefore, indication for neuro-radiation oncology now requires an understanding of molecular diagnosis that will lead to appropriate utilization. Effective complication avoidance strategies employed when prescribing various forms of radiation therapy are more important than ever since patients with primary and secondary tumors of the CNS are now living longer than ever before.

This book is first organized into diseases afflicting the brain, skull base, and spine including benign tumors, vascular disorders and conditions, and malignant tumors. A chapter dealing with palliative radiation therapy of CNS tumors is also included. Then, radiation-related complications involving the brain, spinal cord, optic apparatus, neuroendocrine system, and neuro-cognition performance are covered. Finally, radiation treatment modalities including 3-D conformal therapy, intensity-modulated radiation therapy, LINAC-based radiosurgery, gamma knife, spine SBRT, proton beam therapy, and brachytherapy are addressed. Strategies to avoid CNS complications are covered across multiple chapters when appropriate, and radiation therapy is interwoven as a common theme in all chapters. Chapters include key learning objectives, and will frequently conclude with a highlighted case illustration, and self-assessment questions to help the reader consolidate their learning of the subject matter. It is hoped that this comprehensively organized book will help the reader achieve focused learning according to his/her own educational agenda and gain a thorough and nuanced understanding of specialty discipline of adult CNS radiation oncology.

Los Angeles, CA, USA                    Eric L. Chang, MD, FASTRO
Rochester, MN, USA                          Paul D. Brown, MD
Seattle, WA, USA              Simon S. Lo, MB, ChB, FACR, FASTRO
Toronto, ON, Canada                          Arjun Sahgal, MD
Cleveland, OH, USA              John H. Suh, MD, FACR, FASTRO

# Contents

# Editors and Contributors

## Editors

**Paul D. Brown, MD** Department of Radiation Oncology, Mayo Clinic, Rochester, MN, USA

**Eric L. Chang, MD, FASTRO** Department of Radiation Oncology, Keck School of Medicine of USC, Los Angeles, CA, USA

Radiation Oncology Program, Children's Center for Cancer and Blood Diseases, Children's Hospital Los Angeles, Los Angeles, CA, USA

Department of Radiation Oncology, University of Texas MD Anderson Cancer Center, Houston, TX, USA

**Simon S. Lo, MB, ChB, FACR, FASTRO** Department of Radiation Oncology, University of Washington, Seattle, WA, USA

Department of Neurological Surgery, University of Washington, Seattle, WA, USA

**Arjun Sahgal, MD** Department of Radiation Oncology, University of Toronto, Toronto, ON, Canada

Department of Radiation Oncology, Sunnybrook Odette Cancer Centre, Toronto, ON, Canada

**John H. Suh, MD, FACR, FASTRO** Department of Radiation Oncology, Taussig Cancer Institute, Cleveland Clinic, Cleveland, OH, USA

Rose Ella Burkhardt Brain Tumor and Neuro-oncology Center, Cleveland Clinic, Cleveland, OH, USA

## Contributors

**Chenue Abongwa, MD** Department of Pediatrics, Loma Linda University School of Medicine, Loma Linda, CA, USA

**Nima Alan, MD** Department of Neurological Surgery, University of Pittsburgh Medical Center, Pittsburgh, PA, USA

**Majed Alghamdi, MD** Department of Radiation Oncology, Sunnybrook Odette Cancer Centre, University of Toronto, Toronto, ON, Canada

Faculty of Medicine, Al Baha University, Al Baha, Saudi Arabia

**Andrea L. H. Arnett, MD, PhD** Department of Radiation Oncology, Mayo Clinic, Rochester, MN, USA

**Ehsan H. Balagamwala, MD** Department of Radiation Oncology, Taussig Cancer Institute, Cleveland Clinic, Cleveland, OH, USA

**Sushma Bellamkonda, MD** Department of Neurology, University of Tennessee Health Science Center, Memphis, TN, USA

**Vincent Bernard, MS** Department of Pathology, MD Anderson Cancer Center, Houston, TX, USA

**Jesse L. Berry, MD** USC Roski Eye Institute, Keck School of Medicine of USC, Los Angeles, CA, USA

**Markus Bredel, MD, PhD** Department of Radiation Oncology, University of Alabama at Birmingham, Birmingham, AL, USA

**Lindsay M. Burt, MD** Department of Radiation Oncology, University of Utah School of Medicine, Salt Lake City, UT, USA

Huntsman Cancer Institute, Salt Lake City, UT, USA

**Marc R. Bussière, MSc** Department of Radiation Oncology, Massachusetts General Hospital, Boston, MA, USA

**Alissa M. Butts, PhD** Department of Psychiatry and Psychology, Mayo Clinic, Rochester, MN, USA

**Annie Carbonneau, MD** Department of Radiation Oncology, Jewish General Hospital of Montreal, Montreal, QC, Canada

**Jane H. Cerhan, PhD, ABPP-CN** Department of Psychiatry and Psychology, Mayo Clinic, Rochester, MN, USA

**Samuel T. Chao, MD** Department of Radiation Oncology, Taussig Cancer Institute, Cleveland Clinic, Cleveland, OH, USA

Rose Ella Burkhardt Brain Tumor and Neuro-oncology Center, Cleveland Clinic, Cleveland, OH, USA

**Peter Y. Chen, MD, FACR** Department of Radiation Oncology, Beaumont Health System, Oakland University-William Beaumont School of Medicine, William Beaumont Hospital, Royal Oak, MI, USA

**Raymond Chiu, BS, CMD** Department of Radiation Oncology, Keck School of Medicine of University of Southern California, Los Angeles, CA, USA

**Caroline Chung, MD, MSc, FRCPC, CIP** Department of Radiation Oncology, University of Texas MD Anderson Cancer Center, Houston, TX, USA

**Gil'ad N. Cohen, MS** Department of Medical Physics, Memorial Sloan Kettering Cancer Center, New York, NY, USA

**Stephanie E. Combs, PhD, MD** Department of Radiation Oncology, Klinikum rechts der Isar, Technische Universität München, Munich, Bavaria, Germany

Institute of Innovative Radiotherapy (iRT), Department of Radiation Sciences (DRS), Helmholtz Zentrum München, Oberschleißheim, Bavaria, Germany

**Louis S. Constine, MD, FASTRO** Department of Radiation Oncology, University of Rochester Medical Center, Rochester, NY, USA

Department of Pediatrics, University of Rochester Medical Center, Rochester, NY, USA

**Antonio L. Damato, PhD** Department of Medical Physics, Memorial Sloan Kettering Cancer Center, New York, NY, USA

**Elena De Martin, MSc** Radiotherapy Unit, Department of Neurosurgery, C. Besta Neurological Institute Foundation, Milan, Italy

**Girish Dhall, MD** Neuro-Oncology Program, Children's Center for Cancer and Blood Diseases, Children's Hospital Los Angeles, Los Angeles, CA, USA

Department of Pediatrics, Keck School of Medicine of USC, Los Angeles, CA, USA

**Jorg Dietrich, MD, PhD** Department of Neuro-oncology, Massachusetts General Hospital, Boston, MA, USA

**Richard G. Everson, MD** Department of Neurosurgery, UCLA Medical Center, Los Angeles, CA, USA

**Alysa M. Fairchild, BSc, MD, FRCPC** Department of Radiation Oncology, Cross Cancer Institute, Edmonton, AB, Canada

**Laura Fariselli, MD** Radiotherapy Unit, Department of Neurosurgery, C. Besta Neurological Institute Foundation, Milan, Italy

**Sherise D. Ferguson, MD** Department of Neurosurgery, The University of Texas MD Anderson Cancer Center, Houston, TX, USA

**John B. Fiveash, MD** Department of Radiation Oncology, University of Alabama at Birmingham, Birmingham, AL, USA

**John C. Flickinger, MD** Department of Radiation Oncology, UPMC Presbyterian-Shadyside Hospital, University of Pittsburgh School of Medicine, Pittsburgh, PA, USA

**Senthilkumar Gandhidasan, MD** Department of Radiation Oncology, Illawarra Cancer Care Centre, Wollongong, NSW, Australia

**Peter Carlos Gerszten, MD, MPH, FACS** Department of Neurological Surgery, University of Pittsburgh Medical Center, Pittsburgh, PA, USA

Department of Radiation Oncology, University of Pittsburgh Medical Center, Pittsburgh, PA, USA

**Amol J. Ghia, MD** Department of Radiation Oncology, MD Anderson Cancer Center, Houston, TX, USA

**Lia M. Halasz, MD** Department of Radiation Oncology, University of Washington, Seattle, WA, USA

Department of Neurological Surgery, University of Washington, Seattle, WA, USA

**Sara J. Hardy, MD** Department of Radiation Oncology, University of Rochester Medical Center, Rochester, NY, USA

**Timothy J. Harris, MD, PhD** Department of Radiation Oncology, Virginia Commonwealth University, Richmond, VA, USA

**Richard L. S. Jennelle, MD** Department of Radiation Oncology, Keck School of Medicine of USC, Los Angeles, CA, USA

**Hideyuki Kano, MD, PhD** Department of Neurological Surgery, University of Pittsburgh, Pittsburgh, PA, USA

**Tania Kaprealian, MD** Department of Radiation Oncology, University of California, Los Angeles, Los Angeles, CA, USA

**Timothy J. Kaufmann, MD** Department of Radiology, Mayo Clinic, Rochester, MN, USA

**Jonathan W. Kim, MD** Children's Hospital Los Angeles, Keck School of Medicine of USC, Los Angeles, CA, USA

**Jonathan P. S. Knisely, MD** Department of Radiation Oncology, Weill Cornell School of Medicine, New York Presbyterian Hospital, New York, NY, USA

**Aryavarta M. S. Kumar, MD, PhD** Department of Radiation Oncology, Louis Stokes Cleveland VA Medical Center, Cleveland, OH, USA

**David A. Larson, MD, PhD** Department of Radiation Oncology, University of California San Francisco, San Francisco, CA, USA

**Young Lee, PhD** Department of Radiation Oncology, Sunnybrook Odette Cancer Centre, University of Toronto, Toronto, ON, Canada

**Jay S. Loeffler, MD, FACR, FASTRO** Department of Radiation Oncology, Massachusetts General Hospital, Boston, MA, USA

**L. Dade Lunsford, MD, FACS** Department of Neurological Surgery, University of Pittsburgh, Pittsburgh, PA, USA

**Lijun Ma, PhD** Department of Radiation Oncology, University of California San Francisco, San Francisco, CA, USA

**Marcello Marchetti, MD** Radiotherapy Unit, Department of Neurosurgery, C. Besta Neurological Institute Foundation, Milan, Italy

**G. Laura Masucci, MD** Department of Radiation Oncology, Centre Hospitalier de l'Universite de Montreal (CHUM), Montreal, QC, Canada

**Michael Mayinger, MD, MSc** Department of Radiation Oncology, Klinikum rechts der Isar, Technische Universität München, Munich, Bavaria, Germany

**Nicole McAllister, BS Radiation Health Physics, CMD** Department of Radiation Oncology, Keck School of Medicine of University of Southern California, Los Angeles, CA, USA

**Ian E. McCutcheon, MD** Department of Neurosurgery, The University of Texas MD Anderson Cancer Center, Houston, TX, USA

**Paul Medin, PhD** Department of Radiation Oncology, University of Texas Southwestern, Dallas, TX, USA

**Kenneth Wing Merrell, MD, MS** Department of Radiation Oncology, Mayo Clinic, Rochester, MN, USA

**Michael T. Milano, MD, PhD** Department of Radiation Oncology, University of Rochester Medical Center, Rochester, NY, USA

**Sarah A. Milgrom, MD** Department of Radiation Oncology, MD Anderson Cancer Center, Houston, TX, USA

**Fahad Momin, BS Medical Dosimetry, CMD** Department of Radiation Oncology, Keck School of Medicine of University of Southern California, Los Angeles, CA, USA

**Erin S. Murphy, MD** Department of Radiation Oncology, Taussig Cancer Institute, Cleveland Clinic, Cleveland, OH, USA

Rose Ella Burkhardt Brain Tumor and Neuro-oncology Center, Cleveland Clinic, Cleveland, OH, USA

**Sten Myrehaug, MD** Department of Radiation Oncology, Sunnybrook Odette Cancer Centre, University of Toronto, Toronto, ON, Canada

**Joshua D. Palmer, MD** Department of Radiation Oncology, The James Cancer Hospital and Solove Research Institute at The Ohio State University Wexner Medical Center, Columbus, OH, USA

**Shireen Parsai, MD** Department of Radiation Oncology, Taussig Cancer Institute, Cleveland Clinic, Cleveland, OH, USA

**Michael W. Parsons, PhD** Burkhardt Brain Tumor Center, Cleveland Clinic, Cleveland, OH, USA

**Luke E. Pater, MD** Department of Radiation Oncology, University of Cincinnati, Cincinnati, OH, USA

**Arnold C. Paulino, MD, FACR, FASTRO** Department of Radiation Oncology, MD Anderson Cancer Center, Houston, TX, USA

**David M. Peereboom, MD** Department of Medical Oncology, Taussig Cancer Institute, Cleveland Clinic, Cleveland, OH, USA

Rose Ella Burkhardt Brain Tumor and Neuro-Oncology Center, Cleveland Clinic, Cleveland, OH, USA

**Anthony Pham, MD** Department of Radiation Oncology, Keck School of Medicine of USC, Los Angeles, CA, USA

**Erqi L. Pollom, MD, MS** Department of Radiation Oncology, Stanford University, Stanford, CA, USA

**Richard A. Popple, PhD** Department of Radiation Oncology, University of Alabama at Birmingham, Birmingham, AL, USA

**Dheerendra Prasad, MD, MCh (Neurosurgery), FACRO** Department of Radiation Medicine and Neurosurgery, Roswell Park Comprehensive Cancer Center, Buffalo, NY, USA

**Anussara Prayongrat, MD** Department of Radiation Oncology, King Chulalongkorn Memorial Hospital, Bangkok, Thailand

**Morgan Prust, MD** Department of Neurology, Center for Neuro-Oncology, Massachusetts General Hospital, Harvard Medical School, Boston, MA, USA

**Dirk Rades, MD, PhD** Department of Radiation Oncology, University of Lübeck, Lübeck, Schleswig-Holstein, Germany

**Kristin Janson Redmond, MD, MPH** Department of Radiation Oncology and Molecular Radiation Services, Johns Hopkins University, Baltimore, MD, USA

**David Roberge, MD** Department of Radiation Oncology, Centre Hospitalier de l'Université de Montréal (CHUM), Montreal, QC, Canada

**C. Leland Rogers, MD, FACRO, FACR, FASTRO** Department of Radiation Oncology, Barrow Neurological Institute, Phoenix, AZ, USA

**David M. Routman, MD** Department of Radiation Oncology, Mayo Clinic, Rochester, MN, USA

**Raymond Sawaya, MD** Department of Neurosurgery, The University of Texas MD Anderson Cancer Center, Houston, TX, USA

**Steven E. Schild, MD** Department of Radiation Oncology, Mayo Clinic, Scottsdale, AZ, USA

**Ugur Selek, MD** Koc University, School of Medicine, Department of Radiation Oncology, Istanbul, Turkey

University of Texas, MD Anderson Cancer Center, Radiation Oncology Department, Houston, TX, USA

**Ismat Shafiq, MD** Division of Endocrinology and Metabolism, University of Rochester, Rochester, NY, USA

**Wenyin Shi, MD, PhD** Sidney Kimmel Cancer Center, Thomas Jefferson University, Philadelphia, PA, USA

**Helen A. Shih, MD, MS, MPH** Department of Radiation Oncology, Massachusetts General Hospital, Boston, MA, USA

**Dennis C. Shrieve, MD, PhD** Department of Radiation Oncology, University of Utah School of Medicine, Salt Lake City, UT, USA

Huntsman Cancer Institute, Salt Lake City, UT, USA

**Christina Snider, BA** Cleveland Clinic Lerner College of Medicine, Cleveland, OH, USA

**Hany Soliman, MD** Department of Radiation Oncology, Sunnybrook Odette Cancer Centre, University of Toronto, Toronto, ON, Canada

**Scott G. Soltys, MD** Department of Radiation Oncology, Stanford University, Stanford, CA, USA

**Andrew Song, MD** Sidney Kimmel Cancer Center, Thomas Jefferson University, Philadelphia, PA, USA

**Paul W. Sperduto, MD, MPP, FASTRO** Minneapolis Radiation Oncology and Gamma Knife Center, University of Minnesota Medical Center, Minneapolis, MN, USA

**Timothy D. Struve, MD** Department of Radiation Oncology, University of Cincinnati, Cincinnati, OH, USA

**Gita Suneja, MD, MSHP** Department of Radiation Oncology, Duke University Medical Center, Durham, NC, USA

**Jaipreet S. Suri, MD** Department of Radiation Oncology, University of Rochester Medical Center/James P. Wilmot Cancer Center, Rochester, NY, USA

**Amandeep Singh Taggar, MD, MSC** Department of Radiation Oncology, Sunnybrook Odette Cancer Center, Toronto, ON, Canada

Department of Radiation Oncology, University of Toronto, Toronto, ON, Canada

**Evan M. Thomas, MD, PhD** Department of Radiation Oncology, University of Alabama at Birmingham, Birmingham, AL, USA

**Martin C. Tom, MD** Department of Radiation Oncology, Taussig Cancer Institute, Cleveland Clinic, Cleveland, OH, USA

**Erkan Topkan, MD** Baskent Department of Radiation Oncology, University Adana Medical Faculty, Adana, Turkey

**Nicholas Trakul, MD, PhD** Department of Radiation Oncology, Stanford University, Stanford, CA, USA

**Chia-Lin Tseng, MD** Department of Radiation Oncology, Sunnybrook Odette Cancer Centre, University of Toronto, Toronto, ON, Canada

**Yolanda D. Tseng, MD** Department of Radiation Oncology, University of Washington, Seattle, WA, USA

**Christina I. Tsien, MD** Department of Radiation Oncology, Washington University School of Medicine, St. Louis, MO, USA

**G. Edward Vates, MD, PhD, FACS** Department of Neurosurgery, University of Rochester Medical Center, Rochester, NY, USA

**Balamurugan A. Vellayappan, MBBS, FRANZCR, MCI** Department of Radiation Oncology, National University Cancer Institute, National University Health System, Singapore, Singapore

**Gregory Vlacich, MD, PhD** Department of Radiation Oncology, Washington University in St. Louis, St. Louis, MO, USA

Department of Radiation Oncology, Washington University School of Medicine, St. Louis, St. Louis, MO, USA

**Laszlo Voros, MS, DABR** Department of Medical Physics, Memorial Sloan Kettering Cancer Center, New York, NY, USA

**Kathryn M. Wagner, MD** Department of Neurosurgery, Baylor College of Medicine, Houston, TX, USA

**Paul Y. Windisch** Department of Molecular Genetics, German Cancer Research Center (DKFZ), Heidelberg, Germany

**Kenneth Wong, MD** Department of Radiation Oncology, Keck School of Medicine of USC, Los Angeles, CA, USA

Department of Radiation Oncology, Children's Center for Cancer and Blood Diseases, Children's Hospital Los Angeles, Los Angeles, CA, USA

**Shun Wong, MD** Department of Radiation Oncology, Sunnybrook Odette Cancer Centre, University of Toronto, Toronto, ON, Canada

**Joachim Yahalom, MD** Department of Radiation Oncology, Memorial Sloan Kettering Cancer Center, New York, NY, USA

**Yoshiya Yamada, MD** Department of Radiation Oncology, Memorial Sloan Kettering Cancer Center, New York, NY, USA

**Masaaki Yamamoto, MD, PhD** Department of Neurosurgery, Katsuta Hospital Mito Gamma House, Hitachi-naka, Ibaraki, Japan

**Jenny Yan, MS** Department of Radiation Oncology and Molecular Radiation Services, Johns Hopkins Hospital, Baltimore, MD, USA

**Jason Ye, MD** Department of Radiation Oncology, Keck School of Medicine of USC, Los Angeles, CA, USA

**Debra Nana Yeboa, MD** Department of Radiation Oncology, The University of Texas MD Anderson Cancer Center, Houston, TX, USA

**Divya Yerramilli, MD, MBE** Harvard Radiation Oncology Program, Department of Radiation Oncology, Massachusetts General Hospital, Boston, MA, USA

**Paul Youn, MD** Department of Radiation Oncology, University of Rochester Medical Center/James P. Wilmot Cancer Center, Rochester, NY, USA

**Isabella Zhang, MD** Department of Radiation Medicine, Northwell Health, Lake Success, NY, USA

# Part I

## Brain Tumors: Benign

# Meningioma

1

Timothy J. Harris, Samuel T. Chao, and C. Leland Rogers

## Learning Objectives

- Epidemiology and natural history of meningiomas.
- The role of surgery in the management of meningiomas.
- Various radiation modalities used for meningiomas, specifically external beam radiation therapy and stereotactic radiosurgery.
- Guidelines for utilization of radiation for meningiomas, depending on extent of resection and grade.

## Background

Meningiomas are typically characterized as benign tumors that ostensibly arise from arachnoid cap cells in the dura. However, 20–30% of meningiomas are WHO grade II or III and have aggressive features that result in a higher risk of recurrence, morbidity, and mortality [1]. Symptoms from meningioma may arise from local mass effect on the brain, cranial nerves, or vasculature which, depending upon tumor location and extent, may include motor and sensory deficits, vision loss, diplopia and other cranial nerve deficits, cerebellar dysfunction, headaches, and/or seizure. Surgery and radiation (including conventional and stereotactic radiosurgery) are the mainstays of treatment.

T. J. Harris
Department of Radiation Oncology, Virginia Commonwealth University, Richmond, VA, USA

S. T. Chao
Department of Radiation Oncology, Taussig Cancer Institute, Cleveland Clinic, Cleveland, OH, USA

Rose Ella Burkhardt Brain Tumor and Neuro-oncology Center, Cleveland Clinic, Cleveland, OH, USA

C. L. Rogers (✉)
Department of Radiation Oncology, Barrow Neurological Institute, Phoenix, AZ, USA

Chemotherapy, hormonal therapy, immunotherapy, and targeted therapies are being investigated, but to date, none has been shown to have a frontline role. Some meningiomas persist or recur after multiple surgeries and radiation, and therapeutic advances are clearly needed to optimize management for these challenging patients. Leading the way, trials from the Radiation Therapy Oncology Group (RTOG 0539) and the European Organisation for Research and Treatment of Cancer (EORTC 22042-26042) have helped blaze the path by prospectively studying the role of radiation for meningioma, including patients with recurrence. This chapter will review the practical management of patients with meningioma.

## Epidemiology

It is estimated that 27,000 new cases of meningioma will be diagnosed in the United States in 2017 [2, 3]. This represents 8 cases per 100,000 people, rendering meningioma the most prevalent primary intracranial neoplasm, accounting for approximately 37% of all primary brain tumors [3, 4]. These numbers are likely an underestimate of actual cases as meningioma has been discovered in as many as 2% of people in autopsy studies [5].

Meningiomas, much less common in the pediatric population, are most frequently diagnosed in the sixth and seventh decades of life; however, they remain the second most common CNS tumor in adolescents and young adults (ages 15–30) after tumors of the pituitary gland. With more frequent use of MRIs, particularly in evaluation of uncomplicated headaches, we may find the age at diagnosis, especially for subclinical meningiomas, to decrease [2, 6, 7]. Considering all WHO tumor grades, meningioma is more common in women than men. Nonmalignant meningiomas are identified two- to threefold more frequently in females than males [3, 8, 9]. This predilection is less apparent in childhood and with higher-grade histology. Males may be more likely to develop anaplastic (WHO Grade III) meningioma [3].

## Risk Factors

There are well-documented associations in the development of meningiomas with specific genetic, environmental, and hormonal risk factors; however, the majority is diagnosed without a known cause.

## Genetic Syndromes

Type 2 neurofibromatosis is a rare genetic syndrome that most commonly occurs due to cytogenetic alteration in the NF2 (Merlin) gene found on chromosome 22q12 [10, 11]. Patients with NF2 are more prone to develop schwannomas and meningiomas [12, 13]. Development of meningiomas in patients with NF2 usually occurs at a younger age compared to patients without this germline mutation.

Multiple endocrine neoplasia type 1 (MEN1) is another rare genetic syndrome with a possible association of increased risk of meningioma [13, 14]. Patients usually have a mutation in the MEN1 gene on chromosome 11q13, which encodes the protein menin. Such patients may present with neoplasias of the pituitary, parathyroid, and pancreas, but meningioma were also found in this patient population at a higher frequency than that of the general population.

## Radiation

Exposure to ionizing radiation is an accepted risk factor for meningioma. Data supporting radiation-induced meningioma largely comes from children treated with scalp irradiation for maladies such as tinea capitis, as well as from atomic bomb survivors [15–19]. In one study of children who immigrated to Israel following World War II treated with scalp irradiation for tinea capitis, there was a sevenfold increase in neoplasms of the central nervous system, diagnosed an average of 18 years following radiotherapy. Out of 11,000 patients treated with scalp irradiation, there were 19 incidences of meningioma and 7 of glioma [18]. Another study estimated the risk of developing a radiation-induced meningioma at 0.53% and 8.18% at 5- and 25-year postradiation, respectively [19].

## Staging/Diagnosis

Staging is not used for meningiomas, but diagnosis and pathology are critical to treatment decision-making. The preponderance of data regarding the clinical presentation of meningioma comes from surgical series. This results in a bias toward symptomatic tumors. Symptoms depend largely on the location and size of the tumor and can further be influenced by the presence of cerebral edema. Whereas sphenoid wing meningiomas may present with seizures, skull base meningiomas can present with cranial nerve deficits [20, 21]. With the increasing use of contrast-enhanced CT and MRI for the evaluation of head trauma and headache, the number of incidentally diagnosed meningiomas has risen.

Meningiomas are typically diagnosed or suspected following contrast-enhanced neuroimaging, classically appearing on MRI as an enhancing extra-axial mass with a dural tail [22–25]. Calcifications, which may be present and best visualized on unenhanced CT, have occurred more commonly in lower-grade lesions [26]. Either benign or higher-grade meningiomas can invade the bone. Necrosis or brain invasion may also be noted on MRI and portend higher grade.

Meningiomas can generally be identified by imaging with relatively high reliability. Differential diagnoses include, among other entities, dural-based metastases, schwannoma, and hemangiopericytoma. The majority of cases of dural-based metastases occur in patients with known metastatic cancer. Thus in a patient with no personal history of malignancy, and with no evidence of an extracranial primary lesion or metastatic disease, an isolated dural-based metastasis is rare. Although a consideration, hemangiopericytoma is rare, accounting for less than 1% of CNS tumors. While the common imaging characteristics of meningioma are largely diagnostically predictive, there is far less certainty determining tumor grade by imaging. Appreciating this, WHO Grade I meningiomas, associated with slower growth, more often exhibit homogeneous enhancement, calcifications, iso- or hypo-intense T2 signal, and smooth surface contour [22–25]. Advanced imaging may ultimately predict aggressive features with greater certainty, but to date, multiple studies of MR spectroscopy, diffusion-weighted MR, MR perfusion, and positron-emission tomography have not identified definitive correlations between imaging findings and pathologic grade [27–34].

## Prognostic/Predictive Factors Including Pathology

Meningiomas likely derive from arachnoid cap cells, the epithelioid cells on the outer surface of arachnoid villi. Arachnoid cap cells are cytologically similar to meningioma. Arachnoid cap cells are as well found in greater number at sites where meningioma more commonly occurs, and increase with age in keeping with the age-related incidence of meningioma [1].

The WHO recently published new meningioma grading criteria in 2016. Building upon the prior criteria of 2000 and 2007, the new grading parameters solidify brain invasion as an independent criterion for WHO Grade II, and as with the prior two iterations incorporate mitotic activity, sheet-like growth, hypercellularity, nucleolar prominence, nuclear-to-cytoplasmic ratio, spontaneous necrosis, and certain meningioma variants into the assignment of grade. Strong associations between grade, recurrence-free survival, and overall survival have now been independently validated [35–37].

Before adoption of the 2000 WHO criteria, Grade II histology was identified in approximately 5% of meningiomas. However, with incorporation of the recent criteria, 20–35% of meningiomas are identified as Grade II. Based upon the most recent 2016 definitions, a WHO Grade II (atypical) meningioma has 4–19 mitoses per 10 high-power field (hpf), brain invasion, or exhibits three of five atypical features (sheeting architecture, hypercellularity, prominent nucleoli, high nuclear/cytoplasmic ratio, necrosis). Choroidal and clear cell meningiomas are also defined as WHO Grade II. WHO Grade III, also referred to as malignant or anaplastic, is defined by 20 or greater mitoses per 10 hpf, frank anaplasia, or papillary or rhabdoid meningioma variants. These are aggressive tumors, but with modern grading, only about 1–3% of meningiomas are WHO Grade III. Atypical or malignant histology carries a higher risk of recurrence, morbidity, and mortality and, thus, influences management [1]. Extent of resection may influence risk of recurrence and survival, which will be discussed later in this chapter as part of management.

## Multimodality Management

### WHO Grade I Meningiomas

#### Surgery

Surgery remains the primary therapy for meningiomas, and numerous publications have demonstrated relationship between resection extent and recurrence. Simpson, in 1957, reported on 265 patients managed with surgery and carefully described resection extent [38]. Based on this data, Simpson resection grades, still in common usage, were defined [38]. Table 1.1 summarizes the Simpson resection grades, along with the rate of clinical recurrence he reported for each grade. Contemporary surgical series have generally confirmed the association between the degree of resection of the meningioma, adjacent dura and any involved bone, and local recurrence.

There have been some contemporary surgical series that challenge the Simpson grading scheme. In one study, there was no significant difference in 5-year progression-free survival when comparing Simpson Grades I through IV [39]. Others have reported no significant difference in local progression risk with Simpson Grades I–III, although typically with improved progression-free survival comparing Grades I–III with Grade IV surgery [40, 41]. However, in support of

**Table 1.1** Simpson grade

| Simpson grade | Definition of resection extent | Clinically apparent recurrence risk |
|---|---|---|
| I | Gross total resection of tumor, dural attachments, and abnormal bone | 9% |
| II | Gross total resection of tumor, coagulation of dural attachments | 19% |
| III | Gross total resection of tumor without resection or coagulation of dural attachments or extradural extensions (e.g., invaded or hyperostotic bone) | 29% |
| IV | Partial resection of tumor | 44% |
| V | Simple decompression (biopsy) | N/A |

Definition of Simpson resection grade according to Donald Simpson's initial publication [38]. All recurrences were clinically apparent. Some were confirmed at reoperation or necropsy

**Table 1.2** Local recurrence risk following gross total resection

| First author | Year | n | 5-year (%) | 10-year (%) | 15-year |
|---|---|---|---|---|---|
| Mirimanoff | 1985 | 145 | 7 | 20 | 32% |
| Taylor | 1988 | 90 | 13[a] | 25[a] | 33%[a] |
| Condra | 1997 | 175 | 7 | 20 | 24% |
| Stafford | 1998 | 465 | 12 | 25 | – |
| Soyuer | 2004 | 48 | 23 | 39 | 60%[a] |
| McGovern | 2010 | 124 | 27 | 53[a] | 68%[a] |
| Gousias | 2016 | 901 | 12 | 18 | 21%[a] |
| | Total | 1976 | 7–27 | 18–53 | 21–68% |

Reported risks of local recurrence at 5, 10, and 15 years from several studies with long-term follow-up after gross total resection of a known or presumed Grade I meningioma. Many of these patients were treated predating modern WHO grading criteria
[a]Actuarial data taken from graph

findings from earlier series, a recent, large report by Hasseleid analyzed 391 patients and found a significant difference in progression-free survival comparing outcomes with Simpson Grade I, Grades II and III, and Grades IV and V [42]. Together the majority of reports support the use of Simpson's grading system and suggest that, similar to gliomas, the surgical goal should be maximal safe removal of tumor, which for many convexity meningiomas would be gross total and correspond to Simpson Grades I–III. Indeed, Simpson Grades I–III resection is achieved in up to 95% of convexity tumors and about two-thirds of all meningiomas treated surgically [43]. For WHO Grade I meningioma, a gross total resection is considered definitive therapy; however, with long follow-up, local recurrence after gross total resection is not infrequent. As shown in Table 1.2, single-institution reports with long-term follow-up have identified local recurrence in 7–27% at 5 years, 18–53% at 10 years, and 21–68% at 15 years [37, 40, 44, 45].

As one might expect, subtotal resection (Simpson Grades IV and V) has resulted in considerably higher rates of progression in most studies. As reviewed in Table 1.3,

**Table 1.3** Local recurrence risk following subtotal resection

| Author | Year | n | 5-year (%) | 10-year (%) | 15-year |
|---|---|---|---|---|---|
| Wara (UCSF) | 1975 | 58 | 47 | 62 | – |
| Mirimanoff (MGH) | 1985 | 80 | 37 | 55 | 91% |
| Barbaro (UCSF)[a] | 1987 | 30 | 40 | 100[a] | – |
| Miralbell (MGH)[a] | 1992 | 79 | 40 | 52 | – |
| Condra (U Florida) | 1997 | 55 | 47 | 60 | 70% |
| Stafford (Mayo) | 1998 | 116 | 39 | 61 | – |
| Soyuer (MDA) | 2004 | 32 | 62 | 82[a] | 87%[a] |
| McGovern (MDA) | 2010 | 69 | 63 | 75[a] | 87%[a] |
| | Total | 519 | 37–63 | 52–100 | 70–91% |

Reported progression risks at 5, 10, and 15 years from several studies with long-term follow-up after subtotal resection of a known or presumed Grade I meningioma. Many of these patients were treated predating modern WHO grading criteria
[a]Actuarial data taken from graph

single-institution reports have identified local progression following subtotal resection of benign meningioma in 37–63% of patients at 5 years, 52–100% at 10 years, and 70–91% at 15 years [9, 40, 44–46]. Furthermore, in one study cause-specific survival was significantly decreased in patients receiving subtotal compared to gross total resection, with 15-year cause-specific survival 51% versus 88%, respectively [40].

## Radiotherapy

For WHO Grade I meningioma, gross total resection is considered definitive treatment. However, as detailed in Table 1.2, with extended follow-up, even following gross total resection of a WHO Grade I meningioma, there remains considerable local recurrence risk. In a contemporary study, recurrence following gross total resection was 23% at 5 years, 39% at 10 years, and 60% at 15 years [46]. A more recent report confirmed a high recurrence risk, approximately 65% at 15 years [37]. It can be postulated that the higher rates of recurrence in recent series are the result of improved surveillance imaging. For patients with subtotal resection, the risk of long-term progression is, as expected, greater, 70% or more at 15 years [40, 45, 46].

For a WHO Grade I tumor that either recurs following gross total resection or is not gross totally resected, radiotherapy is the only validated nonsurgical intervention. Radiotherapy is commonly delivered with conventionally fractionated (1.8–2.0 Gy per fraction) external beam approaches or via stereotactic radiosurgery, whether single fraction or hypofractionation.

### External Beam Radiotherapy

Numerous retrospective studies have demonstrated improvement in progression-free survival with conventionally fractionated external beam radiotherapy as a definitive therapy for unresected tumors, as an adjuvant to subtotal resection, and as salvage for recurrence or progression. External beam radiotherapy may also be employed as definitive therapy for tumors diagnosed radiographically or via biopsy. Imaging alone is the appropriate method of diagnosis for optic nerve sheath meningioma, and the diagnosis is commonly reached in this fashion for patients who either refuse biopsy or surgery, or are not appropriate candidates. Imaging has also been used in many series as the sole method of diagnosis preceding radiosurgery. In contemporary studies, 5- to 10-year rates of progression-free survival and local control rates following primary external beam radiation therapy (EBRT) or stereotactic radiosurgery (SRS) have been approximately 90%, readily comparable with local control rates after gross total resection [47–54].

Optic nerve sheath meningiomas are an illustrative subgroup. They arise from the meningeal lining of the optic nerve. Growth rates are typically slow, but eventually the optic nerve and/or its vascular supply may become compromised. Surgical resection is technically possible but is associated with a high risk of vision loss from disruption of blood supply to the optic nerve. The standard therapy for optic nerve sheath meningioma is radiotherapy without biopsy or resection. From multiple clinical experiences, local control with conventionally fractionated radiotherapy is approximately 95%, which is readily comparable to local control of meningioma at other intracranial sites with fractionated EBRT, with radiosurgery, or with gross total resection. Moreover, vision often improves with EBRT [55–58].

### Dose and Toxicities

Recommended doses for external beam radiotherapy for WHO Grade I meningiomas generally range from 45 to 54 Gy in 1.8–2.0 Gy fractions. Goldsmith and colleagues suggested improved 10-year local control with doses greater than 52 Gy; however, in further analysis, this was not established unequivocally [59]. In one study, there was no correlation between the local control and dose ranging from approximately 36 Gy to as high as 79.5 Gy in 1.5–2.0 Gy fractions [60]. In general WHO Grade I meningiomas are treated to approximately 54 Gy in 1.8–2.0 Gy fractions, but this may be reduced (e.g., 50 Gy) when the optic pathway is involved or abuts the gross disease. A total dose in the range of 45–54 Gy has been effective for optic nerve sheath meningioma, appreciating that meningiomas at this site tend to be smaller when diagnosed and treated [55, 57, 58, 61].

Peritumoral edema occurs frequently with intracranial meningioma, whether at diagnosis or following radiation therapy, particularly radiosurgery. The reported rates of edema preceding treatment vary depending upon how it is defined, for instance, by imaging findings alone or by signs or symptoms. A wide range of rates between 11 and 92% have been reported [62–64].

As a sequela of treatment, intracranial edema occurs less frequently following fractionated external beam irradiation than single-fraction radiosurgery [65].

Edema, and in particular symptomatic edema, has been rarely reported following conventionally fractionated external beam radiotherapy and appears to occur in approximately 1% of patients so treated [65]. Selch and colleagues serially evaluated patients for post-external beam radiotherapy edema, and in 45 patients none had developed post treatment edema, with median follow-up of 3 years [66]. In a separate study by Tanzler and colleagues, 2 of 146 patients—or 1.4%—developed edema following external beam radiotherapy [67].

Cranial neuropathies are rare when radiation doses are kept to 54 Gy or less and dose per fraction is 2 Gy or less. One report, evaluating 140 patients, found only five complications related to external beam radiotherapy including retinopathy, optic neuropathy, and brain necrosis [59]. Another found no optic pathway complications when median the dose was 50.4 Gy in 2 Gy fractions or less [68]. Regarding the cavernous sinus, Selch et al. found no cases of cranial neuropathies with doses of 50.4 Gy [66].

## Stereotactic Radiosurgery

Stereotactic radiosurgery is a newer technique than conventionally fractionated radiotherapy but has been utilized extensively in the treatment of meningioma over the past three decades. The reported rates of 5- and 10-year local control have been excellent, commonly 90% or greater [69–71].

Given the excellent local control and limited edema and other side-effect risks with conventionally fractionated external beam radiotherapy, patient selection for stereotactic radiosurgery is crucial. In general, smaller lesions (10 cc and less) with well-defined borders located at a suitable distance (approximately 5 mm or more) from critical structures are good candidates for stereotactic radiosurgery. Parasagittal meningiomas are at higher risk of peritumoral edema, especially those with preexisting edema, so this needs to be considered when deciding on radiation approach [72].

Marginal doses of 12–16 Gy have been found to confer local control of 90% or greater at 5 years and over 80% at 10 years. Ganz and colleagues reported that marginal doses of 10 Gy or less resulted in greater local failure risk than 12 Gy or higher [73, 74]. Stafford and colleagues found no improvement in local control with dose in excess of 16 Gy [7]. Likewise, Kondziolka and colleagues found no benefit in doses above 15 Gy [75].

Regarding tumor size, there does appear to be inferior local control with larger lesions. DiBiase and colleagues reported 92% 5-year local control with lesions ≤10 cc, compared with 68% exceeding 10 cc[76]. Additionally, Pollock et al. found less treatment-related toxicity with smaller lesions (<9.6 cc) [77].

Traditionally stereotactic radiosurgery has been delivered in a single session, but there are now many reports of hypofractionated stereotactic radiotherapy, a common fractionation scheme being 25 Gy in 5 fractions. In multiple studies this appears to have local control similar to single-fraction radiosurgery, potentially with fewer side effects, particularly edema [78, 79].

There remains considerable controversy regarding the management of patients with WHO Grade I meningioma. There is a broad consensus that gross total resection of a newly diagnosed WHO Grade I meningioma is definitive but little consensus regarding the optimal approach to patients following subtotal resection or following recurrence of a benign tumor. Figure 1.1 shows a bar and whiskers plot comparing results from gross total resection (GTR), subtotal resection (STR), STR with fractionated external beam radiation therapy (EBRT), EBRT alone, and stereotactic radiosurgery (SRS). The studies evaluated are those using modern WHO grading parameters.

## WHO Grade II (Atypical) Meningioma

### Surgery

Prior to the year 2000, WHO Grade II meningioma was diagnosed in only approximately 5% of cases; however, with the updated 2000, 2007, and now 2016 WHO criteria, atypical meningioma is now identified in 20–35% of cases. It cannot be overstated that when reviewing the literature for management of atypical meningioma, care must be given to identify what grading system was used to distinguish atypical meningioma and, even if WHO standards were used, whether the criteria predated WHO 2000.

There is a general consensus that postoperative radiotherapy is of benefit following subtotal resection of WHO Grade II meningioma, but this is by no means uniform and is amenable to discussion given the lack of prospective data. In a recent publication from McGill University, only 4 of 30 patients with a subtotally resected WHO Grade II meningioma received postoperative radiation [80]. Goyal and colleagues reported on 22 patients with atypical meningioma, 8 of whom received radiotherapy. Ten-year local control was only 17%, and they found no significant improvement with radiotherapy [81]. However, several recent studies using modern WHO grading parameters have found improvements in progression-free survival with postoperative RT following GTR or STR [42, 80, 82–87].

With respect to adjuvant RT following Simpson Grade I GTR of a WHO Grade II meningioma, Aghi et al. used modern grading criteria and with mean follow-up of 39 months found a 5-year local recurrence risk of 50% in 100 patients after GTR alone [87]. A small cohort ($n = 8$) received adjuvant radiotherapy following GTR, with no recurrences. In a

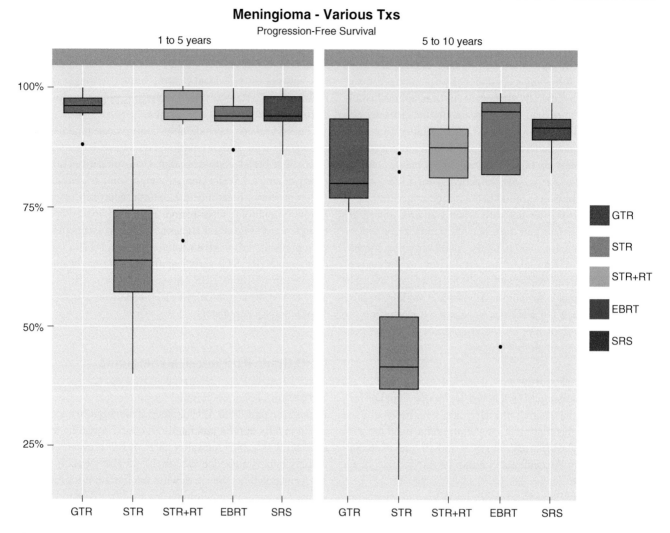

**Fig. 1.1** Progression-free survival (PFS) rates in patients with meningioma in the era of modern microsurgery and/or fractionated radiation therapy (RT) or radiosurgery (RS). The outcomes are grouped by median duration of clinical and radiographic follow-up (1–5 years [left panel] and 5–10 years [right panel]) and mode of treatment (gross total resection [GTR], subtotal resection [STR], STR + RT, RT, and RS). [Courtesy of Igor Barani, Barrow Neurological Institute 2017]

separate contemporary study, GTR alone (Simpson Grades I–II) resulted in 42% recurrence rate at 5 years versus 20% with the addition of adjuvant radiotherapy [85]. In patients with recurrent WHO Grade II meningioma, neither repeat surgery nor salvage radiotherapy reliably provide durable tumor control. Aghi and colleagues noted that following first recurrence, 10-year disease-specific survival was reduced to 69%, even with active treatment interventions [87]. Additionally, Komotar and colleagues concluded that recurrence of a WHO Grade II meningioma resulted in worsened overall survival [85]. Talacchi et al. have shown that, for atypical meningioma, both the disease-free interval and the pattern of progression change with successive recurrence [88]. The mean interval declines from about 33 months with first recurrence down to 5–10 months with fourth or fifth recurrence. This occurs even when histologic grade remains

unchanged. Stable histology grade at recurrence is seen on about 80% of cases [89]. A large retrospective study by Kessel and colleagues found no survivors at 15 years following recurrence of a WHO Grade II meningioma, compared with 64% in patients without recurrence [90]. There is thus compelling justification in a management strategy that decreases recurrence risk if this can be safely achieved.

## Radiotherapy

### External Beam Radiotherapy

Based on the above data demonstrating detriment in survival following recurrence of WHO Grade II meningioma, many clinicians recommend postoperative radiotherapy for atypical meningioma regardless of the extent of resection. However, others, including Goyal [81], Hardesty [91], and

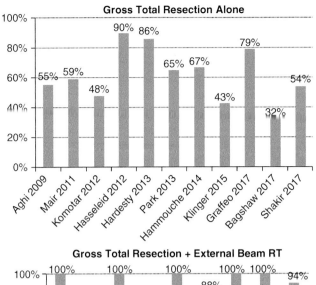

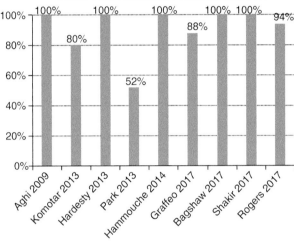

Fig. 1.2 Five-year progression-free survival for gross total resection (GTR) versus GTR and external beam irradiation. Note: in the Park 2013 study the majority of patients (67%) were treated prior to three-dimensional techniques

Jenkinson [92], have found no clear improvement in disease control with postoperative radiotherapy and have concluded that it should not be routinely recommended, especially following GTR. Figure 1.2 compiles recent data with modern grading and compares 5-year PFS following GTR alone or GTR and external beam RT. This suggests a benefit to adjuvant RT, but with the cited data to the contrary, randomized trials are required in order to resolve this important controversy. Two phase III cooperative group studies are currently addressing adjuvant RT following complete resection: the ROAM trial and NRG BN-003.

Based on a completed phase II clinical trial, NRG/RTOG 0539, and the current NRG BN-003 phase III trial, the dose recommendations for patients following GTR are 54–59.4 Gy in 1.8 Gy fractions. Following STR or recurrence, 59.4–60 Gy with standard fractionation (1.8–2.0 Gy) is conventional [93]. More data will be required to better establish

optimal dosing for patients with gross residuum. The phase II EORTC 22042-26042 trial employed a boost to 70 Gy after subtotal surgery.

**Stereotactic Radiosurgery**

Stereotactic radiosurgery (SRS) has generally been employed in the setting of residual/recurrent disease. Stafford and colleagues reported on 13 patients (12 % of their patient cohort) with atypical meningioma treated with radiosurgery. The median marginal dose was 16 Gy and resulted in 5-year local control of 68% compared to 93% for patients with WHO Grade I histology [7]. Harris and colleagues reported on 30 patients with non-benign meningiomas treated with SRS, of which 18 were WHO grade II. Five-year progression-free survival (PFS) was 83% [94]. Huffman and colleagues treated 15 patients with atypical meningioma, median 16 Gy; local control was 60% [95]. Kano et al. reviewed 12 patients with non-benign meningioma (10 WHO Grade II) with SRS, mean margin dose 18 Gy. Five-year PFS was 48%; they found improved PFS with 20 Gy or higher [96].

Attia and colleagues evaluated dose and conformality index, defined as the prescription dose volume divided by the tumor volume. Local recurrence was described as progression within 2 cm of the original tumor margin. With radiosurgery at a median 14 Gy, 5-year local control was 44%. Lower conformality index associated with in-field and marginal failure, but when conformality index was considered, margin dose was not predictive of local control [97]. This raises interesting questions, such as whether higher doses employed for WHO Grade II meningioma in some radiosurgery studies might, in part, be a proxy for a larger conformality index and whether the appropriate target for higher-grade meningiomas exceeds new or residual enhancing tumor alone [98].

Several studies have suggested that atypical meningioma often progresses outside the SRS target yet inside the initial tumor and resection bed. Huffmann reported 15 patients treated with single-fraction radiosurgery to a median 16 Gy. At 18–36 months, 9 were progression-free, for a crude local control rate of 60%. Six (40%) progressed, one (17%) in field, but all within the surgical approach or resection bed [95]. Similarly, Choi reported 25 WHO Grade II patients treated to a median dose of 22 Gy in 1–4 fractions; 9 developed recurrence, 3 (33%) within the targeted region, 5 (56%) elsewhere in the resection bed, and 1 (11%) in both regions [99]. Recently Zhang [100] reported 5-year locoregional control of 36% after SRS for atypical meningioma and Valery [101] a 3-year PFS of 23%. In both these analyses, many of the recurrences were regional. These findings imply that a volume beyond residual or recurrent enhancement is at risk, including the entire tumor and resection bed. Hypofractionated SRS or standard fractionation external beam approaches may safely and effectively address this important issue.

## WHO Grade III (Anaplastic/Malignant) Meningioma

WHO Grade III meningiomas account for about 1–2% of newly diagnosed meningiomas. As a result there are fewer than 500 newly diagnosed malignant meningiomas annually in the United States. There thus is far less data to guide management than for patients with WHO Grade I or II meningioma. However, anaplastic meningiomas behave aggressively, with significantly poorer local control and overall survival than lower-grade meningiomas. In some studies, median overall survival has been less than 3 years. Given the poor prognosis of these tumors, there is a general consensus toward aggressive upfront therapy, including surgery and postoperative radiotherapy regardless of the extent of resection. Moreover, effective systemic therapies are needed and remain a challenge for future investigation.

### Surgery

Surgery is the first-line therapy and indeed is necessary to assign tumor grade. Similar to lower-grade meningiomas, the extent of resection impacts recurrence; however, surgery as a sole modality is insufficient. Jaaskelainen observed a 5-year recurrence rate of 78% following GTR in patients with malignant meningiomas managed with surgery alone. Similarly, Dziuk and colleagues reported a 5-year progression-free survival of 28% following gross total resection and 0% following subtotal resection [102]. Most clinicians recommend adjuvant radiotherapy after initial surgery for a WHO Grade III meningioma, irrespective of resection extent.

Regarding extent of resection, Sughrue and colleagues noted that heroic surgery did not improve survival, rather near total resection (defined as >90% tumor removal) resulted in superior overall survival and neurologic outcomes than gross total resection, provided that adjuvant radiotherapy was given [103]. They also reported that salvage surgery was beneficial with median survival of 53 months with salvage surgery compared to 25 months without [103].

### Radiotherapy

There are yet no published prospective studies regarding multimodality therapy with surgery and adjuvant radiotherapy (RT) in the management of WHO Grade III meningiomas. We await publication of the RTOG-0539 high-risk cohort which includes WHO grade III patients. However, multiple retrospective series, although varying in treatment approach, dose, and definition of malignant meningioma, do strongly suggest benefit with adjuvant RT.

### External Beam Radiotherapy

Milosevic and Dziuk both demonstrated benefit with the addition of RT as a surgical adjuvant, rather than reserving radiotherapy for salvage [102, 104]. This is now, in general, the standard approach for managing malignant meningioma. Milosevic demonstrated that radiation doses of less than 50 Gy were insufficient and associated with poor cause-specific survival [104]. Dziuk reported that adjuvant external beam RT improved 5-year PFS from 28% to 80% for gross totally resection lesions [102]. Regarding salvage radiotherapy, some studies have demonstrated a modest advantage, whereas others have found little to no benefit. Dziuk et al. reported that external beam radiotherapy for recurrent malignant meningioma improved the 2-year progression-free survival from 50% to 89% but had no such impact at 5 years [102]. This corroborates other studies showing poor tumor control even with salvage therapy for non-benign meningioma [82].

Radiation dose appears to correlate with disease control for WHO Grade III meningioma. Milosevic demonstrated improvement with a 5-year cause-specific survival of 42% with 50 Gy or greater and 0% with less than 50 Gy [104]. Likewise, Goldsmith reported that 5-year PFS improved from 17% to 63% with radiation doses exceeding 53 Gy [59]. With protons, DeVries and Hug noted improvement in local control and survival with doses above 60 Gy [16, 105]. Specifically, Hug demonstrated improved overall survival at 5 and 8 years to 87% with at least 60 CGE, compared to 15% with less than 60 CGE [16].

### Recurrent Meningioma

Despite appropriate therapy including surgery and radiotherapy, meningiomas can recur. Tumor volume, grade, location, and other factors have been correlated with recurrence risk following upfront therapy. For a meningioma that recurs following initial therapy, repeat resection should be considered [39]. If radiation has not been given initially, it should be considered after resection of a recurrent meningioma, irrespective of resection extent. Ultimate control of a meningioma is compromised by recurrence [82, 88, 106]. Onodera compared patients with newly diagnosed benign meningioma to those with recurrence. With median 90-month follow-up, they found better overall survival, progression-free survival, and local control in patients who received radiation therapy, 48–54 Gy in 2 Gy fractions with or without surgery as initial compared to salvage therapy. OS, PFS, and LC were 100%, 91.7%, and 100%, respectively, with initial EBRT, versus 90.9%, 68.2%, and 68.2% if radiation was given after relapse. The difference in local control was statistically significant with $p = 0.01$ [106].

For progression outside of previous fields, RT may clearly be considered. Re-irradiation, either external beam RT or SRS, may also be applied judiciously for in-field or marginal failure, particularly if there has been a long disease-free interval.

### Systemic Therapy

Multiple systemic therapy regimens have been evaluated for meningioma, primarily in phase I and II studies. To date there has only been one published phase III clinical trial. The ribonucleotide reductase inhibitor, hydroxyurea, demonstrated 6-month progression-free survival of only 3–10% in nonrandomized studies [107]. Somatostatin analogues (e.g., Sandostatin LAR, octreotide) have demonstrated 29–44% in nonrandomized trials [108, 109]. Tyrosine kinase inhibitors, also in nonrandomized trials, have demonstrated 6-month progression-free survival of 28–61.9% [110, 111]. Bevacizumab in nonrandomized studies demonstrated 6-month progression-free survival of 43.8–85.7% [112].

Yong Ji and colleagues published data from the SWOG S9005 phase III study of mifepristone, the anti-progesterone. To date, this is the only drug with published randomized data in meningioma. In this trial 164 patients with unresectable meningiomas were randomized to receive mifepristone versus placebo. Only one-quarter of the patients had previously received radiotherapy. At 2 years failure-free survival was approximately 30% in both arms [113]. Pharmacological approaches have thus met with limited results, and considerable opportunity exists for the development of systemic or targeted agents for the treatment of recurrent or high-grade meningioma. A current phase II Alliance trial is evaluating SMO, AKT, and NF2 inhibitors for patients with progressive meningioma.

## Contemporary Clinical Trials

### EORTC 22042-26042

This EORTC phase II trial evaluated progression-free survival with WHO Grades II and III meningioma. Patients were stratified by extent of resection and pathologic grade. Patients with gross total resection, defined by Simpson Grades I–III, received postoperative radiotherapy to 60 Gy in 2 Gy fractions, whereas patients with gross residual disease received an additional 5-fraction boost to a total dose of 70 Gy. This study is closed to accrual and data analysis is pending.

### RTOG 0539

The RTOG 0539 clinical trial utilized a risk stratification approach to postoperative management of meningiomas. Low-risk was defined as a gross totally resected or subtotally resected WHO Grade I meningioma, and patients were observed. Intermediate-risk included recurrent/progressive WHO Grade I and gross totally resected WHO Grade II patients. Intermediate-risk patients received radiotherapy, 54 Gy in 1.8 Gy fractions. High-risk was defined as subtotally resected or recurrent WHO Grade II or new or recurrent WHO Grade III regardless of extent of resection. These patients received 60 Gy in 2 Gy fractions. This study has closed to accrual and initial analysis or some of the risk groups is pending. An informative report of pathology concordance from this trial has been published [93].

The results of the intermediate risk arm of RTOG 0539 are in press [114]. The primary endpoint was 3-year PFS, with both progression and death considered as events. With 48 fully evaluable patients 3-year PFS was 93.8%, and 3-year OS was 96%. Only two patients developed local recurrence within 3 years, resulting in 3-year actuarial local failure rate 4.1%. Treatment was well tolerated, with CTCAE adverse events related to protocol therapy limited to Grade 1 or 2.

### NRG Oncology BN003 and ROAM/EORTC1308

Presently, one of the most controversial subjects in meningioma management is the appropriate therapy for a grossly resected WHO Grade II meningioma. This phase III trial, opened in the summer of 2017, will randomize patients with a grossly resected WHO Grade II meningioma to either observation or radiotherapy (59.4 Gy in 33 fractions). Created in concert, a very similar trial ROAM/EORTC1308, is also open internationally. These studies will address one of the most clinically relevant topics in meningioma management and will include, in addition to tumor control outcomes, neurocognitive and quality of life endpoints.

## Treatment Field Design/Target Delineation

### External Beam Radiotherapy

For WHO Grade I meningioma, external beam radiotherapy is generally applicable only for gross residual disease either following subtotal resection or recurrence. Patients are commonly immobilized with a thermoplastic mask, typically with the head in neutral position. A contrast-enhanced T1 sequence MRI is used for delineation of gross tumor volume (GTV). Overlying hyperostotic bone should be included in the GTV as this generally represents tumor invasion; however, the dural tail does not need to be included in the GTV [115]. Clinical tumor volume (CTV) expansion from GTV for WHO Grade I meningioma can range from 0 to 1 cm primarily along dural surface and the hyperostotic bone, with margin restrictions to spare uninvolved normal tissues such as the adjacent brain and respecting natural barriers to tumor growth such as uninvolved falx and bone. The planning target volume (PTV) is a geometric expansion of the CTV and is institutionally defined to account for setup and treatment delivery uncertainties and is usually at least 3 mm. Radiation dose generally ranges from 50.4 to 54 Gy in 1.8–2.0 Gy fractions.

For WHO Grade II meningiomas, as discussed in detail above, radiation is commonly recommended with gross residual but is also an appropriate strategy following a gross total resection (GTR). After GTR, the GTV is defined as the tumor bed. The CTV is the GTV plus an approximately 0.5 cm anatomically constrained expansion. Known or suspected brain invasion with a WHO Grade II meningioma must be addressed, and it is thus reasonable to include a rim

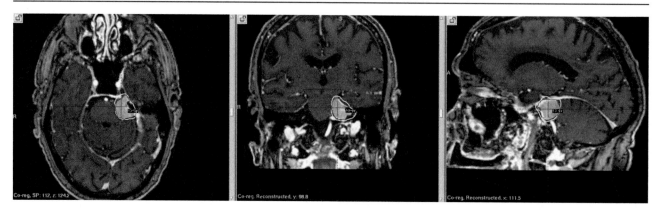

**Fig. 1.3** Petrous apex meningioma stereotactic radiosurgery plan, 13 Gy in 1 fraction

of the adjacent brain in such cases. The PTV expansion is similar to that previously discussed for WHO Grade I meningiomas. Recommended dosing for atypical meningioma following GTR is at least 54 Gy in 1.8–2.0 Gy fractions, some clinicians advocating for 59.4–60 Gy. The NRG Oncology/ RTOG 0539 trial employed 54 Gy in 30 fractions following GTR of a WHO Grade II meningioma; however, supported by several intervening studies, the upcoming second-generation randomized trial stipulates 59.4 Gy in 33 fractions in the same setting [93]. Following subtotal resection (STR) or recurrence, at least 60 Gy in fractions of 1.8–2.0 Gy is recommended, and higher doses in the range of 66 Gy may be considered when organs at risk permit. The EORTC trial (22042, 26042) uses a final 70 Gy for gross residual disease in these settings. Total doses of this extent should be used vigilantly until their utility is confirmed.

For WHO Grade III meningioma, radiation is recommended regardless of resection extent. GTV is defined as T1 post-contrast-enhancing tumor bed and any remaining nodular enhancement and hyperostosis. Based upon NRG Oncology/RTOG 0539, two CTVs may be defined for a simultaneous integrated boost. CTV54Gy is the GTV plus a 2 cm expansion and CTV60Gy is GTV plus a 1 cm expansion. The standard institutional PTV, typically 3–5 mm, is used to expand each of these volumes to define a PTV54Gy and a PTV60Gy. Dose escalation beyond 60, up to 70 Gy— see the separately referenced EORTC trial—have been reported but should be used cautiously, with careful attention to normal tissue (organ at risk) constraints [116].

## Stereotactic Radiosurgery

Stereotactic radiosurgery is an appropriate option with gross residual WHO Grade I and possibly WHO Grade II tumors. Immobilization, or another form of stereotaxis, is required generally resulting in setup uncertainties on the order of a single millimeter. The GTV is defined by the T1 post-contrast MRI. There is commonly no CTV margin, and the PTV is routinely defined as GTV plus 0–2 mm. For a WHO Grade I meningioma, a marginal dose of 12–15 Gy is recommended. Figure 1.3 shows a stereotactic radiosurgery plan for a patient with a left petrous meningioma. For WHO Grade II meningioma, recommended marginal doses from varying reports are 14–20 Gy. This is an important arena additional research to help define optimal dosing for higher-grade meningioma based upon factors such as location, volume, and perhaps even molecular characteristics. For larger (>10 mL) WHO Grade I meningioma, fractionated stereotactic radiotherapy, such as 5 Gy times 5 (total dose 25 Gy), may be considered, and for a WHO Grade II or III tumor 5.5–6 Gy times 5 (27.5–30 Gy).

## Normal Critical Structure Constraints

Restriction of dose to critical structures reduces the risk of toxicities. Table 1.4 summarizes the normal critical structure constraints used in RTOG 0539 and in NRG-BN003. With these considerations, radiation is well tolerated with 5% or less long-term toxicity rate when modern techniques are used [114].

**Table 1.4** Organ-at-risk point dose constraints (point defined as 0.03 cc volume)

| Critical structure | RTOG-0539 group 2 (Gy) | RTOG-0539 group 3 (Gy) | NRG-BN003 (acceptable variation) (Gy) |
|---|---|---|---|
| Lenses | 5 | 7 | ≤7 (>7 to 10) |
| Retinae | 45 | 50 | ≤45 (>45 to 50) |
| Optic nerves | 50 | 55 | ≤54 (>54 to 58) |
| Optic chiasm | 54 | 56 | ≤54 (>54 to 58) |
| Brainstem | 55 | 60 | ≤54 (>54 to 58) |

RTOG-0539 included two groups. Group 2 was defined as intermediate-risk meningioma treated with IMRT, 54 Gy in 30 fractions. Group 3 was high risk, treated to 60 Gy in 30 fractions, with differing organ-at-risk constraints. NRG-BN003 includes patients with a gross totally resected WHO Grade II meningioma, treated to 59.4 Gy in 33 fractions. Note that desirable organ-at-risk doses in patients with WHO Grade I meningioma may indeed be less than those with WHO Grade II or III

Debus et al. reviewed 189 patients treated to a mean 56.8 Gy with fractions of 1.8 Gy and reported that 2.2% developed clinically significant toxicity [48]. In patients without a preexisting neurological deficit, this was even lower (1.7%). Reduced vision, visual field cut, and trigeminal neuropathy were noted as the most common toxicities. Goldsmith et al. reported a 3.6% toxicity rate for subtotally resected meningioma patients who received EBRT. Of the five patients with side effects, retinopathy developed in two, optic neuropathy in one, and radiation necrosis in two [59].

A more recent study by Farzin et al. focused on optic toxicity in 213 treated with radiation for meningiomas [117]. Dry eye developed in 7% and cataracts developed in 11.2%. Two patients developed visual issues due to radiation. They received a maximum and median dose to their neuro-optic structures of 57.3 Gy and 54.6 Gy, respectively.

Selch et al. looked at 45 cavernous sinus meningioma patients who received a total dose of 50.4 Gy at 1.7–1.8 Gy per fraction and found no patients with treatment-related cranial neuropathies [66]. Pituitary dysfunction, cerebrovascular effects, secondary malignancy, orbital fibrosis, and edema have been described but are rare as well.

Cognitive morbidity may occur following radiation. Steinvorth et al. prospectively evaluated patients treated with fractionated radiation for meningioma [118]. By using a comprehensive neurocognitive battery, they found a decline in memory with an increase in attention after the first fraction. There was no cognitive loss with further follow-up. On the other hand, Meyers et al. assessed patients treated to the paranasal sinuses and demonstrated memory impairment in 80% of the patients [119]. This study did use older techniques however.

For stereotactic radiosurgery, optic nerve constraints range from 8 to 12 Gy in the literature. Tishler et al. reported a 24% risk of optic neuropathy with doses greater than 8 Gy to the optic pathways [120]. Other studies have suggested that slightly higher doses than 8 Gy are perhaps safe. Leber et al. looked at 50 patients and did not see radiation optic neuropathy in patients who received less than 10 Gy [121]. Optic neuropathy, however, developed in 26.7% of patient receiving 10 to less than 15 Gy and 77.8% for those receiving 15 Gy or more. According to a series of patients treated at the Mayo Clinic, only 1.1% of the patients developed optic neuropathy at 12 Gy or less to the optic nerves and chiasm [122]. As long as doses are kept reasonably low to the optic nerve and chiasm, risk of vision loss is also low.

## Conclusion

The main management options for meningioma are surgery and radiation. The evidence supporting radiation, up until recently, had relied upon retrospective studies, which made it difficult—especially in an era with considerable revisions in grading criteria—to establish widely acceptable treatment guidelines. Controversy remains over the use and timing of radiation particularly for Grade II atypical meningiomas. With the completion of EORTC 22042-26042 and RTOG 0539, the role of radiation will be better defined. The NRG BN003 and ROAM/EORTC1308 trials, once completed, will further eliminate controversy for patients with gross totally resected atypical meningiomas. While the role of radiosurgery for Grade I meningioma is well supported by retrospective data with long-term follow-up, its use for atypical and anaplastic meningioma is less clear. There remain important questions regarding the optimal target volume. Beyond radiation therapy, more studies are needed for targeted therapies and immunotherapy, especially for patients who fail surgery and radiation therapy.

## Case Study

A 60-year-old woman presented with increasing difficulty with balance. Her past medical and family history were noncontributory. Given her symptoms, her neurologist ordered an MRI of the brain without and with contrast. She was found to have two separate parasagittal masses and a left posterior fossa dural-based mass consistent with multiple meningiomas (Fig. 1.4a). Given the size of her parasagittal meningiomas, she underwent a Simpson Grade II resection of these masses (Fig. 1.4a). Pathology was consistent with WHO Grade II (atypical) meningiomas. After discussion of options which included observation, she elected to proceed with radiation to the resection bed to decrease risk of local recurrence, with plans to watch the posterior fossa meningioma. She received a total dose of 54 Gy (Fig. 1.4b). Given the histologic grade, a CTV margin was included, but given the extent of resection (GTR), the CTV margin was limited to 0.5 cm.

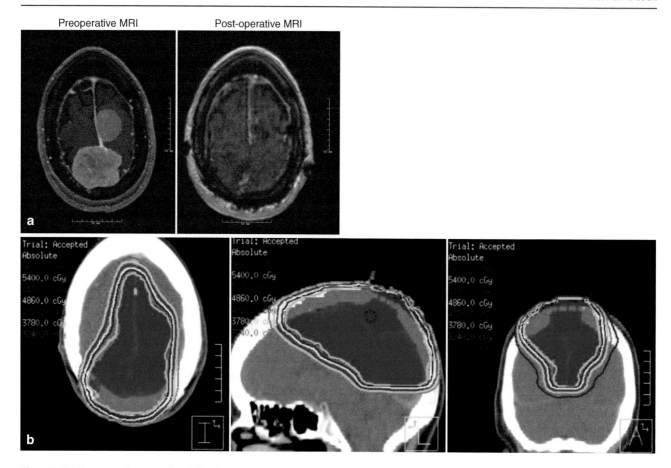

**Fig. 1.4** (**a**) Gross totally resected multifocal parasagittal WHO Grade II meningioma. (**b**) Isodoses in axial, sagittal, and coronal planes for post-operative radiation therapy, 54 Gy in 30 fractions

## Self-Assessment Questions

1. Which of the following statements is true regarding surgical resection of a meningioma?
   A. The extent of surgery is classically defined according to the "Cushing Grade" of resection.
   B. In modern surgical series, gross total resection is accomplished at initial surgery in over three-fourths of patients.
   C. Gross total resection alone results in excellent local control, exceeding 90% at 15 years.
   D. The intracranial primary site with the greatest likelihood of achieving gross total resection is the sphenoid wing.

2. Which of the following is *not* true regarding meningioma cooperative group trials?
   A. Two cooperative group trials evaluating gross total resection (GTR) alone versus GTR and adjuvant frac tionated external beam RT for WHO Grade II meningioma are underway.
   B. Targeted systemic interventions are being evaluated in an Alliance trial.
   C. Mifepristone improved failure-free survival for patients with recurrent or progressive meningioma in a phase III SWOG trial.
   D. The EORTC phase II trial (22042-26042) will report on final RT doses of 70 Gy for patients with subtotally resected high-grade meningioma.

3. Which of the following statements regarding the incidence of meningiomas is *false*?
   A. Historically, the incidence increased following radiation therapy for tinea capitis.
   B. Meningiomas often occur with type 2 neurofibromatosis.
   C. Nonmalignant meningiomas are more common in males than females.
   D. Meningiomas are the second most common primary intracranial tumor, following gliomas.

4. Meningiomas are graded histopathologically by the World Health Organization (WHO) criteria. Which of the following is *false* regarding various WHO grades?
   A. Approximately 70% of meningiomas are benign (WHO Grade I).

15

B. According to WHO 2007–2016 criteria, approximately 25% of meningiomas are atypical (WHO Grade II).
C. Atypical meningiomas treated with surgery alone have 10-year progression-free survival rates exceeding 75%, similar to WHO Grade I.
D. Anaplastic meningiomas (WHO Grade III) carry a median overall survival of less than 3 years.

5. Which of the following is *not* true concerning the use of radiation therapy (RT) in the management of meningioma?
   A. There is a large body of retrospective literature indicating that (RT) improves local control following subtotal resection.
   B. Progression-free survivals following either fractionated RT or stereotactic radiosurgery (SRS) for a known or supposed WHO Grade I meningioma are very similar.
   C. With fractionated RT or SRS, it is necessary to include the "dural tail" within the target volume.
   D. Fractionated RT or SRS may be employed in selected patients diagnosed by imaging criteria, without histopathologic confirmation.

## Answers

1. B
2. C
3. D
4. C
5. C

## References

1. Perry A. Meningiomas. In: Rosenblum M, McLendon R, Bigner DD, editors. Russell & Rubinstein's pathology of tumors of the nervous system. London: Hodder Arnold; 2006. p. 427–74.
2. Claus EB, Bondy ML, Schildkraut JM, et al. Epidemiology of intracranial meningioma. Neurosurgery. 2005;57:1088–95; discussion 1088–95.
3. Ostrom QT, Gittleman H, Xu J, et al. CBTRUS statistical report: primary brain and other central nervous system tumors diagnosed in the United States in 2009–2013. Neuro Oncol. 2016;18:v1–v75. https://doi.org/10.1093/neuonc/now207.
4. Wiemels J, Wrensch M, Claus EB. Epidemiology and etiology of meningioma. J Neurooncol. 2010;99:307–14. https://doi.org/10.1007/s11060-010-0386-3.
5. Nakasu S, Hirano A, Shimura T, et al. Incidental meningiomas in autopsy study. Surg Neurol. 1987;27:319–22.
6. Adegbite AB, Khan MI, Paine KW, et al. The recurrence of intracranial meningiomas after surgical treatment. J Neurosurg. 1983;58:51–6. https://doi.org/10.3171/jns.1983.58.1.0051.
7. Stafford SL1, Pollock BE, Foote RL, et al. Meningioma radiosurgery: tumor control, outcomes, and complications among 190 consecutive patients. Neurosurgery. 2001;49:1029–37; discussion 1037–8.
8. Longstreth WT Jr, Dennis LK, McGuire VM, et al. Epidemiology of intracranial meningioma. Cancer. 1993;72:639–48.
9. Miralbell R, Linggood RM, de la Monte S, et al. The role of radiotherapy in the treatment of subtotally resected benign meningiomas. J Neurooncol. 1992;13:157–64.
10. Louis DN, Ramesh V, Gusella JF. Neuropathology and molecular genetics of neurofibromatosis 2 and related tumors. Brain Pathol. 1995;5:163–72.
11. Riemenschneider MJ, Perry A, Reifenberger G. Histological classification and molecular genetics of meningiomas. Lancet Neurol. 2006;5:1045–54. https://doi.org/10.1016/S1474-4422(06)70625-1.
12. Asthagiri AR1, Parry DM, Butman JA, et al. Neurofibromatosis type 2. Lancet. 2009;373:1974–86. https://doi.org/10.1016/S0140-6736(09)60259-2.
13. Perry A, Dehner LP. Meningeal tumors of childhood and infancy. An update and literature review. Brain Pathol. 2003;13:386–408.
14. Perry A, Giannini C, Raghavan R, et al. Aggressive phenotypic and genotypic features in pediatric and NF2-associated meningiomas: a clinicopathologic study of 53 cases. J Neuropathol Exp Neurol. 2001;60:994–1003.
15. Al-Mefty O, Topsakal C, Pravdenkova S, et al. Radiation-induced meningiomas: clinical, pathological, cytokinetic, and cytogenetic characteristics. J Neurosurg. 2004;100:1002–13. https://doi.org/10.3171/jns.2004.100.6.1002.
16. Hug EB, Devries A, Thornton AF, et al. Management of atypical and malignant meningiomas: role of high-dose, 3D-conformal radiation therapy. J Neurooncol. 2000;48:151–60.
17. Ron E, Modan B, Boice JD Jr. Mortality after radiotherapy for ringworm of the scalp. Am J Epidemiol. 1988;127:713–25.
18. Ron E, Modan B, Boice JD Jr, et al. Tumors of the brain and nervous system after radiotherapy in childhood. N Engl J Med. 1988;319:1033–9. https://doi.org/10.1056/NEJM198810203191601.
19. Strojan P, Popovic M, Jereb B. Secondary intracranial meningiomas after high-dose cranial irradiation: report of five cases and review of the literature. Int J Radiat Oncol Biol Phys. 2000;48:65–73.
20. Bindal R, Goodman JM, Kawasaki A, et al. The natural history of untreated skull base meningiomas. Surg Neurol. 2003;59:87–92; discussion 92.
21. Whittle IR, Smith C, Navoo P, et al. Meningiomas. Lancet. 2004;363:1535–43. https://doi.org/10.1016/S0140-6736(04)16153-9.
22. Ayerbe J, Lobato RD, de la Cruz J, et al. Risk factors predicting recurrence in patients operated on for intracranial meningioma. A multivariate analysis. Acta Neurochir. 1999;141:921–32.
23. Drape JL, Krause D, Tongio J. MRI of aggressive meningiomas. J Neuroradiol. 1992;19:49–62.
24. Rohringer M, Sutherland GR, Louw DF, et al. Incidence and clinicopathological features of meningioma. J Neurosurg. 1989;71:665–72. https://doi.org/10.3171/jns.1989.71.5.0665.
25. Schubeus P, Schorner W, Rottacker C, et al. Intracranial meningiomas: how frequent are indicative findings in CT and MRI? Neuroradiology. 1990;32:467–73.
26. Kuratsu J, Kochi M, Ushio Y. Incidence and clinical features of asymptomatic meningiomas. J Neurosurg. 2000;92:766–70. https://doi.org/10.3171/jns.2000.92.5.0766.
27. Buhl R, Nabavi A, Wolff S, et al. MR spectroscopy in patients with intracranial meningiomas. Neurol Res. 2007;29:43–6. https://doi.org/10.1179/174313206X153824.
28. Demir MK, Iplikcioglu AC, Dincer A, et al. Single voxel proton MR spectroscopy findings of typical and atypical intracra-

nial meningiomas. Eur J Radiol. 2006;60:48–55. https://doi.org/10.1016/j.ejrad.2006.06.002.

29. Ghodsian M, Obrzut SL, Hyde CC, et al. Evaluation of metastatic meningioma with 2-deoxy-2-[18F]fluoro-D-glucose PET/CT. Clin Nucl Med. 2005;30:717–20.

30. Hakyemez B, Yildirim N, Gokalp G, et al. The contribution of diffusion-weighted MR imaging to distinguishing typical from atypical meningiomas. Neuroradiology. 2006;48:513–20. https://doi.org/10.1007/s00234-006-0094-z.

31. Nagar VA, Ye JR, Ng WH, et al. Diffusion-weighted MR imaging: diagnosing atypical or malignant meningiomas and detecting tumor dedifferentiation. AJNR Am J Neuroradiol. 2008;29:1147–52. https://doi.org/10.3174/ajnr.A0996.

32. Ogawa T, Inugami A, Hatazawa J, et al. Clinical positron emission tomography for brain tumors: comparison of fludeoxyglucose F 18 and L-methyl-11C-methionine. AJNR Am J Neuroradiol. 1996;17:345–53.

33. Sibtain NA, Howe FA, Saunders DE. The clinical value of proton magnetic resonance spectroscopy in adult brain tumours. Clin Radiol. 2007;62:109–19. https://doi.org/10.1016/j.crad.2006.09.012.

34. Toh CH, Castillo M, Wong AM, et al. Differentiation between classic and atypical meningiomas with use of diffusion tensor imaging. AJNR Am J Neuroradiol. 2008;29:1630–5. https://doi.org/10.3174/ajnr.A1170.

35. Combs SE, Schulz-Ertner D, Debus J, et al. Improved correlation of the neuropathologic classification according to adapted world health organization classification and outcome after radiotherapy in patients with atypical and anaplastic meningiomas. Int J Radiat Oncol Biol Phys. 2011;81:1415–21. https://doi.org/10.1016/j.ijrobp.2010.07.039.

36. Domingues PH, Sousa P, Otero Á, et al. Proposal for a new risk stratification classification for meningioma based on patient age, WHO tumor grade, size, localization, and karyotype. Neuro Oncol. 2014;16:735–47. https://doi.org/10.1093/neuonc/not325.

37. Olar A, Wani KM, Sulman EP, et al. Mitotic index is an independent predictor of recurrence-free survival in meningioma. Brain Pathol. 2015;25:266–75. https://doi.org/10.1111/bpa.12174.

38. Simpson D. The recurrence of intracranial meningiomas after surgical treatment. J Neurol Neurosurg Psychiatry. 1957;20:22–39.

39. Sughrue ME, Kane AJ, Shangari G, et al. The relevance of Simpson Grade I and II resection in modern neurosurgical treatment of World Health Organization Grade I meningiomas. J Neurosurg. 2010;113:1029–35. https://doi.org/10.3171/2010.3.JNS091971.

40. Condra KS, Buatti JM, Mendenhall WM, et al. Benign meningiomas: primary treatment selection affects survival. Int J Radiat Oncol Biol Phys. 1997;39:427–36.

41. Oya S, Kawai K, Nakatomi H, et al. Significance of Simpson grading system in modern meningioma surgery: integration of the grade with MIB-1 labeling index as a key to predict the recurrence of WHO Grade I meningiomas. J Neurosurg. 2012;117:121–8. https://doi.org/10.3171/2012.3.JNS111945.

42. Hasseleid BF, Meling TR, Ronning P, et al. Surgery for convexity meningioma: Simpson Grade I resection as the goal: clinical article. J Neurosurg. 2012;117:999–1006. https://doi.org/10.3171/2012.9.JNS12294.

43. Morokoff AP, Zauberman J, Black PM. Surgery for convexity meningiomas. Neurosurgery. 2008;63:427–33; discussion 433–4. https://doi.org/10.1227/01.NEU.0000310692.80289.28.

44. Stafford SL, Perry A, Suman VJ, et al. Primarily resected meningiomas: outcome and prognostic factors in 581 Mayo Clinic patients, 1978 through 1988. Mayo Clin Proc. 1998;73:936–42. https://doi.org/10.4065/73.10.936.

45. Mirimanoff RO, Dosoretz DE, Linggood RM, et al. Meningioma: analysis of recurrence and progression following neurosurgical resection. J Neurosurg. 1985;62:18–24. https://doi.org/10.3171/jns.1985.62.1.0018.

46. Soyuer S, Chang EL, Selek U, et al. Radiotherapy after surgery for benign cerebral meningioma. Radiother Oncol. 2004;71:85–90. https://doi.org/10.1016/j.radonc.2004.01.006.

47. Litré CF, Colin P, Noudel R, et al. Fractionated stereotactic radiotherapy treatment of cavernous sinus meningiomas: a study of 100 cases. Int J Radiat Oncol Biol Phys. 2009;74:1012–7. https://doi.org/10.1016/j.ijrobp.2008.09.012.

48. Henzel M, Gross MW, Hamm K, et al. High efficacy of fractionated stereotactic radiotherapy of large base-of-skull meningiomas: long-term results. J Clin Oncol. 2001;19:3547–53. https://doi.org/10.1200/JCO.2001.19.15.3547.

49. Henzel M, Gross MW, Hamm K, et al. Stereotactic radiotherapy of meningiomas: symptomatology, acute and late toxicity. Strahlenther Onkol. 2006;182:382–8. https://doi.org/10.1007/s00066-006-1535-7.

50. Korah MP, Nowlan AW, Johnstone PA, et al. Radiation therapy alone for imaging-defined meningiomas. Int J Radiat Oncol Biol Phys. 2010;76:181–6. https://doi.org/10.1016/j.ijrobp.2009.01.066.

51. Dufour H, Muracciole X, Métellus P, et al. Long-term tumor control and functional outcome in patients with cavernous sinus meningiomas treated by radiotherapy with or without previous surgery: is there an alternative to aggressive tumor removal? Neurosurgery. 2001;48:285–94; discussion 294–6.

52. Pourel N, Auque J, Bracard S, et al. Efficacy of external fractionated radiation therapy in the treatment of meningiomas: a 20-year experience. Radiother Oncol. 2001;61:65–70.

53. Wenkel E, Thornton AF, Finkelstein D, et al. Benign meningioma: partially resected, biopsied, and recurrent intracranial tumors treated with combined proton and photon radiotherapy. Int J Radiat Oncol Biol Phys. 2000;48:1363–70.

54. Maguire PD, Clough R, Friedman AH, et al. Fractionated external-beam radiation therapy for meningiomas of the cavernous sinus. Int J Radiat Oncol Biol Phys. 1999;44:75–9.

55. Liu JK, Forman S, Hershewe GL, et al. Optic nerve sheath meningiomas: visual improvement after stereotactic radiotherapy. Neurosurgery. 2002;50:950–5; discussion 955–7.

56. Pitz S, Becker G, Schiefer U, et al. Stereotactic fractionated irradiation of optic nerve sheath meningioma: a new treatment alternative. Br J Ophthalmol. 2002;86:1265–8.

57. Baumert BG, Villà S, Studer G, et al. Early improvements in vision after fractionated stereotactic radiotherapy for primary optic nerve sheath meningioma. Radiother Oncol. 2004;72:169–74. https://doi.org/10.1016/j.radonc.2004.04.008.

58. Becker G, Jeremic B, Pitz S, et al. Stereotactic fractionated radiotherapy in patients with optic nerve sheath meningioma. Int J Radiat Oncol Biol Phys. 2002;54:1422–9.

59. Goldsmith BJ, Wara WM, Wilson CB, et al. Postoperative irradiation for subtotally resected meningiomas. A retrospective analysis of 140 patients treated from 1967 to 1990. J Neurosurg. 1994;80:195–201. https://doi.org/10.3171/jns.1994.80.2.0195.

60. Winkler C, Dornfeld S, Schwarz R, et al. The results of radiotherapy in meningiomas with a high risk of recurrence. A retrospective analysis. Strahlenther Onkol. 1998;174:624–8.

61. Brower JV, Amdur RJ, Kirwan J, et al. Radiation therapy for optic nerve sheath meningioma. Pract Radiat Oncol. 2013;3:223–8. https://doi.org/10.1016/j.prro.2012.06.010.

62. Otsuka S, Tamiya T, Ono Y, et al. The relationship between peritumoral brain edema and the expression of vascular endothelial growth factor and its receptors in intracranial meningiomas. J Neurooncol. 2004;70:349–57.

63. Cai R, Barnett GH, Novak E, et al. Principal risk of peritumoral edema after stereotactic radiosurgery for intracranial meningioma is tumor-brain contact interface area. Neurosurgery. 2010;66:513–22. https://doi.org/10.1227/01.NEU.0000365366.53337.88.

64. Lee KJ, Joo WI, Rha HK, et al. Peritumoral brain edema in meningiomas: correlations between magnetic resonance imaging, angi-

ography, and pathology. Surg Neurol. 2008;69:350–5; discussion 355. https://doi.org/10.1016/j.surneu.2007.03.027.

65. Rogers L, Barani I, Chamberlain M, et al. Meningiomas: knowledge base, treatment outcomes, and uncertainties. A RANO review. J Neurosurg. 2015;122:4–23. https://doi.org/10.3171/2014.7.JNS131644.

66. Selch MT, Ahn E, Laskari A, et al. Stereotactic radiotherapy for treatment of cavernous sinus meningiomas. Int J Radiat Oncol Biol Phys. 2004;59:101–11. https://doi.org/10.1016/j.ijrobp.2003.09.003.

67. Tanzler E, Morris CG, Kirwan JM, et al. Outcomes of WHO Grade I meningiomas receiving definitive or postoperative radiotherapy. Int J Radiat Oncol Biol Phys. 2011;79:508–13. https://doi.org/10.1016/j.ijrobp.2009.11.032.

68. Uy NW, Woo SY, Teh BS, et al. Intensity-modulated radiation therapy (IMRT) for meningioma. Int J Radiat Oncol Biol Phys. 2002;53:1265–70.

69. Hakim R, Alexander E 3rd, Loeffler JS, et al. Results of linear accelerator-based radiosurgery for intracranial meningiomas. Neurosurgery. 1998;42:446–53; discussion 453–4.

70. Kollová A, Liscák R, Novotný J Jr, et al. Gamma Knife surgery for benign meningioma. J Neurosurg. 2007;107:325–36. https://doi.org/10.3171/JNS-07/08/0325.

71. Skeie BS, Enger PO, Skeie GO, et al. Gamma knife surgery of meningiomas involving the cavernous sinus: long-term follow-up of 100 patients. Neurosurgery. 2010;66:661–8; discussion 668–9. https://doi.org/10.1227/01.NEU.0000366112.04015.E2.

72. Patil CG, Hoang S, Borchers DJ 3rd, et al. Predictors of peritumoral edema after stereotactic radiosurgery of supratentorial meningiomas. Neurosurgery. 2008;63:435–40; discussion 440–2. https://doi.org/10.1227/01.NEU.0000325257.58684.92.

73. Ganz JC, Schrottner O, Pendl G. Radiation-induced edema after Gamma Knife treatment for meningiomas. Stereotact Funct Neurosurg. 1996;66(Suppl 1):129–33.

74. Ganz JC, Backlund EO, Thorsen FA. The results of Gamma Knife surgery of meningiomas, related to size of tumor and dose. Stereotact Funct Neurosurg. 1993;61(Suppl 1):23–9.

75. Kondziolka D, Flickinger JC, Perez B. Judicious resection and/or radiosurgery for parasagittal meningiomas: outcomes from a multicenter review. Gamma Knife Meningioma Study Group. Neurosurgery. 1998;43:405–13; discussion 413–4.

76. DiBiase SJ, Kwok Y, Yovino S. Factors predicting local tumor control after gamma knife stereotactic radiosurgery for benign intracranial meningiomas. Int J Radiat Oncol Biol Phys. 2004;60:1515–9. https://doi.org/10.1016/j.ijrobp.2004.05.073.

77. Pollock BE, Stafford SL, Link MJ, et al. Single-fraction radiosurgery for presumed intracranial meningiomas: efficacy and complications from a 22-year experience. Int J Radiat Oncol Biol Phys. 2012;83:1414–8. https://doi.org/10.1016/j.ijrobp.2011.10.033.

78. Unger KR, Lominska CE, Chanyasulkit J, et al. Risk factors for posttreatment edema in patients treated with stereotactic radiosurgery for meningiomas. Neurosurgery. 2012;70:639–45. https://doi.org/10.1227/NEU.0b013e3182351ae7.

79. Girvigian MR, Chen JC, Rahimian J, et al. Comparison of early complications for patients with convexity and parasagittal meningiomas treated with either stereotactic radiosurgery or fractionated stereotactic radiotherapy. Neurosurgery. 2008;62:A19–27; discussion A27–18. https://doi.org/10.1227/01.neu.0000325933.34154.cb.

80. Shakir SI, Souhami L, Petrecca K, et al. Prognostic factors for progression in atypical meningioma. J Neurosurg. 2018. https://doi.org/10.3171/2017.6.JNS17120.

81. Goyal LK, Suh JH, Mohan DS, et al. Local control and overall survival in atypical meningioma: a retrospective study. Int J Radiat Oncol Biol Phys. 2000;46:57–61.

82. Bagshaw HP, Burt LM, Jensen RL, et al. Adjuvant radiotherapy for atypical meningiomas. J Neurosurg. 2017;126:1822–8. https://doi.org/10.3171/2016.5.JNS152809.

83. Aizer AA, Arvold ND, Catalano P, et al. Adjuvant radiation therapy, local recurrence, and the need for salvage therapy in atypical meningioma. Neuro Oncol. 2014;16:1547–53. https://doi.org/10.1093/neuonc/nou098.

84. Hammouche S, Clark S, Wong AH, et al. Long-term survival analysis of atypical meningiomas: survival rates, prognostic factors, operative and radiotherapy treatment. Acta Neurochir. 2014;156:1475–81. https://doi.org/10.1007/s00701-014-2156-z.

85. Komotar RJ, Iorgulescu JB, Raper DM, et al. The role of radiotherapy following gross-total resection of atypical meningiomas. J Neurosurg. 2012;117:679–86. https://doi.org/10.3171/2012.7.JNS112113.

86. Ohba S, Kobayashi M, Horiguchi T, et al. Long-term surgical outcome and biological prognostic factors in patients with skull base meningiomas. J Neurosurg. 2011;114:1278–87. https://doi.org/10.3171/2010.11.JNS10701.

87. Aghi MK, Carter BS, Cosgrove GR, et al. Long-term recurrence rates of atypical meningiomas after gross total resection with or without postoperative adjuvant radiation. Neurosurgery. 2009;64:56–60; discussion 60. https://doi.org/10.1227/01.NEU.0000330399.55586.63.

88. Talacchi A, Muggiolu F, De Carlo A, et al. Recurrent atypical meningiomas: combining surgery and radiosurgery in one effective multimodal treatment. World Neurosurg. 2016;87:565–72. https://doi.org/10.1016/j.wneu.2015.10.013.

89. McGovern SL, Aldape KD, Munsell MF, et al. A comparison of World Health Organization tumor grades at recurrence in patients with non-skull base and skull base meningiomas. J Neurosurg. 2010;112:925–33. https://doi.org/10.3171/2009.9.JNS09617.

90. Kessel KA, Fischer H, Oechsner M, et al. High-precision radiotherapy for meningiomas: long-term results and patient-reported outcome (PRO). Strahlenther Onkol. 2017. https://doi.org/10.1007/s00066-017-1156-3.

91. Hardesty DA, Wolf AB, Brachman DG, et al. The impact of adjuvant stereotactic radiosurgery on atypical meningioma recurrence following aggressive microsurgical resection. J Neurosurg. 2013;119:475–81. https://doi.org/10.3171/2012.12.JNS12414.

92. Jenkinson MD, Waqar M, Farah JO, et al. Early adjuvant radiotherapy in the treatment of atypical meningioma. J Clin Neurosci. 2016. https://doi.org/10.1016/j.jocn.2015.09.021.

93. Rogers CL, Perry A, Pugh S, et al. Pathology concordance levels for meningioma classification and grading in NRG Oncology RTOG Trial 0539. Neuro Oncol. 2016;18:565–74. https://doi.org/10.1093/neuonc/nov247.

94. Harris AE, Lee JY, Omalu B, et al. The effect of radiosurgery during management of aggressive meningiomas. Surg Neurol. 2003;60:298–305; discussion 305.

95. Huffmann BC, Reinacher PC, Gilsbach JM. Gamma knife surgery for atypical meningiomas. J Neurosurg. 2005;102(Suppl):283–6.

96. Kano H, Takahashi JA, Katsuki T, et al. Stereotactic radiosurgery for atypical and anaplastic meningiomas. J Neurooncol. 2007;84:41–7. https://doi.org/10.1007/s11060-007-9338-y.

97. Attia A, Chan MD, Mott RT, et al. Patterns of failure after treatment of atypical meningioma with gamma knife radiosurgery. J Neurooncol. 2012;108:179–85. https://doi.org/10.1007/s11060-012-0828-1.

98. Rogers L, Jensen R, Perry A. Chasing your dural tail: factors predicting local tumor control after gamma knife stereotactic radiosurgery for benign intracranial meningiomas: In regard to DiBiase et al. (Int J Radiat Oncol Biol Phys 2004;60:1515–1519). Int J Radiat Oncol Biol Phys. 2005;62:616–8; author reply 618–9. https://doi.org/10.1016/j.ijrobp.2005.02.026.

99. Choi CY, Soltys SG, Gibbs IC, et al. Cyberknife stereotactic radiosurgery for treatment of atypical (WHO grade II) cranial meningiomas. Neurosurgery. 2010;67:1180–8. https://doi.org/10.1227/NEU.0b013e3181f2f427.

100. Zhang M, Ho AL, D'Astous M, et al. CyberKnife stereotactic radiosurgery for atypical and malignant meningiomas. World Neurosurg. 2016;91:574–81 e571. https://doi.org/10.1016/j.wneu.2016.04.019.

101. Valery CA, Faillot M, Lamproglou I, et al. Grade II meningiomas and Gamma Knife radiosurgery: analysis of success and failure to improve treatment paradigm. J Neurosurg. 2016;125:89–96. https://doi.org/10.3171/2016.7.GKS161521.

102. Dziuk TW, Woo S, Butler EB, et al. Malignant meningioma: an indication for initial aggressive surgery and adjuvant radiotherapy. J Neurooncol. 1998;37:177–88.

103. Sughrue ME, Sanai N, Shangari G, et al. Outcome and survival following primary and repeat surgery for World Health Organization Grade III meningiomas. J Neurosurg. 2010;113:202–9. https://doi.org/10.3171/2010.1.JNS091114.

104. Milosevic MF, Frost PJ, Laperriere NJ, et al. Radiotherapy for atypical or malignant intracranial meningioma. Int J Radiat Oncol Biol Phys. 1996;34:817–22.

105. DeVries A, Munzenrider JE, Hedley-Whyte T, et al. The role of radiotherapy in the treatment of malignant meningiomas. Strahlenther Onkol. 1999;175:62–7.

106. Onodera S, Aoyama H, Katoh N, et al. Long-term outcomes of fractionated stereotactic radiotherapy for intracranial skull base benign meningiomas in single institution. Jpn J Clin Oncol. 2011;41:462–8. https://doi.org/10.1093/jjco/hyq231.

107. Chamberlain MC. Hydroxyurea for recurrent surgery and radiation refractory high-grade meningioma. lJ Neurooncol. 2012;107:315–21. https://doi.org/10.1007/s11060-011-0741-z.

108. Chamberlain MC, Glantz MJ, Fadul CE. Recurrent meningioma: salvage therapy with long-acting somatostatin analogue. Neurology. 2007;69:969–73. https://doi.org/10.1212/01.wnl.0000271382.62776.b7.

109. Johnson DR, Kimmel DW, Burch PA, et al. Phase II study of subcutaneous octreotide in adults with recurrent or progressive meningioma and meningeal hemangiopericytoma. Neuro Oncol. 2011;13:530–5. https://doi.org/10.1093/neuonc/nor044.

110. Norden AD, Raizer JJ, Abrey LE, et al. Phase II trials of erlotinib or gefitinib in patients with recurrent meningioma. J Neurooncol. 2010;96:211–7. https://doi.org/10.1007/s11060-009-9948-7.

111. Wen PY, Yung WK, Lamborn KR, et al. Phase II study of imatinib mesylate for recurrent meningiomas (North American Brain Tumor Consortium study 01-08). Neuro Oncol. 2009;11:853–60. https://doi.org/10.1215/15228517-2009-010.

112. Kaley T, Barani I, Chamberlain M, et al. Historical benchmarks for medical therapy trials in surgery- and radiation-refractory meningioma: a RANO review. Neuro Oncol. 2014;16:829–40. https://doi.org/10.1093/neuonc/not330.

113. Ji Y, Rankin C, Grunberg S, et al. Double-blind phase III randomized trial of the antiprogestin agent mifepristone in the treatment of unresectable meningioma: SWOG S9005. J Clin Oncol. 2015;33:4093–8. https://doi.org/10.1200/JCO.2015.61.6490.

114. Rogers L, Zhang P, Vogelbaum MA, et al. Intermediate-risk meningioma: initial outcomes from NRG Oncology/RTOG-0539. J Neurosurg. 2017. https://doi.org/10.3171/2016.11.JNS161170.

115. Pieper DR, Al-Mefty O, Hanada Y, et al. Hyperostosis associated with meningioma of the cranial base: secondary changes or tumor invasion. Neurosurgery. 1999;44:742–6; discussion 746–7.

116. Katz TS, Amdur RJ, Yachnis AT, et al. Pushing the limits of radiotherapy for atypical and malignant meningioma. Am J Clin Oncol. 2005;28:70–4.

117. Farzin M, Molls M, Kampfer S, et al. Optic toxicity in radiation treatment of meningioma: a retrospective study in 213 patients. J Neurooncol. 2016;127:597–606. https://doi.org/10.1007/s11060-016-2071-7.

118. Steinvorth S, Welzel G, Fuss M, et al. Neuropsychological outcome after fractionated stereotactic radiotherapy (FSRT) for base of skull meningiomas: a prospective 1-year follow-up. Radiother Oncol. 2003;69:177–82.

119. Meyers CA, Geara F, Wong PF, et al. Neurocognitive effects of therapeutic irradiation for base of skull tumors. Int J Radiat Oncol Biol Phys. 2000;46:51–5.

120. Tishler RB, Loeffler JS, Lunsford LD, et al. Tolerance of cranial nerves of the cavernous sinus to radiosurgery. Int J Radiat Oncol Biol Phys. 1993;27:215–21.

121. Leber KA, Bergloff J, Pendl G. Dose-response tolerance of the visual pathways and cranial nerves of the cavernous sinus to stereotactic radiosurgery. J Neurosurg. 1998;88:43–50. https://doi.org/10.3171/jns.1998.88.1.0043.

122. Stafford SL, Pollock BE, Leavitt JA, et al. A study on the radiation tolerance of the optic nerves and chiasm after stereotactic radiosurgery. Int J Radiat Oncol Biol Phys. 2003;55:1177–81.

# Pituitary Adenoma

**2**

Lindsay M. Burt, Gita Suneja, and Dennis C. Shrieve

## Learning Objectives

- Learn the epidemiology, risk factors, genetics, presentation, and treatment paradigms associated with pituitary adenomas.
- Understand the diagnosis and appropriate workup for pituitary adenomas with imaging, pathology, and labs.
- Know the appropriate medical, surgical, and radiotherapeutic management for both nonfunctioning and functioning pituitary adenomas.
- Recognize indications for various radiotherapy approaches including fractionated radiation or stereotactic radiosurgery.
- Learn appropriate target volumes and doses for both stereotactic radiosurgery and stereotactic fractionated radiation therapy for nonfunctioning and functioning pituitary adenomas.
- Know the local control rates, hormone normalization rates, and side effects associated with treating pituitary adenomas with radiation therapy.

## Epidemiology

Pituitary adenomas account for 16% of all brain tumors diagnosed in the United States (USA), making it the second most common brain tumor in adults. With an average of 11,733 new pituitary adenomas diagnosed annually, the incidence is estimated at 3.66 per 100,000 [1]. The incidence increases with age, peaking in the seventh and eighth decade, and is slightly more common in women than men and African-Americans than Caucasians [2]. Clinically nonfunctioning pituitary adenomas account for 25–30% of pituitary adenomas, of which 80–90% arise from gonadotropic cells. Functioning or secreting adenomas oversecrete a hormone normally produced by the pituitary gland and comprise the remaining 70–75%, with prolactinomas being the most common. Prolactinomas (PRL) account for approximately 32–51% of pituitary adenomas, followed by growth hormone (GH)-secreting adenomas (9–11%) and adrenocorticotropic hormone (ACTH)-secreting adenomas (3–6%.) Less than 1% of pituitary adenomas are thyroid-stimulating secreting or gonadotropin secreting [3].

The etiology of pituitary adenomas is largely unknown. Although studies have examined associations between pituitary adenoma and factors such as cigarette smoking, past diagnosis of head trauma, or prior brain neoplasms, no causal relationship has been identified [4]. There is no successful prevention of, or screening for, pituitary adenomas.

Approximately 60% of pituitary adenomas occur sporadically with no known genetic predisposition. Somatic mutations, including mutations in GNAS, USP8, PIK3CA, and complex I genes, account for almost 40% of pituitary adenomas. Germline mutations and mosaic mutations account for the rest of pituitary adenoma mutations. The most notable germline mutations include a mutation in the MEN1 gene causing multiple endocrine neoplasia type 1 (MEN1). This is associated with the classic triad of parathyroid tumors, pancreatic/gastrointestinal adenomas, and pituitary adenomas. The other mutation is the NF1 gene causing neurofibromatosis type 1 (NF1) which is associated with café-au-lait macules, neurofibromas, freckling, and other clinical features. Mosaic mutations include GNAS and GPR101 [5]. However, underlying genetic mutations do not affect management of pituitary adenomas.

L. M. Burt (✉) · D. C. Shrieve
Department of Radiation Oncology,
University of Utah School of Medicine,
Salt Lake City, UT, USA

Huntsman Cancer Institute, Salt Lake City, UT, USA
e-mail: Lindsay.burt@hci.utah.edu

G. Suneja
Department of Radiation Oncology,
Duke University Medical Center, Durham, NC, USA

© Springer International Publishing AG, part of Springer Nature 2018
E. L. Chang et al. (eds.), *Adult CNS Radiation Oncology*, https://doi.org/10.1007/978-3-319-42878-9_2

## Diagnosis and Prognosis

Early detection and treatment of pituitary adenomas are important. A normal pituitary gland is typically 8 millimeter (mm) by 10 mm by 6–8 mm anterior-posterior, transverse, and cranial-caudal, respectively. Pituitary adenomas that are detected incidentally on imaging studies are often termed incidentalomas and can occur in upward of 20% of CT scans and 38% of MRI scans [6, 7]. If not caught incidentally, nonfunctioning pituitary adenomas often go undiagnosed until they are large enough to cause clinical symptoms due to mass effect. These patients will most commonly present with visual symptoms including loss of temporal fields due to compression of the optic chiasm, followed by headaches and hypopituitarism [8]. Patients with secreting pituitary adenomas present with clinical findings related to hypersecretion of hormones. Prolactin-secreting tumors can cause galactorrhea and hypogonadotropic hypogonadism manifesting as amenorrhea and infertility in females and decreased libido, impotence, infertility, and gynecomastia in men. Growth hormone-secreting adenomas cause acromegaly with clinical findings of coarse facial features including macrognathia, furrowing of the forehead, and enlargement of the nose and ears. In children, gigantism can occur [9]. Adrenocorticotropic hormone-secreting adenomas can cause Cushing's disease with clinical symptoms of central obesity, abdominal stria, buffalo hump, and moon facies. Thyrotropin adenomas can cause signs of hyperthyroidism including warm skin, onycholysis, weight loss, agitation, and urinary frequency [3].

The workup for a suspected pituitary adenoma should include a detailed history and physical examination, referral to an endocrinologist for hormone evaluation and a neuro-ophthalmologist for visual field testing, and pituitary imaging. Hormonal evaluation should include measurements of serum prolactin, insulin-like growth factor-1 (IGF-1), luteinizing hormone (LH), follicle-stimulating hormone (FSH), alpha subunit, thyrotropin-releasing hormone (TRH) when available (currently not available in the US), and a 24-h urine free cortisol measurement.

Magnetic resonance imaging is the most sensitive imaging modality for pituitary adenomas. A dynamic MRI with fat suppression with and without contrast in axial, coronal, and sagittal views should be obtained to evaluate the extent of disease (Fig. 2.1). Thin slices less than 3 mm are recommended as false-negative rates as high as 45–62% have been associated with conventional T1 MR imaging [10]. Pituitary adenomas generally enhance more slowly than the adjacent pituitary and thus will be relatively hypointense compared to the intensely enhancing pituitary gland. Pituitary adenomas are difficult to diagnosis on CT as two-thirds are hypodense on contrast-enhanced images. It is important to try to distinguish pituitary adenomas from other sellar lesions including other tumors such as craniopharyngioma, meningioma, chordoma, primary lymphoma, germ cell tumor, and metastatic disease, as well as other findings in the sella-like Rathke's cleft cyst, infiltrative diseases such as granulomas, lymphocytic hypophysitis and tuberculosis, and inflammatory lesions [10].

The majority of pituitary adenomas are benign neoplasms of adenohypophysial cell origin that do not invade nearby structures or spread systemically. However, there is a spectrum of pituitary neoplasms from benign to malignant. Up to 25% of pituitary adenomas infiltrate and actively invade surrounding sellar structures and may clinically behave more aggressively. Pathologically these tumors show signs of increased proliferation and aggressiveness. Typical pituitary adenomas do not demonstrate mitoses on histology, have low ki-67 labeling indices, and show minimal p53 immunoreactivity and no invasion into other structures, although microscopic dural invasion is common and is not considered an atypical feature. Pituitary adenomas that show signs of increased proliferation rate, invasion, and aggressiveness are termed atypical pituitary adenomas. Distinguishing a typical pituitary adenoma from an atypical pituitary adenoma is not clearly defined. The WHO classification system designates atypical pituitary adenomas as having any of the following features: elevated mitotic count, ki-67 labeling indices >3%, extensive nuclear staining for p53, or invasion into other structures. However, the required degree of increased mitotic count or extensive p53 immunoreactivity is not clearly defined. If metastases are present or the pituitary neoplasm has spread to the cerebrospinal fluid (CSF), it is considered a pituitary carcinoma. Less than 1% of pituitary tumors are pituitary carcinomas [11].

The normal pituitary gland is composed of small acinic cells surrounded by intact reticulin. In cases of pituitary hyperplasia, the reticulin stays intact, while the acini are increased in size. Histologically the hallmark appearance of pituitary adenomas is the monotonous and monomorphous proliferation of neoplastic cells that replaces the normal acinar pattern of the pituitary and disrupts the reticulin fiber (WHO classification). Synaptophysin is consistently positive in pituitary adenomas with a lower percentage immunostaining positive for chromogranin A and low molecular weight keratins. Immunoreactivity for GH, PRL, β-TSH, β-FSH, β-LH, ACTH, and alpha subunit of the glycoproteins (α-SU) aids in pituitary adenoma classification [11].

Pituitary adenomas are now classified by looking at functional characteristics including histology, immunohistochemistry, and ultrastructural features as well as looking at biochemical hormone production, imaging, and surgical features [12]. Functioning pituitary adenomas include GH,

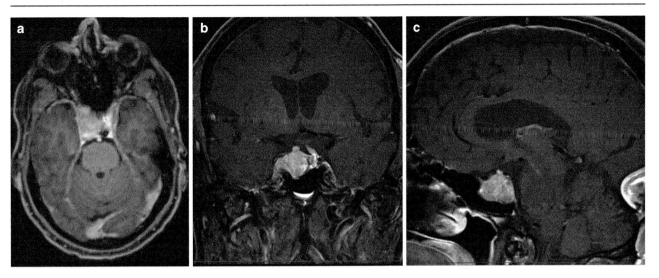

**Fig. 2.1** A fine slice T1 MRI with fat suppression showing the pituitary adenoma within the right sella that extended into the right sphenoid sinuses and posterior clinoid process and displaced the pituitary stalk and pituitary tissue to the left. Views are obtained in the axial (**a**), coronal (**b**), and sagittal (**c**) plane prior to radiation therapy

PRL, thyroid-stimulating hormone (TSH), ACTH, and gonadotropin-producing adenomas; however, most gonadotropin-producing adenomas are classified as nonfunctioning pituitary adenomas. Pituitary adenomas do not always secrete just one hormone; mixed adenomas can occur as well. Plurihormonal adenomas have immunoreactivities for more than one pituitary hormone, and their cytophysiology and developmental mechanisms do not explain their immunoreactivities making them unusual. These do not include common combinations of mixed secreting adenomas like GH, PRL, and TSH or FHS and LH. Nonfunctioning pituitary adenomas are largely composed of gonadotropin adenomas but also include null cell adenomas where no hormone immunoreactivity and no other immunohistochemical or ultrastructural markers of specific adenohypophysial cell differentiation are detected [11].

Pituitary adenomas are often characterized by size with microadenomas being <1 cm and macroadenomas ≥1 cm. One of the most common classification systems initially established by Hardy and later updated by Wilson grades pituitary adenomas on extension and invasion into the sella and sphenoid sinus [13]. Grade 0 has no abnormality of the sphenoid bone, grade I is a normal or focally expanded sella with tumor ≤1 cm, grade II is an enlarged sella with tumor >1 cm, grade III is a localized perforation of the sellar floor, grade IV is a diffuse destruction of the sellar floor, and grade V is spread into the CSF or blood. The extension into the suprasellar region is type A, extension to the anterior recesses of the third ventricle is type B, extension into the whole anterior third ventricle is type C, extension into the intracranial extradural is type D, and extracranial extradural extension is type E [13]. Parasellar extension is also often assessed using a radiographic grading system that looks at the extension of the adenoma into the cavernous sinus in association with the internal carotid artery. These grading systems can assist in surgical planning and determination of the feasibility of resection [14]. The initial grading system proposed in 1993 has more recently been updated to further subdivide the grading system by surgical validation with an endoscopic transnasal transsphenoidal approach [15].

Histologically, pituitary adenomas have been considered benign tumors; however, there is an increased risk of mortality with pituitary adenomas due to mass effect on vascular structures and hormonal imbalances. In nonfunctioning adenomas an increase in mortality has been estimated to be as high as 1.7 (95% confidence interval (CI) 1.34–2.15) compared to the endemic rate, mainly due to hypopituitarism [16]. With secreting pituitary adenomas, if left undiagnosed, there is a significant reduction in life expectancy. Growth hormone-secreting tumors can cause acromegaly. A two- to threefold increased risk of mortality has been demonstrated in patients with acromegaly compared with age- and sex-matched controls [17]. An oversecretion of ACTH can lead to hypercortisolism causing Cushing's disease. If left untreated, Cushing's disease has a median survival of around 5 years [16].

## Overall Treatment Strategy

The management of pituitary adenomas often involves a multimodality approach. An endocrinologist, neurosurgeon, otorhinolaryngologist, radiation oncologist, neuroradiologist, neuro-ophthalmologist, and neuropathologist should be involved in each case. In general, the overall goals of treatment are to preserve or restore normal hormonal function and remove or control any mass effect from the tumor that may be causing neurological or hormonal symptoms. Management can range from observation to a multimodality approach with surgery, radiation therapy, and medical management. Specific treatment recommendations are largely based on the type of pituitary adenoma and extent of disease.

Nonfunctioning "incidentalomas" should undergo a complete workup that includes laboratory evaluation for hormonal hypersecretion or hypopituitarism, appropriate pituitary imaging, and a visual field examination if it is near or abutting the optic chiasm. If there are no signs of visual field deficits, other neurological sequelae, or hormonal imbalances, observation is the recommended management strategy. Those that are less than 1 cm are often managed with close observation. Repeat MRI scans and possible visual field and hormonal evaluation can be performed annually. Many slow-growing tumors may never need further treatment.

The advent of transsphenoidal surgery has provided a less invasive first-line surgical option for many pituitary adenomas that are not appropriate for observation. A transsphenoidal resection can be completed either endoscopically or microscopically through a transnasal, sublabial, transethmoidal, or transantral approach [18]. In cases where there is intracranial extension or a transsphenoidal surgery is not applicable, then a transcranial approach may be used.

In nonfunctioning pituitary adenomas, tumor recurrence/progression has been estimated to be between 10% and 20% after a gross total resection (GTR) and 50% and 60% after a subtotal resection (STR) [19]. With functional pituitary adenomas in the hands of experienced neurosurgeons, GH-secreting adenomas have been found to have normalization of IGF-1 levels in 80–90% of microadenomas and 50% of macroadenomas [20]. In Cushing's disease, surgery has been associated with a 69–98% remission rate but a 3–17% relapse rate. Many studies reporting surgical remission rates of TSH-secreting pituitary adenomas have been poor; however, more recently remission rates with surgical resection have been reported to be as high as 100% for microadenomas and 81% for macroadenomas [21]. Surgery can be a second-line treatment for prolactinomas in those that do not tolerate medical therapy, are unresponsive, and develop visual deficits or for women desiring pregnancy. Surgical resection of prolactinomas has been reported to have curative rates in 74% of microadenomas and 33.9% of macroadenomas [22]. General surgical complications may include bleeding, infection, and thrombosis. Other complications may include CSF leak; damage to surrounding structures including the internal carotid artery, chiasm, and optic nerve; and abnormal secretion of one or more pituitary hormones resulting in symptoms such as diabetes insipidus from decreased antidiuretic hormone (ADH) production and death.

Medical management is the first-line treatment for prolactinomas and often used as adjuvant treatment after surgical resection and radiation therapy for secreting pituitary adenomas if hormonal levels do not normalize. Dopamine is a neuroendocrine inhibitor for secretion of prolactin in the pituitary. A dopamine agonist like bromocriptine or cabergoline has been shown to rapidly normalize prolactin levels and reduce tumor size in 80–90% of patients with prolactinomas [23]. Octreotide and lanreotide are somatostatin analogs that can be used in GH-secreting tumors to lower elevated GH levels before surgery, normalize levels in the latency period after radiation therapy, or treat patients that are not candidates for surgery and/or radiation therapy due to medical comorbidities. Insulin-like growth factor type 1 levels have been shown to decrease in 50–79% of patients and lead to tumor shrinkage in 40–73% patients receiving somatostatin analogs [22]. Growth hormone receptor antagonists like pegvisomant and dopamine analogs, as mentioned above, can also be used to treat acromegaly and aid in normalizing IGF-1 levels. Dopamine agonist and somatostatin analogs have also been found to normalize TSH levels in 79% of patients with TSH hypersecretion [24]. Medical management of ACTH-secreting adenomas is only provided in those that do not have remission after surgical resection and radiation therapy. Medications that inhibit steroidogenesis such as ketoconazole, aminoglutethimide, metyrapone, mitotane, and etomidate can but used for the treatment of persistent ACTH-secreting adenomas [25].

Hypopituitarism resulting from surgical treatment, radiation therapy, or tumor is best managed by an endocrinologist. Treatment may include glucocorticoid replacement with hydrocortisone, thyroid replacement with L-thyroxine, GH replacement in those found to be deficient, and testosterone and estrogen replacement if needed [26].

Although the first-line treatment of pituitary adenomas is typically surgery or medical management, radiation therapy, both fractionated radiation and SRS, can be used in the management of pituitary adenomas. The next sections will discuss in detail the indications, treatment, complications, and outcomes for the treatment of pituitary adenomas with radiation therapy.

## Indications for Radiotherapy

After maximal safe resection, indications for radiation therapy include subtotal surgical resection, recurrent or progressive tumors, hormone refractory disease, and atypical or carcinoma histologies. Hormone normalization and control of tumor growth are the main goals of radiation therapy for functioning adenomas, whereas in nonfunctioning adenomas the primary goal is tumor control. Due to high recurrence rates after a subtotal resection, postoperative radiation therapy is often recommended. However, the timing of postoperative radiation therapy is controversial with some advocating for treatment immediately after the surgery (within 6 months) and others favoring delayed radiotherapy (>6 month or at time of progression). Studies have shown mixed results on control rates and long-term toxicity [19, 27, 28]. Fractionated radiation therapy or SRS after a subtotal resection or debulking surgery can provide excellent local control rates. For atypical pituitary adenomas, there is little data on whether radiation therapy should be administered immediately after surgery or at the first signs of progression. In cases of atypical pituitary adenomas, it is best to assess all clinical data available and weigh the risks of toxicities associated with radiation therapy to the risks associated if the tumor progresses. A lower threshold for radiation therapy treatment should be applied for atypical pituitary adenomas compared to classic pituitary adenomas.

## Treatment Field Design/Target Delineation

Advances in radiation therapy techniques have greatly improved the therapeutic ratio for treatment of pituitary adenomas. Historically, these were treated with opposed laterals or a 3-field technique that delivered large doses of radiation to the temporal and frontal lobes. Advances in radiation delivery systems and the development of stereotactic localization have greatly improved treatment of skull-based tumors. Creating an optimal target volume requires adequate visualization of the pituitary adenoma. This is best obtained with a T1 MRI sequence through the skull base with 1 mm slice thickness. A pre- and post-contrast T1 MRI as well as fat suppression can be helpful in distinguishing post-op changes from residual blood products and fat-packing from the residual tumor. Since the pituitary is located in the sella adjacent to the optic nerves and chiasm, stereotactic localization and image guidance are recommended to allow for precise treatment to the tumor.

When stereotactic localization is used, treatment margins around the tumor can be reduced. A thin slice T1 post-contrast MRI should be fused with the simulation CT scan and used to define the lesion to create the gross tumor volume (GTV) (Fig. 2.2). The CT simulation scan should have slices <3 mm. As pituitary adenomas are typically not infiltrative or invasive, no clinical target volume is needed; however, one may add a small 1–5 mm margin to encompass potential areas of microscopic spread in the cavernous sinus or other areas of concern. The stereotactic headframe originally developed for the Gamma Knife has long been known

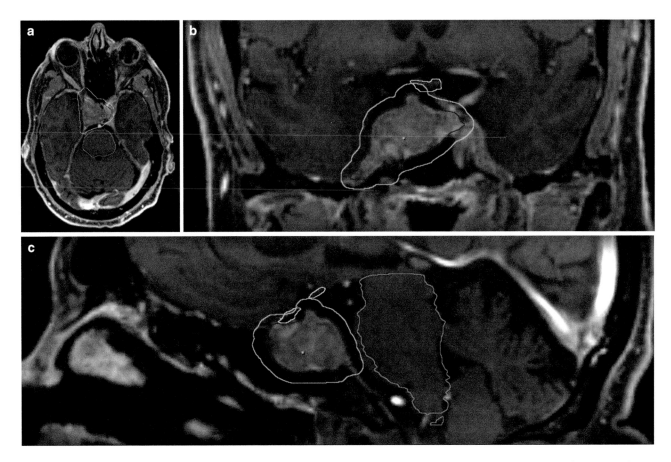

**Fig. 2.2** Axial (**a**), coronal (**b**), and sagittal (**c**) views of the pituitary adenoma contoured to create the GTV followed by a 3 mm expansion to create the PTV. GTV, red; PTV, cyan; eyes, purple

to have submillimeter accuracy [29]. A stereotactic frameless mask along with an image-guided system has been previously reported to obtain geometric accuracy of <0.5 mm [30]. Although up to a 2.8 mm displacement has been reported for fusions using soft tissue, the rigidity of the skull base allows for negligible deviations in position [31]. Due to the precision of setup, no planning treatment volume (PTV) is necessary for SRS. However, some centers may add a 1–3 mm expansion from GTV to PTV.

Due to the proximity of the pituitary to many critical structures, it is important to accurately contour organs at risk (OARs). In this region, OARs should include the optic nerves and chiasm, brainstem, pituitary stalk, and pituitary. Other OARs that could be contoured include the retina, lens, hypothalamus, cranial nerves (CN) within the cavernous sinus (CN III, IV, V1, V2, VI), retina, and hippocampus.

## Radiation Dose Prescription and Organ at Risk Tolerances

For fractionated SRS, doses range from 45 to 50.4 Gy for nonfunctioning adenomas and 50.4 to 54 Gy for functioning adenomas delivered in 1.8 Gy daily fractions (Fig. 2.3). With SRS a dose of 15 Gy is commonly used for nonfunctioning adenomas and 20 Gy for functioning adenomas [32]. Higher doses of radiation therapy are required in secreting pituitary adenomas to obtain hormone normalization. A hypofractionated SRS course of 25 Gy in 5 fractions or 21 Gy in 3 fractions delivered over 5 and 3 days, respectively, is also an acceptable option for pituitary adenomas not meeting dose constraints for single-fraction treatment [33, 34].

Different treatment delivery systems may be used for SRS including Gamma Knife, LINAC-based, and CyberKnife™. Gamma Knife is a frame-based system that utilizes 192 radio-

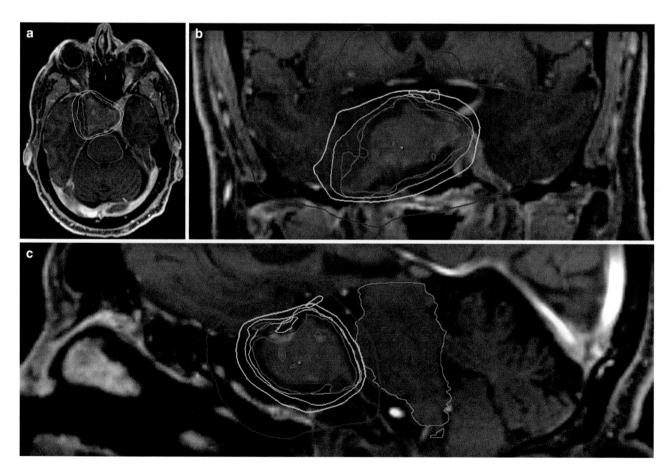

Fig. 2.3 Axial (a), coronal (b), and sagittal (c) views of a treatment plan with a dose of 50.4 Gy in 28 fractions prescribed to the 100% isodose line using an 11-field IMRT technique. Ninety-five percent of the dose is covering 99.4% of the PTV, and 95% of PTV is covered by 99.2% of the dose (D95, 99.4%; V95, 99.2%). The GTV is covered by 97.7% of the dose, and 99.1% of the GTV is getting full dose (D100, 97.7%; V100, 99.1%). The isodose lines are as follows: 100% isodose line, orange; 95% isodose line line, light orange; 80% isodose line, lime green; 30% isodose line, purpur. The 100% coverage is represented by the pink fill

active cobalt-60 sources arranged in a conical shape to create multiple focal beam shots focused at the target. The dose is usually prescribed at the 50% isodose line to maximize the dose within the each pinpoint target and minimize dose at the target edge. A fixed frame or frameless mask can be used in a LINAC-based SRS system, and treatment is often delivered using multiple dynamic conformal arcs or intensity-modulated radiation therapy to focus the dose in the center of the target. CyberKnife™ is a robotic arm with a mobile linear accelerator that has a robotic image-guided system that allows for a frameless mask to be used with SRS. Each delivery method has its benefits and drawbacks with LINAC-based SRS being more homogeneous for large tumors and Gamma Knife providing better conformality with irregular lesions; yet, no one technique has been proven to be superior.

## Complication Avoidance

In planning radiation therapy for pituitary adenomas, it is important to minimize dose to critical structures. Decreasing dose to the normal pituitary gland can avoid radiation-associated neuroendocrine deficits. Limiting the pituitary to a mean dose of ≤15 Gy has been found to decrease hypopituitarism when treating with SRS. It has also been suggested to decrease the infundibulum dose to a mean of ≤17 Gy [35]. It is also important to limit the dose to the optic apparatus. Classically, SRS has been not recommended for tumors within 3 mm of the optic apparatus as it is difficult to obtain enough dose to the tumor and meet the limitations of the optic apparatus. When dose constraints for perioptic tumors cannot be met, a fractionated or hypofractionated SRS course is recommended.

In general, for fractionated radiation therapy, OAR dose tolerances should include a maximum dose of 55 Gy to the optic nerve and chiasm, 54 Gy to the brainstem, 45 Gy to the retina, 7–8 Gy to the lenses, 50 Gy to the hypothalamus, a maximum of 50 Gy to the entire pituitary, and a mean of ≤45 Gy to the cochlea [36–38]. Tolerance doses of CN III, IV, V, VI, and VII are largely unknown but the recommended dose is ≤60 Gy. For SRS, the optic nerve should be limited to a maximum point dose of 10 Gy, the brainstem to a dose of 16 Gy, and the pituitary and distal infundibulum to a mean of ≤15 Gy, the cochlea to a mean dose of ≤3.7 Gy, CN VII ≤12.5–15 Gy, and CN V ≤12.5–13 Gy [35, 39]. Tolerance doses to CN III, IV, and VI are unknown but it is recommended these be kept as low as possible.

## Radiation Toxicity: Acute and Late Effects

Fractionated radiation therapy and SRS are important treatment options for patients with pituitary adenomas; however, they are not without potential acute and long-term side effects. During fractionated radiation therapy, patients may experience temporary alopecia, skin erythema, fatigue, and headaches. It is uncommon to have more severe side effects like vision loss or other cranial nerve deficits. With frame-based SRS, acute side effects may include numbness, tenderness, and bleeding at the frame pin sites. Otherwise, there are minimal side effects associated with SRS, aside from a possible headache and fatigue.

Long-term toxicities include hypopituitarism, optic neuropathy and other cranial neuropathies of the cavernous sinus, radiation necrosis, neurocognitive effects, vascular complications, and secondary malignancies. Hypopituitarism is the most common long-term toxicity and estimated to occur in approximately half of patients undergoing radiation therapy [36]. Hypopituitarism prior to radiation therapy has not been found to be predictive for new or worsening endocrine deficits. The most common hormonal deficiencies after radiation therapy are thyroid and cortisol which can be supplemented with levothyroxine and hydrocortisone [40]. Whether the hypopituitarism is caused by damage to the pituitary, hypothalamus, or both is unknown [41]. As mentioned above minimizing dose to the normal pituitary gland with SRS to a mean of ≤15 Gy and the infundibulum to a mean of ≤17 Gy reduces rates of neuroendocrine deficits.

Another potential long-term toxicity with radiation therapy is optic neuropathy. Keeping the optic apparatus below a dose of 8 Gy has been regarded as extremely safe [42]; however, studies suggest point doses up to 10 Gy results in <2% risk of optic neuropathy [43]. Leber et al. reported no radiation-induced optic neuropathy in patients receiving SRS with a max point dose of <10 Gy and a 26.7% optic neuropathy rate for a point dose of 12–15 Gy [44]. Fractionated external beam radiation carries a very low risk of damage to the optic pathway with an estimated incidence of 0.8% at 10 years [45]. With a hypofractionated course of 5 Gy × 5 fractions, a median maximum chiasm dose of 23.3 Gy (range 18.3–25.1 Gy) was reported with no visual deficits [34]. Excellent results have also been reported for a course of 7 Gy × 3 fractions keeping the mean optic nerve dose to 16.7 Gy and the chiasm to 14.6 Gy [33].

Long-term cranial neuropathies of the cavernous sinus nerves are not common [35]. Newer series assessing SRS for pituitary adenomas have reported new cranial nerve deficits to be below 2% [46]. A dose association has not been found for cranial neuropathies in SRS [42]. Cranial neuropathies with fractionated radiation therapy rarely occur.

Other rare long-term toxicities with radiation therapy include radiation necrosis, vascular complications, and secondary malignancies. Radiation necrosis occurred in 13 of 1567 patients on a meta-analysis of SRS for pituitary adenomas, approximately a 0.8% risk [47]. A fourfold increase in stroke and cerebrovascular accidents has been reported in patients receiving treatment for pituitary adenomas compared to the endemic rate; however, the relative contribution of radiation therapy is debatable [48]. A report from the Netherlands comparing pituitary adenomas treated with radiation therapy and those not irradiated did not show a difference in the incidence of stroke [45, 49]. Meta-analysis data showed a 0.25% rate of cerebrovascular accidents, of which, only 2 of 1567 patients were symptomatic [47]. Lastly, radiation-induced malignancies are always a concern with radiation, although the risk is low with fractionated radiation therapy and negligible with SRS. A review of 426 patients with pituitary adenomas treated at the Royal Marsden Hospital with surgery followed by fractionated radiotherapy found a cumulative risk of secondary brain tumors at 10 years to be 2% and 2.4% at 20 years [50]. The risk of secondary neoplasms at 15 years with SRS has been reported to be around 0.04% [44]. Overall, the risks of long-term side effects can be minimal if appropriate dose constraints are enforced and there appears to be no significant difference in long-term toxicities between SRS and fractionated radiation therapy.

## Outcomes: Tumor Control and Survival

Excellent tumor control rates have been reported for both SRS and fractionated radiation therapy. Fractionated courses of radiation therapy for nonfunctioning and secreting pituitary adenomas have reported rates of tumor control >90% at 5-year follow-up (Table 2.1). A large study of 252 nonfunctioning pituitary adenomas treated with a 3-field conventional plan to doses of 45–50 Gy had 10-year local control rates of 97% and 20-year local control rates of 92% [60]. More recently a large study by Chang et al. found a local control rate of 91% at a median follow-up of 8.4 years in 340 patients with resected nonfunctioning pituitary adenomas [61]. Studies using fractionated SRS have also shown local control rates to be >90% at 10 years. Even in large invasive nonfunctioning pituitary adenomas, postoperative fractionated stereotactic radiotherapy (FSRT) has proven to be effective with local control rates of 97% and 91% at 5 and 10 years, respectively [51].

In secreting pituitary adenomas, control is measured both by tumor growth and secreting hormone normalization. Unfortunately, biochemical control rates are difficult to assess across studies as the interpretation of hormone normalization and biochemical remission values vary among studies. Biochemical normalization of GH-secreting tumors with conventional or stereotactic fractionated radiation therapy may take up to 5–10 years. In a study of 884 patients treated with conventional radiation therapy to a median dose of 45 Gy, normalization of GH levels below 2.5 ng/mL was

**Table 2.1** Selected fractionated stereotactic radiosurgery and hypofractionated radiosurgery studies published since 2010 onward

| Study | # of pts | Type of RT | Tumor volume (mean, cm³) | Fun/ nonfun | Dose/fx (mean) | f/u (median) | LC (5 years) | Hormone control | Visual tox | Hypopitu |
|---|---|---|---|---|---|---|---|---|---|---|
| Minniti [51] | 68 | FSRT | 22.6 (11.1–52.2) | NF | 45 Gy/25fx | 75 | 97% | – | 0% | 26.4% |
| Diallo [52] | 34 | FSRT | 24.5 | GH | 50 Gy /27fx | 152 | 97% | 38.2% | | 39% |
| Puataweepong [53] | 71 (NF) 11 (GH) 9 (PRL) 3 (ACTH) | FSRT | 10 (0.8–45.5) | NF, GH, PRL, ACTH | 45 Gy/25 | 62 | 95% at 6 years | – 26% (GH) 4.3% (PRL) 34.6% ACTH | 3% | 9.6% |
| Kopp [54] | 29 (NF) 8 (F) | FSRT | 22.8 (2.0–78.3) | NF, F | 49.4 Gy/28 | 57 | 91.9% | – | 5% | 5% |
| Kim [55] | 54 (NF) 22 (F) | FSRT | 10.5` (1.5–37.8) | NF, F | 50.4 Gy/28fx | 80 | 97% at 7 years | 63.6% | 0% | 48% |
| Wilson [56] | 53 (CRT) 67 (FSRT) | CRT FSRT | 6.8 (0.2–115.6) | NF | 50.4 Gy/28fx | 53 61 | 86.9% (CRT) 92.8% (FSRT) | – | 11% (CRT) 1.5% (FSRT) | 7% CRT) 32% (FSRT) |
| Sun [57] | 13 (NF) 10 (F) | FSRT | 2 cm (0.5–3.5) | NF, GH, ACTH, PRL | 50.4 Gy/28fx | 39 | 96% (NF)~ 100% (F)~ | 62.5% (F) | 15% (NF) 0% (F) | 0% (NF) 10% (F) |
| Schalin-Jantti [58] | 20 (NF) 10 (F) | FSRT | 8.48` (0.06–65) | NF, F | 45 Gy/25fx | 63 | 100% | All had ↓ in abnormal hormones | 0% | 40% |
| Liao [33] | 21 (NF) 13 (F) | hSRS— 3fx | 5.06 (0.82– 12.69) | NF, F | 21 Gy/3fx | 37 | 100%~ | – 14% | 0% | – |
| Iwata [59] | 83 (3fx) 17 (5fx) | hSRS— 3fx hSRS— 5fx | 5.01` (0.7–64.3) | NF | 21 Gy/3fx 25 Gy/5fx | 33 | 98%° (3fx) 96%° (5fx) | – | 0.1% (3fx) 0% (5fx) | 3.6% (3fx) 0% (5fx) |

`is the median
%° is 3 year local control

**Table 2.2** Select stereotactic radiosurgery studies published since 2010 onward with large patient population (>90 patients)

| Study | # of pts | Type of RT | Tumor volume | Fun/ nonfun | Dose/fx (mean) | f/u | LC (5 years) (%) | Hormone control | Visual tox | Hypopitu (%) |
|---|---|---|---|---|---|---|---|---|---|---|
| Sheehan [69] | 512 | GK | 4.6 ± 4.9 | NF | 16 | 36 | 95 | – | 6.6% | 21 |
| Starke [70] | 140 | GK | 5.6 (0.6–35) | NF | 18 | 50 | 97 | – | 12.8% | 30.3 |
| Park [71] | 125 | GK | 3.5 (0.4–28.1) | NF | 13 | 62 | 94 | – | 0.8% | 24 |
| Franzin [72] | 103 | GK | 1.8 (0.1–7.2) | GH | 22.5 | 71 | 97.3 | 58.5% @5y | 0 | 14 |
| Sheehan [73] | 130 | GK | 1.9 (0.1–27) | GH | 24 | 31 | 93 | 53% | 2.4% | 24.4 |
| Sheehan [40] | 96 | GK | 1.8 (0.2–12.4) | ACTH | 16 | 48 | 98 | 70% | 5.2% | 36 |

median

22%, 63%, 74%, and 77% at 2-, 10-, 15-, and 20-year follow-up, respectively, with IGH-1 dose levels paralleling the GH levels [62]. Another study treating GH-secreting pituitary adenomas with FSRT to a median total dose of 52 Gy found biochemical normalization in 84% of the 25 patients at a median follow-up of 26 months [63]. More recently, a report of 34 patients treated with 50 Gy using FSRT found a 97% normalization rate of IGH-1 at a median follow-up of 12 years. All tumors were locally controlled as well [52].

For ACTH-secreting pituitary adenomas, normalization of cortisol levels usually occurs in the first 2 years. A study reported in the NEJM found a mean radiation dose of 50 Gy (range, 48–54 Gy) to yield biochemical control in 83% of patients at a median follow-up of 42 months [64]. Minniti et al. reported an overall remission rate in cortisol hypersecretion of 80% at median follow-up of 9 years with doses between 45 and 50 Gy. Local tumor control rate was 93% at 10 years. This study also found that biochemical normalization improved with time as 28%, 73%, 78%, and 84% of patients had normalization of cortisol secretion at 1, 3, 5, and 10 years, respectively [65].

Prolactinomas are less commonly treated with radiation therapy as it is a third-line treatment and only used in those resistant to medical management and surgery. Definitive radiation therapy for prolactinomas has been well studied but has historically yielded poor biochemical response in comparison to medical management and surgery [22]. However, more recent studies showed 100% prolactin normalization after FSRT with doses between 45 and 54 Gy [57, 58].

Due to the rarity of TSH-secreting tumors, local control and biochemical control rates after radiation therapy have not been well reported. In a large study of 25 TSH-secreting tumors, 12 received radiation therapy, 2 were treated definitively with radiation therapy. The patients receiving both surgery and radiation therapy with or without medical management had a 57% biochemical remission rate [66]. In another study, 8 of 43 TSH-secreting adenomas had radiation therapy due to uncontrollable tumor after surgery. The dose ranged between 42 and 45 Gy. With a median follow-up of 6.8 years, there were five that had biochemical control at a mean time of 3 years from treatment [67].

Traditionally, pituitary adenomas were treated with conventional radiation therapy. However, more recently conventional radiation therapy has been reserved for cases not amenable to SRS, typically due to the proximity to the optic nerve or large size of the adenoma. The efficacy and safety of SRS appear to be similar to FSRT [68]. Stereotactic radiosurgery in nonfunctioning pituitary adenomas has reported local control rates between 87 and 100% at 5 years assessed by tumor growth (Table 2.2) [74].

Pooling together 15 studies using SRS for 684 patients, the actuarial tumor control rate was 94% at 5 years [75]. In GH-secreting pituitary adenomas, a tumor control rate of 95–100% has been reported in 13 studies using SRS with a median follow-up of 5 years or more [59]. Biochemical remission rates with SRS for GH-secreting pituitary adenomas have been reported in 29 studies for a compiled total of 1215 patients to be 44% (range 15–60%) and 74% (range 46–86%) at 5 and 10 years, respectively [75]. Normalization of IGF-1 levels and biochemical response ranged from 1 to 5.6 years.

In ACTH-secreting pituitary adenomas in studies with a median follow-up of ≥5 years, a tumor control rate with SRS has been reported to be >95% [74]. At a median follow-up of 45 months in 12 studies, 48% of patients with Cushing's disease had biochemical response with a range from 3 months to 3 years for time to response [75].

When radiation is needed for prolactinomas, SRS is a well-utilized option. In studies with a median follow-up of greater than 5 years, the tumor control rate for prolactinomas with SRS was 97–100% but had a biochemical remission rate of 18–46.6% [74]. A pooled analysis of 11 studies utilizing SRS in prolactinomas resistant to medical management and surgery found normalization of PRL levels in 35% of the 338 and patients and the response rate to range between 12 and 66 months [74]. The tumor control rate in this pooled analysis was 99% at a weighted average follow-up of 42 months.

Although hypofractionated courses of SRS have been less studied, local tumor control and biochemical remission appear to be similar to SRS with one fraction [33, 34, 59]. It should be noted that medical therapy for secreting adenomas should be stopped approximately 2 months before radiation therapy as the medications may alter the cell cycle making the tumor less radiosensitive.

## Follow-up

Six to 12 months after the completion of radiation therapy, a baseline MRI of the pituitary and history and physical examination is recommended. Due to the slow-growing nature of most pituitary adenomas, subsequent follow-up imaging is usually on an annual basis. Atypical or carcinoma histology may require more frequent imaging, although the optimal schedule is not known. An MRI with and without contrast and fine slices through the pituitary in all three plans (axial, coronal, and sagittal) is important for assessing tumor recurrence. A history and physical examination should be obtained annually with special attention to visual deficits, cranial nerves that course through the cavernous sinus, panhypopituitarism, and any signs of long-term toxicity from radiation therapy. Follow-up management of treated pituitary adenomas often includes other providers including an endocrinologist, a neuro-ophthalmology, and a skull base/neurosurgeon. For secreting pituitary adenomas, careful attention to normalization of the secreting hormone as well as hypopituitarism of the other pituitary hormones is important. In nonfunctioning adenomas, lab work should be obtained at any concerning finding for hypopituitarism as this is the most common long-term side effect after radiation therapy [73].

## Cases

### Case 1

A 72-year-old male presented with visual symptoms, and an MRI was completed revealing a 3 cm pituitary adenoma that extended superiorly out of the diaphragmatic sella and compressed the optic chiasm as well as invaded the right cavernous sinus. He was seen by an endocrinologist for further workup of his new diagnosis of a pituitary adenoma. Labs were obtained revealing a slightly elevated prolactin level due to compression of the infundibulum. He underwent a transnasal transsphenoidal resection of the pituitary macroadenoma. The pituitary adenoma was markedly debulked, but residual disease remained due to extension into the right cavernous sinus. Pathology revealed a hypercel-

lular, monotonous neoplasm composed of sheets of cells with eosinophilic cytoplasm and oval nuclei with stippled chromatin. There was moderate pleomorphism to the cells consistent with a pituitary adenoma. There were no mitoses or evidence of necrosis. A postoperative brain MRI revealed a debulking of the pituitary adenoma with fat-packing in the nasal cavity and sphenoid sinus. There was residual pituitary adenoma in the right cavernous sinus encasing the right carotid artery measuring 15 × 26 × 15 mm (CC × AP × transverse) in the right cavernous sinus. He developed panhypopituitarism after his surgery and was followed by his endocrinologist. Two years after his surgery, a pituitary protocol MRI revealed interval growth of the pituitary adenoma involving the right cavernous sinus that now measured 36 × 23 × 22 mm in size (Fig. 2.1). He refused any further surgery and therefore was referred to the radiation oncology department. Due to the location next to the right optic nerve, SRS was not possible. Thus, a stereotactic fractionated course of radiation therapy with 50.4 Gy in 28 fractions was recommended. He had a stereotactic fine slice T1 MRI through the pituitary with gadolinium as well as a stereotactic T1 fat suppression through the pituitary region. A CT simulation with a Brainlab mask was completed. The residual tumor was outlined on the T1 fat suppression MRI scan which allowed for better assessment of the disease extent near the orbit and the fat-packing. The GTV was then expanded 3 mm in all directions to create a PTV (Fig. 2.2). A plan was made using an 11-field intensity-modulated radiation therapy (IMRT) technique (Fig. 2.3). The dose-volume histogram illustrates all the normal structures are well below acceptable tolerance doses and the GTV is covered by 97.7% of the dose and 99.1% of the GTV is getting full dose (Fig. 2.4). The patient tolerated the treatment well without difficulty. He is now 3 years out from radiation therapy and has no evidence of disease progression or worsening visual symptoms (Fig. 2.5).

### Case 2

A 21-year-old male presented to his ophthalmologist and was found to have bitemporal hemianopsia. An MRI scan was completed which showed a large enhancing mass expanding out of the sella turcica and into the suprasellar cistern causing compression of the optic chiasm. This was consistent with a pituitary tumor (Fig. 2.6). He was seen by an endocrinologist and on further workup was found to

**Fig. 2.4** Dose-volume histogram showing the brainstem, chiasm, and optic nerves all well below tolerance levels. This was easily achievable due to the prescribed dose being only 50.4 Gy. GTV, red; PTV, cyan; eyes, purple; left optic nerve, pink; right optic nerve, green

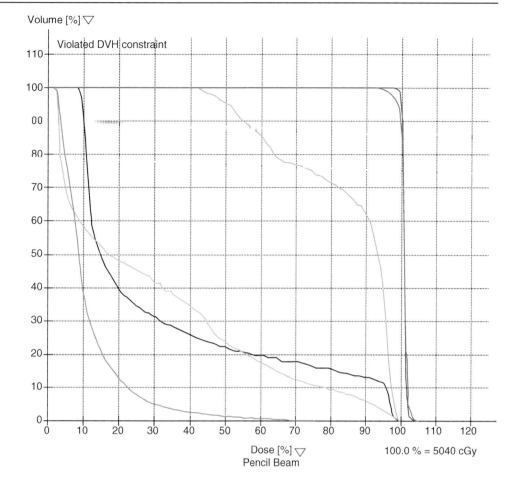

**Fig. 2.5** Axial (**a**), coronal (**b**), and sagittal (**c**) views showing an unchanged pituitary adenoma in the right posterior aspect of the sella that extends into the right cavernous sinus and encases the internal carotid artery

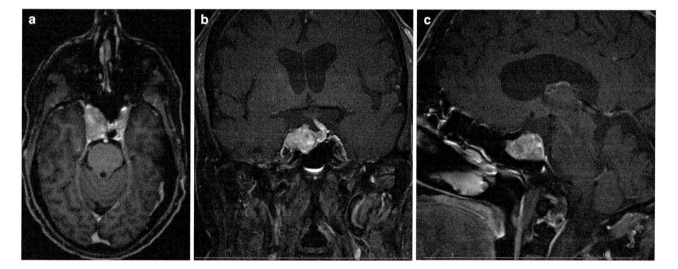

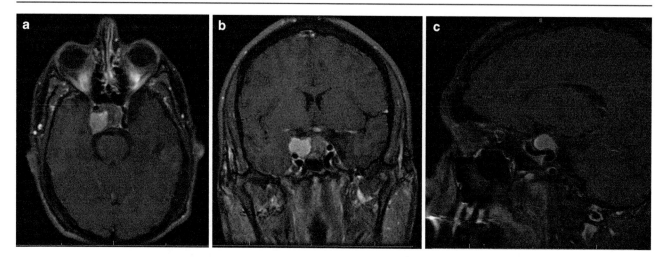

**Fig. 2.6** Axial (**a**), coronal (**b**), and sagittal (**c**) views of the pituitary adenoma extending into the suprasellar cistern, displacing the pituitary stalk and compressing the optic chiasm

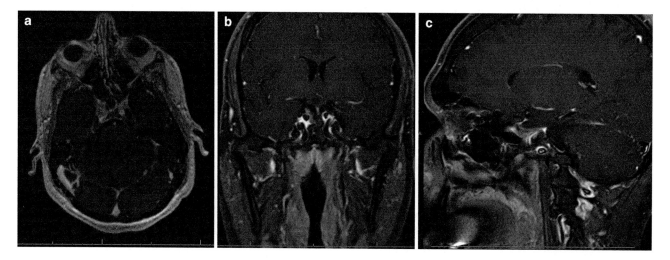

**Fig. 2.7** Axial (**a**), coronal (**b**), and sagittal (**c**) views of the residual pituitary adenoma on the right lateral aspect of the sella turcica after surgical resection

have a GH level of 24 ng/mL and an insulin-like growth factor of 1100. He was taken to the operating room for a transnasal transsphenoidal surgical resection. Pathology revealed a pituitary adenoma with no mitoses. A postoperative MRI showed some residual enhancement within the sella representing either residual tumor or postoperative changes, and his GH and IGF-1 normalized. Unfortunately, over the course of the next year, he had a rise in his GH and IGF-1, and an MRI showed enlargement of an enhancing mass predominantly on the right side of the sella. He was taken back for a redo transsphenoidal resection where pituitary adenoma was resected from the right side of the pituitary gland. Unfortunately, there was adherent tissue along the right lateral aspect of the sella turcica that could not be fully resected. A postoperative MRI revealed residual disease along the right lateral sella turcica (Fig. 2.7). He was then started on Sandostatin by

his endocrinologist. He was followed with stable MRIs and his GH and IGF-1 levels normalized to 0.7 ng/mL and 217 ng/mL, respectively. Unfortunately, 3 years later he was unable to continue Sandostatin. His case was discussed at a multidisciplinary tumor board and it was recommended he undergo SRS. He underwent SRS planning with the GTV encompassing the residual pituitary adenoma on the right lateral sella turcica and no PTV expansions (Fig. 2.8). An 8-field IMRT plan was constructed, prescribing 20 Gy to the GTV (Fig. 2.9). The optic nerves and chiasm were kept well below 8 Gy and the brainstem was limited to 12 Gy. The dose-volume histogram shows that the GTV is covered by 100% of the dose (Fig. 2.10). Prior to SRS, he had been off Sandostatin for over a year and his IGF-1 level rose to 383. He tolerated his SRS treatment well and was seen back in follow-up 6 months later. A brain MRI showed no evidence of progression (Fig. 2.11)

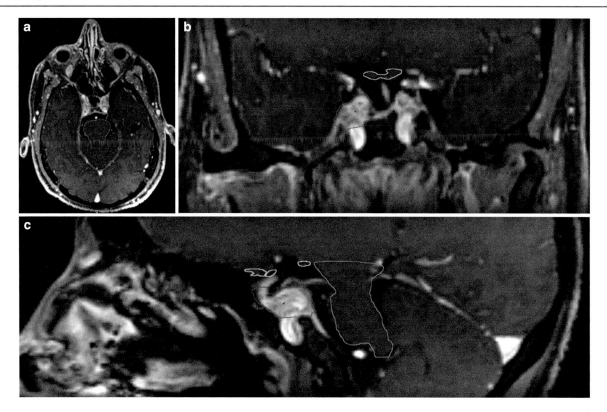

**Fig. 2.8** Axial (**a**), coronal (**b**), and sagittal (**c**) views of the residual pituitary adenoma contoured to create the GTV with no PTV. GTV, red; eyes, purple; right optic nerve, green; chiasm, yellow

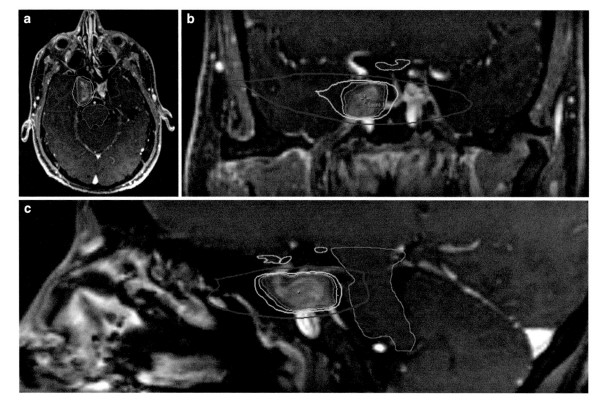

**Fig. 2.9** Axial (**a**), coronal (**b**), and sagittal (**c**) views of the treatment plan. A dose of 20 Gy in a single fraction was prescribed to the 100% isodose line using an 8-field IMRT technique. A three-dimensional conformal arch or volumetric modulated radiation therapy (VMRT) technique may also be utilized. One hundred percent of the GTV covered 100% of the dose which is shown above. The isodose lines are as follows: 100% isodose line, orange; 95% isodose line line, light orange; 80% isodose line, lime green; 30% isodose line, purpur. The 100% coverage is represented by the pink fill

**Fig. 2.10** Dose-volume histogram showing the brainstem, chiasm, and optic nerves all well below tolerance levels. GTV, red; eyes, purple; left optic nerve, pink; right optic nerve, green; pituitary, blue

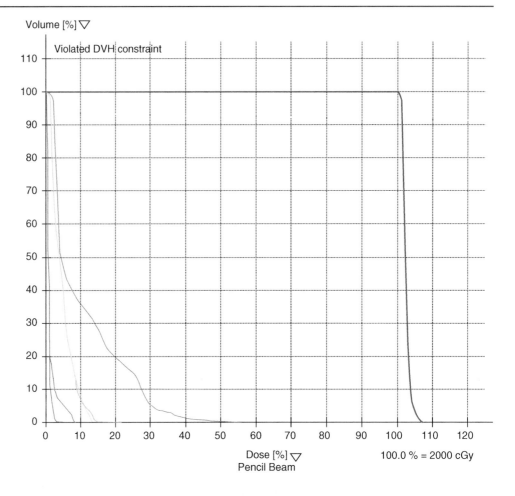

Volume [%] ▽

Violated DVH constraint

Dose [%] ▽
Pencil Beam

100.0 % = 2000 cGy

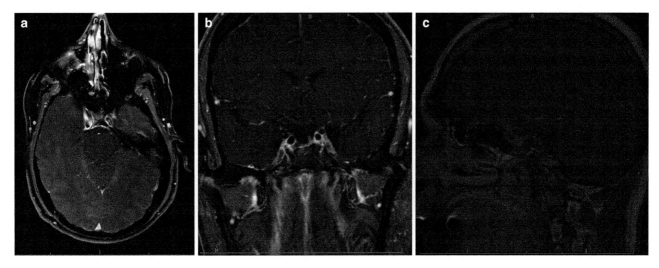

**Fig. 2.11** Axial (**a**), coronal (**b**), and sagittal (**c**) views of the sella showing no evidence of pituitary adenoma

and his IGF-1 level had dropped to 103. He was then followed annually with repeat IGF-1 levels and MRIs. Seven years out from treatment, he is doing well with no evidence of any residual disease progression on MRI, an IGF-1 level of 19, and no radiation-induced toxicities.

## Summary

- Pituitary adenomas are a common benign neoplasm of the brain estimated to represent approximately 15–20% of all intracranial neoplasms.

- Clinically nonfunctioning pituitary adenomas account for 25–30% of pituitary adenomas, while functioning or secreting adenomas oversecrete a hormone normally produced by the pituitary gland and comprise the remaining 70–75%.
- Patients with pituitary adenomas will commonly present with visual symptoms including loss of temporal fields due to compression of the optic chiasm, followed by headaches and hypopituitarism. Patients with secreting pituitary adenomas also present with clinical findings related to hypersecretion of hormones.
- The management of pituitary adenomas involves a multimodality approach with the goals of treatment to preserve or restore normal hormonal function and remove or control any mass effect from the tumor that may be causing neurological or hormonal symptoms.
- Indications for radiation therapy in the treatment of pituitary adenomas include a subtotal resection, recurrent or progressive tumors, hormone refractory disease, and atypical or carcinoma histologies.
- Radiosurgery can be used to treat pituitary adenomas if the optic structures are approximately 3 mm from the pituitary adenoma.
- Fractionated doses of 45–50.4 Gy and radiosurgery doses of 15 Gy are used to treat nonfunctioning pituitary adenomas.
- Secreting pituitary adenomas require slightly higher doses of radiation with fractionated doses of 50.4–54 Gy and radiosurgery doses of 20 Gy.
- Fractionated courses of radiation therapy for nonfunctioning and secreting pituitary adenomas have reported rates of tumor control >90% at 5-year follow-up.
- SRS in nonfunctioning pituitary adenomas have reported local control rates between 87% and 100% at 5 years assessed by tumor growth.
- For secreting pituitary adenomas, biochemical control rates with fractionated radiation and radiosurgery are difficult to assess across studies as the interpretation of hormone normalization and biochemical remission values vary among studies.
- Long-term toxicities with radiation therapy include hypopituitarism, optic neuropathy and other cranial neuropathies of the cavernous sinus, radiation necrosis, neurocognitive effects, vascular complications, and secondary malignancies.

## Self-Assessment Questions

1. Pituitary adenomas are best visualized on which type of imaging scan?
   A. CT scan with and without contrast
   B. T2-weighted brain MRI
   C. T1-weighted brain MRI with gadolinium
   D. PET/CT scan

2. What is the fractionated radiation therapy dose for a secreting pituitary?
   A. 41.4–45 Gy
   B. 45–50.4 Gy
   C. 50.4–54 Gy
   D. 54–59.4 Gy

3. A nonfunctioning pituitary adenoma recurs along the right cavernous sinus and abuts the right optic nerve. The best management would be:
   A. SRS with 15 Gy
   B. SRS with 20 Gy
   C. Fractionated radiation with 45 Gy
   D. Fractionated radiation with 54 Gy

4. The most common side effect from radiation therapy for treatment of a pituitary adenoma is
   A. Visual deficit
   B. Hypopituitarism
   C. Stroke
   D. Secondary malignancies

5. After radiation therapy, repeat imaging should occur:
   A. Every month
   B. Every 3 months
   C. Six months after completing radiation, then annually
   D. Every 2 years

## Answers

1. C
2. C
3. C
4. B
5. C

## References

1. Ostrom QT, Gittleman H, Fulop J, et al. CBTRUS statistical report: primary brain and central nervous system tumors diagnosed in the United States in 2008–2012. Neuro Oncol. 2015;17(Suppl 4):iv1–iv62.
2. Gittleman H, Ostrom QT, Farah PD, et al. Descriptive epidemiology of pituitary tumors in the United States, 2004–2009. J Neurosurg. 2014;121(3):527–35.
3. Mehta GU, Lonser RR. Management of hormone-secreting pituitary adenomas. Neuro Oncol. 2017;19(6):762–73.
4. Schoemaker MJ, Swerdlow AJ. Risk factors for pituitary tumors: a case-control study. Cancer Epidemiol Biomark Prev. 2009;18(5):1492–500.
5. Caimari F, Korbonits M. Novel genetic causes of pituitary adenomas. Clin Cancer Res. 2016;22(20):5030–42.
6. Vasilev V, Rostomyan L, Daly AF, et al. MANAGEMENT OF ENDOCRINE DISEASE: Pituitary 'incidentaloma': neuroradio-

logical assessment and differential diagnosis. Eur J Endocrinol. 2016;175(4):R171–84.

7. Paschou S, Vryonidou A, Goulis DG. Pituitary incidentalomas: a guide to assessment, treatment and follow-up. Maturitas. 2016;92:143–9.

8. Molitch ME. Nonfunctioning pituitary tumors and pituitary incidentalomas. Endocrinol Metab Clin N Am. 2008;37(1):151–71, xi.

9. Vilar L, Naves LA, Azevedo MF, et al. Effectiveness of cabergoline in monotherapy and combined with ketoconazole in the management of Cushing's disease. Pituitary. 2010;13(2):123–9.

10. Ouyang T, Rothfus WE, Ng JM, et al. Imaging of the pituitary. Radiol Clin N Am. 2011;49(3):549–71, vii.

11. DeLellis RA, Lloyd RV, Heitz PU, et al. World Health Organization Classification of Tumors. Pathology and genetics of tumours of endocrine organs. Lyon: IARC; 2004.

12. Kovacs K, Horvath E, Vidal S. Classification of pituitary adenomas. J Neurooncol. 2001;54(2):121–7.

13. Wilson CB. A decade of pituitary microsurgery. The Herbert Olivecrona lecture. J Neurosurg. 1984;61(5):814–33.

14. Knosp E, Steiner E, Kitz K, et al. Pituitary adenomas with invasion of the cavernous sinus space: a magnetic resonance imaging classification compared with surgical findings. Neurosurgery. 1993;33(4):610–7; discussion 7–8.

15. Micko AS, Wohrer A, Wolfsberger S, et al. Invasion of the cavernous sinus space in pituitary adenomas: endoscopic verification and its correlation with an MRI-based classification. J Neurosurg. 2015;122(4):803–11.

16. Sherlock M, Ayuk J, Tomlinson JW, et al. Mortality in patients with pituitary disease. Endocr Rev. 2010;31(3):301–42.

17. Melmed S, Colao A, Barkan A, et al. Guidelines for acromegaly management: an update. J Clin Endocrinol Metab. 2009;94(5):1509–17.

18. Chole RA, Lim C, Dunham B, et al. A novel transnasal transsphenoidal speculum: a design for both microscopic and endoscopic transsphenoidal pituitary surgery. J Neurosurg. 2011;114(5):1380–5.

19. Pomeraniec IJ, Dallapiazza RF, Xu Z, et al. Early versus late Gamma Knife radiosurgery following transsphenoidal resection for nonfunctioning pituitary macroadenomas: a matched cohort study. J Neurosurg. 2016;125(1):202–12.

20. Erturk E, Tuncel E, Kiyici S, et al. Outcome of surgery for acromegaly performed by different surgeons: importance of surgical experience. Pituitary. 2005;8(2):93–7.

21. Yamada S, Fukuhara N, Horiguchi K, et al. Clinicopathological characteristics and therapeutic outcomes in thyrotropin-secreting pituitary adenomas: a single-center study of 90 cases. J Neurosurg. 2014;121(6):1462–73.

22. Platta CS, Mackay C, Welsh JS. Pituitary adenoma: a radiotherapeutic perspective. Am J Clin Oncol. 2010;33(4):408–19.

23. Gillam MP, Molitch ME, Lombardi G, et al. Advances in the treatment of prolactinomas. Endocr Rev. 2006;27(5):485–534.

24. Beck-Peccoz P, Brucker-Davis F, Persani L, et al. Thyrotropin-secreting pituitary tumors. Endocr Rev. 1996;17(6):610–38.

25. Schteingart DE. Drugs in the medical treatment of Cushing's syndrome. Expert Opin Emerg Drugs. 2009;14(4):661–71.

26. Fleseriu M, Hashim IA, Karavitaki N, et al. Hormonal replacement in hypopituitarism in adults: an Endocrine Society clinical practice guideline. J Clin Endocrinol Metab. 2016;101(11):3888–921.

27. Dekkers OM, Pereira AM, Romijn JA. Treatment and follow-up of clinically nonfunctioning pituitary macroadenomas. J Clin Endocrinol Metab. 2008;93(10):3717–26.

28. Sadik ZH, Voormolen EH, Depauw PR, et al. Treatment of non-functional pituitary adenoma post-operative remnants: adjuvant or delayed gamma knife radiosurgery? World Neurosurg. 2017;100:361.

29. Leksell L. The stereotaxic method and radiosurgery of the brain. Acta Chir Scand. 1951;102(4):316–9.

30. Lamba M, Breneman JC, Warnick RE. Evaluation of image-guided positioning for frameless intracranial radiosurgery. Int J Radiat Oncol Biol Phys. 2009;74(3):913–9.

31. Guckenberger M, Baier K, Guenther I, et al. Reliability of the bony anatomy in image-guided stereotactic radiotherapy of brain metastases. Int J Radiat Oncol Biol Phys. 2007;69(1):294–301.

32. Loeffler JS, Shih HA. Radiation therapy in the management of pituitary adenomas. J Clin Endocrinol Metab. 2011;96(7):1992–2003.

33. Liao HI, Wang CC, Wei KC, et al. Fractionated stereotactic radiosurgery using the Novalis system for the management of pituitary adenomas close to the optic apparatus. J Clin Neurosci. 2014;21(1):111–5.

34. Killory BD, Kresl JJ, Wait SD, et al. Hypofractionated CyberKnife™ radiosurgery for perichiasmatic pituitary adenomas: early results. Neurosurgery. 2009;64(2 Suppl):A19.

35. Vladyka V, Liscak R, Novotny J Jr, et al. Radiation tolerance of functioning pituitary tissue in gamma knife surgery for pituitary adenomas. Neurosurgery. 2003;52(2):309–16; discussion 16–7.

36. Pai HH, Thornton A, Katznelson L, et al. Hypothalamic/pituitary function following high-dose conformal radiotherapy to the base of skull: demonstration of a dose-effect relationship using dose-volume histogram analysis. Int J Radiat Oncol Biol Phys. 2001;49(4):1079–92.

37. Emami B, Lyman J, Brown A, et al. Tolerance of normal tissue to therapeutic irradiation. Int J Radiat Oncol Biol Phys. 1991;21(1):109–22.

38. Marks LB, Yorke ED, Jackson A, et al. Use of normal tissue complication probability models in the clinic. Int J Radiat Oncol Biol Phys. 2010;76(3 Suppl):S10–9.

39. Anker CJ, Shrieve DC. Basic principles of radiobiology applied to radiosurgery and radiotherapy of benign skull base tumors. Otolaryngol Clin N Am. 2009;42(4):601–21.

40. Sheehan JP, Xu Z, Salvetti DJ, et al. Results of gamma knife surgery for Cushing's disease. J Neurosurg. 2013;119(6):1486–92.

41. Darzy KH. Radiation-induced hypopituitarism after cancer therapy: who, how and when to test. Nat Clin Pract Endocrinol Metab. 2009;5(2):88–99.

42. Tishler RB, Loeffler JS, Lunsford LD, et al. Tolerance of cranial nerves of the cavernous sinus to radiosurgery. Int J Radiat Oncol Biol Phys. 1993;27(2):215–21.

43. Minniti G, Osti MF, Niyazi M. Target delineation and optimal radiosurgical dose for pituitary tumors. Radiat Oncol. 2016;11(1):135.

44. Patel TR, Chiang VL. Secondary neoplasms after stereotactic radiosurgery. World Neurosurg. 2014;81(3–4):594–9.

45. Erridge SC, Conkey DS, Stockton D, et al. Radiotherapy for pituitary adenomas: long-term efficacy and toxicity. Radiother Oncol. 2009;93(3):597–601.

46. Bir SC, Murray RD, Ambekar S, et al. Clinical and radiologic outcome of gamma knife radiosurgery on nonfunctioning pituitary adenomas. J Neurol Surg B Skull Base. 2015;76(5):351–7.

47. Laws ER, Sheehan JP, Sheehan JM, et al. Stereotactic radiosurgery for pituitary adenomas: a review of the literature. J Neurooncol. 2004;69(1–3):257–72.

48. Brada M, Ashley S, Ford D, et al. Cerebrovascular mortality in patients with pituitary adenoma. Clin Endocrinol. 2002;57(6):713–7.

49. Sattler MG, Vroomen PC, Sluiter WJ, et al. Incidence, causative mechanisms, and anatomic localization of stroke in pituitary adenoma patients treated with postoperative radiation therapy versus surgery alone. Int J Radiat Oncol Biol Phys. 2013;87(1):53–9.

50. Minniti G, Traish D, Ashley S, et al. Risk of second brain tumor after conservative surgery and radiotherapy for pituitary adenoma: update after an additional 10 years. J Clin Endocrinol Metab. 2005;90(2):800–4.

51. Minniti G, Scaringi C, Poggi M, et al. Fractionated stereotactic radiotherapy for large and invasive non-functioning pituitary adenomas: long-term clinical outcomes and volumetric MRI assessment of tumor response. Eur J Endocrinol. 2015;172(4):433–41.

52. Diallo AM, Colin P, Litre CF, et al. Long-term results of fractionated stereotactic radiotherapy as third-line treatment in acromegaly. Endocrine. 2015;50(3):741–8.

53. Puataweepong P, Dhanachai M, Hansasuta A, et al. Outcomes for pituitary adenoma patients treated with Linac-based stereotactic radiosurgery and radiotherapy: a long term experience in Thailand. Asian Pac J Cancer Prev. 2015;16(13):5279–84.

54. Kopp C, Theodorou M, Poullos N, et al. Fractionated stereotactic radiotherapy in the treatment of pituitary adenomas. Strahlenther Onkol. 2013;189(11):932–7.

55. Kim JO, Ma R, Akagami R, et al. Long-term outcomes of fractionated stereotactic radiation therapy for pituitary adenomas at the BC Cancer Agency. Int J Radiat Oncol Biol Phys. 2013;87(3):528–33.

56. Wilson PJ, De-Loyde KJ, Williams JR, et al. A single centre's experience of stereotactic radiosurgery and radiotherapy for non-functioning pituitary adenomas with the Linear Accelerator (Linac). J Clin Neurosci. 2012;19(3):370–4.

57. Sun DQ, Cheng JJ, Frazier JL, et al. Treatment of pituitary adenomas using radiosurgery and radiotherapy: a single center experience and review of literature. Neurosurg Rev. 2010;34(2):181–9.

58. Schalin-Jantti C, Valanne L, Tenhunen M, et al. Outcome of fractionated stereotactic radiotherapy in patients with pituitary adenomas resistant to conventional treatments: a 5.25-year follow-up study. Clin Endocrinol. 2010;73(1):72–7.

59. Iwata H, Sato K, Tatewaki K, et al. Hypofractionated stereotactic radiotherapy with CyberKnife™ for nonfunctioning pituitary adenoma: high local control with low toxicity. Neuro Oncol. 2011;13(8):916–22.

60. Brada M, Rajan B, Traish D, et al. The long-term efficacy of conservative surgery and radiotherapy in the control of pituitary adenomas. Clin Endocrinol. 1993;38(6):571–8.

61. Chang EF, Zada G, Kim S, et al. Long-term recurrence and mortality after surgery and adjuvant radiotherapy for nonfunctional pituitary adenomas. J Neurosurg. 2008;108(4):736–45.

62. Jenkins PJ, Bates P, Carson MN, et al. Conventional pituitary irradiation is effective in lowering serum growth hormone and insulin-like growth factor-I in patients with acromegaly. J Clin Endocrinol Metab. 2006;91(4):1239–45.

63. Milker-Zabel S, Zabel A, Huber P, et al. Stereotactic conformal radiotherapy in patients with growth hormone-secreting pituitary adenoma. Int J Radiat Oncol Biol Phys. 2004;59(4):1088–96.

64. Estrada J, Boronat M, Mielgo M, et al. The long-term outcome of pituitary irradiation after unsuccessful transsphenoidal surgery in Cushing's disease. N Engl J Med. 1997;336(3):172–7.

65. Minniti G, Osti M, Jaffrain-Rea ML, et al. Long-term follow-up results of postoperative radiation therapy for Cushing's disease. J Neurooncol. 2007;84(1):79–84.

66. Brucker-Davis F, Oldfield EH, Skarulis MC, et al. Thyrotropin-secreting pituitary tumors: diagnostic criteria, thyroid hormone sensitivity and treatment outcome in 25 patients followed at the National Institutes of Health. J Clin Endocrinol Metab. 1999;84(2):476–86.

67. Socin HV, Chanson P, Delemer B, et al. The changing spectrum of TSH-secreting pituitary adenomas: diagnosis and management in 43 patients. Eur J Endocrinol. 2003;148(4):433–42.

68. Li X, Li Y, Cao Y, et al. Safety and efficacy of fractionated stereotactic radiotherapy and stereotactic radiosurgery for treatment of pituitary adenomas: a systematic review and meta-analysis. J Neurol Sci. 2017;372:110–6.

69. Sheehan JP, Starke RM, Mathieu D, et al. Gamma Knife radiosurgery for the management of nonfunctioning pituitary adenomas: a multicenter study. J Neurosurg. 2013;119(2):446–56.

70. Starke RM, Williams BJ, Jane JA Jr, et al. Gamma Knife surgery for patients with nonfunctioning pituitary macroadenomas: predictors of tumor control, neurological deficits, and hypopituitarism. J Neurosurg. 2012;117(1):129–35.

71. Park KJ, Kano H, Parry PV, et al. Long-term outcomes after gamma knife stereotactic radiosurgery for nonfunctional pituitary adenomas. Neurosurgery. 2011;69(6):1188–99.

72. Franzin A, Spatola G, Losa M, et al. Results of gamma knife radiosurgery in acromegaly. Int J Endocrinol. 2012;2012:342034.

73. Sheehan J, Pouratian N, Steiner L, et al. Gamma Knife surgery for pituitary adenomas: factors related to radiological and endocrine outcomes. J Neurosurg. 2011;114(2):303–9.

74. Minniti G, Clarke E, Scaringi C, et al. Stereotactic radiotherapy and radiosurgery for non-functioning and secreting pituitary adenomas. Rep Pract Oncol Radiother. 2016;21(4):370–8.

75. Amichetti M, Amelio D, Minniti G. Radiosurgery with photons or protons for benign and malignant tumours of the skull base: a review. Radiat Oncol. 2012;7:210.

# Craniopharyngioma

**3**

Joshua D. Palmer, Andrew Song, and Wenyin Shi

## Learning Objectives

- To be able to describe epidemiology of craniopharyngioma and its treatment outcomes.
- To be able to describe the clinical presentations and imaging findings of craniopharyngioma.
- To understand the pathology and pathogenesis of craniopharyngioma.
- To learn the optimal multidisciplinary treatment management of craniopharyngioma.
- To learn the different radiation techniques for craniopharyngioma.
- To understand the important radiation dose constraints for critical structures in the treatment of craniopharyngioma.
- To become familiar with the sequelae of radiation management of craniopharyngioma.

## Craniopharyngioma

Craniopharyngiomas are rare benign embryonic remnants of the Rathke pouch epithelium that often arise in the sellar and/or suprasellar regions. It has two clinicopathological variants: adamantinomatous and papillary. Craniopharyngioma was first described by Zenker in 1857, as masses of cells resembling squamous epithelium along the pars tuberalis and pars distalis of pituitary [1]. The current terminology of "craniopharyngioma" was introduced by Cushing in 1932 [1].

## Epidemiology

Per the most recent report from the Central Brain Tumor Registry of United States (CBTRUS), the annual average incidence was 0.57/100,000 with an annual average of 586 new cases across age groups, constituting approximately 0.8% of all CNS tumors [2]. Craniopharyngiomas can affect patients of all ages, including the prenatal and neonatal periods. There is a bimodal distribution of adamantinomatous cranipharyngioma, with increased incidence in the 5–14 years old age group and adults aged 50–74 years old [3, 4]. Papillary craniopharyngioma, on the contrary, almost exclusively occurs in adults. The median age is approximately 45 years old [5]. The incidences are similar in males and females [3, 4]. There is some suggestion of international variation in the incidence, with higher rates having been observed in Asia and Africa [3]. There are no known environmental risk factors associated with the disease [3]. The most common location for both subtypes is the suprasellar cistern, while a purely intrasellar location is the least common. Other unusual locations include the nasopharynx, paranasal area, sphenoid bone, ethmoid sinus, intrachiasmatic area, temporal lobe, pineal gland, posterior cranial fossa, cerebellopontine angle, midbrain, and third ventricle [1].

## Diagnosis and Prognosis

The diagnosis of craniopharyngioma is usually based on clinical presentation, radiographic findings, followed by pathologic confirmation. All patients should have a thorough history and physical examination, neuroimaging with MRI and/or CT, laboratory tests including hormonal levels, and a detailed neuro-ophthalmologic evaluation.

## Clinical Presentation

Craniopharyngiomas are usually slow-growing tumors with insidious symptoms. There is often a delay in diagnosis,

J. D. Palmer
Department of Radiation Oncology, The James Cancer Hospital and Solove Research Institute at The Ohio State University Wexner Medical Center, Columbus, OH, USA

A. Song · W. Shi (✉)
Sidney Kimmel Cancer Center, Thomas Jefferson University, Philadelphia, PA, USA
e-mail: wenyin.shi@jefferson.edu

© Springer International Publishing AG, part of Springer Nature 2018
E. L. Chang et al. (eds.), *Adult CNS Radiation Oncology*, https://doi.org/10.1007/978-3-319-42878-9_3

sometimes several years from the initial onset of symptoms. The clinical manifestations are variable and depend on the location, size, growth pattern, and relationship to critical intracranial structures. The most common symptoms are related to increased intracranial pressure, endocrine dysfunction, and visual disturbance. Increased intracranial pressure often initially presents with nonspecific symptoms, such as headache, nausea, vomiting, and lethargy. These symptoms may be induced either from mass effect from the tumor or from hydrocephalus due to obstruction of foramen of Monro, the third ventricle, or the aqueduct [6]. In adult patients with craniopharyngioma, the incidence of hormonal deficits at the time of diagnosis is much higher than pediatric patients. At the time of diagnosis, 40–87% of patients present with at least one hormonal deficit [1, 7]. Hormonal dysfunction usually presents as suppression of endocrine function, such as hypothyroidism, adrenal insufficiency, growth hormone insufficiency, or diabetes insipidus. Occasionally, it may manifest as increased hormone production, such as precocious puberty or obesity. In adult-onset craniopharyngioma patients, the most affected hormones are growth hormone (75%), gonadotropins (40%), ACTH (25%), and TSH (25%) [8]. Diabetes insipidus is observed in 17% of the patients due to compression of pituitary stalk [8]. Significant weight gain from hypothalamic involvement can be observed in 13% of the patients [8]. Visual field impairment is also common in adult patients at the time of initial diagnosis. The rate is reported to be approximately 62–84% [1, 7]. Thus, all patients should have a comprehensive ophthalmological evaluation, including at the minimum testing for visual acuity, visual fields, and a dilated-pupil fundus examination. The most classic finding is a bitemporal hemianopsia from inferior chiasmatic compression.

## Imaging

Non-contrast cranial CT (computer tomography) and MRI (magnetic resonance imaging) with and without contrast are the most important neuroradiologic evaluations for craniopharyngioma patients. The classical appearance of a craniopharyngioma is a suprasellar part solid, part cystic mass with calcification. Though craniopharyngiomas can arise anywhere along the craniopharyngeal canal, the most common locations are the sellar and parasellar regions. In children, the adamantinomatous subtype is most common. They consist of both a cystic and solid component along with calcifications (Fig. 3.1). Calcification is best appreciated on CT imaging (Fig. 3.2). Calcification is more common in children (90%) than in adults (70%), and in adamantinomatous rather than papillary tumors [9]. The solid component of the tumor is usually isointense on T1-weighted non-contrast MRI (Fig. 3.3). It is often characterized by intense heterogeneous enhancement after the administration of contrast (Fig. 3.3). The signal intensity of the cystic component is variable due to proteinaceous content within the cyst. The cystic fluid usually contains cholesterol crystals and protein, which leads to high signal on non-contrast T1-weighted images. It is usually dark in the post-contrast T1 sequences with ring enhancement. Craniopharyngiomas presenting in adulthood are more likely to be the papillary subtype. They may be exclusively solid lesions or have a mixed solid and cystic morphology. As compared to pediatric craniopharyngiomas, they are much less calcified (Fig. 3.4) [9].

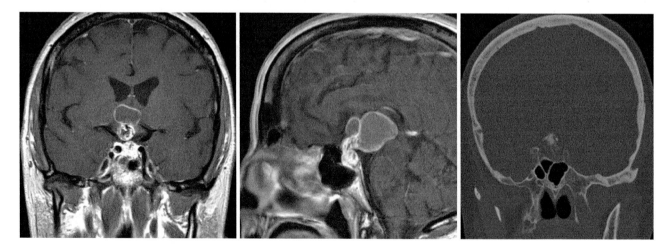

**Fig. 3.1** Classic appearance of adamantinomatous craniopharyngioma in MRI. It has both solid and cystic component. The common location is suprasellar with intrasellar component

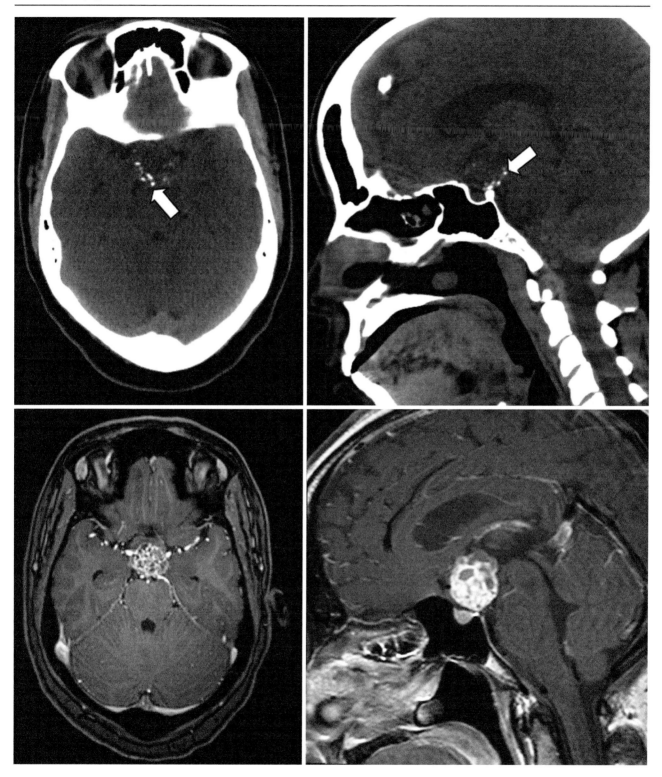

**Fig. 3.2** Corresponding CT scan and MRI demonstrating calcification is best seen on CT scan. Arrow: calcification

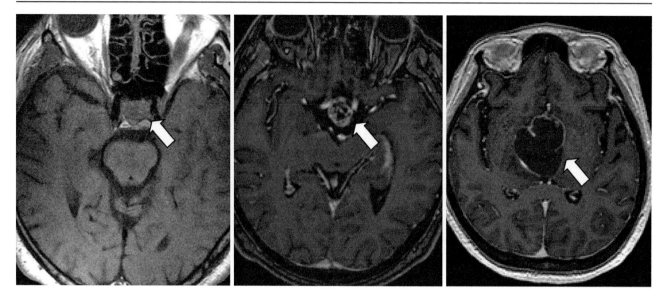

**Fig. 3.3** The solid component of craniopharyngioma is usually isotense on non-enhanced T1 sequence (left, see arrow), brightly enhanced after contrast, and usually heterogeneous (middle, see arrow). The cyst is usually dark on post-contrast T1 with ring enhancement (right, see arrow)

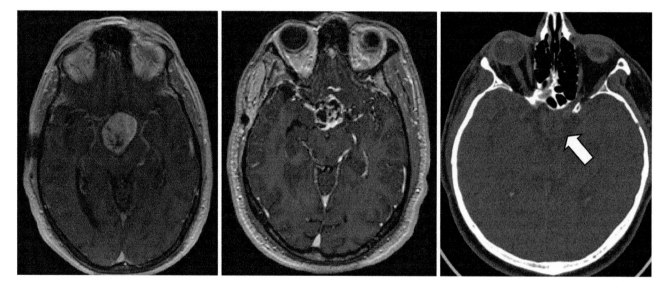

**Fig. 3.4** Classic appearance of two papillary craniopharyngiomas in MRI. They may be exclusively solid lesion (left) or a mixed solid and cystic morphology (middle). They are usually not calcified (right, see arrow)

## Pathology and Pathogenesis

Craniopharygiomas originate from epithelial remnants anywhere along the obscured craniopharyngeal duct from Rathke's cleft to the floor of the third ventricle. There are two theories on the pathogenesis of craniopharyngomas. The first, known as embryonic or embryogenetic, is usually attributed to the adamantinomatous subtype that arises from remnants of Rathke's pouch which undergoes transformation from embryonic squamous cells of the involuted craniopharyngeal duct. This subtype is also associated with the WNT signaling pathway with mutations in

*CTNNB1* which codes for β-catenin [10, 11]. These mutations lead to increased accumulation of β-catenin almost exclusively within the clusters of epithelial nests. These clusters are thought to play a role in tumor invasion as inhibition of the *CTNNB1*, as well as fascin, has resulted in reduced tumor cell migration [12, 13]. Overall, the number of mutations associated with the adamantinomatous subtype is low [10, 13]. Expressions array analysis of methylation profiles has shown relative hypomethylation of the WNT pathway gene AXIN2 and SHH pathway genes GLI2 and PTCH1 when comparing the adamantinomatous vs. papillary subtypes [12]. The molecular pathways which

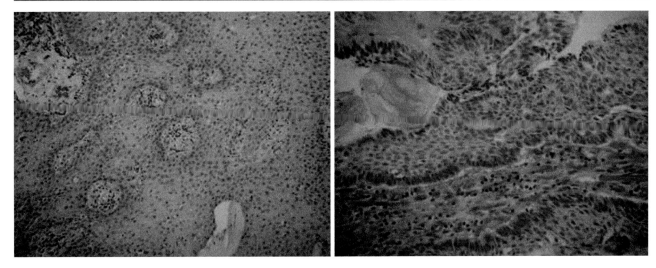

**Fig. 3.5** Representative H&E slides of craniopharyngioma: papillary subtype (left) and adamantinomatous subtype (right). [Courtesy of Dr. Lawrence Kenyon]

have been further characterized as being associated with adamantinomas subtypes include the WNT, SHH, EGFR, and inflammatory pathways [14]. The discovery of the association of these pathways, however, has not yet yielded viable targets for therapy for craniopharyngioma patients at this time.

The metaplastic pathway is attributed to the papillary subtype which is associated with *BRAF*, specifically the BRAF V600E mutation, resulting from metaplasia of adenohypophyseal cells in pars tuberalis of adenohyphophysis, and associated with the formation of squamous cell nests. This is supported by the presence of metaplastic nests in the gland and of hormones contained within the squamous nests [1, 11].

The two subtypes of craniopharyngioma also both differ histologically. The adamintomatous subtype, seen predominantly in the pediatric population, is characterized by squamous epithelial cords, nodules, and irregular trabeculae bordered by palisading columnar epithelium with islands of densely packed cells merged with stellate reticulum. Nodules of wet keratin representing remnants of pale nuclei embedded within an eosinophilic keratinous mass are found in either the compact or looser areas. Cystic cavities containing squamous debris are lined by flattened epithelium. Granulomatous inflammation associated with cholesterol clefts and giant cells may be detectable. Piloid gliosis with abundant Rosenthal fibers is often seen at the infiltrative interface of the tumor (Fig. 3.5). The papillary subtype, more common in adult patients, are rarely calcified, mostly solid, and are better circumscribed. Histologically, they consist of mature squamous epithelium and pseudopapillae with no stellate reticulum or ghost cells (Fig. 3.5) [15]. The papillary subtype also shows increased claudin-1 expression in membranes [16].

## Prognosis

Overall, craniopharyngiomas have relatively high survival rates with 1-, 2-, and 5-year survival rates of 92.1%, 89.5%, and 83.9%, respectively [2]. Children appear to have better survival compared to their adult counterparts with 1-, 2-, and 5-year survival rates of 97.2% vs. 88.3%, 96.3% vs. 84.7%, and 92.7% vs. 77.7%, respectively [2]. The histopathology differs between the age groups, with children often being diagnosed with adamantimatous craniopharyngioma, while adults are more likely to have papillary craniopharyngioma which is a more aggressive disease, which likely contributes to the aforementioned difference in survival. In longer-term follow-up series, best outcomes were seen for those who achieved gross total resections [8]. Patients developed recurrences in approximately 25% of cases, with worse survival at 10 years. Salvage therapy for recurrences was successful in approximately three quarters of patients, with approaches including surgery, radiotherapy, or a combination [8, 17, 18].

## Overall Treatment Strategy

Successfully managing patients with craniopharyngiomas demands close collaboration within a multidisciplinary team and preferably at a specialized center. Optimal treatment for craniopharyngioma is controversial, consisting of either aggressive up-front gross total resection or conservative surgery followed by adjuvant radiotherapy. As this has a benign histology, management should optimize both cure rate and treatment morbidity. Aggressive surgery is associated with significant morbidity, and a noticeable recurrence rate [19, 20]. It has been well established that conservative surgery followed by radiation treatment has excellent local control and significantly reduced complications [19, 21–23]. Thus, treatment paradigms have shifted over the past 20 years from historical series utilizing aggressive complete resection to more modern series utilizing conservative resection followed by adjuvant radiation [20, 21, 24]. The optimal timing of radiation is also controversial as postoperative vs. delayed until recurrence appear to have similar progression-free and overall survival [19, 25–28]. The lack of an apparent difference in overall survival is mainly due to effective salvage treatments at time of recurrence, either with further surgery or radiation treatment [22, 25]. Following a subtotal resection, progression is noted in 70% of patients within 3 years [22, 25, 29]. Repeat surgery is associated with a higher risk of acute complications and adverse cognitive outcomes [30–32]. A recent study further suggests inferior results with delayed radiation [33]. Taken together, for patients with subtotal resection, adjuvant radiation should be considered up front rather than waiting till the time of recurrence.

Management should begin with an ophthalmologic and endocrine functional assessment. Both CT and MRI imaging should be utilized to accurately define the tumor size, character, and proximity to the critical areas including the hypothalamus and optic apparatus. It is critical that an experienced neurosurgeon evaluate the patient for gross total resection, following the known classification systems [34, 35]. The goals of surgical management are fourfold: to establish a tissue diagnosis, relieve symptoms due to mass effect, obtain local control, and decrease tumor burden or proximity to critical structures for adjuvant radiotherapy. Hypothalamic damage is a key long-term morbidity and may be minimized if one utilizes the Puget grading scale for hypothalamic involvement [36]. Typically, a gross total resection is not recommended in situations where the hypothalamus is involved (Puget class II), multiple previous attempts for gross total resection, prior stroke, poor performance status, and/or arterial encasement. In summary, surgical management may be personalized, and a more "radical" surgery may be utilized in patients with prechiasmatic/retrochiasmatic tumors, while more limited surgery may be appropriate for patients with hypothalamic involvement, i.e., large or suprachiasmatic tumors.

## Radiotherapeutic Management

For patients with residual tumor after resection and for recurrent tumor after initial gross total resection, radiation is indicated. Several radiation techniques are useful in the management of patients with craniopharyngiomas.

## Conventional External Beam Radiation

Excellent long-term outcomes of conventional external beam irradiation were reported in many series (Table 3.1) [23, 29, 45, 46]. Several radiation techniques are routinely utilized in clinical treatment of patients with craniopharyngioma, such as three-dimensional conformal radiation treatment (3D-CRT), dynamic conformal arc therapy (DCAT), intensity-modulated radiotherapy (IMRT), and volumetric-modulated arc therapy (VMAT). Since the majority of craniopharyngiomas are in the suprasellar region, close to the optic apparatus, hypothalamus, and hippocampus, IMRT/VMAT may achieve better sparing for the organ at risk (OAR) [47]. Noncoplanar radiation field arrangement is of great importance to improve target conformity and homogeneity in patients with brain tumors [48, 49] (Fig. 3.6). For example, a dosimetric study comparing these radiation techniques showed noncoplanar VMAT can significantly reduce the mean dose to bilateral hippocampus, as compared to dynamic arcs or coplanar VMAT [50].

The radiation gross tumor volume (GTV) is the residual tumor/tumor bed and cystic volume as defined by the postoperative MRI and CT. Craniopharyngiomas are benign tumors, and usually sharply bordered, with less infiltrative growth patterns. As a result, a minimal clinical target volume (CTV) which encompasses subclinical microscopic disease is sufficient. More recent studies employ a 5 mm three-dimensional CTV showed excellent local control justifying its use [31]. A current prospective study at St. Jude is assessing a 3 mm CTV

**Table 3.1** Selected series of radiation treatment for craniopharyngioma

| Series | n | RT dose (Gy) | PFS 5 years | PFS 10 years | PFS 20 years |
|---|---|---|---|---|---|
| Regine [37] | 12 | 55.8 | 83 | 81 | |
| Harrabi [38] | 55 | 52.2 | 95.3 | 92.1 | 88.1 |
| Hetelekidis [29] | 46 | 54.64 | 92 | 89 | |
| Varlotto [39] | 24 | 54 | 95 | 89 | 54 |
| Merchant [31] | 88 | 54 | 83–100 | 60–98 | |
| Rajan [23] | 173 | 50–54 | 92 | 83 | 79 |
| *Alapetite [40] | 49 | 54 (proton) | 90%[a] | | |
| *Indelicato [41] | 40 | 54 (proton) | 100%[a] | | |
| #Fitzek [42] | 15 | 56.9 (proton) | 93% | 85% | |
| ##Kobayashi [43] | 107 | 11.5 (SRS) | 60.8 | 53.8 | |
| ##Xu [44] | 37 | 14.5 (SRS) | 67 | | |

*Two ongoing phase II trials Curie Paris Orsay Institute evaluating dose escalation to 59.5 CGE and (St. Jude) decreasing CTV 3 mm utilizing proton therapy
#RT alone and STR + RT
##Multiple prior therapies including surgeries/prior RT
[a]Local control rate 1 year

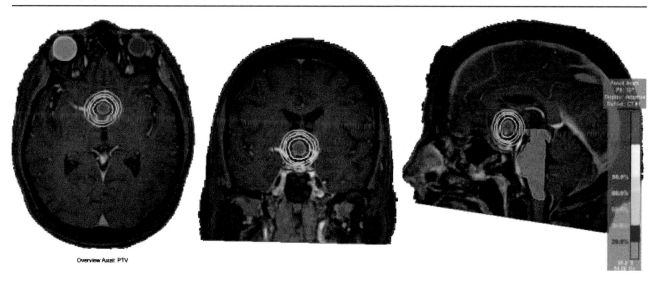

**Fig. 3.6** Example of noncoplanar VMAT plan showing good conformality and steep dose fall off outside PTV

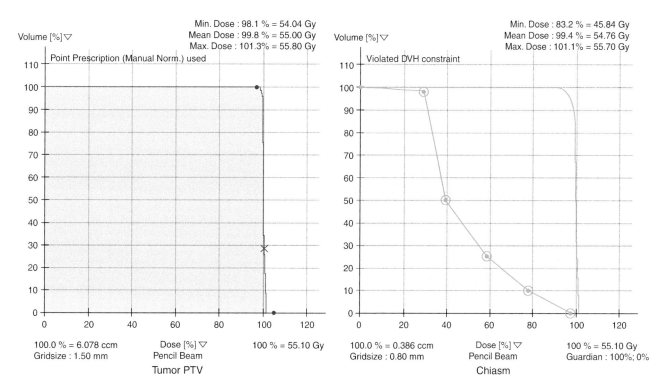

**Fig. 3.7** Dose-volume histogram (DVH) of noncoplanar VMAT plan showing excellent homogeneity of the plan

margin. The planning target volume (PTV) varies depending on patient setup, immobilization, and image guidance techniques and varies between 0 and 1 cm. If stereotactic radiotherapy is used with daily image guidance, a PTV margin of 0–3 mm may be utilized [51]. Due to the location, PTV often abuts or encompasses portion of optic apparatus; effort should be taken to minimize hot spot in the PTV to reduce the risk of radiation optic neuropathy (Fig. 3.7). An important note is that cyst expansion may occur during fractionated radiother-

apy delivery, and periodic MRI imaging should be performed to ensure that the cyst remains adequately covered by the PTV. Recommendations for MRI reimaging vary from weekly, biweekly, to once mid-treatment and depend on resources available at the treatment center [31]. Papillary craniopharyngioma is more common in adult and usually is associated with small cystic component. Mid-treatment MRI is usually sufficient. With the advent of MRI LINACs, more frequent tumor/cyst expansion surveillance imaging may be performed, allowing for more comfort in treatment volumes and potentially a smaller margin for therapy.

Radiation doses of 50–54 Gy in 1.8–2 Gy daily fraction achieve the best overall control, with doses <50 Gy achieving less long-term control [14, 31, 52]. There are not sufficient data to compare the local control for 50 Gy versus 54 Gy. It is important to respect the radiation tolerance of nearby critical structures, such as optic chiasm, optic nerves, and the brainstem. Attempts should be made to maintain the dose to the optic nerves and optic chiasm to <55 Gy, brainstem <60 Gy, and cochlea <40 Gy [53–56].

## Stereotactic Radiosurgery

Stereotactic radiosurgery (SRS) is a relatively recent treatment option for craniopharyngioma. For well-selected patients, SRS offers similar excellent outcomes (Table 3.1). Historically, SRS is largely utilized for minimal residual disease or limited recurrence up to 3 cm and more than 3–5 mm away from the optic apparatus. The volume is usually gross tumor without a margin. Single-fraction doses between 12 and 15 Gy appear sufficient [57]. The optic apparatus should be held to less than 8 Gy, but up to 10–12 Gy is acceptable [54]. The rates for optic neuropathy with doses <8 Gy to the optic apparatus are <1.7%, 8–10 Gy 1.8%, and >12 Gy 10% [54]. In the updated Mayo Clinic experience, doses up to 12 Gy to the optic apparatus were shown to have a very low risk for optic neuropathy <1%; however, great caution should be taken due to the long survival of craniopharyngioma patients and potential for late effects [58].

With the availability of frameless SRS techniques, fractionated SRS in two to five fractions is also utilized for the treatment craniopharyngioma [59, 60]. The $\alpha/\beta$ of craniopharyngioma is assumed to be two [39]. As a result, the dose schedule of 25 Gy in five fractions has equivalent single-fraction dose of 12.3 Gy. Several small series with short follow-up demonstrated favorable clinical outcomes with minimum toxicity [59, 60]. Longer-term follow-up is needed to further validate its utility.

## Proton

Proton therapy has the feature of minimum/no dose beyond the end of the particle range (Bragg peak). As a result, proton therapy may lead to improved dose conformity and potentially expose the normal brain to lesser amounts of low to moderate doses of radiation (Fig. 3.8). The decreased integral dose to the brain is expected to have decreased early and

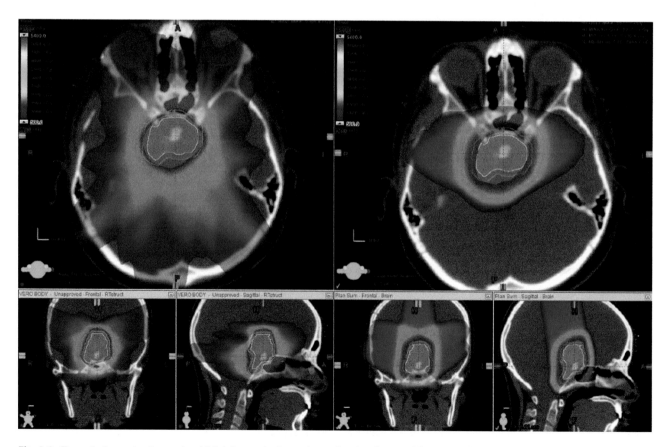

**Fig. 3.8** Example for proton beam plan (right) for craniopharyngioma showing decreased integral brain dose as compared to IMRT plan (left). [Courtesy of Dr. Daniel Indelicato]

late toxicities. Several studies evaluated the efficacy of proton beam radiation for patients with craniopharyngioma and showed favorable 10-year local control of 83–91% (Table 3.1) [42, 61, 62]. A particularly challenging aspect of craniopharyngioma proton treatment is cystic growth during radiation. It is more relevant as compared to photon therapy as the dose distribution is more sensitive to changes in tumor volume. For example, a >5% change in the target volume for IMPT requires replanning compared with >10% for IMRT [63]. Depending on the technique and optimization method, frequent MRI imaging and replanning during the treatment course may be necessary. Close long-term follow-up is warranted to further define the role of proton radiation in the treatment of craniopharyngioma.

## Treatment Outcomes

Disease control rates at 5 years are between 80 and 90% [1]. Pediatric control may be higher with more than 90% control. Late recurrences over 5–10 years have been reported, and long-term follow-up is recommended for surveillance and management of late radiation toxicity. Cyst enlargement within the first year may not herald a true recurrence and may regress with conservative management; however enlargement after 1 year may require additional therapy for improved control (intracavitary β-emitting brachytherapy with [$^{32}$P, $^{186}$Re, $^{90}$Y], bleomycin, or interferon).

## Treatment-Related Toxicity

The acute treatment-related toxicities are characteristic of many brain tumor patients with the most common including fatigue, skin reaction, hair loss, lymphocytopenia, headaches, nausea/vomiting, and cerebral edema. These treatment-related toxicities may be managed conservatively based on severity with medical management.

Late treatment-related toxicity is related to the physical location of these tumors in close proximity to the frontal and temporal lobes, vascular structures, optic apparatus, pituitary gland, and hypothalamus. The white matter in the frontal and temporal lobes are at particular risk for damage, which may contribute to poor cognitive outcomes, disinhibition, and problems with attention/concentration and memory [14, 36, 64–67].

The most common late toxicity is polyendocrinopathy with hypothyroidism (96%), ACTH deficiency (84%), DI (53%), and more than two endocrinopathies in 39% of patients. Common neurologic toxicities include headaches (39%), seizures (27%), abnormal cerebral vessels (37%), cerebrovascular disease (15%), hearing loss (unilateral 6%, bilateral 10%), oculomotor dysfunction (12%), and visual disturbance (unilateral 12%, bilateral 35%). Neurocognitive

sequela includes neurocognitive delay (20%), psychologic problems (30%), academic underachievement, and communication disorders (10%) [68, 69]. Hyperphagia, metabolic syndrome, and hypothalamic obesity may occur in up to half of craniopharyngioma survivors [14, 70]. Risk factors include hypothalamic involvement, weight at diagnosis, growth hormone replacement, and hydrocephalus requiring a shunt. Cardiovascular mortality is significantly higher (up to 19×) compared to the general population [71]. Other adverse effects related with hypothalamic obesity include circadian rhythm dysfunction, abnormal eating behavior, and nonalcoholic fatty liver disease [69].

Local control and overall survival are excellent with this benign histology; however, it has been recently demonstrated that long-term (20 years) survival is significantly, negatively, impacted with the presence of hypothalamic involvement (95% without HI vs. 84% with HI) [72]. Metabolic syndrome and hypothalamic obesity are a major cause of death. A multidisciplinary approach to long-term care is crucial with patients after curative treatment for craniopharyngioma focusing on endocrine dysfunction, neurocognitive training, ophthalmology assessments, management of metabolic syndrome, and cardiovascular as well as cerebrovascular risk factors.

## Conclusions

Optimal management of craniopharyngioma patients has shifted to conservative surgery followed by radiation treatment. Radiation treatment is indicated for patients with residual disease. Despite the overall very favorable treatment outcomes, the long-term sequelae are common and significant. Future efforts in improving radiation treatment, such as proton beam radiation, may further improve the toxicity profile while maintaining excellent local control.

## Case

The patient is a 55-year-old gentleman who presented with bitemporal hemianopsia and headache. He was noted to have bilateral tinnitus and sensorineural hearing loss. TSH, free T4, prolactin, IGF-I, and growth hormone were within normal limits. LH is mildly decreased. Eye examination revealed normal visual acuity and bitemporal hemianopsia. Fundus was undilated without papilledema. The contrast-enhanced brain MRI imaging confirmed a suprasellar enhancing mass measuring 2 × 2 × 1.7 cm. The superior portion of the mass is predominantly cystic with fluid signal and no internal enhancement. The inferior portion of the mass is more heterogeneous, with solid areas of enhancement (Puget class II) (Fig. 3.9). The head CT showed patchy calcification. The imaging findings are most consistent with an adamantinoma-

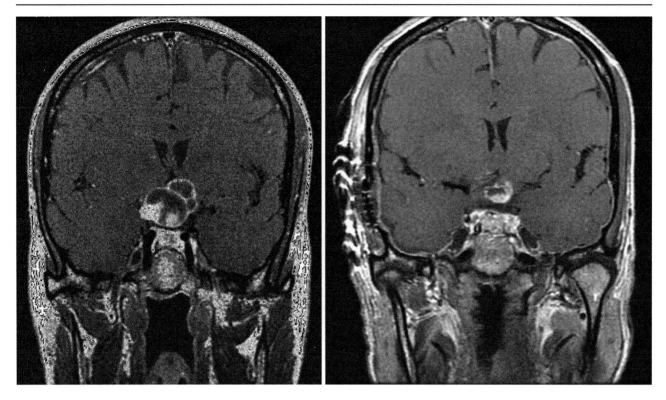

**Fig. 3.9** Imaging finding for sample case. Preoperative MRI (left). MRI after debulk surgery (right)

tous craniopharyngioma. The case was discussed at a multi-disciplinary tumor board. The recommendation is conservative surgery, followed by radiation treatment. He underwent a minimally invasive endoscopic transnasal resection of his craniopharyngioma. Pathology demonstrated an adamantinomatous craniopharyngioma. Postoperative contrast-enhanced brain MRI imaging demonstrated residual disease abutting the optic chiasm (Fig. 3.9). He recovered well from surgery without significant postoperative complications. He started radiation treatment 8-week postsurgery. Due to the close proximity to optic chiasm, fractionated stereotactic radiation treatment was recommended. He received 54 Gy in 1.8 Gy fractions (Fig. 3.10). He tolerated treatment well and remains without evidence of local progression at his last follow-up 6 years postradiation treatment. He has no significant late toxicity.

## Summary

- Craniopharyngiomas arise from Rathke's cleft epithelial remnants on the floor of the third ventricle.

- Craniopharyngiomas have two main histologic subtypes: adamantinomatous which has a bimodal age distribution occurring in children and adults, as well as papillary which occurs in adults.
- Common presenting symptoms include headache, visual field disturbance (bitemporal hemianopsia), hormonal dysfunction, and weight gain.
- Overall survival is between 80% and 90% for adults and children.
- Treatment is multidisciplinary with maximum safe resection followed by radiotherapy for subtotal resections.
- Standard radiotherapy for craniopharyngioma involves fractionated external beam radiotherapy to a dose of 5040–5400 cGy in 180 cGy fractions.
- Improvements in the delivery of radiotherapy with the use of daily image guidance, IMRT/VMAT/proton therapy, and weekly MRI imaging to monitor cyst size (when feasible) have allowed for smaller volumes of radiation.
- Stereotactic radiosurgery and intracavitary brachytherapy are options for treatment recurrence.
- Treatment morbidity may be high for patients with hypothalamic involvement of tumor with hypothalamic obesity and panhypopituitarism leading to early death.

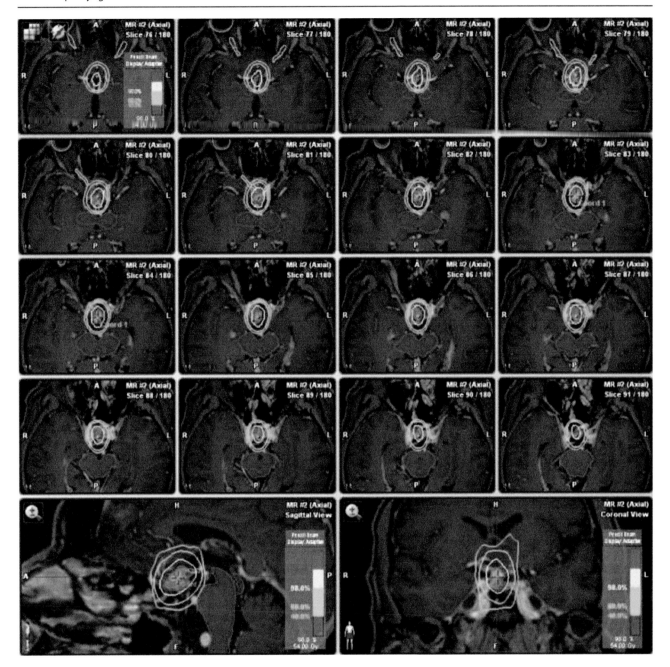

**Fig. 3.10** Stereotactic noncoplanar VMAT plan for the patient

## Self-Assessment Questions

1. Craniopharyngioma patients often present with irregular hormonal function. The most commonly affected hormone is:
   A. Growth hormone (GH)
   B. FSH/LH
   C. TSH
   D. ACTH
   E. Vasopressin

2. What statement about craniopharyngioma is true?
   A. Craniopharyngioma is the most common intracranial neoplasm in children.
   B. Papillary craniopharyngioma is the most common subtype in adult patients.
   C. Craniopharyngioma is often isointense on contrast-enhanced MRI.
   D. The two subtypes of craniopharyngioma are papillary and desmoplastic.
   E. BRAF mutations are often seen in adamantinomatous-type craniopharyngioma.

3. A 17-year-old girl presented with cold intolerance, easy fatigability, and polyuria. A physical examination revealed bilateral papilledema. Lab work showed abnormal thyroid function. An MRI shows an enhancing multilobulated suprasellar mass with ring calcification in the region of the sella turcica. If the lesion represents a primary intracranial neoplasm, which of the following is the most likely diagnosis?
   A. Germinoma
   B. Craniopharyngioma
   C. Ependymoma
   D. Hemangioblastoma
   E. Prolactinoma

4. Which statement regarding radiation treatment for craniopharyngioma is true?
   A. Craniopharyngioma is a benign tumor and well controlled with low-dose radiation treatment. A conventional fractionated treatment course of 36 Gy is sufficient.
   B. Optimal treatment of subtotal resected craniopharyngioma is craniospinal irradiation, followed by tumor bed boost to 54 Gy.
   C. Hormonal dysfunction as a late side effect of radiation treatment for craniopharyngioma is rare.
   D. Radiosurgery is ideal for small craniopharyngioma abutting the optic chiasm.
   E. A patient with adamantinomatous craniopharyngioma after gross total resection can be safely observed.

5. Which statement regarding the management of craniopharyngioma is true?
   A. In order to minimize treatment toxicity, highly aggressive surgery should be used to avoid adjuvant radiation treatment.
   B. Cyst decompression for nonresectable lesions prior to RT may ease sparing of critical structures.
   C. Long-term event-free survival of radiation is far inferior to radical surgery.
   D. Due to excellent overall survival of craniopharyngioma patients treated with radiation, routine follow-up may not be necessary.
   E. In order to prevent tumor recurrence or progression, postoperative radiation should start right after surgery.

## Answers

1. A
2. B
3. B
4. E
5. B

## References

1. Muller HL. Craniopharyngioma. Endocr Rev. 2014;35(3):513–43.
2. Ostrom QT, Gittleman H, Xu J, et al. CBTRUS statistical report: primary brain and other central nervous system tumors diagnosed in the United States in 2009–2013. Neuro-Oncology. 2016;18(Suppl_5):v1–v75.
3. Haupt R, Magnani C, Pavanello M, et al. Epidemiological aspects of craniopharyngioma. J Pediatr Endocrinol Metab. 2006;19(Suppl 1):289–93.
4. Bunin GR, Surawicz TS, Witman PA, et al. The descriptive epidemiology of craniopharyngioma. J Neurosurg. 1998;89(4):547–51.
5. Crotty TB, Scheithauer BW, Young WF Jr, et al. Papillary craniopharyngioma: a clinicopathological study of 48 cases. J Neurosurg. 1995;83(2):206–14.
6. Garnett MR, Puget S, Grill J, et al. Craniopharyngioma. Orphanet J Rare Dis. 2007;2:18.
7. Zoicas F, Schofl C. Craniopharyngioma in adults. Front Endocrinol (Lausanne). 2012;3:46.
8. Karavitaki N, Brufani C, Warner JT, et al. Craniopharyngiomas in children and adults: systematic analysis of 121 cases with long-term follow-up. Clin Endocrinol. 2005;62(4):397–409.
9. Lee IH, Zan E, Bell WR, et al. Craniopharyngiomas: radiological differentiation of two types. J Korean Neurosurg Soc. 2016;59(5):466–70.
10. Brastianos PK, Taylor-Weiner A, Manley PE, et al. Exome sequencing identifies BRAF mutations in papillary craniopharyngiomas. Nat Genet. 2014;46(2):161–5.
11. Garre ML, Cama A. Craniopharyngioma: modern concepts in pathogenesis and treatment. Curr Opin Pediatr. 2007;19(4):471–9.
12. Hölsken A, Buchfelder M, Fahlbusch R, et al. cell migration in adamantinomatous craniopharyngiomas is promoted by activated Wnt-signalling. Acta Neuropathol. 2010;119(5):631–9.

13. Goschzik T, Gessi M, Dreschmann V, et al. Genomic alterations of adamantinomatous and papillary craniopharyngioma.
J Neuropathol Exp Neurol. 2017;76(2):126–34.

14. Müller HL, Merchant TE, Puget S, et al. New outlook on the diagnosis, treatment and follow-up of childhood-onset craniopharyngioma. Nat Rev Endocrinol. 2017;13(5):299–312.

15. Lubuulwa J, Lei T. Pathological and topographical classification
of craniopharyngiomas: a literature review. J Neurol Surg Rep.
2016;77(3):e121–7

16. Louis DN, Perry A, Reifenberger G, et al. The 2016 World Health
Organization classification of tumors of the central nervous system:
a summary. Acta Neuropathol. 2016;131(6):803–20.

17. Van Effenterre R, Boch AL. Craniopharyngioma in adults and children: a study of 122 surgical cases. J Neurosurg. 2002;97(1):3–11.

18. Mortini P, Losa M, Pozzobon G, et al. Neurosurgical treatment of craniopharyngioma in adults and children: early
and long-term results in a large case series. J Neurosurg.
2011;114(5):1350–9.

19. Lin LL, El Naqa I, Leonard JR, et al. Long-term outcome in children treated for craniopharyngioma with and without radiotherapy.
J Neurosurg Pediatr. 2008;1(2):126–30.

20. Rao YJ, Hassanzadeh C, Fischer-Valuck B, et al. Patterns of care
and treatment outcomes of patients with Craniopharyngioma in the
national cancer database. J Neurooncol. 2017;132(1):109–17.

21. Schoenfeld A, Pekmezci M, Barnes MJ, et al. The superiority of
conservative resection and adjuvant radiation for craniopharyngiomas. J Neurooncol. 2012;108(1):133–9.

22. Merchant TE, Kiehna EN, Sanford RA, et al. Craniopharyngioma:
the St. Jude Children's Research Hospital experience 1984–2001.
Int J Radiat Oncol Biol Phys. 2002;53(3):533–42.

23. Rajan B, Ashley S, Gorman C, et al. Craniopharyngioma--a long-
term results following limited surgery and radiotherapy. Radiother
Oncol. 1993;26(1):1–10.

24. Zacharia BE, Bruce SS, Goldstein H, et al. Incidence, treatment
and survival of patients with craniopharyngioma in the surveillance, epidemiology and end results program. Neuro Oncol.
2012;14(8):1070–8.

25. Stripp DC, Maity A, Janss AJ, et al. Surgery with or without radiation therapy in the management of craniopharyngiomas in children
and young adults. Int J Radiat Oncol Biol Phys. 2004;58(3):714–20.

26. Regine WF, Mohiuddin M, Kramer S. Long-term results of pediatric and adult craniopharyngiomas treated with combined surgery
and radiation. Radiother Oncol. 1993;27(1):13–21.

27. Tomita T, Bowman RM. Craniopharyngiomas in children: surgical experience at Children's Memorial Hospital. Childs Nerv Syst.
2005;21(8–9):729–46.

28. Moon SH, Kim IH, Park SW, et al. Early adjuvant radiotherapy
toward long-term survival and better quality of life for cranio-
pharyngiomas--a study in single institute. Childs Nerv Syst.
2005;21(8–9):799–807.

29. Hetelekidis S, Barnes PD, Tao ML, et al. 20-year experience in
childhood craniopharyngioma. Int J Radiat Oncol Biol Phys.
1993;27(2):189–95.

30. Netson KL, Conklin HM, Wu S, et al. Longitudinal investigation of
adaptive functioning following conformal irradiation for pediatric
craniopharyngioma and low-grade glioma. Int J Radiat Oncol Biol
Phys. 2013;85(5):1301–6.

31. Merchant TE, Kiehna EN, Kun LE, et al. Phase II trial of conformal
radiation therapy for pediatric patients with craniopharyngioma and
correlation of surgical factors and radiation dosimetry with change
in cognitive function. J Neurosurg. 2006;104(2 Suppl):94–102.

32. Merchant TE. Craniopharyngioma radiotherapy: endocrine and
cognitive effects. J Pediatr Endocrinol Metab. 2006;19(Suppl
1):439–46.

33. Kalapurakal JA, Goldman S, Hsieh YC, et al. Clinical outcome
in children with craniopharyngioma treated with primary surgery and radiotherapy deferred until relapse. Med Pediatr Oncol.
2003;40(4):214–8.

34. Kassam AB, Gardner PA, Snyderman CH, et al. Expanded endonasal approach, a fully endoscopic transnasal approach for the resection of midline suprasellar craniopharyngiomas: a new classification
based on the infundibulum. J Neurosurg. 2008;108(4):715–28.

35. Wen DY, Seljeskog EL, Haines SJ. Microsurgical management of
craniopharyngiomas. Br J Neurosurg. 1992;6(5):467–74.

36. Puget S, Garnett M, Wray A, et al. craniopharyngiomas: classification and treatment according to the degree of hypothalamic involvement. J Neurosurg. 2007;106(1 Suppl):3–12.

37. Regine WF, Kramer S. Pediatric craniopharyngiomas: long term
results of combined treatment with surgery and radiation. Int J
Radiat Oncol Biol Phys. 1992;24(4):611–7.

38. Harrabi SB, Adeberg S, Welzel T, et al. Long term results after
fractionated stereotactic radiotherapy (FSRT) in patients with craniopharyngioma: maximal tumor control with minimal side effects.
Radiat Oncol. 2014;9:203.

39. Varlotto JM, Flickinger JC, Kondziolka D, et al. External beam irradiation of craniopharyngiomas: long-term analysis of tumor control
and morbidity. Int J Radiat Oncol Biol Phys. 2002;54(2):492–9.

40. Alapetite C, Puget S, Ruffier A, et al. Proton therapy for craniopharyngioma in children: update of the Orsay proton center experience.
Neuro Oncol. 2012;14(i22–i5):CR-09.

41. Indelicato DJ, Rotondo R, Flampouri S, et al. Proton therapy for
craniopharyngioma: early clinical outcomes. Int J Radiat Oncol
Biol Phys. 2012;84:S634.

42. Fitzek MM, Linggood RM, Adams J, et al. Rotondo R, Flampouri
S, et al. Combined proton and photon irradiation for craniopharyngioma: long-term results of the early cohort of patients treated
at Harvard Cyclotron Laboratory and Massachusetts General
Hospital. Int J Radiat Oncol Biol Phys. 2006;64(5):1348–54.

43. Kobayashi T. Long-term results of gamma knife radiosurgery for
100 consecutive cases of craniopharyngioma and a treatment strategy. Prog Neurol Surg. 2009;22:63–76.

44. Xu Z, Yen CP, Schlesinger D, et al. Outcomes of Gamma
Knife surgery for craniopharyngiomas. J Neurooncol.
2011;104(1):305–13.

45. Pemberton LS, Dougal M, Magee B, et al. Experience of external
beam radiotherapy given adjuvantly or at relapse following surgery
for craniopharyngioma. Radiother Oncol. 2005;77(1):99–104.

46. Combs SE, Thilmann C, Huber PE, et al. Achievement of long-term
local control in patients with craniopharyngiomas using high precision stereotactic radiotherapy. Cancer. 2007;109(11):2308–14.

47. Wiggenraad RG, Petoukhova AL, Versluis L, et al. Stereotactic
radiotherapy of intracranial tumors: a comparison of intensity
modulated radiotherapy and dynamic conformal arc. Int J Radiat
Oncol Biol Phys. 2009;74(4):1018–26.

48. Aggarwal A, Fersht N, Brada M. Radiotherapy for craniopharyngioma. Pituitary. 2013;16(1):26–33.

49. Martin F, Magnier F, Berger L, et al. Fractionated stereotactic
radiotherapy of benign skull-base tumors: a dosimetric comparison
of volumetric modulated arc therapy with Rapidarc(R) versus noncoplanar dynamic arcs. Radiat Oncol. 2016;11:58.

50. Uto M, Mizowaki T, Ogura K, et al. Non-coplanar volumetric-
modulated arc therapy (VMAT) for craniopharyngiomas reduces
radiation doses to the bilateral hippocampus: a planning study comparing dynamic conformal arc therapy, coplanar VMAT, and noncoplanar VMAT. Radiat Oncol. 2016;11:86.

51. Schulz-Ertner D, Frank C, Herfarth KK, et al. Fractionated stereotactic radiotherapy for craniopharyngiomas. Int J Radiat Oncol Biol
Phys. 2002;54(4):1114–20.

52. Minniti G, Esposito V, Amichetti M, et al. The role of fractionated
radiotherapy and radiosurgery in the management of patients with
craniopharyngioma. Neurosurg Rev. 2009;32(2):125–32; discussion 132.

53. Lawrence YR, Li XA, el Naqa I, et al. Radiation dose-volume effects in the brain. Int J Radiat Oncol Biol Phys. 2010;76(3 Suppl):S20–7.
54. Mayo C, Martel MK, Marks LB, et al. Radiation dose-volume effects of optic nerves and chiasm. Int J Radiat Oncol Biol Phys. 2010;76(3 Suppl):S28–35.
55. Mayo C, Yorke E, Merchant TE. Radiation associated brainstem injury. Int J Radiat Oncol Biol Phys. 2010;76(3 Suppl):S36–41.
56. Bhandare N, Jackson A, Eisbruch A, et al. Radiation therapy and hearing loss. Int J Radiat Oncol Biol Phys. 2010;76(3 Suppl):S50–7.
57. Veeravagu A, Lee M, Jiang B, et al. The role of radiosurgery in the treatment of craniopharyngiomas. Neurosurg Focus. 2010;28(4):E11.
58. Pollock BE, Link MJ, Leavitt JA, et al. Dose-volume analysis of radiation-induced optic neuropathy after single-fraction stereotactic radiosurgery. Neurosurgery. 2014;75(4):456–60; discussion 460.
59. Iwata H, Tatewaki K, Inoue M, et al. Single and hypofractionated stereotactic radiotherapy with CyberKnife for craniopharyngioma. J Neurooncol. 2012;106(3):571–7.
60. Lee M, Kalani MY, Cheshier S, et al. Radiation therapy and CyberKnife radiosurgery in the management of craniopharyngiomas. Neurosurg Focus. 2008;24(5):E4.
61. Winkfield KM, Linsenmeier C, Yock TI, et al. Surveillance of craniopharyngioma cyst growth in children treated with proton radiotherapy. Int J Radiat Oncol Biol Phys. 2009;73(3):716–21.
62. Luu QT, Loredo LN, Archambeau JO, et al. Fractionated proton radiation treatment for pediatric craniopharyngioma: preliminary report. Cancer J. 2006;12(2):155–9.
63. Beltran C, Naik M, Merchant TE. Dosimetric effect of target expansion and setup uncertainty during radiation therapy in pediatric craniopharyngioma. Radiother Oncol. 2010;97(3):399–403.
64. Sughrue ME, Yang I, Kane AJ, et al. Endocrinologic, neurologic, and visual morbidity after treatment for craniopharyngioma. J Neurooncol. 2011;101(3):463–76.
65. Pierre-Kahn A, Recassens C, Pinto G, et al. Social and psycho-intellectual outcome following radical removal of craniopharyngiomas in childhood. A prospective series. Childs Nerv Syst. 2005;21(8–9):817–24.
66. Poretti A, Grotzer MA, Ribi K, et al. of craniopharyngioma in children: long-term complications and quality of life. Dev Med Child Neurol. 2004;46(4):220–9.
67. Cavazzuti V, Fischer EG, Welch K, et al. Neurological and psychophysiological sequelae following different treatments of craniopharyngioma in children. J Neurosurg. 1983;59(3):409–17.
68. Crom DB. Metabolic abnormalities in an adult survivor of pediatric craniopharyngioma. Oncology (Williston Park). 2008;22(8 Suppl Nurse Ed):43–6.
69. Crom DB, Smith D, Xiong Z, et al. Health status in long-term survivors of pediatric craniopharyngiomas. J Neurosci Nurs. 2010;42(6):323–8; quiz 329–30.
70. Tan TS, Patel L, Gopal-Kothandapani JS, et al. The neuroendocrine sequelae of paediatric craniopharyngioma: a 40-year meta-data analysis of 185 cases from three UK centres. Eur J Endocrinol. 2017;176(3):359–69.
71. Muller HL. Diagnostics, treatment, and follow-up in craniopharyngioma. Front Endocrinol (Lausanne). 2011;2:70.
72. Sterkenburg AS, Hoffmann A, Gebhardt U, et al. Survival, hypothalamic obesity, and neuropsychological/psychosocial status after childhood-onset craniopharyngioma: newly reported long-term outcomes. Neuro Oncol. 2015;17(7):1029–38.

# Vestibular Schwannoma

**4**

## Michael Mayinger and Stephanie E. Combs

## Learning Objectives

In this chapter, one will learn about:

- Schwannoma and its types.
- Epidemiological factors that influence this condition.
- The risk factors and pathogenesis of unilateral as well as bilateral vestibular schwannoma.
- Staging vestibular schwannoma according to its size, tumor volume and invasion, and tumor growth.
- Conservative, surgical, and radiological management of vestibular schwannoma and their complications.
- Predictive factors and long-term outcomes of different methods of vestibular schwannoma management.

## Background

Vestibular schwannoma, which is a benign tumor derived from Schwann cells, is also known as acoustic neuroma, acoustic schwannoma, and vestibular neurilemoma.

Schwann cells are cells that normally wrap around the supporting nerve fibers. An overgrowth of these Schwann cells will form this non-cancerous tumor, which mostly originate from the vestibular part of the eighth cranial nerve. Even though these tumors are benign, they can disturb the normal functions of the cranial nerves and, if they are large and compress normal tissue, the brain and the brainstem. Typical symptoms of vestibular schwannomas are hearing impairment, gait disturbances, dizziness, and tinnitus [1]. These symptoms can be present even with very small lesions of only a few millimeters. As the tumor increases in size, it can press on the cochlear and vestibular nerves causing increasing auditory disturbances and disturbances in the body balance. A large tumor can press on the facial nerve or other surrounding brain structures causing serious symptoms.

There are two types of vestibular schwannomas:

1. *Unilateral Vestibular Schwannoma.* This is the most common form (95%) of vestibular schwannoma and affects only one ear. This benign tumor may be caused by nerve damage from environmental factors [2]. However, the patients who present with unilateral acoustic neuromas at a young age must be suspected of having a neurofibromatosis 2 (NF2) gene mutation, and they are at a high risk of developing bilateral condition later in life [3].
2. *Bilateral Vestibular Schwannoma.* This type of vestibular schwannoma affects bilateral VIII nerves and is an inherited condition known as NF2. It is a genetic condition resulted by a mutation of the NF2 gene. Moreover, these patients have a higher risk of developing other tumors of the nervous system [3].

Acoustic neuromas or vestibular schwannomas account for about 5–6% of intracranial tumors and about 80–90% of tumors that are located in the cerebellopontine angle (CPA) [4].

## Epidemiology

Statistics show that the incidence of vestibular schwannoma is almost 1:100,000 persons per year [5, 6]. The incidence rate is increasing and is believed to be due to incidental findings with the increased use of MRI and CT diagnostic techniques. Therefore, the prevalence of vestibular schwannoma could be higher than that is indicated. Each year, about 5000 cases are diagnosed in the United States, and majority of them are reported as incidental findings during a MRI or a

M. Mayinger
Department of Radiation Oncology, Klinikum rechts der Isar, Technische Universität München, Munich, Bavaria, Germany

S. E. Combs (✉)
Department of Radiation Oncology, Klinikum rechts der Isar, Technische Universität München, Munich, Bavaria, Germany

Institute of Innovative Radiotherapy (iRT), Department of Radiation Sciences (DRS), Helmholtz Zentrum München, Oberschleißheim, Bavaria, Germany
e-mail: Stephanie.combs@tum.de

© Springer International Publishing AG, part of Springer Nature 2018
E. L. Chang et al. (eds.), *Adult CNS Radiation Oncology*, https://doi.org/10.1007/978-3-319-42878-9_4

CT, which are carried out in the aim of ruling out or diagnosing another disease [5].

Based on race, Caucasians seem to have a higher prevalence (83.16%), while African-Americans and Hispanics show the lowest incidence [7]. Most vestibular schwannoma cases are diagnosed in patients who are at the age of 30–60 years, and the median age of diagnosis is 50 years [8]. For unknown reasons, more Caucasian patients are diagnosed at an older age (mean age of 56 years), compared to Hispanics (mean age of 50 years) [9].

Although the white populations are diagnosed at an older age, more black, Hispanic, and Asian patients present with larger tumors. However, there were no racial differences with regard to the treatment modality. The prognosis and survival rate are inferior in Hispanics and African-Americans compared to those in Caucasians following the surgical treatment [9].

## Pathogenesis and Risk Factors

Generally, there are no established risk factors for the development of sporadic vestibular schwannoma. In patients with NF2, there is mutation of a single gene which is named as neurofibromin 2. Neurofibromin 2 is located on chromosome 22 and is responsible in producing merlin, which is also known as schwannomin. Schwannomin is a cell membrane-related protein that suppresses tumor formation. A mutation of this gene leads to a dysfunction of the merlin protein [10].

A biallelic mutation of NF2 gene was found in most (50%) of the sporadic vestibular schwannomas. But, otherwise, some epigenetic factors or protease cascade activation may also contribute to the non-expression of merlin or schwannomin. Mostly, patients with NF2 develop bilateral vestibular schwannomas [11].

Other than NF2 gene mutation, there are many other risk factors that are discussed controversially; however, for most cases, no data is available to support these hypotheses:

- Exposure to low-dose radiation in the childhood to treat certain benign conditions of the head and the neck has been shown to increase the risk [12, 13]. Furthermore, the dose of the radiation given to the cerebellopontine angle (CPA) during these treatments is proportional to the exponential risk of developing acoustic neuromas [13].
- Long-term use of mobile phones may significantly increase the risk of developing this condition [14]. According to a research study, it was found that acoustic neuromas due to cell phone use, located mostly on the contralateral side than the ipsilateral side of the head [15]. Therefore, there is now a clear link between cell phone use and the development of benign tumors of the neurocranium.
- Some groups discuss that exposure to loud noises in occupational and leisure settings increases the risk for

acoustic neuroma [16]. However, many groups and their studies oppose this theory, making a controversy probably supported mostly by the fear and uncomfort of loud noise.
- A history of parathyroid adenoma is considered to be another risk factor [17]. However, the mechanism of developing acoustic neuroma due to this condition is not yet known and therefore remains a hypothesis.
- A history of chicken pox and a history of more than one cranial X-ray can contribute to the formation of acoustic neuroma [18]. These hypotheses require further validation to understand their mechanism.

In conclusion, this list provides many factors that are discussed in the framework of vestibular schwannoma development. However, besides NF2, no established risk factors have been identified. Importantly, patients with bilateral vestibular schwannoma should be counseled regarding the potential genetic background since genetic testing is available and can be offered based on the patient's preference. Children of affected patients are considered to be at 50% risk of NF2. Formal screening for vestibular schwannoma should start at 10 years, as it is rare for tumors to become symptomatic before that time even in severely affected families. Annual audiological tests, including auditory brainstem response, as well as an MRI scan at around 12 years of age are recommended [19].

## Staging

### Staging of Acoustic Neuroma/Vestibular Schwannoma

Acoustic neuroma can be staged through three different characteristics:

1. Jackler staging system [20]—classified according to the size of the tumor (Table 4.1)
2. Koos classification—classified according to the extent of the tumor invasion or tumor volume [21] (Table 4.2)
3. Jackler classification [22]—classified according to the tumor growth:

**Table 4.1** Jackler staging system—classified according to the size of the tumor

| Stage | Tumor size |
|---|---|
| Intracanalicular | Tumor only within internal auditory canal |
| I (small) | <10 mm |
| II (medium) | 11–25 mm |
| III (large) | 25–40 mm |
| IV (giant) | >40 mm |

Based on data from Ref. [20]

**Table 4.2** Koos classification—classified according to the extent of the tumor invasion or tumor volume

| Stage | Tumor invasion/volume |
|---|---|
| Stage I | Intracanalicular tumor |
| Stage II | Tumor spreading in the cerebellopontine angle but not reaching pons |
| Stage III | Tumor reaching the pons, perhaps deforming it but not shifting it |
| Stage IV | Tumor deforming the pons and shifting the fourth ventricle |

Based on data from Ref. [21]

(a) Intracanalicular phase—The tumor compresses the auditory and vestibular nerves, and the patient complains of tinnitus and hearing loss (unilateral).
(b) Cisternal phase—The tumor protrudes through internal auditory canal into cerebellopontine angle. There are severe hearing loss and disequilibrium (severe vertigo).
(c) Compressive phase—The tumor makes contact with the cerebellum or brainstem, but without compressing them. However, the tumor compresses the V nerve (trigeminal nerve) and causes corneal hypesthesia, loss of sensation of the midface, and occipital headache.
(d) Hydrocephalic phase—The tumor deforms the cerebellum or brainstem and can cause CSF flow blockage and can lead to hydrocephalus. The common symptoms of this phase are headache, visual changes, and altered mental status. If this phase is not treated, the growing hydrocephalus leads to coma and possible death.

## Diagnosis

The diagnostic work-up is usually prompted by asymmetric sensorineural hearing loss which is to be evaluated by audiometry. This is followed by diagnostic imaging either with MRI or with CT. MRI scanning should be performed both with and without gadolinium. The thickness of the slices should be 3 mm in maximum but ideally 1.0–1.5 mm [23]. An MRI dedicated to the internal auditory canal can demonstrate more details of the tumors. High-resolution CT scans with contrast can be used if MRI is contraindicated. Typically, MRI and CT will show a round or oval lesion in the CPA with relatively homogenous contrast enhancement [24]. MRI can detect lesions with the size of 1–2 mm [25]. T2-weighted scans are to be performed in order to detect surrounding edema in normal brain tissue. CT scans with bone windows can provide a more accurate view of the internal auditory canal allowing for evaluation of the extent of its widening [24].

## Pathology

Schwannomas arise from perineural elements of the Schwann cell. They occur with equal frequency on the superior and inferior branches of the vestibular nerve; however, only rarely are they derived from the cochlear portion of the VIII nerve. Pathohistologically, zones of alternately dense and sparse cellularity, referred to as Antoni A and B areas, respectively, are characteristic of vestibular schwannoma. Immunohistochemical staining for S100 protein is usually positive [26].

## Prognosis

The rate of tumor recurrence after treatment with surgery or radiotherapy is generally very low, ranging from <1% to 9% [27–29]. An increased risk of residual or recurrent tumor is seen with the suboccipital approach due to relatively blind dissection of the IAC fundus. Residual tumor is deliberately left in approximately 1–2% of patients if dissection is complicated or vital structures such as the facial nerve are at risk for injury [30]. Recurrence rate can be as high as 20% in 10 years for partially or incompletely resected tumors [10].

Tumor size and location directly correlate to the general outcome of the carried-out treatment [22, 31, 32].

## Overall Treatment Strategy

The management of acoustic neuroma is a complex process, and the options include radiation therapy, surgical excision of the tumor, and observation. Interdisciplinary decision-making is recommended. Patients should be offered all treatment alternatives and should be counseled regarding the respective treatment methods and outcome, including toxicity. In general, vestibular schwannomas are characterized by a slow growth kinetic, and a growth of 1–2 mm per year is usually observed. Therefore, not every tumor requires immediate treatment, and in some cases, a wait-and-see strategy can be followed.

## Observation

With vestibular schwannomas being benign lesions, they are characterized by slow growth patterns [7, 9, 10]. In the literature, growth rates of 1–3 mm are described [7, 9], and in many patients, the lesions do not get larger over many years. Thus, for small and asymptomatic lesions, wait-and-see strategy may be offered in selected cases, especially in elderly patients. Observation with frequent follow-up MRI scans (every 6–12 months) can be considered. Follow-up should also include close clinical observation to detect early symptoms such as gait disturbances, hearing impairment, or facial weakness/numbness. A wait-and-see strategy can be justified, especially in elderly patients with asymptomatic lesions.

In patients with tumors with rapid growth or progressive symptoms such as hearing loss and VII and V nerve deficits, surgery or radiotherapy should be considered. Additionally, one should consider that the preservation of hearing with radiotherapy is better in early stages. To improve the chance for maximal possible hearing preservation, treatment should not be delayed.

## Surgery

Surgery is generally regarded as the standard of treatment. Compared to radiotherapy, surgery also yields satisfactory long-term local control. However, the recurrence rate can be as high as 20% in 10 years for partially or incompletely resected tumors [10].

There are three main surgical approaches for surgical resection of vestibular schwannoma. These approaches are based on the size of the tumor, without consideration of hearing preservation. The surgical approaches are:

Retrosigmoid or retromastoid suboccipital approach—This approach can be used for tumors of any size with or without considering hearing preservation [10].
Translabyrinthine approach—This approach is for tumors >3 cm and also for tumors <3 cm, when there is no consideration about hearing preservation [33].
Middle fossa approach—This approach is for small tumors which are less than 1.5 cm (<1.5 cm), and the main aim of the surgery is to preserve hearing [10].

## Complications

The major complications of surgical approach are damage to cranial nerve VII and VIII (cranial nerve palsies), mortality, cerebrospinal fluid leakage, hemorrhage, and infections [34]. Patients must be informed about the different surgical possibilities as well as the prevalent risk of side effects. In patients with large lesions with brainstem compression, however, surgery should be recommended for surgical decompression. Depending on the anatomical situation and surgeon's and patient's preference, partial resections can be planned prior to planned radiotherapy of the tumor remnant. This multimodal approach can be beneficial in terms of reduction of risk of complications.

## Radiation Therapy

The major goal of radiation therapy is to terminate the tumor growth without injuring critical structures adjacent to the vestibular schwannoma [6]. In some cases, radiation therapy can also lead to reduction of tumor volume. High-precision radiotherapy is recommended, either in the form of stereotactic radiosurgery (SRS), hypofractionated SRT (HSRT), or fractionated stereotactic radiotherapy (FSRT). Since the risk of side effects with SRS is closely correlated to tumor volume, in general, SRS is offered to patients with smaller tumors. With FSRT, the beneficial effect of fractionation is exploited, and this can potentially reduce the risk of complications. Moreover, FSRT can be applied safely independently of volume. Comparing the outcomes from the literature and considering the volume-dependent choices, both modalities appear to be comparable [32].

## Indications for Irradiation

Indications for radiotherapy include newly diagnosed vestibular schwannomas, residual vestibular schwannomas after surgery, and recurrent vestibular schwannomas. Patients should present without symptomatic brainstem compression, and tumor size should be less than 3 cm in diameter [35].

## Target Volume Delineation

The delineation of the target volume is based on MRI scans (see– Fig. 4.1a). The gross tumor volume (GTV) should be defined as the contrast enhancement in T1-weighted MRI scans. In FSRT the GTV is increased by 1–2 mm for every direction, generating a planning target volume (PTV). For SRS, no PTV expansion is used. Computed tomography-magnetic resonance imaging fusion is performed for treatment planning (Fig. 4.1b). Patients should be immobilized and have to be treated with an individually manufactured mask system, as thermoplastic face masks (Fig. 4.2a, b).

Depending on the volume and the anatomical situation, coplanar and noncoplanar beams are used. For FSRT, at least 95% of the volume of PTV should receive the prescription dose (45–54) Gy. At least 98% of the volume of the GTV should receive the prescription dose [36].

SRS dosing is 12–13 Gy in a single fraction prescribed to at least the 50% isodose line, and for radiosurgery cases, three planning calculations are performed [37]:

1. Conformality index: prescription isodose volume/tumor volume $\leq 1.2$–1.5
2. Selectivity index: target volume covered by prescribed isodose/prescribed isodose volume $> 0.9$

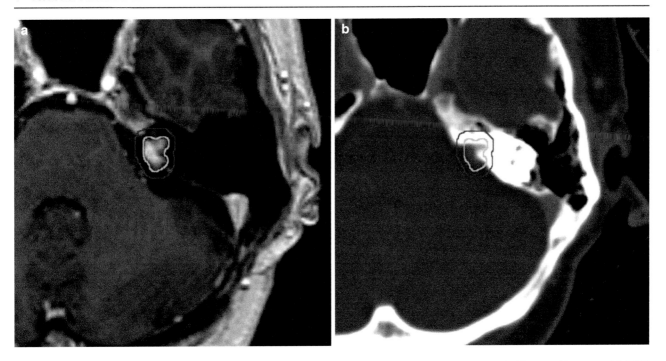

**Fig. 4.1** Gross tumor volume (GTV) (green) and planning target volume (PTV) (red) delineated on T1-weighted MRI scan with contrast (**a**). GTV and PTV on registered computed tomography scan (**b**)

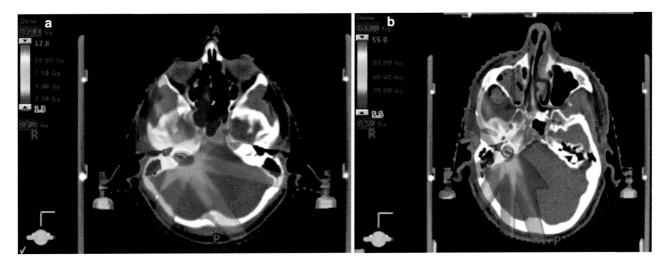

**Fig. 4.2** Radiation dose prescription and organ-at-risk tolerances. Stereotactic radiosurgery treatment plan (**a**) and stereotactic fractionated plan (**b**)

3. Gradient index: ratio of the volume receiving half the prescription of isodose to the volume receiving the full prescription of isodose <3

## Complication Avoidance

To avoid complications normal tissue dose constraints must be complied with (Table 4.3). Daily positioning controls are required.

## Radiation Toxicity: Acute and Late

Hearing can be lost despite the stability of tumor on scans. Risk factors for worse hearing outcomes include older age, larger tumor volume, and greater degree of baseline hearing loss [22, 31, 32]. The impact of cochlear radiation dose alone as a predictive parameter for hearing outcomes remains controversial.

Delayed cystic degeneration has been reported in 2% of patients, occurring at a median of 6 years after SRS and requiring craniotomy for symptomatic management in a small minority [40].

Postirradiation tumor expansion, defined as an increase in tumor diameter of >2 mm (with median tumor volume increase of 75%), has been reported in 14% of patients at a median of 9 months following SRS, of which one-third remain enlarged with no sequential growth [41]. A decrease in central enhancement was observed in 93% of patients. Postirradiation expansion may be more likely in tumors with a greater pre-irradiation growth rate [42].

Radiation injury to the facial nerve may rarely cause facial palsy and may be associated with dryness of the ipsilateral eye and altered taste sensation [43]. Recovery usually occurs over many months with conservative management [42]. There is a concern that scarring following SRS may complicate subsequent microsurgery should the tumor recur. In a series of 20 cases in which surgical salvage was performed following recurrence after radiosur-

gery, approximately one-half were determined to have greater difficulty for resection or facial nerve preservation [44]. Malignant transformation has been described in case reports [45–47]. In a single-center series of 440 patients that included over 5000 patient-years of follow-up, one patient developed a malignant peripheral nerve sheath tumor 5.5 years after SRS, resulting in a malignant transformation rate of 0.3% [40]. Secondary malignancies occur at a low rate of <1 in 1000 patients, often many years after the treatment [48].

## Outcomes: Tumor Control

Treated with current techniques, patients have a very good prognosis with minimal complications. Tumors treated with focused radiation have a control rate of >90%.

If baseline hearing is near normal, depending on radiation technique, 60–80% of hearing is preserved. FSRT is associated with higher rates of hearing preservation compared to RS (Table 4.4). Facial nerve preservation rates are very high with radiation. However, outcomes may be dependent on tumor size and center experience [28, 56, 59, 60].

### Fractionated Stereotactic Radiotherapy

With FSRT, fractionated dose of radiation is given over a series of several sessions using stereotactic techniques. The goal of this technique also aimed at the preservation of neural structures from radiation and effective tumor growth control. This technique is proved to be more effective and safe through a number of studies, especially in case of topographic proximity of the tumor to sensory cranial nerves. With fractionation, the radiobiological repair mechanisms of

**Table 4.3** Intensity-modulated radiation therapy and radiosurgery normal tissue dose constraints

| Critical structures | Recommended constraints[a] |
|---|---|
| Lens | Dmax <5 Gy[b] |
| Retinae | Dmax <45 Gy[b] |
| Optic nerves | Dmax <50 Gy[b] |
| Optic chiasm | Dmax <54 Gy[b] |
| | Dmax for SRS dosing: 8 Gy [38] |
| Spinal cord | Dmax <50 Gy[c] |
| Brainstem | Dmax <54 Gy[c] |
| Cochlea | Dmean <45 Gy[c] |
| | Dmean for SRS <4 Gy [39] |

[a]Maximum point dose defined as a volume greater than 0.03 cc
[b]Constraints based on RTOG 0539
[c]Constraints based on QUANTEC

**Table 4.4** Summary of treatment outcomes for SRS, FSRT, and HSRT

| Author and publication year | Design | Treatment type (n) | Follow-up (range) | Tumor recurrence | Facial intact | Loss of useful hearing |
|---|---|---|---|---|---|---|
| Chopra et al. 2007 [49] | Retrospective | SRS (216) | 68 months (range –143) | 5/102 | 100% | 45/106 |
| Fukuoka et al. 2009 [50] | Retrospective | SRS (152) | >5 years | 92.4% | 152/152 | 17/59 |
| Sun et al. 2012 [51] | Prospective | SRS (190) | 109 months (range 8–195) | 14/190 | 162/190 | 4/22 |
| Yomo et al. 2012 [52] | Retrospective | SRS (154) | 60 months (range 7–123) | 8/154 | 153/154 | 46/110 |
| Hasegawa et al. 2012 [22] | Retrospective | SRS (440) | 12.5 years | 36/440 | 433/440 | 46/135 |
| Weber et al. 2003 [53] | Retrospective | Proton beam SRS (88) | 38.7 months (12–102.6 months) | 5% | 90% | 66.7% |
| Aoyama et al. 2013 [54] | Retrospective | FSRT (201) | 72 months (range 2–175) | 13/201 | 182/201 | 34/77 |
| Litre et al. 2013 [55] | Retrospective | FSRT (155) | 60 months (range 24–192) | 4/155 | 134/155 | 28/61 |
| Combs et al. 2015 [56] | Retrospective | SRS FSRT (449) | 67 months (2–252 months) | 3% 3% | 97% 99% | 16% 14% |
| Song et al. 1999 [57] | Retrospective | HSRT (31) | 6 months (6–44 months) | 0/31 | 31/31 | 3/12 |
| Lederman et al. 1997 [58] | Retrospective | HSRT (38) | 27.1 months | 0/38 | 38/38 | – |

*SRS* stereotactic radiosurgery, *FSRT* fractionated stereotactic radiotherapy, *HSRT* hypofractionated stereotactic radiotherapy

normal tissue can be exploited to reduce treatment-related side effects.

In a study of 200 patients, 202 vestibular schwannomas were treated with fractionated stereotactic radiation therapy (172 patients) and stereotactic radiosurgery (30 patients). The average dose of 57.6 Gy in the form of 1.8 Gy fractions was given. The follow-up of 75 months showed a tumor growth control (96%) with no distinctive differences between fractionated stereotactic radiation therapy and stereotactic radiosurgery. Stereotactic radiation therapy showed 78% of hearing preservation in a 5-year period [56].

In another study of 101 vestibular schwannomas, patients were given 40–50 Gy of fractionated stereotactic radiation therapy in 20–25 fractions for 5–6-year period. The average follow-up of 45 months showed 91.4% tumor growth control and 71% hearing preservation. However, the rates for facial nerve palsies, trigeminal neuropathy, and balance disturbance were 4%, 14%, and 17%, respectively. In addition, 11% of the patients required surgical intervention to place a shunt to reduce the hydrocephalus after the stereotactic radiation therapy [61].

Besides, especially in case of bilateral vestibular schwannoma, stereotactic radiotherapy is preferred over stereotactic radiosurgery, as neurofibromatosis 2 is characterized by a highly impaired tolerance against radiation side effects.

### Stereotactic Radiosurgery

This technique uses Gamma Knife or linear accelerator to converge multiple beams of radiation to a specific target volume. This approach delivers an ablative dose of radiation to the target volume while limiting the radiation exposure to adjacent tissues and structures. Stereotactic radiosurgery is indicated for patients with tumor <3 cm or progressive tumor growth in patients who are contraindicated for a surgical approach.

For target delineation, there is no PTV expansion from the GTV (defined as the enhancing mass on post-contrast T1-weighted MRI scan) given the fact that in most cases, rigid skull fixation is used.

Early studies in the 1980s used high-radiation doses of 18–20 Gy in single-center experiences and reported a tumor growth control by >95% [62, 63]. However, about one-third of the patients suffered from cranial nerve palsies of trigeminal and facial nerve. Therefore, the prescribed dose has been lowered to improve the therapeutic ratio [64–67].

Studies with marginal doses of 12–14 Gy in tumors <3 cm report 90–99% tumor control rates (Table 4.4). Five-year hearing preservation was 60–70%; facial and trigeminal nerve preservation rates are 95–100% and 79–100% [22, 49–52].

The effective delivery of SRS relies on optimal tumor imaging, thoughtful treatment planning, and appropriate dose prescription. With a highly conformal plan and appro-priate dosing, the risk of damage to the trigeminal nerve, the facial nerve, and the cochlea can be minimized. Apart from the marginal dose prescribed to the tumor, the maximum dose is also evaluated. The typical prescribed dose of radiation with SRS is 12–13 Gy to at least 50% isodose line.

## Comparison of Stereotactic Radiosurgery and Fractionated Stereotactic Radiotherapy

It is generally known that the risk for treatment-related side effects in SRS is strongly associated with tumor volume and dose. For vestibular schwannoma, most lesions treated with SRS are smaller and independent of the technique used. For dose, it has been shown that doses above 12–13 Gy significantly increase the rate of cranial nerve toxicity. With doses of 12–13 Gy and in smaller-volume tumors, the rate of cranial nerve toxicity is comparable between SRS and FSRT [68]. In a large pooled analysis where FSRT and SRS were compared, there was no significant difference in local control ($p = 0.39$), loss of useful hearing (FSRT = 14%; SRS = 16%), or other side effects like trigeminal and facial nerve toxicity. However, PTV in SRS group was smaller than in FSRT patients (SRS = 1.1 ml; FSRT = 2.7 ml) [56].

### Hypofractionated Stereotactic Radiotherapy

HSRT schedules typically range from two to six fractions. Hypofractionation provides some of the advantages of fractionation in terms of sparing normal tissues but with the convenience of a more limited treatment time. Optimal dose/fractionation schedule for HSRT with the best therapeutic ratio is yet to be determined. HSRT was first described by Lederman et al. in 1997 with four or five weekly fractions to a total dose of 20 Gy [58]. The authors reported 100% tumor control and no permanent cranial neuropathies. Meijer et al. and Song et al. reported similar results delivering doses of 5 × 4–5 Gy [57, 69]. Hansasuta et al. showed that HSRT delivering a total dose of 18 Gy in three fractions resulted in 96% tumor control with a 76% hearing preservation rate at a median follow-up interval of 3.6 years (range 1–10 years) [70]. Limited data with short-term follow-up show that HSRT, like FSRT, can yield similar outcomes as single-fraction SRS, but a longer follow-up is required to determine the long-term efficacy of this approach.

### Proton Beam Therapy

This technique is associated with distinct physical properties reducing the integral dose: Normal tissue can be spared, and the dose is focused mainly on the tumor with a high effective dose of radiation. This is possible by the so-called Bragg peak, enabling a highly conformal dose distribution with high-dose deposit in the target volume and an increased sparing of the OARs [71]. Weber et al.

**Table 4.5** Summary of treatment outcomes for surgery

| Author publication year | Design | Treatment type (n) | Follow-up (range) | Tumor recurrence | Facial intact | Loss of useful hearing | QoL (results) |
|---|---|---|---|---|---|---|---|
| Sughrue et al. 2011 [10] | Prospective predefined incl. crit. | Surg. (727) | 37 months mean (3–266 months) | 58/727 | – | – | – |
| Gormley et al. 1997 [59] | Retrospective | Surg. (178) | 70 months mean (3–171 months) | 1/178 | 96% | 38% | – |
| Regis et al. 2002 [28] | Retrospective non-matched controls | Surg. (110) RS (97) | 3 years median (2.1–4 years) | 9% 3% | 67% 100% | 63% 30% | ↓39% ↓9% |
| Myrseth et al. 2005 [60] | Retrospective matched controls | Surg. (86) RS (103) | 5.9 years mean (1–14.2 years) | 6% 5% | 80% 95% | – | ↓ = |

*QoL* quality of life, *RS* radiosurgery, *FSRT* fractionated stereotactic radiotherapy

reported on 88 patients who received proton beam radiosurgery (median dose 12 Gy; range 10–18 Gy) that tumor growth control was approximately 95% and around 90% cranial nerve preservation [53]. Hash et al. observed similar results in 68 patients after proton beam radiosurgery (dose 12 Gy; local control 84%; cranial nerve preservation 100%) [72].

Bush et al. evaluated fractionated proton beam radiotherapy with 54–60 daily doses of 1.8–2.0 Gy in 30 patients and reported no disease progression on magnetic resonance imaging scans during follow-up (mean 34 month). Of the 13 patients with pretreatment Gardner-Robertson grades I–II hearing, 4 (31%) maintained useful hearing [73].

To date, however, the published data on proton therapy for vestibular schwannoma report inferior hearing preservation rates and not an increase in local control. The explanation for the higher rate of side effects may be due to uncertainties in calculation of the relative biological effectiveness (RBE), however, to date not fully explained. Additionally, for smaller volumes dose distributions are generally more conformal using stereotactic photon radiotherapy. Therefore, no benefit of proton therapy in this indication has been documented to date. Moreover, for smaller lesions, proton treatment plans in some cases show an inferior dose distribution compared to advanced photons (Table 4.5).

## Predictive Factors of Tumor Growth and Course of the Disease

There are several factors that predict the course and severity of the disease in vestibular schwannoma. As mentioned earlier, a presentation of unilateral vestibular schwannoma at a young age could predict a future development of the bilateral disease. Such a presentation could also suggest the presence of neurofibromatosis type 2 [3].

Tumor growth can be predicted by the size of the tumor at presentation. A large tumor size at diagnosis is associated with higher chances of tumor growth. A 1 mm increment of the size of the tumor at presentation increases the possibility of tumor growth nearly by 20% [74].

Further, there were some symptom markers recognized in certain studies that helped in predicting the tumor growth in acoustic neuroma. The presence of tinnitus at the time of diagnosis remarkably increased the likelihood of tumor growth by three times [17].

Shorter symptom duration and also a younger age at the presentation suggest a fast tumor growth and a high possibility of having a large vestibular schwannoma [17].

## Predictive Factors of Treatment Outcomes of Vestibular Schwannoma

As the above features suggest and help the diagnosis and to predict the course of the disease, there are also certain features that help in predicting treatment outcomes and the overall prognosis of acoustic neuroma. Other than the tumor size and location which directly correlate to the general outcome of the carried-out treatment, here are few more predictive factors that can determine the outcomes of certain possible complications.

1. The predictive factors for long-term facial nerve function:
   (a) If the facial nerve is left intact during the surgical treatment and if a perioperative graft repair is not performed, the treatment can yield a better outcome [75].
   (b) The rate of recovery during the first postoperative year is a very useful early predictor of long-term facial nerve function [76].
   (c) Poor long-term function of the facial nerve can also be predicted by the use of intraoperative nerve monitoring, and this can also be used to determine the length of the duration of postoperative rehabilitation of the patients [77].
2. The predictive factors for hearing preservations:
   (a) Tumor size is a good predictive factor of hearing preservation after the removal of the tumor. Patients with small-volume tumors have a better chance of hearing preservation [78].

(b) Surgical removal of intracanalicular schwannomas and schwannomas that extend to the cerebellopontine angle (CPA) more than 1 cm using middle fossa (MF) approach yields more favorable hearing outcomes compared to retrosigmoid approach [79].

(c) Radiation injury to the cochlea or a high-radiation dose delivered to auditory canal or both can lead to deterioration of hearing [80].

(d) Unilateral vestibular schwannoma, young age at presentation, and low-dose radiation to the cochlea predict better preservation of hearing [81].

3. Compared to surgical approaches, radiotherapy can be a better method of managing a vestibular schwannoma of a lesser volume. Stereotactic radiotherapy gives really favorable outcomes with minimal toxicity [82]. Patients who have prior surgical treatments are at a higher risk of developing trigeminal neuropathy [82]. Also, patients who undergo stereotactic radiotherapy for large tumors are more likely to require a neurosurgical intervention afterwards [82].

Early treatment outcomes of stereotactic radiotherapy are better for patients with small- to medium-sized vestibular schwannomas [83]. SRT also provides a high rate of hearing preservation, especially in case of little impairment of hearing prior to treatment [61]. But, if a frequent tumor progression was indicated in long-term follow-up, radiosurgery should be considered as the best management of the condition [83].

## Follow-Up: Radiographic Assessment

Posttreatment imaging for recurrent or residual tumor varies among different treatment centers and is debated in the literature [84]. Surveillance with follow-up MRI scans every 6–12 months is recommended. Follow-up should also include close clinical observation to detect early symptoms such as gait disturbances, hearing impairment, or facial weakness/numbness.

## Case Study

A 45-year-old woman had a routine hearing test for work, and a sensorineural hearing loss is detected. She has no signs or symptoms. She had type 2 diabetes mellitus and arterial hypertension. Her current medications included metformin, nifedipine, and a multivitamin. She appeared well. Vital signs were within normal limits. Physical examination showed no abnormalities. When informed about her test result, she reported a history of progressively decreased hearing in her left ear over the past few years. She noticed the hearing deficit when trying to use the phone with the left ear compared to her right. She had no signs or symptoms of dizziness, tinnitus, facial numbness, or vague headaches.

Cranial gadolinium-enhanced MRI revealed a 1.1 cm, uniformly enhanced, dense mass extending into internal acoustic meatus, with absence of a dural tail (Fig. 4.3a).

She was informed about the effective treatment options of proceeding with surgery or radiation to ensure best chance of preserving hearing.

The patient decided to undergo FSRT in accordance with her local physician as she wanted to avoid surgery and minimize possible risks for side effects. She was informed that to date superiority of SFRT compared to RC was not confirmed. She underwent daily treatment with 54 Gy total dose in 30 fractions (Fig. 4.3b). The patient did not experience any acute side effects, while left-side hearing remained slightly worse than the right side. Follow-up MRI after 3 months revealed a slight decrease of enhancement and in size (0.8 cm) (Fig. 4.3c).

## Summary

• Vestibular schwannoma has two types: unilateral vestibular schwannoma and bilateral vestibular schwannoma.
• Vestibular schwannoma prevalence is about 1:100,000, but it is considered to be higher than predicted.

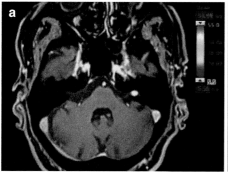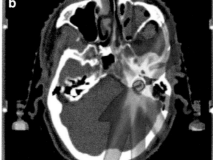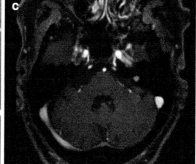

**Fig. 4.3** MRI T1 sequence with gadolinium showed a contrast-enhanced lesion in the left internal acoustic meatus compatible with left vestibular schwannoma (**a**) CT-based treatment plan (**b**) and 3 months posttreatment follow-up MRI T1 with gadolinium showed tumor shrinkage (**c**)

- There are genetic factors (neurofibromatosis or NF2 gene mutation) and environmental factors that increase the risk of acoustic neuroma.
- Staging is performed according to the size of the tumor (Jackler staging method), volume or extent of tumor invasion (Koos classification), and tumor growth (Jackler classification of phases of tumor growth).
- Management of vestibular schwannoma includes radiotherapy, surgical approach, or observation.
- Radiation therapy is a highly effective treatment for vestibular schwannomas.
- Stereotactic radiosurgery and fractionated stereotactic radiotherapy (FSRT) can be considered equieffective. Larger volumes are treated preferentially with fractionated regimens.

## Self-Assessment Questions

1. What are the typical early symptoms of vestibular schwannoma?
   A. Unilateral sensorineural hearing loss
   B. Tinnitus
   C. Dizziness and disequilibrium
   D. All of the above

2. What is the rate of tumor control after surgery or radiation therapy?
   A. >90%
   B. 80–90%
   C. 60–80%
   D. 40–60%

3. Next to close clinical observation, which of the following can be included in follow-up of vestibular schwannoma patients?
   A. Follow-up MRI scans
   B. Follow-up CT scans
   C. Short increment sensitivity index test
   D. Stenger test

4. What are first-line treatment options for tumor sizes from 1.5 to 3 cm?
   A. Stereotactic radiosurgery
   B. Stereotactic radiotherapy
   C. Surgery
   D. All of the above

5. Which of the following are predictive factors for hearing preservation?
   A. Tumor size
   B. Irradiation dose delivered to auditory canal

C. Young age of presentation
D. All of the above

## Answers

1. D [1]
2. A [28, 56, 59, 60]
3. A [84]
4. D [10, 34, 40, 56]
5. D [78–80, 85]

## References

1. Park JK, Vernick DM, Ramakrishna N. Vestibular schwannoma (acoustic neuroma). 2016. http://www. uptodate.com/contents/vestibular-schwannoma-acoustic-neuroma
2. Schlehofer B, Schlaefer K, Blettner M, et al. Environmental risk factors for sporadic acoustic neuroma (Interphone Study Group, Germany). Eur J Cancer. 2007;43(11):1741–7.
3. Mohyuddin A, Neary WJ, Wallace A, et al. Molecular genetic analysis of the NF2 gene in young patients with unilateral vestibular schwannomas. J Med Genet. 2002;39(5):315–22.
4. Schüz J, Steding-Jessen M, Hansen S, et al. Sociodemographic factors and vestibular schwannoma: a Danish nationwide cohort study. Neuro Oncol. 2010;12(12):1291–9.
5. Lin D, Hegarty JL, Fischbein NJ, et al. The prevalence of "incidental" acoustic neuroma. Arch Otolaryngol Head Neck Surg. 2005;131(3):241–4.
6. Propp JM, McCarthy BJ, Davis FG, et al. Descriptive epidemiology of vestibular schwannomas. Neuro Oncol. 2006;8(1):1–11.
7. Babu R, Sharma R, Bagley JH, et al. Vestibular schwannomas in the modern era: epidemiology, treatment trends, and disparities in management. J Neurosurg. 2013;119(1):121–30.
8. ANA. What is an acoustic neuroma? - Acoustic Neuroma Association. Anausa.org [cited 12 November 2017]. Available from: anausa.org/overview/what-is-acoustic-neuroma
9. Curry, W.T., Jr. and F.G. Barker, II, Racial, ethnic and socioeconomic disparities in the treatment of brain tumors. J Neurooncol, 2009. 93(1): p. 25–39.
10. Sughrue ME, Kaur R, Rutkowski MJ, et al. Extent of resection and the long-term durability of vestibular schwannoma surgery. J Neurosurg. 2011;114(5):1218–23.
11. Roche PH, Bouvier C, Chinot O, et al. Genesis and biology of vestibular schwannomas. Prog Neurol Surg. 2008;21:24–31.
12. Schneider AB, Ron E, Lubin J, et al. Acoustic neuromas following childhood radiation treatment for benign conditions of the head and neck. Neuro Oncol. 2008;10(1):73–8.
13. Shore-Freedman E, Abrahams C, Recant W, et al. Neurilemomas and salivary gland tumors of the head and neck following childhood irradiation. Cancer. 1983;51(12):2159–63.
14. De Vocht F. The case of acoustic neuroma: comment on: mobile phone use and risk of brain neoplasms and other cancers. Int J Epidemiol. 2014;43(1):273–4.
15. Muscat JE, Malkin MG, Shore RE, et al. Handheld cellular telephones and risk of acoustic neuroma. Neurology. 2002;58(8):1304–6.
16. Hours M, Bernard M, Arslan M, et al. Can loud noise cause acoustic neuroma? Analysis of the INTERPHONE study in France. Occup Environ Med. 2009;66(7):480–6.

17. Bäcklund LM, Grandér D, Brandt L, et al. Parathyroid adenoma and primary CNS tumors. Int J Cancer. 2005;113(6):866–9.

18. Corona AP, Ferrite S, Lopes Mda S, et al. Risk factors associated with vestibular nerve schwannomas. Otol Neurotol. 2012;33(3):459–65.

19. Evans DG, Newton V, Neary W, et al. Use of MRI and audiological tests in presymptomatic diagnosis of type 2 neurofibromatosis (NF2). J Med Genet. 2000;37(12):944–7.

20. Jackler RK, Driscoll CLW. Tumors of the ear and temporal bone. Philadelphia, PA: Lippincott Williams & Wilkins; 2000.

21. Régis J, Carron R, Delsanti C, et al. Radiosurgery for vestibular schwannomas. Neurosurg Clin N Am. 2013;24(4):521–30.

22. Hasegawa T, Kida Y, Kato T, et al. Long-term safety and efficacy of stereotactic radiosurgery for vestibular schwannomas: evaluation of 440 patients more than 10 years after treatment with Gamma Knife surgery. J Neurosurg. 2013;118(3):557–65.

23. Wilson DF, Hodgson RS, Gustafson MF, et al. The sensitivity of auditory brainstem response testing in small acoustic neuromas. Laryngoscope. 1992;102(9):961–4.

24. Matthies C, Samii M, Krebs S. Management of vestibular schwannomas (acoustic neuromas): radiological features in 202 cases--their value for diagnosis and their predictive importance. Neurosurgery. 1997;40(3):469–81; discussion 481–2.

25. Marx SV, Langman AW, Crane RC. Accuracy of fast spin echo magnetic resonance imaging in the diagnosis of vestibular schwannoma. Am J Otolaryngol. 1999;20(4):211–6.

26. Rouleau GA, Merel P, Lutchman M, et al. Alteration in a new gene encoding a putative membrane-organizing protein causes neurofibromatosis type 2. Nature. 1993;363(6429):515–21.

27. Combs SE, Welzel T, Schulz-Ertner D, et al. Differences in clinical results after LINAC-based single-dose radiosurgery versus fractionated stereotactic radiotherapy for patients with vestibular schwannomas. Int J Radiat Oncol Biol Phys. 2010;76(1):193–200.

28. Régis J, Pellet W, Delsanti C, et al. Functional outcome after gamma knife surgery or microsurgery for vestibular schwannomas. J Neurosurg. 2002;97(5):1091–100.

29. Schmerber S, Palombi O, Boubagra K, et al. Long-term control of vestibular schwannoma after a translabyrinthine complete removal. Neurosurgery. 2005;57(4):693–8; discussion 693–8.

30. Larson TL. Understanding the posttreatment imaging appearance of the internal auditory canal and cerebellopontine angle. Semin Ultrasound CT MR. 2003;24(3):133–46.

31. Carlson ML, Jacob JT, Pollock BE, et al. Long-term hearing outcomes following stereotactic radiosurgery for vestibular schwannoma: patterns of hearing loss and variables influencing audiometric decline. J Neurosurg. 2013;118(3):579–87.

32. Roos DE, Potter AE, Zacest AC. Hearing preservation after low dose linac radiosurgery for acoustic neuroma depends on initial hearing and time. Radiother Oncol. 2011;101(3):420–4.

33. Lanman TH, Brackmann DE, Hitselberger WE, et al. Report of 190 consecutive cases of large acoustic tumors (vestibular schwannoma) removed via the translabyrinthine approach. J Neurosurg. 1999;90(4):617–23.

34. Sughrue ME, Yang I, Aranda D, et al. Beyond audiofacial morbidity after vestibular schwannoma surgery. J Neurosurg. 2011;114(2):367–74.

35. Golfinos JG, Hill TC, Rokosh R, et al. A matched cohort comparison of clinical outcomes following microsurgical resection or stereotactic radiosurgery for patients with small- and medium-sized vestibular schwannomas. J Neurosurg. 2016;125(6):1472–82.

36. Lee NY, Riaz N, Lu J. Target volume delineation for conformal and intensity-modulated radiation therapy. New York: Springer; 2015.

37. Yomo S, Tamura M, Carron R, et al. A quantitative comparison of radiosurgical treatment parameters in vestibular schwannomas: the Leksell Gamma Knife Perfexion versus Model 4C. Acta Neurochir. 2010;152(1):47–55.

38. Leber KA, Bergloff J, Pendl G. Dose-response tolerance of the visual pathways and cranial nerves of the cavernous sinus to stereotactic radiosurgery. J Neurosurg. 1998;88(1):43–50.

39. Kano H, Kondziolka D, Khan A, et al. Predictors of hearing preservation after stereotactic radiosurgery for acoustic neuroma. J Neurosurg. 2009;111(4):863–73.

40. Roos DE, Potter AE, Brophy BP. Stereotactic radiosurgery for acoustic neuromas: what happens long term? Int J Radiat Oncol Biol Phys. 2012;82(4):1352–5.

41. Jacob JT, Carlson ML, Schiefer TK, et al. Significance of cochlear dose in the radiosurgical treatment of vestibular schwannoma: controversies and unanswered questions. Neurosurgery. 2014;74(5):466–74; discussion 474.

42. Pollock BE. Management of vestibular schwannomas that enlarge after stereotactic radiosurgery: treatment recommendations based on a 15 year experience. Neurosurgery. 2006;58(2):241–8; discussion 241–8.

43. Yang I, Sughrue ME, Han SJ, et al. A comprehensive analysis of hearing preservation after radiosurgery for vestibular schwannoma. J Neurosurg. 2010;112(4):851–9.

44. Tanbouzi Husseini S, Piccirillo E, Taibah A, et al. Malignancy in vestibular schwannoma after stereotactic radiotherapy: a case report and review of the literature. Laryngoscope. 2011;121(5):923–8.

45. Link MJ, Cohen PL, Breneman JC, et al. Malignant squamous degeneration of a cerebellopontine angle epidermoid tumor. Case report. J Neurosurg. 2002;97(5):1237–43.

46. Niu NN, Niemierko A, Larvie M, et al. Pretreatment growth rate predicts radiation response in vestibular schwannomas. Int J Radiat Oncol Biol Phys. 2014;89(1):113–9.

47. Shin M, Ueki K, Kurita H, et al. Malignant transformation of a vestibular schwannoma after gamma knife radiosurgery. Lancet. 2002;360(9329):309–10.

48. Muracciole X, Regis J. Radiosurgery and carcinogenesis risk. Prog Neurol Surg. 2008;21:207–13.

49. Chopra R, Kondziolka D, Niranjan A, et al. Long-term follow-up of acoustic schwannoma radiosurgery with marginal tumor doses of 12 to 13 Gy. Int J Radiat Oncol Biol Phys. 2007;68(3):845–51.

50. Fukuoka S, Takanashi M, Hojyo A, et al. Gamma knife radiosurgery for vestibular schwannomas. Prog Neurol Surg. 2009;22:45–62.

51. Sun S, Liu A. Long-term follow-up studies of Gamma Knife surgery with a low margin dose for vestibular schwannoma. J Neurosurg. 2012;117(Suppl):57–62.

52. Yomo S, Carron R, Thomassin JM, et al. Longitudinal analysis of hearing before and after radiosurgery for vestibular schwannoma. J Neurosurg. 2012;117(5):877–85.

53. Weber DC, Chan AW, Bussiere MR, et al. Proton beam radiosurgery for vestibular schwannoma: tumor control and cranial nerve toxicity. Neurosurgery. 2003;53(3):577–86; discussion 586–8.

54. Aoyama H, Onodera S, Takeichi N, et al. Symptomatic outcomes in relation to tumor expansion after fractionated stereotactic radiation therapy for vestibular schwannomas: single-institutional long-term experience. Int J Radiat Oncol Biol Phys. 2013;85(2):329–34.

55. Litre F, Rousseaux P, Jovenin N, et al. Fractionated stereotactic radiotherapy for acoustic neuromas: a prospective monocenter study of about 158 cases. Radiother Oncol. 2013;106(2):169–74.

56. Combs SE, Engelhard C, Kopp C, et al. Long-term outcome after highly advanced single-dose or fractionated radiotherapy in patients with vestibular schwannomas - pooled results from 3 large German centers. Radiother Oncol. 2015;114(3):378–83.

57. Song DY, Williams JA. Fractionated stereotactic radiosurgery for treatment of acoustic neuromas. Stereotact Funct Neurosurg. 1999;73(1–4):45–9.

58. Lederman G, Lowry J, Wertheim S, et al. Acoustic neuroma: potential benefits of fractionated stereotactic radiosurgery. Stereotact Funct Neurosurg. 1997;69(1–4 Pt 2):175–82.

59. Gormley WB, Sekhar LN, Wright DC, et al. Acoustic neuromas: results of current surgical management. Neurosurgery. 1997;41(1):50–8; discussion 58–60.

60. Myrseth E, Møller P, Pedersen PH, et al. Vestibular schwannomas: clinical results and quality of life after microsurgery or gamma knife radiosurgery. Neurosurgery. 2005;56(5):927–35; discussion 927–35.

61. Sawamura Y, Shirato H, Sakamoto T, et al. Management of vestibular schwannoma by fractionated stereotactic radiotherapy and associated cerebrospinal fluid malabsorption. J Neurosurg. 2003;99(4):685–92.

62. Noren G, Arndt J, Hindmarsh T. Stereotactic radiosurgery in cases of acoustic neurinoma: further experiences. Neurosurgery. 1983;13(1):12–22.

63. Kondziolka D, Nathoo N, Flickinger JC, et al. Long-term results after radiosurgery for benign intracranial tumors. Neurosurgery. 2003;53(4):815–21; discussion 821–2.

64. Flickinger JC, Lunsford LD, Linskey ME, et al. Gamma knife radiosurgery for acoustic tumors: multivariate analysis of four year results. Radiother Oncol. 1993;27(2):91–8.

65. Foote RL, Coffey RJ, Swanson JW, et al. Stereotactic radiosurgery using the gamma knife for acoustic neuromas. Int J Radiat Oncol Biol Phys. 1995;32(4):1153–60.

66. Kondziolka D, Lunsford LD, McLaughlin MR, et al. Long-term outcomes after radiosurgery for acoustic neuromas. N Engl J Med. 1998;339(20):1426–33.

67. Mendenhall WM, Friedman WA, Buatti JM, et al. Preliminary results of linear accelerator radiosurgery for acoustic schwannomas. J Neurosurg. 1996;85(6):1013–9.

68. Anderson BM, Khuntia D, Bentzen SM, et al. Single institution experience treating 104 vestibular schwannomas with fractionated stereotactic radiation therapy or stereotactic radiosurgery. J Neurooncol. 2014;116(1):187–93.

69. Meijer OW, Wolbers JG, Baayen JC, et al. Fractionated stereotactic radiation therapy and single high-dose radiosurgery for acoustic neuroma: early results of a prospective clinical study. Int J Radiat Oncol Biol Phys. 2000;46(1):45–9.

70. Hansasuta A, Choi CY, Gibbs IC, et al. Multisession stereotactic radiosurgery for vestibular schwannomas: single-institution experience with 383 cases. Neurosurgery. 2011;69(6):1200–9.

71. Suit H, DeLaney T, Goldberg S, et al. Proton vs carbon ion beams in the definitive radiation treatment of cancer patients. Radiother Oncol. 2010;95(1):3–22.

72. Harsh GR, Thornton AF, Chapman PH, et al. Proton beam stereotactic radiosurgery of vestibular schwannomas. Int J Radiat Oncol Biol Phys. 2002;54(1):35–44.

73. Bush DA, McAllister CJ, Loredo LN, et al. Fractionated proton beam radiotherapy for acoustic neuroma. Neurosurgery. 2002;50(2):270–3; discussion 273–5.

74. Agrawal Y, Clark JH, Limb CJ, et al. Predictors of vestibular schwannoma growth and clinical implications. Otol Neurotol. 2010;31(5):807–12.

75. Fenton JE, Chin RY, Fagan PA, et al. Facial nerve outcome in non-vestibular schwannoma tumour surgery. Acta Otorhinolaryngol Belg. 2004;58(2):103–7.

76. Rivas A, Boahene KD, Bravo HC, et al. A model for early prediction of facial nerve recovery after vestibular schwannoma surgery. Otol Neurotol. 2011;32(5):826–33.

77. Isaacson B, Kileny PR, El-Kashlan H, et al. Intraoperative monitoring and facial nerve outcomes after vestibular schwannoma resection. Otol Neurotol. 2003;24(5):812–7.

78. Gjuric M, Mitrecic MZ, Greess H, et al. Vestibular schwannoma volume as a predictor of hearing outcome after surgery. Otol Neurotol. 2007;28(6):822–7.

79. Irving RM, Jackler RK, Pitts LH. Hearing preservation in patients undergoing vestibular schwannoma surgery: comparison of middle fossa and retrosigmoid approaches. J Neurosurg. 1998;88(5):840–5.

80. Massager N, Nissim O, Delbrouck C, et al. Irradiation of cochlear structures during vestibular schwannoma radiosurgery and associated hearing outcome. J Neurosurg. 2007;107(4):733–9.

81. Thomas C, Di Maio S, Ma R, et al. Hearing preservation following fractionated stereotactic radiotherapy for vestibular schwannomas: prognostic implications of cochlear dose. J Neurosurg. 2007;107(5):917–26.

82. Chan AW, Black P, Ojemann RG, et al. Stereotactic radiotherapy for vestibular schwannomas: favorable outcome with minimal toxicity. Neurosurgery. 2005;57(1):60–70; discussion 60–70.

83. Pollock BE, Driscoll CL, Foote RL, et al. Patient outcomes after vestibular schwannoma management: a prospective comparison of microsurgical resection and stereotactic radiosurgery. Neurosurgery. 2006;59(1):77–85; discussion 77–85.

84. Doherty JK, Friedman RA. Controversies in building a management algorithm for vestibular schwannomas. Curr Opin Otolaryngol Head Neck Surg. 2006;14(5):305–13.

85. Tamura M, Carron R, Yomo S, et al. Hearing preservation after gamma knife radiosurgery for vestibular schwannomas presenting with high-level hearing. Neurosurgery. 2009;64(2):289–96; discussion 296.

# Part II

# Brain Tumors: Malignant Gliomas

# Low-Grade Glioma

**5**

David M. Routman and Paul D. Brown

## Learning Objectives

After reading the chapter, the reader will be able to:

- Describe the incidence, presenting symptoms, natural history, and common radiologic findings of LGG.
- Understand histologic and molecular features used in the diagnosis and classification of diffuse grade II gliomas, including the WHO 2016 classification system for astrocytoma and oligodendroglioma.
- Identify the key molecular markers in LGG and their impact on prognosis, including IDH mutations and 1p19q codeletions.
- Describe the evidence and considerations for maximal safe resection of LGG versus observation.
- Outline the key trials providing evidence for adjuvant radiation, radiation doses, and chemotherapy.
- List high-risk features of LGG including those used in RTOG 9802.
- Describe target delineation and treatment volumes, setup, and delivery of RT in LGG.
- Name the most common side effects of treatment and dose constraints for organs at risk.

## Background Epidemiology

Statistics on the incidence and prevalence of low-grade glioma vary given limitations of epidemiologic data in the setting of a heterogeneous group of tumors and evolving categorization of primary tumors of the CNS. An estimated 24,000 CNS tumors will be diagnosed annually in the United

States [1]. Approximately 21,000 of these will arise in the brain, the majority of which will be high-grade glioma [2].

Gliomas in general have an annual incidence of approximately 6.0 per 100,000. Low-grade gliomas represent up to 10% of all malignant brain tumors and are a heterogeneous group with around 3000 incident cases annually. Within diffuse (grade II) LGG, the estimated annual incidence of diffuse *astrocytoma* is 0.51 per 100,000, which would equate to approximately 1700 expected cases for a US population of 325 million without age adjustment. The estimated annual incidence of *oligodendroglioma* is 0.25 per 100,000, for estimated incidence of 700–800 cases yearly [2]. With incorporation of molecular information, *oligoastrocytoma* has essentially been eliminated as a diagnosis based on WHO 2016 criteria.

## Risk Factors

The risk factors and etiologic factors of LGG remain largely undetermined. There are rare but noted syndromic associations with LGG including in neurofibromatosis type 1 (von Recklinghausen disease) and neurofibromatosis type 2, with pilocytic astrocytoma being most common. Additionally, patients with tuberous sclerosis have an increased risk of subependymal giant cell astrocytoma, a rare type of grade I astrocytoma.

## Diagnosis, Staging, Pathology, and Prognosis

### Symptoms and Presentation

Diffuse LGG can present at nearly any age in adulthood, but the most common incidence is in the 30–50 age range with an estimated mean age of presentation of 41 and median age ranging from 38–48 years old depending on the series [2, 3]. The diagnosis is more common in males compared to females

D. M. Routman · P. D. Brown (✉)
Department of Radiation Oncology, Mayo Clinic, Rochester, MN, USA
e-mail: brown.paul@mayo.edu

with a ratio of approximately 1.5:1. Seizure secondary to diffuse cortical involvement is the most common presenting symptom in an estimated 60–80% of patients, with patients presenting with focal seizures more commonly than generalized ones. Seizures may be more common for LGGs with an IDH mutation [4, 5]. Other symptoms can include headache, weakness or altered sensation, visual change or other focal neurologic symptoms, behavioral changes including altered mental status, and symptoms related to increased intracranial pressure such as nausea and vomiting. Less than 5% of LGGs are discovered incidentally, and these patients have an improved outcome likely due to a lead time bias [6].

Symptomatology is important as a prognostic factor. Brown et al. showed that patients with an abnormal Mini Mental Status exam had worse PFS and OS in comparison to patients with normal mental status [7]. Conversely, seizures alone at presentation portend a better prognosis compared to patients with neurocognitive deficits or neurologic symptoms described above, as these symptoms may be associated with more aggressive tumors, different molecular characteristics or histology, and more eloquent locations less amenable to resection. Seizure symptoms can impact quality of life and may be a proxy for response to therapy [5]. With a question of whether or not to initiate treatment in lower-risk patients at the time of presentation versus at progression, symptoms and their impact on quality of life are an important consideration.

## Radiographic Findings

CT findings in diffuse LGG include a non-enhancing tumor with a poorly defined area of low attenuation. Lesions are round to oval and are most commonly seen in the frontal and temporal lobes, as much as 70% of the time [8]. Magnetic resonance imaging (MRI) better visualizes diffuse LGG compared to CT, including T1- and T2-weighted images with and without contrast as well as FLAIR sequences. LGGs most commonly appear hypointense on T1 and hyperintense on T2 images, often with heterogeneity. While oligodendrogliomas and astrocytomas have some characteristic radiologic findings, they cannot be distinguished reliably on imaging alone.

Astrocytomas typically spread along white matter tracts, while oligodendrogliomas are more likely to involve the cortex. Astrocytomas may be less likely to present in the frontal lobe than oligodendrogliomas, though lobar location is the most common site for both [8, 9]. Furthermore, IDH-mutated gliomas are more likely to occur in the frontal lobe compared to IDH wild-type tumors [10]. Perfusion-weighted imaging on MRI may be helpful to distinguish astrocytomas from oligodendrogliomas given differences in microvascular density resulting in differences in vascularity detected by relative

cerebral blood volume (rCBV) measurements. Oligodendrogliomas typically have a higher rCBV max value than their astrocytic counterparts, and specificity as high as 87.5% may be possible in distinguishing the two based on an rCBV max value cutoff of 3.0 [11].

Oligodendrogliomas are the primary brain tumor most likely to calcify, with retrospective series noting a rate as low as 20% and other estimates ranging as high as 70% [12, 13]. However, calcification can also be found in astrocytoma as much as 10–20% of the time, and given that astrocytomas are a more common histology, calcification is therefore not a distinguishing characteristic of oligodendroglioma versus astrocytoma.

Imaging characteristics of oligodendrogliomas such as calcification, enhancement, apparent diffusion coefficient (ADC), and rCBV have been correlated to lesion grade as well as prognosis. Khalid et al. found lesions with any contrast enhancement versus no enhancement were more likely to be grade III than grade II. Additionally, oligodendrogliomas with a low ADC were much more likely to be high grade. Edema, hemorrhage, and cystic degeneration have also been correlated to higher-grade anaplastic lesions [14]. Enhancement in LGG has not consistently been shown to portend a worse prognosis, including in prospective trials, possibly due to the difficulty of defining the contrast enhancement (i.e., nodular, trace) on multicenter clinical trials [15]. However, a number of studies have shown enhancement to correspond to a worse prognosis and further correlated enhancement to an increased chance of malignant transformation [16].

Advances in imaging and molecular characterization of LGGs may lead to the ability to utilize known common mutations of LGG for the purposes of diagnostic imaging and response to treatment (Fig. 5.1, below). For example, with magnetic resonance spectroscopy, radiologists have quantified the oncometabolite 2-hydroxyglutarate (2HG) that is found in tumors with known IDH mutations and have shown correlation to tumor grade as well as to increase in concentration at time of progression. Furthermore, mass spec could be used to assess response to treatment by quantification of 2HG [17].

## Pathology

Low-grade gliomas represent a heterogeneous group of tumors, and grading and classification continues to evolve with incorporation of molecular features. Bailey and Cushing initially devised a grading system in the 1920s dividing tumors based on known glial types and correlating histology to outcomes, defining a subset of astrocytoma with a more favorable prognosis [19]. More grading systems followed including Kernohan, St. Anne-Mayo, and

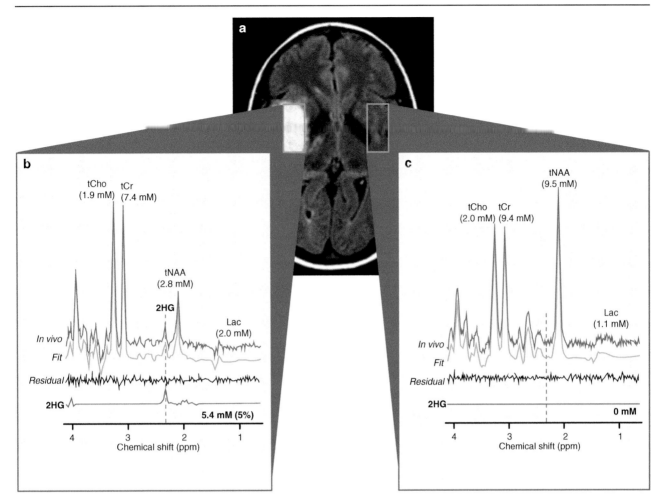

**Fig. 5.1** Detection of 2-hydroxyglutarate (2HG) in IDH mutated tumors using MR spectroscopy. Vertical dashed red line drawn at 2.5 parts per million (ppm). (**a**) MRI demonstrating T2 changes of a right-sided IDH1 mutated oligodendroglioma. Mass spectroscopic comparison of the tumor to the normal appearing contralateral left side. Mass spec after correction for noise in the area of the lesion (**b**) revealed a 2HG peak of 5.4 mM (5%), while in the normal appearing left side (**c**), there was no detectable 2HG. *tCho* total choline, *tCr* total creatine, *tNAA* total *N*-acetylasparate, *LAC* lactate. [Reprinted from An Z, et al. Detection of 2-hydroxyglutarate in brain tumors by triple-refocusing MR spectroscopy at 3T in vivo. Magn Reson Med. 2017;78(1):40–48. With permission from John Wiley & Sons, Inc.] [18]

Renertz. Over the course of nearly a century, classification and grading systems have continued to utilize light microscopy with staining such as hematoxylin and eosin to attempt to distinguish cells of origin and identify grades of differentiation [20]. Additional features such as mitotic activity as measured by Ki-67/MIB-1 labeling indices were found to correlate to prognosis and used to help more reliably distinguish grades [21–23]. In addition to mitotic activity, presence of anaplasia, endothelial proliferation, and necrosis was ultimately incorporated into the most commonly accepted glioma grading system—the World Health Organization Classification of Tumors of the Central Nervous System [20]. Generally, grade I is reserved for tumors with low proliferative potential which are well circumscribed. Grade II tumors are infiltrative neoplasms with recurrent potential and can progress to higher-grade lesions becoming anaplastic with increasing proliferative activity.

Grade II tumors do not display mitotic activity, endothelial proliferation, or necrosis in comparison to high-grade lesions [8, 20].

Traditionally, low-grade glioma has been defined as any grade I or II tumor. Limitations of this classification include a lack of interrater reliability and the fact that the distinction between grades such as grade II and grade III astrocytoma in actuality represent a somewhat artificial demarcation along a continuum [24]. Nevertheless, this system has been historically useful in forming prognostic groups and has been the basis of inclusion criteria for clinical trials [25–27]. However, with the increased recognition of molecular subtypes, the 2016 WHO classification incorporates parameters based on molecular analysis and represents a major restructuring of diffuse gliomas [28]. For the purposes of this chapter, we will consider pilocytic astrocytoma separately as well as other grade I lesions and focus on diffuse gliomas and genetic-based profiles (according to the WHO 2016 criteria), with the understanding that genetic profiles may be more important in certain instances than histologic grading. Indeed, per Louis et al., "diffuse astrocytoma and oligodendrogliomas are now nosologically more similar than are diffuse astrocytoma and pilocytic astrocytoma; the family trees have been redrawn [28]." For example, pilocytic astrocytomas generally do not show an IDH gene alteration (as do most grade II gliomas), commonly have BRAF alterations, are well circumscribed, and are non-infiltrating lesions with distinct treatment recommendations. Similarly, subependymal giant cell astrocytoma likely represents a separate entity from diffuse grade II glioma, also with distinct molecular alterations.

## Molecular Classification

As displayed in Fig. 5.2, histologic subtype in the WHO grading scheme is followed by a comma, with either genetic profile or NOS in the case of limited or inconclusive genetic information. For genetically profiled tumors, the designations are diffuse astrocytoma, IDH wild type; diffuse astrocytoma, IDH mutant; and oligodendroglioma, IDH mutant and 1p19q codeleted. Molecular classification depends mainly on 1p/19q codeletion and IDH mutational status. Other molecular characteristics including ATRX mutation, TP53 mutation, and MGMT methylation are not required for diagnosis but are important markers as described below.

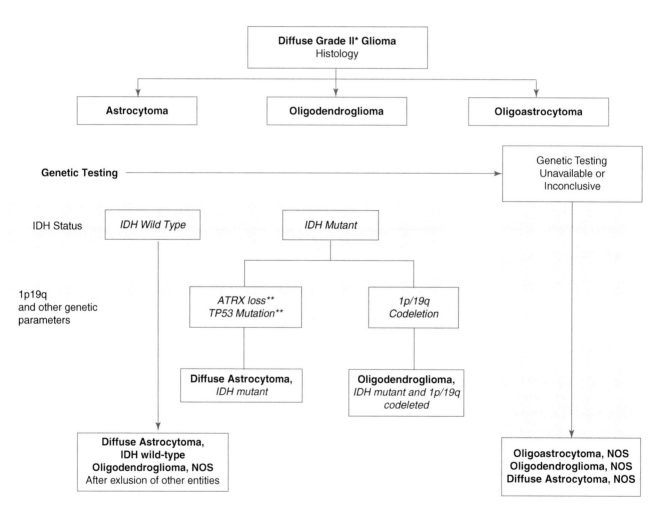

\* Grade II tumors are infiltrative but lack the nuclear atypia and mitotic activity distinguishing Grade III lesion
\*\* Characteristic but not required for diagnosis

**Fig. 5.2** Grade II glioma classification algorithm per the WHO 2016 classification system. [Adapted from Louis D.N. et al. *The 2016 World Health Organization Classification of Tumors of the Central Nervous* *System: a summary*. Acta Neuropathol 2016 131(6): p. 803–20. With permission from Springer-Verlag]

## 1p/19q Codeletion

1p/19q represents an unbalanced [t(1;19)(p10;q10)] centromeric or peri-centromeric translocation at a breakpoint with highly repeated sequences. The aberrant chromosome after translocation is lost with deletion of the short arm of chromosome 1 and the long arm of chromosome 19. The genes specifically associated with this breakpoint have yet to be identified [29, 30]. Several candidate tumor suppressor genes may be implicated in the oncogenic nature of this deletion, including capicua transcriptional repressor (CIC) on chromosome 19 and far upstream element-binding protein 1 (FUBP1) on chromosome 1 [31–33]. 1p/19q codeletion co-occurs with IDH mutations the vast majority of the time, and IDH mutation appears to be an early event in the development of oligodendroglioma, likely preceding 1p/19q codeletion [34, 35].

1p/19q codeletion is necessary for the diagnosis of oligodendroglioma as described above, with formerly designated mixed origin oligoastrocytomas to not be a diagnosed entity in the molecular era. For example, on review of 43 oligoastrocytomas, Sahm et al. found only one case molecularly consistent with a potentially mixed etiology. Thirty-one of the 43 were found to have profiles consistent with oligodendroglioma, while in 11 of 43, a typical pattern for astrocytoma was seen. By investigating staining including IDH1 R132H at the cellular level, the regions formerly called astrocytoma in the setting of 1p/19q codeletion more likely represented reactive gliosis [36]. Finally, diagnosis of oligodendroglioma and 1p/19q codeletion has prognostic and potentially predictive implications described later in this chapter.

## Isocitrate Dehydrogenase (IDH 1 and IDH 2)

IDH 1 and IDH 2 are enzymes involved in the citric acid cycle that convert isocitrate to alpha-ketoglutarate and when mutated have oncogenic potential, likely mediated by the accumulation of the oncometabolite 2HG described above. Mutations in IDH are thought be the primary event in development of diffuse gliomas or are at least one of the earliest discovered events. IDH mutation was originally identified at R132 in a genomic analysis of glioblastomas in 2008 and subsequently found to be present in LGG [37]. Up to 80% of LGG have mutations in IDH1 and even more when IDH2 is analyzed [38]. This rate of IDH mutation includes both astrocytomas with TP53 mutations and oligodendroglioma with loss of 1p/19q. IDH mutations are associated with a better prognosis than IDH wild-type tumors. IDH mutations may also be predictive of response to chemotherapy and are associated with MGMT methylation in the vast majority of cases [39].

For LGG classification, IDH wild-type tumors based on WHO 2016 criteria include astrocytoma, IDH wild type, and oligodendroglioma, NOS. IDH mutant tumors include astrocytoma, IDH mutant and oligodendroglioma, IDH mutant and 1p/19q codeleted.

## Alpha-Thalassemia/Mental Retardation Syndrome X-Linked (ATRX)

ATRX is involved in transcriptional regulation and chromatin remodeling, and in astrocytoma mutation may lead to a phenotype of telomere instability [40]. ATRX mutations are mutually exclusive with 1p/19q codeletion but are characteristic of IDH mutant astrocytoma along with TP53 mutation. However ATRX, per WHO 2016 criteria, is not required for diagnosis of astrocytoma, IDH mutant.

## TP53

The TP53 gene is a well-known tumor suppressor gene implicated in multiple malignancies. It encodes P53, a protein that has been described as the guardian of the genome. P53 has multiple roles including DNA repair, cell cycle arrest, apoptosis, and senescence response to shortened telomeres. TP53 mutation is mutually exclusive with 1p/19q codeletion just as ATRX above [41]. Also, like ATRX, although TP53 mutation is characteristic of astrocytoma, IDH mutant, it is not required for diagnosis.

## Methyl Guanine Methyl Transferase (MGMT)

MGMT is a DNA repair enzyme. It is responsible for removing alkyl groups at the $O_6$ position of guanine. MGMT is able to repair damage from alkylating agents, such as TMZ. When the MGMT promoter is hypermethylated, MGMT is silenced, and tumor cells are more susceptible to alkylation. MGMT hypermethylation has been shown to be prognostic and potentially predictive of response to alkylating agents, though controversy regarding prediction of response remains [42]. Furthermore, the effect may be dependent upon coexisting mutations such as IDH1 [43]. MGMT is further discussed in the high-grade glioma chapter (Chap. 6).

## Telomerase Reverse Transcriptase (TERT)

TERT is an enzyme that is a part of the telomerase complex, which is involved in stabilization and lengthening of telomeres. Mutation in the TERT promoter (outside of the coding region of the gene) leads to an increase in the length of telomeres via increased telomerase production and activity. This can increase cell survival and ultimately promote malignancy [44]. TERT mutation has prognostic implications in LGG, and its impact on OS may depend on presence or absence of other molecular features as described in the section below [45].

## Prognosis

Compared to age- and sex-matched healthy controls, patients with LGG have decreased survival. Prognostic factors historically have been based on histology, tumor characteristics, a patient's age, performance status, and neurologic status.

Pignatti et al. investigated factors predicting a poor prognosis in a construction set of 322 patients in EORTC 22844 and validated these factors in a cohort of 288 patients in EORTC 22845 [46]. Poor prognosis was associated with tumors ≥6 cm, astrocytoma histology, tumor crossing midline, age greater than 40, and neurologic deficit at presentation. Based on this classification system, patients at high risk (classified as those with three to five of these factors) had a median OS of 3.7 years in comparison to low-risk patients (zero to two risk factors) who had a median OS of 7.8 years [46]. As previously mentioned, patients with abnormal Mini Mental Status exam have worse PFS and OS in comparison to those with a normal one [7].

Molecular profile has additionally been found to be an important prognostic factor. Patients with 1p19q codeletion appear to have a more favorable prognosis. This has been shown on numerous analyses, with one series finding a median OS of 9.1 years for 1p19q intact versus 13.0 years for those with 1p19q codeletion [30]. Extrapolating from studies of higher-grade lesions, IDH mutation confers a better prognosis than IDH wild type, irrespective of 1p19q status and potentially irrespective of treatment [47]. The interplay of these factors has yet to be fully elucidated, and many pertinent findings are from trials of higher-grade lesions. MGMT hypermethylation has been found to have both prognostic and predictive values. Wick et al. investigated the prognostic versus predictive value of MGMT status in association with IDH and 1p19q status. MGMT hypermethylation was found to be associated with a better prognosis for IDH mutant tumors (increased PFS regardless of type of adjuvant therapy) but not predictive of response to treatment. However, for IDH wild-type tumors, MGMT was found to be predictive of response to therapy but not prognostic—MGMT hypermethylated IDH wild-type tumors had increased PFS when treated with chemotherapy with no difference in PFS when treated with RT [43].

Eckel-Passow et al. investigated traditional factors and molecular markers including the role of TERT mutation on prognosis of grade II and grade III gliomas, in a combined retrospective series of patients from the Cancer Genome Atlas, University of California, San Francisco, and Mayo Clinic. A multivariate cox proportional model was performed. Histologic subtype was significant for worse prognosis on univariate but not multivariate analysis for astrocytoma compared to oligodendroglioma. Age at diagnosis and grade were associated with survival on multivariate analysis. When controlling for the above factors, molecular subgroup remained significantly associated with OS. Patients that were "triple positive," with 1p/19q codeletion and IDH and TERT mutations, had the highest median OS, followed by combined IDH and TERT mutations, IDH mutation only, and "triple negative," respectively. Patients that had TERT mutation alone had the lowest median OS with a HR of 11.74 ($p < 0.05$). However, there were very few grade II gliomas in this group as 85% in this category, TERT mutation alone, were diagnosed as GBM. TERT mutation alone represented only 10% or 7 of 74 of the grade II tumors analyzed [45].

In summary, a patient's OS is impacted by diagnosis of LGG in comparison to a healthy age-matched cohort. Factors including age and extent of resection along with tumor characteristics impact prognosis. Molecular subtyping can further stratify groups. Patients with IDH mutations along with codeletion of 1p/19q have the best prognosis. Of IDH mutants that are not codeleted, TERT mutation appears to confer a better prognosis. The predictive role of these factors and the most effective treatment selection by group and risk category have yet to be established.

## Treatment Strategy: A Multimodality Management Approach for Diffuse LGG

The overall treatment strategy for LGG is evolving, and work remains to delineate clear indications for primary surgical and adjuvant therapy. Prior studies have failed to adequately assess overall quality of life against the morbidity of treatment, given the relatively favorable natural history of LGG. Treatment strategies can be stratified by risk categories and include observation, surgery alone, and surgery with adjuvant therapy such as RT, chemotherapy (CT), or chemoradiation (CRT).

### Observation

Optimal timing of treatment for patients with LGG is controversial as observation remains a potential strategy for select patients. Prior to development of molecular subtypes, observational studies showed marked variability in the natural history of LGG due to inclusion of what are now considered distinct clinical entities. The lack of definitive evidence favoring invasive interventional modalities including surgical resection and RT and the associated morbidities of treatment, along with the relatively favorable prognosis of LGG, make observation a potentially justifiable strategy. However, with a median age of onset in the 30s to 40s, the natural history for all pathologic and molecular subtypes is significantly worse than appropriately matched controls [48]. Retrospective series have additionally shown that extent of resection (EOR) correlates to survival. Furthermore, recent studies including RTOG 9802 have provided prospective evidence that treatment in higher-risk patients can improve survival; however, when to initiate this treatment remains an open consideration.

## Surgery

There are no randomized trials comparing extensive resection versus subtotal resection or biopsy alone in LGG. Patients with intractable seizures or other symptomatology including symptoms secondary to mass effect have an indication for surgery. Controversy remains regarding optimal treatment strategy for the patient with controlled symptoms. However, many retrospective series as well as prospective observational trials have suggested that a greater EOR improves OS.

Jakola et al. compared two centers in Norway with different treatment strategies, allowing for distinct population-based cohorts, with one center favoring a biopsy and watchful waiting strategy and one favoring maximal safe resection. The median OS for grade II astrocytomas was 5.6 years for the center favoring watchful waiting versus 9.7 years at the center favoring resection [49]. Additional retrospective studies have compared STR to gross total resection (GTR) and found that greater EOR improves OS and decreases rate of malignant transformation to higher-grade lesions [50, 51].

In a study investigating 216 patients treated at the University of California, San Francisco, patients with LGG were analyzed and categorized based on EOR of greater than or less than 90%. Tumor volumes pre- and postoperatively were measured on FLAIR MRI sequences. Greater than 90% resection correlated to an OS at 5 years and 8 years of 97% and 91% in comparison to a 5- and 8-year OS of 76% and 60% for patients with less than 90% resected. Of note, no mortality related to surgery was identified, and new permanent neurologic deficits as a result of surgery were identified in less than 2% of patients [51]. After adjusting for age, KPS, tumor location, and tumor subtype, EOR remained predictive of OS. Longer-term follow-up from a Mayo Clinic series of over 300 patients similarly found on multivariate analyses that GTR significantly improved OS [52].

Limitations of such series include the potential inherent biases associated with EOR analyses. Namely, more favorably located lesions are more likely to be resectable versus unfavorable lesions in eloquent locations such as the brainstem. Additionally, neurosurgeons may be more likely to pursue aggressive surgery in patients with better performance status at baseline. Nevertheless, prospective studies have confirmed the above retrospective findings. RTOG 9802 observed 111 patients defined as low risk—age less than 40 and with GTR. Residual tumor based on MRI postoperatively was associated with risk of recurrence. At a median follow-up of 4.4 years, 26% of patients recurred that had residual tumor less than 1 cm compared to 68% of patients with 1–2 cm residual disease [53].

Current neurosurgical guidelines generally recommend resection over observation but do not definitively do so, given a lack of level I evidence favoring intervention and level II evidence that biopsy alone is an alternative. In the absence of randomized prospective evidence, the above studies suggest EOR is associated with improved survival and maximal safe resection is likely indicated for LGG, understanding that in LGG minimization of morbidity and impact of surgery on quality of life warrants careful consideration given a favorable natural history [54].

## Radiation

Postoperative radiation therapy can benefit patients by controlling symptoms, delaying tumor recurrence, and improving OS (in combination with chemotherapy) in select patients. Questions remain regarding optimal timing of RT (immediately after surgery versus at time of recurrence), optimal dosing, and optimal treatment volumes.

The timing of RT was addressed in EORTC 22845 which randomized patients with supratentorial LGG to RT of 54 Gy versus deferred radiation until the time of progression. This study found no difference in median survival, 7.4 years in the treatment arm and 7.2 years in observation arm, even though early RT improved progression-free survival to 5.3 years compared to 3.4 years in delayed RT group. Seizures were better controlled at 1 year in the early RT group. In patients who were progression-free at 2 years, there were no differences in performance or cognitive status, though overall quality of life was not measured temporally. Thus, whether delayed median progression of 1.9 years resulted in improved quality of life could not be assessed [27]. Further evidence of the potential for RT to improve symptoms comes from studies investigating patients with medically intractable seizures resulting from LGG. Patients in multiple series achieved a significant reduction in frequency of seizures compared to baseline after fractionated RT [55, 56]. The rate of malignant transformation after radiation was a concern also addressed by EORTC 22845. There were no differences in the malignant transformation between study arms at the time of progression. While rate of dedifferentiation may be decreased by surgical resection, RT appears to have no effect on the likelihood of transformation [27].

In a practice-changing study, RTOG 9802 showed an overall survival benefit on long-term follow-up for high-risk patients with the addition of six cycles of procarbazine, lomustine, and vincristine (PCV) after RT compared to RT alone. High-risk patients were defined as patients 40 or older with diffuse grade II gliomas undergoing any extent of resection and adults under age 40 who had undergone STR. High-risk patients with RT + PCV had a statistically significant improved median OS of 13.3 years versus

7.8 years for those undergoing RT alone [25]. This study is a paradigm shifting for high risk-patients and is the first study in WHO grade II glioma to show a positive impact on OS.

While the results of RTOG 9802 will likely change practice for the treatment of LGG, controversy regarding potential observation remains for low-risk LGG. Comparison studies involving temozolomide (TMZ) are underway as described below. Additionally, whether to treat with RT + PCV at the time of progression for low-risk patients remains unclear. In the low risk LGG Phase II portion of RTOG 9802, with age less than 40 and GTR (extent of resection as defined by the neurosurgeon), 5 year PFS was 48%; and preoperative tumor diameter >4 cm, astrocytoma histologic subtype, and residual tumor on MRI >1 cm were associated with decreased PFS [25, 53]. Thus, it is quite possible that a substantially larger subset of patients would have a survival benefit from RT + PCV in LGG than those defined by RTOG 9802, but this risk group remains to be identified based on clinical, pathologic, and molecular factors.

Figure 5.3 incorporates the above information into a treatment algorithm for grade II LGG.

## Chemotherapy

The addition of chemotherapy to radiation has been shown to improve OS in high-grade glioma and in high-risk LGG, e.g., addition of PCV in RTOG 9802 as described previously. Besides this clearly defined group of high-risk patients (age ≥40 or <40 with a STR), questions remain regarding the type of chemotherapy, the benefit to lower-risk patients, and whether in select patients chemotherapy can be used alone.

EORTC 22033-26033 was a phase III randomized trial that investigated chemotherapy alone. Four hundred seventy-seven patients with high-risk features defined as age ≥40, progressive disease, tumor size ≥5 cm, tumor crossing midline, or neurologic symptoms were randomized to TMZ versus

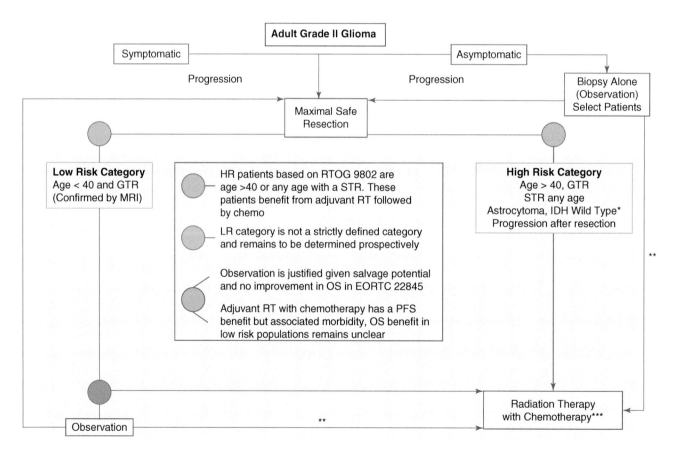

* Based on generally poorer prognosis, No Level 1 evidence
** Progression and not a surgical candidate
*** PCV or TMZ

**Fig. 5.3** Treatment algorithm of adult diffuse grade II glioma including maximal safe resection followed by observation or adjuvant therapy, stratified by RTOG 9802 risk category. *HR* high risk, *LR* low risk, *GTR* gross total resection, *STR* subtotal resection, *OS* overall survival, *PFS* progression-free survival, *RT* radiotherapy, *PCV* procarbazine, lomustine, and vincristine, *TMZ* temozolomide

RT. Overall, there was no significant difference in the primary endpoint of PFS between the two groups. Post hoc subgroup analysis showed that patients with IDH mutation, 1p19q intact, had significantly longer PFS when treated with RT as opposed to TMZ [57]. Overall toxicity was higher in the TMZ arm mainly due to hematologic effects though this did not translate into differences in health-related quality of life. There were no differences in cognitive function, as measured by the Mini Mental State Examination, between the two arms after 36 months of follow-up [58]. Patients with IDH mutation and 1p19q codeletion as well as IDH wild-type tumors did not show any difference in PFS by treatment type. This study confirmed the poor prognosis associated with IDH wild-type gliomas [57].

The combination of RT and TMZ has been demonstrated by Stupp et al. in higher-grade lesions to improve OS, and RTOG 0424 investigated this regimen in the phase II setting for LGG [59]. Patients with three or more high-risk features (age $\geq$40 years, astrocytoma histology, bihemispherical tumor, preoperative tumor diameter of $\geq$6 cm, or a preoperative neurological function status of >1) were enrolled. Chemotherapy consisted of concurrent oral and 12 cycles of adjuvant TMZ. The study's primary endpoint was comparison to a historic control—pre-specified 3 year OS of 54%. The OS at 3 years was 73.1% and was significant in comparison to the pre-specified endpoint [60]. Subgroup analysis according to molecular profile has not yet been presented.

Best practice in LGG requires clinical judgment in the setting of a multidisciplinary approach, and decisions for adjuvant radiation therapy and chemotherapy will need to be made in the absence of level I evidence, as improvement in survival with TMZ or PCV for low-risk patients after radiation therapy could take more than 10 years to establish prospectively in a randomized trial. Furthermore, no high-level evidence exists for comparison of PCV and TMZ, and the interplay of molecular profiles with these agents alone or in combination with RT is under investigation.

## Future Trials

The Alliance-sponsored N0577 study known as the CODEL trial (NCT00887146) is a phase III intergroup study of RT with concomitant and adjuvant TMZ versus RT with adjuvant PCV in patients with 1p/19q codeleted LGG or anaplastic (grade III) glioma. This study was originally designed to investigate treatment in WHO grade III glioma that was 1p19q codeleted, randomizing adults to RT alone, RT + TMZ, or TMZ alone. The results of RTOG 9402 which found improved OS for 1p19q codeleted grade III gliomas with adjuvant PCV versus RT alone were presented during the accrual phase of CODEL [61]. This finding was similar to EORTC 26951 which also showed

improved OS with the addition of PCV [62]. Given these findings, the RT alone and the TMZ alone arms were dropped.

All patients enrolled to date were analyzed which equaled 12 patients in each arm. The TMZ alone group fared worse compared to RT alone or RT + TMZ in terms of progress and OS [63]. The trial was temporarily closed. It reopened with RT + PCV as the control arm and RT with TMZ as the experimental arm. The primary endpoint is PFS. Ideally, and long term, this trial will answer the question of whether adjuvant PCV versus concomitant and adjuvant TMZ is superior in terms of OS for codeleted tumors. The trial now includes LGG (adding 1p19q grade II oligodendroglioma). If these treatment regimens prove equivalent, the secondary endpoints of neurocognitive effects, toxicity, and quality of life will be most important [64].

## Radiation Dosing and Treatment Volumes

Recommended RT dosing is generally 45–54 Gy in 1.8–2.0 Gy fractions. Studies have failed to show improved outcome with dose escalation. EORTC 22844 randomized patients to a moderate dose of 45 Gy versus a higher dose of 59.4 Gy. This study found no difference in OS but found worse QOL in patients receiving higher doses, including increased fatigue, malaise, and insomnia. The Intergroup Trial NCCTG 86-72-51 randomized 203 patients and compared 50.4 Gy to 64.8 Gy. This trial also found no difference in OS. Furthermore, there was no difference in time to progression, and there was higher toxicity in the 64.8 Gy arm. EORTC 22844 and NCCTG 86-72-51 in combination with EORTC 22845 have led to guidelines recommending dosing of 45–54 Gy for LGG, including the National Comprehensive Care Network guidelines [65].

Analyses of failure patterns in LGG have revealed that tumor progression occurs at the primary site the majority of the time, most commonly within the treated volume. While this provided a rational for consideration for dose escalation as above, it also means that expanding volumes beyond partial irradiation of the brain will likely not benefit patients. NCCTG 86-72-51 prospectively confirmed this predominance in field failure, with 92% of failures occurring in the treated field [15]. Treatment volumes are therefore limited to the tumor extent and resection cavity on postoperative T2 and T1 post-gadolinium images. Current protocols recommend treating the tumor based on these sequences with a 1 cm margin (CODEL trial) or 1–1.5 cm margin (EORTC 22033-26033) on the gross tumor volume (GTV) to generate a clinical target volume (CTV), covering microscopic disease [57, 64]. The CTV is an anatomical expansion, respecting bone, tentorium, meninges, and only crossing to the contralateral hemisphere with invasion of a midline structure such as the corpus callosum. Postoperative MRIs are helpful for determining residual disease and the resection cavity and should be fused for contouring if possible.

## Radiation Therapy: General Principles of Simulation and Target Delineation

- CT simulation with a thermoplast mask for immobilization.
- Obtain volumetric thin slice MRI with T1 pre- and post-gadolinium and T2 and FLAIR for target delineation. The target volume for low-grade gliomas is the non-enhancing mass which is best visualized on FLAIR sequences.
- Ideally, fuse both the preoperative and postoperative T2/FLAIR and post-gadolinium MRIs to help delineate target volume as described in Table 5.1.
- If patient has contraindications to MRI, use CT with and without contrast.
- In cases of partial or complete lobectomy, the region anterior to the resection edge where no brain tissue is present does not necessarily need to be included in the GTV or CTV.
- 3D conformal, IMRT, or proton therapy can be considered.

## Radiation Dose Prescription, Organ-At-Risk Tolerances, and Toxicities

- 50.4–54.0 Gy in 1.8–2.0 Gy fractions.

**Table 5.1** Suggested target volumes

| Target volumes | Definition and description |
|---|---|
| GTV | Tumor extent and resection cavity on postoperative T2/FLAIR and T1 post-gadolinium images. Preoperative MRIs are helpful for determining residual disease and resection cavity |
| CTV | GTV + 1 cm. This should be an anatomical expansion and constrained around anatomic boundaries such as bone and dura |
| PTV | CTV + 0.3–0.5 cm depending on comfort of patient positioning, mask fit, and image guidance technique (AP/lateral imaging or cone beam CT) |

*GTV* gross tumor volume, *CTV* clinical target volume, *PTV* planning target volume

**Table 5.2** Recommended normal tissue constraints for 1.8 Gy/day

| Object at risk | Suggested dose constraints |
|---|---|
| Optic nerves and chiasm | <54 Gy[a] |
| Brainstem | <55 Gy |
| Brain (uninvolved contralateral) | <50–60% of total dose[b] |
| Retinae | <40 Gy[a] |
| Lenses | <5 Gy[a] |
| Lacrimal glands | <30 Gy, mean <25 Gy without compromising tumor coverage[c] |
| Hippocampi | Beam angles and planning techniques (e.g., IMRT or proton therapy) to minimize dose to hippocampi |
| Pituitary gland | Beam angles and planning techniques (e.g., IMRT or proton therapy) to minimize dose to pituitary |

[a]N0577 (CODEL) trial
[b]EORTC 22033-26033
[c]Batth SS, et al. Clinical-dosimetric relationship between lacrimal gland dose and ocular toxicity after intensity-modulated radiotherapy for sinonasal tumors [66]

**Table 5.3** Acute and late toxicities for patients undergoing radiation therapy for low-grade glioma

| Acute | Hair loss, fatigue, headaches, nausea, and cerebral edema causing neurological symptoms |
|---|---|
| Long term | Neurocognitive decline and hypopituitarism |
| Uncommon or rare risks | Radiation necrosis, pseudoprogression causing neurological symptoms, vision loss, hearing loss, secondary malignancies |

- Recommended normal tissue constraints for 1.8 Gy/day fractionation schemes are presented in Table 5.2.

## Radiation Toxicity, Acute and Late: Complication Avoidance

Brain irradiation can cause a number of toxicities including acute and long-term effects (Table 5.3). Acute side effects generally resolve, but long-term side effects such as neurocognitive decline, hypopituitarism, and radiation necrosis can cause significant morbidity and in rare instances mortality. Toxicity related to RT has been a rational to delay treatment after surgical resection, as described earlier in this chapter, though the extent to which 45–54 Gy of partial brain RT with modern techniques causes cognitive decline is debatable.

LGG itself can cause decreased cognition and impact quality of life [67]. Furthermore, surgery can further impact cognitive function and performance status. Studies evaluating neurocognitive effects of radiation therefore must take into account a pre-RT baseline neurocognitive status. Prospective trials serially assessing cognitive function in

**Fig. 5.4** Schematic of NRG-BN005 protocol for proton versus photon radiation for grade II and grade III glioma. *IMRT* intensity-modulated radiation therapy, *KPS* Karnofsky performance status

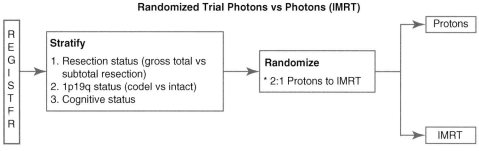

\* Eligibility criteria: IDH mutant WHO grade II or III glioma, KPS ≥70, age >18, no history of psychiatric or neurologic disease

patients treated with RT have not seen any significant decline in intellectual function or memory up to 5 years after receiving RT [68, 69].

Radiation necrosis has a low incidence but can be life threatening. Rates of radiation necrosis correspond to dose, with rates varying from 1% to 5% in studies of LGG. For example, NCCTG 86-72-51 had a 2-year actuarial rate of grade III or higher radiation necrosis of 2.5% in the 50.4 Gy arm compared to 5% in 64.8 Gy arm [15]. QUANTEC suggests partial brain RT to 72 Gy carries a 5% risk of symptomatic radiation necrosis [70]. With most patients receiving advanced imaging including MRI for follow-up, rates of detection of asymptomatic radiation necrosis are likely more frequently detected today compared to previous trials. By decreasing dose to organs at risk and potentially decreasing mean or low dose to the normal brain, proton therapy may decrease rates of toxicity in LGG in select cases.

## Proton Therapy

Given that many LGG patients treated with RT have expected median survivals of 10 years or more, radiation treatment with protons is of interest as it has properties that allow for reduced doses to organs at risk in comparison to photon therapy. Therefore, it may be possible to decrease late toxicities and provide for a better quality of life after treatment in comparison to photons. Proton therapy for LGG has been evaluated prospectively to assess for morbidity and outcomes, including neurocognitive function and hypothalamus-pituitary axis (HPA) dysfunction. Shih et al. reported on 20 patients treated serially with close follow-up. Proton therapy was feasible and effective with OS of 84% at 5 years, comparable to prior trials. There was no noted neurocognitive decline in patients treated with proton RT at a median follow-up of 3.2 years after thorough testing, including intellectual functioning, visuospatial ability, attention and working memory, processing speed, executive functions, language, and verbal and visual memory. Cumulative risk of *new* HPA dysfunctions was 30% at 5 years. The authors analyzed doses of <30 Gy (RBE) to the pituitary. Fourteen (of 20) patients had a dose less than 30 Gy, although

not all patients necessarily required protons to achieve this dose. Additionally, the 6 (of 20) remaining patients not meeting RBE <30 Gy to the pituitary were not preventable with protons given tumor proximity [71].

Based on the results of this trial and other trials, the NRG (PI Dr. David Grosshans) has planned a randomized trial of protons versus photons in IDH mutant LGG and grade III gliomas (Fig. 5.4) with cognitive function being the primary endpoint. The overall impact of protons for LGG will take long-term follow-up and quantification of the impact of toxicity such as HPA dysfunction on patients' QOL. For example, growth hormone secretion is sensitive to RT, with notable cardiovascular, immune, and metabolic effects likely impacted by deficiency and improved with replacement [72, 73].

## Follow-Up and Recurrence

### Follow-Up: Radiographic Assessment

The gold standard for follow-up is MRI. Postoperative MRI should be performed 24–72 h after surgery in order to determine the extent of resection [65]. During initial follow-up, MRI is generally performed every 3–6 months with longer intervals further out from treatment [74]. PET/CT including F-DOPA PET may be useful to potentially differentiate tumor from radiation necrosis, to correlate with tumor grade, or to potentially localize the best location for biopsy [65]. MR spectroscopy and perfusion MRI can also have utility.

### Recurrent Disease

Given the natural history of LGG, most patients will unfortunately recur at some point in their course. Recurrence may be detected clinically secondary to progressive symptoms or based on follow-up imaging. Treatment options depend on the patient's functional status and prior treatments received. Generally, surgery, radiation including re-irradiation, and chemotherapy remain as options.

Recurrent lesions may have dedifferentiated to more aggressive, higher-grade lesions which are associated with a poorer prognosis. Biopsy is generally recommended followed by maximal safe resection if the patient is a surgical candidate. For patients that have not received radiation, treatment with radiation followed by chemotherapy is generally recommended. For re-irradiation, doses such as 35 Gy in 10 fractions have been shown to be effective and tolerable in higher-grade lesions and can be applied to LGG [75].

## Case Presentation

A 42-year-old male patient initially presented with a rash on his torso present for 7 days and coincident encephalopathy, ultimately found to have C3 deposition consistent with a leukoclastic vasculitis. The patient underwent an MRI to evaluate his encephalopathy and was incidentally found to have a right frontal FLAIR abnormality, as demonstrated in Fig. 5.5. The lesion on MRI measured approximately 1.4 cm and was non-enhancing and centrally located at the anterior aspect of the right superior frontal gyrus, centered in the subcortical white matter. Perfusion images suggested mildly elevated cerebral blood volume associated with this lesion.

He was initially observed, and after his encephalopathy improved, he ultimately underwent GTR circa 1 year after presentation. Pathology revealed WHO grade II diffuse astrocytoma, 1p19q intact, MGMT promoter methylated. IDH testing was not performed at this time.

The patient underwent serial MRI every 3 months demonstrating stable disease for the first year and then MRI every 6 months for 2 years when he was found to have an increasing signal abnormality at the margin of the resection bed concerning for progressive disease, eventually presenting to our institution for consult 39 months after initial resection.

**Fig. 5.5** Select MR images from initial patient presentation. (**a**) Non-enhancing lesion on T1 post-gadolinium, (**b**) frontal gyrus lesion with edema noted on T2 (**c**), redemonstrated on T2 axial FLAIR, (**d**) sagittal image of frontal lesion

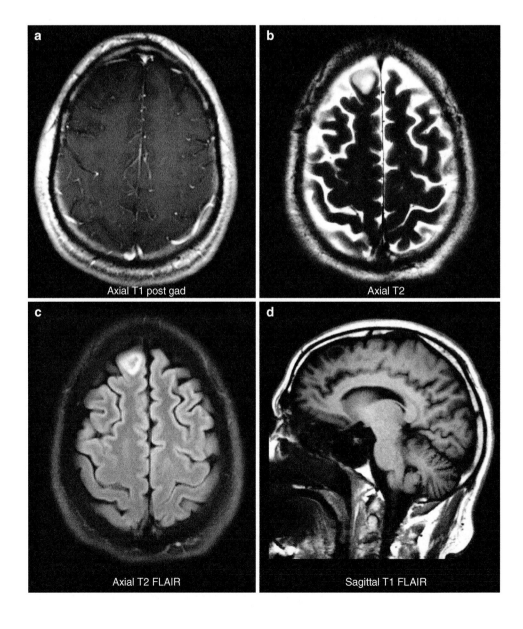

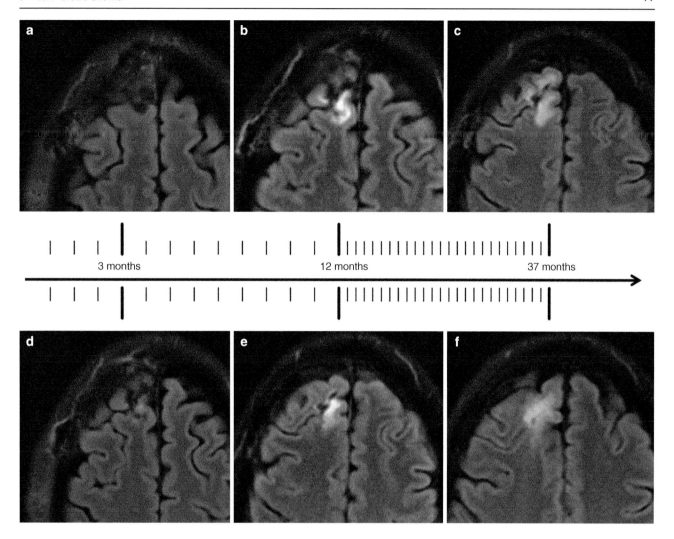

**Fig. 5.6** Follow-up MRIs. (**a, d**) 3 months postoperatively, (**b, e**) 12 months postoperatively, and (**c, f**) 37 months postoperatively demonstrating increased T2 hypertintensity changes concerning for recurrence

A review of his MRIs showed initial interval right frontal craniotomy with resection of the mass as well as expected postoperative changes about the surgical margins. Over the course of the subsequent exams, there was a progression of T2/FLAIR signal abnormality about the margins of the resection bed concerning for tumor progression (Fig. 5.6). No clear restricted diffusion was associated with the region of new signal abnormality.

Per neurosurgery, he underwent biopsy: the lesion was IDH1-R132H negative, though with a loss of ATRX expression, suggesting the possibility of the glioma harboring another less common IDH mutation. Immunohistochemistry revealed an IDH1 R132C mutation. The path report noted "mitotic activity is inconspicuous, and there is no definite microvascular proliferation or tumor necrosis, supporting a WHO grade II designation." The patient subsequently underwent a right frontal craniotomy with re-resection circa 40 months after his initial resection and 52 months after initial presentation (Fig. 5.7).

Radiation oncology was consulted, and the patient was ultimately planned for RT to 50.4 Gy in 28 fractions using proton therapy. Postoperatively the patient had a mild-to-moderate headache and lethargy that improved by the time he was seen for simulation, at which point he had no focal neurologic deficits with cranial nerves II through XII intact, sensation generally intact though with developing complaints of numbness, and five out of five strength noted bilaterally for upper and lower extremities. Treatment was initiated circa 7 weeks after re-resection. He was also seen by medical oncology with a plan for PCV chemotherapy after RT (Fig. 5.8).

## Summary

- Timing of intervention remains an open consideration for grade II gliomas.
- Treatment paradigms are evolving based on molecular subtyping and risk categorization.
- Grade II oligodendroglioma are generally defined by 1p/19q codeletion and most often are IDH mutants.

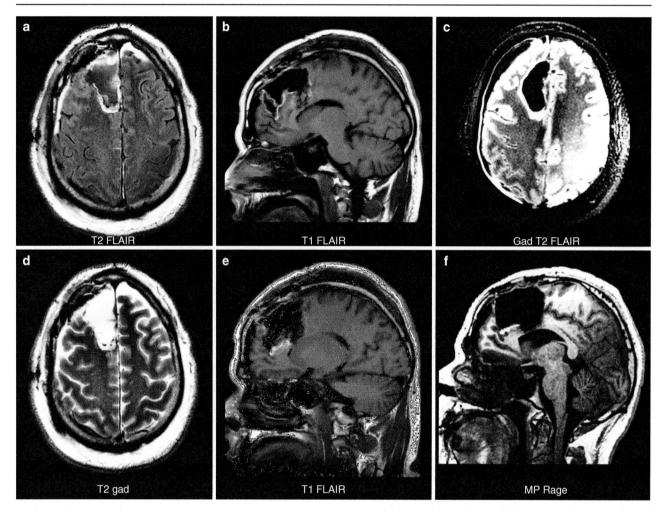

**Fig. 5.7** MRIs postoperatively after re-resection. Immediate postoperative MRIs, (**a**) axial T2 FLAIR, (**b**) sagittal T1 FLAIR, (**d**) axial T2 with gadolinium (gad), and (**e**) T1 FLAIR sagittal, all demonstrating resection cavity. One month postoperative MRIs, (**c**) axial T2 FLAIR and (**f**) sagittal MP-RAGE, also demonstrating re-resection

- Grade II astrocytomas are most commonly IDH mutants, and ATRX and TP53 mutations are characteristic.
- Observation, maximal safe resection alone, and maximal safe resection followed by adjuvant therapy are all treatment options for low-risk patients.
- No randomized trials have demonstrated benefit for early surgical intervention though retrospective and prospective observational studies have shown EOR correlates to OS.
- RT alone improves PFS with no effect on OS.
- Treatment with adjuvant RT followed by PCV is indicated for grade II glioma patients at high risk as defined by age older than 40 or those less than 40 with a STR and improved OS.
- Precisely which lower-risk patients may derive improvement in OS from the addition of PCV after RT remains to be determined along with impact on long-term quality of life.
- Adjuvant RT dosing is 50.4–54 Gy in 1.8–2.0 Gy fractions.
- For target volume, GTV includes tumor extent and resection cavity on postoperative T2/FLAIR and T1 post-gadolinium images.

- CTV is generally GTV + 1–1.5 cm. This should be an anatomical expansion and constrained around anatomic boundaries such as the bone and dura. PTV is 0.3–0.5 cm expansion of the CTV depending on setup, institutional protocol, and image guidance.
- Proton therapy can reduce dose to OARS and may be clinically meaningful depending on tumor location.
- Treatment of recurrent disease will be dictated by prior treatment and performance status, with a biopsy recommended to assess for more malignant transformation.
- Future studies must assess the interplay of molecular markers and type of treatment and evaluate RT with PCV versus RT with TMZ.

## Self-Assessment Questions

1. Which statement is true regarding adult patients with newly diagnosed low-grade gliomas?
   A. Radiotherapy after surgery achieves improved progression-free survival but no overall survival

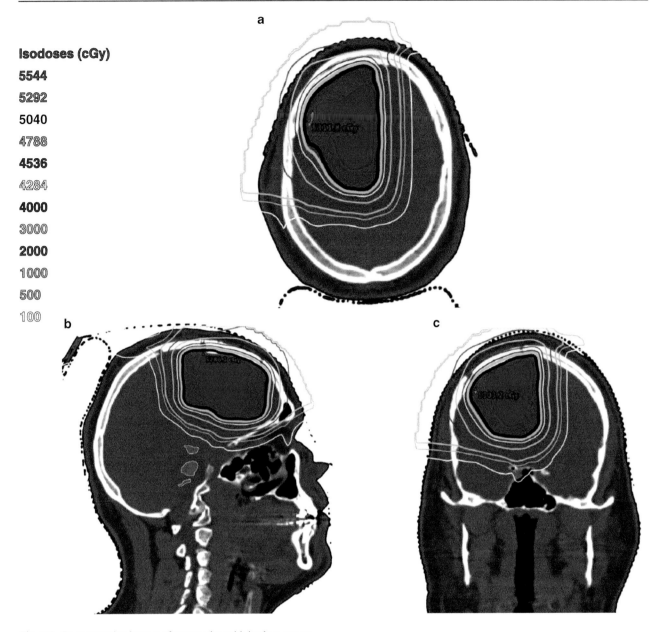

Isodoses (cGy)

5544

5292

5040

4788

4536

4284

4000

3000

2000

1000

500

100

a

b

c

**Fig. 5.8** Representative images of proton plan with isodose curves

advantage compared to delayed radiotherapy at time of progression.

B. Higher doses of radiation such as 59.4 Gy achieves superior survival compared to lower doses such as 45 Gy.

C. Radiotherapy induces more seizure over time in patients with low-grade glioma.

D. Tumor progression after radiotherapy tends to occur outside the high-dose region of the radiotherapy.

E. Procarbazine, lomustine, and vincristine in addition to radiotherapy improve progression-free survival but not overall survival compared to radiotherapy alone in high-risk patients.

2. Which statement is true regarding molecular classification for adult patients with low-grade tumors according to the WHO 2016 criteria?

A. It is expected oligoastrocytoma will be a more frequent diagnosis with the current criteria than in the past.

B. For a small subset of diffuse astrocytoma, IDH mutant, there is both 1p/19q codeletion and ATRX loss.

C. TP53 mutation is required for a diagnosis of diffuse astrocytoma, IDH mutant.

D. Only a minority of low-grade gliomas have IDH 1 mutations.

E. For the diagnosis of oligodendroglioma, 1p/19q codeletion is necessary.

3. Which statement is true regarding surgery for adult patients with newly diagnosed low-grade gliomas?
    A. Randomized trials comparing gross total resection to biopsy have shown an overall survival advantage for gross total resection.
    B. Surgeon defined gross total resection is the most powerful predictor of risk of recurrence.
    C. Greater extent of resection has been associated with decreased rates of malignant transformation to higher grade.
    D. Location of the low-grade glioma does not influence extent of resection.
    E. Gross total resection of a low-grade glioma is specifically defined as complete resection of the contrast-enhancing tumor.

4. Which statement is true regarding signs, symptoms, and presentation of adult patients with newly diagnosed low-grade gliomas?
    A. The mean age is 55 years old.
    B. Seizures are the most common presenting symptom.
    C. A large proportion of low-grade gliomas are discovered incidentally.
    D. Seizures alone at presentation portend a worse prognosis compared to patients with neurocognitive deficits or neurologic symptoms.
    E. Incidentally discovered low-grade gliomas have a worse prognosis.

5. Which statement is true regarding treatment of adult patients with newly diagnosed low-grade gliomas?
    A. Treatment with temozolomide alone has better median overall survival than radiotherapy alone.
    B. There is level I evidence that temozolomide combined with radiotherapy improves overall survival compared to radiotherapy alone.
    C. IDH mutant, non-1p19q codeleted tumors have a progression-free survival benefit for temozolomide alone compared to radiotherapy alone.
    D. Leucopenia is a common toxicity during and after cranial radiotherapy.
    E. Procarbazine, lomustine, and vincristine in addition to radiotherapy improve overall survival compared to radiotherapy alone in high-risk patients.

## Answers

1. A
Feedback: As reported in the phase III trial by van den Bent et al., radiotherapy after surgery achieves improved progression-free survival but no overall survival advantage compared to delayed radiotherapy at time of progression. In this trial seizures were almost half in the radiated arm compared to the observation arm at 1 year. As reported in the phase III trials by Karim et al. and Shaw et al., there is no evidence that higher doses (e.g., 59.4 and 64.8 Gy) of radiation achieve superior survival results compared to moderate doses of radiotherapy (e.g., 45 and 50.4 Gy). Multiple studies including the trial by Shaw et al. show the vast majority (~90%) of failures after radiotherapy occurs in field. RTOG 9802 showed procarbazine, lomustine, and vincristine in addition to radiotherapy improve progression-free survival *and* overall survival compared to radiotherapy alone in high-risk patients.
References: [15, 25–27]

2. E
Feedback: It is expected oligoastrocytoma will become a very infrequent diagnosis with the current criteria. 1p/19q codeletion and ATRX loss are mutually exclusive. Although TP53 is characteristic of astrocytoma, IDH mutant, it is not required for diagnosis. Up to 80% of low-grade gliomas have IDH 1 mutations.
Reference: [28]

3. C
Feedback: To date there have been no randomized trials comparing gross total resection to biopsy in adults with low-grade glioma. RTOG 9802 found the amount of residual tumor on postoperative MRI (after a surgeon defined "gross total resection") to be the strongest predictor of risk of recurrence. There are a number of biases in retrospective studies noting lobar lesions are often completely resected, while infiltrative brainstem tumors cannot be completely resected. Gross total resection of a low-grade glioma is defined as complete resection of the tumor as defined on FLAIR imaging as a substantial proportion of low-grade gliomas are not contrast enhancing.
References: [49–51]

4. B
Feedback: The mean age of presentation is 41. Less than 5% of LGGs are discovered incidentally and have an improved outcome possibly due to a lead time bias. Seizures alone at presentation portend a better prognosis.
Reference: [6]

5. E
Feedback: For the trial EORTC 22033-26033 randomizing patients to radiotherapy or temozolomide, median overall survival has not been reached, and further data maturation is needed for overall survival analyses. Also IDHmt/non-codel tumors treated with radiotherapy had a longer progression-free survival than those treated with temozolomide. In EORTC 22033-26033, leucopenia was very uncommon after radiotherapy, and only 5% of patients experienced grades I–II and no patients with grades III–IV. RTOG 0424 trial of temozolomide-based chemoradiation therapy for high-risk low-grade gliomas suggested a survival benefit compared to historical controls and was a phase II trial.
References: [25, 57, 60]

# References

1. Siegel RL, Miller KD, Jemal A. Cancer statistics, 2016. CA Cancer J Clin. 2016;66(1):7–30.
2. Ostrom QT, Gittleman H, Xu J, et al. CBTRUS statistical report: primary brain and other central nervous system tumors diagnosed in the United States in 2009–2013. Neuro-Oncology. 2016;18(Suppl_5):v1–v75.
3. Claus EB, Walsh KM, Wiencke JK, et al. Survival and low-grade glioma: the emergence of genetic information. Neurosurg Focus. 2015;38(1):E6.
4. Stockhammer F, Misch M, Helms HJ, et al. IDH1/2 mutations in WHO grade II astrocytomas associated with localization and seizure as the initial symptom. Seizure. 2012;21(3):194–7.
5. Avila EK, Chamberlain M, Schiff D, et al. Seizure control as a new metric in assessing efficacy of tumor treatment in low-grade glioma trials. Neuro Oncol. 2017;19(1):12–21.
6. Potts MB, Smith JS, Molinaro AM, et al. Natural history and surgical management of incidentally discovered low-grade gliomas. J Neurosurg. 2012;116(2):365–72.
7. Brown PD, Buckner JC, O'Fallon JR, et al. Importance of baseline mini-mental state examination as a prognostic factor for patients with low-grade glioma. Int J Radiat Oncol Biol Phys. 2004;59(1):117–25.
8. Brown PD, Chan MD, Shaw EG, et al. Chapter 26 - Low-grade gliomas. In: Gunderson L, Tepper JE, editors. Clinical radiation oncology. 4th ed. Philadelphia: Elsevier; 2016. p. 452–68.e3.
9. Zlatescu MC, TehraniYazdi A, Sasaki H, et al. Tumor location and growth pattern correlate with genetic signature in oligodendroglial neoplasms. Cancer Res. 2001;61(18):6713–5.
10. Lai A, Kharbanda S, Pope WB, et al. Evidence for sequenced molecular evolution of IDH1 mutant glioblastoma from a distinct cell of origin. J Clin Oncol. 2011;29(34):4482–90.
11. Saito T, Yamasaki F, Kajiwara Y, et al. Role of perfusion-weighted imaging at 3T in the histopathological differentiation between astrocytic and oligodendroglial tumors. Eur J Radiol. 2012;81(8):1863–9.
12. Olson JD, Riedel E, DeAngelis LM. Long-term outcome of low-grade oligodendroglioma and mixed glioma. Neurology. 2000;54(7):1442–8.
13. Jenkinson MD, du Plessis DG, Smith TS, et al. Histological growth patterns and genotype in oligodendroglial tumours: correlation with MRI features. Brain. 2006;129(Pt 7):1884–91.
14. Khalid L, Carone M, Dumrongpisutikul N, et al. Imaging characteristics of oligodendrogliomas that predict grade. AJNR Am J Neuroradiol. 2012;33(5):852–7.
15. Shaw E, Arusell R, Scheithauer B, et al. Prospective randomized trial of low- versus high-dose radiation therapy in adults with supratentorial low-grade glioma: initial report of a North Central Cancer Treatment Group/Radiation Therapy Oncology Group/Eastern Cooperative Oncology Group study. J Clin Oncol. 2002;20(9):2267–76.
16. Chaichana KL, McGirt MJ, Niranjan A, et al. Prognostic significance of contrast-enhancing low-grade gliomas in adults and a review of the literature. Neurol Res. 2009;31(9):931–9.
17. Choi C, Raisanen JM, Ganji SK, et al. Prospective longitudinal analysis of 2-hydroxyglutarate magnetic resonance spectroscopy identifies broad clinical utility for the management of patients with IDH-mutant glioma. J Clin Oncol. 2016;34(33):4030–9.
18. An Z, Ganji SK, Tiwari V, et al. Detection of 2-hydroxyglutarate in brain tumors by triple-refocusing MR spectroscopy at 3T in vivo. Magn Reson Med. 2017;78(1):40–8.
19. Bailey P, Cushing HW. A classification of the tumors of the glioma group on a histo-genetic basis with a correlated study of prognosis. Philadelphia: J.B. Lippincott; 1926.
20. Louis DN, Ohgaki H, Wiestler OD, et al. The 2007 WHO classification of tumours of the central nervous system. Acta Neuropathol. 2007;114(2):97–109.
21. Johannessen AL, Torp SH. The clinical value of Ki-67/MIB-1 labeling index in human astrocytomas. Pathol Oncol Res. 2006;12(3):143–7.
22. Kros JM, Hop WC, Godschalk JJ, et al. Prognostic value of the proliferation-related antigen Ki-67 in oligodendrogliomas. Cancer. 1996;78(5):1107–13.
23. Neder L, Colli BO, Machado HR, et al. MIB-1 labeling index in astrocytic tumors--a clinicopathologic study. Clin Neuropathol. 2004;23(6):262–70.
24. van den Bent MJ. Interobserver variation of the histopathological diagnosis in clinical trials on glioma: a clinician's perspective. Acta Neuropathol. 2010;120(3):297–304.
25. Buckner JC, Shaw EG, Pugh SL, et al. Radiation plus procarbazine, CCNU, and vincristine in low-grade glioma. N Engl J Med. 2016;374(14):1344–55.
26. Karim AB, Maat B, Hatlevoll R, et al. A randomized trial on dose-response in radiation therapy of low-grade cerebral glioma: European Organization for Research and Treatment of Cancer (EORTC) Study 22844. Int J Radiat Oncol Biol Phys. 1996;36(3):549–56.
27. van den Bent MJ, Afra D, de Witte O, et al. Long-term efficacy of early versus delayed radiotherapy for low-grade astrocytoma and oligodendroglioma in adults: the EORTC 22845 randomised trial. Lancet. 2005;366(9490):985–90.
28. Louis DN, Perry A, Reifenberger G, et al. The 2016 World Health Organization Classification of Tumors of the Central Nervous System: a summary. Acta Neuropathol. 2016;131(6):803–20.
29. Ducray F, Idbaih A, de Reyniès A, et al. Anaplastic oligodendrogliomas with 1p19q codeletion have a proneural gene expression profile. Mol Cancer. 2008;7:41.
30. Jenkins RB, Blair H, Ballman KV, et al. A t(1;19)(q10;p10) mediates the combined deletions of 1p and 19q and predicts a better prognosis of patients with oligodendroglioma. Cancer Res. 2006;66(20):9852–61.
31. Bettegowda C, Agrawal N, Jiao Y, et al. Mutations in CIC and FUBP1 contribute to human oligodendroglioma. Science. 2011;333(6048):1453–5.
32. Jiao Y, Killela PJ, Reitman ZJ, et al. Frequent ATRX, CIC, FUBP1 and IDH1 mutations refine the classification of malignant gliomas. Oncotarget. 2012;3(7):709–22.
33. Yip S, Butterfield YS, Morozova O, et al. Concurrent CIC mutations, IDH mutations, and 1p/19q loss distinguish oligodendrogliomas from other cancers. J Pathol. 2012;226(1):7–16.
34. Labussière M, Idbaih A, Wang XW, et al. All the 1p19q codeleted gliomas are mutated on IDH1 or IDH2. Neurology. 2010;74(23):1886–90.
35. Watanabe T, Nobusawa S, Kleihues P, et al. IDH1 mutations are early events in the development of astrocytomas and oligodendrogliomas. Am J Pathol. 2009;174(4):1149–53.
36. Sahm F, Reuss D, Koelsche C, et al. Farewell to oligoastrocytoma: in situ molecular genetics favor classification as either oligodendroglioma or astrocytoma. Acta Neuropathol. 2014;128(4):551–9.
37. Parsons DW, Jones S, Zhang X, et al. An integrated genomic analysis of human glioblastoma multiforme. Science. 2008;321(5897):1807–12.
38. Ichimura K, Pearson DM, Kocialkowski S, et al. IDH1 mutations are present in the majority of common adult gliomas but rare in primary glioblastomas. Neuro Oncol. 2009;11(4):341–7.
39. Mulholland S, Pearson DM, Hamoudi RA, et al. MGMT CpG island is invariably methylated in adult astrocytic and oligodendroglial tumors with IDH1 or IDH2 mutations. Int J Cancer. 2012;131(5):1104–13.
40. Abedalthagafi M, Phillips JJ, Kim GE, et al. The alternative lengthening of telomere phenotype is significantly associated with loss of ATRX expression in high-grade pediatric and adult astrocytomas: a multi-institutional study of 214 astrocytomas. Mod Pathol. 2013;26(11):1425–32.

41. Brat DJ, Verhaak RG, Aldape KD, et al. Comprehensive, integrative genomic analysis of diffuse lower-grade gliomas. N Engl J Med. 2015;372(26):2481–98.

42. van den Bent MJ, Dubbink HJ, Sanson M, et al. MGMT promoter methylation is prognostic but not predictive for outcome to adjuvant PCV chemotherapy in anaplastic oligodendroglial tumors: a report from EORTC Brain Tumor Group Study 26951. J Clin Oncol. 2009;27(35):5881–6.

43. Wick W, Meisner C, Hentschel B, et al. Prognostic or predictive value of MGMT promoter methylation in gliomas depends on IDH1 mutation. Neurology. 2013;81(17):1515–22.

44. Reitman ZJ, Pirozzi CJ, Yan H. Promoting a new brain tumor mutation: TERT promoter mutations in CNS tumors. Acta Neuropathol. 2013;126(6):789–92.

45. Eckel-Passow JE, Lachance DH, Molinaro AM, et al. Glioma groups based on 1p/19q, IDH, and TERT promoter mutations in tumors. N Engl J Med. 2015;372(26):2499–508.

46. Pignatti F, van den Bent M, Curran D, et al. Prognostic factors for survival in adult patients with cerebral low-grade glioma. J Clin Oncol. 2002;20(8):2076–84.

47. van den Bent MJ, Dubbink HJ, Marie Y, et al. IDH1 and IDH2 mutations are prognostic but not predictive for outcome in anaplastic oligodendroglial tumors: a report of the European Organization for Research and Treatment of Cancer Brain Tumor Group. Clin Cancer Res. 2010;16(5):1597–604.

48. Shaw EG. The low-grade glioma debate: evidence defending the position of early radiation therapy. Clin Neurosurg. 1995;42:488–94.

49. Jakola AS, Myrmel KS, Kloster R, et al. Comparison of a strategy favoring early surgical resection vs a strategy favoring watchful waiting in low-grade gliomas. JAMA. 2012;308(18):1881–8.

50. Pallud J, Capelle L, Taillandier L, et al. Prognostic significance of imaging contrast enhancement for WHO grade II gliomas. Neuro Oncol. 2009;11(2):176–82.

51. Smith JS, Chang EF, Lamborn KR, et al. Role of extent of resection in the long-term outcome of low-grade hemispheric gliomas. J Clin Oncol. 2008;26(8):1338–45.

52. Schomas DA, Laack NN, Rao RD, et al. Intracranial low-grade gliomas in adults: 30-year experience with long-term follow-up at Mayo Clinic. Neuro Oncol. 2009;11(4):437–45.

53. Shaw EG, Berkey B, Coons SW, et al. Recurrence following neurosurgeon-determined gross-total resection of adult supratentorial low-grade glioma: results of a prospective clinical trial. J Neurosurg. 2008;109(5):835–41.

54. Aghi MK, Nahed BV, Sloan AE, et al. The role of surgery in the management of patients with diffuse low grade glioma: a systematic review and evidence-based clinical practice guideline. J Neurooncol. 2015;125(3):503–30.

55. Rogers LR, Morris HH, Lupica K. Effect of cranial irradiation on seizure frequency in adults with low-grade astrocytoma and medically intractable epilepsy. Neurology. 1993;43(8):1599–601.

56. Rudà R, Bello L, Duffau H, et al. Seizures in low-grade gliomas: natural history, pathogenesis, and outcome after treatments. Neuro Oncol. 2012;14(Suppl 4):iv55–64.

57. Baumert BG, Hegi ME, van den Bent MJ, et al. Temozolomide chemotherapy versus radiotherapy in high-risk low-grade glioma (EORTC 22033-26033): a randomised, open-label, phase 3 intergroup study. Lancet Oncol. 2016;17(11):1521–32.

58. Reijneveld JC, Taphoorn MJ, Coens C, et al. Health-related quality of life in patients with high-risk low-grade glioma (EORTC 22033-26033): a randomised, open-label, phase 3 intergroup study. Lancet Oncol. 2016;17(11):1533–42.

59. Stupp R, Mason WP, van den Bent MJ, et al. Radiotherapy plus concomitant and adjuvant temozolomide for glioblastoma. N Engl J Med. 2005;352(10):987–96.

60. Fisher BJ, Hu C, Macdonald DR, et al. Phase 2 study of temozolomide-based chemoradiation therapy for high-risk low-grade gliomas: preliminary results of Radiation Therapy Oncology Group 0424. Int J Radiat Oncol Biol Phys. 2015;91(3):497–504.

61. Fisher BJ, Hu C, Macdonald DR, et al. Phase III trial of chemoradiotherapy for anaplastic oligodendroglioma: long-term results of RTOG 9402. J Clin Oncol. 2013;31(3):337–43.

62. van den Bent MJ, Brandes AA, Taphoorn MJ, et al. Adjuvant procarbazine, lomustine, and vincristine chemotherapy in newly diagnosed anaplastic oligodendroglioma: long-term follow-up of EORTC brain tumor group study 26951. J Clin Oncol. 2013;31(3):344–50.

63. Jaeckle K, Vogelbaum M, Ballman K, et al. CODEL (Alliance-N0577; EORTC-26081/22086; NRG-1071; NCIC-CEC-2): phase III randomized study of RT vs. RT+TMZ vs. TMZ for newly diagnosed 1p/19q-codeleted anaplastic oligodendroglial tumors. Analysis of patients treated on the original protocol design in American Academy of Neurology PL02.005. Neurology. 2016;86 Suppl 16:Abstract PL02.005.

64. Jaeckle K, et al. N0577 (CODEL) clinical trial protocol: phase III intergroup study of radiotherapy with concomitant and adjuvant temozolomide versus radiotherapy with adjuvant PCV chemotherapy in patients with 1p/19q co-deleted anaplastic glioma or low grade glioma. 2017 [3/12/2017]. Available from: https://clinicaltrials.gov/ct2/show/NCT00887146.

65. NCCN. NCCN clinical practice guidelines in oncology central nervous system cancers. 2017. Available from: https://www.nccn.org/professionals/physician_gls/pdf/cns.pdf.

66. Batth SS, Sreeraman R, Dienes E, et al. Clinical-dosimetric relationship between lacrimal gland dose and ocular toxicity after intensity-modulated radiotherapy for sinonasal tumours. Br J Radiol. 2013;86(1032):20130459.

67. Reijneveld JC, Sitskoorn MM, Klein M, et al. Cognitive status and quality of life in patients with suspected versus proven low-grade gliomas. Neurology. 2001;56(5):618–23.

68. Armstrong CL, Hunter JV, Ledakis GE, et al. Late cognitive and radiographic changes related to radiotherapy: initial prospective findings. Neurology. 2002;59(1):40–8.

69. Laack NN, Brown PD, Ivnik RJ, et al. Cognitive function after radiotherapy for supratentorial low-grade glioma: a North Central Cancer Treatment Group prospective study. Int J Radiat Oncol Biol Phys. 2005;63(4):1175–83.

70. Lawrence YR, Li XA, el Naqa I, et al. Radiation dose-volume effects in the brain. Int J Radiat Oncol Biol Phys. 2010;76(3 Suppl):S20–7.

71. Shih HA, Sherman JC, Nachtigall LB, et al. Proton therapy for low-grade gliomas: results from a prospective trial. Cancer. 2015;121(10):1712–9.

72. Salomon F, Cuneo RC, Hesp R, et al. The effects of treatment with recombinant human growth hormone on body composition and metabolism in adults with growth hormone deficiency. N Engl J Med. 1989;321(26):1797–803.

73. Carroll PV, Christ ER, Bengtsson BA, et al. Growth hormone deficiency in adulthood and the effects of growth hormone replacement: a review. Growth Hormone Research Society Scientific Committee. J Clin Endocrinol Metab. 1998;83(2):382–95.

74. Soffietti R, Baumert BG, Bello L, et al. Guidelines on management of low-grade gliomas: report of an EFNS-EANO Task Force. Eur J Neurol. 2010;17(9):1124–33.

75. Fogh SE, Andrews DW, Glass J, et al. Hypofractionated stereotactic radiation therapy: an effective therapy for recurrent high-grade gliomas. J Clin Oncol. 2010;28(18):3048–53.

# High-Grade Gliomas

**6**

Gregory Vlacich and Christina I. Tsien

## Learning Objectives

- Understand the natural history and prognostic factors associated with high-grade gliomas and the emerging role of molecular markers in identifying and refining subgroups within this population.
- Understand the current treatment paradigm for high-grade gliomas and how treatment is being tailored to subpopulations based on clinical (e.g., elderly) and/or molecular factors (e.g., 1p/19q co-deletion).
- Understand the radiation treatment approaches for high-grade glioma and when and how each is implemented.
- Understand patterns of failure in high-grade glioma and treatment approaches for recurrent disease.

## Diagnosis and Prognosis

High-grade gliomas are the most common malignant tumors arising in the central nervous system (CNS), comprising approximately 40% of all primary brain tumors [1]. Based on the World Health Organization (WHO) classification system, they include WHO grade III tumors such as anaplastic oligodendroglioma and anaplastic astrocytoma and WHO grade IV tumors such as glioblastoma multiforme (GBM) and diffuse midline glioma [2]. The incidence of high-grade gliomas in adults in North America is about 5 per 100,000 per year, accounting for approximately 2% of all adult tumors [3]. Nearly 80% of these cases are GBMs. The incidence increases with age, and the median age at presentation is about 45 years for grade III tumors and 60 years for grade

G. Vlacich • C. I. Tsien (✉)
Department of Radiation Oncology, Washington University School of Medicine, St. Louis, MO, USA
e-mail: ctsien@wustl.edu

IV tumors [3]. Men are more commonly affected than women with a 1.6:1 ratio, and the incidence is also much higher among Caucasians compared to Asians/Pacific Islanders and other races [4]. The etiologic factors for high-grade gliomas are largely unknown. The vast majority of these tumors are sporadic and likely result from a complex mix of genetic and environmental influences. High-grade gliomas may arise either de novo or may progress from low-grade gliomas. The latter are termed secondary gliomas and are more common in younger patients and generally carry a more favorable prognosis [5].

The most common presenting symptom is headache (50%) [6]. This symptom is the result of increased intracranial pressure (ICP) due to vasogenic edema. Headaches are often worse in the morning due to further increased ICP with prolonged recumbency from sleep and may be accompanied by nausea, vomiting, or changes in vision. Seizures are present in 30% of patients, and a lesser number experience focal neurologic dysfunction or mental status changes depending on the precise location of the tumor [6]. Elderly patients are more likely to present with neurocognitive decline and memory impairment secondary to involvement of the frontotemporal lobe. Anticonvulsants should only be used if there is a clear history of seizures [7]. Dexamethasone can be given before and after surgery as clinically indicated, but should be tapered gradually and maintained at the lowest dose possible [7].

After initial presentation, a clinical diagnosis is often first made radiographically. On computed tomography (CT) scans, high-grade gliomas typically appear as a hypodensity on non-contrasted imaging and mixed hyper- and hypodensities following contrast administration. Magnetic resonance (MR) imaging is strongly preferred for better tumor characterization. On T1-weighted MRI, high-grade gliomas appear hypodense relative to the surrounding parenchyma and show a heterogeneous enhancement after gadolinium

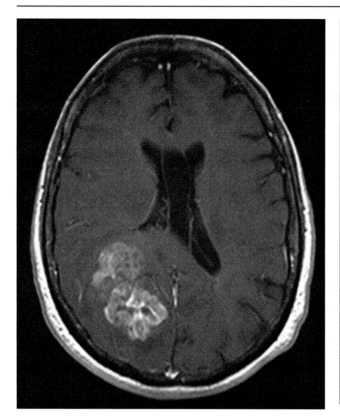

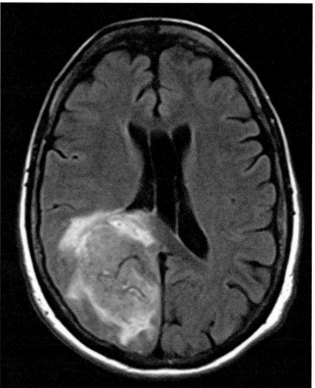

**Fig. 6.1** Post-gadolinium MRI T1 sequence demonstrating heterogeneous enhancement of a right parietal glioblastoma multiforme

**Fig. 6.2** MRI FLAIR sequence, axial slice, demonstrating a right parietal glioblastoma multiforme with associated vasogenic edema and mass effect on the right lateral ventricle

administration (see Fig. 6.1). These masses have the propensity to cross midline and may appear in a "butterfly pattern." T2 or FLAIR MRI sequences will frequently reveal substantial peritumoral edema (see Fig. 6.2). These imaging findings can mimic those of brain metastases; therefore, if there is suspicion for an occult extracranial malignancy, systemic imaging should also be performed.

Pathologically, gliomas have classically been diagnosed by their clinical and histologic characteristics. High-grade gliomas are considered infiltrating tumors. The majority is described as "diffuse" and generally invades the parenchyma of the cerebral hemispheres. These tumors commonly track along the white matter but may also occur primarily in the gray matter and even spread to other parts of the central nervous system [8]. Apart from infiltration, another frequent pathologic feature of high-grade gliomas is their high mitotic activity as well as microvascular proliferation. Grade IV tumors additionally exhibit necrosis [2].

Astrocytic tumors, which include anaplastic astrocytomas and GBMs, are composed of cells with elongated or irregular hyperchromatic nuclei. They stain positive for glial fibrillary acidic protein (GFAP). Oligodendrogliomas have round nuclei with perinuclear halos, often described as a "fried-egg" appearance. They often display calcifications and branching "chicken-

wire" blood vessels. High-grade gliomas are thought to arise from neural progenitor cells and contain multipotent tumor stem cells that are responsible for populating and repopulating the tumors [9].

Despite being the subject of numerous clinical trials over the last several decades, the prognosis for patients with high-grade glioma remains poor with a median survival of 3 years for anaplastic astrocytomas and only 16 months for GBM [1]. Historically, clinical prognostic factors included patient age, histology, Karnofsky performance status (KPS), and the duration of symptoms [7, 10]. Their prognostic significance was highlighted in the RTOG RPA classification system, developed to predict survival for patients with high-grade gliomas, and this is summarized in Table 6.1. As would be expected, patients who are younger, with a higher performance status, and less aggressive histology have an improved survival.

Extent of surgical resection has been identified as a prognostic factor for high-grade glioma. Previous studies have demonstrated that a greater extent of surgery as defined by the percentage of enhancing tumor resected on post-gadolinium T1 imaging is associated with improved outcomes. Recent modeling data indicates that a maximum safe resection is preferred with the survival benefit estimated for the specific extent of resection and not with an arbitrary threshold [10].

**Table 6.1**  RTOG RPA classes for high-grade glioma

| I and II | Anaplastic astrocytoma, age ≤50, normal MS, OR age >50, KPS >70, symptoms >3 months | MS 40–60 months |
|---|---|---|
| III and IV | Anaplastic astrocytoma, age ≤50, abnormal MS, OR age >50, symptoms <3 months, GBM, age <50, OR age >50 and KPS ≥70 | MS 11–18 months |
| V and VI | GBM, age >50, and KPS ≥70, OR abnormal MS | MS 5–9 months |

Increasingly, molecular markers have become important adjuncts to clinical determinants of prognosis for high-grade glioma and are continuing to play a larger role as our knowledge of established markers expands and new markers are identified. Current clinical trials are often stratifying patients based on these markers as well. One of the more established prognostic molecular markers is methyl-guanine methyltransferase (MGMT) promoter methylation status. MGMT is a DNA repair enzyme that removes alkyl groups from the O6 position of guanine, and when its promoter is methylated, this leads to epigenetic silencing of the gene and loss of expression. The presence of methylation and subsequent reduced expression of MGMT improves the effectiveness of alkylating agents such as temozolomide (TMZ) as well as an associated improvement in median survival [11–13].

Another important prognostic molecular marker includes the mutational status of isocitrate dehydrogenase 1 and 2 (IDH1 and IDH2). Several large prospective studies have shown that patients with IDH mutated gliomas are associated with a significantly prolonged progression-free survival (PFS) and overall survival (OS) compared to wild-type tumors [14]. These mutations are thought to be associated with younger patients with secondary GBM that progressed from lower-grade lesions. In anaplastic oligodendroglial tumors specifically, 1p/19q chromosomal co-deletion is an important prognostic factor. Specifically, the presence of 1p19q co-deletion confers a favorable prognosis and is predictive of a favorable response to the addition of alkylating agents to radiation therapy [15, 16].

## World Health Organization Pathologic Criteria 2016 Edition

Classically, gliomas have been categorized by their clinical and histologic characteristics alone. With the most recent World Health Organization (WHO) 2016 classification [17], molecular signatures have been integrated into the classification system. Genetic signatures have not replaced histologic evaluation, which is still the determinant of grade, but highlight the increasingly important role of the molecular phenotype in high-grade gliomas. Specifically, the mutational status of IDH plays a prominent role in the new classification

system. Diffuse gliomas include WHO grade II and III astrocytomas, grade II and III oligodendrogliomas, and grade IV GBM. For WHO grade III anaplastic astrocytomas, the mutational status of IDH (i.e., wild type, mutant, or NOS if unable to be determined) has been added to the classification. A determination of an IDH-wild-type grade III anaplastic astrocytoma should be interpreted with caution given the rarity of this genotype/phenotype combination and may be more consistent with an IDH-wild-type GBM [18]. Anaplastic oligodendrogliomas in the new classification system are evaluated for both IDH mutational status (wild type, mutant, NOS) and 1p/19q co-deletional status (co-deleted or not). The new classification also strongly discourages the diagnosis of oligoastrocytoma suggesting that classification as one or the other can be achieved with genetic testing in most circumstances [17]. For grade IV GBM, IDH mutational status (wild type, mutant, NOS) has been added to the classification.

## Overall Treatment Strategy

Although our understanding of high-grade gliomas continues to evolve, management of these patients has been relatively consistent and involves a combined modality treatment approach incorporating surgery and adjuvant chemoradiation as the standard of care.

## Surgery

Surgery has several major roles in the treatment of this disease. First, a tissue diagnosis is generally needed to confirm the diagnosis prior to treatment. This can be obtained at the time of a more extensive gross total resection or via a stereotactic biopsy in the case of a lesion that is not amenable to resection or for patients too debilitated for a more extensive surgery. Stereotactic image-guided biopsy with either CT or MRI has developed into an accurate and relatively safe procedure [19]. Recently, PET and magnetic resonance spectroscopy (MRS) have also been increasingly utilized to improve localization and diagnostic yield [20, 21].

Second, surgical resection of a tumor can offer substantial palliative benefit. Surgery can reduce the mass effect associated with the tumor and improve symptoms with a rapidity that other treatments cannot match. Surgery is considered for any cases of life-threatening elevated intracranial pressure or for severe symptoms including midline shift related to mass effect.

Finally, the extent of surgical resection has been associated with improved outcomes in patients with high-grade glioma. Several retrospective reviews have demonstrated improved overall survival for patients undergoing surgical resection of their tumor compared to a biopsy and longer survival with more complete resections [22, 23].

To aid in the resection of these lesions, preoperative MRI is an essential component of the initial workup. Additional studies have been performed to understand the role of PET imaging in the surgical management of high-grade gliomas [24]. Preoperative tumor mapping using both functional MRI (fMRI) to map out the location of tumors with respect to both "eloquent" cortical regions, motor and language strips, and other areas of critical functionality and diffusion tractography has become an essential workup in the surgical management of these patients [25].

Intraoperative CT and MRI have also been developed to provide intraoperative guidance and increase the rates of complete resection. In addition, awake craniotomies with intraoperative cortical stimulation and repetitive neurologic assessments can also be performed in cases where the patient is at high risk for postoperative neurologic impairment [26, 27]. Attention has also been directed toward using enhanced endogenous fluorescence in malignant glioma cells to improve the likelihood of a gross total resection. Elevated levels of the naturally occurring amino acid precursor 5-ALA and upregulation of the heme biosynthesis pathway in malignant glioma cells lead to an enhanced production of fluorescent porphyrins. Therefore, fluorescence-guided surgery using 5-ALA allows for better illumination of these tumors intraoperatively. This has been shown to significantly improve the extent of a gross total resection as determined by postoperative contrast-enhanced MRI [28]. However, despite these efforts, local recurrence is exceedingly common even in cases of apparently complete resection.

## Radiation

Because of the infiltrative nature of high-grade gliomas, adjuvant radiation therapy (RT) is indicated after surgery regardless of the extent of resection. Adjuvant RT has been shown to improve both local control and overall survival. This was initially demonstrated with whole brain radiation (WBRT) in several randomized controlled trials in the 1970s [29, 30]. Over the last few decades, more conformal techniques such as three-dimensional conformal RT and intensity-modulated RT (IMRT) partial brain irradiation have now become the standard of care.

Sufficient radiation doses are required to maximize the survival benefit as demonstrated by the Brain Tumor Study Group. A retrospective review of 91 patients with high-grade gliomas who had a stereotactic biopsy followed by RT showed that patients who had RT doses of 50–60 Gy had a longer median survival than those who received lower postoperative doses (19 vs 11 weeks for patients with GBM and 27 vs 11 weeks for anaplastic astrocytoma) [31]. However,

radiation dose escalation alone above 60 Gy has not been shown to be beneficial with trials using modern, 3D-conformal techniques with no additional benefit to doses of 70, 80, or 90 Gy in 2 Gy fractions [32]. Concurrent temozolomide and dose-escalated intensity-modulated radiation therapy of 75 Gy in 30 fractions has been shown to be safe [33]. Currently, the large phase II multi-institutional randomized study NRG Oncology BN001 (NCT02179086) is being completed to determine if this regimen has improved efficacy.

Additionally, radiation treatment volumes have changed significantly over time. Whereas whole brain radiotherapy had initially been the standard of care, studies have since demonstrated that most recurrent disease occurred within 2–3 cm of the initial margin of gross disease, and treating these smaller volumes results in equivalent survival compared to the treatment of the whole brain.

## Chemotherapy

Chemotherapy has also been shown to provide a survival benefit in patients with high-grade gliomas. This was initially demonstrated with the use of nitrosoureas such as carmustine. Meta-analyses demonstrated that this agent, in conjunction with RT, improved PFS as well as OS. Therefore, it remained the standard of care until the more recent trials have established the effectiveness of temozolomide.

Temozolomide (TMZ), an oral alkylating agent, is now the preferred chemotherapeutic agent in patients with high-grade gliomas. Stupp et al.'s landmark phase III trial of 573 patients with GBM demonstrated the benefits of concurrent and adjuvant temozolomide [12]. Patients were randomly assigned to receive either postoperative involved field RT (IFRT) with 60 Gy in 30 fractions or 60 Gy IFRT with concomitant temozolomide (75 mg/m$^2$ daily up to 49 days) followed by six cycles of high-dose adjuvant temozolomide (150–200 mg/m$^2$ for 5 days, every 28 days). At a median follow-up of over 5 years, the study found that the combination of temozolomide plus RT was associated with a statistically significant prolongation of survival (27% vs 11% at 1 year and 10% vs 2% at 5 years). Subsequent analyses showed that methylation of the MGMT promoter region was a major prognostic factor for improved survival and was predictive of benefit from chemotherapy. Specifically, patients with MGMT methylation experienced 2-year survival rates of 49% with combination therapy versus 24% with RT alone. The percentages for unmethylated patients were only 15% and 2%, respectively [34]. More recently, the Radiation Therapy Oncology Group (RTOG) 0525 trial compared different treatment schedules of temozolomide but found no statistically significant difference in either overall or progression-free survival. This prospective study did, however, confirm the importance of MGMT methylation as an important prognostic factor [35]. Given the evidence that MGMT promoter methylation is associated with improved survival, inhibitors of the MGMT enzyme, such as O6-benzylguanine (O6-B6), are being evaluated as a way to restore sensitivity to alkylating agents in patients who have previously progressed on therapy [36, 37].

Bevacizumab, a vascular endothelial growth factor inhibitor, has also been used in the treatment of GBM. In a multicenter phase II study of patients newly diagnosed with GBM, 70 patients were treated with bevacizumab (10 mg/kg every 2 weeks) in combination with a standard regimen of TMZ plus RT [38]. The median overall and progression-free survival was 19.6 and 13.6 months, respectively. The addition of bevacizumab to standard adjuvant therapy was then tested in the phase III RTOG 0825 study, which evaluated approximately 978 patients with GBMs. All patients received adjuvant radiation therapy and TMZ and were subsequently randomized to receive concurrent bevacizumab versus placebo. Preliminary results show no benefit to OS or PFS but did show that the treatment arm had worse neurocognitive symptoms and quality of life scores. These results have since discouraged the routine use of bevacizumab in the upfront setting.

Additional studies regarding the role of adjuvant chemotherapy in anaplastic astrocytomas have been reported. A phase III randomized trial comparing RT and temozolomide versus RT and nitrosourea in patients with anaplastic astrocytoma did not appear to show a significant improvement in overall survival or time to tumor progression. However, the RT and TMZ regimen was much better tolerated. The study also confirmed that the IDH1-R132H mutation is an important prognostic factor for overall survival [39]. Retrospective analyses of patients with anaplastic astrocytomas showed that adjuvant temozolomide was as effective and less toxic than using the PCV (procarbazine, lomustine, and vincristine) regimen [40]; therefore, European Organisation for Research and Treatment of Cancer (EORTC) trial 26053 (NCT00626990) is investigating the role of concurrent and adjuvant temozolomide in patients with anaplastic gliomas.

This prospective trial is a 2 × 2 randomization and investigated the role of adjuvant temozolomide following RT versus RT alone in anaplastic gliomas without 1p/19q co-deletion [41]. The four arms of the study include radiotherapy alone, radiotherapy plus 12 months of adjuvant TMZ, radiotherapy plus concurrent TMZ, or radiotherapy plus concurrent TMZ plus 12 months of adjuvant TMZ. Initial results showed an overall survival benefit with the addition of 12 cycles of adjuvant temozolomide following RT compared to RT alone. Further follow-up is required to determine the additional role of concurrent temozolomide. Correlative molecular analyses are ongoing.

EORTC 26951 investigated the role of radiation alone versus radiotherapy followed by adjuvant PCV in anaplastic oligodendroglial tumors. Long-term follow-up demonstrated that the addition of six cycles of PCV following RT (59.4 Gy) increased both PFS and OS [42]. This study demonstrated 1p/19q co-deletion as an important molecular biomarker predictive of treatment response. Anaplastic oligodendroglial tumors with 1p/19q co-deletion derived a greater benefit from adjuvant PCV compared with non-1p/19q-deleted tumors [42]. RTOG 9402 similarly examined the role of PCV, this time followed by radiation (59.4 Gy), versus radiation alone in anaplastic oligodendrogliomas or oligoastrocytomas, and confirmed the clinical significance of 1p/19q co-deletion. Specifically, patients with 1p/19q co-deletion demonstrated significantly improved survival in both arms compared to non-co-deleted patients, and the addition of PCV in the 1p/19q co-deletion patients improved survival by approximately 7 years compared to radiation alone [15]. As with astrocytomas, the possibility of substituting PCV for the generally less toxic TMZ and adding it concurrently with radiation was evaluated for oligodendroglial tumors in RTOG BR0131 [43]. Dose-intense temozolomide was given before chemoradiation therapy, and the pre-RT rate of progression was acceptable (10% vs 20% with PCV as reported in RTOG 9402) but was associated with unexpectedly high-grade III–IV toxicity.

Additional evidence supporting the use of TMZ compared to the PCV regimen is based on a phase III trial of 447 patients with high-grade gliomas at first recurrence following initial treatment with RT alone. There was no statistically significant difference in either progression-free survival or overall survival with the use of TMZ [44]. Patients on TMZ were assigned to either 200 mg/m$^2$ for 5 days or 100 mg/m$^2$ for 21 days, each repeated every 4 weeks for 9 months. Patients on the 5-day regimen had a significantly longer median progression-free and overall survival compared to those on the 21-day regimen [44]. However, whether the results are applicable to newly diagnosed anaplastic gliomas is yet to be determined.

## Treatment of Elderly Patients

Special attention has been given to identifying the optimal therapy in the elderly given their especially poor prognosis and often limited functional status. From a radiation therapy standpoint, the approach in the elderly has been to reduce treatment time while attempting to maintain treatment efficacy. To this effect, Roa et al. randomized 100 patients 60 years or older with a poor performance status (KPS <70) to 60 Gy given over 6 weeks versus 40 Gy given over 3 weeks and found no difference in survival between these two regimens [45]. In addition, patients in the shorter course arm required steroids less often. Subsequent studies in elderly patients have affirmed this finding with dose-fractionation regimens of 40 Gy in 15 fractions, 30 Gy in 10 fractions, and 34 Gy in 10 fractions, all showing non-inferiority compared to the standard 60 Gy regimen. Interestingly, more recent data from Roa et al. suggest that an even more hypofractionated regimen of 25 Gy in 5 fractions may be no less inferior to the previously mentioned hypofractionated regimen (40 Gy in 15 fractions) in a particular poor prognosis subgroup of patients (median survival 7.9 months and 6.4 months, respectively) [46].

More recently, the NOA-08 randomized trial studied 373 high-grade glioma patients >65 years of age with a KPS of at least 60 and compared radiotherapy alone with 60 Gy versus dose-intensive temozolomide therapy (100 mg/m² temozolomide given on days 1–7 with a 1-week-on followed by 1-week-off cycle). This trial found that overall survival was nearly equivalent (8.6 months versus 9.6 months, respectively) between the two arms [47]. Of note, in the elderly patient population, MGMT methylation appears to be an important biomarker of improved survival with TMZ. MGMT-methylated patients showed an improved survival with TMZ only, while non-MGMT methylated patients showed an improved survival with RT. This finding suggests that temozolomide alone may be an option in elderly and frail patients with MGMT methylated tumors who may not tolerate concurrent chemoradiation or for whom daily radiation treatments are not feasible. Unfortunately, neither the Roa et al. study nor the NOA-08 study included an arm with combination chemoradiation. However, recent data from the EORTC 26062-22061/NCIC CTG CE.6 phase III randomized trial comparing hypofractionated RT with concurrent and adjuvant temozolomide to hypofractionated RT regimen alone in elderly patients showed an improvement in OS and PFS with the addition of concurrent and adjuvant temozolomide [48]. The largest benefit was noted in patients with MGMT promoter methylation. Ultimately, quality of life remains an important consideration in the optimal management of this patient population.

## Indications for Irradiation

Radiation therapy, unless performance status precludes treatment, is almost uniformly indicated after maximal safe resection in the treatment of high-grade gliomas to improve local control and survival. For anaplastic astrocytoma and oligodendroglioma, conventional fractionation is delivered either sequentially with PCV or concurrently with temozolomide. For GBM, most patients also receive conventionally fractionated radiation therapy with concurrent temozolomide. Hypofractionated radiation can be considered for elderly patients (>70 years old) with GBM or with any high-

grade glioma patient who has a poor performance status but can tolerate a short course of therapy. In the setting of local recurrence, re-irradiation can be considered to help improve local control with variable reported effects on progression-free and overall survival. Radiation therapy techniques employed are generally guided by the intent of treatment and proximity of the treatment volume to critical normal structures. These include 3D conformal radiation therapy, intensity-modulated radiation therapy (IMRT), stereotactic radiosurgery (SRS), and brachytherapy and will be described in more detail below.

## Target Volume Delineation

Generally speaking, radiation therapy targets for high-grade glioma are similar to most radiation treatments and are generated from (smallest to largest) a gross tumor volume (GTV), clinical target value (CTV), and planning target volume (PTV). The GTV encompasses any gross tumor remaining after maximal safe resection as well as the surgical cavity as determined by postoperative imaging. The CTV is an expansion on the GTV to account for subclinical disease, and this is then expanded to a PTV to account for setup error. The GTV volume is generally consistent regardless of mode and intent of radiation therapy, while there can be more variability in CTV and PTV delineation.

For conventionally fractionated radiation for grade III and IV tumors, the GTV specifically consists of the T1 contrast-enhancing volume on postoperative MRI and the surgical cavity. A low- and high-dose CTV are then generated. The low-dose CTV is first generated by including the GTV as well as any additional hyperintense volume on T2 or FLAIR sequences on postoperative MRI in a preliminary structure. An expansion of 2 cm on this preliminary volume then accounts for the final low-dose CTV. In this expansion, the final volume should be reduced around natural barriers to tumor spread including the ventricles and falx. The high-dose CTV is a 2.0 expansion (accounting for natural barriers) on the GTV alone for GBM with a smaller expansion (1 cm) considered for grade III tumors. In both cases, this expansion is intended to account for the infiltrative nature of high-grade gliomas and the extent of pathologic spread based on postmortem studies [49]. If there is no surrounding edema on imaging as seen on T2 or FLAIR, then generally a high-dose CTV is sufficient or a 2.5 cm expansion on the GTV can be used instead for the low-dose CTV. PTV expansion is generally 0.3–0.5 cm in all directions to account for daily setup errors and is individualized based on numerous factors effecting setup reproducibility (e.g., image guidance). Typical expansions for GBM are illustrated in Fig. 6.3.

For hypofractionated radiation, a low-dose CTV is not employed. Instead, a single CTV with a 1.5–2.0 cm expansion

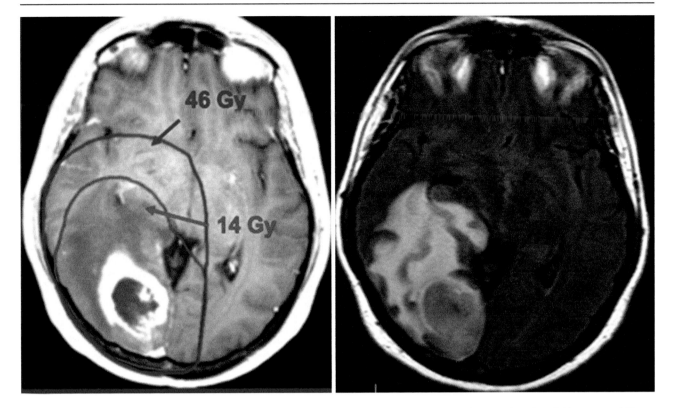

**Fig. 6.3** Target delineation for conventional fractionated radiation for GBM. Postoperative targets after resection of a glioblastoma multiforme are shown with PTV1 in blue and PTV2 in red. The PTV1 is the initial plan to 46 Gy and the PTV2 is the 14 Gy boost to a total of 60 Gy

(accounting for anatomic boundaries) on the GTV is utilized. PTV expansion again is generally 0.3–0.5 cm.

Target delineation for SRS cases is more simplified and is generally similar to that for brain metastases, namely, gross disease as determined by contrast enhancement on T1-weighted images and the surgical cavity (if applicable) with no additional expansion.

## Radiation Dose Prescription and Organ at Risk Tolerances

### Conventional and Hypofractionated Radiation

For conventionally fractionated treatment of GBM, the total dose of 60 Gy in 2 Gy fractions is divided into an initial dose of 46 Gy given to the low-dose PTV followed by a boost of 14 Gy to the high-dose PTV (as both described above). RTOG guidelines recommend MRI fusion for appropriate target delineation. Radiation therapy typically begins within 4–6 weeks after surgery assuming the incision is adequately healed.

Anaplastic oligodendroglial tumors are conventionally treated to a similar dose. Given the improved prognosis in these patients, radiation treatments are generally administered in a lower dose per fraction (1.8 Gy/fraction versus 2.0 Gy/fraction) to theoretically decrease the risk of late side effects. Accordingly, as per the most recent RTOG and EORTC trials, these gliomas are treated to 50.4 Gy in 1.8 Gy fractions for 28 fractions followed by an five-fraction boost of 1.8 Gy/fraction to a total of 59.4 Gy.

Hypofractionated radiation dose and fractionations are varied and include 40 Gy in 15 fractions, 30 Gy in 10 fractions, 34 Gy in 10 fractions, and 25 Gy in 5 fractions [45–48]. If concurrent chemotherapy with temozolomide is anticipated, the 40 Gy in 15 fraction regimen is indicated [48].

For conventionally fractionated treatments, the goal for PTV coverage (initial volume and boost) is ≥95% receiving 100% of the prescribed dose and a maximum point dose (0.03 cc) ≤110%. For normal structures, constraints are generally characterized by maximum point doses as follows: optic nerve, ≤54 Gy; optic chiasm, ≤54 Gy; brainstem, ≤60 Gy; spinal cord, ≤45–50 Gy; lens, ≤7 Gy; and retina, ≤45 Gy. For the optic nerves and chiasm, constraints are typically applied to a planning risk volume (PRV), which is a 3 mm expansion on the anatomic structures. The lacrimal gland dose may also be considered in treatment planning. A specific constraint has not been well established, but keeping maximum dose to 36–40 Gy or less appears to lower the risk of severe dry eye [50]. When PTV volumes extend into critical structures, coverage goals may need to be modified to respect normal tissue constraints. To ensure/confirm acceptable PTV coverage away from these critical structures, one option is to generate a sub-PTV volume that encompasses the PTV outside of the normal structures to ensure that this area is adequately covered by the prescription dose.

For hypofractionated treatment to 40 Gy as used in elderly patients, dose constraints have not been uniformly established, but the prospective trials aimed to keep dose to any organ at risk (e.g., brainstem, optic nerve, optic chiasm) to ≤40 Gy and dose to the lens <4 Gy. Additional planning goals included keeping the PTV hotspot and hotspot to any normal tissue ≤105% [48].

## Stereotactic Radiation Therapy

Stereotactic radiosurgery (SRS) uses 3D planning techniques to precisely deliver narrow collimated beams of radiation in a single high dose fraction to small targets. By using a large number of beams (typically 9–12 beams) that converge on a single target, a steep dose gradient can be achieved around the PTV with a high central, ablative dose. Stereotactic radiotherapy uses the same techniques to deliver hypofractionated radiation therapy in a small number of large doses (commonly 3–5 fractions delivered over 1–2 weeks). Several single institution series have reported a survival benefit with the addition of a radiosurgical boost after fractionated radiation therapy in newly diagnosed GBM [51]. However, RTOG 93-05, which was a randomized trial of 203 patients that employed a radiosurgery boost prior to fractionated RT with concurrent carmustine, did not confirm this survival benefit [52]. Currently, stereotactic treatments are used primarily for recurrent disease in previously treated patients with promising single institution reports supporting its safety and efficacy [53].

Stereotactic radiosurgery doses when delivered as a boost are prescribed based on size. Specifically, tumors up to 2 cm are treated with a single fraction of 24 Gy, between 2 and 3 cm to 18 Gy, and between 3 and 4 cm to 15 Gy to the 50–90% isodose surface [52]. This is similar to the dose prescription for brain metastases per RTOG 90-05 [54]. Per RTOG guidelines, maximum point dose to the optic nerves, optic chiasm, and brainstem should not exceed 8 Gy, and dose to the motor strip should not exceed 15 Gy. SRS in the retreatment setting is more variable and has been delivered as a single fraction or fractionated in published studies [55–57]. As a consequence, prescription dose and normal tissue constraints in the retreatment setting are less standardized. In 2005, ASTRO published an evidence-based review on the role of SRS in high-grade gliomas in the boost and retreatment setting. Consensus option was that a boost delivered before external beam radiation therapy in the manner delivered in RTOG 93-05 showed no survival, local control, or quality of life benefit but that further study into alternative boost approaches such as timing and dose

and with more modern concurrent chemotherapy is warranted. Additionally, there was insufficient evidence to assess either the benefit or harm of SRS for recurrence or fractionated SRS in the newly diagnosed or recurrent setting [58].

## Brachytherapy

Brachytherapy is thought to have several potential advantages in the treatment of high-grade gliomas. The intraoperative placement of radioisotopes (either radioactive seeds coated with Iodine-125 or Iridium-192 or a liquid infusion with Iodine-125 in a GliaSite catheter) into the tumor or resection cavity permits the delivery of a large radiation dose to the target, with rapid falloff in the surrounding tissues [59]. It provides continuous rather than intermittent delivery, which decreases repair of sublethal damage and increases tumor susceptibility. However, despite these theoretical advantages, brachytherapy has shown little benefit in the treatment of high-grade gliomas despite several promising single institution reports. In a trial of 299 patients with high-grade astrocytomas randomized to either IFRT plus carmustine with or without interstitial brachytherapy, there was no statistically significant difference in median survival [60].

Brachytherapy carries an increased risk of radionecrosis and is contraindicated in many patients, particularly when the tumor is in close proximity to organs at risk or with recent administration of bevacizumab [61]. Thus, interest in brachytherapy has diminished relative to 3D-CRT, IMRT, and stereotactic techniques.

## Treatment Planning Complication Avoidances

Treatment delivery historically had been performed with two-dimensional planning, which then evolved to three-dimensional CT-based treatment planning (or 3D conformal radiation therapy (3D-CRT)). Fusion of the planning CT with either MRI or PET data is helpful in target definition [62]. Photons of 6 MV are most commonly used with typically three to four separate beam angles. Depending on the location of the PTV, non-coplanar beams such as a vertex field can also be utilized to further spare organs at risk. Therefore, the advantage of 3D-CRT techniques is the ability to decrease the radiation dose to uninvolved brain tissue when compared to 2D techniques. In this technique, block edges are typically around 1 cm from the PTV edge to ensure adequate PTV coverage.

Intensity-modulated RT (IMRT) provides additional beam modification beyond 3D-conformal radiation therapy to vary the radiation intensity across each treatment field (see Fig. 6.4). Its use has become increasingly prevalent in the treatment of high-grade gliomas since it offers the advantage of decreasing

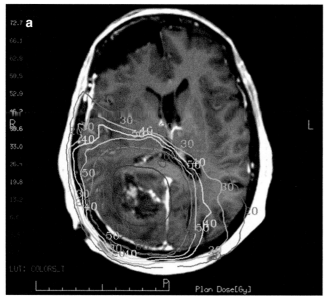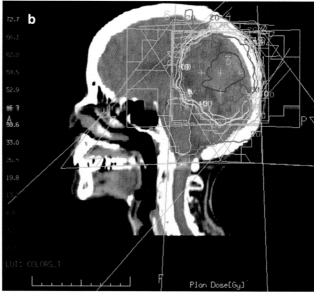

**Fig. 6.4** IMRT treatment planning images. The PTV1 (violet) is the initial plan to 46 Gy, and the PTV2 (red) is the 14 Gy boost to a total of 60 Gy for a resected GBM. (**a**) Isodose lines displayed on the diagnostic postoperative MRI used for treatment planning. (**b**) Sagittal image of treatment planning CT with isodose lines and beams displayed

radiation-related adverse effects [63]. IMRT is especially useful when the tumor abuts radiation-sensitive structures such as the eyes, optic nerves, optic chiasm, cochlea, and brainstem because of its ability to shape dose around these structures. There may be less advantage to IMRT when the tumor is distant from any avoidance structures. IMRT is also accompanied by the obvious disadvantage of increased cost, complexity in treatment planning, adaptation of linear accelerator hardware, need for additional planning time for physics quality assurance, and increased treatment times.

Volumetric modulated arc therapy (VMAT) is a novel radiation technique also currently used for treatment planning of CNS tumors. One or more multiple arc(s) are utilized for treatment delivery and, therefore, has the additional benefit of reduced monitor units (MU) and treatment delivery time compared to IMRT plans. This technique allows the simultaneous variation of three parameters during treatment delivery, i.e., gantry rotation speed, dose rate, and treatment aperture shape via multi-leaf collimator (MLC) positions [64]. The preferred method for treatment delivery should be reviewed on an individual basis in regard to optimal PTV coverage, dose delivered to the critical organs at risk, and the extent of normal brain irradiated.

## Radiation Toxicity, Acute and Late

Fatigue, headaches, nausea, and vomiting are common acute adverse effects. Patients are also at risk for transient worsening of neurologic symptoms or seizure secondary to cerebral edema, which may require steroid use [65]. Lesions near the surface of the brain may also result in patchy alopecia. Patients receiving concurrent chemotherapy and steroids are at risk for infections related to immunosuppression such as oral candidiasis, pneumocystis carinii pneumonia requiring prophylaxis, as well as cytopenias with aplastic anemia being a possible consequence of temozolomide use. Long-term, all patients are at risk for cognitive decline and short-term memory impairment. Patients are also at risk for cerebral radionecrosis and pituitary dysfunction. Treatment of lesions near the optic pathways, cochlea, or eloquent brain such as the primary sensory or motor cortex can result in permanent focal deficits in these areas. In addition, any treatment with radiation carries with it a small long-term risk of secondary malignancy, but this is rarely a concern in this patient population given the poor prognosis associated with this disease.

## Outcomes: Tumor Control and Survival

Despite aggressive multimodality therapy, long-term tumor control and outcomes, with few exceptions, are poor. Grade III tumors generally have a more favorable outcome than grade IV tumors, though subsets of each can fare significantly better than others. Median survival for anaplastic astrocytomas is 3 years, but only 16 months for GBM [1]. For GBM, the median progression-free survival and overall survival are 6.9 months and 14.6 months, respectively, for patients receiving adjuvant therapy with radiation and temozolomide [12].

Patients with tumors exhibiting MGMT promoter methylation show an improvement in survival with this standard regimen with a median progression-free survival and overall survival of 10.3 months and 21.7 months, respectively [11]. For grade III tumors, oligodendrogliomas have a better prognosis, particularly those that exhibit co-deletion of 1p/19q. After treatment with chemotherapy (PCV) and radiation, the median survival for non-co-deleted patients was approximately 2.7 years compared to 14.7 years for co-deleted patients [15].

## Follow-Up: Radiographic Assessment

The majority of patients who fail standard therapy will recur locally within or near the original site of disease. A smaller percentage will develop recurrent disease in other portions of the brain parenchyma outside the original treatment area. Despite their malignant potential, however, extracranial failure is exceedingly rare. Therefore, surveillance after therapy consists of periodic clinical evaluation and radiographic imaging of the brain. Follow-up imaging is typically initiated within 4–6 weeks after completing RT and every 2–3 months thereafter with an increasing interval between studies for the rare patient with prolonged disease-free survival (Fig. 6.5).

A well-known phenomenon that complicates early post-treatment surveillance typically within 3 months from completion of chemoradiation is that of pseudoprogression. This is when imaging demonstrates increased contrast enhancement and increased T2 FLAIR hyperintensity that can mimic disease progression but is in fact the result of treatment effect and resolves spontaneously without further intervention. Pseudoprogression occurs in upward of 15–30% of all GBM patients treated with combined chemoradiation and often leads to unwarranted treatment adjustments that may compromise efficacy. Indeed, there is evidence to suggest that further dose intensification leads to higher rates of pseudoprogression [33]. Factors that favor pseudoprogression include the absence of symptoms and MGMT methylation as true progression is more often symptomatic and seen in those with an unmethylated MGMT status. Additionally, the use of complimentary imaging techniques has been studied to better distinguish pseudoprogression from true progression. Perfusion imaging provides evidence of tumor viability and is sensitive to tumor vascular properties and transport kinetics following therapy [66] (Fig. 6.6).

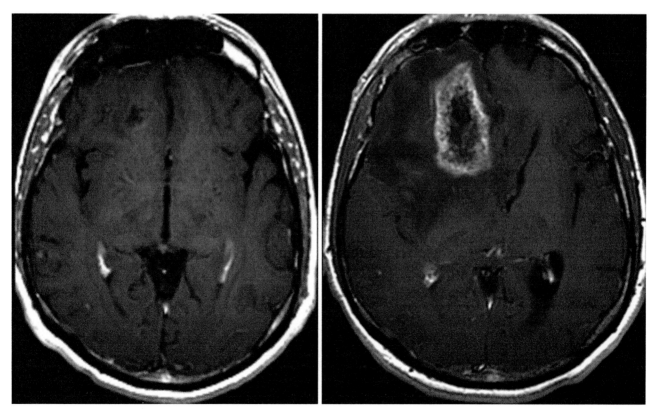

**Fig. 6.5** Post-operative MRI confirms gross total resection of a right frontal GBM with no evidence of residual tumor. One month following completion of concurrent temozolomide and 60 Gy RT in 30 fractions, an MRI shows substantial contrast enhancement with imaging characteristics such as "spreading wavefront" and "swiss cheese" enhancement pattern suggestive of treatment-related changes. Surgical resection confirmed pathologic diagnosis of gliosis and RT related vascular changes

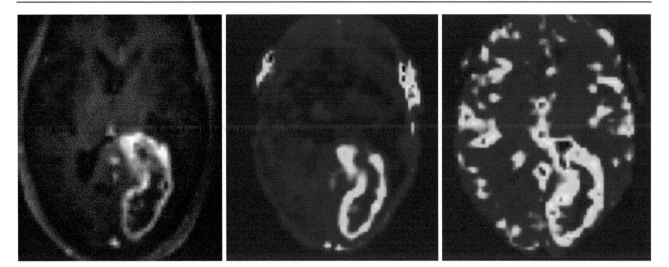

**Fig. 6.6** Conventional MR T1 post-gadolinium (left panel) demonstrating a contrast-enhancing left parietal GBM. Physiologic MR imaging including elevated ktrans as a measure of vascular permeability (middle panel) and increased rCBV (right panel) as a measure of increased perfusion provides additional tools to distinguish recurrent tumor and treatment-associated changes. Contrast-enhancing GBM left parietal occipital region with elevated ktrans and increased rCBV consistent with tumor progression

In a preliminary study, early MR perfusion changes improved response assessments in patients receiving chemoradiotherapy [67]. MR spectroscopy may also help distinguish true progression from pseudoprogression as higher choline-to-creatine and choline-to-NAA (*N*-acetylaspartate) ratios are noted in tumor recurrence [68]. Ultimately, if pseudoprogression is suspected, continuation of chemotherapy with short-term interval imaging is recommended.

PET allows for noninvasive quantitative measurements of metabolism and biochemical processes that are complementary to MRI. The most widely used tracer in the clinic is 2-deoxy-2-[$^{18}$F]fluoro-D-glucose (FDG), which provides a measure of glycolysis, with increased glycolytic rates noted in tumors. MR perfusion and FDG-PET are often used to distinguish radionecrosis from recurrent brain tumors, but diagnostic accuracy is limited by both the high physiologic uptake of FDG by normal brain tissue and false-positive results due to uptake by inflammatory cells. Dynamic PET imaging acquisition and kinetic modeling can provide additional physiologic information useful for improving imaging biomarker specificity to further improve specificity in distinguishing tumor progression from radionecrosis (Fig. 6.7).

## Recurrent Disease

Treatment options for recurrent disease are limited and effectively palliative in nature. Median overall survival after recurrence is less than 1 year. For diffuse or multifocal recurrence, systemic therapy is considered for patients with acceptable performance status with surgery reserved for palliation of particularly large and/or symptomatic lesions.

Otherwise, best supportive care is indicated. For patients with local-only recurrence, particularly with a longer interval between primary treatment and recurrence, focal therapy such as re-resection or re-irradiation can be considered.

## Chemotherapy

Typical systemic agents in the recurrent setting include bevacizumab, nitrosoureas, and rechallenging with temozolomide. Bevacizumab in this setting results in a radiographic response as a single agent or in combination with irinotecan or lomustine, but there has not been a proven overall survival benefit. Nevertheless, prospective studies have shown a potential steroid-sparing benefit with single and combined therapy and a progression-free survival benefit for combined therapy over bevacizumab alone [69, 70]. For patients not amenable to bevacizumab, single agent or combined nitrosoureas are an alternative systemic therapy option. Response rates and median progression-free survival with single-agent lomustine, however, are modest [71, 72], and combined therapy appears to be comparable to temozolomide alone [44]. Finally, repeat treatment with temozolomide has been studied with various dosing regimens, and results have been mixed but have generally demonstrated the most benefit for patients with tumors positive for MGMT promoter methylation and with longer intervals between treatment completion and relapse [73, 74].

## Re-irradiation

Salvage re-irradiation for recurrent GBM has been used as a potential treatment option [57, 75–77]. Re-irradiation is associated with an increased risk of late radiation-related side effects such as neurocognitive deficits and radiation

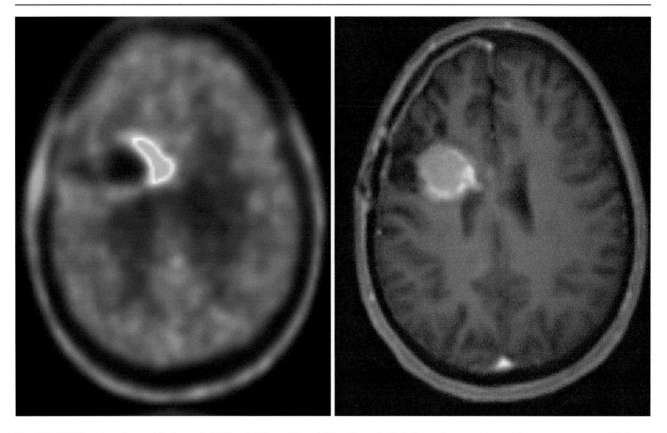

**Fig. 6.7** PET imaging along with elevated rCBV on MRI provides additional metabolic information consistent with recurrent tumor and helps to distinguish from postoperative enhancement changes

necrosis. Despite these risks, results from over 300 GBM patients confirm a 6-month progression-free survival (PFS) from 28% to 39% and a median 1-year overall survival (OS) of 26% [78–80]. Reports demonstrate an acceptable risk of cerebral necrosis if the total cumulative dose from all treatments remains under approximately 100 Gy [81], and recent RT technologic advances including protons, IMRT, and fractionated stereotactic radiotherapy (FSRT) allow for highly conformal treatment to significantly reduce late CNS toxicity [80]. Several studies also report an improvement in functional status and discontinuation of corticosteroid usage [57, 76, 79]. Late CNS toxicity was uncommon especially following fractionated stereotactic radiotherapy (FSRT).

Combs et al. reported on 172 recurrent gliomas treated with FSRT 36 Gy in 2 Gy fractions. Median time to re-irradiation was 10 months. Median OS was 8 months. Median GBM tumor size was 47.7 cc. Factors associated with improved outcome include extent of initial resection and younger age [78]. Fogh et al. reported on 147 high-grade gliomas treated with FSRT 35 Gy in 10 fractions. Median time to re-irradiation was 8 months. Median survival was 11 months. Median tumor volume was 22 cc. Eighty-four patients underwent salvage surgery, and 48 patients received concurrent chemotherapy. Multivariate analysis suggested younger age and smaller tumor volumes were associated

with improved outcome [80]. Gutin et al. reported median OS of 12.5 months in 25 recurrent glioma (grade III–IV) patients using FSRT 30 Gy in 6 fractions with concurrent and adjuvant bevacizumab. Median time to re-irradiation was 15 months. Enhancing tumor volume was ≤3.5 cm. No cases of late radionecrosis were reported [82]. RTOG 1205, a multi-institutional phase II randomized trial (NCT01730950) of bevacizumab and re-irradiation compared to bevacizumab alone in bevacizumab-naïve patients, has recently been completed with a primary objective to confirm the efficacy and safety of re-irradiation in recurrent GBM.

Re-irradiation is frequently associated with a higher risk of CNS radiation necrosis. A small randomized double-blind placebo-controlled trial of bevacizumab therapy for treatment of CNS radiation necrosis showed imaging response only in patients receiving bevacizumab. These initial trial results have established this as an effective treatment option for patients presenting with radiation necrosis along with corticosteroids and surgical resection.

## Key Studies

Tables 6.2, 6.3 and 6.4.

**Table 6.2** Glioblastoma multiforme

| Study | Inclusion criteria | Randomization | RT dose | Chemotherapy | Patient characteristics | Outcomes | Comments |
|---|---|---|---|---|---|---|---|
| **Conventional RT** | | | | | | | |
| *EORTC 26981/22981-NCIC CE.3* Stupp et al. NEJM, 2005 Update—Stupp et al. Lancet Oncol 2009 | 18–70 years old; newly diagnosed pathology confirmed GBM; WHO PS 0–2 | Radiation alone *vs* concurrent chemoradiation and adjuvant chemotherapy | 60 Gy in 30 fx | Daily temozolomide (75 mg/m², 7 days/week) with radiation, adjuvant temozolomide 150–200 mg/m² (5 days/week) q28 days × 6 cycles | 573 patients, median age 56, GTR 39%, STR 44%, biopsy only 16% | *Median survival:* RT alone: 12.1 months ChemoRT: 14.6 months (SS) HR 0.63 (95% CI, 0.52–0.75) *5-year OS:* RT alone 1.9% vs ChemoRT 9.8% *Toxicity:* 7% with grade III/IV hematologic toxicity with concurrent temozolomide and 14% with adjuvant temozolomide | Survival improved for all subgroups except those with biopsy alone and poor PS Update shows methylation of *MGMT* promoter strongest predictor for outcome and benefit to temozolomide |
| *MGMT Analysis—EORTC/NCIC Trial* Hegi et al. NEJM, 2005 | Known *MGMT* promoter methylation status from larger EORTC/NCIC cohort | Same as above | Same as above | Same as above | 206 patients (36% of full cohort) with methylation status evaluated. 43% (92 pts) positive for *MGMT* methylation | *Median survival (all SS)* RT alone Methylated: 16 months Unmethylated: 11.8 months ChemoRT Methylated: 21.7 months Unmethylated: 12.7 months *Median PFS* RT alone Methylated: 5.9 months Unmethylated: 4.4 months ChemoRT Methylated: 10.3 months Unmethylated: 5.3 months | >70% pts. in RT alone group received salvage chemotherapy |

(continued)

**Table 6.2** (continued)

| Study | Inclusion criteria | Randomization | RT dose | Chemotherapy | Patient characteristics | Outcomes | Comments |
|---|---|---|---|---|---|---|---|
| **Hypofractionated RT** | | | | | | | |
| *Canada Multi-Institutional* Roa et al., JCC 2004 | Histologically confirmed GBM; age ≥60; KPS ≥50 | Standard adjuvant RT vs hypofractionated RT | Standard arm: 60 Gy in 30 fx (46 Gy in 23 fx followed by 14 Gy boost) Hypofractionated arm: 40 Gy in 15 fx (no boost) | None | 95 patients; median age: 71–72; median KPS: 70; GTR 9.5%, STR 51.5%, biopsy only 39% | *Median survival* Standard arm: 5.1 months Hypofrac arm: 5.6 months ($p = 0.57$) Quality of life measures (KPS and FACT-Br) comparable between two groups | |
| *IAEA Trial* Rao et al., JCO 2015 | Histologically confirmed GBM; frail (age ≥50, KPS 50–70), elderly (age ≥65, KPS 80–100), or both (age ≥65, KPS 50–70) | 15 fraction adjuvant RT vs 5 fraction RT | Control arm: 40 Gy in 15 fx Experimental arm: 25 Gy in 5 fx | None | 98 patients; 38% age 50–65, 62% age >65; GTR 16%, STR 65%, biopsy only 13%, 6% missing | *Median survival* 15 fx arm: 6.4 months 5 fx arm: 7.9 months ($p = 0.988$) *Median PFS* 4.2 months in both groups ($p = 0.716$) | Post-RT QoL measurement comparable |
| *EORTC 26062/22061— NCIC CE.6— TROG 08.02* Perry et al., NEJM 2017 | Histologically confirmed GBM; age ≥65; not suitable for conventional chemoRT; ECOG PS 0–2 | Adjuvant hypofractionated RT alone vs concurrent hypofractionated chemoRT and adjuvant chemotherapy | 40.05 Gy in 15 fx | Daily temozolomide (75 mg/m², 7 days/week) with radiation, adjuvant temozolomide 150–200 mg/m² (5 days/week) q28 days × 6 cycles | 562 patients; median age 73; GTR or STR 68%, biopsy alone 32%; 47% MGMT promoter methylated | *Median survival* RT alone: 7.6 months ChemoRT: 9.3 months ($p < 0.001$) *MGMT-positive pts.* RT alone: 7.7 months ChemoRT: 13.5 months ($p < 0.001$) Hematologic toxicity worse with chemoRT with grade III/IV lymphopenia (27% vs 10%) and thrombocytopenia (11% vs 0.4%) | MGMT status not a prognostic factor in RT alone group |

| | Eligibility criteria | Objective | Radiation | Treatment | Patients | Results | Notes |
|---|---|---|---|---|---|---|---|
| **Targeted therapy** | | | | | | | |
| *RTOG 0825* Gilbert et al., NEJM 2014 | Age ≥18 years old; KPS ≥70; histologically confirmed GBM; no evidence of intracranial hemorrhage on imaging; no active cardiac disease or recent stroke | The addition of bevacizumab vs placebo to conventional chemoRT with temozolomide | 60 Gy in 30 fx (46 Gy in 23 fx followed by 14 Gy boost) | Both arms: daily temozolomide (75 mg/m², 7 days/week) with radiation, adjuvant temozolomide 150–200 mg/m² (5 days/week) q28 days × 6 cycles. Experimental arm: addition of bevacizumab (10 mg/kg q 2wk) starting at week 4 of RT and until either disease progression, severe toxicity, or completion of adjuvant therapy | 637 patients; 80% age ≥50; GTR 61%, STR 36%, biopsy alone ineligible; 28% *MGMT* promoter methylated | *Median survival* Placebo: 16.1 months; Bevacizumab: 15.7 months ($p = 0.21$). *Median PFS* Placebo: 7.3 months; Bevacizumab: 10.7 months ($p = 0.007$). *Toxicity:* bevacizumab associated with worse thromboembolic events (7.7% vs 4.7%), intestinal perforation (1.2% vs 0.4%), and hemorrhage (1.5% vs 0.9%). Greater decline in neurocognitive function and worse QoL with bevacizumab | Treatment group revealed at time of progression and bevacizumab could be continued/started. *MGMT* methylation status prognostic regardless of treatment group |

**Table 6.3** Anaplastic astrocytoma

| Study | Inclusion criteria | Randomization | RT dose | Chemotherapy | Patient characteristics | Outcomes | Comments |
|---|---|---|---|---|---|---|---|
| *RTOG 9813* Chang et al., Neuro Oncol 2016 | Histologically confirmed, newly diagnosed anaplastic astrocytoma; Age ≥18 years; KPS ≥60 | Adjuvant chemoRT with temozolomide vs chemoRT with nitrosourea | 59.4 Gy in 33 fx (50.4 Gy in 28 fx followed by 9 Gy boost) | Temozolomide: 200 mg/m² days 1–5 on first week of RT, q28 days × 12 cycles Nitrosourea: BCNU (80 mg/m²) days 1, 2, and 3 on first week of RT; then days 56, 57, and 58; and then q8 weeks ×4. CCNU (130 mg/m²) q8 weeks ×6 | 196 patients; median age 42–43; GTR/STR 64%, biopsy only 36%; *IDH1-R132H* mutation positive 44.1%, negative 48.6%, 7.2% not scored | *Median survival* Temozolomide: 3.9 years Nitrosurea: 3.8 years (*p* = 0.36) Median PFS statistically similar *Toxicity*: All grade ≥3 toxicity worse in nitrosourea arm (76% vs 48%, *p* < 0.001), primarily hematologic. Only 21% completed chemo as planned in nitrosourea group (vs 60% in temozolomide group, *p* < 0.001) | Study did not meet target accrual *IDH1* mutant-positive patients had improved OS (HR 0.42; CI, 0.25–0.72) and PFS (HR 0.53, CI, 0.32–0.86) on multivariate analysis |

## Case Study

A 65-year-old retired teacher presents with a 3-week history of mild confusion and difficulties with memory and word finding. An MRI is obtained that shows a right, contrast-enhancing temporal lesion. He is started on steroids with improvement in his symptoms. He is evaluated by neurosurgery and undergoes a right temporal craniotomy surgical resection. Pathology is consistent with GBM, IDH wild-type, MGMT methylated, and EGFR non-amplified. After discussion of the risks and benefits of treatment, he elects to proceed with concurrent temozolomide and RT 60 Gy in 30 fractions (see Fig. 6.3).

## Summary

- High-grade gliomas are the most common primary malignant tumor of the CNS, comprising 40% of all primary brain tumors.
- Glioblastoma multiforme has a universally poor prognosis with a median survival of 14.6 months with multimodality therapy. Improved outcomes are seen for anaplastic gliomas, and median survival ranges from over 2 years to almost 15 years depending on the histologic and molecular subtype.
- Recently updated WHO pathologic criteria integrate the molecular phenotype into histologic evaluation, particularly IDH-1 mutational status and the presence or absence of 1p/19q co-deletion.

- Standard of care for GBM continues to be maximally safe resection followed by adjuvant chemoradiation with temozolomide. Improved outcomes are seen with tumors exhibiting *MGMT* promoter methylation. Elderly patients or those with poor performance status are more often treated with hypofractionated radiation therapy alone or with concurrent temozolomide.
- For anaplastic gliomas, most studies support the use of sequential adjuvant radiation and PCV chemotherapy. The role of temozolomide is under investigation; however, available studies suggest this is a reasonable alternative to PCV.
- Radiation treatment volumes for high-grade gliomas consist of residual contrast-enhancing tumor and/or the postoperative cavity with a 1–2 cm expansion within anatomical constraints to account for subclinical disease. Expansions are to account for the infiltrative nature of these tumors and are larger for GBMs.
- Depending on tumor location, IMRT is often considered to reduce radiation dose to adjacent critical structures including the optic nerves, optic chiasm, and brainstem.
- Posttreatment surveillance can be complicated by the phenomenon of pseudoprogression which can mimic tumor progression radiographically. Additional radiologic studies have been utilized to try and distinguish pseudoprogression from true progression with varying accuracy.
- The majority of patients will develop a local failure after primary treatment. Treatment options for recurrent disease are limited and can include systemic therapy and/or re irradiation for select patients.

**Table 6.4** Anaplastic oligodendroglioma

| Study | Inclusion criteria | Randomization | RT dose | Chemotherapy | Patient characteristics | Outcomes | Comments |
|---|---|---|---|---|---|---|---|
| *EORTC 26951* Van den Bent et al., JCO 2006 Update—van den Bent et al., JCO 2012 | Histologically confirmed, newly diagnosed anaplastic oligodendroglioma (AO) or mixed oligoastrocytoma (AOA) (≥25% oligo); age 16–70 years old; ECOG PS 0–2 | Adjuvant RT alone vs RT followed by chemotherapy | 59.4 Gy in 33 fx (45 Gy in 25 fx followed by 14.4 Gy boost) | PCV: procarbazine (60 mg/m$^2$) days 8–21, lomustine (110 mg/m$^2$) day 1, vincristine (1.4 mg/m$^2$) days 8 and 29, q6 weeks ×6. Started within 4 weeks after completion of RT | 368 patients; median age 49–50; GTR 36%, STR 50%, biopsy alone 14%; AO 72%, AOA 27%, 1% missing; co-deletion 1p/19q—21% (25% of evaluable patients) | *Median survival* RT alone: 30.6 months RT → PCV: 42.3 months (SS) *Median PFS* RT alone: 13.2 months RT → PCV: 24.3 months (SS) 1p/19q co-deleted pts.: median OS not reached with 140 months median f/u in PCV group. Median PFS 157 months vs 50 months w/ RT alone (SS) *Toxicity*: PCV resulted in significant grade III/IV hematologic toxicity. Median cycles administered: 3 of 6 | In RT alone group, 65% received salvage PCV at time of progression Updated report evaluated *MGMT* methylation and *IDH1*-mutant status. Multivariate analysis showed *IDH1* and 1p/19q but not *MGMT*, status independently prognostic for OS |
| *RTOG 9402* Cairncross et al., JCO 2006 Update—Cairncross et al., JCO 2013 | Histologically confirmed, newly diagnosed anaplastic oligodendroglioma (AO) or mixed oligoastrocytoma (AOA) (≥25% oligo); age ≥18 years old; KPS ≥60 | Adjuvant RT alone vs adjuvant chemotherapy followed by RT | 59.4 Gy in 33 fx (50.4 Gy in 28 fx followed by 9 Gy boost). Started within 6 weeks of final chemotherapy | PCV: procarbazine (75 mg/m$^2$) day 8–21, lomustine (130 mg/m$^2$) day 1, vincristine (1.4 mg/m$^2$) days 8 and 29, q6 weeks ×4 | 291 patients; median age 43; GTR 32%, STR 55%, biopsy only 12%; AO 52%, AOA 48%, Co-deletion 1p/19q 43% (48% of evaluable patients) | *Median survival* RT alone: 4.7 years PCV → RT: 4.6 years (NS) 1p/19q co-deleted pts.: median OS 14.7 years in PCV group vs 7.3 years with RT alone (SS). In non-co-deleted pts., median survival comparable between groups (2.6 years vs 2.7 years, $p = 0.39$) *Toxicity*: PCV resulted in 65% grade III/IV toxicity. 54% received four cycles | In RT alone group, 79% received salvage chemotherapy at time of progression (vs 41% in PCV group, $p < 0.001$) Higher percentage of mixed tumors than EORTC 26951, 13% astrocytoma dominant |

## Self-Assessment Questions

1. When is the most common time for pseudoprogression to occur?
   A. At the start of radiotherapy
   B. In the first 3 months after completion of radiotherapy
   C. 4–6 months after completion of radiotherapy
   D. 1 year after completion of radiotherapy

2. What molecular features are likely to be associated with an anaplastic oligodendroglioma?
   A. IDH1 mutation and 1p19q co-deletion
   B. BRAF mutation
   C. EGFR amplification
   D. ATRX mutation

3. Prospective, randomized data indicate that use of 5-ALA during craniotomy for GBM produces which of the following benefits:
   A. Improved neurological outcome
   B. Improved overall survival
   C. Improved progression-free survival
   D. Improved neurocognitive function

4. IDH1-positive tumors are associated with which of the following?
   A. Worse patient prognosis
   B. Contrast-enhancing tumors
   C. Small size tumors at time of diagnosis
   D. Secondary glioblastoma
   E. Susceptibility to temozolomide treatment

5. In addition to corticosteroids and surgery, effective treatments for radiation necrosis include:
   A. Pentoxifylline
   B. Hyperbaric oxygen
   C. Anticoagulation
   D. Bevacizumab

## Answers

1. B
   References: [83, 84]
2. A
   References: [85–87]
3. C
   Reference: [28]
4. D
   Reference: [88]
5. D
   Reference: [89]

## References

1. Wen PY, Kesari S. Malignant gliomas in adults. N Engl J Med. 2008;359:492.
2. Kleihues P, Cavenee WK. Pathology and genetics of tumours of the nervous system. In: Louis DN, Ohgaki H, Wiestler OD, Cavenee WK, editors. World Health Organization Classification of Tumours of the Nervous System, Editorial and Consensus Conference Working Group. Lyon, France: IARS Press; 2007.
3. Ostrum QT, Gittleman H, Fulop J, et al. CBTRUS statistical report: primary brain and central nervous system tumors diagnosed in 2008–2012. Neuro Oncol. 2015;17(Suppl 4):iv1.
4. Dubrow R, Darefsky AS. Demographic variation in incidence of adult glioma by subtype, United States, 1992–2007. BMC Cancer. 2011;11:325.
5. Louis DN, Pomeroy SL, Cairncross JG. Focus on central nervous system neoplasia. Cancer Cell. 2002;1:125.
6. Chang SM, Parney IF, Huang W, et al. Patterns of care for adults with newly diagnosed malignant glioma. JAMA. 2005;293:557.
7. Hansen EK, Roach M, editors. Handbook of evidence-based radiation oncology. 2nd ed. New York, NY: Springer Science + Business Media; 2010.
8. Ironside JW, Moss TH, Louis DN, et al. Diagnostic pathology of the nervous system tumours. London: Churchill Livingstone; 2002.
9. Galli R, Binda E, Orfanelli U, et al. Isolation and characterization of tumorigenic, stem-like neural precursors from human glioblastoma. Cancer Res. 2004;64:7011.
10. Marko NF, Weil RJ, Schroeder JL, et al. Extent of resection of glioblastoma revisited: personalized survival modeling facilitates more accurate survival prediction and supports a maximum-safe-resection approach to surgery. J Clin Oncol. 2014;32:774.
11. Hegi ME, Diserens AC, Gorila T, et al. MGMT gene silencing and benefit from temozolomide in glioblastoma. N Engl J Med. 2005;352:997.
12. Stupp R, Mason WP, van den Bent MJ, et al. Radiotherapy plus concomitant and adjuvant temozolomide for glioblastoma. N Engl J Med. 2005;352:987.
13. Gerstner ER, Yip S, Wang DL, et al. Mgmt methylation is a prognostic biomarker in elderly patients with newly diagnosed glioblastoma. Neurology. 2009;73:1509.
14. Kloosterhof NK, Bralten LB, Dubbink HJ, et al. Isocitrate dehydrogenase-1 mutations: a fundamentally new understanding of diffuse glioma? Lancet Oncol. 2011;12:83.
15. Cairncross G, Wang M, Shaw E, et al. Phase III trial of chemoradiotherapy for anaplastic oligodendroglioma: long-term results of RTOG 9402. J Clin Oncol. 2013;31:337.
16. van den Bent MJ, Brandes AA, Taphoorn MJ, et al. Adjuvant procarbazine, lomustine, and vincristine chemotherapy in newly diagnosed oligodendroglioma: long-term follow-up of EORTC brain tumor group study 26951. J Clin Oncol. 2013;31:344.
17. Louis DN, Perry A, Reifenberger G, et al. The 2016 world health organization classification of tumors of the central nervous system: a summary. Acta Neuropathol. 2016;131:803.
18. Reuss DE, Kratz A, Sahm F, et al. Adult IDH wildtype astrocytomas biologically and clinically resolve into other tumor entities. Acta Neuropathol. 2015;130:407.
19. Paleologos TS, Dorward NL, Wadley JP, et al. Clinical validation of true frameless stereotactic biopsy: analysis of the first 125 consecutive cases. Neurosurgery. 2001;49:830.
20. Pirotte B, Goldman S, Massager N, et al. Comparison of 18F-FDG and 11C-methionine for PET-guided stereotactic brain biopsy of gliomas. J Nucl Med. 2004;45:1293.
21. McKnight TR, von dem Bussche MH, Vigneron DB, et al. Histopathological validation of a three-dimensional magnetic resonance spectroscopy index as a predictor of tumor presence. J Neurosurg. 2002;97:794.

22. Laws ER, Parney IF, Huang W, et al. Survival following surgery and prognostic factors for recently diagnosed malignant glioma: data from the Glioma Outcomes Project. J Neurosurg. 2003;99:467.

23. Lacroix M, Abi-Said D, Fourney DR, et al. A multivariate analysis of 416 patients with glioblastoma multiforme: prognosis, extent of resection, and survival. J Neurosurg. 2001;95:190.

24. Pirotte B, Goldman S, Dewitte O, et al. Integrated positron emission tomography and magnetic resonance imaging-guided resection of brain tumors: a report of 103 consecutive procedures. J Neurosurg. 2006;104:238.

25. Krishnan R, Raabe A, Hattingen E, et al. Functional magnetic resonance imaging-integrated neuronavigation: correlation between lesion-to-motor cortex distance and outcome. Neurosurgery. 2004;55:904.

26. Meyer FB, Bates LM, Goerss SJ, et al. Awake craniotomy for aggressive resection of primary gliomas located in eloquent brain. Mayo Clin Proc. 2001;76:677.

27. Sanai N, Mirzadeh Z, Berger MS. Functional outcome after language mapping for glioma resection. N Engl J Med. 2008;358:18.

28. Stummer W, Pichlmeier U, Meinel T, et al. Fluorescence-guided surgery with 5-animolevulinic acid for resection of malignant glioma: a randomized controlled multicenter phase III trial. Lancet Oncol. 2006;7:392–401.

29. Walker MD, Green SB, Byar DP, et al. Randomized comparisons of radiotherapy and nitrosureas for the treatment of malignant glioma after surgery. N Engl J Med. 1980;303:1323.

30. Andersen AP. Postoperative irradiation of glioblastomas. Results in a randomized series. Acta Radiol Oncol Radiat Phys Biol. 1978;17:475.

31. Coffey RJ, Lunsford LD, Taylor FH. Survival after stereotactic biopsy of malignant gliomas. Neurosurgery. 1988;22:465.

32. Chan JL, Lee SW, Sandler HM, et al. Survival and failure patterns of high-grade gliomas after three-dimensional conformal radiotherapy. J Clin Oncol. 2002;20:1635.

33. Tsien CI, Brown D, Normolle D, et al. Concurrent temozolomide and dose-escalated intensity-modulated radiation therapy in newly diagnosed glioblastoma. Clin Cancer Res. 2012;18:273.

34. Stupp R, Hegi ME, Mason WP, et al. Effects of radiotherapy with concomitant and adjuvant temozolomide versus radiotherapy alone on survival in glioblastoma in a randomized phase III study: 5-year analysis of the EORTC-NCIC trial. Lancet Oncol. 2009;10:459.

35. Gilbert MR, Wang M, Aldape KD, et al. RTOG 0525: a randomized phase III trial comparing standard adjuvant temozolomide with a dose-dense schedule in newly diagnosed glioblastoma. J Clin Oncol. 2011;15(Suppl):141s.

36. Quinn JA, Jiang SX, Rearden DA, et al. Phase II trial of temozolomide plus O6-benzylguanine in adults with recurrent, temozolomide-resistant malignant glioma. J Clin Oncol. 2009;27:1262.

37. Quinn JA, Jiang SX, Carter J, et al. Phase II trial of Gliadel plus O6-benzylguanine in adults with recurrent glioblastoma multiforme. Clin Cancer Res. 2009;15:1064.

38. Lai A, Tran A, Nghiemphu PL, et al. Phase II study of bevacizumab plus temozolomide during and after radiation therapy for patients with newly diagnosed glioblastoma multiforme. J Clin Oncol. 2011;29:142.

39. Chang S, Zhang P, Cairncross JG, et al. Phase III randomized study of radiation and temozolomide versus radiation and nitrosourea therapy for anaplastic astrocytoma: results of NRG oncology RTOG 9813. Neuro Oncol. 2016;19:252.

40. Brandes AA, Nicolardi L, Tosoni A, et al. Survival following adjuvant PCV or temozolomide for anaplastic astrocytoma. Neuro Oncol. 2006;8:253.

41. van den Bent M, Erridge S, Vogelbaum MA, et al. Results of the interim analysis of the EORTC randomized phase III CANTON trial on concurrent and adjuvant temozolomide in anaplastic glioma without 1p/19q co-deletion: an intergroup trial. J Clin Oncol. 2016;34(Suppl):abstr LBA2000.

42. van den Bent MJ, Carpentier AF, Brandes AA, et al. Adjuvant procarbazine, lomustine, and vincristine improves progression-free survival but not overall survival in newly diagnosed anaplastic oligodendrogliomas and oligoastrocytomas: a randomized European Organisation for Research and Treatment of Cancer phase III trial. J Clin Oncol. 2006;24:2715.

43. Vogelbaum MA, Berkey B, Peereboom D, et al. Phase II trial of preirradiation and concurrent temozolomide in patients with newly diagnosed anaplastic oligodendrogliomas and mixed anaplastic oligoastrocytomas: RTOG BR0131. Neuro Oncol. 2009;11:167.

44. Brada M, Stenning S, Gabe R, et al. Temozolomide versus procarbazine, lomustine, and vincristine in recurrent high-grade glioma. J Clin Oncol. 2010;28:4601.

45. Roa W, Brasher PM, Bauman G, et al. Abbreviated course of radiation therapy in older patients with glioblastoma multiforme: a prospective randomized clinical trial. J Clin Oncol. 2004;22:1583.

46. Roa W, Kepka L, Kumar N, et al. International Atomic Energy Agency randomized phase III study of radiation therapy in elderly and/or frail patients with newly diagnosed glioblastoma multiforme. J Clin Oncol. 2015;33:4145.

47. Wick W, Platten M, Mesiner C, et al. Temozolomide chemotherapy alone versus radiotherapy alone for malignant astrocytoma in the elderly: the NOA-08 randomised, phase 3 trial. Lancet Oncol. 2012;13:707.

48. Perry JR, Laperriere N, O'Callaghan CJ, et al. Short-course radiation plus temozolomide in elderly patients with glioblastoma. N Engl J Med. 2017;376:1027.

49. Halperin EC, Bentel G, Heinz ER, et al. Radiation therapy treatment planning in supratentorial glioblastoma multiforme: an analysis based on post morten topographic anatomy with CT correlations. Int J Radiat Oncol Biol Phys. 1989;17:1347–50.

50. Parsons JT, Bova FJ, Fitzgerald CR, et al. Severe dry-eye syndrome following external beam irradiation. Int J Radiat Oncol Biol Phys. 1994;30:775.

51. Nwokedi EC, DiBiase SJ, Jabbour S, et al. Gamma knife stereotactic radiosurgery for patients with glioblastoma multiforme. Neurosurgery. 2002;50:41.

52. Souhami L, Seiferheld W, Brachman D, et al. Randomized comparison of stereotactic radiosurgery followed by conventional radiotherapy with carmustine to conventional radiotherapy with carmustine for patients with glioblastoma multiforme: report of Radiation Therapy Oncology Group 93-05 protocol. Int J Radiat Oncol Biol Phys. 2004;60:853.

53. Minniti G, Armosini V, Salvati M, et al. Fractionated stereotactic reirradiation and concurrent temozolomide in patients with recurrent glioblastoma. J Neurooncol. 2001;103:683.

54. Shaw E, Scott C, Souhami L, et al. Single dose radiosurgical treatment of recurrent previously irradiated primary brain tumors and brain metastases: final report of RTOG protocol 90-05. Int J Radiat Oncol Biol Phys. 2000;47:291.

55. Combs SE, Widmer V, Thilmann C, et al. Stereotactic radiosurgery (SRS): treatment option for recurrent glioblastoma multiforme (GBM). Cancer. 2005;104:2168.

56. Hall WA, Djalilian HR, Lamborn KR, et al. Stereotactic radiosurgery for recurrent malignant gliomas. J Clin Oncol. 1995;13:1642.

57. Laing RW, Warrington AP, Graham J, et al. Efficacy and toxicity of fractionated stereotactic radiotherapy in the treatment of recurrent gliomas (phase I/II study). Radiother Oncol. 1993;27:22.

58. Tsao MN, Mehta MP, Whelan TJ, et al. The American Society for Therapeutic Radiology and Oncology (ASTRO) evidence-based review of the role of radiosurgery for malignant glioma. Int J Radiat Oncol Biol Phys. 2005;63:47.

59. Sneed PK, Lamborn KR, Larson DA, et al. Demonstration of brachytherapy boost dose-response relationships in glioblastoma multiforme. Int J Radiat Oncol Biol Phys. 1996;35:37.

60. Selker RG, Shapiro WR, Burger P, et al. The Brain Tumor Cooperative Group NIH Trial 87-01: a randomized comparison of surgery, external radiotherapy, and carmustine versus surgery, interstitial radiotherapy boost, external radiation therapy, and carmustine. Neurosurgery. 2002;51:343.

61. Wilson CB, Larson DA, Gutin PH. Radiosurgery: a new application? J Clin Oncol. 1992;10:1373.

62. Ten Haken RK, Thornton AF Jr, Sandler HM, et al. A quantitative assessment of the addition of MRI to CT-based, 3-D treatment planning of brain tumors. Radiother Oncol. 1992;25:121.

63. Narayana A, Yamada J, Berry S, et al. Intensity-modulated radiotherapy in high-grade gliomas: clinical and dosimetric results. Int J Radiat Oncol Biol Phys. 2006;64:892.

64. Teoh M, Clark CH, Wood K, et al. Volumetric modulated arc therapy: a review of current literature and clinical use in practice. Br J Radiol. 2011;84:967.

65. Valk PE, Dillon WP. Radiation injury of the brain. AJNR Am J Neuroradiol. 1991;12:45.

66. Galban CJ, Chenevert TL, Meyer CR, et al. The parametric response map is an imaging biomarker for early cancer treatment outcome. Nat Med. 2009;15:572.

67. Tsien C, Galban CJ, Chenevert TL, et al. Parametric response map as an imaging biomarker to distinguish progression from pseudoprogression in high-grade glioma. J Clin Oncol. 2010;28:2293.

68. Verma N, Cowperthwaite MC, Burnett MG, et al. Differentiating tumor recurrence from treatment necrosis: a review of neurooncologic imaging strategies. Neuro Oncol. 2013;15:515.

69. Friedman HS, Prados MD, Wen PY, et al. Bevacizumab alone and in combination with irinotecan in recurrent glioblastoma. J Clin Oncol. 2009;27:4733.

70. Wick W, Brandes AA, Gorlia T, et al. EORTC 26101 phase III trial exploring the combination of bevacizumab and lomustine in patients with first progression of glioblastoma. J Clin Oncol. 2016;34(Suppl):abstr 2001.

71. Wick W, Puduvalli VK, Chamberlain MC, et al. Phase III study of enzastaurin compared with lomistine in the treatment of recurrent intracranial glioblastoma. J Clin Oncol. 2010;28:1168.

72. Batchelor TT, Mulholland P, Neyns B, et al. Phase III randomized trial comparing the efficacy of cediranib as monotherapy, and in combination with lomustine, versus lomustine alone in patients with recurrent glioblastoma. J Clin Oncol. 2013;31:3212.

73. Perry JR, Belanger K, Mason WP, et al. Phase II continuous dose-dense temozolmide in recurrent malignant glioma: RESCUE study. J Clin Oncol. 2051;2010:28.

74. Weller M, Tabatabai G, Kastner B, et al. MGMT promoter methylation is a strong prognostic biomarker for benefit from dose-intensified temozolomide rechallenge in progressive glioblastoma: the DIRECTOR trial. Clin Cancer Res. 2015;21:2057.

75. Hudes RS, Corn BW, Werner-Wasik M, et al. A phase I dose escalation study of hypofractionated stereotactic radiotherapy as salvage therapy for persistent or recurrent malignant glioma. Int J Radiat Oncol Biol Phys. 1999;43:293.

76. Kim HK, Thornton AF, Greenberg HS, et al. Results of re-irradiation of primary intracranial neoplasms with three-dimensional conformal therapy. Am J Clin Oncol. 1997;20:358.

77. Lederman G, Wronski M, Arbit E, et al. Treatment of recurrent glioblastoma multiforme using fractionated stereotactic radiosurgery and concurrent paclitaxel. Am J Clin Oncol. 2000;23:155.

78. Combs SE, Thilmann C, Edler L, et al. Efficacy of fractionated stereotactic reirradiation in recurrent gliomas: long-term results in 172 patients treated in a single institution. J Clin Oncol. 2005;23:8863.

79. Nieder C, Astner ST, Mehta MP, et al. Improvement, clinical course and quality of life after palliative radiotherapy for recurrent glioblastoma. Am J Clin Oncol. 2008;31:300.

80. Fogh SE, Andrews DW, Glass J, et al. Hypofractionated stereotactic radiation therapy: an effective therapy for recurrent high-grade gliomas. J Clin Oncol. 2010;28:3048.

81. Mayer R, Sminia P. Reirradiation tolerance of the human brain. Int J Radiat Oncol Biol Phys. 2008;70:1350.

82. Gutin PH, Iwamoto FM, Beal K, et al. Safety and efficacy of bevacizumab with hypofractionated stereotactic irradiation for recurrent malignant gliomas. Int J Radiat Oncol Biol Phys. 2009;75:156.

83. Brandsma D, Stalpers L, Taal W, et al. Clinical features, mechanisms, and management of pseudoprogression in malignant gliomas. Lancet Oncol. 2008;9(5):453–61.

84. Wen PY, Macdonald DR, Reardon DA, et al. Updated response assessment criteria for high-grade gliomas: response assessment in neuro-oncology working group. J Clin Oncol. 2010;28(11):1963–72.

85. Jiao Y, Killela PJ, Reitman ZJ, et al. Frequent ATRX, CIC, FUBP1 and IDH1 mutations refine the classification of malignant gliomas. Oncotarget. 2012;3(7):709–22.

86. Bettegowda C, Agrawal N, Jiao Y, et al. Mutations in CIC and FUBP1 contribute to human oligodendroglioma Science. 2011;333(6048):1453–5.

87. Van den Bent MJ, Gravendeel LA, Gorlia T, et al. A hypermethylated phenotype is a better predictor of survival than MGMT methylation in anaplastic oligodendroglial brain tumors: a report from EORTC study 26951. Clin Cancer Res. 2011;17(22):7148–55.

88. Carrillo JA, Lai A, Nghiemphu PL, et al. Relationship between tumor enhancement, edema, IDH1 mutational status, MGMT promoter methylation, and survival in glioblastoma. AJNR Am J Neuroradiol. 2012;33(7):1349–55.

89. Levin VA, Bidaut L, Hou P, et al. Randomized double-blind placebo-controlled trial of bevacizumab therapy for radiation necrosis of the central nervous system. Int J Radiat Oncol Biol Phys. 2011;79(5):1487–95.

# Part III

# Spine: Benign

# Schwannomas and Neurofibromas

# 7

## Marcello Marchetti, Elena De Martin, and Laura Fariselli

## Learning Objectives

- To understand the epidemiology, the pathology, the anatomical relationship, and the prognosis of spinal schwannomas and neurofibromas.
- To evaluate patients affected by spinal schwannomas and neurofibromas with a special emphasis on the clinical presentation and the radiology features.
- To understand the multimodal management of spinal schwannomas and neurofibromas.
- To understand the radiosurgical planning including dose, fractionation, and target delineation for patients with spinal schwannomas and neurofibromas.
- To understand the state of the art of the knowledge about radiosurgery for spinal schwannomas and neurofibromas.

## Epidemiology

Intradural tumors of the spine are rare, accounting overall for 10% of central nervous system (CNS) neoplasms in adults. Two thirds of these tumors are extramedullary, and they are usually benign with well-defined boundaries. Eighty percent are meningiomas or nerve sheath tumors [1–4].

Nerve sheath tumors include both schwannoma and neurofibroma. These account for almost one third of spinal neoplasms and approximately for the 25% of the intradural spinal tumors in adult patients. The main part of these is sporadic schwannomas [5–7]. They occur most frequently between the fourth and the sixth decades. Males and females are equally affected. Most schwannomas and neurofibromas are benign lesions, and treatment intent should be curative.

About the 2.5% of nerve sheath tumors are malignant, and about one half of these occur in neurofibromatosis patients. These tumors are not responsive to any treatment modality and the prognosis is extremely poor. They have to be distinguished from cellular schwannomas which have a locally aggressive behavior but a good prognosis [8].

Nerve sheath tumors are in general solitary, but multiple neurofibromas are relatively common in case of neurofibromatosis and represent an extremely challenging population to manage.

## Diagnosis

### Pathology, Anatomical Considerations, and Prognosis

Nerve sheath tumors include both schwannomas and neurofibromas. Electron microscopy, tissue culture studies, and immunohistochemistry demonstrate that both schwannomas and neurofibromas arise from Schwann cells that normally produce the insulating myelin sheath covering of the nerves. Under a morphological point of view, neurofibromas are more heterogeneous, and other perineural cells as well as fibroblasts are probably involved in their development.

Schwannomas and neurofibromas may have different histological and biological features.

Schwannomas in general appear as a smooth and globoid mass. They grow eccentrically from a single fiber of the nerve. Under a histological point of view, schwannomas (see Fig. 7.1) consist of elongated bipolar cells with fusiform, darkly staining nuclei usually arranged in compact interlacing fascicles that tend to palisade (Antoni A pattern) or that more rarely arrange in a stellate fashion (Antoni B pattern) [4].

Two rare types of schwannomas are the cellular schwannomas and the plexiform schwannomas.

The cellular type, also defined as hypercellular schwannoma, is a benign tumor, but it may have a high mitotic

M. Marchetti · E. De Martin · L. Fariselli (✉)
Radiotherapy Unit, Department of Neurosurgery,
C. Besta Neurological Institute Foundation, Milan, Italy
e-mail: laura.fariselli@istituto-besta.it

© Springer International Publishing AG, part of Springer Nature 2018
E. L. Chang et al. (eds.), *Adult CNS Radiation Oncology*, https://doi.org/10.1007/978-3-319-42878-9_7

**Fig. 7.1** Schwannoma: typical elements, with elongated nuclei in a different way oriented, are represented. [Courtesy of Bianca Pollo, MD, Neuropathology Unit, Foundation Neurological Institute, Milan, Italy.]

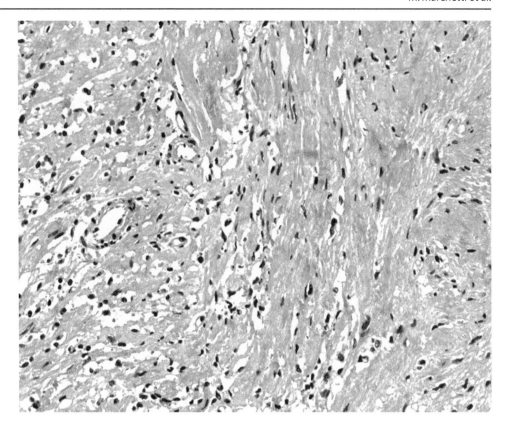

activity (also ≥10 mitoses per 10 HPF). For this type of schwannoma, recurrences and local aggressiveness are not uncommon clinical features, and the most common location is at a paravertebral site. Plexiform schwannomas generally involve multiple nerve fascicles or the nerve plexus. Despite the high rate of growth, the hypercellularity, and the increased mitotic activity, the behavior of these tumors is benign. A rare association with the neurofibromatosis type 2 is known, and the location along the spine is uncommon.

The neurofibroma stroma, different from the schwannomas, consists of abundant fibrous tissue and nervous fibers [9]. Moreover, neurofibromas usually determine a fusiform enlargement of the involved nerve root. In general, it is nearly impossible to distinguish between the normal nerve and the tumor (Fig. 7.2).

The prognosis of neurofibromas is in general good, but the potential transformation of such lesions into malignant peripheral nerve sheath tumors (about 5% of the total) has to be considered. Although most of the nerve sheath tumors arise from the dorsal root, a ventral origin is relatively more frequent for the neurofibromas. Although these tumors are usually completely intradural, a percentage in the order of 10% to the 15% may have an intradural-extradural characteristic (i.e., dumbbell-shaped tumors) [5].

Only 1% of the nerve sheath tumors are intramedullary. In such cases, the tumor probably arises from the nerves accompanying the spinal cord vasculature. Among them, about 10% are epidural or paravertebral. Subpial extension is rare and more frequently observed in those cases of plexiform neurofibromas.

## Clinical Features

The signs and the symptoms from spinal nerve sheath tumors can be extremely variable, and it is not rare that patients are asymptomatic. Pain is the more common symptom. If present, the level at which it is perceived, as well as its distribution, is characteristic for the tumor site. Neurologic symptoms are less frequent and generally follow the pain development.

Cervical tumors are usually associated with cervical pain irradiating along the arm of the lesion side. Arm weakness and numbness are also possible. Thoracic tumors may produce long-tract signs with the corticospinal tract more commonly affected. Progressive paraparesis, spasticity, and sensory gait ataxia can be observed, and in the case of thoracic spinal involvement, the pain typically has a typical dermatomal distribution. Lumbosacral tumors are in general responsible for back pain with or without a radiating component involving the

**Fig. 7.2** Neurofibroma: the cytology varies from cells with spindle-shaped nuclei to cells with relatively rounded nuclei. Presence of some collagen bundles. [Courtesy of Bianca Pollo, MD, Neuropathology Unit, Foundation Neurological Institute, Milan, Italy.]

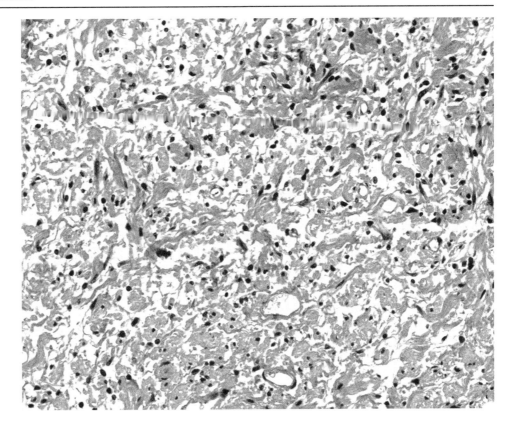

legs. Distal weakness and numbness of one leg usually follow initial pain.

## Radiology

At the state of art, the diagnosis of nerve sheath tumors of the spine is most likely based on magnetic resonance imaging (MRI). Indeed, MRI provides an optimal spatial and contrast resolution of neural and perineural structures. Computerized tomography (CT) images may be useful to integrate the MRI ones (e.g., to search for calcifications in order to differentiate a meningioma from a schwannoma). CT may be useful as in the presence of bone remodeling; this can help diagnose an indolent type of nerve sheath tumor. Radiographs as well as myelography are nowadays generally considered as outdated.

In general, nerve sheath tumors are hypo-isointense relatively to the spinal cord on T1-weighted MR images and hyperintense on T2-weighted MR images. After gadolinium injection, they usually show a more or less homogenous enhancement (Fig. 7.3).

Despite the availability of MR imaging, the distinction between schwannomas and neurofibromas can nonetheless be difficult. Cysts, hemorrhages, and a heterogeneous con-trast enhancement are more common in cases of schwanno-mas. A more homogeneous contrast enhancement, the "target sign," and the presence of multiple lesions may be more sug-gestive of neurofibroma.

Other pathologies which have to be considered for the differential diagnosis are meningiomas, myxopapillary ependy-moma, meningocele, extruded disc fragment, chronic inflammatory demyelinating polyneuropathy (CIDP), and, in general, all the other causes of multiple enlarged enhancing spinal nerve (Fig. 7.4).

## Treatment Strategy

The treatment strategy for nerve sheath tumors of the spine includes surgery and radiotherapy. There has yet to be any evidence to support systemic chemotherapy, and efficacy with some novel targeted agents like bevacizumab can be only speculated.

The first-choice treatment for most benign intradural extramedullary spinal lesions, including nerve sheath tumors, is microsurgical resection, the safety and effectiveness of which are well documented in literature [7, 10–13]. Despite this, in selected cases, the most appropriate treatment option is yet to be defined. In particular, in cases of recurrent, resid-

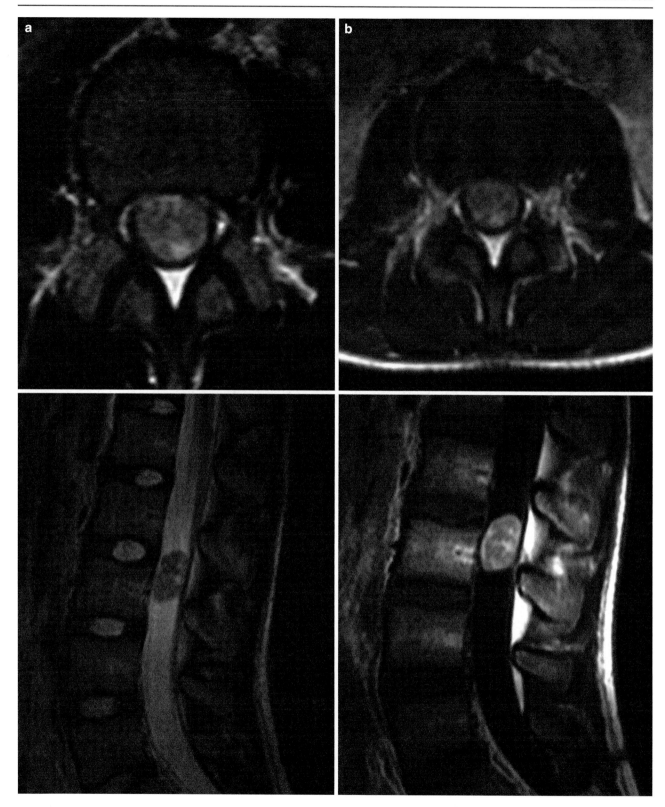

**Fig. 7.3** L3 schwannoma Axial and sagittal T2-weighted images (**a**) show relative hyperintense signal of the lumbar neuroma. The axial and sagittal T1 gadolinium images (**b**) show the relatively homogeneous contrast enhancement

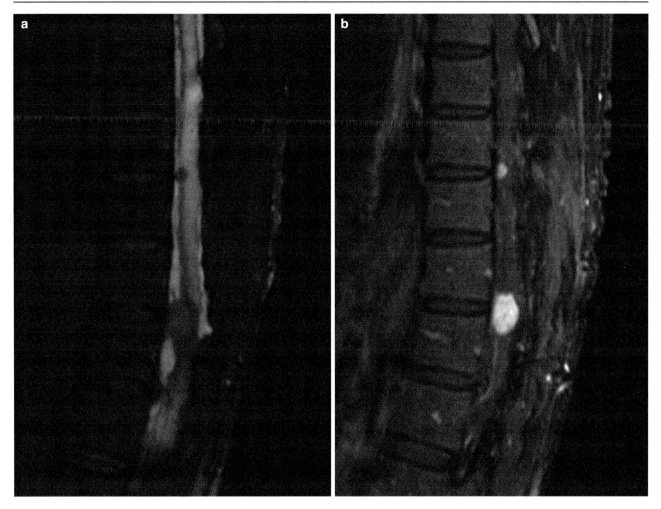

**Fig. 7.4** Multiple thoracic neurofibromas. The MRI distinction between schwannomas and neurofibromas can be often extremely difficult if not impossible. A more homogeneous contrast enhancement and the presence of multiple lesions usually suggest the diagnosis of neurofibroma. T2-weighted image is presented in **a** and T1 contrast-enhanced image in **b**

ual, or multiple lesions (as for family phakomatoses), or when a patient has undergone a previous conventional fractionated radiotherapy course, the appropriateness of a surgical approach may be debated. Moreover, some patients are less than ideal candidates for an open surgical procedure, due to comorbidity or poor clinical condition.

In these cases, radiotherapy and radiosurgery could represent an interesting treatment alternative.

## Radiotherapy

The role of the radiotherapy for many malignancies of the spine is well established. However, there is always concern about radiation myelopathy especially when radiating the spine as to spinal cord tolerance. With improved understanding of the tolerance, it is well known that radiation can be delivered safely to the spine with a low risk (<1%) of radiation myelopathy especially for nerve sheath tumors that do

not need dose escalation beyond 45 Gy to 54 Gy in 1.8 Gy/day fraction sizes [14–20]. A dedicated chapter to radiation tolerance is presented in this book (see Chap. 37). However, the risk of radiation-induced secondary malignancies is always concerning especially in younger patients with benign disorders. Lastly, there is always a small risk of radiation-induced transformation, and this may be more relevant to those with neurofibromatosis.

## Radiosurgery

In 1994, Flickinger defined radiosurgery as a technique which utilizes multiple narrow radiation beams directed stereotactically to produce radiobiological effects within a carefully defined and small volume [21]. At present, it is generally accepted that radiosurgery allows the delivery of high doses of radiation also for targets which develop in close proximity to radiosensitive critical organs at risk. Stereotactic radiosur-

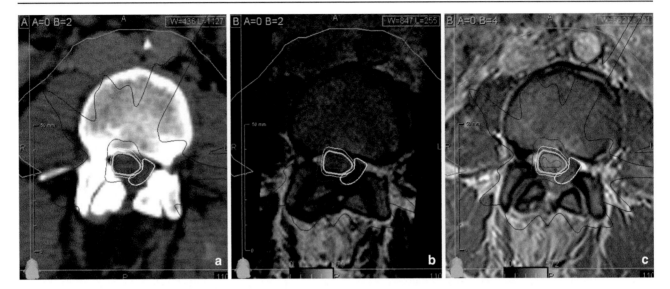

**Fig. 7.5** Target and OAR definition. The treatment plans are, in general, CT based (**a**). One or more MRI sequences are usually fused to the primary exam to optimize the definition of both the planning target vol-ume (PTV) and the OARs. In **b** and **c** T2 1 mm 3D MRI and T1 contrast-enhanced 1 mm 3D MRI sequences are, respectively, showed

gery has proven safe and effective in treating many benign neoplasms of the skull base [22–25].

In this sense, radiosurgery appears to be the ideal treatment alternative for the patients affected by a benign intradural extramedullary tumor who are not suitable for an open surgery or who present recurrences or remnants. In selected cases, radiosurgery can be considered also as a primary treatment modality. In these cases radiosurgery could represent an interesting treatment alternative.

The first radiosurgical delivery systems were frame-based and therefore unable to treat extracranial targets, but, more recently, the problems related to the positioning/repositioning of the patients and the problems related to the precision of the treatment delivery have been, at least in part, overtaken by many systems. Studies inherent to the precision of the different radiosurgical devices suggest that all are able to deliver radiosurgery to the spine with a high degree of precision [26–28]. A dedicated chapter to spine radiosurgery, also referred to stereotactic body radiotherapy (SBRT), is presented in this book (see Chap. 46).

Given that the procedure is not based on an invasive frame for immobilization, like most skull-based radiosurgery procedures, and the spinal cord is adjacent to the tumor, radiosurgery for benign intradural extramedullary spinal lesions has received much less attention. In particular, little was known as to the tolerance of the spinal cord with radiosurgery and with the long life expectancy of these patients, concern about delayed radiation myelopathy was of primary importance. With a far greater understanding of safe doses of radiation to the spinal cord with radiosurgery, there has been increasing, but limited, experience for nerve sheath tumors [29–37] that suggests both safety and efficacy specific to schwannomas and neurofibromas of the spine.

## Indications

Radiosurgery should be considered in cases of residual or recurrent intradural extramedullary lesions of the spine. Radiosurgery can also be considered for patients that are less than optimal candidates for an open surgery due to comorbidities, previous radiotherapy, or age-related limits. Finally, in the light of the results from the most recent clinical series, radiosurgery could be considered as a primary treatment modality, after a multidisciplinary discussion, in case of tumors for which a complete removal is not achievable, or it could be considered also to take into account a patient's preference. Contraindications to radiosurgery are rapidly progressing neurological deficit due to spinal cord compression and/or a clear vertebral instability.

## Target Delineation and Treatment Schedule

Definitive guidelines for contouring the treatment targets and the organs at risk (OARs) are not yet established. In general, treatment plans are CT based with one or more MRI sequences fused to the primary exam to better define the gross tumor volume (GTV), planning target volume (PTV), and the OARs. In such cases, volumetric sequences are generally preferred (Figs. 7.5 and 7.6).

Many authors define the PTV as the tumor volume without margins, while some others prefer to apply a minimal margin (1–3 mm) to compensate for the setup errors.

There is also no general consensus about the treatment schedule. At present experience varies with respect to a single (sRS) or a multisession radiosurgery (mRS). sRS may be

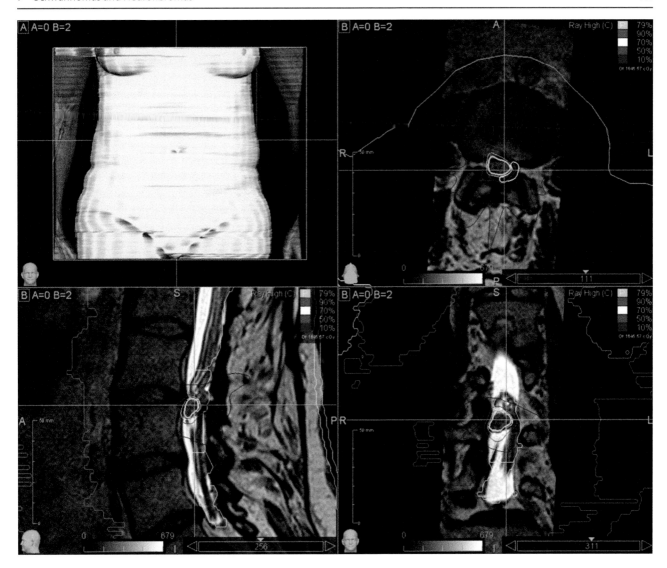

**Fig. 7.6** Treatment plan. A L3 schwannoma together with the dose distribution is presented on the three T2 MRI plans

useful to overcome repositioning-related uncertainty, while mRS may optimize the ratio between the dose to the target and the OAR sparing. At the state of the art, there are no comparative studies about sRS and mRS.

## Clinical Experiences

The literature regarding radiosurgery for the spinal schwannomas and neurofibromas is still extremely poor but growing slowly. In general, the data are limited in terms of follow-up and in the number of patients. Moreover, the studies generally include a mixed cohort of benign intradural extramedullary tumors of the spine as opposed to only nerve sheath tumors. Despite these limits, the first experiences confirm the short-term efficacy and safety of radiosurgery and suggest a potential interest also for the long-term results.

In 2007, Sahgal et al. [29] reported their first series of 16 consecutive patients with 19 benign spinal tumors, including 11 neurofibromas, treated with radiosurgery. The mean dose

was 26,7 Gy delivered in 1–5 fractions. After a median follow-up period of 25 months, tumor control was quite good. Two neurofibromas in two neurofibromatosis type 1 patients were not controlled by the treatment, confirming a worse prognosis for such patients. After a detailed dose/volume analysis, the authors suggest that the traditional dose limit to the spinal cord appears too restrictive and that the maximum dose to a small volume can be increased.

The results from the 2008 Pittsburg series [30] confirmed optimal tumor growth control. The authors reported on 73 benign tumors, including 35 schwannomas and 25 neurofibromas. All but one patient had single-fraction treatment, with a mean prescription dose of 21 Gy. In this experience, all the tumors were stable or reduced in size after a mean period of 37 months. Considering the patients treated specifically for a schwannoma, the authors report that of the 17 patients for whom pain was the primary indication, 14 experienced significant pain improvement based on the visual analog score. A single patient underwent an open surgical removal of a C8 tumor because of significant numbness in the dominant hand. Of the seven lesions for which radiosurgery was used as the primary treatment, a single patient underwent open surgical resection of the lesion at another institution after the development of significant numbness in the S1 nerve root distribution territory. None of the lesions treated for radiological progression after open surgical resection showed further radiological progression. Finally, for the five patients who were treated for neurological deficits, three improved, one stabilized, and one patient with NF and a large C1 tumor underwent open surgical resection. With respect to the neurofibroma cases, the authors report that 20 out of 25 cases were associated with NF1. Tumor progression was not demonstrated in a single case. Of the 13 patients treated for pain resulting from a specific neurofibroma, eight patients experienced improvement. In three cases, all with NF type 1, two demonstrated temporary improvement in their pain, and one patient subsequently underwent the placement of a morphine pump. For the four patients treated with radiosurgery for myelopathy caused by a cervical neurofibroma (all suffering for NF1), two patients had a clear improvement in walking ability, and two patients had stabilization of their myelopathy. In this study and in many others, NF was predictive of a worse outcome. Three patients (two schwannomas) experienced radiation-induced myelopathy, but it was not possible to identify specific prognostic factors.

Selch et al. [32] described the experience of the University of California, Los Angeles (UCLA) specific to benign peripheral nerve sheath tumors treated with radiosurgery with a median follow-up period of 18 months. Twenty-five tumors had a radiosurgery treatment with a mean marginal dose of 12 G delivered in a single session. The authors didn't split the tumors per histology, but they indicated that eight patients suffered for a neurofibromatosis (four NF1 and four NF2). The observation period is short, but the local control appears to be excellent and the toxicity only transient.

In 2011, the Stanford group [34] updated their previous publication [33]. The authors reported on 130 benign intradural extramedullary tumors of the spine of which 47 were schwannomas and 24 neurofibromas. The delivered dose ranged from 14 to 30 Gy in 1 to 5 fractions. Nine patients had a diagnosis of NF1 and 14 patients of NF2. During the mean follow-up of 33 months, only one schwannoma showed a radiological progression 73 months after radiosurgery and underwent open surgery. Seven other patients from the series (one meningioma, two neurofibromas, and four schwannomas) underwent a surgical resection mainly due to the persistency of the symptoms. Four out of these seven patients (one neurofibroma and three schwannomas) reported some degree of improvement. Only one patient developed a transient myelitis.

In 2012, Gerszten et al. [35] reported a further series, but, in this case, a second radiosurgical device was utilized. From this series of 45 tumors, 16 were schwannomas and 14 were neurofibromas. The dose if a sRS was delivered ranged from 11 to 17 Gy; the dose ranged from 18 to 21 Gy if three fractions were delivered. Nine patients had a diagnosis of NF. No tumor progressed given a mean follow-up of 43 months. The authors did not report any complications.

Our group reported our first series of patients treated because of a benign lesion of the spine in 2013 [36]. The dose ranged from 10 to 13 Gy for the sRS patients and from 20 to 25 Gy when a mRS was delivered. This series include nine schwannomas and one neurofibroma, and none of these (including the five patients affected by NF) showed tumor progression at the site of the treatment (mean follow-up of 43 months). Clinical outcomes with respect to neurological symptoms and pain were favorable, and toxicity was not observed.

Shin et al. in 2015 [37] reported a series of 58 patients (110 tumors) treated by radiosurgery. Of these, 92 were benign neurogenic lesions (69 schwannomas and 23 neurofibromas). The mean prescribed dose was 13 Gy for the sRS and 25 Gy for the mRS (up to five fractions). Sixty-five out of these 92 lesions had a radiological volumetric evaluation which revealed that only three lesions increased in volume after radiosurgery. One out of these three patients showed a good tumor control for 4 years but eventually developed a late-onset intratumoral necrotic cyst enlargement during an 8-year follow-up. In the other cases, progression was observed earlier.

The main features of the presented studies are summarized in Table 7.1.

## Toxicity

While we are waiting for more definitive data with respect to spinal cord tolerance, the results from the clinical series (see Table 7.1) indicate a very low rate of radiation-induced toxicity. Interestingly, the reported experiences suggest that the toxicity is not always related to a high level of delivered radiation dose. A dedicated chapter to radiation myelopathy and dose limits for radiosurgery is presented in this book (Chap. 37).

## Case Study

A 38-year-old lady came to our attention in 2012 because of a right C3 neurofibroma. The MRI at the presentation time showed an initial spinal cord compression but without spinal cord alterations on the T2-weighted sequences (see Fig. 7.7a). Other lesions were observed along the lower cranial nerve and at C1 level. The neurological assessment evidenced a very mild paraparesis. A Babinski's sign was not elicitable. Due to the relatively large volume (about 1 cc) and the relationship

**Table 7.1** The main literature series data are reported

| Authors | Schwannomas Neurofibromas (#) | NF (pts) | Mean F-UP range (months) | Volume mean median range (cc) | System | Mean prescription dose (Gy) | Fraction (#) | Local control (%) | Toxicity |
|---|---|---|---|---|---|---|---|---|---|
| Sahgal et al. (2007) [29] | 0 schwannoma 11 neurofibromas | NF1 (3) | 25 | – | CK | 26,7 (15,4–59,7) | 1–5 | Three cases PD (two neurofibromas in NF1) | – |
| Gerszten et al. (2008) [30] | 35 schwannomas 25 neurofibromas | NF1 (21) NF2 (9) | 37 | 10,5 4,11 0,3–93,4 | CK | 21 (15–25) | 1 | 100 | 3 pts |
| Selch et al. (2009) [32] | All PNST | NF1 (4) NF2 (4) | 18 (median) 12–58 | – 2,1 0,9–4,1 | Novalis | 12 (marginal dose) | 1 | 100 (28% PR) | 2 pts. (transitory) |
| Sachdev et al. (2011) [34] | 47 schwannomas 24 neurofibromas | NF1 (11) NF2 (20) | 33 | 5,2 2,2 0,05–54,5 | CK | 19,4 (14–30) | 1–5 | 99 one schwannoma | 1 pt. transient myelitis |
| Gerszten et al. (2012) [35] | 16 schwannomas 14 neurofibromas | 9 NF | 26 (median) | 13,2 5,1 0,37–94,5 | Synergy | sRS 14 (11–17) mSRS 18–21 | 1 (or 3) | 100 | 0 |
| Marchetti et al. (2013) [36] | 9 schwannomas 1 neurofibroma | NF1 (2) NF2 (3) | 43 32–73 | 11,8 2,6 0,2–138 | CK | sRS 10–13 mSRS 20–25 | 1–6 | 100 (25% PR) | 0 |
| Shin et al. (2015) [37] | 69 schwannomas 23 neurofibromas | NF1 (7) | 43 12–137 | 12 0.03–340 | Novalis | sRS 13 mRS 25 | 1–5 | 95.4 | 0 |

The literature regarding radiosurgery for the spinal schwannomas has been increasing during the last few years. The mean follow-up is still too short (range 18–43 months) to lead to conclusive data. Despite this, preliminary results are at least interesting, being the local control always higher than 85% and the toxicity very limited or absent

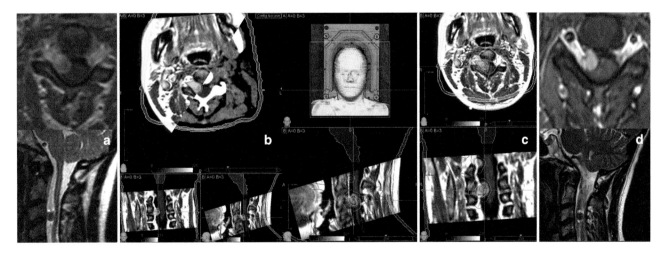

**Fig. 7.7** The MRI images and the treatment plan of the case study are represented. The MRI at the presentation time showed C3–C4 and C1 neurofibromas. The main tumor (C3–C4) was characterized by an initial spinal cord compression but without spinal cord alterations on the T2-weighted sequences (see **a**). The tumors and the OARs were drawn by fusing the CT and the MRI images, and the PTV was defined as the tumor volume without margins (see **b**). The calculated treatment plan and dose distribution are presented in section **c**. In section **d**, the 48-month posttreatment MRI suggests a stabilization of the disease

between the lesion and the spinal cord, we decided to administer a radiosurgical treatment also in the absence of clear evidence of tumor progression. Due to the relative proximity of the little C1 lesion, we decided to treat both the neurofibromas in order to obtain a better control of the sum of the doses.

The tumors and the OARs were drawn by fusing the CT and the MRI images. The PTV was defined as the tumor volume without margins (see Fig. 7.7b). 25 Gy in five fractions to the 80% (including the 95% of the PTV) were then administered. The max point dose per fraction to the spinal cord was 4.9 Gy; the D1.2 cc, D1.0 cc, and D0.25 cc, per fraction, were, respectively, 1.2 Gy, 1.3 Gy, and 3 Gy. The treatment plan and dose distribution are presented in section c. About 48 months posttreatment, the tumor volume was stable (see Fig. 7.7d), and so the neurological conditions were maintained. No acute or delayed toxicity was detected.

## Summary

- Although there is a general low level of evidence, the current literature suggests that radiosurgery is effective to control both schwannomas and neurofibromas of the spine.
- The effective doses, both for sRS and mRS, have to be better defined.
- While we are waiting for more definitive results about the spinal cord tolerance, the published series suggest an acceptable rate of radiation-induced myelopathy.
- Long- and very long-term studies (10 and 20 years) are needed to definitively support the results, in terms of both effectiveness and safety. Despite this, radiosurgery may be considered in the range of treatment options used to manage benign tumors of the spine, including schwannomas and neurofibromas, also as a primary treatment modality.
- Almost all the studies indicate that radiosurgery is effective to control the pain associated with these tumors.
- The impact of radiosurgery on neurological symptoms has to be better explored. It is well known that radiosurgery may improve the clinical condition, and this is true also when the response to the treatment is a stabilization of the lesions. On the other hand, we do not know the specific prognostic factors useful to identify which patients will improve. Moreover, the neurological outcome is more difficult to characterize. Most patients may have undergone surgery prior to radiosurgery, which complicates the differentiation between disease progression-related symptoms, surgical sequelae, and radiosurgical complications. Other patients (e.g., those with neurofibromatosis) suffer from progressive disease and progressive neurology, which again makes it difficult to isolate the cause of a neurological worsening.

- Neurofibromatosis patients tend to have a worse prognosis. The impact of radiosurgery on the treated lesions in these patients shows some differences among the various studies and has to be better investigated. However, the generally good results, also when compared to the open surgery, together with its low invasive nature, make radiosurgery particularly suitable for these subjects.

## Self-Assessment Questions

1. When do the schwannomas occur more frequently?
   A. In the childhood
   B. Between the fourth and the sixth decades
   C. Between the second and the third decades
   D. After the seventh decade
   E. None of the above mentioned

2. Which of the following statement is true?
   A. The nerve sheath tumors include both the schwannomas and the neurofibromas.
   B. The schwannomas grow eccentrically from a single fiber of the nerve. They consist of elongated bipolar cells with fusiform, darkly staining nuclei usually arranged in compact interlacing fascicles that tend to palisade (Antoni A pattern) or that more rarely arrange in a stellate fashion (Antoni B pattern).
   C. The plexiform schwannomas generally involve multiple nerve fascicles or the nerve plexus.
   D. The neurofibroma stroma consists of abundant fibrous tissue and nervous fibers.
   E. All the above mentioned.

3. What about the hypercellular schwannomas?
   A. They do not exist.
   B. They are a rare type of schwannomas. They are benign tumors, but they may have a high mitotic activity (also ≥10 mitoses per 10 HPF).
   C. The recurrences are impossible.
   D. They are malignant nerve sheath tumors.
   E. They usually are intramedullary.

4. Which are the MRI differences between schwannomas and neurofibromas?
   A. The MRI signal is hyperintense in the T1-weighted images for the schwannomas, and it is hypo-intense in case of neurofibromas.
   B. The schwannomas uptake the MRI contrast agent, while the neurofibromas don't uptake the contrast.
   C. The MRI distinction between schwannomas and neurofibromas can be often extremely difficult if not impossible. A more homogeneous contrast enhance-

ment and the presence of multiple lesions usually suggest the diagnosis of neurofibromas.

D. Radiograph and myelography are nowadays more specific to distinguish between schwannomas and neurofibromas.

E. None of the above mentioned.

5. Which kind of treatments should be considered to treat the schwannomas and neurofibromas of the spine?
   A. Surgery and radiosurgery.
   B. Only the multisession radiosurgery.
   C. Surgery and adjuvant radiotherapy.
   D. They do not require any treatments.
   E. None of the above mentioned.

## Answers

1. B
2. E
3. B
4. C
5. A

## References

1. Guidetti B, Fortuna A. Differential diagnosis of intramedullary and extramedullary tumours. In: Vinken PJ, Bruyn JW, editors. Handbook of clinical neurology. Amsterdam: Elsevier; 1975. p. 51–75.
2. Guidetti B, Mercuri S, Vagnozzi R. Long term results of the surgical treatment of 129 intramedullary spinal gliomas. J Neurosurg. 1981;54:323–30.
3. Weinstein JN, McLain RF. Tumor of the spine. In: Rothman RH, Simeone FA, editors. The spine, vol 1, vol. 1992. Philadelphia: WB Saunders; 1992. p. 1639–54.
4. Kernohan JW, Sayre GP. Tumours of the central nervous system. Fascicle 35. Washington, DC: Armed Forces, Institute of Pathology; 1952.
5. Nittner K. Spinal meningiomas, neurinomas and neurofibromas, and hourglass tumours. In: Vinken PH, Bruyn GW, editors. Handbook of clinical neurology. New York: Elsevier; 1976. p. 177–322.
6. Levy WJ, Latchaw J, Hahn JF. Spinal neurofibromas: a report of 66 cases and a comparison with meningiomas. Neurosurgery. 1986;18:331–4.
7. Seppala M, Haltia M, Sankila R, et al. Long term outcome after removal of spinal schwannoma: a clinicopathological study of 187 cases. J Neurosurg. 1995;83:621–6.
8. Seppala MT, Haltia MJJ. Spinal malignant nerve sheath tumor or cellular schwannoma? A striking difference in prognosis. J Neurosurg. 1993;79:528–32.
9. Russel DS, Rubinstein LJ. Pathology of tumors of the central nervous system. Baltimore: Williams & Wilkins; 1989. p. 192–214.
10. Conti P, Pansini G, Mouchaty H, et al. Spinal neurinomas retrospective analysis and long-term outcome of 179 consecutively operated cases and review of the literature. Surg Neurol. 2004;61:34–43.
11. Klekamp J, Samii M. Surgery of spinal nerve sheath tumors with special reference to neurofibromatosis. Neurosurgery. 1998;42(2):279–89.
12. Parsa A, Lee J, Parney I, et al. Spinal cord and intradural–extraparenchymal spinal tumors: current best care practices and strategies. J Neurooncol. 2004;69:291–318.
13. Seppala M, Haltia M, Sankila R, et al. Long-term outcome after removal of spinal neurofibroma. J Neurosurg. 1995;82(4):572–7.
14. Abbatucci JS, Delozier T, Quint R, et al. Radiation myelopathy of the spinal cervical cord: time, dose and volume factors. Int J Radiat Oncol Biol Phys. 1978;4:239–48.
15. Burman C, Kutcher GJ, Emami B, et al. Fitting of normal tissue tolerance data to an analytic function. Int J Radiat Oncol Biol Phys. 1991;21(1):123–35.
16. Kopelson G, Linggood RM, Keinman GM, et al. Management of intramedullary spinal cord tumors. Radiology. 1980;135:473–9.
17. McCunnif AJ, Liang MJ. Radiation tolerance of the cervical spinal cord. Int J Radiat Oncol Biol Phys. 1989;16:675–8.
18. Phillips TL, Buschke F. Radiation tolerance of the thoracic spinal cord. Am J Roentgenol Radium Ther Nucl Med. 1969;105(3):659–64.
19. Schultheiss TE, Kun LE, Ang KK, et al. Radiation response of the central nervous system. Int J Radiat Oncol Biol Phys. 1995;31:1093–112.
20. Kirkpatrick JP, van der Kogel AJ, Schultheiss TE. Radiation dose-volume effects in the spinal cord. Int J Radiat Oncol Biol Phys. 2010;76(3 Suppl):S42–9.
21. Flickinger JC, Loeffler JS, Larson DA. Stereotactic radiosurgery for intracranial malignancies. Oncology (Williston Park). 1994;8(1):81–6.
22. Kondziolka D, Nathoo N, Flickinger JC. Long term results after radiosurgery for benign intracranial tumors. Neurosurgery. 2003;53:815–22.
23. Murphy ES, Barnett GH, Vogelbaum MA, et al. Long-term outcomes of Gamma Knife radiosurgery in patients with vestibular schwannomas. J Neurosurg. 2011;114(2):432–40.
24. Santacroce A, Walier M, Régis J, et al. Long-term tumor control of benign intracranial meningiomas after radiosurgery in a series of 4565 patients. Neurosurgery. 2012;70(1):32–9.
25. Tamura M, Carron R, Yomo S, et al. Hearing preservation after gamma knife radiosurgery for vestibular schwannomas presenting with high-level hearing. Neurosurgery. 2009;64(2):289–96.
26. Yu C, Main W, Taylor D, et al. An anthropomorphic phantom study of the accuracy of Cyberknife spinal radiosurgery. Neurosurgery. 2004;55(5):1138–49.
27. Yin FF, Ryu S, Ajlouni M, et al. A technique of intensity-modulated radiosurgery (IMRS) for spinal tumors. Med Phys. 2002;29:2815–22.
28. Gerszten PC, Novotny J Jr, Quader M, et al. Prospective evaluation of a dedicated spine radiosurgery program using the Elekta Synergy S system. J Neurosurg. 2010;113(Suppl):236–421.
29. Sahgal A, Chou D, Ames C, et al. Image-guided robotic stereotactic body radiotherapy for benign spinal tumors: the University of California San Francisco preliminary experience. Technol Cancer Res Treat. 2007;6(6):595–604.
30. Gerszten PC, Burton SA, Ozhasoglu C, et al. Radiosurgery for benign intradural spinal tumors. Neurosurgery. 2008;62(4):887–95.
31. Gerszten PC, Quader M, Novotny et al. Radiosurgery for benign tumors of the spine: clinical experience and current trends. Technol Cancer Res Treat. 2012;11(2):133–9.
32. Selch MT, Lin K, Agazaryan N, et al. Initial clinical experience with image-guided linear accelerator-based spinal radiosurgery for treatment of benign nerve sheath tumors. Surg Neurol. 2009;72(6):668–74.

33. Dodd RL, Ryu MR, Kamnerdsupaphon P, et al. CyberKnife radiosurgery for benign intradural extramedullary spinal tumors. Neurosurgery. 2006;58(4):674–85.

34. Sachdev S, Dodd RL, Chang SD, et al. Stereotactic radiosurgery yields long-term control for benign intradural, extramedullary spinal tumors. Neurosurgery. 2011;69(3):533–9.

35. Gerszten PC, Chen S, Quader M, et al. Radiosurgery for benign tumors of the spine using the Synergy S with cone-beam computed tomography image guidance. J Neurosurg. 2012;117(Suppl):197–202.

36. Marchetti M, De Martin E, Milanesi I, et al. Intradural extramedullary benign spinal lesions radiosurgery. Medium- to long-term results from a single institution experience. Acta Neurochir. 2013;155(7):1215–22.

37. Shin DW, Sohn MJ, Kim HS, et al. Clinical analysis of spinal stereotactic radiosurgery in the treatment of neurogenic tumors. J Neurosurg Spine. 2015;23(4):429–37.

# Spinal Meningioma

**8**

Nima Alan, John C. Flickinger, and Peter Carlos Gerszten

## Learning Objectives

- Understand the epidemiology, risk factors, and natural history of spinal meningiomas.
- Evaluate patients for multimodal management of spinal meningiomas.
- Understand the radiosurgical planning including dose, fractionation, and target delineation for patients with spinal meningiomas.
- Evaluate patients with spinal meningiomas for complications associated with radiosurgery.

## Epidemiology

Tumors of the spine are classified based on their anatomic relationship with the dura and the spinal cord. Spinal meningiomas are benign intradural extramedullary tumors of the spine accounting for up to 25–46% of primary spinal neoplasms [1]. They may also have an extradural component. Spinal meningiomas derive from the arachnoid cap cells, similar to their intracranial counterparts, and comprise 7.5–12.7% of all meningiomas [2]. They usually present in the fifth to seventh decade of life and are more common in women with a female/male ratio between 3 and 4.2:1 [3]. This preponderance in females has been attributed to sex hormones, as suggested by the presence of various hormone receptors in meningiomas [4]. After accounting for the relative length of the thoracic spine to the entire human spine, spinal meningiomas predominantly occur in the thoracic spine (up to 75%), with the cervical spine being the second most common location (20%). The tendency to involve the thoracic spine is true for women; in men, the thoracic and cervical location of spinal meningiomas are almost equally represented [5].

Complete or partial loss of chromosome 22 has been reported in patients with spinal meningioma. Although patients with neurofibromatosis type 2 have a mutation or deletion of the NF2 gene located on chromosome 22, and despite a propensity for these patients to develop intracranial meningiomas, spinal meningiomas are uncommon in this patient population [6].

## Diagnosis and Prognosis

Due to the slow growth of spinal meningiomas, patients often present with symptoms that may have had persisted for various periods of time, with a mean duration of symptoms of 1–2 years [3, 6, 7]. Presenting symptoms of spinal meningiomas are due to local compressive effect on neural elements (e.g., spinal cord, cauda equina, or nerve roots) manifesting as localized back pain, myelopathy, or sensorimotor radiculopathy depending upon the level of the tumor within the spine.

The diagnosis of spinal meningiomas is made most easily by magnetic resonance (MR) imaging. Spinal meningiomas are isointense to spinal cord on T1 and T2 sequences with homogenous contrast enhancement with gadolinium [8, 9]. Subtle imaging characteristics allow one to distinguish spinal meningiomas from schwannomas and neurofibromas, as the former characteristically has a "dural tail," best observed on coronal

N. Alan
Department of Neurological Surgery, University of Pittsburgh
Medical Center, Pittsburgh, PA, USA

J. C. Flickinger
Department of Radiation Oncology, UPMC Presbyterian-
Shadyside Hospital, University of Pittsburgh School of Medicine,
Pittsburgh, PA, USA

P. C. Gerszten (✉)
Department of Neurological Surgery, University of Pittsburgh
Medical Center, Pittsburgh, PA, USA

Department of Radiation Oncology, University of Pittsburgh
Medical Center, Pittsburgh, PA, USA
e-mail: gersztenpc@upmc.edu

© Springer International Publishing AG, part of Springer Nature 2018
E. L. Chang et al. (eds.), *Adult CNS Radiation Oncology*, https://doi.org/10.1007/978-3-319-42878-9_8

**Table 8.1** World Health Organization (WHO) classification of meningiomas

| WHO grade I Benign | WHO grade II Atypical | WHO grade III Malignant |
|---|---|---|
| Meningothelial | Chordoid | Papillary |
| Fibrous | Clear cell | Rhabdoid |
| Transitional | Atypical | Anaplastic |
| Psammomatous | | |
| Microcystic | | |
| Secretory | | |
| Lymphoplasmacytic | | |
| Metaplastic | | |

images. Unlike schwannomas and neurofibromas, meningiomas rarely exit through the neural foramen [6–8]. In addition, spinal meningiomas enhance less avidly compared to the other aforementioned intradural extramedullary tumors [6–8].

The definitive diagnosis of spinal meningioma, much like any other tumor of the central nervous system, is made by histopathological examination. The World Health Organization (WHO) classification of meningiomas, last updated in 2016 [10], is summarized in Table 8.1. No changes were made to the most recent classification system of meningiomas [10]. Of note, no difference is made between intracranial or spinal meningiomas with respect to their histological subtypes. The most common histological subtype of spinal meningiomas are meningothelial, fibroblastic, transitional, and psammomatous, which are all WHO grade I tumors [7, 8]. Unless malignant features are present, the histological subtype has not been shown to affect prognosis [11, 12]. Patients with spinal meningiomas have excellent prognosis if complete surgical resection can be achieved. This is due to the fact that malignant subtypes for spinal meningiomas are relatively rare, and these tumors are frequently amenable to complete surgical resection without incurring neurologic deficits [11–17].

## Overall Treatment Strategy

The mainstay of management for spinal meningiomas is open surgical resection aimed at gross total resection using microsurgical technique [12–15]. These tumors are noninfiltrative and hence, amenable to safe and complete surgical resection which has been reported in 82–99% of cases [3, 11, 12, 16, 17]. However, these tumors have a recurrence rate of 4–8% with a mean time to recurrence of 5 years [2, 11, 17, 18]. Progression-free survival at 5, 10, and 15 years has been reported to be 93%, 80%, and 68% for gross total resection and 63%, 45%, and 9% for subtotal resection, respectively [19].

## Indications for Radiotherapy

Surgery aimed at gross total resection is the standard of care and best initial management strategy for spinal meningiomas. However, some patients are not ideal surgical candidates due to age, medical comorbidities, recurrence of tumor after prior surgery, location of the tumor ventral to the spinal cord, or presence of multiple tumors [20–23]. It is in such clinical settings that radiotherapy may serve as an important tool in the armamentarium of the multimodal management of spinal meningiomas.

The National Comprehensive Cancer Network has published recommended treatment algorithms for spinal meningiomas that include conventional fractionated radiotherapy techniques [24]. WHO grade I meningiomas may be treated by fractionated conformal radiotherapy with doses of 45–54 Gy. Stereotactic or image-guided therapy is recommended when using tight margins or when close to critical structures. Conformal radiation therapy (e.g., 3D-CRT, IMRT, VMAT) is recommended to spare critical structures and uninvolved tissue. WHO grade I meningiomas may also be treated with radiosurgery doses of 12–16 Gy in a single fraction when appropriate.

WHO grade II and grade III meningiomas of the spine are considered much more aggressive than grade I meningiomas and are therefore treated accordingly. For WHO grade II meningiomas undergoing radiation, treatment should be directed to the gross tumor (if present) and surgical bed plus a margin (1–2 cm) to a dose of 54–60 Gy in 1.8–2.0 Gy fractions. WHO grade III meningiomas should be treated as malignant tumors with treatment directed to the gross tumor (if present) and surgical bed plus a margin (2–3 cm) receiving 59.4–60 Gy in 1.8–2.0 Gy fractions.

## Indications for Radiosurgery

The role of radiosurgery has been explored for WHO grade I meningiomas of the spine. The following discussion refers exclusively to grade I meningiomas. The current indications for hypofractionated radiosurgery for the management of spinal meningioma include tumors whose location pose significant surgical challenges, tumors that have recurred after prior open surgical extirpation, and patients who have significant medical comorbidities that preclude open surgical intervention. Several relative contraindications to radiosurgery for spinal meningiomas include tumors without well-defined margins with invagination of the spinal cord, patients with significant neurologic deficits due to spinal cord or nerve root compression that warrant decompression of neural elements, and tumors that are amenable to safe surgical resection [25, 26].

In theory, similar to the case for intracranial meningiomas, the initial management for spinal meningiomas with radiosurgery over open surgery has several significant benefits. This would be the case only for smaller tumors with little neural compression in which the clinician has confidence in the diagnosis based upon high-quality imaging. Radiosurgery would obviate the need for open surgery, avoiding all of the risks of surgery, including iatrogenic spinal instability, spinal cord injury, cerebrospinal fluid leakage, and wound healing problems, among others. Perhaps most importantly, radiosurgery is a minimally invasive technique that can be performed entirely in an outpatient setting with absolutely no recovery time, sparing the patient the extended pain, hospitalization, and convalescence associated with open surgery. Radiosurgery also has significant benefits over conventional fractionated radiotherapy for spinal meningiomas. By delivering dose only to the intended tumor target, there is a limit to dose that is delivered to normal tissues including the spinal cord and adjacent bone marrow.

## Target Volume Delineation

Accurate target delineation and contouring is essential for conformal radiosurgery. Although spinal meningiomas are conspicuous by their abundant contrast enhancement, the large size and irregular shape of these tumors make contouring difficult in many cases. As mentioned previously, the diagnostic imaging modality of choice is MRI. However, MR imaging fusion with CT-based radiosurgical guidance for radiosurgical planning, as is common in most current radiosurgery platforms, has its challenges. The quality of MR spinal imaging often requires that the patient's imaging position closely matches the intended treatment position and the patient's position during CT simulation. Issues of spatial distortion need to be considered if MRI is used directly for tumor contouring. Since signal intensities of MR images do not reflect a direct relationship with electron densities, unless attenuation coefficiencies are manually assigned to the region of interest, spatial distortion limits the accuracy of using MRI directly in radiosurgery [25]. Alternatively, spinal meningiomas enhance avidly on contrasted computed tomography (CT) which may allow for adequate visualization. However, for these cases, MRI is still much better for the delineation of the spinal cord compared to its appearance on CT imaging. At our institution, fusion of fine cut MR imaging with images acquired during CT imaging is the preferred method for radiosurgical planning for intradural extramedullary tumors.

## Radiation Dose Prescription

The objective of radiosurgery treatment for spinal meningiomas is to deliver a clinically significant radiation dose to the tumor via a plan that respects the radiation dose tolerance limits of the nearby spinal cord, cauda equina, and surrounding organs such as the bowel, esophagus, kidneys, larynx, and liver. Similar to radiosurgery for intracranial tumors, spine radiosurgery doses generally range from 12 to 16 Gy in a single fraction and 18 Gy in three fractions, and doses as high as 30 Gy have been delivered when the treatment was hypofractionated in five sessions [20, 22, 23, 27–30]. Although spinal radiosurgery is frequently delivered using a single-radiation fraction technique, the formal definition includes hypofractionated dosing plans with a maximum of five treatment sessions. The linear quadratic equation remains the most accepted mathematical model of cell kill secondary to ionizing radiation [31]. Given that spinal meningiomas are by definition intradural and frequently adjacent to the spinal cord or nerve roots, there is a tendency to hypofractionate these cases in order to limit total dose to the neural elements and avoid unwanted toxicity.

For spinal meningiomas of the cervical and thoracic spine, the spinal cord is usually the organ at risk that limits dose to the targeted tumor. However, using current prescriptions, the dose to the spinal cord can be successfully limited. Some data point to a less than 5% probability of myelopathy at 5 years the cord receives a 60 Gy dose using standard fractionation [31]. Most centers ensure that the spinal cord is not exposed to more than 50 Gy during fractionated therapy [32].

In contrast to patients with metastatic cancer and other malignant primary tumors of the spine, patients receiving radiosurgery for spinal meningiomas are expected to survive longer with higher functional status. Therefore, it is prudent that planning for spinal meningiomas err on the underestimating spinal cord tolerance in case radiation-induced myelopathy may manifest over decades.

## Radiation Toxicity and Complication Avoidance

For spine radiosurgery, the spinal cord and cauda equina are the organs at risk that most frequently limit the prescribed target dose. Spinal cord injury is the most feared complication of radiosurgery and has historically limited the aggressiveness of spinal tumor treatment, whether benign or malignant [33].

Dodd and colleagues [20] reported one of the first cases of radiation-induced myelopathy in a 29-year-old woman with cervicothoracic meningioma who developed myelopathic symptoms 8 months after radiosurgery to a dose of 24 Gy delivered in three sessions. The authors discussed that the relatively large volume of spinal cord (1.7 cm³) irradiated above 18 Gy (over three sessions of 6 Gy each) may have been the contributing factor [20].

In the updated case series reported by Sachdev et al. from Stanford University [30] which included 103 benign extramedullary spinal tumors, 32 of which were meningiomas, one patient developed transient radiation myelitis 9 months after treatment. The affected patient had a C7–T2 recurrent, previously resected, meningioma (7.6 cm³) with no previous radiation to the area and received 24 Gy in three fractions with an intratumoral maximum dose of 34.3 Gy. The volume of spinal cord irradiated included 4.7 cm³ over 8 Gy and 0.1 cm³ over 27 Gy. The maximum spinal cord dosage was 29.9 Gy. The patient was treated with corticosteroids which stabilized his neurologic symptoms. The tumor volume had decreased at the time of intervention, and the tumor remained radiographically controlled at the last follow-up. In a series of 19 benign spine tumors, two of which were meningiomas, Sahgal et al. [29] reported no late toxicity including myelopathy.

In our initial series of 73 benign spinal tumors from the University of Pittsburgh Medical Center [23], 1 patient with a meningioma, out of 13 total, developed radiosurgery-related spinal cord injury manifesting as Brown-Sequard syndrome at 12 months posttreatment. The patient was treated with corticosteroids, vitamin E, and gabapentin. The patient had undergone previous attempt at surgical resection which may have caused a predisposition of the spinal cord to radiation injury. In our most recent series of 40 consecutive benign spinal tumors treated using cone-beam CT image guidance and newer devices for radiosurgery delivery, no subacute or long-term spinal cord or cauda equina toxicity at a median follow-up of 32 months occurred [21]. This series included eight spinal meningiomas. The mean maximum dose received by the gross total volume (GTV) was 16 Gy (range 12–24 Gy) delivered in a single fraction in 39 cases. The mean lowest dose received by the GTV was 12 Gy

(range 8–16 Gy). The GTV ranged from 0.37 to 94.5 cm³ (mean 13.7 cm³). In the majority of cases, a planning target volume expansion of 2 mm was used. The risk of radiation-induced spinal cord injury is a function of initial dose, fraction size, length of spinal cord exposed, and duration of treatment [34, 35]. These factors should be considered to avoid complications of radiosurgery.

The technique used at our institution may serve as an important reference for treating spinal meningiomas, specifically, and benign spinal tumors, generally, with a high safety profile. Our prescribed dose to the target volume for benign spine tumors has decreased over time as we have become more comfortable with the successful long-term radiographic control of these lower doses and reinforced by the absence of radiation-induced toxicity.

A detailed overview of radiation myelopathy and dose limits for both conventional and radiosurgery is presented in this book for the interested reader.

## Outcomes and Radiographic Assessment

There has been a relative paucity of reports detailing clinical outcomes of spinal meningiomas specifically, and benign spinal tumors generally, compared to spine malignancies treated with radiosurgery. One contributing factor is that the evaluation of radiosurgery for benign spinal tumors requires longer follow-up to confirm durable safety and efficacy than for malignant tumors of the spine. Furthermore, the incidence of spinal metastases is far greater than benign tumors of the spine.

Dodd and colleagues [20] reported 16 treated spinal meningiomas (mean dose 20 Gy, mean tumor volume 2.4 cm³, mean follow-up 27 months) and demonstrated radiologic stabilization in 67% and radiologic tumor decrease in 33% of the 15 who had radiographic follow-up (Table 8.2). One patient required surgery and another sustained the only complication reported in series, as described earlier. Seventy

**Table 8.2** Select series of radiosurgery for spinal meningiomas

| Series | N (meningioma) | N (total) | Mean age (years) | Indication | Dose per fractions | Length of follow-up (months) | Outcome |
|---|---|---|---|---|---|---|---|
| Dodd et al. (2006) [20] | 16 | 51 | 46 | Postsurgical | 16–30 Gy/1–5 fractions | 25 | 96% stable/ decreased 1 repeat surgery 1 myelopathy |
| Sahgal et al. (2007) [29] | 2 | 13 | 58 | Postsurgical | 21 Gy/3 fractions | 25 | Stable |
| Gerszten et al. (2008) [23] | 13 | 73 | 44 | 11 postsurgical 2 primary treatment | 12–20 Gy/1 fraction | 37 | Stable |
| Sachdev et al. (2011) [30] | 32 | 87 | 53 | Surgery contraindicated | 14–30 Gy/1–5 fractions | 33 | Stable/ decreased |
| Gerszten et al. (2012) [21, 22] | 10 | 45 | 52 | Postsurgical or primary treatment | 12–24 Gy | 32 | 100% control |

percent of meningiomas treated in this series were symptomatically stable or improved. Most patient experience an improvement in pain and strength with radiosurgery.

From our institution's initial published series [23], 13 spinal meningiomas were treated using a single-fraction technique (mean dose 21 Gy, mean tumor volume 4.9 cm³). Eleven of 13 patients received radiosurgery as an adjunct treatment for residual or recurrent tumor following surgical resection. Radiographic tumor control was demonstrated in all cases with median follow-up of 17 months [23]. Of the 11 patients who had undergone previous surgical resection, none demonstrated radiographic tumor progression on subsequent serial imaging after the radiosurgery treatment. Radiographic tumor control was also demonstrated for those two patients in whom radiosurgery was used as a primary treatment modality with median follow-up imaging at 14 months.

In the updated series by Sachdev and colleagues [30], all 32 meningiomas with radiographic follow-up were controlled at a mean follow-up of 33 months (range 6–87 months). At the last follow-up, 47% of meningiomas were stable, while 53% had decreased in volume. In another series, Sahgal and coauthors [29] reported treating two spinal meningiomas with radiosurgery (mean dose 23 Gy delivered in two fractions, mean tumor volume 1.6 cm³) with no evidence of radiographic tumor progression. Benzil et al. [28] and De Salles et al. [27] also reported their respective experience with treating spinal meningiomas with good long-term radiographic follow-up.

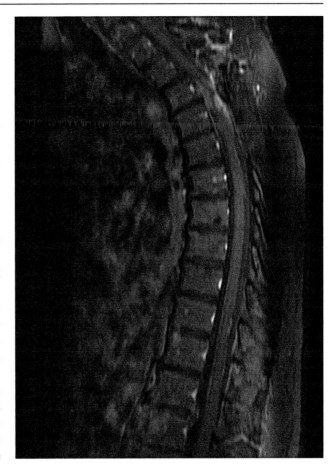

**Fig. 8.1** Gadolinium-enhanced sagittal magnetic resonance imaging demonstrates a recurrence of the T3–T4 meningioma

## Case Presentation

A representative case of an 86-year-old woman who previously underwent open resection for a WHO grade I meningioma at the T3–T4 level. Fourteen years after her initial surgery, she developed symptomatic spinal cord compression resulting in progressive difficulty with ambulation. Magnetic resonance imaging revealed tumor recurrence. Given her age and medical comorbidities, she was felt to be a poor candidate for repeat open surgical resection of the tumor and spinal cord compression. It was decided to treat the tumor with hypofractionated radiosurgery.

Magnetic resonance imaging demonstrated a recurrence of the T3–T4 meningioma at the same level as the laminectomy defect from the prior surgical resection (Figs. 8.1, 8.2, 8.3, and 8.4). 1.2 mm slide thickness MR axial images were fused with the planning CT for contouring purposes. The tumor was contoured using gadolinium-enhanced MR axial imaging. The spinal cord margin was defined using T2-weighted axial imaging. The tumor was treated with a prescribed dose of 18 Gy delivered in three fractions prescribed to the 77% isodose line. The GTV (gross tumor vol-

ume) was 3.7 cm³. The $D_{max}$ to the GTV was 23.4 Gy, and the $D_{min}$ was 16.7 Gy (mean 20.7 Gy, median 21.0 Gy). No PTV (planning target volume) was employed. The volume of the delineated spinal cord was 3.1 cm³. The $D_{max}$ to the spinal cord was 18.1 Gy, and the $D_{min}$ was 0.5 Gy (mean 11.1 Gy, median 14.4 Gy). The $D_{max}$ to the skin was 4.0 Gy. The carina was also carefully delineated as another organ at risk. The $D_{max}$ to the carina was 4.5 Gy (Figs. 8.4, 8.5, 8.6, and 8.7).

The treatment was delivered using two arcs of volumetric-modulated arc therapy (Fig. 8.8). Each treatment lasted less than 30 min. All treatments were well tolerated by the patient, and no acute nor subacute toxicities occurred.

## Summary

- Spinal meningiomas are benign extramedullary tumors affecting predominantly females in fifth to seventh decade of life and occurring mainly in the thoracic spine.
- MRI is the imaging modality of choice for diagnosis showing avid homogenous enhancement of extramedul-

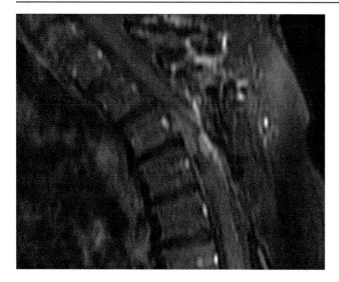

**Fig. 8.2** Gadolinium-enhanced sagittal magnetic resonance imaging demonstrates that the tumor has recurred both ventral and dorsal to the spinal cord at the level of the laminectomy defect

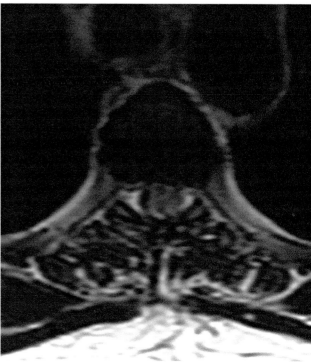

**Fig. 8.4** T2-weighted axial magnetic resonance imaging demonstrates compression of the spinal cord by the tumor

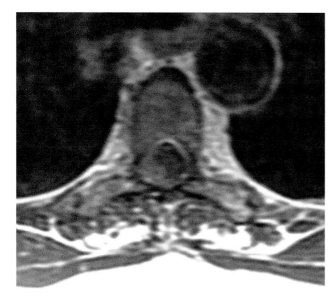

**Fig. 8.3** Gadolinium-enhanced axial magnetic resonance imaging demonstrates the tumor extrinsic to the right side of the spinal cord

lary with or without both intra- and extradural components.
- Surgical resection remains the mainstay of treatment of spinal meningiomas.
- WHO grade I meningiomas may be treated with fractionated conformal radiotherapy with doses of 45–54 Gy.
- Radiosurgery is recommended when target requires, or in patients with residual or recurrent tumors, or in those whose tumors are not amenable to surgical resection, or are poor surgical candidates. Clinical experience with this technique is limited.

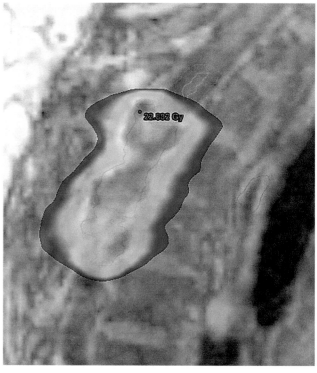

**Fig. 8.5** Sagittal projections of the isodose lines of the treatment plan. The tumor was treated with a prescribed dose of 18 Gy in three fractions to a volume of 3.7 cm³

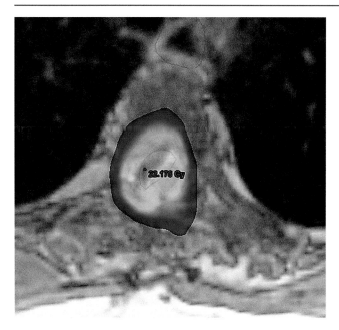

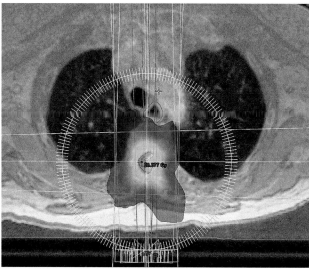

**Fig. 8.7** Dose volume histogram of the treatment plan

**Fig. 8.6** Axial projection of the isodose lines of the treatment plan. The $D_{max}$ to the spinal cord was 18.1 Gy

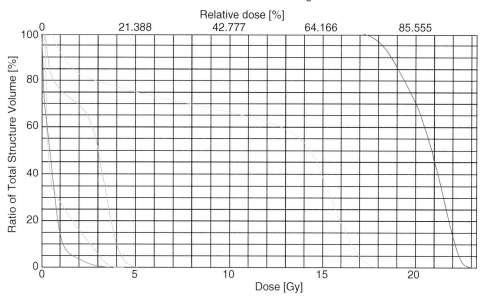

**Fig. 8.8** The treatment was delivered using two arcs of volumetric-modulated arc therapy

| Structure | Coverage [%/%] | Volume | Min Dose | Max Dose | Mean Dose | Modal Dose | Median Dose | Std Dev |
|---|---|---|---|---|---|---|---|---|
| cordFinal | 100.0/100.0 | 3.1 cm³ | 0.5 Gy | 18.1 Gy | 11.1 Gy | 15.2 Gy | 14.4 Gy | 6.0 Gy |
| gtvFinal | 100.0/99.7 | 3.7 cm³ | 16.7 Gy | 23.4 Gy | 20.7 Gy | 21.8 Gy | 21.0 Gy | 1.3 Gy |
| carina | 100.0/99.8 | 9.6 cm³ | 0.1 Gy | 4.5 Gy | 0.9 Gy | 0.3 Gy | 0.4 Gy | 1.0 Gy |
| Esophagus | 100.0/99.9 | 12.8 cm³ | 0.2 Gy | 5.4 Gy | 2.6 Gy | 0.3 Gy | 3.0 Gy | 1.4 Gy |
| Skin | 100.0/101.7 | 434.9 cm³ | 0.0 Gy | 4.0 Gy | 0.6 Gy | 0.1 Gy | 0.4 Gy | 0.5 Gy |

- WHO grade I meningiomas may be treated with radiosurgery doses of 12–16 Gy in a single fraction, 18 Gy in three fractions, or 25–30 Gy in five fractions when appropriate.
- MRI is the imaging modality of choice for radiosurgical planning.
- Radiosurgical management of spinal meningioma results in stable or improved size of tumor with long-term radiographic assessment; however, clinical experience is still limited.

## Self-Assessment Questions

Answer True or False for the following statements.

1. Complete surgical resection is now replaced by radiosurgery as the preferred primary treatment option for symptomatic spinal meningiomas.
2. Doses of 45–54 Gy using fractions of 1.8 Gy/day is a treatment strategy for grade 1 spinal meningiomas.
3. Doses of 12–16 Gy in a single fraction have been reported as safe and effective for grade 1 spinal meningiomas using radiosurgery techniques.
4. The radiation treatment for WHO grade II meningiomas should be directed to the gross tumor and surgical bed plus a margin using fractionated daily radiotherapy.
5. WHO grade III meningiomas are considered malignant and may be treated in a similar fashion to WHO grade 1 and grade II meningiomas using fractionated daily radiotherapy.

## Answers

1. False
2. True
3. True
4. True
5. False

## References

1. Helseth A, Mork SJ. Primary intraspinal neoplasms in Norway, 1955 to 1986. A population-based survey of 467 patients. J Neurosurg. 1989;71:842–5.
2. Solero CL, Fornari M, Giombini S, et al. Spinal meningiomas: review of 174 operated cases. Neurosurgery. 1989;25:153–60.
3. Gottfried ON, Gluf W, Quinones-Hinojosa A, et al. Spinal meningiomas: surgical management and outcome. Neurosurg Focus. 2003;14(6):e2.
4. Parisi JE, Mena H. Nonglial tumors. In: Nelson JS, Parisi JE, Schochet Jr SS, editors. Principles and practice of neuropathology. St. Louis: Mosby; 1993. p. 203–66.
5. Levy WJ, Latchaw J, Hahn JF, et al. Spinal neurofibromas: a report of 66 cases and a comparison with meningiomas. Neurosurgery. 1986;18(3):331–4.
6. Dickman CA, Fehlings MG, Gokaslan ZL. Spinal column and spinal column tumors: principles and practice. New York: Thieme Medical Publishers; 2006. p. 335–48.
7. King AT, Sharr MM, Gullan RW, et al. Spinal meningiomas: a 20-year review. Br J Neurosurg. 1998;12:521–6.
8. Gezen F, Kahraman S, Canakci Z, et al. Review of 36 cases of spinal cord meningioma. Spine. 2000;25:727–31.
9. Matsumoto S, Hasuo K, Uchino A, et al. MRI of intradural extramedullary spinal neurinomas and meningiomas. Clin Imaging. 1993;17:46–52.
10. Louis DN, Perry A, Reifenberger G, et al. The 2016 World Health Organization Classification of tumors of the central nervous system: a summary. Acta Neruopathol. 2016;131:803–20.
11. Roux FX, Nataf F, Pinaudeau M, et al. Intraspinal meningiomas: review of 54 cases with discussion of poor prognosis factors and modern therapeutic management. Surg Neurol. 1996;46:458–64.
12. McCormick P. Surgical management of dumbbell tumors of the thoracic and lumbar spine. Neurosurgery. 1996;38:67–74.
13. McCormick P. Surgical management of dumbbell tumors of the cervical spine. Neurosurgery. 1996;38:294–300.
14. Parsa A, Lee J, Parney I, et al. Spinal cord and intraductal-extraparenchymal spine tumors: current base care practices and strategies. J Neurooncol. 2004;69:219–318.
15. Asazuma T, Toyama Y, Maruiwa H, et al. Surgical strategy for cervical dumbbell tumors based on a three-dimensional classification. Spine. 2004;29:E10–4.
16. Klekamp J, Samii M. Surgical results for spinal meningiomas. Surg Neurol. 1999;52:552–62.
17. Levy WJ Jr, Bay J, Dohn D. Spinal cord meningioma. J Neurosurg. 1982;57:804–12.
18. Schick U, Marquardt G, Lorenz R. Recurrence of benign spinal neoplasms. Neurosurg Rev. 2001;24:20–5.
19. Mirimanoff R, Dosretz D, Lingood R, et al. Meningioma: analysis of recurrence and progression following neurosurgical resection. J Neurosurg. 1985;62:18–24.
20. Dodd RL, Ryu MR, Kamnerdsupaphon P, et al. CyberKnife radiosurgery for benign intradural extramedullary spinal tumors. Neurosurgery. 2006;58(4):674–85.
21. Gerszten PC, Chen S, Quader M, et al. Radiosurgery for benign tumors of the spine using the Synergy S with cone-beam computed tomography image guidance. J Neurosurg. 2012;117(Suppl):197–202.
22. Gerszten PC, Quader M, Novotny J Jr, et al. Radiosurgery for benign tumors of the spine: clinical experience and current trends. Technol Cancer Res Treat. 2012;11(2):133–9.
23. Gerszten PC, Burton SA, Ozhasoglu C, et al. Radiosurgery for benign intradural spinal tumors. Neurosurgery. 2008;62(4):887–95.
24. Nabors LB, Portnow J, Ammirati M, et al. Central nervous system cancers, version 1.2015. J Natl Compr Cancer Netw. 2016;13(10):1191–202.
25. Gibbs I, Chang S, Dodd R, et al. Radiosurgery for benign extramedullary tumors of the spine. In: Gerszten P, Ryu S, editors. Spine radiosurgery. New York: Thieme; 2015.
26. Gerszten P. The role of minimally invasive techniques in the management of spine tumors: percutaneous bone cement augmentation, radiosurgery, and microendoscopic approaches. Orthop Clin North Am. 2007;38:441–50.
27. De Salles AA, Pedroso AG, Medin P, et al. Spinal lesions treated with Novalis shaped beam intensity-modulated radiosurgery and stereotactic radiotherapy. J Neurosurg. 2004;101(Suppl 3):435–40.
28. Benzil DL, Saboori M, Mogilner AY, et al. Safety and efficacy of stereotactic radiosurgery for tumors of the spine. J Neurosurg. 2004;101(Suppl 3):413–8.

29. Sahgal A, Chou D, Ames C, et al. Image-guided robotic stereotactic body radiotherapy for benign spinal tumors: The University of California San Francisco preliminary experience. Technol Cancer Res Treat. 2007;6:595–604.

30. Sachdev S, Dodd RL, Chang SD, et al. Stereotactic radiosurgery yields long-term control for benign intradural, extramedullary spinal tumors. Neurosurgery. 2011;69(3):533–9.

31. Yamada Y, Lovelock DM, Bilsky MH. A review of image-guided intensity-modulated radiotherapy for spinal tumors. Neurosurgery. 2007;61(2):226–35.

32. Gerszten P, Bilsky MH. Spine radiosurgery. Contemp Neurosurg. 2006;28:1–8.

33. Gibbs IC, Patil C, Gerszten PC, et al. Delayed radiation-induced myelopathy after spinal radiosurgery. Neurosurgery. 2009;64(2 Suppl):A67–72.

34. Rampling R, Symonds P. Radiation myelopathy. Curr Opin Neruol. 1998;11:627–32.

35. Isaacson S. Radiation therapy and the management of intramedullary spinal cord tumors. J Neurooncol. 2000;47:231–8.

# Astrocytic Tumors of the Spinal Cord

# 9

Tania Kaprealian

## Abbreviations

| | |
|---|---|
| 2-D | Two-dimensional |
| 3-D | Three-dimensional |
| AA | Anaplastic astrocytoma |
| AP-PA | Anterior/posterior-posterior/anterior |
| Cm | Centimeters |
| CNS | Central nervous system |
| CSF | Cerebrospinal fluid |
| CT | Computerized tomography |
| CTV | Clinical target volume |
| CTx | Chemotherapy |
| GBM | Glioblastoma |
| GTV | Gross tumor volume |
| HGA | High-grade astrocytoma |
| IMRT | Intensity-modulated radiation therapy |
| LGA | Low-grade astrocytoma |
| MS | Median survival |
| MV | Megavoltage |
| NR | Not reported |
| OS | Overall survival |
| PCV | Procarbazine, lomustine, and vincristine |
| PFS | Progression-free survival |
| PTV | Planning target volume |
| RFS | Recurrence-free survival |
| RT | Radiation therapy |
| RTOG | Radiation Therapy Oncology Group |
| TD | Tolerance dose |
| VEGF | Vascular endothelial growth factor |
| WHO | World Health Organization |

## Learning Objectives

- Know the incidence of spinal cord astrocytomas.
- Understand the classic signs and symptoms of spinal cord astrocytomas as well as the risk factors associated with developing these tumors.
- Learn the histology and grading of spinal cord astrocytomas.
- Understand the prognostic indicators and molecular marker correlations.
- Learn the multimodality treatment management of spinal cord astrocytomas.
- Know the outcomes in survival and local control of spinal cord astrocytomas.

## Background Epidemiology

Primary spinal cord tumors comprise 2–4% of all adult central nervous system (CNS) tumors of which astrocytomas account for approximately 6–8% of all spinal cord tumors. Astrocytomas are the second most common primary spinal cord tumor next to ependymomas [1, 2], which is opposite of that found in children with spinal astrocytomas being more common than spinal ependymomas. Astrocytomas along with ependymomas comprise the intradural intramedullary tumors of the spine and tend to be infiltrative. Intramedullary tumors comprise 8–10% of all primary spinal cord tumors of which 30–40% are astrocytomas [1]. The ratio of intracranial to spinal astrocytomas is 10:1 [3].

Astrocytic tumors of the spine consist of juvenile pilocytic astrocytoma (World Health Organization [WHO] grade I), diffuse or low-grade astrocytoma (WHO grade II), anaplastic astrocytoma (WHO grade III), and glioblastoma (WHO grade IV), with the majority consisting of low-grade (WHO grade 2) diffuse or fibrillary astrocytomas (75%) [1, 4]. Glioblastoma of the spine is very aggres-

T. Kaprealian
Department of Radiation Oncology, University of California, Los Angeles, Los Angeles, CA, USA
e-mail: tkaprealian@mednet.ucla.edu

sive and has the worst prognosis of all the spinal astrocytomas, often not responsive to any treatment modality. There is a high risk of leptomeningeal dissemination with spinal cord malignant astrocytomas unlike cerebral malignant astrocytomas. The proximity of the tumor to the subarachnoid space and cerebrospinal (CSF) fluid may explain this increased risk. Fortunately, spinal cord glioblastomas are quite rare. In general, primary spinal cord astrocytomas are more common in males and Caucasians [2, 5], and they tend to occur in the cervical and thoracic spinal cord.

## Risk Factors

There are no established risk factors for astrocytic spinal cord tumors. There may be an association between allelic losses on chromosome arm 22q and the development of these tumors [6]. Prior radiation therapy to the spine may increase the risk for developing spinal cord astrocytomas, but the extent of risk associated with prior irradiation is unknown. There are various genetic mutations associated with astrocytomas both intracranially and within the spinal cord [7]. The following mutations are associated with spinal pilocytic astrocytomas: BRAF (7q34), CDKN2A (9q21), NF1 (17q11.2), and PTEN (10q23.3). The following mutations are associated with spinal astrocytomas and glioblastomas: H3F3A (17q25) and IDH1 (2q33.3).

## Staging

Currently, there is not an established staging system for spinal cord astrocytic tumors.

## Diagnosis

Patients can present with a variety of symptoms including back pain, radicular symptoms, bowel and bladder dysfunction, impotence, gait difficulties, or slowly progressive motor and sensory deficits. Typically sensory and pain deficits precede the onset of motor weakness by months; however, in some instances, depending on the location of the tumor, motor weakness may precede any other symptomatic complaints, particularly in tumors located centrally in the spinal cord. In general, symptoms develop and progress over months to years in low-grade astrocytomas before a patient is diagnosed. However, in high-grade tumors, progression is on the order of months with rapid deterioration often seen. The modified McCormick scale is used to assess patients' functional status both preoperatively and postoperatively as follows:

Grade I: neurologically intact, normal gait, and minimal dysesthesia.
Grade II: mild motor or sensory deficit; patient is still functionally independent.
Grade III: moderate motor or sensory deficit; patient has limitation of function but is independent with an external aid.
Grade IV: severe motor or sensory deficit; patient has limited function and is not capable of functioning independently.
Grade V: paraplegia or quadriplegia [4, 8].

Clonus, hyperreflexia, and Babinski are common signs but not diagnostic.

Appropriate imaging is necessary to help make an accurate diagnosis. MRI with and without contrast is the primary imaging modality used to diagnose intramedullary spinal tumors. Astrocytomas are typically asymmetrical and present with irregular tumor margins as well as possible cystic components of the tumor with a focal fusiform expansion on the cord [9]. On T1-weighted images they can appear hypo- or isointense, while on T2-weighted images they are hyperintense. Syrinxes, which are fluid-filled cavities, are commonly associated with spinal cord astrocytomas, particularly in pilocytic astrocytomas [10]. A syrinx within the spinal cord is called a syringomyelia. Astrocytomas located higher in the spinal column are more prone to developing syringomyelia. T2-weighted MRI sequences can detect syringomyelia [11]. Most astrocytomas have some degree of enhancement with contrast. However, both WHO grade I and II astrocytomas can present with patchy or no enhancement at all with contrast, Fig. 9.1. Spinal astrocytomas are difficult to distinguish from other intramedullary spinal tumors, particularly ependymomas, using MRI alone; and thus, pathological tissue diagnosis is necessary. Relative to ependymomas, astrocytomas tend not to have well-defined margins and are less likely to be centrally located within the spinal cord.

The WHO revised the classification of CNS tumors in 2016 using both histological and molecular characteristics to define the classification. The tumors are still graded WHO 1–4; however, now there are distinct classifications based on molecular findings.

The role of the molecular markers in spinal astrocytomas is less certain than in the intracranial setting and needs further studies. Grade I astrocytomas consist of pilocytic astrocytoma and subependymal giant cell astrocytoma. Grade II astrocytomas consist of diffuse astrocytoma, IDH mutant; diffuse astrocytoma, IDH-wild type; and pleomorphic xanthoastrocytoma. Grade III astrocytomas consist of anaplastic astrocytoma, IDH mutant; anaplastic astrocytoma, IDH-wild type; and anaplastic pleomorphic xanthoastrocytoma. Grade IV astrocytomas consist of glioblastoma, IDH mutant; glioblastoma, IDH-wild type; and diffuse midline gli-

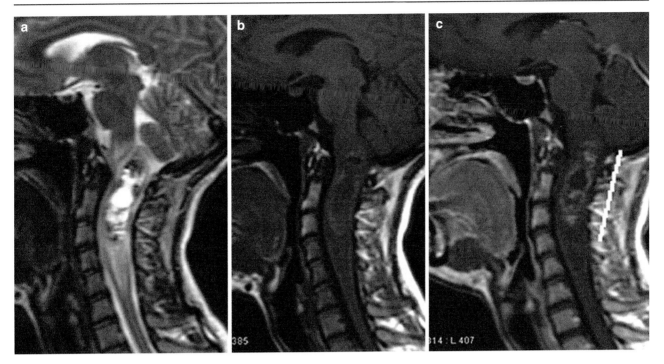

**Fig. 9.1** Fibrillary astrocytoma. (**a**) Sagittal T2-weighted image demonstrates a heterogeneously hyperintense lesion in the cervical cord. (**b**) Unenhanced T1-weighted image shows an isointense lesion with mild heterogeneous hyperintensity in the periphery that may represent blood products. (**c**) Contrast-enhanced T1-weighted image shows marked heterogeneous enhancement. Histopathology confirmed fibrillary astrocytoma. [Reprinted from Abul-Kasim K, Thurnher MM, McKeever, Sundgren PC. Intradural spinal tumors: current classification and MRI features. Neuroradiology. 2008 April;50(4):301–14. With permission from Springer]

oma, H3 K27M mutant (which can occur in the brain stem, thalamus, or spinal cord). In the setting of unknown molecular markers, there are classifications of diffuse astrocytoma, NOS; anaplastic astrocytoma, NOS; anaplastic oligoastrocytoma, NOS; oligodendroglioma, NOS; and anaplastic oligodendroglioma, NOS. With known molecular markers, there is no longer a classification of oligoastrocytoma. There are classifications for grade II oligodendroglioma, IDH mutant, 1p/19q co-deleted, and grade III anaplastic oligodendroglioma, IDH mutant, 1p/19q co-deleted [12].

## Prognostic and Predictive Factors

Tumor histology and grade are the most significant prognostic factors of primary spinal cord astrocytomas (Fig. 9.2) [13–16]. Pilocytic tumors and lower-grade tumors are associated with improved survival. Within the grade II astrocytomas, the gemistocytic tumors lead to a worse median survival (50 months) compared to fibrillary and protoplasmatic astrocytomas [15]. The 5- and 10-year overall survival by grade is listed in Table 9.1 [16]. Male sex has also been shown to lead to improved survival in several studies [14, 17]. There is data to suggest that both younger age [2] and more advanced age are negative prognostic indicators [16, 18–22]. Extent of resection has also been found to have

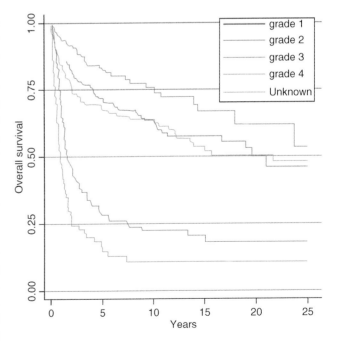

**Fig. 9.2** Kaplan-Meier overall survival of spinal cord astrocytoma by grade. Beyond 25 years, the total number of patients at risk is small (31), so survival is shown only up to 25 years. [Reprinted from Milano MT, Johnson MD, Sul J, Mohile NA, Korones DN, Okunieff P, et al. Primary spinal cord glioma: a Surveillance, Epidemiology, and End Results database study. J Neurooncol. 2010 May;98(1):83–92. With permission from Springer]

**Table 9.1** Overall survival of spinal cord astrocytomas by grade

| Grade (per SEER database) | 5-Year overall survival | 10-Year overall survival |
|---|---|---|
| Well differentiated, grade I | 80% | 68% |
| Moderately differentiated, grade II | 71% | 65% |
| Poorly differentiated, grade III | 36% | 31% |
| Undifferentiated, anaplastic grade IV | 23% | 17% |

Based on data from Ref. [16]

mixed results with some data suggesting resection affects prognosis with lower mortality and improved progression-free survival seen in those undergoing gross total resection [4, 13, 14, 23–25], while other studies suggest that biopsy alone portends for better survival [2, 15, 18, 26, 27]. It is possible that older surgical techniques used in many of the studies are the reason behind the differences seen in the various studies. With more advanced resection modalities, it is probable that extent of resection will have a clearer benefit in terms of survival and outcome. Performance status has been shown to affect prognosis both in the preoperative and postoperative setting [4, 13, 15] with higher performance status leading to better survival outcomes and neurologic outcome. Increased survival has been shown in patients with greater than 6–12 month interval from the appearance of the first symptoms to diagnosis [2, 15]. Overall 5-year survival was found to be 71% with a longer symptom interval vs. 42% for a shorter interval [15]. Adjuvant radiation therapy leads to a better prognosis in many studies, particularly in the non-pilocytic tumors [2, 22]. However, this finding is also controversial, and there have been mixed results in the literature.

## Multimodality Management Approach

### Surgery

Surgery is considered the mainstay of treatment for intramedullary spinal tumors in general; however, the specific role in the management of spinal cord astrocytomas is less evident. For infiltrative tumors such as astrocytomas, a gross total resection and even a subtotal resection can be very difficult to achieve due to the involvement of the spinal cord itself. In order to decrease the risk of injury to the spinal cord, often only biopsies or limited subtotal resections are accomplished. Tumor histology predicts for resectability and recurrence [28], while intraoperative identification of a clear tumor plane for resection has prognostic significance and higher incidence of long-term neurological function improvement [26]. The data has been mixed with some studies finding a benefit to resection in the management of spinal cord astrocytomas, while others finding no difference

between biopsy and resection in all grades of astrocytomas. Older surgical techniques may explain the discrepancies in the data. Over the last decade, due to the introduction of microsurgical techniques, use of intraoperative neurophysiologic monitoring and intraoperative ultrasound, and advances in MRI technology, there has been a shift with an increasing role for surgery in the management of intramedullary astrocytomas. Historically, in the setting of low-grade astrocytomas, gross total resection was associated with low morbidity and excellent long-term prognosis in patients with good preoperative performance status [29]. High-grade astrocytomas do not have well-demarcated boundaries and are thus harder to resect safely. Most studies reveal that a gross total resection is not possible for higher-grade astrocytomas [30]. However, even in the setting of grade II astrocytomas, gross total resection can be difficult to achieve and is on the order of 12–20% of tumors, whereas it is up to 80% in the setting of grade I pilocytic astrocytomas (Fig. 9.3) [4, 7, 26, 27].

To limit postoperative morbidity and achieve the best resection possible, it is ideal to diagnose and operate before a patient develops severe neurological deficits and to have an experienced neurosurgeon operate on the patient using modern technology given the rarity of these tumors. Postoperative morbidities include pain, hemorrhages, wound healing, infections, cord tethering, and cerebrospinal fluid fistulas. Patients will very often experience postoperative sensory deficits, including impairment of sensations for light touch, temperature, and pain. The extent of sensory deficits depends on the extent and location of the myelotomy and the use of somatosensory potential monitoring intraoperatively. There is often some improvement of sensory symptoms, but typically it is incomplete improvement. Patients may also experience worsening of motor skills, gait and sphincter function, or sexual dysfunction, either transient or permanent. Transient motor deficits are found to be worse in those who are older and those who underwent gross total resections, due to spinal cord plasticity and dissection along tumor boundaries, respectively. Time and physical rehabilitation are required for the symptoms to improve, though rates and extent of improvement vary throughout the literature. It can take days to months for a patient to recover, and generally sensory deficits recover before motor deficits. Risk of permanent deficits has ranged from 20% to 35% for surgical resection of all intramedullary spinal cord tumors, with patients over 60 having near double the rate of permanent morbidity compared to younger patients [26, 31]. The risk of any surgical morbidity is influenced by the spinal level of the tumor, preoperative neurological state, tumor hemorrhages, surgical experience, use of newer surgical modalities, and the rate of reoperation [31, 32]. Care must be taken both in counseling the patient and giving the patient proper postoperative rehabilitation.

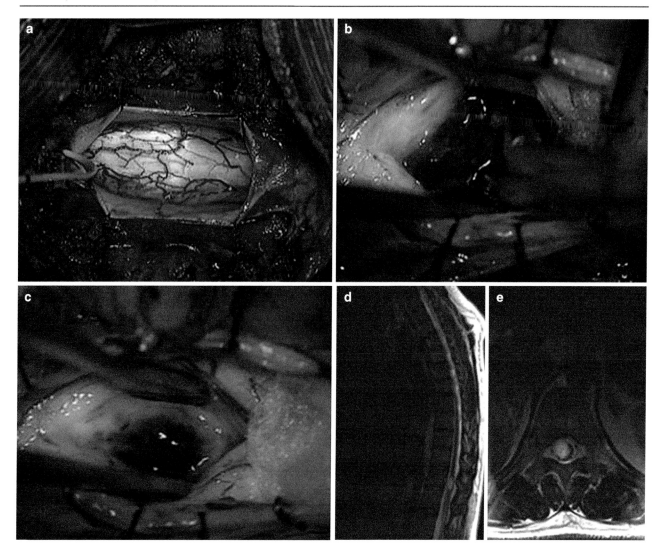

**Fig. 9.3** Surgery and imaging in spinal cord astrocytoma. (a–c) Intraoperative images showing the excision of a diffuse intramedullary astrocytoma in the spinal cord from a posterior approach. The spinal cord appears enlarged, and thus surgical approach begins with a midline myelotomy to separate the dorsal columns (a).The tumor is then exposed and excised via careful dissection (b). Gliosis and hyperemia can be seen in the resection cavity (c). (d, e) Preoperative sagittal (d) and axial (e) T2-weighted MRI reveal hyperintensity and expansion of the spinal cord. [Reprinted from Zadnik PL, Gokaslan ZL, Burger PC, Bettegowda C. Spinal cord tumors: advances in genetics and their implications for treatment. Nat Rev. Neurol. 2013 May;9(5):257–66. With permission from Nature Publishing Group]

Postoperative MRI with and without contrast is necessary to determine the extent of resection of intramedullary spinal tumors, despite the surgeon's observation intraoperatively. Even with what appears a gross total resection on imaging, there very likely may be tumor tissue left behind, particularly in the setting of astrocytomas, which are infiltrative and have less distinct tumor boundaries.

## Radiation Therapy

Adjuvant radiation therapy is a useful treatment modality in the treatment of spinal cord astrocytomas given the low rates of gross total resection. However, the use of radiation ther-apy remains controversial as several studies have failed to show a clear benefit in the use of postoperative radiation therapy in both low- and high-grade spinal cord astrocyto-mas [14, 16, 17, 20, 26].

There are studies, however, that do show a clear benefit to the use of radiation therapy [2, 22, 24, 33, 34]. Radiation therapy is indicated or is encouraged in patients with grade III–IV spinal cord astrocytomas, progressive tumors, and tumors that have undergone subtotal resections. The role of radiation therapy in the treatment of gross totally resected grade II spinal cord astrocytomas is more controversial, with several studies showing no benefit to the addition of postop-erative radiation therapy in this setting [23, 29, 35], while others do show a benefit either in progression-free survival or overall survival or both [21, 36]. These same studies show a benefit to the use of postoperative radiation therapy in subtotally resected grade II astrocytomas and some subtotally resected grade I astrocytomas. The role of radiation therapy in the treatment of pilocytic astrocytomas in the spinal cord is limited, with data suggesting a lack of benefit to the use of postoperative radiation therapy, particularly in the setting of a gross total resection [22]. Thus, use of radiation therapy typically should not precede tissue diagnosis through biopsy or resection. Despite the lack of benefit seen with the use of radiation therapy to treat pilocytic astrocytomas, there does appear to be a benefit in survival with postoperative radiation therapy in the treatment of patients with infiltrative astrocytomas. In the setting of spinal cord pilocytic astrocytomas and gross total resection of grade II spinal cord astrocytomas, postoperative observation may be considered rather than immediate postoperative radiation therapy to minimize any radiation-related morbidities. There are several studies to suggest and recommend that patients undergo maximal safe resection followed by observation for low-grade spinal cord astrocytomas [15, 21, 23, 29].

## Radiation Techniques

As with surgery, there have been advances in the field of radiation oncology through the years. There are more precise delivery techniques available now, including intensity-modulated radiation therapy, conventionally fractionated stereotactic radiotherapy and radiosurgery, and proton beam radiation therapy. A breadth of the data that is available for the treatment of spinal astrocytomas with radiation therapy has been conducted with the use of two-dimensional (2-D) radiation therapy and three-dimensional (3-D) conformal therapy. Particularly with 2-D radiation therapy, there is more dose spillage to the nearby tissues, including the surrounding organs. However, the dose-limiting structures are often the spinal cord or cauda equina itself; and thus, dose escalation beyond the tolerance of these structures is often not possible.

There may be limitations with the use of stereotactic radiosurgery and proton beam therapy as they both have sharper dose falloff. Given astrocytomas are infiltrative tumors, the marginal dose may become critical. Proton beam therapy has a decreased entrance dose and almost no exit dose, thus decreasing the amount of radiation to normal tissues surrounding the treatment target. Improved results have not been shown with the use of proton beam radiotherapy [37], although further studies are warranted. Stereotactic radiosurgery delivers a high dose of radiation in one to five treatments, also limiting dose to the surrounding normal structures with high-precision radiation delivery. Hotspots are typically found in the PTV of tumors treated with stereotactic radiosurgery. Thus, portions of the tumor are receiving higher doses than the actual prescription. In addition, dose and the margins used in the treatment of tumors are limited with the use of stereotactic radiosurgery, and thus, without further studies, the use of radiosurgery in the treatment of spinal cord astrocytomas may not be appropriate as part of the primary treatment.

Conventionally fractionated stereotactic radiotherapy, intensity-modulated radiation therapy, dynamic conformal radiation therapy, and 3-D conformal therapy techniques are the most commonly used radiation treatment techniques in the delivery of radiation therapy for spinal cord astrocytomas. The more conformal techniques allow for better dose distribution and sparing of surrounding normal tissues, thus limiting toxicity. Daily image guidance such as cone beam CT has also improved our delivery of radiation therapy and allows for use of smaller margins and more conformal treatment plans, minimizing dose spillage and toxicity. Generally, radiation therapy should be delivered within 4–6 weeks postoperative.

## Prescribed Dose and Fractionation

Several studies have shown a dose-dependent response in the treatment of spinal astrocytomas with radiation therapy. Figure 9.4 shows a dose-dependent response comparing

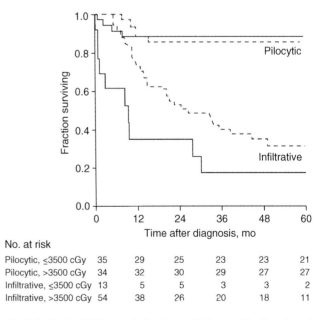

| No. at risk | | | | | | |
|---|---|---|---|---|---|---|
| Pilocytic, ≤3500 cGy | 35 | 29 | 25 | 23 | 23 | 21 |
| Pilocytic, >3500 cGy | 34 | 32 | 30 | 29 | 27 | 27 |
| Infiltrative, ≤3500 cGy | 13 | 5 | 5 | 3 | 3 | 2 |
| Infiltrative, >3500 cGy | 54 | 38 | 26 | 20 | 18 | 11 |

**Fig. 9.4** Kaplan-Meier survival estimate. Patients with pilocytic and infiltrative tumors treated with postoperative radiotherapy to dose of 0–3500 cGy (solid lines) vs. >3500 cGy (dashed lines) (pilocytic, $p = 0.52$; infiltrative, $p = 0.04$). [Reprinted from Minehan KJ, Brown PD, Scheithauer BW, Krauss WE, Wright MP. Prognosis and treatment of spinal cord astrocytoma. Int J Radiat Oncol Biol Phys. 2009 March 1;73(3):727–733. With permission from Elsevier]

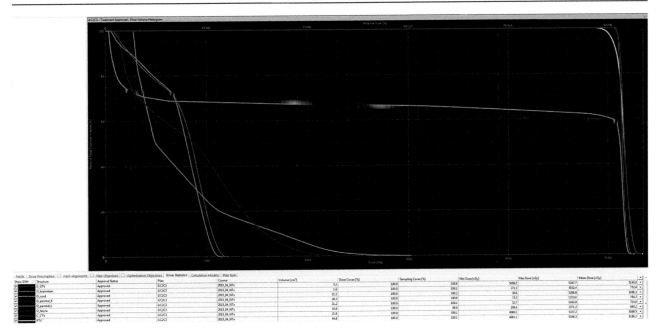

**Fig. 9.5** Dose-volume histogram showing dose to the normal structures as well as the GTV, CTV, and PTV. *GTV* gross tumor volume, *CTV* clinical target volume, *PTV* planning target volume. Red = GTV; blue = CTV; yellow = PTV. [Courtesy of University of California, Los Angeles Department of Radiation Oncology]

patients with infiltrative astrocytomas who received >35 Gy having better survival outcomes compared to those with lower doses [22]. Another study indicates that patients who received >40 Gy had better local control of their intramedullary spinal cord tumors, including both astrocytomas and ependymomas [38]. However, several studies have failed to show a benefit in survival or local control with doses greater than 50.4 Gy [34–37, 39].

Various dosing and fractionation regimens have been tried in the past, ranging from 30 to 55 Gy delivered in 1–3 Gy per fraction in daily or twice-daily treatments. Doses of 65–100 Gy, which exceed the spinal cord tolerance (termed radiocordectomy), have been used in patients who already had poor motor function, and the tumors were located in the thoracic or lumbar region of the spinal cord [34, 40, 41]. Due to the small number of patients in these studies, a dose-response relationship was not established, though there is suggestion that radiocordectomy can lead to long-term survival for patients with high-grade spinal astrocytomas. However, the ethical use of radiocordectomy is questioned, and it is not advocated in the modern era.

The current accepted fractionation is 45–50.4 Gy in 1.8–2 Gy daily fractions for the spinal cord and up to 54 Gy in the region of the cauda equina or in cases of high-grade astrocytomas, 5 days a week, respecting spinal cord and cauda equina tolerances. Various photon energies can be used and have been used in the literature including cobalt (1.25 megavoltage [MV]) and photon energies ranging from 4 to 25 MV photons. The most commonly used energies in

the modern era are 4–10 MV X-ray photons. It is important to take into account the dose to the entire spinal cord in the planning target volume (PTV). The length of the field plus the difference in the contour of the body and spine can create dose inhomogeneity and hot spots on the spinal cord.

A dose-volume histogram (DVH) can accurately account for the dose to the critical normal structures such as the spinal cord and allow for correction and adjustment of dose in the plan accordingly, Fig. 9.5.

Hyperfractionation may increase spinal cord tolerance due to lower fraction sizes, allowing for sublethal damage repair. Thus, the total dose to the spinal cord may be increased without causing increased toxicity. Hyperfractionation has been used in several retrospective studies; however, further studies are needed to elucidate the actual benefit of its use and whether higher total doses can be employed [39].

## Treatment Field Design/Target Delineation

Focal radiation therapy rather than complete neuraxis irradiation is used in the treatment of spinal astrocytomas. Historically with 2-D/3-D radiation therapy, patients were treated either in the supine or prone position using single posterior field, anterior-posterior/posterior-anterior fields (AP-PA), three-field technique, lateral or oblique wedged pairs, or a combination of multiple fields including oblique fields. The field encompassed one to two vertebral bodies above and below the level of the preoperative tumor volume

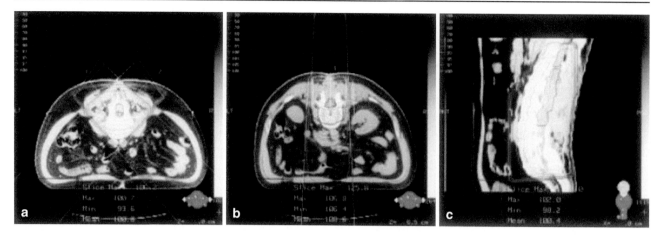

**Fig. 9.6** (**a**) Posterior wedge pair technique with less exit dose to normal tissues and better conformation to spinal target. (**b**) Direct posterior technique is simple applied but has increased exit dose to normal tissues. (**c**) Direct opposed lateral fields for cervical or lumbosacral sites sparing normal tissues. [Reprinted from Isaacson SR. Radiation therapy and the management of intramedullary spinal cord tumors. J Neurooncol. 2000 May;47(3):231–238. With permission from Springer]

or 2–5 centimeter (cm) margins circumferentially [42, 43]. Parallel opposed lateral fields were typically used for cervical spinal lesions to minimize dose to the larynx and pharynx. Thoracic tumor fields were typically treated with direct posterior or posterior wedged fields to minimize dose to the normal structures surrounding the area of involvement. Lumbar and cauda equina tumors were treated with AP-PA fields. Lateral fields were used if there was a need to minimize dose to the organs of the pelvis. Appropriate arm position to avoid beams through the arm and the use of wedges are important to be able to spare pelvic organs such as the ovaries and uterus. The width of the field was established between the tips of the lateral processes of the vertebral bodies or 2 cm on each side of the vertebral body; thus, the average width of the field was 7–8 cm. In the sacral region, the field did not need to extend beyond the sacroiliac joint laterally and does not need to go caudally beyond the S3 vertebral body. Larger fields in the sacral region have not shown to be of benefit [41, 43]. Figure 9.6 depicts various conventional field arrangements in the treatment of spinal cord astrocytomas [43].

With advanced radiation techniques, patients undergo computerized tomography (CT) simulation in the supine or prone position using an immobilization device for setup, including thermoplastic head and neck masks going down to the upper chest for lesions in the cervical spine. The pre- and postoperative post-contrast T1-weighted and T2-weighted fluid-attenuated inversion recovery (FLAIR) MRIs can be fused to the CT for planning. Intensity-modulated radiation therapy (IMRT) or sophisticated dynamic conformal planning techniques are ideal to provide a homogenous dose distribution to the target while minimizing dose to the nearby organs, including the larynx, pharynx, heart, lungs, kidneys, liver, esophagus, and bowel (Fig. 9.7). The gross tumor

volume (GTV) encompasses the resection cavity and residual disease as seen on T1-weighted post-contrast MRI scans plus any non-enhancing tumor seen on T2-weighted FLAIR MRI. Both pre- and postoperative images are used to determine the location and extent of the tumor. A clinical target volume (CTV) margin accounting for microscopic disease is used. Generally, 1–3 cm may be used for low-grade tumors depending on the accuracy of setup and daily image guidance available, whereas a CTV margin of 2–4 cm may be used for high-grade tumors. The CTV is drawn in the rostral and caudal direction, while laterally the CTV may be shaved off natural anatomic boundaries such as the vertebral bodies. Depending on the level of cervical cord involvement in some cases of high cervical spine lesions, a portion of the brain stem will be in the CTV. As discussed, syringomyelias can frequently be seen in spinal cord gliomas and do not need to be included in the treatment volumes. A PTV of 3–5 millimeters (mm) will be added to all CTVs, accounting for the accuracy of setup.

Due to the difficulty in controlling the tumor locally, craniospinal irradiation is not recommended in the setting of high-grade astrocytomas, even though leptomeningeal dissemination is common. Failure is typically local; and thus, the toxicity of craniospinal irradiation outweighs any benefit of controlling any disseminated microscopic disease.

## Normal Critical Structure Tolerance Constraints

In the setting of spinal cord astrocytomas, the dose-limiting structures are the spinal cord and cauda equina themselves. The cauda equina and peripheral nerves have a higher dose tolerance than the spinal cord and are more resistant to radiation toxicity.

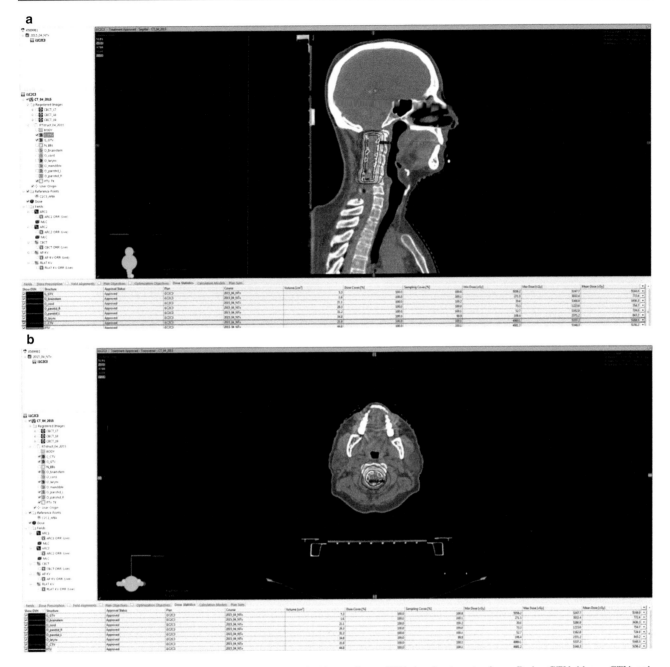

**Fig. 9.7** (**a**) Sagittal view of IMRT plan showing dose sparing of critical structures while maximizing dose to the target. (**b**) Axial view of IMRT plan showing dose sparing of critical structures while maximizing dose to the target. *GTV* gross tumor volume, *CTV* clinical target volume, *PTV* planning target volume. Red = GTV; blue = CTV; yellow = PTV. [Courtesy of University of California, Los Angeles Department of Radiation Oncology]

The spinal cord tolerance depends on the daily fraction, the location of the spinal cord being treated, the length of the spinal cord being irradiated, as well as the use of chemotherapy and prior surgeries. The traditionally accepted dose tolerance for the spinal cord is 45–50 Gy in 1.8–2 Gy daily fractions, with a 5% radiotoxicity at 5 years (tolerated dose [TD] 5/5) [44, 45]. However data has suggested that there is very minimal to no risk of myelopathy with doses of 45 Gy delivered in conventional fractionation and that the TD 5/5 is more likely in the range of 57–61 Gy [46–48]. Thus, the spinal cord may be safely irradiated to doses up to 55 Gy without increased risk with reported rates of myelopathy of 0.2–0.5% with 50 Gy in conventional fractionation and 1–6% with 60 Gy [49–51].

There is minimal data to support reducing the dose with increased target volume of the spinal cord as well as differences in spinal cord tolerance based on location of cervical, thoracic, and lumbar regions [52, 53]. The same dose tolerances are used for the entire spinal cord independent of the volume treated. Maximum point dose for the spinal cord is 50 Gy with a 0.2% risk of myelopathy and 60 Gy with a 6% risk of myelopathy [54].

There are additional organs at risk depending on the location of the tumor within the spinal cord. These organs include the larynx (mean 44 Gy or V50 < 27%), pharynx (mean < 50 Gy), esophagus (mean < 34 Gy), heart (V25 < 10%), lungs (V20 $\leq$ 30%), liver (mean < 30–32 Gy), kidneys (mean < 15–18 Gy for both kidneys), and bowel (V15 < 120 cc for individual small-bowel loops) [54]. With the use of modern conformal treatment planning techniques, doses to these structures can be minimized and are well below their tolerances.

## Radiation Toxicity, Acute and Late

Radiation toxicities are dependent on the region of the spinal canal that is irradiated. For cervical and high thoracic lesions, acute toxicities can include dysphagia, odynophagia, and possibly cough. For mid-thoracic and lumbar lesions, acute toxicities can include nausea, vomiting, and diarrhea. For lesions in all locations, hyperpigmentation or erythema of the skin in the treatment field, fatigue, bone marrow suppression, and transient worsening of patient's neurological symptoms or pain due to edema are all possible. Steroid prescription can help alleviate any transient worsening of neurological symptoms or pain due to edema. Long-term toxicities, though rare, include radiation myelopathy, permanent worsening of present neurological deficits, radiation necrosis, permanent hyperpigmentation of the skin in the treatment field, vertebral body compression fracture or collapse, radiation-induced malignancy, hypothyroidism (for cervical spinal level lesions), permanent dysphagia (for high spinal level lesions), radiation pneumonitis (for thoracic spinal level lesions), and renal or hepatic dysfunction (for lower spinal level lesions).

## Chemotherapy

There is limited data regarding the use of chemotherapy in the treatment of spinal cord astrocytomas. With benefit seen in the use of chemotherapy to treat intracranial astrocytomas, particularly high-grade astrocytomas, chemotherapy is often given to patients with high-grade spinal astrocytomas given their overall poor outcomes with surgery and radiation therapy. Extrapolating from data on the benefit of temozolomide, an oral alkylating agent, for the treatment of high-grade intracranial astrocytomas, temozolomide has been used to treat recurrent low-grade spinal or primary and recurrent high-grade spinal cord gliomas [55–57]. Recurrent low-grade spinal cord gliomas have shown a modest response to temozolomide with a median time to tumor progression of 14.5 months (range 2–28 months) and median survival 23 months (range 4–39 months) [57]. Use of temozolomide in high-grade spinal cord astrocytomas has mixed results with some patients failing to respond to the treatment while others exceeding median survival time of 9 months with 12–16 month survival times as reported in several studies [20, 24, 41, 56].

Temozolomide is administered concurrently with radiation therapy for high-grade spinal cord gliomas at a dose of 75 mg/m$^2$/day as well as adjuvantly for 12 cycles at a dose of 150–200 mg/m$^2$/day for 5 consecutive days every 4 weeks [54–56]. If progression is noted sooner than the completion of the 12 adjuvant cycles, patients can be treated with alternative salvage treatments. For patients with recurrent low-grade spinal cord gliomas who had already undergone prior radiation therapy, temozolomide was administered at a dose of 150–200 mg/m$^2$/day for 5 consecutive days every 4 weeks for a median of 14 cycles [57].

One review stratified the various data available with the use of temozolomide for spinal cord glioblastomas into two groups: those that used temozolomide and those that did not. The group using temozolomide were presented in nine articles for a total of 19 patients. Those that did not use temozolomide were presented in 19 articles with 45 patients. Though not statistically significant, the group of patients treated with temozolomide had a median overall survival of 16 months, compared to a median overall survival of 10 months in the group of patients not treated with temozolomide [58] (Fig. 9.8).

The data, once again, has been mixed with the use of chemotherapy in the treatment of spinal cord astrocytomas with several studies showing a lack of benefit in the use of chemotherapy while others showing a modest and often not statistically significant benefit. In addition, there is minimal data available for adult patients in general. The rarity of these tumors, combined with the low number of patients in these studies, makes it difficult to draw a clear conclusion. However, given temozolomide is well-tolerated often with minimal toxicities, it is generally used in the cases of high-grade spinal gliomas and recurrent low- and high-grade spinal cord gliomas with minimal other treatment options.

Toxicity of temozolomide includes neutropenia, anemia, thrombocytopenia, lymphopenia, nausea, vomiting, fatigue, constipation, insomnia, rash, pruritus, and possible alopecia.

Patients with high-grade spinal cord gliomas who fail temozolomide have been treated with bevacizumab, an antiangiogenic agent and vascular endothelial growth factor (VEGF) inhibitor (10 mg/kg administered once every

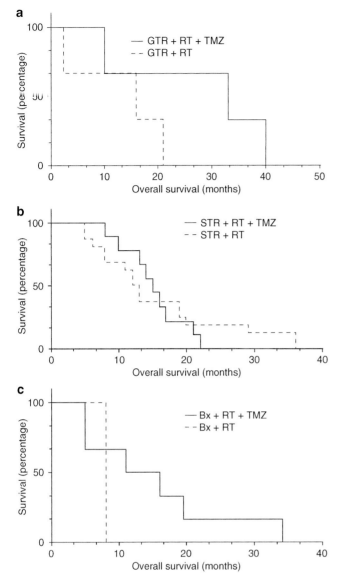

**Fig. 9.8** Kaplan-Meier curves showing overall survival in months according to the treatment received. (**a**) Patients treated with GTR + RT + TMZ compared to those treated with GTR + RT only. (**b**) Patients treated with STR + RT + TMZ compared to those treated with STR + RT only. (**c**) Patients treated with Bx + RT + TMZ compared to those treated with Bx + RT only. *Bx* biopsy, *GTR* gross total resection, *RT* radiotherapy, *STR* subtotal resection, *TMZ* temozolomide. [Reprinted from Hernández-Durán S, Bergy A, Shah AH, Hanft S, Komotar RJ, Manzano GR. Primary spinal cord glioblastoma multiforme treated with temozolomide. J Clin Neurosci. 2015 Dec;22(12):1877–1882. With permission from Elsevier]

2 weeks with two treatments equating one cycle) with overall median disease-free progression of 7 months (range 3–11 months) and an overall survival of 9 months (range 5–13 months) [59]. The effect of bevacizumab to decrease peritumoral edema and mass effect also makes it ideal in the treatment of spinal cord gliomas, particularly when given concurrently with radiation therapy. Its direct

effect on the tumor as well as the edema and mass effect not only can contribute to a survival benefit but can also improve neurological symptoms that a patient has developed secondary to edema and mass effect either from the tumor itself or from radiation therapy. Another review evaluated eight patients with high-grade spinal cord astrocytomas treated with temozolomide at varying doses and schedules in both the upfront and recurrent settings and six patients treated with bevacizumab all treated at the time of recurrence. Both the use of temozolomide and bevacizumab showed an improvement in radiographic and clinical findings [60]. Bevacizumab (10 mg/kg) can be also be used concurrently with temozolomide and radiation therapy in the management of spinal cord astrocytomas [61].

Toxicity of bevacizumab includes anemia, leukopenia, thrombosis/embolism, intratumoral hemorrhage, epistaxis, infection without neutropenia, fatigue, hypertension, proteinuria, and possible wound dehiscence.

Other agents that have been used in children include lomustine, carboplatin, and vincristine; chemotherapy which includes procarbazine, lomustine, and vincristine (PCV); and 8-in-1 chemotherapy which includes vincristine, carmustine, procarbazine, hydroxyurea, cisplatin, cytarabine, prednisone, and cyclophosphamide. There has been a varied response to these regimens, though the 8-in-1 did not show benefit compared to less inclusive regimens. These various drugs can be tried in individual cases with minimal to no other treatment options [1]. Long-term results of Radiation Therapy Oncology Group (RTOG) 9402 evaluating the use of PCV in the treatment of intracranial anaplastic oligodendrogliomas showed a benefit to the use of PCV plus radiation therapy in the treatment of tumors that had the 1p/19q co-deletion [62]. Perhaps there can be a benefit to the use of PCV in the treatment of high-grade spinal cord astrocytomas as one case report suggests [63].

The toxicities of PCV chemotherapy are more intense and the regimen is harder to complete. Side effects include myelosuppression, cognitive or mood change, peripheral or autonomic neuropathy, vomiting, hepatic dysfunction, and rash [62].

Larger, prospective studies are needed to determine the true efficacy of chemotherapy in the treatment of spinal cord astrocytomas as well as the use of radiosensitizers, targeted therapy, or immunotherapy. There are ongoing studies evaluating the use of various agents in the treatment of intracranial high-grade gliomas; however, studies are needed to specifically evaluate the role of these agents in the management of spinal cord gliomas. Evaluating therapies that can cross the blood-brain barrier and deliver the drug to specific regions of the spinal cord involved may also improve results with systemic treatment. Intrathecal delivery of chemotherapy or systemic agents bypasses the blood-brain barrier; however, there is still the issue of penetrating the spinal cord tissue [64]. In addition, intrathecal therapy can lead to unnecessary side effects as the drug distributes throughout the entire central nervous system.

## Failure Pattern

Local recurrence is the dominant failure pattern [65]. Recurrence outside the radiation or surgical treatment area is rare and typically only seen in cases of high-grade spinal cord astrocytomas, which do have a tendency for leptomeningeal dissemination. High-grade spinal cord astrocytomas have a rate of 50–60% distant spread in some studies [33]. Intracranial metastases have been reported in several studies [35, 41, 42] as well as extraneural metastases in the liver and spleen [21].

## Outcomes: Tumor Control and Survival

Tumor control and survival are moderate for low-grade spinal cord astrocytomas but quite poor in the setting of high-grade astrocytomas (Fig. 9.9) [36]. There is a significant difference in the control and survival rates when comparing anaplastic astrocytomas and glioblastoma; however, many of the reports in the literature do not separate the two diagnoses in their analyses. Five-year survival rates are on the order of 50–60% for most low-grade spinal cord astrocytomas treated with biopsy, surgery, and often adjuvant radiation therapy (Table 9.2), whereas the median survival for most high-grade spinal astrocytomas is on the order of 6–15 months with trimodality therapy: surgery, radiation therapy, and chemotherapy (Table 9.3).

## Follow-Up

Follow-up should consist of radiographic assessment and clinical exam to assess for disease progression every 3–4 months during the first year. Increasing intervals may be used for low-grade astrocytomas, whereas continued close monitoring of high-grade astrocytomas is necessary due to the high relapse rate and poor survival.

## Case Presentation

A 42-year-old man presented with a several month history of left-sided numbness and paresthesia. MRI of the cervical spine revealed a heterogeneously enhancing intramedullary 1.0 cm lesion at the C4–C5 level with an associated syrinx extending from C1 to C5. He underwent C4–C5

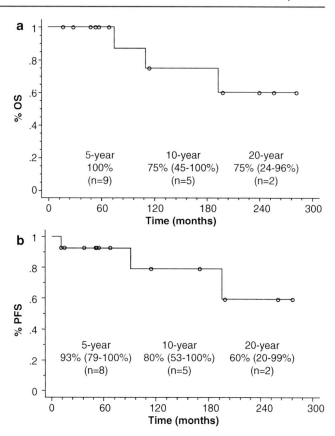

**Fig. 9.9** Kaplan-Meier survival curves for: (**a**) Overall survival (OS) and (**b**) Progression-free survival (PFS) for all patients with low-grade astrocytoma of the spinal cord. Survival data for all patients with 5-, 10-, and 20-year survival rates reported and 95% confidence intervals in parentheses. [Reprinted from Robinson CG, Prayson RA, Hahn JF, Kalfas IH, Whitfield MD, Lee SY et al. Int J Radiat Oncol Biol Phys. Sept 1;63(1):91–100. With permission from Elsevier]

complete bilateral laminectomy with microscopic piecemeal resection of the tumor. The surgery was a near gross total resection, and pathology revealed infiltrative astrocytoma, WHO grade II. Ki-67 revealed rare positive tumor cell nuclei. The cells were minimally pleomorphic and mitoses were inconspicuous. There were rare Rosenthal fibers seen. Postoperative MRI 2 months later revealed postoperative changes and the resection cavity with myelomalacia of the cervical cord with uncertain evidence of residual disease (Fig. 9.10). The remainder of his spine as well as his brain were imaged 2 months later without evidence of disease.

Postoperatively, the patient had some residual left-sided numbness in the arm, torso, and legs but otherwise had no deficits. Patient was presented at the multidisciplinary tumor board. Given the infiltrative nature of the tumor, it was thought that the resection was subtotal, at least microscopically, and that there would be a high risk of relapse. Recommendation was made for adjuvant focal radiation therapy. He received 5040 cGy in 28 fractions of 180 cGy

**Table 9.2** Outcomes of spinal cord astrocytomas treated with postoperative radiation therapy

| Author/study | Tumor histology | 5-Year actuarial OS (%) | 10-Year actuarial OS (%) | 5-Year RFS (%) | 10-Year RFS (%) | 5-Year PFS (%) | 10-Year PFS (%) |
|---|---|---|---|---|---|---|---|
| Garcia (1985) [36] | LGA | 60 | 50 | NR | NR | NR | NR |
| Linstadt (1989) [37] | LGA | 91 | 91 | 66 | 53 | – | – |
| Chun (1990) [63] | LGA | 60 | 40 | 40 | 25 | – | – |
| Sandler (1992) [15] | LGA | 57 | 57 | 44 | 30 | – | – |
| Huddart (1993) [32] | Mixed LGA/HGA | 59 | 52 | – | – | 38 | 26 |
| Shirato (1995) [35] | Mixed LGA/HGA | 50 | NR | NR | NR | NR | NR |
| Jyothirmaryi (1997) [31] | Mixed LGA/HGA | 55 | 39 | – | – | 75 | 55 |
| Rodrigues (2000) [16] | Mixed LGA/HGA | 54 | 45 | – | – | 58 | 43 |
| Robinson (2005) [34] | LGA | 100 | 75 | – | – | 93 | 80 |
| AbdelWahab (2006) [18] | Mixed LGA/HGA | 59 | 53 | – | – | 42 | 29 |
| Minehan (2009) [19] | Mixed LGA/HGA | 29 | 17 | – | – | LGG-64 HGG-20 | NR |

*OS* overall survival, *RFS* recurrence-free survival, *PFS* progression-free survival, *LGA* low-grade astrocytoma, *HGA* high-grade astrocytoma, *NR* not reported

**Table 9.3** Outcomes of high-grade spinal cord astrocytomas

| Author/study | MS (months) | Treatment | 1-Year OS (%) | 5-Year OS (%) |
|---|---|---|---|---|
| Cohen (1989) [39] | 6 | Surgery + RT + CTx | NR | NR |
| Linstadt (1989) [37] | <8 | Surgery + RT | – | 0 |
| Jyothirmaryi (1997) [31] | 10 | Surgery + RT | NR | NR |
| Kim (2001) [40] | AA: 107 GBM: 14 | Surgery + RT | NR | NR |
| Santi (2003) [17] | 10–13 | Surgery + RT + CTx | NR | NR |
| Raco (2005) [4] | 15.5 | Surgery | NR | NR |
| McGirt (2008) [22] | 43 AA: 72 GBM: 9 | Surgery + RT + CTx | 75 AA: 85 GBM: 31 | 45 AA: 59 GBM: 0 |

*MS* median survival, *RT* radiation therapy, *CTx* chemotherapy, *NR* not reported, *AA* anaplastic astrocytoma, *GBM* glioblastoma

per fraction to the cervical cord from C1 to C6 using IMRT (Fig. 9.11). He tolerated the treatment well without any side effects. He has been followed for 7 years with stable neck tension and numbness in his left third and fourth distal fingers. He has yearly surveillance MRIs which have been without evidence of disease.

## Summary

- Primary spinal cord tumors comprise 2–4% of all adult central nervous system tumors of which astrocytomas account for approximately 6–8% of all spinal cord tumors.
- Intramedullary tumors comprise 8–10% of all primary spinal cord tumors of which 30–40% are astrocytomas.

- Astrocytic tumors of the spinal cord consist of juvenile pilocytic astrocytoma (World Health Organization [WHO] grade I), diffuse or low-grade astrocytoma (WHO grade II), anaplastic astrocytoma (WHO grade III), and glioblastoma (WHO grade IV), with the majority consisting of low-grade (WHO grade 2) diffuse or fibrillary astrocytomas.
- There are no established risk factors of astrocytic spinal cord tumors.
- Symptoms including back pain, radicular symptoms, bowel and bladder dysfunction, impotence, gait difficulties, or slowly progressive motor and sensory deficits.
- The modified McCormick scale is used to assess patients' functional status both preoperatively and postoperatively.
- Tumor histology and grade are the most significant prognostic factors of primary spinal cord astrocytomas. Sex, age, extent of resection, performance status, and adjuvant therapy are additional prognostic factors.
- Surgery is considered the mainstay of treatment for intramedullary spinal tumors in general; however, the specific role in the management of spinal cord astrocytomas is less evident. For infiltrative tumors such as astrocytomas, a gross total resection and even a subtotal resection can be very difficult to achieve due to the involvement of the spinal cord itself. Maximal safe resection or biopsy leads to diagnosis, relief of symptoms, and possible improved survival in some patients.
- Tumor histology predicts for resectability and recurrence, while intraoperative identification of a clear tumor plane for resection has prognostic significance and higher incidence of long-term neurological function improvement.
- Radiation therapy is indicated or is encouraged in patients with grade III–IV spinal cord astrocytomas, progressive

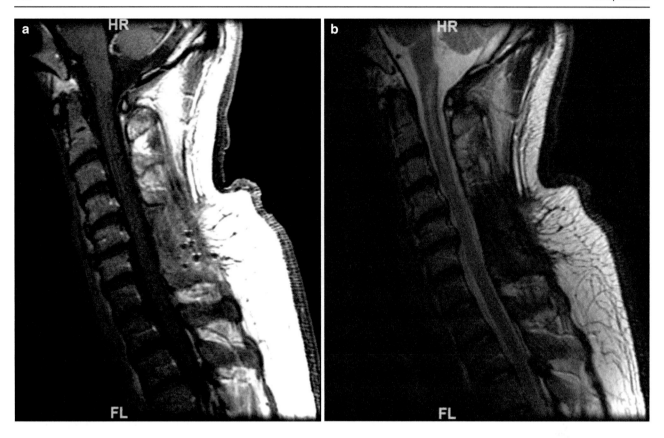

**Fig. 9.10** (**a**) Two-month postoperative sagittal T1 contrast-enhanced spine MRI demonstrating myelomalacia with no clear evidence of gross residual disease. (**b**) Two-month postoperative sagittal T2 spine MRI

tumors, and tumors that have undergone subtotal resections.

- There are several studies to suggest and recommend that patients undergo maximal safe resection followed by observation for low-grade spinal cord astrocytomas, whereas other studies show a benefit to postoperative radiation therapy in subtotally resected low-grade spinal cord astrocytomas. Observation of resected pilocytic spinal astrocytomas is recommended.

- Conventionally fractionated stereotactic radiotherapy, intensity-modulated radiation therapy, dynamic conformal radiation therapy, and 3-D conformal therapy techniques are the most commonly used radiation treatment techniques in the delivery of radiation therapy for spinal cord astrocytomas in the modern era.

- The current accepted fractionation is 45–50.4 Gy in 1.8–2 Gy daily fractions for the spinal cord and up to 54 Gy in the region of the cauda equina or in cases of high-grade astrocytomas, 5 days a week, respecting spinal cord and cauda equina tolerances.

- Extrapolating from data for the treatment of high-grade intracranial astrocytomas, temozolomide and bevacizumab have been used to treat recurrent low-grade spinal gliomas or primary and recurrent high-grade spinal gliomas. Further studies are needed to understand the full potential and benefit of chemotherapy in the treatment of spinal cord astrocytomas.

- Local recurrence is the dominant failure pattern. High-grade astrocytomas have a tendency for leptomeningeal dissemination.

- Five-year survival rates are on the order of 50–60% for most low-grade spinal cord astrocytomas treated with biopsy, surgery, and often adjuvant radiation therapy, whereas the median survival for most high-grade spinal cord astrocytomas is on the order of 6–15 months.

- Follow-up should consist of radiographic assessment and clinical exam to assess for disease progression every 3–4 months during the first year for low-grade astrocytomas and greater intervals thereafter, whereas for high-grade astrocytomas, continued monitoring every 3–4 months is ideal.

## Self-Assessment Questions

1. The most common spinal cord tumor in adults is:
   A. Ependymoma
   B. Astrocytoma
   C. Hemangioblastoma
   D. Meningioma

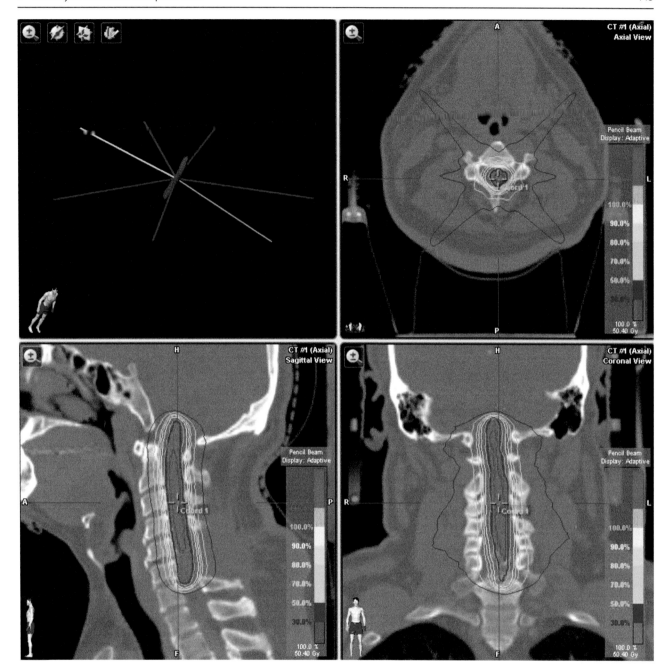

**Fig. 9.11** Axial, sagittal, and coronal plane of a postoperative intensity-modulated radiation therapy (IMRT) plan for spinal grade II astrocytoma status post near gross total piecemeal resection; 5040 cGy (orange isodose line) in 28 fractions delivered to the spinal cord and canal from C1 to C6

2. Which of the following molecular markers are not part of the 2016 WHO grading of CNS tumors:
   A. IDH
   B. H3 K27M
   C. PTEN
   D. 1p/19q

3. Five-year overall survival for grade I spinal astrocytomas is:
   A. 90%
   B. 80%

   C. 70%
   D. 60%

4. The rate of achieving a gross total resection in a grade II spinal astrocytoma is:
   A. Up to 50%
   B. Up to 80%
   C. Up to 10%
   D. Up to 20%

5. Which of the following radiation treatment modalities would be the most effective in the management of spinal astrocytomas:
   A. Hyperfractionation
   B. Hypofractionation
   C. Stereotactic radiosurgery
   D. Intensity-modulated radiation therapy

## Answers

1. A [1, 2]
2. C [10]
3. B [14]
4. D [4, 7, 21, 24]
5. D [21, 36–41]

## References

1. Chamberlain MC, Tredway TL. Adult primary intradural spinal cord tumors: a review. Curr Neurol Neurosci Rep. 2011;11(3):320–8.
2. Minehan KJ, Shaw EG, Scheithauer BW, et al. Spinal cord astrocytoma: pathological and treatment considerations. J Neurosurg. 1995;83(4):590–5.
3. Parsa AT, Chi JH, Acosta FL Jr, et al. Intramedullary spinal cord tumors: molecular insights and surgical innovation. Clin Neurosurg. 2005;52:76–84.
4. Raco A, Esposito V, Lenzi J, et al. Long-term follow-up of intramedullary spinal cord tumors: a series of 202 cases. Neurosurgery. 2005;56(5):972–81.
5. Hsu S, Quattrone M, Ostrom Q, et al. Incidence patterns for primary malignant spinal cord gliomas: a Surveillance, Epidemiology and End Results (SEER) study. J Neurosurg Spine. 2011;14(6):742–7.
6. Huang B, Starostik P, Kühl J, et al. Loss of heterozygosity on chromosome 22 in human ependymomas. Acta Neuropathol. 2002;103(4):415–20.
7. Zadnik PL, Gokaslan ZL, Burger PC, et al. Spinal cord tumours: advances in genetics and their implications for treatment. Nat Rev Neurol. 2013;9(5):257–66.
8. Manzano G, Green BA, Vanni S, et al. Contemporary management of adult intramedullary spinal tumors—pathology and neurological outcomes related to surgery. Spinal Cord. 2008;46(8):540–6.
9. Abul-Kasim K, Thurnher MM, McKeever, et al. Intradural spinal tumors: current classification and MRI features. Neuroradiology. 2008;50(4):301–14.
10. Koeller KK, Rosenblum RS, Morrison AL. Neoplasms of the spinal cord and filum terminale: radiologic-pathologic correlation. Radiographics. 2000;20(6):1721–49.
11. Timpone VM, Patel SH. MRI of a syrinx: is contrast material always necessary? Am J Roentgenol. 2015;204(5):1082–5.
12. Louis DN, Perry A, Reifenberger G, et al. The 2016 World Health Organization classification of tumors of the central nervous system: a summary. Acta Neuropathol. 2016;131(6):803–20.
13. Seki T, Hida K, Yano S, et al. Clinical factors for prognosis and treatment guidance of spinal cord astrocytoma. Asian Spine J. 2016;10(4):748–54.
14. Wong AP, Dahdaleh NS, Fessler RG, et al. Risk factors and long-term survival in adult patients with primary malignant spinal cord astrocytomas. J Neurooncol. 2013;115(3):493–503.
15. Innocenzi G, Salvati M, Cervoni L, et al. Prognostic factors in intramedullary astrocytomas. Clin Neurol Neurosurg. 1997;99(1):1–5.
16. Milano MT, Johnson MD, Sul J, et al. Primary spinal cord glioma: a surveillance, epidemiology, and end results database study. J Neurooncol. 2010;98(1):83–92.
17. Adams H, Avendano J, Raza SM, et al. Prognostic factors and survival in primary malignant astrocytomas of the spinal cord: a population-based analysis from 1973 to 2007. Spine. 2012;37(12):1–20.
18. Sandler HM, Papadopoulos SM, Thornton AF Jr, et al. Spinal cord astrocytomas: results of therapy. Neurosurgery. 1992;30(4):490–3.
19. Rodrigues GB, Waldron JN, Wong CS, et al. A retrospective analysis of 52 cases of spinal cord glioma managed with radiation therapy. Int J Radiat Oncol Biol Phys. 2000;48(3):837–42.
20. Santi M, Mena H, Wong K, et al. Spinal cord malignant astrocytomas. Clinicopathologic features in 36 cases. Cancer. 2003;98(3):554–61.
21. Abdel-Wahab M, Etuk B, Palermo J, et al. Spinal cord gliomas: a multi-institutional retrospective analysis. Int J Radiat Oncol Biol Phys. 2006;64(4):1060–71.
22. Minehan KJ, Brown PD, Scheithauer BW, et al. Prognosis and treatment of spinal cord astrocytoma. Int J Radiat Oncol Biol Phys. 2009;73(3):727–33.
23. Constantini S, Miller DC, Allen JC, et al. Radical excision of intramedullary spinal cord tumors: surgical morbidity and long-term follow-up evaluation in 164 children and young adults. J Neurosurg. 2000;93(2 Suppl):183–93.
24. McGirt MJ, Goldstein IM, Chaichana KL, et al. Extent of surgical resection of malignant astrocytomas of the spinal cord: outcome analysis of 35 patients. Neurosurgery. 2008;63(1):55–60.
25. Babu R, Karikari IO, Owens TR, et al. Spinal cord astrocytomas: a modern 20-year experience at a single institution. Spine. 2014;39(7):533–40.
26. Garcés-Ambrossi GL, McGirt MJ, Mehta VA, et al. Factors associated with progression-free survival and long-term neurological outcome after resection of intramedullary spinal cord tumors: analysis of 101 consecutive cases. J Neurosurg Spine. 2009;11(5):591–9.
27. Babu R, Karikari IO, Owens TR, et al. Spinal cord astrocytomas. Spine. 2014;39(7):533–40.
28. Karikari IO, Nimjee SM, Hodges TR, et al. Impact of tumor histology on resectability and neurological outcome in primary intramedullary spinal cord tumors: a single-center experience with 102 patients. Neurosurgery. 2015;68(1):188–97.
29. Epstein FJ, Farmer J, Freed D. Adult intramedullary astrocytomas of the spinal cord. J Neurosurg. 1992;77(3):355–9.
30. Juthani RG, Bilsky MH, Vogelbaum MA. Current management and treatment modalities for intramedullary spinal cord tumors. Curr Treat Options Oncol. 2015;16(8):39.
31. Klekamp J. Treatment of intramedullary tumors: analysis of surgical morbidity and long-term results. J Neurosurg Spine. 2013;19(1):12–26.
32. Boström A, Kanther N-C, Grote A, et al. Management and outcome in adult intramedullary spinal cord tumours: a 20-year single institution experience. BMC Res Notes. 2014;7:908.
33. Huddart R, Traish D, Ashley S, et al. Management of spinal astrocytoma with conservative surgery and radiotherapy. Br J Neurosurg. 1993;7(5):473–81.
34. Shirato H, Kamada T, Hida K, et al. The role of radiotherapy in the management of spinal cord glioma. Int J Radiat Oncol Biol Phys. 1995;33(2):323–8.
35. Jyothirmayi R, Madhavan J, Nair MK, et al. Conservative surgery and radiotherapy in the treatment of spinal cord astrocytoma. J Neurooncol. 1997;33(3):205–11.
36. Robinson CG, Prayson RA, Hahn JF, et al. Long-term survival and functional status of patients with low-grade astrocytoma of spinal cord. Int J Radiat Oncol Biol Phys. 2005;63(1):91–100.

37. Kahn J, Loeffler JS, Niemierko A, et al. Long-term outcomes of patients with spinal cord gliomas treated by modern conformal radiation techniques. Int J Radiat Oncol Biol Phys. 2011;81(1):232–8.

38. Garcia D. Primary spinal cord tumors treated with surgery and postoperative irradiation. Int J Radiat Oncol Biol Phys. 1985;11(11):1933–9.

39. Linstadt D, Wara WW, Leibel SA, et al. Postoperative radiotherapy of primary spinal cord tumors. Int J Radiat Oncol Biol Phys. 1989;16(6):1397–403.

40. Nowak-Sadzikowska J, Gliński B. The value of postoperative radiotherapy of primary spinal cord glioma. Rep Pract Oncol Radiother. 2002;7(4):139–47.

41. Cohen AR, Wisof JH, Allen JC, et al. Malignant astrocytomas of the spinal cord. J Neurosurg. 1989;70(1):50–4.

42. Kim MS, Chung CK, Choe G, et al. Intramedullary spinal cord astrocytoma in adult: postoperative outcome. J Neurooncol. 2001;52(1):85–94.

43. Isaacson SR. Radiation therapy and the management of intramedullary spinal cord tumors. J Neurooncol. 2000;47(3):231–8.

44. Wara WM, Phillips TL, Sheline GE, et al. Radiation tolerance of the spinal cord. Cancer. 1975;35(6):1558–62.

45. Phillips TL, Buschke F. Radiation tolerance of the thoracic spinal cord. Am J Roentgenol Radium Ther Nucl Med. 1969;105(3):659–64.

46. Schultheiss TE, Stephens LC. The pathogenesis of radiation myelopathy: widening the circle. Int J Radiat Oncol Biol Phys. 1995;23(5):1089–93.

47. Schultheiss TE, Kun LE, Ang KK, et al. Radiation response of the central nervous system. Int J Radiat Oncol Biol Phys. 1995;31(5):1093–112.

48. Schultheiss TE. The radiation dose-response of the human spinal cord. Int J Radiat Oncol Biol Phys. 2008;71(5):145–1459.

49. Kirkpatrick JP, van der Kogel AJ, Schultheiss TE. Radiation dose-volume effects in the spinal cord. Int J Radiat Oncol Biol Phys. 2010;76(3 Suppl):S42–9.

50. Marcus RB Jr, Million RR. The incidence of myelitis after irradiation of the cervical spinal cord. Int J Radiat Oncol Biol Phys. 1990;19(1):3–8.

51. Rampling R, Symonds P. Radiation myelopathy. Curr Opin Neurol. 1998;11(6):627–32.

52. Schultheiss TE, Stephens LC, Ang KK, et al. Volume effects in rhesus monkey spinal cord. Int J Radiat Oncol Biol Phys. 1994;29(1):67–72.

53. Schultheiss TE, Stephens LC, Jiang GL, et al. Radiation myelopathy in primates treated with conventional fractionation. Int J Radiat Oncol Biol Phys. 1990;19(4):935–40.

54. Marks LB, Yorke ED, Jackson A, et al. Use of normal tissue complication probability models in the clinic. Int J Radiat Oncol Biol Phys. 2010;76(3 Suppl):S10–9.

55. Stupp R, Mason WP, van den Bent MJ, et al. Radiotherapy plus concomitant and adjuvant temozolomide for glioblastoma. N Engl J Med. 2005;352(10):987–96.

56. Kim WH, Yoon SH, Kim CY, et al. Temozolomide for malignant primary spinal cord glioma: an experience of six cases and a literature review. J Neurooncol. 2011;101(2):247–54.

57. Chamberlain MC. Temozolomide for recurrent low-grade spinal cord gliomas in adults. Cancer. 2008;113(5):1019–24.

58. Hernández-Durán S, Bergy A, Shah AH, et al. Primary spinal cord glioblastoma multiforme treated with temozolomide. J Clin Neurosci. 2015;22(12):1877–82.

59. Chamberlain MC, Johnston SK. Recurrent spinal cord glioblastoma: salvage therapy with bevacizumab. J Neurooncol. 2011;102(3):427–32.

60. Kaley TJ, Mondesire-Crump I, Gavrilovic IT. Temozolomide or bevacizumab for spinal high-grade gliomas. J Neurooncol. 2012;109(2):385–9.

61. Yanamadala V, Koffie RM, Shankar GM, et al. Spinal cord glioblastoma: 25years of experience from a single institution. J Clin Neurosci. 2016;27:138–41.

62. Cairncross G, Wang M, Shaw E, et al. Phase III trial of chemoradiotherapy for anaplastic oligodendroglioma: long-term results of RTOG 9402. J Clin Oncol. 2013;31(3):337–42.

63. Henson JW, Thornton AF, Louis DN. Spinal cord astrocytoma: response to PCV chemotherapy. Neurology. 2000;54(2):518–20.

64. Tobin MK, Geraghty JR, Engelhard HH, et al. Intramedullary spinal cord tumors: a review of current and future treatment strategies. Neurosurg Focus. 2015;39(2):E14.

65. Chun HC, Schmidt-Ullrich RK, Wolfson A, et al. External beam radiotherapy for primary spinal cord tumors. J Neurooncol. 1990;9(3):211–7.

# Spinal Cord Ependymoma

Martin C. Tom, Ehsan H. Balagamwala, John H. Suh, and Samuel T. Chao

## Learning Objectives

- Understand the epidemiology and risk factors for spinal cord ependymomas.
- Describe the clinical presentation and subtypes for spinal cord ependymomas.
- Review the associated prognostic and predictive factors for spinal cord ependymomas.
- Describe the overall management strategy, including indications for radiotherapy and associated treatment planning for spinal cord ependymomas.
- Summarize the expected outcomes for spinal cord ependymomas.

## Background Epidemiology

Ependymomas are glial tumors arising from ependymal cells and most commonly occur in the white matter adjacent to the ventricular surface, along the central canal of the spinal cord, or in the filum terminale. They are frequently divided into three sites, including the supratentorial region, the infratentorial region, and the spinal cord. Large population databases report that ependymomas occur in the spinal cord 52% of the time [1]. This was corroborated in a large series of pathologically confirmed adult ependymoma, where the majority occurred in the spinal cord (46%), followed by the infratentorial region (35%), and supratentorial region (19%) [2]. Ependymomas occur in the spinal cord more commonly in adults (50–60%) as com-

pared to children (21.3%) [1]. However, among all spinal cord tumors in adults, ependymomas are only the third most common histology accounting for 20.5%, behind meningeal tumors (37.6%) and nerve sheath tumors (23.1%). Among all spinal cord tumors in ages 0–19, ependymomas are actually the most common histology (21.6%) [3].

Overall, spinal cord ependymomas occur at an annual age adjusted rate of 0.22 per 100,000 [1]. Among central nervous system (CNS) tumors, ependymal tumors have a higher incidence rate in males than females (1.3 times) and in whites than blacks (1.7 times) [3]. The most common age at diagnosis is between 40 and 44 years [2, 4–6].

Myxopapillary ependymoma (MPE) is a morphological variant and subset of ependymoma with distinct characteristics that have been studied independently. A recent Surveillance, Epidemiology, and End Results (SEER) Program analysis reported an incidence of 1 per million person-years, with higher incidence among men and Caucasians. Incidence peaks among those ages 25–29 and 45–59 [7]. About 2.2% present with spinal cord dissemination [8].

## Familial Syndromes and Risk Factors

Neurofibromatosis type 2 (NF2) is a dominant heritable syndrome caused by abnormalities in the NF2 gene and is manifested by multiple tumors of the nervous system. In addition to the hallmark bilateral vestibular schwannomas, many individuals with the syndrome will develop spinal cord tumors. Whereas schwannomas of the dorsal root are the most commonly associated spinal cord tumors of NF2, imaging evidence of ependymomas is seen in 33–53% of these patients with the most common location being the cervical cord or cervicomedullary junction [9–11]. In contrast to sporadic spinal cord ependymomas, those associated with NF2 tend to display an indolent growth pattern, and some advocate that they can be reasonably observed if found incidentally [11]. No risk factors for the development of spinal cord ependymomas have been identified.

M. C. Tom · E. H. Balagamwala
Department of Radiation Oncology, Taussig Cancer Institute, Cleveland Clinic, Cleveland, OH, USA
e-mail: chaos@ccf.org

J. H. Suh · S. T. Chao (✉)
Department of Radiation Oncology, Taussig Cancer Institute, Cleveland Clinic, Cleveland, OH, USA

Rose Ella Burkhardt Brain Tumor and Neuro-oncology Center, Cleveland Clinic, Cleveland, OH, USA

© Springer International Publishing AG, part of Springer Nature 2018
E. L. Chang et al. (eds.), *Adult CNS Radiation Oncology*, https://doi.org/10.1007/978-3-319-42878-9_10

## Presentation and Diagnosis

In a survey of adult spinal cord ependymoma patients, the most common self-reported presenting symptoms included numbness/tingling (67%), back pain (58%), weakness (51%), and radiating back pain (46%). Twenty-nine percent of these patients endorsed moderate to severe symptoms, and the majority were symptomatic for over 6 months prior to surgery [12]. Tumor location within the spinal cord often dictates symptomatology, with the most common location being cervical (32%), followed by conus/cauda equina (26.8%), thoracic (16.3%), cervicothoracic (16.3%), thoracolumbar (5.1%), and cervicomedullary (3.4%). Limb weakness is the most common symptom for upper spinal cord (cervical and thoracic) ependymomas, whereas back pain is more common in lower spinal cord lesions (thoracolumbar and conus/cauda equina). Bowel or bladder dysfunction and abnormal gait are fairly evenly distributed among different spinal cord locations. Grade II ependymomas are more commonly found in the upper spinal cord, while myxopapillary ependymomas make up the majority of lower spinal cord ependymomas. Grade III (anaplastic) ependymomas appear to be relatively evenly distributed along the spinal cord [13].

## Classification, Pathology, and Imaging

The 2016 World Health Organization (WHO) classification of CNS tumors divides ependymal tumors into five groups based on cellular density, degree of variability of cellular pleomorphism, number of mitotic figures, degree of tumor infiltration, and now includes genetic markers. Grade I tumors are either subependymoma or myxopapillary ependymoma. Grade II tumors are designated ependymoma and are further subclassified into papillary, clear cell, and tanycytic subtypes. Grade III tumors are called anaplastic or malignant ependymoma. A new group for the 2016 classification is called ependymoma RELA fusion positive, which can be grade II or III and relates to most supratentorial ependymomas in children [14].

Subependymomas (grade I) occur most commonly in the fourth ventricle followed by the lateral ventricles. On MRI, they typically appear as well-demarcated, nonenhancing, nodular masses. Histologic characteristics include hypocellular clusters of cells with bland nuclei set within abundant glial matrix commonly accompanied by microcystic changes [15].

Myxopapillary ependymomas (grade I) represent a biologically and morphologically distinct subtype compared to other ependymomas. They generally occur in the region of the conus medullaris, cauda equina, and filum terminale. Less commonly they are found in the cervical or thoracic cord and rarely in the ventricles or brain parenchyma. On

MRI they appear as well-circumscribed, gadolinium-enhancing, sausage-shaped masses. Histological characteristics include pseudopapillary structures, mucin-rich microcysts, collagen balls or balloons, and tumor cells surrounded by mucoid material [15].

Ependymoma (grade II) is the most common subtype among intramedullary spinal cord tumors. They are further subclassified based on histopathologic appearance into papillary (central vascular core surrounded by cylindrical cells), clear cell (regularly arranged cells with clear cytoplasm and inconspicuous perivascular rosettes), or tanycytic (elongated spindle-shaped cells with eosinophilic fibrillary processes arranged in fascicles and prominent pseudorosettes) [15]. The cellular subtype has been removed from the 2016 classification [14].

Anaplastic ependymomas (grade III) are less common and display anaplastic features of abundant mitosis, hypercellularity, hyperchromatic and pleomorphic nuclei, pseudopalisading necrosis, microvascular proliferation, and the lack of ependymal rosettes [15].

## Prognostic and Predictive Factors

Given the rarity of spinal cord ependymomas, data regarding prognostic factors are limited to population-based databases and retrospective analyses with fairly low sample sizes. Smaller analyses have identified tumor size, length of clinical history, preoperative neurologic status, and presence of metastasis as prognostic factors [16–22]. Larger studies have identified location, grade, and age as prognosticators. Predictive factors include extent of resection and, controversially, postoperative radiation therapy (RT). A summary is located in Table 10.1.

Among all ependymomas, spinal cord location is associated with significantly improved median 5-year progression-free survival (PFS) (87%), as compared to the supratentorial

**Table 10.1** Summary of prognostic and predictive factors among spinal cord ependymomas in the literature

| | N | Prognostic and predictive factors |
|---|---|---|
| Vera-Bolanos et al. [2] | 129 | GTR had improved PFS over STR + RT |
| Tarapore et al. [6] | 134 | GTR improved PFS over STR + RT Grade II had longest PFS (followed by grade I and then grade III) |
| Abdel-Wahab et al. [23] | 126 | Complete resection improved OS Increasing age improved OS and PFS |
| Lee et al. [4] | 88 | Extent of resection improved PFS Anaplastic histology had worse PFS |
| Oh et al. [5] | 348 | STR + RT improved PFS vs. STR alone GTR improved OS vs. STR + RT WHO grade III had worse PFS than grade II |

*GTR* gross total resection, *OS* overall survival, *PFS* progression-free survival, *RT* radiation therapy, *STR* subtotal resection

(38%) and infratentorial locations (78%) [2]. Molecular studies suggest spinal cord ependymomas have genetics distinct from their intracranial counterparts [24, 25]. Additionally, in a large pathologic study, histologic characteristics predicted outcomes for intracranial ependymomas, whereas none of these characteristics were found to be predictive among spinal cord ependymomas [26]. Ependymomas of the upper spinal cord (i.e., cervicothoracic, cervical, cervicomedullary) appear to have more favorable 5-year recurrence rates (11%) compared to lower spinal cord (i.e., conus/cauda equina, thoracolumbar, thoracic) lesions (29.7%) [13]. Furthermore, tumor grade predicts outcomes, although not designedly. Median PFS is most favorable for grade II spinal cord ependymomas (14.9 years), followed by grade I (6 years) and grade III (3.7 years) [6]. Additionally, increasing age appears to decrease the risk of disease progression [23].

The strongest predictor of outcomes is the extent of surgical resection. Up to 77% of patients achieve gross total resection (GTR), which provides the best chance of cure and has consistently demonstrated an improvement in PFS [2, 4–6, 23, 27]. Furthermore, a compilation of the literature demonstrated an overall survival (OS) benefit for those who achieved GTR [5]. This may explain why grade II ependymomas have improved outcomes since they are more likely to occur in the upper spinal cord and are thus more amenable to GTR, as opposed to MPE which tend to involve the cauda equina.

The role of postoperative radiation is unclear, despite several studies attempting to address this question. Evidence in support of adjuvant radiation comes from an extensive literature review compiling data from 348 patients, which appropriately excluded myxopapillary ependymomas (as well as all WHO grade I ependymomas). Of the 80 patients who underwent subtotal resection (STR), 47 received postoperative radiation. Five-year PFS was significantly improved with the receipt of adjuvant RT after STR (65.3%) compared to STR alone (45.1%), which remained significant on multivariate analysis (HR = 2.26, $p = 0.047$). PFS with STR and RT was still inferior to GTR, and the addition of RT did not demonstrate an OS benefit. A summary of these results is located in Table 10.2. Of note, radiation doses of 50 Gy or more did not

improve outcomes compared to doses less than 50 Gy [5], which was counter to earlier suggestions by Shaw et al. [28].

Despite these findings, several single- and multi-institutional studies have not demonstrated a benefit with the addition of radiation after any extent of resection. The Rare Cancer Network reviewed 129 spinal cord ependymoma patients (30 with MPE) and found no difference in PFS between patients who underwent STR alone and those who underwent STR plus RT. Similarly, outcomes were no different after treatment with GTR alone versus GTR plus RT [2]. Likewise, a Korean study of 88 spinal cord ependymoma patients (24 with MPE) found adjuvant RT after STR or GTR did not significantly decrease recurrence rates [4]. Moreover, the University of California, San Francisco, group reviewed 134 cases of spinal cord ependymoma and found that the addition of RT to STR did not significantly improve PFS among grade II ependymomas [6]. In general, there appears to be enough data to not support routine use of RT, especially after a GTR.

## Spinal Cord Myxopapillary Ependymoma, A Unique Subset

Myxopapillary ependymoma is often included among studies of spinal cord ependymoma; however, it has a distinct biology. As a result, it has periodically been studied exclusively as a subset of ependymoma. A summary of identified prognostic and predictive factors is located in Table 10.3.

Age appears to predict outcomes in spinal cord MPE. In the largest series inclusive of 183 patients, those age 36 years and above had a more favorable 10-year PFS of 85% compared to about 40% for those younger than 36 years [8]. This was reflected in an early Mayo Clinic study which demonstrated younger patients appearing to have more frequent local recurrences [31]. Interestingly, patients below the age of 36 years trended to having improved OS [8]. A SEER

**Table 10.2** Summary of outcomes reported by Oh et al. [5] for spinal cord ependymomas

|  | GTR | STR | STR + RT | p value |
|---|---|---|---|---|
| n | 268 of 348 (77%) | 33 (41.3%) | 47 (58.8%) | NA |
| Median PFS | Not reached | 48 months | 96 months | $p = 0.047$ (for STR vs. STR + RT) |
| 5-Year PFS | 97.9% | 45.1% | 65.3% | |
| 5-Year OS | 98.8% | 73.7% | 79.3% | $p = 0.99$ (for STR vs. STR + RT) |

*GTR* gross total resection, *NA* not applicable, *RT* radiation therapy, *STR* subtotal resection

**Table 10.3** Summary of prognostic and predictive factors among myxopapillary spinal cord ependymomas in the literature

|  | N | Favorable prognostic and predictive factors |
|---|---|---|
| Weber et al. [8] | 183 | Gross total resection<br>Age ≥ 36 years old<br>Surgery + RT (compared to surgery alone) |
| Kotecha et al. [29] | 59 | Gross total resection<br>At time of recurrence, adjuvant RT (compared to surgery alone) |
| Klekamp et al. [30] | 42 | Gross total resection<br>Encapsulated tumor<br>Surgery + RT (compared to surgery alone)<br>Short preoperative history |
| Sonneland et al. [31] | 77 | Gross total resection<br>Encapsulated tumor<br>En bloc removal |

*RT* radiation therapy

analysis revealed similar findings in that patients under the age of 30 years had improved survival [7]. It is suggested that although spinal cord MPE tends to recur more frequently in younger patients, it does not significantly impact the survival of otherwise young and healthy patients.

Gross total resection has consistently demonstrated improved outcomes and is achieved in 54 to 77% of cases [8, 29, 31]. An early study from the Mayo Clinic reported significantly better OS after GTR (19 years) than after STR (14 years), also with a reduction in treatment failure from 34% to 10% [31]. Similarly, data from the Cleveland Clinic demonstrated improved 5-year relapse-free survival (RFS) after GTR (86.3%) compared to STR (50.3%). Median RFS was 17 years following GTR versus 5.5 years after STR [29, 32]. In the largest study of spinal cord MPE, patients undergoing GTR had significantly improved local control (LC) and PFS [8].

Even with GTR, an en bloc resection appears to improve LC. In the Mayo Clinic series, patients who underwent a GTR had higher recurrence rates with piecemeal resections (19%) compared to en bloc resections (10%) [31]. A separate study reviewed 107 patients and found that capsular violation was significantly associated with higher recurrence rates [33]. Furthermore, unencapsulated tumors are at higher risk of subarachnoid dissemination [30].

Postoperative radiation may decrease the rate of local recurrence in spinal cord MPE, but its role remains controversial. In 2006, MD Anderson Cancer Center initially reported on 35 patients with spinal cord MPE and found that adjuvant RT reduced the rate of tumor progression regardless of extent of resection [34]. Their results were updated in 2014 with similar findings. Among patients who received STR alone, 10-year LC was 0% compared to 65% with RT ($p = 0.008$). Among those who achieved GTR, 10-year LC was 56% after GTR alone versus 92% after GTR plus RT ($p = 0.14$). Median time of LC was 10.5 years with GTR plus RT versus 4.75 years with GTR alone ($p = 0.03$) [35]. In 2009 the Rare Cancer Network reported on 85 patients with spinal cord MPE and similarly found that adjuvant radiation improved 5-year PFS from 50.4% to 74.8%. Furthermore, on MVA high-dose adjuvant RT ($\geq$50.4 Gy) independently predicted for improved PFS [36]. In 2015, these groups pooled their databases to report on 183 patients with spine cord MPE. Receipt of adjuvant RT improved 10-year PFS from <40% to 70% as compared to those treated with surgery alone [8].

Contrary to these findings, an analysis from the Cleveland Clinic initially reported outcomes of 37 patients with spinal cord MPE, with a subsequent update including 59 patients affirming the initial study. Adjuvant RT did not significantly improve RFS after STR or GTR. However, of the patients who recurred, adjuvant RT at the time of initial recurrence was associated with significantly longer RFS (114.6 months vs. 18.9 months) [29, 32]. A recent SEER analysis found that receipt of radiation correlated with worse OS. However, receipt of RT was associated with significantly larger tumors, which suggested a selection bias in using RT in tumors that are more difficult to remove [7].

## Overall Treatment Strategy

Imaging of the entire neuraxis is strongly recommended to evaluate for separate sites of disease. Afterwards, surgical resection is the mainstay of treatment. In addition to achieving rapid symptomatic relief, histopathologic identification is essential for further management. As such, if resection is not feasible, biopsy is strongly recommended. Even with tissue, between 7% and 15% of patients are misdiagnosed with a nonependymoma [2, 18]. Every attempt should be made to achieve GTR by an experienced surgeon. For spinal cord MPE, an en bloc resection should be endeavored. An MRI with and without contrast is generally performed 6 to 8 weeks following surgery to assess for residual disease while allowing for postoperative changes to subside. This should also include the entire brain and spinal cord to evaluate for distant seeding. If there is concern for seeding of the cerebrospinal fluid or leptomeningeal spread, a lumbar puncture can be considered. Postoperative radiation may be considered as discussed below. There is no established evidence to support the use of chemotherapy.

## Indications for Irradiation

The role of postoperative radiation is controversial as previously discussed. Typical indications for radiation treatment include subtotal resection (STR), grade III (anaplastic) ependymomas, or after re-resection for recurrent disease. As demonstrated by the literature review above, there may be a role for radiation following GTR of spinal cord MPE, as resection is difficult and often piecemeal, but the data is open to interpretation. For grade II ependymomas, the data is more suggestive that radiation does not need to be routinely employed subsequent to GTR. Although spinal cord MPE can potentially seed along the cord, ependymomas are typically localized, and radiation therapy, if employed, should be local.

## Target Volume Delineation

While historically 2D techniques were used, given that disease is typically limited and does not extend beyond the spinal canal/thecal sac, conformal treatment is favored. Intensity-modulated radiation therapy (IMRT) or volumetric-modulated arc therapy (VMAT) is more standardly employed. Since these techniques allow for tighter margins, immobilization should be employed with either a five-point head mask for cervical and upper thoracic spinal cord tumors or a vacuum-locked bag for lesions involving the middle to lower thoracic cord, lumbar cord, or sacrum. If available, image guidance should be considered to account for setup uncertainty.

There is no established consensus regarding contouring and margins. The authors typically fuse the preoperative and postoperative MRI scans to delineate where the tumor was located and to define the extent of the resection bed (inclusive of any residual disease), which represents the gross tumor volume (GTV). A 1.5 cm clinical target volume (CTV) margin is placed around the GTV, allowing the CTV margin to include nerve roots, while shaving the margin through the bone to 0.5 cm, as this is a natural barrier to spread. A 0.5 cm margin is placed around the CTV as a planning target volume (PTV) margin to account for setup errors. Daily image guidance (IGRT) such as cone beam CT (CBCT) is advised. During treatment planning, because the cord or cauda is included, hotspots in the treatment volume should be limited to 105% of the prescribed dose, if possible.

## Radiation Dose Prescription and Organ at Risk Tolerances

The recommended prescription doses range from 50.4 to 54 Gy, using 1.8 Gy per fraction. Since the cord and/or cauda equina is within the treatment volume and will receive at least prescription dose, the authors recommend keeping the prescription dose relatively homogeneous by limiting hotspots as previously mentioned. With conventional fractionation of 1.8–2 Gy per fraction, the 5-year incidence of myelopathy is 5% ($TD_{5/5}$) for doses of 57–61 Gy, whereas the incidence is 50% at 5 years ($TD_{50/5}$) with doses of 68–73 Gy [37]. Lumbosacral nerve roots appear to have a higher tolerance, with 0% complication rates using conventional fractionation up to 70 Gy [38]. That said, it is best to restrict the dose to no greater than 54 Gy as there is no strong evidence to suggest administering higher doses results in better outcomes.

The lungs can be difficult to spare depending on the length of spinal cord within the treatment field. They should be limited so that less than 35% of the total lung volume receives more than 20 Gy to minimize the risk of radiation pneumonitis, which is adopted from dose tolerances used in lung cancer. Similarly, the kidneys can be difficult to avoid, especially when using IMRT or VMAT. No more than 50% of the total kidneys should receive 20 Gy or more, again adopting the dose restrictions used in abdominal radiation. Since the bowel is usually outside of the PTV volume, it should never go beyond tolerance. By the same token, the esophagus is usually outside of the PTV, and the amount of prescription dose to this organ should also be limited.

## Complication Avoidance, Radiation Toxicity, Acute and Late

As previously described, being that most ependymomas do not extend beyond the spinal canal, most organs at risk can be avoided with modern conformal radiation techniques. However, contingent upon the size and location of the tumor, toxicities can be anticipated. Mild acute gastrointestinal side effects are not uncommon. Prophylaxis with a 5-HT3 antagonist is usually not necessary, but these drugs can be employed if the patient develops nausea or vomiting. Esophagitis can be managed with viscous lidocaine alone or in formulated combinations with antacid and anticholinergic medications. Diarrhea can generally be treated with over-the-counter or prescription antidiarrheal medications (i.e., loperamide or Lomotil). In the subacute to chronic setting, if radiation pneumonitis is diagnosed, the typical treatment consists of glucocorticoids followed by a gradual taper.

Radiation myelopathy is a concerning, although very uncommon, late effect as described above. Early presentation (2–6 months following spinal cord irradiation) may manifest as a self-limited Lhermitte's syndrome (transient, nonpainful, electric shock-like sensation shooting down the spine with neck flexion) and is generally not thought to be a precursor for chronic myelitis [39]. In general, no treatment is indicated other than reassurance that symptoms are likely temporary. Unlike early radiation myelopathy, late radiation-induced myelopathy (>6 months following RT) is typically irreversible unless treated early. Symptoms are insidious and can include a multitude of sensory or motor deficits (e.g., decreased temperature sensation, diminished proprioception, numbness, leg weakness, incontinence), the severity of which tends to progress but may stabilize. With time, symptoms may advance owing to involvement of higher anatomical levels within the spinal cord. Diagnosis depends upon characteristic symptoms, a concordant radiation dose and latency period (>6 months), and exclusion of other etiologies. There is no robust clinical data regarding treatment, but the condition is generally managed with glucocorticoids [37].

## Outcomes: Tumor Control and Survival

For spinal cord ependymomas, population-based databases report relative OS rates at 1, 3, 5, and 10 years to be 98.5%, 96.1%, 94.3%, and 91.0%, respectively [1]. A summary of outcomes from larger retrospective studies is listed in Table 10.4. Overall, between 17% and 30% of patients with spinal cord ependymoma will recur and not uncommonly arising several years following treatment [2, 4–6, 23, 27]. Of those who recur, 67% will be local, 14% will be in a different location, and 10% will be both local and distant [2].

**Table 10.4** Review of spinal cord ependymomas in the literature

| Year of publication | Author | Number of cases | Number of MPE included (% of all cases) | Years included | Age at diagnosis (years) | Follow-up (years) | GTR rate | OS | PFS | Treatment failure rate | Adjuvant RT improved outcomes? |
|---|---|---|---|---|---|---|---|---|---|---|---|
| 2014 | Vera-Bolanos et al. [2] | 129 | 30 (23%) | 1972–2011 | 44 (mean) | NA | 74% | 5 years; 97% | 5 years; 87% | 19% | No |
| 2013 | Tarapore et al. [6] | 134 | 28 (21%) | 1985–2010 | 41 (median) | NA | 56% | NA | 12.8 years (median) | 22% | No |
| 2006 | Abdel-Wahab et al. [23] | 126 | 17 (13%) | 1953–2000 | NA | 5.7 | 50% | 5, 10, and 15 years; 91%, 84%, and 75% | 5, 10, and 15 years; 74%, 60%, and 35% | 30% | No |
| 2013 | Lee et al. [4] | 88 | 24 (27%) | 1989–2009 | 40.2 (median) | 6.1 | 82% | NA | 5 and 10 years; 87% and 80% | 17% | No |
| 2013 | Oh et al. [5] | 348 | 0 (0%) | 1965–2011 | 41 (mean) | 4 | 77% | See Table 10.2 | See Table 10.2 | NA | Yes, see Table 10.2 |

*MPE* myxopapillary ependymoma, *NA* not applicable, *RT* radiation therapy

**Table 10.5** Review of myxopapillary spinal cord ependymomas in the literature

| Year | Author | Number of patients | Years included | Age at diagnosis (years) | Follow-up (years) | GTR rate | OS | PFS | Treatment failure rate | Time to recurrence | Adjuvant RT improved outcomes? |
|---|---|---|---|---|---|---|---|---|---|---|---|
| 2014 | Weber et al. [8] | 183 | 1968–2012 | 35.5 (median) | 5 (median) | 54.1% | 10 years, 92.4% | 5 and 10 years; 69.5% and 61.2% | 31.7% | 2.2 years (median) | Yes |
| 2016 | Kotecha et al. [29] | 59 | 1974–2015 | 34 (median) | 6.2 (median) | 66.1% | NA | 5 and 10 years; 74.5% and 54.7% | 34% | NA | Only at time of recurrence |
| 2015 | Klekamp et al. [30] | 42 | 1980–2014 | 38 (mean) | 10 (mean) | 77.7% | 20 years, 88.9% | NA | 37% | NA | Yes |
| 1985 | Sonneland et al. [31] | 77 | 1924–1983 | 36.4 (mean) | NA | 58.4% | 17.1 years (mean) | NA | 17% | 5.8 years (mean) | NA |

*NA* not applicable, *RT* radiation therapy

For spinal cord MPE, SEER data reports 3-, 5-, and 9-year OS to be 96.9%, 95.4%, and 93.8%, respectively. The 3-, 5-, and 9-year cause-specific survival (CSS) is 99.1%, 98.6%, and 98.6%, respectively [7]. A summary of outcomes from larger retrospective series is included in Table 10.5. Recurrence occurs in 17 to 37% of patients, with the most common site of failure being local (26.8%) and less commonly distantly in the spinal cord (9.3%) or in the brain (6%). Among those who recur, estimated 10-year OS is 90.3%, which is not significantly different from those who do not recur (97.2%) [8]. In children, spinal cord MPE tends to be more aggressive with higher rates of local recurrence [40].

## Follow-Up: Radiographic Assessment

Since the median time to progression is over years, the authors typically obtain the first follow-up 3 months after completion of radiation to assess for toxicity. The second follow-up is 6 months later and, subsequently, every year for the first 5 years. Afterward, consideration may be made for follow-up every 2 years. At each follow-up, MRI of the involved spine with and without contrast should be obtained to assess for local recurrence. Although MPE can disseminate elsewhere in the spinal cord, the authors do not routinely image the entire craniospinal axis. However, any suspicious neurological symptoms should be imaged to rule out distant recurrence or dissemination.

## Case Presentation: Highlight RT Management with Neuroimaging and Thought Process

A 34-year-old female presented with 3 months of progressive low back pain, bilateral lower extremity weakness, and episodic urinary and bowel incontinence. MRI of the lumbar spine revealed a T1 isointense heterogeneously enhancing mass centered about the conus extending from T11 to L3, measuring 12.6 cm, and also with T2 hyperintensity (Fig. 10.1a). She underwent T11–L3 laminectomies and subtotal piecemeal resection of the intradural tumor. Pathology returned spindled cells varied in cellularity, arranged around blood vessels in a rosette-like configuration. There was no significant anaplasia, and mitotic figures were difficult to identify. The findings suggested a diagnosis of ependymoma. Postoperative MRI at 6 weeks revealed multiple areas of abnormal enhancement in the area of prior neoplasm, likely from postoperative changes, but residual disease could not be ruled out (Fig. 10.1b). The

remainder of the spine was unremarkable. She was seen in consultation, and surgical pathology was sent for review, which returned myxopapillary ependymoma, WHO grade I. She was recommended to undergo postoperative radiation to improve local control given the subtotal piecemeal resection and concern for residual disease on imaging.

She agreed to treatment and received 4860 cGy in 27 fractions of 180 cGy per fraction to the spinal cord and canal from levels T10 to S2 with a simultaneous integrated boost to 5130 cGy (at 190 cGy per fraction) to areas of residual disease using IMRT (Fig. 10.2). She tolerated treatment well with mild fatigue and nausea which was controlled with scheduled ondansetron. After treatment and rehabilitation, she ultimately regained full neurologic function with only occasional mild lower back pain. She has been followed for 5 years with no evidence of disease on yearly surveillance MRI.

## Summary

- Spinal cord ependymomas typically have a more indolent course compared to their intracranial counterparts.

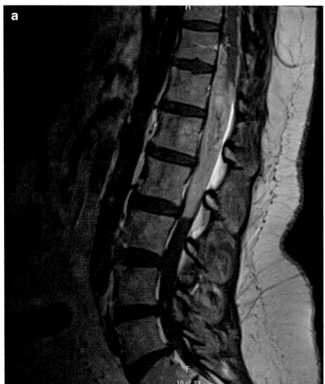 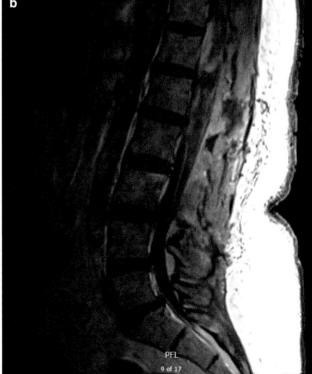

**Fig. 10.1** (**a**) Sagittal T1 contrast-enhanced spine MRI demonstrating an enhancing mass centered about the conus extending from the level of T11 to the L2–L3 interspace, representative of a myxopapillary spinal cord ependymoma. (**b**) Six-week postoperative sagittal T1 contrast-enhanced spine MRI demonstrating multiple areas of abnormal enhancement in the area of prior neoplasm, most prominent at T11/T12, suspicious for residual disease

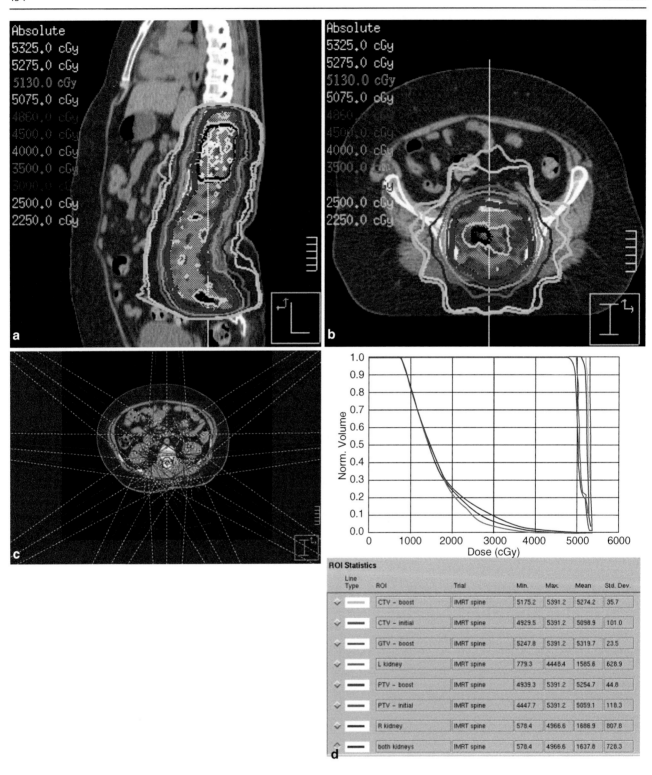

**Fig. 10.2** (a) Sagittal plane of a postoperative intensity-modulated radiation therapy (IMRT) plan for myxopapillary spinal cord ependymoma status post subtotal piecemeal resection; 4860 cGy (navy isodose line) in 27 fractions delivered to the spinal cord and canal from T10 to S2 with a simultaneous integrated boost to 5130 cGy (black isodose line) to gross residual disease. (b) Axial plane of IMRT plan with boost to area of residual disease. (c) IMRT beam arrangement. (d) Dose volume histogram

- Gross total resection is associated with better local control.
- The use of radiation is controversial given the lack of strong data. Postoperative radiation may be considered for patients with subtotal resection (STR), grade III (anaplastic) ependymomas, or after re-resection for recurrent disease.
- Recommended doses for spinal cord ependymoma range from 50.4 to 54 Gy when given at 1.8 Gy per fraction.

## Self-Assessment Questions

1. What is the treatment volume for ependymoma involving the spinal cord and/or cauda equina?
   A. Entire craniospinal axis
   B. Residual disease alone without CTV margin
   C. Residual disease and resection bed with CTV and PTV margins
   D. None, as there is no role for radiation

2. Where is myxopapillary ependymoma most commonly located?
   A. Brain
   B. Cervical spinal cord
   C. Thoracic spinal cord
   D. Cauda equina

3. Which patients can be observed following resection of spinal cord ependymoma?
   A. Gross totally resected WHO grade II spinal cord ependymoma
   B. Subtotally resected WHO grade I cauda equina ependymoma
   C. Gross totally resected WHO grade II ependymoma involving the posterior fossa
   D. Re-resected, recurrent spinal myxopapillary ependymoma, with no residual disease on postoperative imaging

4. Following resection of spinal cord ependymomas, when should postoperative MRI with and without contrast be performed?
   A. 24–72 h
   B. Within 2 weeks
   C. 6–8 weeks
   D. After 6 months

5. What is strongest predictor of outcomes among patients with spinal cord ependymoma?
   A. Age at diagnosis
   B. Receipt of adjuvant radiation therapy
   C. Location of tumor
   D. Extent of resection

## Answers

1. C
2. D
3. A
4. C
5. D

## References

1. Villano JL, Parker CK, Dolecek TA. Descriptive epidemiology of ependymal tumours in the United States. Br J Cancer. 2013;108(11):2367–71.
2. Vera-Bolanos E, Aldape K, Yuan Y, Wu J, et al. Clinical course and progression-free survival of adult intracranial and spinal ependymoma patients. Neuro Oncol. 2015;17(3):440–7.
3. Ostrom QT, Gittleman H, Fulop J, et al. CBTRUS statistical report: primary brain and central nervous system tumors diagnosed in the United States in 2008–2012. Neuro Oncol. 2015;17(Suppl 4):iv1–iv62.
4. Lee SH, Chung CK, Kim CH, et al. Long-term outcomes of surgical resection with or without adjuvant radiation therapy for treatment of spinal ependymoma: a retrospective multicenter study by the Korea Spinal Oncology Research Group. Neuro Oncol. 2013;15(7):921–9.
5. Oh MC, Ivan ME, Sun MZ, et al. Adjuvant radiotherapy delays recurrence following subtotal resection of spinal cord ependymomas. Neuro Oncol. 2013;15(2):208–15.
6. Tarapore PE, Modera P, Naujokas A, et al. Pathology of spinal ependymomas: an institutional experience over 25 years in 134 patients. Neurosurgery. 2013;73(2):247–55. discussion 55
7. Bates JE, Choi G, Milano MT. Myxopapillary ependymoma: a SEER analysis of epidemiology and outcomes. J Neurooncol. 2016;129(2):251–8.
8. Weber DC, Wang Y, Miller R, et al. Long-term outcome of patients with spinal myxopapillary ependymoma: treatment results from the MD Anderson Cancer Center and institutions from the Rare Cancer Network. Neuro Oncol. 2015;17(4):588–95.
9. Mautner VF, Tatagiba M, Lindenau M, et al. Spinal tumors in patients with neurofibromatosis type 2: MR imaging study of frequency, multiplicity, and variety. AJR Am J Roentgenol. 1995;165(4):951–5.
10. Patronas NJ, Courcoutsakis N, Bromley CM, et al. Intramedullary and spinal canal tumors in patients with neurofibromatosis 2: MR imaging findings and correlation with genotype. Radiology. 2001;218(2):434–42.
11. Plotkin SR, O'Donnell CC, Curry WT, et al. Spinal ependymomas in neurofibromatosis type 2: a retrospective analysis of 55 patients. J Neurosurg Spine. 2011;14(4):543–7.
12. Acquaye AA, Vera E, Gilbert MR, et al. Clinical presentation and outcomes for adult ependymoma patients. Cancer. 2017;123(3):494–501.
13. Oh MC, Kim JM, Kaur G, et al. Prognosis by tumor location in adults with spinal ependymomas. J Neurosurg Spine. 2013;18(3):226–35.
14. Louis DN, Perry A, Reifenberger et al. The 2016 World Health Organization classification of tumors of the central nervous system: a summary. Acta Neuropathol. 2016;131(6):803–20.

15. Wu J, Armstrong TS, Gilbert MR. Biology and management of ependymomas. Neuro Oncol. 2016;18(7):902–13.

16. Waldron JN, Laperriere NJ, Jaakkimainen L, Simpson WJ, Payne D, Milosevic M, et al. Spinal cord ependymomas: a retrospective analysis of 59 cases. Int J Radiat Oncol Biol Phys. 1993;27(2):223–9.

17. Mork SJ, Loken AC. Ependymoma: a follow-up study of 101 cases. Cancer. 1977;40(2):907–15.

18. Armstrong TS, Vera-Bolanos E, Bekele BN, et al. Adult ependymal tumors: prognosis and the M. D. Anderson Cancer Center experience. Neuro Oncol. 2010;12(8):862–70.

19. Wahab SH, Simpson JR, Michalski JM, et al. Long term outcome with post-operative radiation therapy for spinal canal ependymoma. J Neurooncol. 2007;83(1):85–9.

20. Cervoni L, Celli P, Fortuna A, et al. Recurrence of spinal ependymoma. Risk factors and long-term survival. Spine (Phila Pa 1976). 1994;19(24):2838–41.

21. Hanbali F, Fourney DR, Marmor E, et al. Spinal cord ependymoma: radical surgical resection and outcome. Neurosurgery. 2002;51(5):1162–72. discussion 72–4

22. Marks JE, Adler SJ. A comparative study of ependymomas by site of origin. Int J Radiat Oncol Biol Phys. 1982;8(1):37–43.

23. Abdel-Wahab M, Etuk B, Palermo J, et al. Spinal cord gliomas: a multi-institutional retrospective analysis. Int J Radiat Oncol Biol Phys. 2006;64(4):1060–71.

24. Lee CH, Chung CK, Ohn JH, et al. The similarities and differences between intracranial and spinal ependymomas: a review from a genetic research perspective. J Korean Neurosurg Soc. 2016;59(2):83–90.

25. Lee CH, Chung CK, Kim CH. Genetic differences on intracranial versus spinal cord ependymal tumors: a meta-analysis of genetic researches. Eur Spine J. 2016;25(12):3942–51.

26. Raghunathan A, Wani K, Armstrong TS, et al. Histological predictors of outcome in ependymoma are dependent on anatomic site within the central nervous system. Brain Pathol. 2013;23(5):584–94.

27. Gomez DR, Missett BT, Wara WM, et al. High failure rate in spinal ependymomas with long-term follow-up. Neuro Oncol. 2005;7(3):254–9.

28. Shaw EG, Evans RG, Scheithauer BW, et al. Radiotherapeutic management of adult intraspinal ependymomas. Int J Radiat Oncol Biol Phys. 1986;12(3):323–7.

29. Kotecha R, Modugula S, Angelov L, et al. The role of adjuvant radiation therapy in patients with myxopapillary ependymomas. Int J Radiat Oncol Biol Phys. 2016;96((2):E112.

30. Klekamp J. Spinal ependymomas. Part 2: Ependymomas of the filum terminale. Neurosurg Focus. 2015;39(2):E7.

31. Sonneland PR, Scheithauer BW, Onofrio BM. Myxopapillary ependymoma. A clinicopathologic and immunocytochemical study of 77 cases. Cancer. 1985;56(4):883–93.

32. Chao ST, Kobayashi T, Benzel E, et al. The role of adjuvant radiation therapy in the treatment of spinal myxopapillary ependymomas. J Neurosurg Spine. 2011;14(1):59–64.

33. Abdulaziz M, Mallory GW, Bydon M, et al. Outcomes following myxopapillary ependymoma resection: the importance of capsule integrity. Neurosurg Focus. 2015;39(2):E8.

34. Akyurek S, Chang EL, Yu TK, et al. Spinal myxopapillary ependymoma outcomes in patients treated with surgery and radiotherapy at M.D. Anderson Cancer Center. J Neurooncol. 2006;80(2):177–83.

35. Tsai CJ, Wang Y, Allen PK, et al. Outcomes after surgery and radiotherapy for spinal myxopapillary ependymoma: update of the MD Anderson Cancer Center experience. Neurosurgery. 2014;75(3):205–14. discussion 13–4

36. Pica A, Miller R, Villa S, et al. The results of surgery, with or without radiotherapy, for primary spinal myxopapillary ependymoma: a retrospective study from the rare cancer network. Int J Radiat Oncol Biol Phys. 2009;74(4):1114–20.

37. Schultheiss TE, Kun LE, Ang KK, et al. Radiation response of the central nervous system. Int J Radiat Oncol Biol Phys. 1995;31(5):1093–112.

38. Pieters RS, Niemierko A, Fullerton BC, et al. Cauda equina tolerance to high-dose fractionated irradiation. Int J Radiat Oncol Biol Phys. 2006;64(1):251–7.

39. Fein DA, Marcus RB Jr, Parsons JT, et al. Lhermitte's sign: incidence and treatment variables influencing risk after irradiation of the cervical spinal cord. Int J Radiat Oncol Biol Phys. 1993;27(5):1029–33.

40. Feldman WB, Clark AJ, Safaee M, et al. Tumor control after surgery for spinal myxopapillary ependymomas: distinct outcomes in adults versus children: a systematic review. J Neurosurg Spine. 2013;19(4):471–6.

# Metastatic Epidural Spinal Cord Compression: Conventional Radiotherapy

# 11

Dirk Rades and Steven E. Schild

## Learning Objectives

This chapter focuses solely on conventional radiotherapy for metastatic epidural spinal cord compression (MESCC). The role of stereotactic body radiation therapy is discussed elsewhere. This chapter summarizes prognostic factors with respect to different endpoints including the effect of radiotherapy on motor function, ambulatory status, local control of MESCC, and overall survival. Treatment modalities that may be administered in addition to radiotherapy and potential indications are described. The most commonly used dose-fractionation regimens of radiotherapy ranging from single-fraction to longer-course multi-fraction programs are presented. With the help of scoring systems developed to estimate the remaining life span of patients with MESCC, personalized treatment approaches are emphasized and recommendations made regarding the optimal treatment for individual patients who are considered suitable candidates for conventional radiotherapy for MESCC.

## Background

### Epidemiology

In 1925, metastatic epidural spinal cord compression (MESCC) had been described for the first time [1]. It was defined as comprehensive indentation, displacement, or encasement (by epidural metastatic lesions) of the thecal sac, which encompasses the spinal cord or the cauda equina. If the metastatic lesions have not yet led to neurologic (mainly motor) deficits, it would be more appropriately called impending MESCC.

Up to 10% of all adult cancer patients will develop MESCC over the course of their malignant disease [2–4]. The incidence of MESCC becomes lower with increasing age. Incidences are 4.4% in patients 40–50 years of age and 0.5% in those aged 70–80 years [3]. The three most common primary tumors associated with MESCC are breast, prostate, and lung cancer, each accounting for 20–25% of MESCC cases [2, 4]. Involvement of the cervical spinal cord occurs in less than 10% of the patients, involvement of the thoracic spine in 60–80% of the patients, and the lumbar spine in 15–30% of the patients, respectively. In about 50% of affected patients, two or more spinal segments are involved by MESCC [2–4]. Since MESCC is considered an oncologic emergency, treatment should be started as soon as possible, ideally within 24 h after presentation with neurologic deficits due to MESCC [3].

## Pathophysiological Aspects

In more than 80% of the cases, MESCC is caused by metastases of the vertebral body after destruction of the posterior edge of the vertebral body followed by posterior extension of the metastatic mass (Fig. 11.1). Such a mass can impinge on the thecal sac, the spinal cord, or the epidural venous plexus. Furthermore, MESCC may be caused by pathological fractures of the involved vertebrae that may be associated with a collapse of the vertebral body or dislocation of bone fragments into the epidural space.

According to animal studies performed 30–40 years ago, pathophysiological processes associated with MESCC include edema of the white-matter and axonal swelling resulting in white-matter necrosis and gliosis [5–7]. The blood circulation of both spinal arteries and spinal veins can be impaired, depending also on the dynamics of the development of MESCC. It has been reported that a faster progression of MESCC is not infrequently associated with disruption

D. Rades (✉)
Department of Radiation Oncology, University of Lübeck, Lübeck, Schleswig-Holstein, Germany

S. E. Schild
Department of Radiation Oncology, Mayo Clinic, Scottsdale, AZ, USA

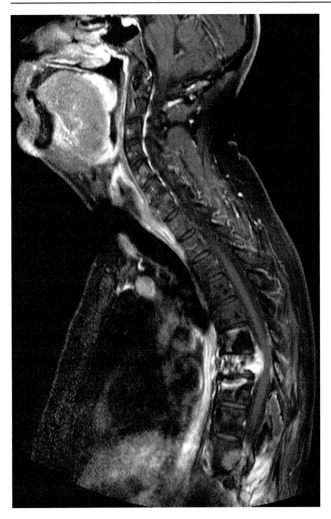

**Fig. 11.1** Example of MESCC caused by destruction of the posterior edge of the vertebral body and posterior extension of the metastatic mass at two levels of the thoracic spinal cord (Th 6–8 and Th 10–11)

of the arterial blood flow, which can lead to ischemia of the spinal cord or even spinal cord infarction. Particularly in the latter case, existing motor deficits are often irreversible. The motor deficits are much more likely to be reversible if the progression of MESCC occurs slowly, since the functional impact of MESCC is mainly caused by venous congestion and white-matter edema. These pathophysiological considerations have been supported by animal studies that were performed in the 1950s [8, 9]. Rapid progression of MESCC requires rapid decompression of the spinal cord within 10 h, whereas successful treatment of slowly developing neurologic deficits was possible even after 7 days. The findings of these animal studies were supported by the results of two clinical studies that investigated the impact of the time developing motor deficits on the effect of radiotherapy on motor function. In 2001, a retrospective study of 131 patients compared three groups of patients designed according to the time their motor deficits developed, namely, 1–7 days, 8–14 days,

and more than 14 days [10]. Two weeks following irradiation, improvement of motor deficits was observed in 4%, 32.5%, and 65% of patients, respectively ($p < 0.001$). According to the results of a subsequent prospective non-randomized study of 98 patients using the same three groups, development of motor deficits >14 days before start of radiotherapy resulted in a higher improvement rate of motor dysfunction than 8–14 days and 1–7 days [11]. Improvement rates were 86%, 29%, and 10%, respectively ($p < 0.001$), post-radiotherapy ambulatory rates 86%, 55%, and 35%, respectively ($p = 0.026$).

## Clinical Symptoms

The most frequently observed clinical symptoms are pain (70–96% of patients) and motor dysfunction (61–91%) [12–15]. Less common symptoms include sensory deficits (46–90%) and sphincter dysfunction (40–57%). Motor dysfunction can be considered the hallmark symptom of MESCC. Major goals of radiotherapy of MESCC include maintaining or regaining the patients' ability to walk, and decreasing the often agonizing pain. About 20 years ago, more than 50% of the patients with MESCC were unable to walk prior to treatment [16, 17]. Due to greater awareness of MESCC, the proportion of patients who were ambulatory at diagnosis has increased considerably.

With a major focus on ambulatory status, the motor function of patients with MESCC can be graded with a 5-point scale modified according to the scale developed by Tomita et al. [18]: 0 normal strength, 1 patient is ambulatory without aid, 2 patient is ambulatory but requires a walking aid, 3 patient is not ambulatory, and 4 patient has complete paraplegia. A more differentiated approach offers an 8-point scale developed from and modified according to the scales presented by the American Spinal Injury Association and the International Medical Society of Paraplegia [19]: 0 total paralysis; 1 palpable or visible muscle contractions; 2 active movement of the leg, gravity eliminated; 3 active movement against gravity; 4 active movement against mild resistance; 5 active movement against moderate resistance; 6 active movement against severe resistance; and 7 normal strength.

## Diagnostic Procedures

Magnetic resonance imaging (MRI) is considered the diagnostic procedure of choice [20–22]. If a MRI cannot be performed, other procedures including computed tomography with or without positron emission tomography may be used to confirm the diagnosis of MESCC. In an early MRI study from 1988, sensitivity and specificity rates of 93% and 97%, respectively, with respect to the correct diagnosis of MESCC were reported [20]. In that study, sensitivity and specificity rates with respect to distinguishing between a benign cause of spinal cord compression (mainly spondylodiscitis) and MESCC were 98% and 100%, respectively. The possibility of the differential diagnosis of spondylodiscitis may not be underestimated and could be a pitfall for radiation oncologists. In a retrospective study of 170 patients, who were presented to a radiation oncologist for treatment of MESCC with only plain radiographs and computed tomography, an additional MRI resulted in a correction of the diagnosis from MESCC to benign spondylodiscitis in ten (6%) patients [22].

## Prognostic and Predictive Factors

### Prognostic Factors for the Effect of Radiotherapy on Motor Deficits and Ambulatory Status

Earlier studies published 20 years ago identified two prognostic factors significantly associated with the effect of conventional radiotherapy on motor dysfunction, the type of primary tumor and pretreatment ambulatory status [16, 23, 24]. In 1993, Kim et al. presented a retrospective series of 25 patients irradiated with 20 Gy in 5 fractions ($n = 4$), 30 Gy in 10 fractions ($n = 14$), or 40 Gy in 16 fractions ($n = 7$) for MESCC associated with a paravertebral mass [23]. Functional outcome was significantly better in patients with MESCC from a very radiosensitive tumor (i.e., lymphoma) than in other patients. Furthermore, none of the 15 non-ambulatory patients regained the ability to walk after irradiation, whereas five of six ambulatory patients maintained their gait function. In the same year, Leviov et al. reported on 70 patients receiving 30–45 Gy of radiotherapy alone [24]. In this retrospective study, pretreatment ambulatory status was found to be the most important predictor of response to irradiation. Of the previously ambulatory patients, 66% were able to walk following radiotherapy compared to 30% of paraparetic non-ambulatory patients and 16% of the patients who had complete paraplegia prior to radiotherapy. The type of primary tumor was another important predictor of response; 70% of lymphoma patients and 46% of breast cancer patients showed complete response. In 1995, Maranzano et al. presented data on 209 patients irradiated with 30 Gy in 10 fractions over 2 weeks or a split-course regimen of 15 Gy in 3 daily fractions followed by 4 days rest and another 15 Gy in 5 daily fractions [16]. Recovery or preservation of ambulation was observed in all of the 73 patients (100%) who were ambulatory without aid before radiotherapy, in 34 of 36 patients (94%) who were ambulatory with aid, in 49 of 82 non-ambulatory patients (60%), and only in 2 of 18 patients (11%) who were

paraplegic. In addition, patients with paresis or paraplegia who had primary tumor histology considered favorable, i.e., lymphoma, myeloma, breast cancer, or prostate cancer, experienced a significantly better response than other patients. Of those 51 non-ambulatory or paraplegic patients who regained their ability to walk, 36 patients (71%) had such a favorable primary tumor type. The largest study reporting on prognostic factors regarding the response to radiotherapy of MESCC, was published 10 years later in 2005 [25]. The authors presented a retrospective series of 1304 patients irradiate with 8 Gy in 1 fraction ($n = 261$), 20 Gy in 5 fractions ($n = 279$), 30 Gy in 10 fractions ($n = 274$), 27.5 Gy in 15 fractions ($n = 233$), or 40 Gy in 20 fractions ($n = 257$). In the multivariate analysis of this study, better functional outcome was significantly associated with age $\leq 63$ years ($p = 0.026$), an Eastern Cooperative Oncology Group (ECOG) performance score of 1–2 ($p < 0.001$), involvement of only one to two vertebrae by MESCC ($p = 0.001$), a favorable tumor entity (myeloma/lymphoma, breast cancer, and prostate cancer; $p < 0.001$), pre-radiotherapy ambulatory status ($p < 0.001$), time developing motor deficits prior to the start of radiotherapy of >14 days ($p < 0.001$), and an interval between the first diagnosis of the malignant disease and radiotherapy of MESCC of >24 months ($p < 0.001$).

Being ambulatory following radiotherapy is very important for patients treated for MESCC. In the multivariate analysis of a retrospective study including 2096 patients with MESCC, an ECOG performance status of 1–2 (risk ratio [RR] 14.28; 95% confidence interval [CI] 4.38–46.54; $p < 0.001$), a favorable type of primary tumor (RR 7.75; 95% CI 3.48–16.06; $p < 0.001$), an interval between tumor diagnosis and MESCC of >15 months (RR 1.81; 95% CI 1.29–2.54; $p = 0.001$), absence of visceral metastases at the time of radiotherapy (RR 1.58; 95% CI 1.14–2.20; $p = 0.007$), ambulatory status before radiotherapy (RR 21.41; 95% CI 7.72–59.40; $p < 0.001$), and a slower (>14 days) development of motor deficits before radiotherapy (RR 8.20; 95% CI 5.59–12.05; $p < 0.001$) were significantly associated with the ambulatory status following radiotherapy [26]. Based on these prognostic factors, a scoring system was created that allows one to predict the probability of being ambulatory after radiotherapy of MESCC. However, the ECOG performance score was not included, since motor function (ambulatory status) and ECOG performance status are considered confounding variables. For each of the five prognostic factors, the post-radiotherapy ambulatory rate in % was divided by 10. The score for each patient represented the sum of the scoring points of the five prognostic factors included. The patient scores did range between 21 and 44 points, and five prognostic groups were designed, i.e., 21–28 points ($n = 389$), 29–31 points ($n = 278$), 32–34 points ($n = 303$), 35–37 points ($n = 366$), and 38–44 points ($n = 760$).

The corresponding post-radiotherapy ambulatory rates were 6% for patients with 21–28 points, 44% for 29–31 points, 70% for 32–34 points, 86% for 35–37 points, and 99% for 38–44 points ($p < 0.001$). This scoring system has been validated in patients with MESCC who were prospectively followed [27]. The post-radiotherapy ambulatory rates were similar in the different prognostic groups of both studies [26, 27]. Furthermore, the scoring system was simplified by reducing the number of prognostic groups from five to three. Post-radiotherapy ambulatory rates in the validation study were 11% in the 21–28 points group, 71% in the 29–37 points group, and 99% in the 38–44 points group ($p < 0.001$). The ambulatory rates in the preceding retrospective series were 6%, 68%, and 99%, respectively ($p < 0.001$).

## Prognostic Factors for Local Control of MESCC

On univariate analysis of a retrospective study of 1852 patients, improved local control of MESCC (defined as freedom from an in-field recurrence of MESCC in the previously irradiated part of the spine) was significantly associated with favorable type of primary tumor (i.e., breast cancer, prostate cancer, or lymphoma/myeloma) ($p < 0.001$), absence of visceral metastases at the time of radiotherapy ($p < 0.001$), and longer-course radiotherapy (30–40 Gy in 10–20 fractions over 2–4 weeks) ($p < 0.001$) [28]. In the subsequent multivariate analysis, the absence of visceral metastases (RR 2.64; 95% CI 1.76–3.90; $p < 0.001$) and longer-course radiotherapy (RR 1.85; 95% CI 1.54–2.22; $p < 0.001$) were significant. A favorable primary tumor was no longer significant and showed a trend (RR 1.09; 95% CI 0.97–1.21; $p = 0.14$).

## Prognostic Factors for Overall Survival

In the retrospective study of 1852 patients with MESCC, several predictors of survival have been identified [28]. On univariate analysis, improved survival was associated with female gender ($p < 0.001$), an ECOG performance score of 1–2 ($p < 0.001$), a favorable primary tumor (myeloma/lymphoma, breast cancer, prostate cancer) ($p < 0.001$), involvement of only one to two vertebrae by MESCC ($p < 0.001$), absence of other bone metastases at the time of radiotherapy ($p < 0.001$), absence of visceral metastases at the time of radiotherapy ($p < 0.001$), an interval between the first diagnosis of the malignant disease and MESCC of >15 months ($p < 0.001$), ability to walk prior to radiotherapy ($p < 0.001$), and a slower development of motor deficits (>14 days) prior to the start of radiotherapy ($p < 0.001$). On multivariate analysis, favorable primary tumor type (RR 1.23; 95% CI 1.18–1.29; $p < 0.001$), absence of other bone

metastases (RR 1.29; 95% CI 1.04–1.59; $p = 0.018$), absence of visceral metastases (RR 4.89; 95% CI 4.26–5.60; $p < 0.001$), an interval from first diagnosis of the malignant disease until MESCC of >15 months (RR 1.25; 95% CI 1.18–1.33; $p < 0.001$), the ability to walk prior to radiotherapy (RR 2.13; 95% CI 1.79–2.56; $p < 0.001$), and a slower development of motor deficits prior to the start of radiotherapy (RR 1.39; 95% CI 1.30–1.47; $p < 0.001$) remained significant and, therefore, were independent predictors of survival.

Based on the 6-month survival rates associated with these six independent prognostic factors, a scoring system was developed that allows to predict the survival of patients with MESCC [29]. The scoring points for each prognostic factor were obtained by dividing the corresponding 6-month survival rate in % by 10. The total scores for individual patients were received by adding the scores of the six prognostic factors and ranged between 20 and 45 points. Five prognostic groups were created, i.e., 20–25 points, 26–30 points, 31–35 points, 36–40 points, and 41–45 points. The 6-month survival rates of these five groups were 4%, 11%, 48%, 87%, and 99%, respectively ($p < 0.001$). This scoring system has been validated in a cohort of 439 patients [30]. In this validation cohort, the 6-month survival rates were 7% (20–25 points), 19% (26–30 points), 56% (31–35 points), 73% (36–40 points), and 90% (41–45 points), respectively ($p < 0.001$). The group-by-group comparisons of the test cohort and the validation cohort did not reveal a significant difference, which demonstrates reproducibility and validity of the scoring system [30]. In addition, the scoring system was simplified by reducing the prognostic groups from five to three. The three new groups were 20–30 points, 31–35 points, and 36–45 points. The corresponding 6-month survival rates were 14%, 56%, and 80%, respectively ($p < 0.001$). Again, no significant difference was observed when each of the three prognostic groups of the validation cohort was compared to its corresponding group of the previously reported test cohort [29, 30].

In addition to this scoring system that included patients with MESCC from many different primary tumors, separate survival scores were designed for most tumor entities that account for more than 5% of all patients who develop MESCC during their disease course such as breast cancer, prostate cancer, lung cancer, myeloma, cancer of unknown primary (CUP), renal cell carcinoma, and colorectal cancer [31–37] (Table 11.1). The scoring systems for the four largest series of patients with MESCC from a particular type of primary tumor are described in the following paragraphs.

The scoring tool for breast cancer patients was developed and validated in a series of 510 patients, who were divided in a test cohort ($n = 255$) and a validation cohort ($n = 255$) [31]. On multivariate analysis of the test cohort, an ECOG performance score of 1–2, the ability to walk prior to radiotherapy, absence of further bone metastases at the time

**Table 11.1** Survival scores designed for particular primary tumor types: prognostic factors that were significantly associated with overall survival and, therefore, included in the corresponding scoring system

| Primary tumor type | Ambulatory status prior to radiotherapy | Other bone lesions at the time of radiotherapy | Visceral metastases at the time of radiotherapy | Interval from initial tumor diagnosis to MESCC | Time developing motor deficits prior to radiotherapy |
|---|---|---|---|---|---|
| Breast cancer [31] | × | × | × | × | × |
| Prostate cancer [32] | × | × | × | × | |
| Non-small cell lung cancer [33] | × | | × | | × |
| Myeloma [34] | × | × | | | |
| Cancer of unknown primary [35] | × | | × | | × |
| Renal cell carcinoma [36] | × | | × | × | × |
| Colorectal cancer [37] | × | | × | | × |

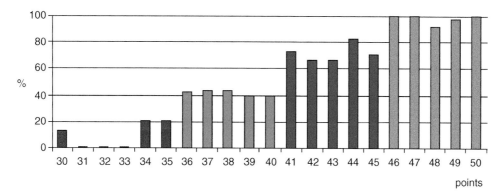

**Fig. 11.2** Scoring system to estimate the survival of patients with MESCC from breast cancer: scoring points ranging from 30 to 50 points and the corresponding 6-month survival rates given in %. Four prognostic groups were formed, 30–35 points (red columns), 36–40 points (green columns), 41–45 points (blue), and 46–50 points (orange). [Adapted from Rades D et al. A validated survival score for breast cancer patients with metastatic spinal cord compression. Strahlenther Onkol 2013;189:41–46. With permission from Springer Verlag]

of radiotherapy, absence of visceral metastases at the time of radiotherapy, an interval between breast cancer diagnosis and radiotherapy of MESCC of >15 months, and a slower development (>7 days) of motor dysfunction prior to radiotherapy proved to be independent positive predictors of survival. Total patient scores, which were obtained from the addition of 6-month survival rates of these six factors divided by 10, ranged from 30 to 50 points (Fig. 11.2). Four prognostic groups were formed: 30–35 points, 36–40 points, 41–45 points, and 46–50 points. In the test cohort, the corresponding 6-month survival rates were 12%, 41%, 74%, and 98%, respectively ($p < 0.001$) (Fig. 11.3). In the validation cohort, the 6-month survival rates were quite similar being 14%, 46%, 77%, and 99%, respectively ($p < 0.001$). Thus, this score proved to be valid and reproducible.

The study, in which the survival score for patients with MESCC from prostate cancer was developed, included a total of 436 patients [32]. Of these patients, 218 patients were assigned to the test cohort and 218 patients to the vali-

dation cohort. On multivariate analysis of the test group, improved 6-month survival probability was significantly related to an ECOG performance score of 1–2, the ability to walk prior to radiotherapy, absence of further bone metastases at the time of radiotherapy, absence of visceral metastases at the time of radiotherapy, and an interval between prostate cancer diagnosis and radiotherapy of MESCC of >15 months. The procedure of calculating the scoring points was the same as for the previously described survival scores. This tool included three prognostic groups, namely, 20–24 points, 26–33 points, and 35–39 points (Fig. 11.4). In the test group, the 6-month survival rates were 7%, 45%, and 96%, respectively ($p < 0.001$) (Fig. 11.5). In the validation group, the 6-month survival rates were almost identical with 7%, 45%, and 95%, respectively ($p < 0.001$). Thus, also this scoring system could be considered valid and reproducible.

Another study was performed in 356 patients with MESCC from non-small cell lung cancer (NSCLC) [33]. Similar to the scoring tools created for breast cancer and prostate cancer patients, the cohort was equally divided in a test group ($n = 178$) and a validation group ($n = 178$). On the multivariate analysis performed in the test group, an ECOG performance score of 1–2, being able to walk prior to radiotherapy, absence of visceral metastases at the time of radiotherapy, and a slower development (>7 days) of motor deficits prior to radiotherapy showed a significantly positive association with survival at 6 months. The total scores obtained from the addition of the scoring points (6-month survival rates divided by

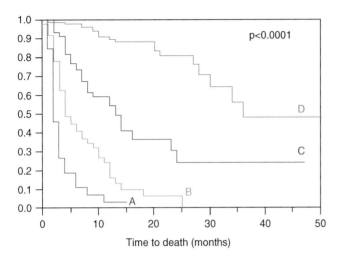

**Fig. 11.3** Scoring system to estimate the survival of patients with MESCC from breast cancer: Kaplan-Meier curves of the four prognostic groups 30–35 points (**A**), 36–40 points (**B**), 41–45 points (**C**), and 46–50 points (**D**). [Adapted from Rades D et al. A validated survival score for breast cancer patients with metastatic spinal cord compression. Strahlenther Onkol 2013;189:41–46. With permission from Springer Verlag]

10) of these four independent predictors of survival ranged from 6 to 19 points (Fig. 11.6). The 6-month survival rates of the three prognostic groups 6–10 points, 11–15 points, and 16–19 points were 6%, 29%, and 78%, respectively, in the test group ($p < 0.001$), and this compared to 4%, 24%, and 76%, respectively, in the validation group ($p < 0.001$) (Fig. 11.7). Since the 6-month survival rates in both the test group and the validation group were quite similar, also this scoring tool was considered valid and reproducible.

The fourth largest series of patients with MESCC from a specific tumor type included 216 myeloma patients [34]. Also this series was divided in a test cohort ($n = 108$) and a validation cohort ($n = 108$). According to the multivariate analysis of the test cohort, an ECOG performance score of 1–2 and ambulatory status prior to radiotherapy were independent significant predictors of survival. In addition, absence of other osseous lesions showed a strong trend toward improved survival. Therefore, these three factors were included in the scoring tool. Since patients with MESCC from myeloma have a much more favorable survival prognosis than patients with MESCC from a solid tumor, this scoring tool was designed to predict the 12-month rather than the 6-month survival probability. Therefore, the scoring points from the three predictive factors were calculated by dividing the 12-month survival rate (in %) by 10. When adding the scoring points of the three factors, sum scores of 19–24 points were received (Fig. 11.8). These scores allowed the creation of three prognostic groups, namely, 19–20 points, 21–23, points and 24 points. The corresponding 12-month survival rates were 49%, 74%, and 93%, respectively ($p = 0.002$) (Fig. 11.9). In the validation group,

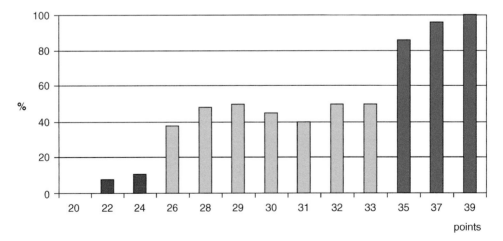

**Fig. 11.4** Scoring system to estimate the survival of patients with MESCC from prostate cancer: scoring points ranging from 20 to 39 points and the corresponding 6-month survival rates given in %. Three prognostic groups were designed, 20–24 points (red columns), 26–33 points (green columns), and 35–39 points (blue). [Adapted from Rades D et al. A survival score for patients with metastatic spinal cord compression from prostate cancer. Strahlenther Onkol 2012;188:802–806. With permission from Springer Verlag]

**Fig. 11.5** Scoring system to estimate the survival of patients with MESCC from prostate cancer: Kaplan-Meier curves of the three prognostic groups 20–24 points (group I), 26–33 points (group II), and 35–39 points (group III). [Adapted from Rades D et al. A survival score for patients with metastatic spinal cord compression from prostate cancer. Strahlenther Onkol 2012;188:802–806. With permission from Springer Verlag]

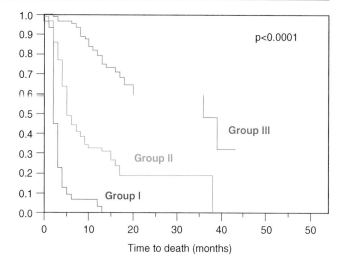

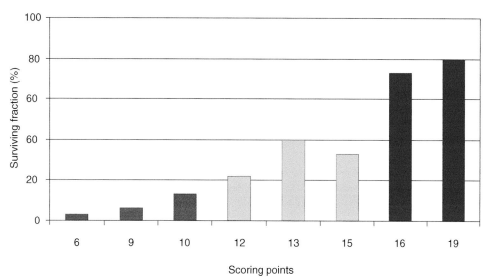

**Fig. 11.6** Scoring system to estimate the survival of patients with MESCC from non-small cell lung cancer (NSCLC): scoring points ranging from 6 to 19 points and the corresponding 6-month survival rates given in %. Three prognostic groups were created, 6–10 points (red columns), 12–15 points (green columns), and 16–19 points (blue).

[Adapted from Rades D et al. A validated survival score for patients with metastatic spinal cord compression from non-small cell lung cancer. BMC Cancer 2012;12:302. With permission from Creative Commons: https://creativecommons.org/licenses/by/2.0/]

the rates were 51%, 80%, and 93%, respectively ($p < 0.001$). Like the scoring systems described before, the tool designed to predict the survival of patients with MESCC from myeloma was valid and reproducible.

All these prognostic scores help physicians estimate an individual patient's remaining life span and contribute to an improved personalization of the treatment for MESCC. Personalization of treatment may include the decision to use radiotherapy alone or to combine radiotherapy with other treatments such as corticosteroids, bisphosphonates or denosumab, chemotherapy, and decompressive surgery.

## Multi-Modality Management Approach

### Radiotherapy Supplemented by Corticosteroids

One important effect of the administration of corticosteroids is the decrease of vasogenic edema [38]. In addition, corticosteroids lead to a reduction of lipid peroxidation and hydrolysis, ischemia as well as intracellular calcium accumulation. In patients with MESCC, the most frequently used type of corticosteroids is dexamethasone which has been reported to be able to contribute to improvement or maintaining of a patient's motor function. The most appropriate regimen of dexamethasone administration is controversial. A small randomized trial from Denmark ($n = 57$) compared high daily doses of dexamethasone to no corticosteroids [39]. Initially, an intravenous bolus of 96 mg dexamethasone was administered, followed by 3 days of oral administration of 96 mg per day (if possible given in four fractions per day) and, thereafter, tapering the dose to zero within 10 days. The total dose of radiotherapy was 28 Gy given in seven fractions on 7 consecutive days. Following treatment, 81% of those patients treated with dexamethasone and 63% of those patients not corticosteroids during radiotherapy, respectively, were ambulatory. Six months following treat-

ment, ambulatory rates were 59% and 33%, respectively. Severe dexamethasone-related toxicity was observed in three patients (11%). One patient became hypomanic, one patient developed a manifest psychosis, and one patient required surgical intervention for a perforated gastric ulcer. The latter two patients had to discontinue the treatment with dexamethasone, and in another patient dexamethasone treatment was stopped due to systemic infection. In another prospective study of 37 patients that compared an initial intravenous bolus of high-dose (100 mg) dexamethasone followed by daily oral doses of 16 mg, to initial intravenous administration of 10 mg followed by daily oral doses of 16 mg, motor function improved in 25% and 8% of the patients, respectively ($p = 0.22$).

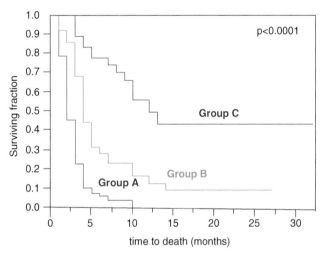

**Fig. 11.7** Scoring system to estimate the survival of patients with MESCC from non-small cell lung cancer (NSCLC): Kaplan-Meier curves of the three prognostic groups 6–10 points (**A**), 12–15 points (**B**), and 16–19 points (**C**). [Adapted from Rades D et al. A validated survival score for patients with metastatic spinal cord compression from non-small cell lung cancer. BMC Cancer 2012;12:302. With permission With permission from Creative Commons: https://creativecommons.org/licenses/by/2.0/]

**Fig. 11.9** Scoring system to estimate the survival of patients with spinal cord compression from myeloma: Kaplan-Meier curves of the three prognostic groups 19–20 points (**A**), 21–23 points (**B**), and 24 points (**C**). [Adapted from Douglas S et al. A new score predicting the survival of patients with spinal cord compression from myeloma. BMC Cancer 2012;12:425. With permission from Creative Commons: https://creativecommons.org/licenses/by/2.0/]

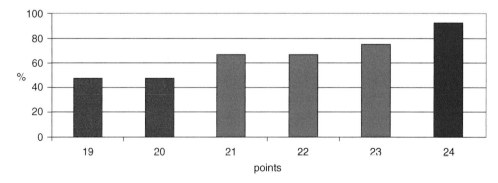

**Fig. 11.8** Scoring system to estimate the survival of patients with spinal cord compression from myeloma: scoring points ranging from 19 to 24 points and the corresponding 12-month survival rates given in %. Three prognostic groups were created, 19–20 points (red columns), 21–23 points (green columns), and 24 points (blue). [Adapted from

Douglas S et al. A new score predicting the survival of patients with spinal cord compression from myeloma. BMC Cancer 2012;12:425. With permission from Creative Commons: https://creativecommons.org/licenses/by/2.0/]

A historical case-control study series of patients irradiated for MESCC compared 28 patients additionally treated with initial intravenous administration 96 mg of dexamethasone tapered to zero within 14 days to 38 consecutive patients receiving in addition to radiotherapy an initial dose of 16 mg dexamethasone also tapered to zero within 14 days [40]. In the high-dose dexamethasone group, eight patients (28.6%) experienced a dexamethasone-related toxicity, which was considered serious (one fatal ulcer with hemorrhage, one rectal bleeding, and two gastrointestinal perforations) in four patients (14.3%). In three patients of the low-dose dexamethasone group (7.9%), a dexamethasone-related toxicity was observed but not considered serious (0%). The differences between both groups regarding the rates of overall toxicities and serious toxicities were significant, whereas the posttreatment ambulatory rates were not.

When selecting the appropriate dexamethasone dose for patients irradiated for MESCC, both the effect on motor function and dexamethasone-related toxicity must be considered. It appears appropriate to start dexamethasone treatment with intermediate doses of 12–32 mg per day and tapering down as tolerated over weeks. Prophylactic treatment with proton pump inhibitors is strongly recommended at least during the period of dexamethasone administration.

## The Role of Bisphosphonates and Denosumab

In 2002, a randomized placebo-controlled trial of 643 patients with hormone-refractory prostate cancer and a history of bone metastases compared 4 mg of zoledronic acid ($n$ = 214) versus 8 mg of zoledronic acid, subsequently reduced to 4 mg ($n$ = 221) versus placebo ($n$ = 208), given every 3 weeks for a total of 15 months [41]. The primary endpoint was the proportion of "skeletal-related events" (pathological fractures, MESCC, requirement of radiotherapy or surgery). In the three groups compared, the study was completed by 38%, 28% and 31% of patients, respectively. Skeletal-related events were observed in 44% of patients in the placebo group, in 33% of patients receiving 4 mg zoledronic acid ($p$ = 0.21 versus placebo), and in 39% of patients receiving 8/4 mg zoledronic acid ($p$ = 0.22 versus placebo). In a follow-up report in 2004, the proportions of patients who had at least one skeletal-related event at 2 years were 38% in patients who received 4 mg zoledronic acid versus 49% in those who receive a placebo ($p$ = 0.028) [42]. Thus, 4 mg zoledronic acid every 3 weeks can significantly decrease the risk of skeletal-related events including MESCC. In 2011, a prospective non-randomized study that compared different radiotherapy regimens for local control of MESCC showed a trend toward improved local control with bisphosphonate (mainly zoledronic acid) administration [43]. One-year local control rates were 79% with, and 68% without, bisphosphonates ($p$ = 0.068). However, the study was not powered to detect a significant advantage with administration of bisphosphonates. In a subsequent matched-pair study of 294 patients irradiated for MESCC, 98 patients who received zoledronic acid in addition to radiotherapy were matched 1:2, to 196 patients treated with radiotherapy alone for ten potential prognostic factors [44]. One-year rates of local control of MESCC were 90% and 81%, respectively ($p$ = 0.042). Bisphosphonates should be used with caution in patients with abnormal white blood cells, dental disease, or with high parathyroid hormone [2]. Potential adverse events include fever, transient leucopenia, hypocalcemia, increase of parathyroid hormone, eye inflammation, renal failure, bone pain, skin rash, and osteonecrosis of the jaw.

More recently, denosumab, an IgG2-anti-RANKL antibody (RANKL = receptor activator of nuclear factor kappa B ligand), has been introduced in the treatment of cancer patients. This antibody inhibits the formation of a RANKL-RANK complex, which leads to activation of osteoclasts and subsequent increase of bone resorption and release of tumor cell-stimulating growth factors [45]. Randomized trials that compared denosumab to zoledronic acid with respect to delaying the time to the first skeletal-related event have been performed. In two of these trials, denosumab was significantly superior to zoledronic acid in breast cancer patients (hazard ratio [HR] 0.82; $p$ = 0.01 [46]) and prostate cancer patients (HR 0.82; $p$ = 0.008 [47]). The third trial was performed for tumors other than breast and prostate cancer and found a trend for higher efficacy of denosumab (HR 0.84; $p$ = 0.06 [48]). According to its subgroup analysis, the difference between both drugs was not significant for NSCLC (HR 0.84; $p$ = 0.20) and for myeloma (HR 1.03; $p$ = 0.89), but for other tumors (HR 0.79; $p$ = 0.04). In the three randomized trials, the incidence of osteonecrosis of the jaw in the bisphosphonate groups ranged between 1.1% and 1.4%, compared to 1.3–2.3% in the denosumab groups [46–48]. In each of the three trials, the difference between both drugs was not significant.

Thus, both bisphosphonates and denosumab are effective in delaying the time to skeletal-related events. Denosumab has been demonstrated to be more effective, at least with breast cancer or prostate cancer.

## Chemotherapy in Addition to Radiotherapy

The role of systemic chemotherapy for the treatment of MESCC is very limited. Adding chemotherapy to radiotherapy can be considered for spinal cord compression from chemosensitive tumors including lymphoma, myeloma, and germ cell tumors. In the study of Aviles et al. that compared radiotherapy alone, chemotherapy alone, and the combination of both treatments in 48 patients with spinal cord compression from lymphoma, recovery of neurologic deficits was similar in the three groups [49]. However, the 10-year local control rates were nonsignificantly different in favor of the combined approach (76% versus 50% after radiotherapy alone and 46% after chemotherapy alone). Another small study of 48 patients with spinal cord compression from lymphoma or myeloma investigated radiotherapy with and without chemotherapy [50]. Progression of neurologic deficits considered as response was achieved in 75% of patients with combined radio-chemotherapy and in 58% of patients with radiotherapy alone. The difference was not significant, possibly due to the small number of patients. Larger prospective randomized trials are required to properly define the role of chemotherapy in the treatment of malignant spinal cord compression.

## Decompressive Surgery Followed by Radiotherapy

Indications for decompressive surgery in patients with MESCC include bony fragments that compromise the spinal cord, instability of the spinal segment involved by metastases, impending or present autonomic dysfunction, no response to radiotherapy, and in-field recurrence of MESCC within 6 months after previous longer-course radiotherapy, precluding the safe administration of a second radiotherapy course [2, 4, 51].

Decompressive surgical procedures include a simple laminectomy and more sophisticated approaches including stabilization of the spinal segment involved by MESCC and replacement of a vertebral body (Fig. 11.10). If MESCC is caused by posterior extension of a metastatic mass arising from the vertebral body, which is by far the most common situation leasing to MESCC, a simple laminectomy without stabilization of the involved vertebrae is not indicated [51–53]. Since the laminae and spinous processes form the last of three pillars providing the stability of the involved spinal segment, a laminectomy, which includes the removal of these structures, can result in even greater instability, and neurologic function may become worse after laminectomy and transient improvement. Instead of performing a laminectomy, surgical approaches should include decompression followed by direct stabilization and replacement of the vertebral body if appropriate. If spinal surgery is performed, it must be followed by postoperative radiotherapy to the residual tumor.

The benefit of upfront decompressive surgery in addition radiotherapy is controversial. In 1980, a small randomized trial of 29 patients compared radiotherapy alone (*n* = 13) to decompressive laminectomy followed by radiotherapy

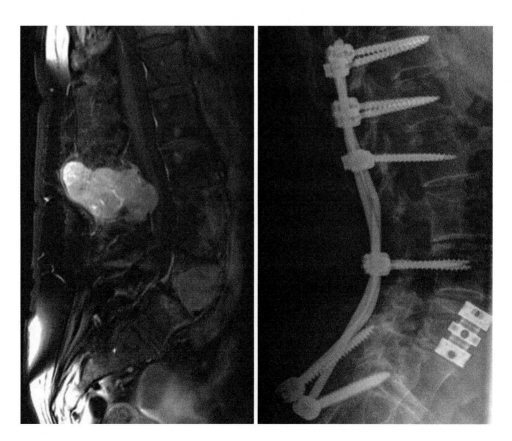

**Fig. 11.10** Example of a sophisticated surgical approach including both dorsal stabilization and replacement of a vertebral body in the lumbar spine

($n = 16$) [54]. Posttreatment ambulatory rates were 38% and 38%, respectively (not significant). In 1990, a retrospective study of 345 patients from Denmark compared radiotherapy alone ($n = 149$), decompressive laminectomy alone ($n = 105$), and laminectomy followed by radiotherapy ($n = 91$) [55]. Posttreatment ambulatory rates were 38%, 34%, and 53%, respectively. However, when motor function prior to the start of treatment was considered, no significant difference was observed between the three treatments regarding their effect on functional outcome. In 2003, Klimo et al. presented a review article and defined success of treatment as ambulatory status following treatment for MESCC [56]. They reported mean success rates of 47% after radiotherapy alone (11 reports, $n = 841$), 47% after surgery plus adjuvant radiotherapy (nine reports, $n = 866$), and 30% after surgery alone (13 reports, $n = 1003$) in patients treated for MESCC between 1957 and 1990. However, surgery performed was laminectomy, not decompressive surgery plus direct stabilization. A meta-analysis by the same group published in 2005 included also patients surgically treated with stabilization of the involved spinal segments [57]. The authors compared 999 patients from 24 studies treated with decompressive surgery with most receiving postoperative radiotherapy to a cohort of 543 patients from four studies treated with radiotherapy alone. In this meta-analysis, the ambulatory rates following treatment of MESCC were 64% after radiotherapy alone and 85% after decompressive surgery with or without radiotherapy. Of those patients who were not ambulatory prior to treatment, 59% (228 of 384 patients) in the surgery group and only 30% (79 of 265 patients) in the radiotherapy alone group were ambulatory after treatment. However, these results were likely to be confounded by selection biases, since the significantly more patients who received decompressive surgery had favorable characteristics including ambulatory status before treatment, better performance status, younger age, and involvement of fewer vertebrae by MESCC. Other important predictors of functional outcome including the time developing motor deficits prior to treatment of MESCC and the interval between first diagnosis of cancer and MESCC were not examined. Therefore, the conclusions drawn from of this meta-analysis in favor of decompressive surgery in addition to radiotherapy should be interpreted with caution [57]. A randomized trial was required to better define the role of upfront decompressive surgery in addition to radiotherapy for the treatment of MESCC.

In 2005, Patchell et al. compared 30 Gy in ten fractions of radiotherapy alone to the same regimen supplemented by upfront decompressive surgery including direct stabilization of the involved vertebrae [51]. According to the results of this trial, the combined approach resulted in a significantly higher proportion of patients being ambulatory following their treatment when compared to the radiotherapy alone

group (84% versus 57%, $p = 0.001$). In addition, those patients receiving additional surgery maintained their walking ability significantly longer (122 versus 13 days, $p = 0.003$). Of the previously non-ambulatory patients, 10 of 16 patients after combined treatment and 3 of 16 patients after radiotherapy alone, respectively, regained ambulatory status ($p = 0.01$). Moreover, overall survival was significantly longer in those patients receiving the combined treatment than in those treated with radiotherapy alone (126 versus 100 days, $p = 0.033$). However, concerns were expressed regarding methodological problems of this trial [58, 59]. Since it took 10 years to accrue 101 patients, which means an average recruitment of only ten patients per year, it appeared plausible that only highly selected and not all eligible patients were included. Furthermore, the results in the radiotherapy alone group appeared much less favorable than in other reports. The inclusion criteria did not reflect the ordinary patients with MESCC. Only patients with an estimated survival of at least 3 months, a Karnofsky performance score of 70 or higher, and involvement of only one spinal by MESCC area were included. Furthermore, patients with very radiosensitive tumors (e.g., myeloma, lymphoma, or germ cell tumors), with brain metastases, with complete paraplegia lasting for longer than 48 hours, or with cauda equina compression were excluded. Therefore, the select eligible population included in this trial represented about 10% of patients with MESCC, and the findings may not properly address the therapy of the majority of patients with MESCC. However, it was a randomized trial that demonstrated significant benefits for the addition of upfront surgery to radiotherapy, and another larger randomized trial including less selected patients would be difficult to justify and perform.

Instead of another randomized trial, a large matched-pair study including 324 less selected patients with MESCC was presented in 2010 [60]. In this study, 108 patients treated with decompressive surgery followed by radiotherapy were matched 1:2 to 216 patients treated with radiotherapy alone. These patients were matched for 11 patient characteristics including age, gender, ECOG performance score, primary tumor type, no of vertebrae involved by MESCC, presence of further bone metastases at the start of radiotherapy, presence of visceral metastases at the start of radiotherapy, interval between first diagnosis of the malignant disease and MESCC, pretreatment ambulatory status, time developing motor deficits, and the dose-fractionation regimen of radiotherapy. Each triple of matched patients should match for a least 10 of these 11 characteristics. The treatment regimens, surgery plus radiotherapy and radiotherapy alone, were not significantly different with respect to improvement of motor function (27% versus 26%, $p = 0.92$), posttreatment ambulatory rate (69% versus 68%, $p = 0.99$), regaining the ability to walk (30% versus 26%, $p = 0.86$), 1-year local control of MESCC (90% versus 91%, $p = 0.48$), and 1-year overall survival (47% versus 40%, $p = 0.50$). Since decompressive surgery plus direct stabilization is defined as the appropriate surgical technique, a subgroup analysis was performed of the 70 patients receiving this type of surgery who were matched 1:2 to 140 patients receiving radiotherapy alone. Also in this subgroup analysis, both treatment regimens were not significantly different with respect to posttreatment motor function ($p = 0.65$; improvement rates 29% versus 29%), posttreatment ambulatory status (84% versus 78%, $p = 0.68$), regaining the ability to walk (42% versus 34%, $p = 0.81$), 1-year local control of MESCC (97% versus 91%, $p = 0.64$), and 1-year overall survival (55% versus 49%, $p = 0.53$).

In 2011, a subsequent matched-pair study was reported that was limited to patients with MESCC from an unfavorable primary tumor type, namely, NSCLC, cancer of unknown primary, kidney cancer, and colorectal cancer [61]. Sixty-seven patients receiving decompressive surgery plus radiotherapy were matched 1:2, to 134 patients receiving radiotherapy alone for ten characteristics, i.e., for the same characteristics as in the previous study [60] except the dose-fractionation regimen, since all patients had received longer-course radiotherapy with 30 Gy in 10 fractions, 37.5 Gy in 15 fractions, or 40 Gy in 20 fractions. In this additional study, both treatment regimens were not significantly different with respect to improvement of motor function (27% versus 26%, $p = 0.92$), posttreatment ambulatory rate (69% versus 68%, $p = 0.99$), regain of the ability to walk (30% versus 26%, $p = 0.86$), 1-year local control of MESCC (90% versus 91%, $p = 0.48$), and 1-year overall survival (47% versus 40%, $p = 0.50$). Like in the previous matched-pair study, a subgroup analysis was performed for the 43 patients receiving adequate surgery (decompression plus stabilization) who were matched 1:2, to 86 patients treated with radiotherapy alone. In this subgroup analysis, both treatment regimens were not significantly different with respect to posttreatment ambulatory status (86% versus 67%, $p = 0.30$), regaining the ability to walk (45% versus 18%, $p = 0.86$), 1-year local control of MESCC (94% versus 88%, $p = 0.78$), and 1-year overall survival (45% versus 29%, $p = 0.18$). However, improvement of motor function occurred significantly more frequently after the combined approach than after radiotherapy alone (28% versus 19%, $p = 0.024$). Also ambulatory status after treatment including regaining the ability to walk was observed more often following surgery plus radiotherapy, although significance was not achieved, maybe due to the relatively small number of patients available for this subgroup analysis. Regarding the contradictory results of the studies that compared decompressive surgery followed by radiotherapy to radiotherapy alone, it appears that additional randomized trials with an appropriately large sample size are required to properly define the role of upfront decompressive surgery plus stabilization in addition to radiotherapy for the more common subgroups of patients with MESCC should be performed [51, 54, 55, 60, 61].

## Radiation Techniques and Dose Fractionation of Conventional Radiotherapy

### Radiotherapy Techniques

Nowadays, radiotherapy of MESCC is performed most frequently with photon beams from a linear accelerator. Since MESCC is an oncologic emergency and requires an urgent start of radiotherapy, CT- or MRI-based treatment planning is not often feasible. Less time-consuming, simple techniques include delivery of radiotherapy through a single posterior (PA) field or parallel opposed fields taking into account the distance between the patient's surface and the spinal cord. If this distance is greater than 5.5 cm, the dose maximum can be more than 115% of the prescribed dose with a single PA field. This applies to both total dose and dose per fraction leading to a significant increase in the equivalent dose in 2 Gy fractions (EQD2) [62]. In these patients, radiotherapy with parallel-opposed fields results in a more appropriate dose distribution with a lower dose maximum and, therefore, a decreased risk of radiation myelopathy and subcutaneous tissue fibrosis. In obese patients, the distance between the surface and the spinal cord may exceed 11.5 cm. In these patients, the photon energy of both parallel opposed fields should be $\geq 10$ MV or more fields can be used. The doses of radiotherapy are generally prescribed to the posterior part of the vertebral body (single posterior field) or the midplane (parallel opposed fields). In general, the treatment volume encompasses one normal vertebra above and below those vertebrae involved by MESCC. If the non-affected vertebrae attached to those involved by MESCC belong to the cervical spine, the treatment volume encompasses two cervical vertebrae in addition to those affected by MESCC.

If there is sufficient time, radiotherapy should be performed in a more sophisticated way with 3D-conformal radiotherapy and CT- or MRI-based treatment planning (Fig. 11.11) or even with modern techniques such as intensity-modulated radiation therapy (IMRT) and volumetric modulated arc therapy (VMAT) (Fig. 11.12). However, there are no absolute standards regarding target volume delineation. In many institutions, the clinical target volume (CTV) includes the vertebral and soft tissue tumor as seen on the planning computed tomography and diagnostic magnetic resonance imaging, the spinal canal, the width of the involved vertebrae, and half a vertebra above and below the vertebrae affected by MESCC. The planning target volume (PTV)

**Fig. 11.11** Example of 3D-conformal radiotherapy for MESCC including the arrangement of radiation fields and the distribution of the isodoses

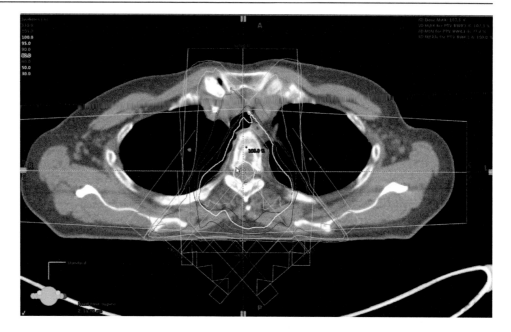

**Fig. 11.12** Example of volumetric modulated arc therapy (VMAT) for MESCC including the distribution of the isodoses. The maximum dose to the spinal cord is only 101% of the prescribed dose

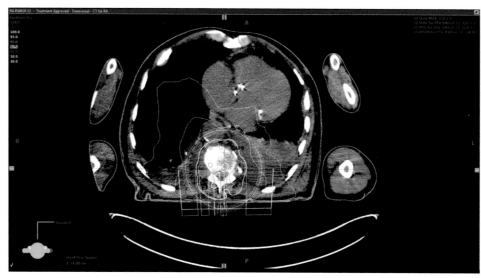

should include the CTV plus a margin of 0.8 cm and should ideally be covered by the 95% isodose. The EQD2 taking into account total dose and doses per fraction should not exceed the tolerance dose of the spinal cord generally considered to be 45–50 Gy [63, 64]. MESCC may affect single or multiple sites of the spinal cord. All sites should be treated following these prescriptions.

## Dose-Fractionation Regimens of Conventional Radiotherapy

Many dose-fractionation regimens are available worldwide including single fractions of 8 or 10 Gy and short-course regimens of 4–6 fractions lasting about 1 week and longer-course regimens with higher total doses such as of 30–40 Gy

given in 10–20 fractions over a period of 2–4 weeks [2, 4]. The appropriate dose-fractionation regimen for an individual patient depends on the goals of the treatment.

The most important goal of the treatment of MESCC is the improvement of motor function resulting in maintaining or regaining the ability to walk. A few prospective studies are available that investigated the effect of different radiotherapy programs on motor function and walking ability. Almost 20 years ago, a prospective Italian study from Italy compared a split-course program, which consisted of 15 Gy in three fractions followed by 4 days rest and another 15 Gy in five fractions, to 16 Gy given in two fractions of 8 Gy with a week rest between both fractions [65]. In this non-randomized study of 44 prostate cancer patients developing MESCC from prostate cancer, the response rates (i.e., improvement or no further progression of motor dysfunction) were not significantly different in both groups. In 2004, our group presented a prospective multicenter study of 214 patients that compared two longer-course radiotherapy programs, namely, 30 Gy in 10 fractions ($n = 110$) and 40 Gy in 20 fractions ($n = 104$) [66]. Directly after the end of radiotherapy, in the 30 Gy group, the rates of improvement, no further progression, and deterioration of motor function were 43%, 30%, and 27%, respectively. In the 40 Gy group, the corresponding rates were 41%, 36%, and 23%, respectively. When applying the ordered logit model, the effect of both programs on motor function was not significantly different ($p = 0.799$). At 3 months following radiotherapy, 93 patients in the 30 Gy group and 91 patients in the 40 Gy group were evaluable. Improvement of motor function was observed in 49% and 46% of patients, respectively, no further progression in 28% and 36% of patients, respectively, and deterioration in 23% and 18%, respectively ($p = 0.580$). Directly after radiotherapy, ambulatory rates were 60% after 30 Gy in 10 fractions and 64% after 40 Gy in 20 fractions, respectively ($p = 0.708$). At 3 months following radiotherapy, the ambulatory rates were 68% and 71%, respectively ($p = 0.791$). One year later, a randomized phase III trial from Italy was reported that included 276 patients irradiated for MESCC and compared the same programs used in the previous non-randomized study of 44 prostate cancer patients with MESCC [65], i.e., a split-course regimen (15 Gy in three fractions followed by 4 days rest and 15 Gy in five fractions), to 16 Gy in two fractions with 1 week rest in between [67]. The post-radiotherapy ambulatory rates were 71% and 68%, respectively ($p$-value not stated), and median duration for improvement of motor function was 3.5 months in both groups. Since the short-course program (16 Gy in two fractions) was not inferior to the more time-consuming split-course regimen, another randomized trial was initiated to investigate a potential further reduction of the overall treatment time from 8 days (16 Gy in two fractions with a week rest between both fractions) to 1 day (single fraction of 8 Gy) [68]. This new phase III trial including 303 eligible patients was published in 2009. This trial did not demonstrate a significant difference between the two investigated radiotherapy programs with respect to their effect on functional outcome. Median duration times of response to radiotherapy were 5 months in the 16 Gy/2-group and 4.5 months in the 8 Gy/1-group, respectively ($p = 0.4$). In 2011, the final results of the SCORE-1 study, a prospective non-randomized binational study including patients from the Netherlands and Germany, were reported [43]. This study compared short-course radiotherapy ($n = 131$), defined as 8 Gy in 1 fraction or 20 Gy in 5 fractions, to long-course radiotherapy ($n = 134$) consisting of 30 Gy in 10 fractions, 37.5 Gy in 15 fractions, or 40 Gy in 20 fractions. One of the secondary endpoints of this study was the effect of the radiotherapy program on motor function, which was not

significantly different between both groups ($p = 0.95$). Improvement of motor function occurred in 28% of patients in the short-course radiotherapy group and 29% in the long-course radiotherapy group, respectively. Further progression of motor dysfunction was stopped in additional 56% and 55% of patients, respectively, whereas motor function further deteriorated in 15% and 16% of patients, respectively. In 2016, another randomized phase III trial, the SCORE-2 trial, was published [69]. This trial was limited to patients with a poor or intermediate survival prognosis according to the previously developed survival score [29, 30] and compared 101 patients receiving 20 Gy in five fractions over 1 week to 102 patients receiving 30 Gy in 2 weeks. The primary endpoint was overall response at 1 month following radiotherapy defined as improvement or no further progression of motor deficits. The overall response rates were 87.2% after 20 Gy and 89.6% after 30 Gy, respectively ($p = 0.73$). Improvement of motor function was observed in 38.5% and 44.2% of patients, respectively, no further progression in 48.7% and 45.5% of patients, respectively, and deterioration of motor function in 12.8% and 10.4% of patients, respectively ($p = 0.44$). At 1 month following radiotherapy, 71.8% and 74.0% of the patients, respectively, were able to walk ($p = 0.86$).

Thus, all prospective studies and trials that compared various radiotherapy programs used for MESCC with respect to functional outcome in terms of overall response, improvement of motor function, and post-radiotherapy ambulatory status were unable to demonstrate that a particular program was superior.

Another important goal of conventional radiotherapy for MESCC is the prolongation of the time to an in-field recurrence of MESCC in the initially irradiated spinal parts. As the tolerance dose of the spinal cord regarding radiation myelopathy is 45–50 Gy (when conventionally fractionated), re-irradiation for a local recurrence of MESCC with a sufficient EQD2 often cannot be performed [63, 64]. Local control of MESCC is important. However, the risk of developing an in-field recurrence of MESCC depends on the dose-fractionation regimen used for the initial (primary) treatment of MESCC. A large retrospective study including 1304 patients with MESCC treated with conventional radiotherapy alone plus dexamethasone compared five dose-fractionation regimens including 8 Gy in 1 fraction, 20 Gy in 5 fractions over 1 week, 30 Gy in 10 fractions over 2 weeks, 37.5 Gy in 15 fractions over 3 weeks, and 40 Gy in 20 fractions over 4 weeks [25]. In this study, the 24%, 26%, 14%, 9%, and 7% of the patients, respectively, experience an in-field recurrence up to 2 years following primary radiotherapy of MESCC ($p < 0.001$). Neither the difference between the two short-course programs 8 Gy in 1 fraction and 20 Gy in 5 fractions ($p = 0.44$) nor the difference between the three long-course programs 30 Gy in 10 fractions,

37.5 Gy in 15 fractions, and 40 Gy in 20 fractions ($p = 0.71$) was significant. The results of this retrospective study led to the prospective SCORE-1 study that compared short-course radiotherapy (8 Gy in 1 fraction or 20 Gy in 5 fractions) to long-course radiotherapy (30 Gy in 10 fractions, 37.5 Gy in 15 fractions, or 40 Gy in 20 fractions) in 265 patients irradiated for MESCC [43]. The local control rates of MESCC at 1 year were 61% after short-course compared to 81% after long-course radiotherapy ($p = 0.005$). An additional retrospective study compared 30 Gy in 10 fractions to two long-course regimens including a higher total dose (37.5 Gy in 15 fractions and 40 Gy in 20 fractions) in patients with a favorable survival prognosis according to the scoring system developed to predict the 6-month survival of patients irradiated for MESCC [29, 30, 70]. This study was performed as a matched-pair study matching 191 patients receiving 30 Gy in 10 fractions over 2 weeks 1:1 for ten potential prognostic factors, to 191 patients treated with higher doses (37.5 Gy in 15 fractions or 40 Gy in 20 fractions) [70]. The local control rates at 2 years were 71% and 92%, respectively ($p = 0.012$).

If re-irradiation for an in-field recurrence of MESCC is required, the treatment appears safe if the cumulative biologically effective dose (BED) of the primary radiotherapy and re-irradiation not exceeds 100 Gy$_2$ [71]. The risk of radiation-induced myelopathy appears small if the cumulative BED is 135.5 Gy$_2$ or less and the interval between both treatments is 6 months or longer [72]. The BED can be calculated with the following equation: $\text{BED} = D \times [1 + (d/\alpha/\beta)]$ [62]. In the equation, $D$ stands for total dose, $d$ for dose per fraction, $\alpha$ for the linear and $\beta$ for the quadratic component of cell killing, and $\alpha/\beta$-ratio for the dose at which both cell killing components are equal. The $\alpha/\beta$-ratio depends on the endpoint considered and is 2 Gy for radiation-induced myelopathy. A dedicated chapter to spinal cord tolerance is presented in this book for the interested reader.

An in-field recurrence of MESCC usually occurs only several months following radiotherapy. Its risk increases with the patient's life span [28, 43]. Therefore, patients with a poor survival prognosis should be irradiated with a short course of radiotherapy in order to avoid these patients spending more time than necessary of their limited life span receiving radiotherapy. Since local control of MESCC becomes more important with increasing life span and can be improved with the use of longer-course radiotherapy programs, these patients should not receive single-fraction or short-course multi-fraction radiotherapy. Patients with an intermediate survival prognosis appear more appropriately treated with the worldwide most commonly used regimen 30 Gy in ten fractions. Since patients with a very favorable survival prognosis appear to benefit from an escalation of the radiotherapy dose beyond 30 Gy in terms of better local control of MESCC, these patients appear more appropriately

treated with 37.5 Gy in 15 fractions or 40 Gy in 20 fractions. These considerations show that it is very important to be able to predict the survival prognosis of an individual patient with MESCC assigned to receive conventional radiotherapy as precisely as possible. The estimation of a patient's remaining life span can be facilitated using the survival scores mentioned previously described under "Prognostic and Predictive Factors."

## Case Presentation

A 74-year-old male was first diagnosed with stage IV non-small lung cancer 6 months ago with pulmonary and adrenal metastases. He now presents with severe back pain and progressive motor deficits (onset 10 day ago) of both legs. The patient was no longer able to walk and had an ECOG performance score of 4. On clinical examination, active movement against gravity of both legs was still possible. Spinal MRI revealed disseminated vertebral metastases and MESCC affecting T4–5 and T10–11. The patient received dexamethasone treatment and was presented to a neurosurgeon, who decided that upfront surgery was not reasonable. The patient was assigned to receive palliative radiotherapy. According to a survival score, the patient's probability to survive for 6 months was only about 5%. Therefore, the patient received short-course radiotherapy with a single fraction of 8 Gy. At 4 weeks following radiotherapy, both pain and motor function had improved. The previously bedbound patient became ambulatory and was able to walk a distance of 100 m with a walker. Unfortunately, the patient died another 6 weeks later due to progression of visceral metastases.

## Summary

- The majority of patients with MESCC are treated with radiotherapy supplemented by corticosteroids.
- Typical fractionation regimens include short-course programs such as 8 Gy in 1 fraction or 20 Gy in 5 fractions and longer-course programs such as 30 Gy in 10 fractions, 37.5 Gy in 15 fractions, or 40 Gy in 20 fractions.
- Short-course programs have a similar effect on motor function as longer-course programs and should be preferred in patients with a short expected survival time.
- Longer-course programs result in better local control of MESCC than short-course programs and should be preferred in patients with more favorable survival prognoses.
- An individual patient's survival prognosis can be estimated with the available scoring tools prior to the start of radiotherapy to optimally personalize the treatment.

## Self-Assessment Questions

1. What can be considered the hallmark symptom of MESCC?
   A. Pain
   B. Fatigue
   C. Sensory deficits
   D. Motor deficits
   E. Sphincter dysfunction

2. What is generally considered the diagnostic procedure of choice for detection of MESCC?
   A. Plain radiographs
   B. Myelography
   C. Computed tomography (CT) with contrast medium
   D. Positron emission tomography (PET)
   E. Magnetic resonance imaging (MRI)

3. Spinal surgery for MESCC…
   A. …is indicated for the vast majority of patients with MESCC.
   B. …generally does not require post-operative radiotherapy.
   C. … should ideally be performed as a simple laminectomy without direct stabilization.
   D. …is indicated in case of bony fragments that compromise the spinal cord or instability of the involved spinal segment.
   E. …is generally performed in the middle of a radiotherapy course.

4. When aiming to assign the best available radiotherapy program to a patient with MESCC, one should keep in mind that…
   A. …in patients with a short expected survival time, short course programs are inferior to longer-course programs regarding the effect on motor function.
   B. …the addition of corticosteroids is generally not indicated because of the toxicity profile.
   C. …additional treatment with bisphosphonates should be given particularly in patients with a poor prognosis due to the remarkable synergistic effect of bisphosphonates and radiotherapy in improving motor function.
   D. …longer-course programs result in fewer in-field recurrences of MESCC when compared to short-course and single-fraction programs.
   E. …particularly in patients with MESCC from a solid tumor and a poor survival prognosis, the addition of chemotherapy to radiotherapy should be strongly considered.

5. If re-irradiation for an in-field recurrence of MESCC is required,
   A. …the cumulative biologically effective dose (BED) of the primary radiotherapy and re-irradiation should not exceed 50 $Gy_2$.
   B. …the risk of radiation-induced myelopathy is not acceptable if the cumulative BED is 50 $Gy_2$ and the interval between both treatments is longer than 6 months.
   C. …the BED can be calculated with the equation: $BED = D \times [1 + (d/\alpha/\beta)]$.
   D. …re-irradiation of MESCC after single-fraction radiotherapy with $1 \times 8$ Gy must always be performed as stereotactic body radiation therapy.
   E. …salvage decompressive surgery is generally added to re-irradiation.

## Answers

1. D
2. E
3. D
4. D
5. C

## References

1. Spiller WG. Rapidly progressive paralysis associated with carcinoma. AMA Arch Neurol Psychiatry. 1925;13:471–7.
2. Rades D, Abrahm JL. The role of radiotherapy for metastatic epidural spinal cord compression. Nat Rev Clin Oncol. 2010;7:590–8.
3. Loblaw DA, Laperriere NJ, Mackillop WJ. A population-based study of malignant spinal cord compression in Ontario. Clin Oncol. 2003;15:211–7.
4. Prasad D, Schiff D. Malignant spinal-cord compression. Lancet Oncol. 2005;6:15–24.
5. Ushio Y, Posner R, Posner JB, et al. Experimental spinal cord compression by epidural neoplasms. Neurology. 1977;27:422–9.
6. Kato A, Ushio Y, Hayakawa T, et al. Circulatory disturbance of the spinal cord with epidural neoplasms in rats. J Neurosurg. 1985;63:260–5.
7. Manabe S, Tanaka H, Hogo Y, et al. Experimental analysis of the spinal cord compressed by spinal metastasis. Spine. 1989;14:1308–15.
8. Tarlov I, Klinger H, Vitale S. Spinal cord compression studies: I. Experimental techniques to produce acute and gradual compression. AMA Arch Neurol Psychiatry. 1953;70:813–9.
9. Tarlov I, Klinger H. Spinal cord compression studies: II. Time limits for recovery after acute compression in dogs. AMA Arch Neurol Psychiatry. 1954;71:271–90.
10. Rades D, Heidenreich F, Bremer M, et al. Time of developing motor deficits before radiotherapy as a new and relevant prognostic factor in metastatic spinal cord compression: final results of a retrospective analysis. Eur Neurol. 2001;45:266–9.
11. Rades D, Heidenreich F, Karstens JH. Final results of a prospective study of the prognostic value of the time to develop motor defi-

cits before irradiation in metastatic spinal cord compression. Int J Radiat Oncol Biol Phys. 2002;53;975–9.

12. Gilbert RW, Kim JH, Posner RB. Epidural spinal cord compression from metastatic tumor: diagnosis and treatment. Ann Neurol. 1978;3:40–51.

13. Bach F, Larsen BH, Rohde K, et al. Metastatic spinal cord compression. Occurrence, symptoms, clinical presentations, and prognosis in 398 patients with spinal cord compression. Acta Neurochir. 1990;107:37–43.

14. Kovner F, Spigel S, Rider I, et al. Radiation therapy of metastatic spinal cord compression. Multidisciplinary team diagnosis and treatment. J Neurooncol. 1999;42:85–92.

15. Helweg-Larsen S, Sørensen PS, Kreiner S. Prognostic factors in metastatic spinal cord compression: a prospective study using multivariate analysis of variables influencing survival and gait function in 153 patients. Int J Radiat Oncol Biol Phys. 2000;46:1163–9.

16. Maranzano E, Latini P. Effectiveness of radiation therapy without surgery in metastatic spinal cord compression: final results from a prospective trial. Int J Radiat Oncol Biol Phys. 1995;32:959–67.

17. Husband DJ. Malignant spinal cord compression: prospective study of delays in referral and treatment. BMJ. 1998;317:18–21.

18. Tomita T, Galicich JH, Sundaresan N. Radiation therapy for spinal epidural metastases with complete block. Acta Radiol Oncol. 1983;22:135–43.

19. Baskin DS. Spinal cord injury. In: Ewans RW, editor. Neurology and trauma. Philadelphia: Saunders; 1996. p. 276–99.

20. Li KC, Poon PY. Sensitivity and specificity of MRI in detecting malignant spinal cord compression and in distinguishing malignant from benign compression fractures of vertebrae. Magn Reson Imaging. 1988;6:547–56.

21. Colletti PM, Siegel HJ, Woo MY, et al. The impact on treatment planning of MRI of the spine in patients suspected of vertebral metastasis: an efficacy study. Comput Med Imaging Graph. 1996;20:159–62.

22. Rades D, Bremer M, Goehde S, et al. Spondylodiscitis in patients with spinal cord compression: a possible pitfall in radiation oncology. Radiother Oncol. 2001;59:307–9.

23. Kim RY, Smith JW, Spencer SA, et al. Malignant epidural spinal cord compression associated with a paravertebral mass: its radiotherapeutic outcome on radiosensitivity. Int J Radiat Oncol Biol Phys. 1993;27:1079–83.

24. Leviov M, Dale J, Stein M, et al. The management of metastatic spinal cord compression: a radiotherapeutic success ceiling. Int J Radiat Oncol Biol Phys. 1993;27:231–4.

25. Rades D, Stalpers LJ, Veninga T, et al. Evaluation of five radiation schedules and prognostic factors for metastatic spinal cord compression. J Clin Oncol. 2005;23:3366–75.

26. Rades D, Rudat V, Veninga T, et al. A score predicting posttreatment ambulatory status in patients irradiated for metastatic spinal cord compression. Int J Radiat Oncol Biol Phys. 2008;72:905–8.

27. Rades D, Douglas S, Huttenlocher S, et al. Validation of a score predicting post-treatment ambulatory status after radiotherapy for metastatic spinal cord compression. Int J Radiat Oncol Biol Phys. 2011;79:1503–6.

28. Rades D, Fehlauer F, Schulte R, et al. Prognostic factors for local control and survival after radiotherapy of metastatic spinal cord compression. J Clin Oncol. 2006;24:3388–93.

29. Rades D, Dunst J, Schild SE. The first score predicting overall survival in patients with metastatic spinal cord compression. Cancer. 2008;112:157–61.

30. Rades D, Douglas S, Veninga T, et al. Validation and simplification of a score predicting survival in patients irradiated for metastatic spinal cord compression. Cancer. 2010;116:3670–3.

31. Rades D, Douglas S, Schild SE. A validated survival score for breast cancer patients with metastatic spinal cord compression. Strahlenther Onkol. 2013;189:41–6.

32. Rades D, Douglas S, Veninga T, et al. A survival score for patients with metastatic spinal cord compression from prostate cancer. Strahlenther Onkol. 2012;188:802–6.

33. Rades D, Douglas S, Veninga T, et al. A validated survival score for patients with metastatic spinal cord compression from non-small cell lung cancer. BMC Cancer. 2012;12:302.

34. Douglas S, Schild SE, Rades D. A new score predicting the survival of patients with spinal cord compression from myeloma. BMC Cancer. 2012;12:425.

35. Douglas S, Schild SE, Rades D. Metastatic spinal cord compression in patients with cancer of unknown primary. Estimating the survival prognosis with a validated score. Strahlenther Onkol. 2012;188:1048–51.

36. Rades D, Douglas S, Veninga T, et al. Prognostic factors and a survival score for patients with metastatic spinal cord compression (MSCC) from renal cell carcinoma (RCC). Australasian J Cancer. 2012;11:169–74.

37. Rades D, Douglas S, Huttenlocher S, et al. Prognostic factors and a survival score for patients with metastatic spinal cord compression from colorectal cancer. Strahlenther Onkol. 2012;188:1114–8.

38. Amar AP, Levy ML. Pathogenesis and pharmacological strategies for mitigating secondary damage in acute spinal cord injury. Neurosurgery. 1999;44:1027–40.

39. Sørensen PS, Helweg-Larsen S, Mouridsen H, et al. Effect of high-dose dexamethasone in carcinomatous metastatic spinal cord compression treated with radiotherapy: a randomized trial. Eur J Cancer. 1994;30A:22–7.

40. Heimdal K, Hirschberg H, Slettebo H, et al. High incidence of serious side effects of high-dose dexamethasone treatment in patients with epidural spinal cord compression. J Neurooncol. 1992;12:141–4.

41. Saad F, Gleason DM, Murrey R, et al. A randomized, placebo-controlled trial of zoledronic acid in patients with hormone-refractory metastatic prostate carcinoma. J Natl Cancer Inst. 2002;94:1458–68.

42. Saad F, Gleason DM, Murray R, et al. Long-term efficacy of zoledronic acid for the prevention of skeletal complications in patients with metastatic hormone-refractory prostate cancer. J Natl Cancer Inst. 2004;96:879–82.

43. Rades D, Lange M, Veninga T, et al. Final results of a prospective study comparing the local control of short-course and long-course radiotherapy for metastatic spinal cord compression. Int J Radiat Oncol Biol Phys. 2011;79:524–30.

44. Rades D, Hakim SG, Bajrovic A, et al. Impact of zoledronic acid on control of metastatic spinal cord compression. Strahlenther Onkol. 2012;188:910–6.

45. Roodman GD. Mechanisms of bone metastasis. N Engl J Med. 2004;350:1655–64.

46. Stopeck AT, Lipton A, Body JJ, et al. Denosumab compared with zoledronic acid for the treatment of bone metastases in patients with advanced breast cancer: a randomized, double-blind study. J Clin Oncol. 2010;28:5132–9.

47. Fizazi K, Carducci M, Smith M, et al. Denosumab versus zoledronic acid for treatment of bone metastases in men with castration-resistant prostate cancer: a randomised, double-blind study. Lancet. 2011;377:813–22.

48. Henry DH, Costa L, Goldwasser F, et al. Randomized, double-blind study of denosumab versus zoledronic acid in the treatment of bone metastases in patients with advanced cancer (excluding breast and prostate cancer) or multiple myeloma. J Clin Oncol. 2011;29:1125–32.

49. Aviles A, Fernandez R, Gonzalez JL, et al. Spinal cord compression as a primary manifestation of aggressive malignant lymphomas:

long-term analysis of treatments with radiotherapy, chemotherapy or combined therapy. Leuk Lymphoma. 2002;43:355–9.

50. Wallington M, Mendis S, Premawardhana U, et al. Local control and survival in spinal cord compression from lymphoma and myeloma. Radiother Oncol. 1997;42:43–7.

51. Patchell R, Tibbs PA, Regine WF, et al. Direct decompressive surgical resection in the treatment of spinal cord compression caused by metastatic cancer: a randomised trial. Lancet. 2005;366:643–8.

52. Yen D, Kuriachan V, Yach J, et al. Long-term outcome of anterior decompression and spinal fixation after placement of the Welesley Wedge for thoracic and lumbar spinal metastasis. J Neurosurg. 2002;96(Suppl 1):6–9.

53. Klimo P Jr, Dailey AT, Fessler RG. Posterior surgical approaches and outcomes in metastatic spine-disease. Neurosurg Clin N Am. 2004;15:425–35.

54. Young RF, Post EM, King GA. Treatment of spinal epidural metastases. Randomized prospective comparison of laminectomy and radiotherapy. J Neurosurg. 1980;53:741–8.

55. Sørensen PS, Borgesen SE, Rohde K, et al. Metastatic epidural spinal cord compression: results of treatment and survival. Cancer. 1990;65:1502–8.

56. Klimo P Jr, Kestle JR, Schmidt MH. Treatment of metastatic spinal epidural disease: a review of the literature. Neurosurg Focus. 2003;15:E1.

57. Klimo P Jr, Thompson CJ, Kestle JR, et al. A meta-analysis of surgery versus conventional radiotherapy for the treatment of metastatic spinal epidural disease. Neuro Oncol. 2005;7:64–76.

58. Kunkler I. Surgical resection in metastatic spinal cord compression. Lancet. 2006;367:109.

59. Knisely J, Strugar J. Can decompressive surgery improve outcome in patients with metastatic epidural spinal-cord compression? Nat Clin Pract Oncol. 2006;3:14–5.

60. Rades D, Huttenlocher S, Dunst J, et al. Matched pair analysis comparing surgery followed by radiotherapy and radiotherapy alone for metastatic spinal cord compression. J Clin Oncol. 2010;28:3597–604.

61. Rades D, Huttenlocher S, Bajrovic A, et al. Surgery followed by radiotherapy versus radiotherapy alone for metastatic spinal cord compression from unfavorable tumors. Int J Radiat Oncol Biol Phys. 2011;81:e861–8.

62. Joiner MC, Van der Kogel AJ. The linear-quadratic approach to fractionation and calculation of isoeffect relationships. In: Steel GG, editor. Basic clinical radiobiology. New York: Oxford University Press; 1997. p. 106–12.

63. Emami B, Lyman J, Brown A, et al. Tolerance of normal tissue to therapeutic irradiation. Int J Radiat Oncol Biol Phys. 1991;21:109–22.

64. Marks LB, Yorke ED, Jackson A, et al. Use of normal tissue complication probability models in the clinic. Int J Radiat Oncol Biol Phys. 2010;76(3 Suppl):S10–9.

65. Maranzano E, Latini P, Beneventi S, et al. Comparison of two different radiotherapy schedules for spinal cord compression in prostate cancer. Tumori. 1998;84:472–7.

66. Rades D, Fehlauer F, Stalpers LJA, et al. A prospective evaluation of two radiation schedules with 10 versus 20 fractions for the treatment of metastatic spinal cord compression: final results of a multicenter study. Cancer. 2004;101:2687–92.

67. Maranzano E, Bellavita R, Rossi R, et al. Short-course versus split-course radiotherapy in metastatic spinal cord compression: results of a phase III, randomized, multicenter trial. J Clin Oncol. 2005;23:3358–65.

68. Maranzano E, Trippa F, Casale M, et al. 8Gy single-dose radiotherapy is effective in metastatic spinal cord compression: results of a phase III randomized multicentre Italian trial. Radiother Oncol. 2009;93:174–9.

69. Rades D, Šegedin B, Conde-Moreno AJ, et al. Radiotherapy with 4 Gy × 5 versus 3 Gy × 10 for metastatic epidural spinal cord compression: final results of the SCORE-2 trial (ARO 2009/01). J Clin Oncol. 2016;34:597–602.

70. Rades D, Panzner A, Rudat V, et al. Dose escalation of radiotherapy for metastatic spinal cord compression (MSCC) in patients with relatively favorable survival prognosis. Strahlenther Onkol. 2011;187:729–35.

71. Rades D, Stalpers LJ, Veninga T, et al. Spinal reirradiation after short-course RT for metastatic spinal cord compression. Int J Radiat Oncol Biol Phys. 2005;63:872–5.

72. Nieder C, Grosu AL, Andratschke NH, et al. Update of human spinal cord reirradiation tolerance based on additional data from 38 patients. Int J Radiat Oncol Biol Phys. 2006;66:1446–9.

# Vertebral Body Metastasis

Amol J. Ghia and Anussara Prayongrat

## Abbreviations

| | |
|---|---|
| AAPM | The American Association of Physicists in Medicine |
| ASTRO | American Society for Radiation Oncology |
| BED | Biological equivalent dose |
| CBCT | Cone beam CT |
| cEBRT | Conventional external beam radiation treatment |
| CT | Computed tomography |
| CTV | Clinical target volume |
| EPID | Electronic portal imaging device |
| GTV | Gross target volume |
| IGRT | Image-guidance radiotherapy |
| KPS | Karnofsky performance status |
| KV | Kilovoltage |
| LINAC | Linear accelerator |
| LQ model | Linear-quadratic model |
| MESCC | Metastatic epidural spinal cord compression |
| MLC | Multileaf collimator |
| MRI | Magnetic resonance imaging |
| MV | Megavoltage |
| OARs | Organs at risk |
| OS | Overall survival |
| $P_{max}$ | Maximal point dose |
| PRISM | Prognostic index for spine metastasis |
| PRV | Planning organ-at-risk volume |
| PTV | Planning target volume |
| QUANTEC | Quantitative analysis of normal tissue effects in the clinic |
| RCC | Renal cell carcinoma |
| RM | Radiation myelopathy |
| RPA | Recursive partitioning analysis |
| RT | Radiotherapy |
| RTOG | Radiation Therapy Oncology Group |
| SBRT | Stereotactic body radiotherapy |
| SINS | Spine Instability Neoplastic Score |
| TPD | Time from primary diagnosis |
| VCF | Vertebral compression fracture |

## Learning Objectives

- Outline a treatment approach for patients with vertebral body metastasis based on individual prognostic and predictive factors.
- Justify the use of radiation treatment in vertebral body metastasis, and identify patients who gain benefit from stereotactic body radiotherapy.
- Describe the radiotherapy techniques including simulation and immobilization, target delineation, dose prescription and fractionation, and normal tissue constraints.
- Evaluate possible toxicities from stereotactic body radiotherapy.

## Epidemiology

Osseous metastatic disease is the third most common form of dissemination behind pulmonary and hepatic metastatic disease. The spine is the most common anatomical distribution of bone metastases due to vascular access and host factors [1]. In fact, spinal metastases develop in 30–90% of cancer patients based on autopsy, and 5–30% of patients suffer from neurological deficit [2]. The most common clinical symptom related to spinal metastasis is progressive axial pain which frequently is nocturnal. Neurological compromise may range from occasional radiculopathy to spinal cord compression.

A. J. Ghia (✉)
Department of Radiation Oncology, MD Anderson Cancer Center, Houston, TX, USA
e-mail: AJGhia@mdanderson.org

A. Prayongrat
Department of Radiation Oncology, King Chulalongkorn Memorial Hospital, Bangkok, Thailand

## Risk Factors

No risk factors have been associated with vertebral body metastasis.

## Prognostic and Predictive Factors

Historical scoring systems have been designed in an attempt to select the proper treatment modality for each individual patient with spinal metastasis incorporating prognostic factors such as primary tumor characteristics, number of visceral metastases, number of bone lesions, performance status, and neurological status [3–6]. Patients with favorable prognoses may be better suited for locally aggressive approaches whereas those with unfavorable prognoses were selected for less locally aggressive approaches. These prognostic scoring systems allow surgeons and oncologists to better estimate patients' prognosis and select proper management.

## Multimodality Management Approach

Currently, several treatment modalities are available for patients with spinal metastases, and a multidisciplinary approach to decision-making is essential for optimal management. Level 1 evidence supports the role of surgical decompression in patients with symptomatic spinal cord compression as it improves ambulatory rates. Modern surgical techniques range from a spinal decompression with spinal stabilization using instrumental fixation to a separation surgery involving clearance of epidural disease in conjunction with stabilization. Historical indications for surgery included intractable mechanical pain unresponsive to nonoperative measures; existence of a growing tumor that is resistant to radiotherapy (RT), chemotherapy, or hormonal therapy; patients who have reached full spinal cord tolerance after prior RT; spinal instability manifested as pathologic fracture, progressive deformity, or neurologic deficit; and/or clinically significant neural compression, especially by the bone or bone debris [7].

In addition to surgical intervention, local radiotherapy is a noninvasive treatment modality which may be administered in the primary or postoperative setting as well as in the salvage setting as detailed below. Medical treatments including systemic chemotherapy, hormonal treatment, corticosteroids, bisphosphonates, and pain medications should also be considered [4]. Clearly, a multidisciplinary

decision-making approach is preferred involving a team consisting of spine surgeons, neuroradiologists, medical oncologists, pain specialists, and radiation oncologists.

The Memorial Sloan Kettering Cancer Center has developed a multidisciplinary decision framework for metastatic spine disease, *NOMS* (neurologic, oncologic, mechanical instability, and systemic disease assessment), to facilitate physicians' decision-making on the optimal treatment modality for the individual patient [8]. *Neurologic* assessment includes a clinical and radiographic assessment of tumor extent. Bilsky et al. proposed an MRI-based grading system for metastatic epidural spinal cord compression (ESCC) [9]. In general, patients with low-grade ESCC such as grade 0 (bone involvement only) and grade 1 (epidural impingement without spinal cord compression, classified into grades 1a to 1c) in the absence of mechanical instability are considered for radiation therapy. Those with higher-grade compression such as grade 2 (partial ESCC) and grade 3 (complete ESCC) may be suited for surgical decompression followed by radiation. Recently, Ryu et al. proposed a scoring system to determine the use of surgery versus advance radiation technique using stereotactic body radiotherapy (SBRT) based on radiographic (MRI) and neurological criteria [10]. Patients with progressive neurological deterioration in concert with a significant epidural metastatic lesion should be considered for surgical decompression followed by radiotherapy when feasible.

*Oncologic* assessment focuses on the responsiveness of tumor and duration of tumor control to the available treatments and the natural history of primary tumor histology, usually determined by the intrinsic radiosensitivity of the tumor. Radiosensitive solid tumors include breast, prostate, ovarian, and neuroendocrine carcinoma, while renal cell carcinoma (RCC), sarcoma, and melanoma are considered radioresistant tumors which may require higher radiation dose to achieve local control.

*Mechanical instability* serves as an indication for surgical intervention and requires both clinical and radiographic assessment. The Spine Instability Neoplastic Score (SINS) is a validated tool to assess for instability with high reliability using a comprehensive set of factors including spinal location of tumor, pain, bone lesion, spinal alignment, vertebral body collapse, and posterior involvement. SINS of greater than 7 indicates a potentially unstable spine, and surgical stabilization may be considered [11, 12].

*Systemic disease* assessment depends on the extent of tumor dissemination, available systemic options, medical comorbidities, and tumor histology determining patients' treatment tolerability.

## Radiation Treatment

The American Society for Radiation Oncology (ASTRO) provided evidence-based guidelines on the treatment of bone metastasis (including but not limited to spinal metastases) and summarized the historical role of palliative radiotherapy for bone metastases [13]. RT has been recommended as a treatment of choice in patients with symptomatic spinal metastases and asymptomatic spinal metastases with epidural encroachment with or without surgical decompression/stabilization. The combined modality approach to local disease in the spine depends on factors such as the intrinsic radiosensitivity of the lesion, neurological stability, degree of spinal cord compression by epidural soft tissue disease, and those with inoperable medical condition, disseminated systemic disease, or poor survival.

## Conventional Radiotherapy

Conventional external beam radiation treatment (cEBRT) has been the mainstay spinal metastasis treatment for many decades with intent to palliate painful bone metastases and prevent progression of metastatic spinal cord compression. Various radiotherapy schedules and dose fractionation are used, ranging from 8 Gy in single fraction, 20 Gy in 5 fractions, 30 Gy in 10 fractions, 37.5 Gy in 15 fractions, and 40 Gy in 20 fractions. The palliative efficacy among these different schedules was similar though retreatment rate and pathologic fracture rates seemed to be higher in short fractionation regimen [14–17]. In the postoperative setting, 30 Gy in ten fractions is a common fractionation schedule and is also used frequently in the palliative setting as well.

## Stereotactic Body Radiotherapy

SBRT is an emerging treatment modality combining advanced technologies such as computerized planning software, advanced imaging (such as MRI), rigid immobilization devices, treatment delivery with beam intensity or beam gantry modulation, and image-guidance radiotherapy (IGRT). The goal of SBRT in spinal metastases is to alleviate pain, improve local control, and prevent or improve neurological dysfunction as well as maintain good quality of life while minimizing possible toxicities. The advantages of SBRT may be characterized in terms of physical aspects, biological aspect, and clinical aspects:

1. *Physical aspects*: Excellent dose conformity can be achieved by complicated beam arrangement and beam intensity modulation as well as precise and accurate targeting localization with the advances in image-guidance and treatment delivery systems contributing to tumor dose escalation and adjacent normal tissue sparing. This allows for the delivery of ablative doses of radiation (e.g., 24 Gy in a single fraction) within millimeters of the spinal cord while preserving neurologic function.

2. *Biological aspects*: SBRT delivers concentrated radiation usually in one to five fractions leading to a higher biological equivalent dose (BED) than cEBRT, with the goal of improving durable rates of local control with minimal toxicity. The BED, approximated using linear-quadratic (LQ) model, is as high as $41.6$–$81.6$ $Gy_{10}$ in SBRT (16–24 Gy in single fraction to 24–27 Gy in three fractions) compared with $14.4$–$39$ $Gy_{10}$ in cEBRT (8 Gy in single fraction to 30 Gy in ten fractions). This likely translates to improved local tumor control through direct (e.g., DNA damage) and indirect mechanisms. Although the precise biologic mechanisms of tumor cell death in response to SBRT have not been fully established, some have proposed changes in the vascular environment as well as immune environment may contribute to the enhanced efficacy of SBRT even beyond that predicted by the LQ model [18–21].

3. *Clinical aspects*: Temporary palliation is effectively accomplished by the use of cEBRT; however, in well-selected patients, durable palliation and local control may be further improved with IGRT and SBRT technology. Image-guided SBRT allows delivery of an ablative radiation dose with minimal toxicity and potentially improves local tumor control, particularly for radioresistant tumors. However, further understanding of long-term normal tissue toxicity is still lacking [22], and the potential risks of SBRT must be weighed against the aforementioned potential benefits. The excellent conformality of dose delivery lends this tool as particularly useful in the salvage radiation setting. Moreover, the brevity of treatment and targeted treatment leading to bone marrow preservation may provide the benefit of prompt systemic treatment with minimal side effect [23]. To summarize, SBRT is a noninvasive procedure and can be applied in a single fraction as an outpatient treatment offering an ablative alternative to surgical intervention or extended fractionated radiotherapy.

## Indication for Spine SBRT

Patient selection cannot be underestimated when considering spinal SBRT. Clinical consideration and judgment should be based on specific patient and disease characteristics in a multidisciplinary fashion. The risks of spinal SBRT must be weighed against the potential long-term benefits. There are several guidelines and reviews that summarize the inclusion and exclusion criteria acquired from many published trials [13, 24–29]. At MD Anderson Cancer Center (MDACC), patients are considered for spinal SBRT if they have oligometastatic/oligoprogressive disease, have radioresistant disease, or have received prior radiotherapy at the site.

Two study groups assessed the survival after SBRT treatment for spinal metastases and proposed SBRT-specific prognostic models: recursive partitioning analysis (RPA) index and prognostic index for spine metastasis (PRISM) [30, 31].

RPA index for patients undergoing spine SBRT developed by Chao et al. classifies patients into three classes: Class 1 defined as patients with a time from primary diagnosis (TPD) of >30 months and a KPS of >70, Class 2 defined as those with a TPD of >30 months and a KPS of ≤70 or a TPD of <30 months and age <70 years, and Class 3 defined as a TPD of ≤30 months and age ≥70 years. Median overall survivals (OS) were 21.1 months, 8.7 months, and 2.4 months for Classes 1, 2, and 3, respectively [30]. A more recent model called the PRognostic Index for Spinal Metatases (PRISM) was developed by Tang et al. using seven pretreatment parameters to stratify patients into four groups with excellent (Group 1) and poor (Group 4) prognosis after spine SBRT with the median OS of >70 months and 9.1 months, respectively [31]. Neither prognostic model has been externally validated to this point.

## Clinical Application of Spine SBRT

Spine SBRT in clinical practice can be classified into three categories according to variety of patients, treatment characteristics, and predicted treatment outcomes [24].

### 1. Primary Treatment in Unirradiated Patients

Patients may be considered for spinal SBRT if they have oligometastatic disease or symptomatic radioresistant disease. Studies reported tumor and/or pain control in patients treated with SBRT for spinal metastases of 80–100% in unirradiated patients [32–38] as described in Table 12.1. The median duration of tumor/pain control was 6.5–13.3 months. Radioresistant tumors also benefit from SBRT as previous studies reported the promising outcome of 89–96% pain control in spinal metastases from RCC, melanoma, and sarcoma [33, 42, 49]. This compares very favorably to historical data in the use of fractionated radiation for radioresistant metastases [50].

### 2. Salvage Treatment in Previously Irradiated Patients

Following radiation treatment for spinal metastasis, local recurrence of disease is a challenging clinical scenario [51, 52]. The historical goal of treatment in these patients is palliation and prevention of further complication due to tumor progression without inducing radiation myelopathy (RM). As a result, historical treatment options in this setting have included surgical decompression or low dose cEBRT alone with minimal data regarding durable local control. Spinal SBRT offers a safe and effective noninvasive salvage approach. Many studies demonstrate the efficacy of re-irradiated spine SBRT on tumor and/or pain control of 77–100% [39–44, 53] as shown in Table 12.1.

### 3. Combined Treatment with Surgery

Based on the promising results from definitive treatment, SBRT has been applied selectively in the postoperative setting usually in patients with radioresistant disease or in patients previously irradiated with resultant tumor control of 81–94.4% [45–47] compared with 60% in cEBRT patients [54, 55]. SBRT is usually performed in 1–2 weeks after surgery. A systematic review suggested that timing between SBRT and surgery should be at least 1 week to minimize wound complications [56, 57], which is often earlier than that of conventional RT. Unlike cEBRT, accumulated skin dose from SBRT plan is rarely of concern by virtue of multi-directional beam arrangement and highly focused, precise targeting around the involved vertebrae as demonstrated in Fig. 12.1. Salvage surgery after SBRT in recurrent cases could also be safely performed based on this.

For patients with significant epidural disease, spinal cord constraints limit tumor coverage near the spinal cord in spinal SBRT cases. In fact, a common pattern of failure in spinal SBRT is within this epidural space. "Separation surgery" has emerged as a treatment strategy by which the epidural tumor is selectively removed and the remaining disease is treated with spinal SBRT. This strategy allows for minimal surgery and optimal radiation dose to the remaining tumor with SBRT. Studies reported a 1-year local failure rate of 9.5–16.4% (6.3–9% for 24 Gy single fraction) without any cases of myelopathy using this multimodality approach [47, 48].

## Radiotherapy Techniques

### Simulation and Immobilization

Computed tomography (CT) simulation with slice thickness of 1–2 mm is required. The patient must be immobilized comfortably with a stereotactic immobilization device in order to allow reproducibility of positioning and minimize unnecessary movement during treatment (see Fig. 12.2). Li et al. reported minimal intrafraction motion using image-guidance, near-rigid body immobilization with vacuum fixation, justify-

**Table 12.1** Treatment outcomes among various studies on stereotactic body radiotherapy for treatment of spine metastases

| Study | Number of patient | Median FU (months) | Radiation treatment | Pain relief[a] | Tumor control | Overall survival (months) | Toxicity |
|---|---|---|---|---|---|---|---|
| *Primary treatment in unirradiated patients* | | | | | | | |
| Ryu [32] | 49 | 6.4 | 10–16 Gy single fraction | 85% TPR = 14 days DPR = 13.6 months | NA | 1Y = 74.3% | No RM |
| Gerzten [33] | 48 RCC | 37 | 20 Gy single fraction (median) | 89% | 87.5% | NA | NA |
| Yamada [34] | 93 | 15 | 18–24 Gy single fraction | NA | 15m = 100% | 15 | No RM |
| Chang [35] | 63 | 21.3 | 27 Gy in three fractions (median) | NA | 1Y = 84% | 16.3 | No RM |
| Garg [36] | 61 | 17.8 | 16–24 Gy single fraction | 87% | 1Y = 100% 18m = 88% | 30.4 | RM 3% VF 3% |
| Guckenberger [37] | 301 | 11.8 | 24 Gy in three fractions (median) | 76.8% | 1Y = 89.9% 2Y = 83.9% TLF = 9 months | 19.5 | No RM VF = 7.8% |
| Bishop [38] | 285 | 19 | 27 Gy in three fractions (median) | NA | 1Y = 88% 3Y = 82% TLF = 6 months | 23 | NA |
| *Salvage treatment in irradiated patients* | | | | | | | |
| Milker [39] | 18 | 12.3 | 39.6 Gy (median) (previous dose 38 Gy) | 81.3% | 1Y = 94.7% TLF = 17.7 months | 10.5 | No RM |
| Yamada [40] | 35 | 7 | 20 Gy in five fractions (previous dose 30 Gy) | 90% | 81% TLF = 5.5 months | 7 | No RM |
| Wang [41] | 149 | | 27–30 Gy in three fractions | 92.9% | 1Y = 80.5% 2Y = 72.4% TLF = 13 months | 23 | No RM |
| Gerzten [42] | 36 Melanoma 64% prior RT | | 21.7 Gy single fraction (median) | 96% | 75% | NA | NA |
| Gerzten [43] | 393 68% prior RT | 21 | 12.5–25 Gy single fraction | 86% | 1Y = 90% | NA | No RM |
| Gibbs [44] | 74 74% prior RT | 9 | 16–25 Gy in 1–5 fractions | 83.9% | NA | 11 | RM 4% |
| *Combined treatments* | | | | | | | |
| Gerzten [45] | 26 | 16 | 16–20 Gy single fraction | 92% | NA | NA | NA |
| Rock [46] | 18 | 7 | 6–16 Gy single fraction | NA | NA | NA | RM 5.6% |
| Moulding [47] | 21 | | 18–24 Gy single fraction | NA | 90.5% | 10.3 | No RM |
| Laufer [48] | 186 | | 24–30 Gy in 1–3 fractions | NA | 95.9% | NA | NA |
| | | | 18–36 Gy in 5–6 fractions | NA | 77.4% | NA | NA |

Abbreviation: *FU* follow-up, *TPR* time to pain relief, *DPR* duration of pain relief, *TLF* time to local failure, *RM* radiation myelopathy, *VF* vertebral fracture, *RCC* renal cell carcinoma, *NA* not applicable
[a]Pain relief, defined by complete and partial pain relief or pain improvement or pain control, varied by studies

ing 2 mm margin for setup error [58]. In clinical practice, PTV margins range from 0 to 2 mm. CT simulation images are then transferred to the treatment planning computers.

## Target Delineation

MRI-based planning is recommended for identification of gross tumor as well as critical normal tissue such as the spinal cord. T1-weighted images with and without contrast as well as T2-weighted images may be used. Gross target volume (GTV) is defined as radiographically visible tumor on CT or MRI. Clinical target volume (CTV) is contoured based on potential anatomical extension according to routes of spread [35, 59]. A 5 mm margin in the soft tissue may be applied in cases of paraspinal soft tissue involvement [60]. The development of metastatic disease at adjacent levels has been found to be only 5% [59]; therefore, it is not necessary to include adjacent levels in the radiation target [24]. The Radiation Therapy Oncology Group (RTOG) 0631 and the

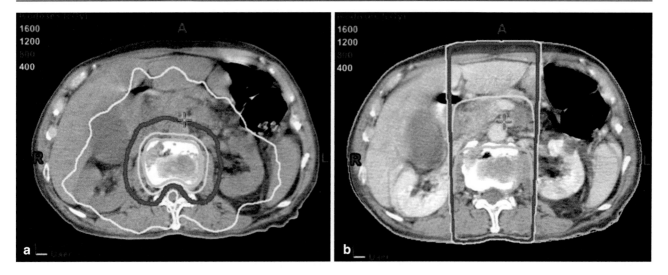

**Fig. 12.1** Comparing skin dose between two different radiation techniques: stereotactic body radiotherapy (**a**) and conventional radiotherapy (**b**) (*green = isodose line of 16 Gy; cyan = isodose line of 12 Gy; purple = isodose line of 8 Gy; and yellow = isodose line of 4 Gy*)

**Fig. 12.2** Rigid immobilization utilizing a BodyFix apparatus

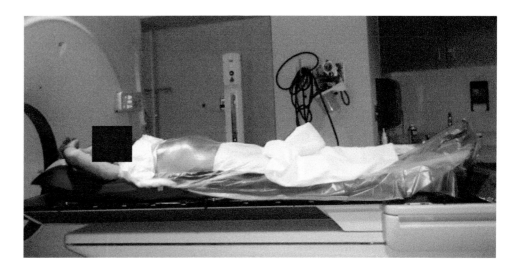

International Spine Radiosurgery Consortium have proposed similar approach [29, 61]. For postoperative SBRT, GTV is the area of residual disease in postoperative imaging. The CTV encompasses GTV and tumor bed based on preoperative imaging and surgical findings. It is not suggested to include the surgical track and scar which are frequently included in the conventional EBRT portal. A PTV margin ranging between 0 and 2 mm may be applied to account for setup error, image fusion errors, contouring uncertainty, potential intrafraction motion, and mechanical errors associated with IGRT system [60].

## Organs-at-Risk Delineation and Dose-Volume Constraints

The true spinal cord is most commonly the dose-limiting structure in spinal SBRT planning. Dose constraints vary depending on the institution and source. The quantitative analysis of normal tissue effects in the clinic (QUANTEC) study demonstrated that conventional fractionation (1.8–2 Gy per fraction) to the full-thickness cord to 54 and 61 Gy resulted in the estimated risk of myelopathy of <1% and <10%, respectively, and recommended to limit the maximal spinal cord dose to 13 Gy in single fraction for the spine SBRT treatment [62], similar to the 14 Gy cord constraint used in RTOG 0631 [29], American Association of Physicists in Medicine Task Group (AAPM TG) 101 [63], and study by Sahgal et al. [64, 65]. Partial spinal cord volume, defined from 5–6 mm above and below the target spine based on contrast-enhancing T1-weighted and T2-weighted image, is limited to 10 Gy in single fraction or 18 Gy in three fractions to no more than 10% volume [29, 63]. At MDACC, our current practice is to allow 0.01 cc of the spinal cord to receive 10–12 Gy when single fraction SBRT is delivered in the radiation naïve setting. A 1.5–2.0 mm margin could be applied to the OAR, so-called

**Table 12.2**  Dose constraints recommended in RTOG 0631 [29] and AAPM TG 101 [63]

| Normal critical tissues | Max critical volume | RTOG 0631 One fraction $D_{max}$ (Gy) | AAPM TG101 One fraction $D_{max}$ (Gy) | Three fractions $D_{max}$ (Gy) | Five fractions $D_{max}$ (Gy) |
|---|---|---|---|---|---|
| Spinal cord | ≤0.35 cc | 10 | 10 | 18 | 23 |
| | ≤10% of partial spinal cord | 10 | 10 | 18 | 23 |
| | <1.2 cc | – | 7 | 12.3 | 14.5 |
| | Point dose[a] | 14 | 14 | 21.9 | 30 |
| Cauda equina | <5 cc | 14 | 14 | 21.9 | 30 |
| | Point dose[a] | 16 | 16 | 24 | 32 |
| Sacral plexus | <5 cc | 14.4 | 14.4 | 22.5 | 30 |
| | Point dose[a] | 18 | 16 | 24 | 32 |
| Esophagus | <3 cc | 11.9 | 11.9 | 17.7 | 19.5 |
| | Point dose[a] | 16 | 15.4 | 25.2 | 35 |
| Trachea/larynx | <4 cc | 10.5 | 10.5 | 15 | 16.5 |
| | Point dose[a] | 20.2 | 20.2 | 30 | 40 |
| Brachial plexus | <3 cc | 14 | 14 | 20.4 | 27 |
| | Point dose[a] | 17.5 | 17.5 | 24 | 30.5 |
| Skin | <10 cc | 23 | 23 | 30 | 36.5 |
| | Point dose[a] | 26 | 26 | 33 | 39.5 |

[a]Point dose = 0.03 cc in RTOG 0631 and 0.035 cc in AAPM TG 101

planning organ at risk volume (PRV), to account for variations in patient position due to the same reasons as the PTV margin [66], but this is not required and at the discretion of the treating institution. Normal critical tissue tolerance constraints recommended in RTOG 0631 [29] and AAPM TG 101 [63] are summarized in Table 12.2.

In the context of re-irradiation, the spinal cord constraint must be more conservative to respect cumulative dose tolerance. Re-irradiation data in animals and humans suggested that partial repair of radiation-induced subclinical damage of the spinal cord occurred at approximately 6 months after RT and increased over 2 years [62]. The clinical study in re-irradiated patients with and without radiation myelopathy offered the following recommendations: (1) maximal retreatment point dose ($P_{max}$) to the thecal sac of ≤25.5 $Gy_{2/2}$ (2 Gy equivalent with $\alpha/\beta = 2$), (2) thecal sac $P_{max}$ cumulative dose of ≤70 $Gy_{2/2}$, (3) ratio of thecal sac $P_{max}$ retreatment dose to thecal sac $P_{max}$ cumulative dose of ≤0.5, and (4) minimum interval time to re-irradiation of ≥5 months [67]. Our current clinical practice is to limit the true spinal cord $D_{max}$ to 10 Gy over three fractions in the re-irradiation setting, but this is an active area of investigation.

## Dose Prescription

Various dose prescriptions for spine SBRT have been reported. Common fractionation schemes varies from a single fraction of 16–24 Gy or multiple hypofractionation regimens consisting of 24–27 Gy in three fractions and 30–35 Gy in five fractions. The determining factors include tumor histology, extent of disease, location of disease, and prior treatment. The dose-response relationship was demonstrated by

the significant high local control rate of 90% associated with dose of >23–24 Gy [34]. At our institution, simultaneous integrated boost is typically performed; for example, 16 Gy is prescribed to CTV, and 18–24 Gy is prescribed to the GTV in single fraction regimen. According to RTOG 0631, the optimal treatment plan includes at least 90% of the target volume which was covered by the prescription dose with dose constraints of OARs met. A minimum dose to the GTV of 14–15 Gy in a single fraction has been correlated with optimal local control [38]. At MDACC, a simultaneous integrated boost is commonly utilized whereby the GTV receives a higher prescription dose than the CTV as seen in Fig. 12.3.

## Treatment Planning and Delivery

There are various treatment planning systems and delivery for spine SBRT dose optimization including linear accelerator (LINAC)-based, tomotherapy-based, and CyberKnife-based systems. Regarding postoperative SBRT, one particular challenge is poor image quality for tumor and normal organ delineation due to metallic artifacts. As a result, CT myelogram might offer an additional benefit to MRI in these cases. At our institution, a LINAC-based approach is used with nine posteriorly oriented beams and step-and-shoot IMRT technique [68].

## Treatment Verification

Recent development of in-room and onboard imaging system has improved accuracy on target localization under IGRT to ensure accuracy prior to the treatment initiation (setup and

**a**

**b**

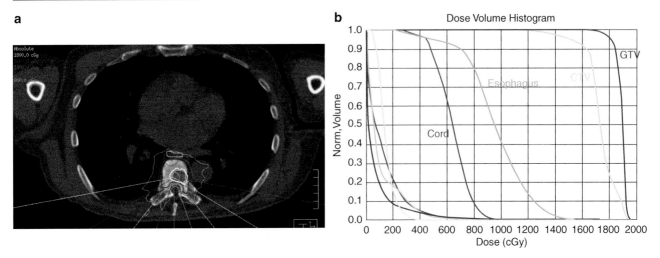

**Fig. 12.3** Spinal SBRT example for a 68-year-old with oligometastatic disease at T8 from papillary thyroid carcinoma

interfraction) as well as during treatment delivery (intrafraction). The image-guided techniques can be divided to:

1. *Stereoscopic X-ray-based system* consists of (a) electronic portal imaging device (EPID) using treatment megavoltage (MV) X-ray and (b) kilovoltage (KV) X-ray source with opposed imaging panel mounted on the ceiling/floor of the treatment room. Adjustment of patient position is done according to marker locations between current images and reference images using treatment couch or the robotic arm of the CyberKnife.
2. *CT-based systems* include cone beam CT (CBCT) attached to the LINAC using the KV X-ray head for image acquisition and reconstruction, spiral MV CT using the treatment beam in the helical tomotherapy machine, and diagnostic quality (KV) CT scanners in the treatment room on the same treatment couch, known as CT on rails.

To account for interfraction motion, just prior to each radiation treatment, every patient is immobilized on the treatment couch and undergoes image verification. During radiation delivery, the multileaf collimator (MLC)-based LINAC system uses a 6D robotic couch and imaging guidance based on stereoscopic X-ray- and/or CT-based imaging to detect intrafraction motion. Stereoscopic X-ray images may have residual rotational errors, and additional CT verification may correct for this [68]. The X-ray image can be taken within seconds allowing near-real-time image acquisition and correction, while CT imaging provides high quality volumetric images with the cost of increased image acquisition time and radiation exposure.

Unlike MLC-based LINAC, CyberKnife uses robotic arm to manipulate the LINAC position itself according to the orthogonal image acquired by near-real-time stereoscopic KV X-ray which is mounted on the floor in the treatment room. Thus CyberKnife treatment has the ability to correct the position of the target, while the beam is on [60].

## Toxicity of SBRT

Acute toxicity is relatively uncommon from spine SBRT. Pain flare, defined as a temporary increase in pain immediately after radiation, occurred in 23–68.3% of patients treated with SBRT [69, 70]. The mechanism for pain flare is unclear, but some have postulated that edema inducing nerve compression or release of inflammatory cytokines as a mediator; thus dexamethasone can be administered (and rapidly tapered) on an as-needed basis [69]. The use of prophylactic steroids in this patient population is an active area of investigation.

Overall late toxicity from spine SBRT is not common, but patients are at risk for developing radiation myelopathy and vertebral compression fracture (VCF). RM can occur 3–25 months after treatment but is very rare occurring in <1% of cases. VCF caused by tumor-induced demineralization through abnormal bone turnover and architectural changes as well as radiation-induced collagen damage and osteoradionecrosis of bone and tumor tissue [71] is more likely to occur with SBRT, 11–39% compared with approximately 5% after conventional radiotherapy. The time to fracture peaks at around 3–4 months posttreatment with a second peak around 14 months posttreatment [72–75]. Many studies reported the predictive factors of fracture, including tumor location at or below T10, lytic lesions especially involving >40% of the vertebral body, kyphotic deformity, radiation dose ≥20 Gy per fraction, age >55 years, preexisting fracture, baseline pain [72–75], or high SINS [11, 12]. Most radiographic fractures do not require invasive intervention. Surgical management for VCF includes percutaneous cement augmentation procedures, such as vertebroplasty and kyphoplasty, as well as open stabilization generally required in one-third of patients with radiographic fractures. However, no consensus for prophylactic spine stabilization in high-risk patients has been made, and this is an active area of investigation.

## Case Presentation

A 57-year-old male with metastatic renal cell carcinoma developed neck pain and limited neck range of motion. An MRI scan revealed a contrast-enhancing metastatic focus involving the C1 arch (Fig. 12.4). He underwent single fraction spinal SBRT to a dose of 24 Gy delivered to the GTV and 16 Gy delivered to the CTV.

Following treatment, his pain completely resolved and he regained full range of motion. He did not report toxicity after the treatment. Four months following treatment, his MRI scan revealed a complete imaging response.

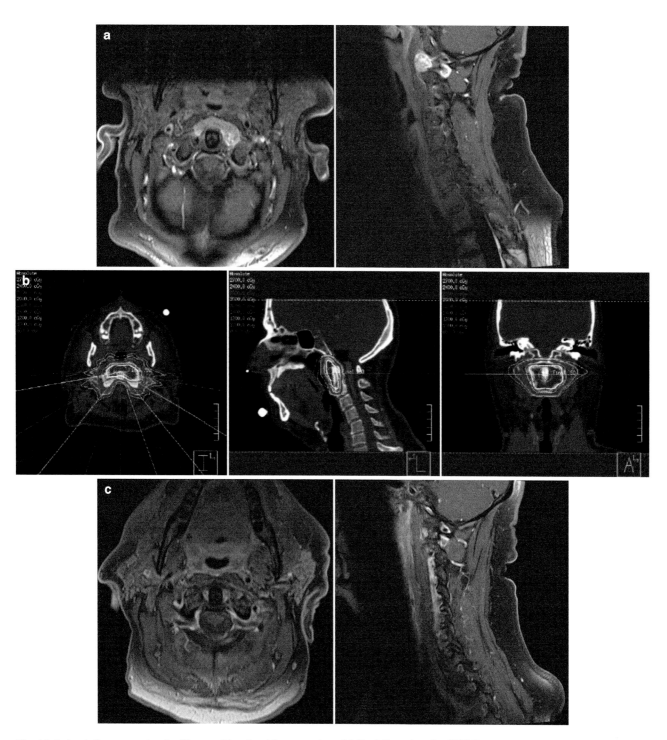

**Fig. 12.4** (a–c) Case example of a 57-year-old male with metastatic renal cell carcinoma and a symptomatic C1 vertebral metastasis treated with single fraction SBRT to a dose of 24 Gy delivered to the GTV and 16 Gy delivered to the CTV. Four months later, surveillance imaging revealed a complete radiographic response

## Summary

- Spinal metastasis is a common manifestation among cancer patients and requires multimodality treatment including surgical intervention, radiation treatment, and medical treatment.
- Stereotactic body radiotherapy (SBRT) can be implemented as (1) primary treatment in unirradiated patients, (2) salvage treatment in previously irradiated patients, and (3) postoperative treatment with excellent outcomes and minimal toxicity.
- Appropriate patient selection and radiation techniques are crucial for achieving good tumor control and minimal toxicity.

## Self-Assessment Questions

1. Which factor should be LEAST considered for decision-making on the optimal treatment modality in spine metastasis?
   A. Primary tumor histology
   B. Extent of tumor dissemination
   C. Duration of spinal metastasis
   D. Radiological evaluation of tumor extent using MRI
   E. Radiological evaluation of spinal instability using MRI

2. Which option should be considered for patients with progressive neurological deterioration with a significant epidural metastatic lesion in order to maximize tumor control?
   A. Surgery
   B. Conventional radiation
   C. Stereotactic body radiotherapy
   D. Surgery followed by postoperative radiation
   E. Surgery followed by systemic treatment

3. According to an Update of an ASTRO Evidence-Based Guideline: Palliative radiation therapy for bone metastases [76], which is the incorrect answer?
   A. Single fraction (8 Gy single fraction) provides equivalent pain relief to multiple fraction (20 Gy in five fractions, 24 Gy in six fractions, 30 Gy in ten fractions) in painful peripheral bone metastases.
   B. Single 8 Gy fraction provides noninferior pain relief compared with prolonged RT course in painful spinal metastases.
   C. Retreatment with radiation could be performed in patient who had persistent or recurrent bone metastases after 1 month of initial treatment.

D. Stereotactic body radiotherapy (SBRT) is strongly recommended for retreatment of peripheral and spinal metastases.
E. None of above.

## Answers

1. C
2. D
3. D

## References

1. Kakhki VR, Anvari K, Sadeghi R, et al. Pattern and distribution of bone metastases in common malignant tumors. Nucl Med Rev Cent East Eur. 2013;16(2):66–9.
2. Lee CS, Jung CH. Metastatic spinal tumor. Asian Spine J. 2012;6(1):71–87.
3. Tomita K, Kawahara N, Kobayashi T, et al. Surgical strategy for spinal metastases. Spine. 2001;26(3):298–306.
4. Tokuhashi Y, Matsuzaki H, Toriyama S, et al. Scoring system for the preoperative evaluation of metastatic spine tumor prognosis. Spine. 1990;15(11):1110–3.
5. Tokuhashi Y, Matsuzaki H, Oda H, et al. A revised scoring system for preoperative evaluation of metastatic spine tumor prognosis. Spine. 2005;30(19):2186–91.
6. Wang M, Bunger CE, Li HS, et al. Predictive value of Tokuhashi scoring Systems in spinal metastases, focusing on various primary tumor groups evaluation of 448 patients in the Aarhus spinal metastases database. Spine. 2012;37(7):573–82.
7. Asdourian P. Metastatic disease of the spine. In: Bridwell KH, Dewald RL, editors. The textbook of spinal surgery. 2nd ed. Philaderphia, PA: Lippincott–Raven Publishers; 1997. p. 2007–50.
8. Laufer I, Rubin DG, Lis E, et al. The NOMS framework: approach to the treatment of spinal metastatic tumors. Oncologist. 2013;18(6):744–51.
9. Bilsky MH, Laufer I, Fourney DR, et al. Reliability analysis of the epidural spinal cord compression scale. J Neurosurg Spine. 2010;13(3):324–8.
10. Ryu S, Rock J, Jain R, et al. Radiosurgical decompression of metastatic epidural compression. Cancer. 2010;116(9):2250–7.
11. Fisher CG, DiPaola CP, Ryken TC, et al. A novel classification system for spinal instability in neoplastic disease: an evidence-based approach and expert consensus from the Spine Oncology Study Group. Spine. 2010;35(22):E1221–9.
12. Fourney DR, Frangou EM, Ryken TC, et al. Spinal instability neoplastic score: an analysis of reliability and validity from the spine oncology study group. J Clin Oncol. 2011;29(22):3072–7.
13. Lutz S, Berk L, Chang E, et al. Palliative radiotherapy for bone metastases: an ASTRO evidence-based guideline. Int J Radiat Oncol Biol Phys. 2011;79(4):965–76.
14. Wu JS, Wong R, Johnston M, et al. Cancer Care Ontario Practice Guidelines Initiative Supportive Care G. Meta-analysis of dose-fractionation radiotherapy trials for the palliation of painful bone metastases. Int J Radiat Oncol Biol Phys. 2003;55(3):594–605.
15. Rades D, Stalpers LJ, Veninga T, et al. Evaluation of five radiation schedules and prognostic factors for metastatic spinal cord compression. J Clin Oncol. 2005;23(15):3366–75.

16. Hartsell WF, Scott CB, Bruner DW, et al. Randomized trial of short- versus long-course radiotherapy for palliation of painful bone metastases. J Natl Cancer Inst. 2005;97(11):798–804.
17. Sze WM, Shelley MD, Held I, et al. Palliation of metastatic bone pain: single fraction versus multifraction radiotherapy—a systematic review of randomised trials. Clin Oncol (R Coll Radiol). 2003;15(6):345–52.
18. Brown JM, Carison DJ, Brenner DJ. The tumor radiobiology of SRS and SBRT: are more than the 5 Rs involved? Int J Radiat Oncol Biol Phys. 2014;88(2):254–62.
19. Song CW, Kim MS, Cho LC, et al. Radiobiological basis of SBRT and SRS. Int J Clin Oncol. 2014;19(4):570–8.
20. Song CW, Cho LC, Yuan J, et al. Radiobiology of stereotactic body radiation therapy/stereotactic radiosurgery and the linear-quadratic model. Int J Radiat Oncol Biol Phys. 2013;87(1):18–9.
21. Kirkpatrick JP, Meyer JJ, Marks LB. The linear-quadratic model is inappropriate to model high dose per fraction effects in radiosurgery. Semin Radiat Oncol. 2008;18(4):240–3.
22. Yu HH, Hoffe SE. Beyond the conventional role of external-beam radiation therapy for skeletal metastases: new technologies and stereotactic directions. Cancer Control. 2012;19(2):129–36.
23. Regine WF, Ryu S, Chang EL. Spine radiosurgery for spinal cord compression: the radiation oncologist's perspective. J Radiosurg SBRT. 2011;1:55–61.
24. Sahgal A, Larson DA, Chang EL. Stereotactic body radiosurgery for spinal metastases: a critical review. Int J Radiat Oncol Biol Phys. 2008;71(3):652–65.
25. Park HJ, Kim HJ, Won JH, et al. Stereotactic body radiotherapy (SBRT) for spinal metastases: who will benefit the most from SBRT? Technol Cancer Res Treat. 2015;14(2):159–67.
26. Chawla S, Schell MC, Milano MT. Stereotactic body radiation for the spine: a review. Am J Clin Oncol. 2013;36(6):630–6.
27. Harel R, Zach L. Spine radiosurgery for spinal metastases: indications, technique and outcome. Neurol Res. 2014;36(6):550–6.
28. Hall WA, Stapleford LJ, Hadjipanayis CG, et al. Stereotactic body radiosurgery for spinal metastatic disease: an evidence-based review. Int J Surg Oncol. 2011;2011(2090-1410 (Electronic)):979214.
29. Ryu S, Pugh SL, Gerszten PC, et al. RTOG 0631 phase 2/3 study of image guided stereotactic radiosurgery for localized (1-3) spine metastases: phase 2 results. Pract Radiat Oncol. 2014;4(2):76–81.
30. Chao ST, Koyfman SA, Woody N, et al. Recursive partitioning analysis index is predictive for overall survival in patients undergoing spine stereotactic body radiation therapy for spinal metastases. Int J Radiat Oncol Biol Phys. 2012;82(5):1738–43.
31. Tang C, Hess K, Bishop AJ, et al. Creation of a prognostic index for spine metastasis to stratify survival in patients treated with spinal stereotactic radiosurgery: secondary analysis of mature prospective trials. Int J Radiat Oncol Biol Phys. 2015;93(1):118–25.
32. Ryu S, Jin R, Jin JY, et al. Pain control by image-guided radiosurgery for solitary spinal metastasis. J Pain Symptom Manag. 2008;35(3):292–8.
33. Gerszten PC, Burton SA, Ozhasoglu C, et al. Stereotactic radiosurgery for spinal metastases from renal cell carcinoma. J Neurosurg Spine. 2005;3(4):288–95.
34. Yamada Y, Bilsky MH, Lovelock DM, et al. High-dose, single-fraction image-guided intensity-modulated radiotherapy for metastatic spinal lesions. Int J Radiat Oncol Biol Phys. 2008;71(2):484–90.
35. Chang EL, Shiu AS, Mendel E, et al. Phase I/II study of stereotactic body radiotherapy for spinal metastasis and its pattern of failure. J Neurosurg Spine. 2007;7(2):151–60.
36. Garg AK, Shiu AS, Yang J, et al. Phase 1/2 trial of single-session stereotactic body radiotherapy for previously unirradiated spinal metastases. Cancer. 2012;118(20):5069–77.
37. Guckenberger M, Mantel F, Gerszten PC, et al. Safety and efficacy of stereotactic body radiotherapy as primary treatment for vertebral metastases: a multi-institutional analysis. Radiat Oncol. 2014;9:226.
38. Bishop AJ, Tao R, Rebueno NC, et al. Outcomes for spine stereotactic body radiation therapy and an analysis of predictors of local recurrence. Int J Radiat Oncol Biol Phys. 2015;92(5):1016–26.
39. Milker-Zabel S, Zabel A, Thilmann C, et al. Clinical results of retreatment of vertebral bone metastases by stereotactic conformal radiotherapy and intensity-modulated radiotherapy. Int J Radiat Oncol Biol Phys. 2003;55(1):162–7.
40. Yamada Y, Lovelock DM, Yenice KM, et al. Multifractionated image-guided and stereotactic intensity-modulated radiotherapy of paraspinal tumors: a preliminary report. Int J Radiat Oncol Biol Phys. 2005;62(1):53–61.
41. Wang XS, Rhines LD, Shiu AS, et al. Stereotactic body radiation therapy for management of spinal metastases in patients without spinal cord compression: a phase 1-2 trial. Lancet Oncol. 2012;13(4):395–402.
42. Gerszten PC, Burton SA, Quinn AE, et al. Radiosurgery for the treatment of spinal melanoma metastases. Stereotact Funct Neurosurg. 2005;83(5–6):213–21.
43. Gerszten PC, Burton SA, Ozhasoglu C, et al. Radiosurgery for spinal metastases: clinical experience in 500 cases from a single institution. Spine. 2007;32(2):193–9.
44. Gibbs IC, Kamnerdsupaphon P, Ryu MR, et al. Image-guided robotic radiosurgery for spinal metastases. Radiother Oncol. 2007;82(2):185–90.
45. Gerszten PC, Burton SA, Welch WC, et al. Combination kyphoplasty and spinal radiosurgery: a new treatment paradigm for pathological fractures. J Neurosurg Spine. 2005;3(4):296–301.
46. Rock JP, Ryu S, Shukairy MS, et al. Postoperative radiosurgery for malignant spinal tumors. Neurosurgery. 2006;58(5):891–8. discussion −8
47. Moulding HD, Elder JB, Lis E, et al. Local disease control after decompressive surgery and adjuvant high-dose single-fraction radiosurgery for spine metastases. J Neurosurg Spine. 2010;13(1):87–93.
48. Laufer I, Iorgulescu JB, Chapman T, et al. Local disease control for spinal metastases following "separation surgery" and adjuvant hypofractionated or high-dose single-fraction stereotactic radiosurgery: outcome analysis in 186 patients. J Neurosurg Spine. 2013;18(3):207–14.
49. Chang UK, Cho WI, Lee DH, et al. Stereotactic radiosurgery for primary and metastatic sarcomas involving the spine. J Neurooncol. 2012;107(3):551–7.
50. Greco C, Pares O, Pimentel N, et al. Spinal metastases: from conventional fractionated radiotherapy to single-dose SBRT. Rep Pract Oncol Radiother. 2015;20(6):454–63.
51. Maranzano E, Trippa F, Pacchiarini D, et al. Re-irradiation of brain metastases and metastatic spinal cord compression: clinical practice suggestions. Tumori. 2005;91(4):325–30.
52. Nieder C, Grosu AL, Andratschke NH, et al. Update of human spinal cord reirradiation tolerance based on additional data from 38 patients. Int J Radiat Oncol Biol Phys. 2006;66(5):1446–9.
53. Hamilton AJ, Lulu BA, Fosmire H, et al. Preliminary clinical experience with linear accelerator-based spinal stereotactic radiosurgery. Neurosurgery. 1995;36(2):311–9.
54. Klekamp J, Samii H. Surgical results for spinal metastases. Acta Neurochir. 1998;140(9):957–67.
55. Gerszten PC, Mendel E, Yamada Y. Radiotherapy and radiosurgery for metastatic spine disease: what are the options, indications, and outcomes? Spine. 2009;34(22 Suppl):S78–92.
56. Itshayek E, Cohen JE, Yamada Y, et al. Timing of stereotactic radiosurgery and surgery and wound healing in patients with

spinal tumors: a systematic review and expert opinions. Neurol Res. 2014;36(6):510–23.

57. Itshayek E, Yamada J, Bilsky M, et al. Timing of surgery and radiotherapy in the management of metastatic spine disease: a systematic review. Int J Oncol. 2010;36(3):533–44.

58. Li W, Sahgal A, Foote M, et al. Impact of immobilization on intrafraction motion for spine stereotactic body radiotherapy using cone beam computed tomography. Int J Radiat Oncol Biol Phys. 2012;84(2):520–6.

59. Ryu S, Rock J, Rosenblum M, et al. Patterns of failure after single-dose radiosurgery for spinal metastasis. J Neurosurg. 2004;101(Suppl 3, 0022-3085 (Print)):402–405.

60. Sahgal A, Bilsky M, Chang EL, et al. Stereotactic body radiotherapy for spinal metastases: current status, with a focus on its application in the postoperative patient. J Neurosurg Spine. 2011;14(2):151–66.

61. Cox BW, Spratt DE, Lovelock M, et al. International Spine Radiosurgery Consortium consensus guidelines for target volume definition in spinal stereotactic radiosurgery. Int J Radiat Oncol Biol Phys. 2012;83(5):e597–605.

62. Kirkpatrick JP, van der Kogel AJ, Schultheiss TE. Radiation dose-volume effects in the spinal cord. Int J Radiat Oncol Biol Phys. 2010;76(3 Suppl):S42–9.

63. Benedict SH, Yenice KM, Followill D, et al. Stereotactic body radiation therapy: the report of AAPM Task Group 101. Med Phys. 2010;37(8):4078–101.

64. Sahgal A, Ma L, Gibbs I, et al. Spinal cord tolerance for stereotactic body radiotherapy. Int J Radiat Oncol Biol Phys. 2010;77(2):548–53.

65. Sahgal A, Weinberg V, Ma L, et al. Probabilities of radiation myelopathy specific to stereotactic body radiation therapy to guide safe practice. Int J Radiat Oncol Biol Phys. 2013;85(2):341–7.

66. Lo SS, Sahgal A, Wang JZ, et al. Stereotactic body radiation therapy for spinal metastases. Discov Med. 2010;9(47):289–96.

67. Sahgal A, Ma L, Weinberg V, et al. Reirradiation human spinal cord tolerance for stereotactic body radiotherapy. Int J Radiat Oncol Biol Phys. 2012;82(1):107–16.

68. Weksberg DC, Palmer MB, Vu KN, et al. Generalizable class solutions for treatment planning of spinal stereotactic body radiation therapy. Int J Radiat Oncol Biol Phys. 2012;84(3):847–53.

69. Pan HY, Allen PK, Wang XS, et al. Incidence and predictive factors of pain flare after spine stereotactic body radiation therapy: secondary analysis of phase 1/2 trials. Int J Radiat Oncol Biol Phys. 2014;90(4):870–6.

70. Chiang A, Zeng L, Zhang L, et al. Pain flare is a common adverse event in steroid-naive patients after spine stereotactic body radiation therapy: a prospective clinical trial. Int J Radiat Oncol Biol Phys. 2013;86(4):638–42.

71. Sahgal A, Whyne CM, Ma L, et al. Vertebral compression fracture after stereotactic body radiotherapy for spinal metastases. Lancet Oncol. 2013;14(8):e310–20.

72. Rose PS, Laufer I, Boland PJ, et al. Risk of fracture after single fraction image-guided intensity-modulated radiation therapy to spinal metastases. J Clin Oncol. 2009;27(30):5075–9.

73. Cunha MV, Al-Omair A, Atenafu EG, et al. Vertebral compression fracture (VCF) after spine stereotactic body radiation therapy (SBRT): analysis of predictive factors. Int J Radiat Oncol Biol Phys. 2012;84(3):e343–9.

74. Boehling NS, Grosshans DR, Allen PK, et al. Vertebral compression fracture risk after stereotactic body radiotherapy for spinal metastases. J Neurosurg Spine. 2012;16(4):379–86.

75. Thibault I, Al-Omair A, Masucci GL, et al. Spine stereotactic body radiotherapy for renal cell cancer spinal metastases: analysis of outcomes and risk of vertebral compression fracture. J Neurosurg Spine. 2014;21(5):711–8.

76. Lutz S, Balboni T, Jones J, et al. Palliative radiation therapy for bone metastases: update of an ASTRO evidence-based guideline. Pract Radiat Oncol. 2017;7(1):4–12.

# Part VI

# Leptomeningeal Disease

# Evaluation and Workup of Leptomeningeal Disease

# 13

Sushma Bellamkonda and David M. Peereboom

## Learning Objectives

- Describe the incidence and pathophysiology of leptomeningeal disease.
- Determine key factors and steps involved in the evaluation and workup of leptomeningeal disease.
- Understand the strengths and weaknesses of available techniques used in the evaluation of leptomeningeal disease.
- Identify potential pitfalls and challenges to the diagnosis of leptomeningeal disease.

## Introduction

Leptomeningeal disease (LMD), the spread of cancer to the leptomeninges, can arise from solid tumors as well as hematological malignancies such as lymphoma or leukemia. LMD is synonymous with neoplastic meningitis. Leptomeningeal carcinomatosis or carcinomatous meningitis refers to LMD specifically from carcinomas—i.e., epithelial malignancies such as breast or lung cancers. Lymphomatous meningitis or leptomeningeal lymphoma refers to LMD caused by lymphoma, while the analogous terms—leukemic meningitis or leptomeningeal leukemia—pertain to LMD from leukemia [1]. The presentation is often subacute with variable and multifocal symptoms and hence is easily missed. A timely diagnosis leads to treatment, which, though not curative, can preserve function and maintain the quality of life.

S. Bellamkonda
Department of Neurology, University of Tennessee
Health Science Center, Memphis, TN, USA

D. M. Peereboom (✉)
Department of Medical Oncology, Taussig Cancer Institute,
Cleveland Clinic, Cleveland, OH, USA

Rose Ella Burkhardt Brain Tumor and Neuro-oncology Center,
Cleveland Clinic, Cleveland, OH, USA
e-mail: peerebd@ccf.org

## Incidence

LMD occurs in approximately 3–5% of patients with cancer [2]. The incidence is increasing as patients are living longer due to advances in cancer treatment [3]. LMD occurs most commonly in breast cancer, lung cancer, especially small cell, and melanoma [4]. Primary brain tumors can rarely lead to LMD, which is most likely due to either infiltration of leptomeninges or dissemination into the CSF [5, 6]. In children, retinoblastomas and embryonal rhabdomyosarcomas may occasionally spread to leptomeninges as well. Most patients have a diagnosis of cancer at the time of presentation, but in rare cases, LMD can be their initial presentation with no other evidence of systemic disease [7].

## Anatomy

The three membranes covering the brain are dura mater, arachnoid mater, and pia mater (Fig. 13.1). Another term for dura mater is pachymeninges, whereas arachnoid mater and pia mater are together referred to as leptomeninges. Invasion of leptomeninges by malignant cells via CSF leads to leptomeningeal disease or neoplastic meningitis.

## Pathogenesis

The spread of tumor cells to the leptomeninges can occur via various mechanisms [8, 9].

- Hematogenous spread
- Direct extension from lesions in the parenchyma, dura, or bone
- Perineural spread followed by dissemination into CSF
- Seeding of subarachnoid space during resection of brain metastases

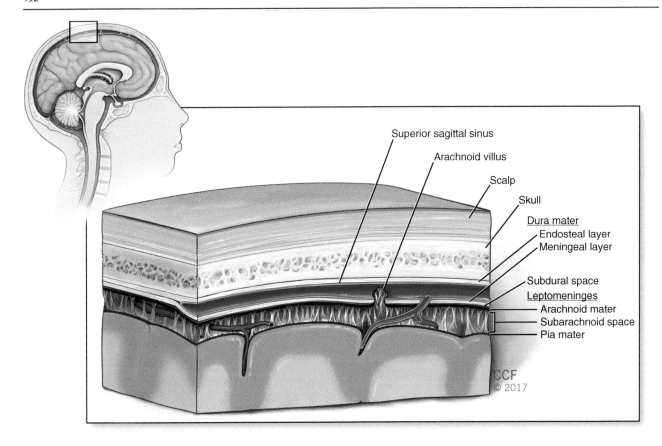

**Fig. 13.1** Anatomy of the leptomeninges. [Reprinted with permission, Cleveland Clinic Center for Medical Art & Photography © 2017. All Rights Reserved]

## Clinical Presentation

Since LMD can affect any level of the neuraxis, the presentation can be multifocal and the diagnosis challenging, requiring a high index of suspicion [7, 10].

Common sites of involvement are the basilar cisterns, the posterior fossa, and the cauda equina. Slow CSF flow in these sites along with gravity leads to deposition of tumor cells in these sites [4].

Signs and symptoms (Table 13.1) can be attributed to local tumor infiltration leading to focal neurological deficits and seizures, obstruction of CSF flow leading to increased intracranial pressure (ICP), and alteration of CNS metabolism leading to altered mental status that ranges from slowing of thought processes to encephalopathy. Signs are noted to be much more prominent than symptoms [4, 5, 7, 11–14].

## Prognosis

Left untreated, the median survival for LMD is 4–6 weeks, and with treatment, the median survival improves to 3–6 months [3]. LMD secondary to lymphoma and leukemia has the best prognosis, and the recommendation in these

**Table 13.1** Clinical features in LMD

| Cerebral and cerebellar hemispheres | Headache, encephalopathy, seizures, motor weakness, ataxia, plateau waves (paroxysmal neurological symptoms in the setting of elevated intracranial pressure, typically with positional changes), papilledema |
|---|---|
| Cranial nerves | Diplopia (III, IV, VI), facial weakness (VII), hearing impairment (VII), "numb chin syndrome" (V3), tongue weakness (XII) |
| Spinal roots and nerves | Pain, weakness, cauda equina syndrome |

Based on data from [4, 5, 7, 11–14]

patients is aggressive treatment [15, 16]. Among the solid tumor-associated LMD, breast cancer has a better prognosis than lung cancer or melanoma [17, 18]. The performance status, extent of systemic disease, histological and molecular characteristics, and prior treatment history all factor into the prognosis of the patient [18–21]. It is often challenging to decide whom to treat and how to treat them. The goal of treatment is to palliate symptoms, maintain function, and prolong survival. Per National Comprehensive Cancer Network (NCCN) guidelines, one can classify patients as poor risk and good risk. Poor-risk patients are those with Karnofsky Performance Status (KPS) < 60, major neurological deficits, extensive systemic disease with few treatment options, bulky CNS disease, and encephalopathy. Palliative care is recommended for those who are poor risk, while directed therapy to the leptomeninges should be recommended for those patients with good risk [22].

## Evaluation

Evaluation of LMD includes neuroimaging followed by CSF analysis. The overall evaluation is outlined in Fig. 13.2. Neuroimaging is more sensitive than CSF analysis, whereas the latter is more specific for the diagnosis of LMD [23, 24]. The specificity approaches 100%, with a sensitivity of 75% for

CSF cytology, while gadolinium-enhanced MRI (Gd-MRI) has a specificity of 77% and sensitivity of 76% [24].

## Neuroimaging

Gd-MRI of the brain and spine is recommended. If MRI is contraindicated, then a CT with contrast is recommended though it will be less sensitive [11, 25]. A myelogram does not have a role in the evaluation of LMD.

[18]F-fluorodeoxyglucose positron emission tomography/computed tomography ([18]F-FDG PET/CT) could be considered as an alternative method for diagnosing LMD in

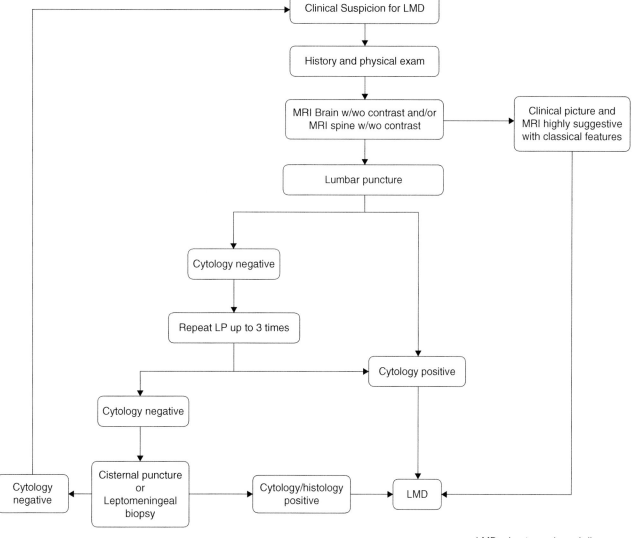

LMD = Leptomeningeal diasease

CCF@2017

**Fig. 13.2** Algorithm for evaluation of suspected leptomeningeal disease. [Reprinted with permission, Cleveland Clinic Center for Medical Art & Photography © 2017. All Rights Reserved]

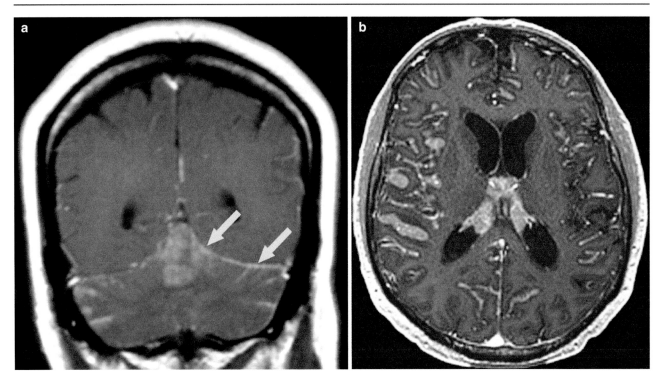

**Fig. 13.3** Radiographic appearance of leptomeningeal disease in the brain. (**a**) Coronal T1-weighted MRI with gadolinium enhancement. Note the "frosted" appearance of the cerebellar folia (arrows). (**b**) Axial

T1-weighted MRI with gadolinium enhancement. Note the thick leptomeningeal enhancement

the patients who test negative with initial imaging as well as CSF analysis [26]. In general, however, we do not recommend this study as part of the routine evaluation of LMD.

## MRI Brain

The typical finding is thin diffuse leptomeningeal enhancement along the gyri and sulci, creating a "frosted" appearance. Common sites of involvement are cerebellar folia, basal cisterns including ventral brainstem, and cortical surfaces (Fig. 13.3). Cranial nerves along the brainstem may enhance and appear thickened. Hydrocephalus—obstructive or communicating—and subarachnoid masses can be seen [4, 16].

## MRI Spine

Linear or nodular enhancement along the cord or cauda equina, nerve root thickening, cord enlargement, clumping of nerve roots, and spinal cord pial enhancement (described as "sugar coating" by Kramer et al.) are suggestive of LMD (Fig. 13.4) [27, 28].

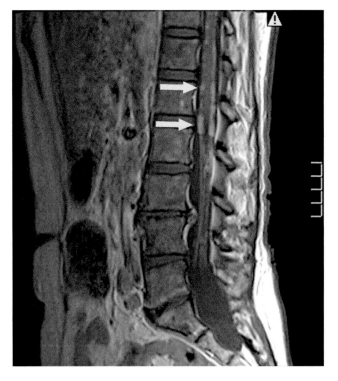

**Fig. 13.4** MRI spine—enhancing leptomeningeal nodules (arrows). [Reprinted with permission, Cleveland Clinic Center for Medical Art & Photography © 2017. All Rights Reserved]

## Pitfalls

It is best to obtain neuroimaging prior to lumbar puncture to avoid post-lumbar puncture imaging artifacts. Lumbar puncture can sometimes lead to enhancement of leptomeninges which could interfere with the diagnostic evaluation [16].

Bevacizumab is an anti angiogenic drug that can minimize or eliminate the expected leptomeningeal enhancement making the MRI less sensitive [29].

## CSF Flow Study

CSF flow has a complex flow pattern with several sites vulnerable to obstruction by bulky LMD (Fig. 13.5). An [111]indium-diethylenetriamine pentaacetate (DTPA) CSF flow study is recommended prior to the administration of intrathecal therapy to detect any interruption in CSF flow. CSF flow

obstructions can be seen in up to 70% of patients with LMD and are not limited to those patients with bulky metastases [11]. It is most commonly seen at the base of the brain, along the spine, or over the cortical convexities. These areas of obstruction will decrease the efficacy and increase the potential toxicity of chemotherapy. Involved field irradiation can reverse the flow abnormalities caused by CSF blocks [11, 16, 30–32].

## Cerebrospinal Fluid Analysis

The analysis of CSF is most commonly performed by lumbar puncture. It is important that the proper specimens are obtained to help with diagnosis. CSF analysis should include basic parameters such as measurement of opening pressure, cell count including differential, glucose, protein, cytology (Fig. 13.6), review of a sample stained with hematoxylin and

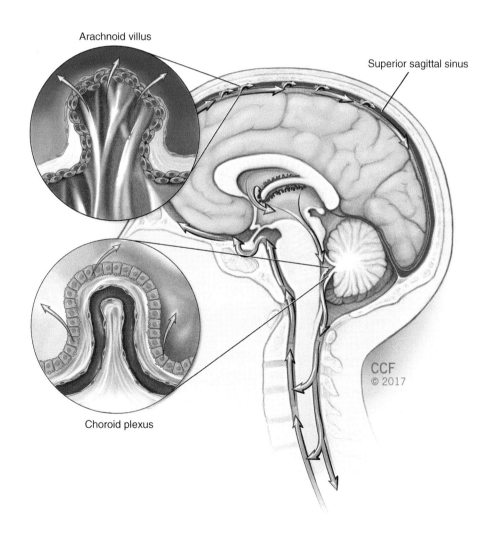

**Fig. 13.5** CSF flow diagram—yellow arrows depict the CSF as it is produced by the choroid plexus, flows through the CSF space, and is reabsorbed through the arachnoid villi. [Reprinted with permission, Cleveland Clinic Center for Medical Art & Photography © 2017. All Rights Reserved]

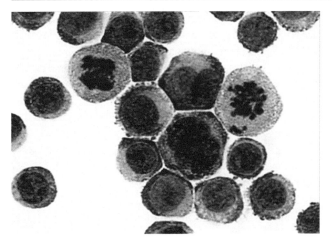

**Fig. 13.6** CSF cytology. Note the large nuclei and two mitotic figures. [Reprinted with permission, Cleveland Clinic Center for Medical Art & Photography © 2017. All Rights Reserved]

**Table 13.2** Features of CSF in LMD

| | |
|---|---|
| Elevated opening pressure | Non-specific, not diagnostic |
| Mildly elevated white blood cell count, usually lymphocytes | |
| Elevated protein | |
| Decreased glucose | |
| Malignant cells on cytology | Specific, diagnostic |
| Flow cytometry | Specific, diagnostic (hematologic malignancies) |

Based on data from [7, 12, 13]

**Table 13.3** Practical pearls to increase sensitivity and minimize false negatives

– High volume tap (>10 ml) designated for cytology
– Immediate processing of specimen. Avoid letting the specimen sit overnight even if refrigerated
– Site of CSF sampling is important as yield differs based on the site. Obtaining CSF from a site of known leptomeningeal disease increased the likelihood of positive results[a]
– Repeat LP up to three times. The third lumbar puncture can increase the yield to 90% [7]
– The patient should be off steroids prior to LP if lymphoma is in the differential diagnosis

Based on data from [7, 10, 12, 14, 34]
[a]If signs/symptoms are cranial, ventricular sample is more likely to be positive, and if signs/symptoms are spinal, lumbar puncture is more likely to be positive [35]

eosin, and flow cytometry in hematological malignancies. Flow cytometry improves the sensitivity of conventional cytology quite significantly in hematological malignancies associated with LMD, especially in paucicellular samples [33]. While several tubes are collected for the various assays, it is critical that at least 10 ml in one tube be designated specifically for cytology in order to maximize the yield.

The multifocal and diffuse nature of this disease makes extensive sampling a necessity for diagnosis [13].

## Typical CSF Picture for LMD

See Table 13.2.

CSF analysis has a high specificity, but sensitivity is low with a rate of high false-negative results (see Table 13.3).

It is not recommended to repeat lumbar punctures beyond three times. If LP is negative after three attempts, cisternal puncture may be considered in patients whose symptoms are intracranial or cervical in nature, and if still inconclusive, leptomeningeal biopsy is the next recommended option [10, 36].

Despite all these methods, CSF studies may continue to be inconclusive. If so, positive neuroimaging in the presence of typical clinical features is adequate to make the diagnosis of leptomeningeal metastasis [23, 24].

## CSF Biomarkers

Though not done routinely, CSF biomarkers can help in the early detection of LMD. Tumor markers such as CEA, AFP, Beta-hCG, and CA-125 in the CSF can be useful and, in cases where the lab values return higher than serum levels,

can be considered diagnostic [37]. However, levels should be obtained from the serum and CSF simultaneously so as to determine whether the elevation is due to LMD or as a result of passive diffusion [16]. As the cells become more dependent on anaerobic metabolism during the malignant transformation, an abnormal pattern of LDH isoenzymes is noted with an elevation of LDH-5 fraction and a relative reduction of LDH-1 fraction [38]. An elevation of LDH-5 isoenzyme as a percentage of total LDH in the absence of infection is indicative of LMD and if used in conjunction with other biomarkers such as beta-glucuronidase can help in the early diagnosis of LMD secondary to solid tumors [39]. Beta 2 microglobulin is a useful marker for LMD in hematological malignancies. The hope is that in the future, these CSF biomarkers, in addition to aiding with early diagnosis, will also help to assess the response to therapy and predict the disease course [40, 41].

## Novel Techniques

### Circulating Tumor Cells (CTC)

Detection of CTCs in the blood (Veridex CellSearch® technology) is used in the follow-up and prognosis of breast, prostate, colorectal, and lung cancer, which express epithelial cell adhesion molecule (EpCAM) markers. There is an ongoing effort to adapt this method to identify CTCs in the CSF. This strategy could potentially lead to an earlier diagnosis even with delayed processing and a smaller sample [40–44]. Recent data demonstrated the ability of this technology to achieve a positive predictive value of 90% and negative predictive value of 97%.

## Cell-Stabilizing Agents

Immediate processing of CSF samples is recommended, especially for flow cytometry, preferably within 60 min after withdrawal as cells appear to decrease rapidly ex vivo [45, 46]. However, this is not practical in many institutions. Several studies have evaluated cell-stabilizing agents such as Transfix™ and serum-containing medium. Serum-containing medium can prevent cellular loss for up to 5 h of storage, but it is not commercially available and has a lim-

ited shelf life of 3 months [45, 47]. Transfix™ CSF storage tubes are available commercially and have a longer shelf life of up to 1 year. In a comparison between Transfix™, serum-containing medium, and native CSF, Transfix™ enhanced flow cytometric detection of LMD even after 18 h of storage [47]

## Case Study

A 41-year-old woman with metastatic ER/PR-negative/HER2-positive breast cancer received chemotherapy, followed by maintenance trastuzumab and pertuzumab. Four years into her disease course, she presented with generalized seizures and was found on MRI to have multiple brain metastases in the parenchyma as well as right cerebellar leptomeningeal metastases (Fig. 13.7). At the time she had a normal neurological exam and a Karnofsky Performance Status (KPS) of 90. The diagnosis of leptomeningeal disease was based on sulcal enhancement along the folia of the right cerebellum. Given this typical appearance for lep-

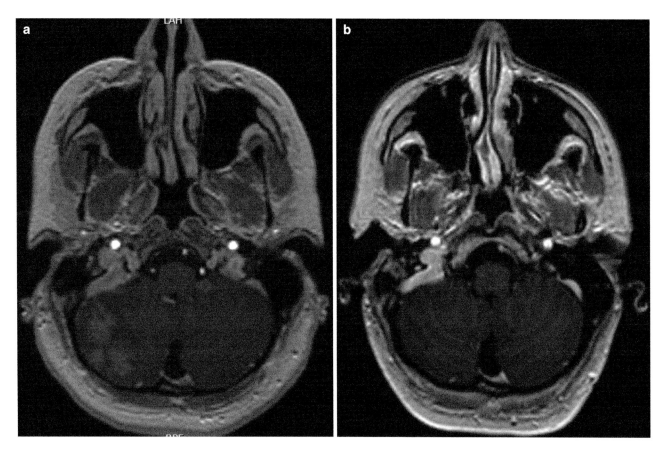

**Fig. 13.7** (a) Leptomeningeal disease involving right cerebellum (b) MRI 4 months later with excellent response to whole-brain radiation therapy

tomeningeal disease, cytological confirmation was felt not to be necessary. MRI of the spine with gadolinium did not show visible leptomeningeal disease. The patient received whole-brain radiation therapy 3000 cGy in 10 fractions. MRI 4 months later demonstrated an excellent response to therapy. She remained neurologically intact at that time with a KPS of 90. Leptomeningeal disease can be diagnosed radiographically but may require histological conformation if clinical suspicion exists.

## Summary

- LMD is an elusive condition whose incidence is on the rise. A high index of suspicion on the clinician's part is required to initiate the appropriate workup. A prompt diagnosis can palliate symptoms, preserve the quality of life, and prolong survival.
- A subacute onset with multifocal neurological signs and symptoms is the classical presentation of LMD where signs may be more prominent than symptoms.
- Gadolinium-enhanced MRI brain and spine and CSF analysis are the cornerstones in the evaluation of LMD, though they are of variable yield. Consequently, it is sometimes challenging to make a definitive diagnosis with one test alone.
- The MRI should be performed prior to the CSF analysis to avoid post-LP imaging artifacts.
- Gd-MRI shows diffuse linear or nodular enhancement of the leptomeninges most commonly in the cerebellar folia, basal cisterns, cortical surfaces, and cauda equina. In selected cases where suspicion for LMD is high, MRI with typical features may be adequate for diagnosis.
- CSF in LMD has non-specific but suggestive features such as elevated opening pressure, mild pleocytosis, elevated protein, and decreased glucose.
- CSF flow cytometry is recommended if hematological malignancies are suspected.
- CSF cytology is the more specific test and traditionally considered the gold standard in the diagnosis of LMD.
- CSF biomarkers, though not routinely done, may be helpful in cases where cytology is repeatedly negative and imaging is atypical. However, given the high percentage of false negatives, the lumbar puncture may need to be repeated up to three times. We recommend a high-volume tap along with the immediate processing of the specimen.
- Given the variable yield of the currently recommended diagnostic tests, there is an elevated need for tests that can help with an early diagnosis and prognostic assessment. There is much promising research on this subject, and hopefully these novel techniques will improve the evaluation and management of patients with LMD.

## Self-Assessment Questions

1. Which of the following is the order of frequency from most common to least common causes for LMD?
   A. Breast, lung, melanoma
   B. Lung, breast, colon
   C. Breast, colon, melanoma
   D. Lung, colon, breast

2. Which of the following is the recommended evaluation in the diagnosis of LMD?
   A. Gd-MRI with $^{18}$F-FDG PET/CT
   B. CSF analysis followed by Gd-MRI
   C. Gd-MRI followed by CSF analysis
   D. CSF analysis with $^{18}$F-FDG PET/CT

3. Which of the following is correct regarding the CSF analysis in suspected LMD?
   A. Sensitivity can be improved by repeating the LP up to three times.
   B. CSF sample should be immediately refrigerated to improve the yield.
   C. Volume of the sample collected does not affect the sensitivity of the test.
   D. Steroids may be continued and do not alter the CSF findings.

4. Which of the following statements is false?
   A. Positive Gd-MRI in the presence of typical clinical features is adequate for a definitive diagnosis of LMD.
   B. CSF flow cytometry is helpful in LMD secondary to hematological malignancies.
   C. Prognosis is better for LMD from hematological malignancies than from solid malignancies.
   D. The site of CSF sampling is not important in the diagnosis of LMD.

5. Which of the following depicts the typical CSF picture in LMD?
   A. Elevated glucose, elevated protein, decreased opening pressure
   B. Decreased glucose, elevated protein, elevated opening pressure
   C. Decreased glucose, decreased protein, decreased opening pressure
   D. Elevated glucose, decreased protein, normal opening pressure

## Answers

1. A
2. C
3. A
4. D
5. D

## References

1. Clarke JL. Leptomeningeal metastasis from systemic cancer. Continuum (Minneap Minn). 2012;18(2):328–42.
2. Suh JH, Chao ST, Peereboom DP, et al. Metastatic cancer to brain. In Devita, Hellman, and Rosenberg's Cancer: Principles and Practice of Oncology, 10th edition. Eds. DeVita V, Lawrence T, Rosenberg S. Philadelphia, Wolters Kluwer. p. 1832–44. 2015.
3. Gleissner B, Chamberlain MC. Neoplastic meningitis. Lancet Neurol. 2006;5(5):443–52.
4. Grossman SA, Krabak MJ. Leptomeningeal carcinomatosis. Cancer Treat Rev. 1999;25(2):103–19.
5. Boyle R, Thomas M, Adams JH. Diffuse involvement of the leptomeninges by tumour—a clinical and pathological study of 63 cases. Postgrad Med J. 1980;56(653):149–58.
6. Saito R, Kumabe T, Jokura H, et al. Symptomatic spinal dissemination of malignant astrocytoma. J Neurooncol. 2003;61(3):227–35.
7. Wasserstrom WR, Glass JP, Posner JB. Diagnosis and treatment of leptomeningeal metastases from solid tumors: experience with 90 patients. Cancer. 1982;49(4):759–72.
8. Kokkoris CP. Leptomeningeal carcinomatosis. How does cancer reach the pia-arachnoid? Cancer. 1983;51(1):154–60.
9. Norris LK, Grossman SA, Olivi A. Neoplastic meningitis following surgical resection of isolated cerebellar metastasis: a potentially preventable complication. J Neurooncol. 1997;32(3):215–23.
10. Balm M, Hammack J. Leptomeningeal carcinomatosis. Presenting features and prognostic factors. Arch Neurol. 1996;53(7):626–32.
11. Bomgaars L, Chamberlain MC, Poplack DG, et al. Leptomeningeal metastases. In Cancer in the nervous system, 2nd edition. Ed. Levin VA. New York, Oxford University Press. p. 375–93. 2002.
12. Little JR, Dale AJ, Okazaki H. Meningeal carcinomatosis. Clinical manifestations. Arch Neurol. 1974;30(2):138–43.
13. Olson ME, Chernik NL, Posner JB. Infiltration of the leptomeninges by systemic cancer. A clinical and pathologic study. Arch Neurol. 1974;30(2):122–37.
14. Twijnstra A, Ongerboer de Visser BW, Van Zanten AP. Diagnosis of leptomeningeal metastasis. Clin Neurol Neurosurg. 1987;89(2):79–85.
15. Siegal T, Lossos A, Pfeffer MR. Leptomeningeal metastases: analysis of 31 patients with sustained off-therapy response following combined-modality therapy. Neurology. 1994;44(8):1463–9.
16. DeAngelis LM. Current diagnosis and treatment of leptomeningeal metastasis. J Neurooncol. 1998;38(2–3):245–52.
17. Harstad L, Hess KR, Groves MD. Prognostic factors and outcomes in patients with leptomeningeal melanomatosis. Neurooncology. 2008;10(6):1010–8.
18. Le Rhun E, Taillibert S, Chamberlain MC. Carcinomatous meningitis: leptomeningeal metastases in solid tumors. Surg Neurol Int. 2013;4(Suppl 4):S265–88.
19. Le Rhun E, Galanis E. Leptomeningeal metastases of solid cancer. Curr Opin Neurol. 2016;29(6):797–805.
20. Scott BJ, Oberheim-Bush NA, Kesari S. Leptomeningeal metastasis in breast cancer – a systematic review. Oncotarget. 2016;7(4):3740–7.
21. Le Rhun ET, Taillibert S, Chamberlain MC. Neoplastic meningitis due to lung, breast and melanoma metastases. Cancer Control. 2017;24(1):22–32.
22. National Comprehensive Cancer Network (NCCN). NCCN Clinical Practice Guidelines in Oncology: Central Nervous System Cancers. https://www.nccn.org/professionals/physician_gls/pdf/cns.pdf. 2016.
23. Freilich RJ, Krol G, DeAngelis LM. Neuroimaging and cerebrospinal fluid cytology in the diagnosis of leptomeningeal metastasis. Ann Neurol. 1995;38(1):51–7.
24. Straathof CS, de Bruin HG, Dippel DW, et al. The diagnostic accuracy of magnetic resonance imaging and cerebrospinal fluid cytology in leptomeningeal metastasis. J Neurol. 1999;246(9):810–4.
25. Chamberlain MC, Sandy AD, Press GA. Leptomeningeal metastasis: a comparison of gadolinium-enhanced MR and contrast-enhanced CT of the brain. Neurology. 1990;40(3 Pt 1):435–8.
26. Short RG, Bal S, German JP, et al. Potential of F-18 PET/CT in the detection of leptomeningeal metastasis. Neuroradiol J. 2014;27(6):685–9.
27. Chamberlain MC. Comparative spine imaging in leptomeningeal metastases. J Neurooncol. 1995;23(3):233–8.
28. Kramer ED, Rafto S, Packer RJ, et al. Comparison of myelography with CT follow-up versus gadolinium MRI for subarachnoid metastatic disease in children. Neurology. 1991;41(1):46–50.
29. Kleinschmidt-DeMasters BK, Damek DM. The imaging and neuropathological effects of Bevacizumab (Avastin) in patients with leptomeningeal carcinomatosis. J Neurooncol. 2010;96(3):375–84.
30. Glantz MJ, Hall WA, Cole BF, et al. Diagnosis, management, and survival of patients with leptomeningeal cancer based on cerebrospinal fluid-flow status. Cancer. 1995;75(12):2919–31.
31. Grossman SA, Trump DL, Chen DC, et al. Cerebrospinal fluid flow abnormalities in patients with neoplastic meningitis. An evaluation using 111indium-DTPA ventriculography. Am J Med. 1982;73(5):641–7.
32. Chamberlain MC, Corey-Bloom J. Leptomeningeal metastases: 111indium-DTPA CSF flow studies. Neurology. 1991;41(11):1765–9.
33. Quijano S, Lopez A, Manuel Sancho J, et al. Identification of leptomeningeal disease in aggressive B-cell non-Hodgkin's lymphoma: improved sensitivity of flow cytometry. J Clin Oncol. 2009;27(9):1462–9.
34. Glantz MJ, Cole BF, Glantz LK, et al. Cerebrospinal fluid cytology in patients with cancer: minimizing false-negative results. Cancer. 1998;82(4):733–9.
35. Chamberlain MC, Kormanik PA, Glantz MJ. A comparison between ventricular and lumbar cerebrospinal fluid cytology in adult patients with leptomeningeal metastases. Neurooncology. 2001;3(1):42–5.
36. Rogers LR, Duchesneau PM, Nunez C, et al. Comparison of cisternal and lumbar CSF examination in leptomeningeal metastasis. Neurology. 1992;42(6):1239–41.
37. Schold SC, Wasserstrom WR, Fleisher M, et al. Cerebrospinal fluid biochemical markers of central nervous system metastases. Ann Neurol. 1980;8(6):597–604.
38. Sherwin AL, LeBlanc FE, McCann WP. Altered LDH isoenzymes in brain tumors. Arch Neurol. 1968;18(3):311–5.
39. Fleisher M, Wasserstrom WR, Schold SC, et al. Lactic dehydrogenase isoenzymes in the cerebrospinal fluid of patients with systemic cancer. Cancer. 1981;47(11):2654–9.
40. van Zanten AP, Twijnstra A, Ongerboer de Visser BW, et al. Cerebrospinal fluid tumour markers in patients treated for meningeal malignancy. J Neurol Neurosurg Psychiatry. 1991;54(2):119–23.

41. Walbert T, Groves MD. Known and emerging biomarkers of lepto-meningeal metastasis and its response to treatment. Future Oncol. 2010;6(2):287–97.
42. Le Rhun E, Massin F, Tu Q, et al. Development of a new method for identification and quantification in cerebrospinal fluid of malignant cells from breast carcinoma leptomeningeal metastasis. BMC Clin Pathol. 2012;12:21.
43. Le Rhun E, Tu Q, De Carvalho Bittencourt M, et al. Detection and quantification of CSF malignant cells by the CellSearch technology in patients with melanoma leptomeningeal metastasis. Med Oncol. 2013;30(2):538.
44. Nayak L, Fleisher M, Gonzalez-Espinoza R, et al. Rare cell capture technology for the diagnosis of leptomeningeal metastasis in solid tumors. Neurology. 2013;80(17):1598–605. discussion 603
45. Lin X, Fleisher M, Rosenblum M, et al. Cerebrospinal fluid circulating tumor cells: a novel tool to diagnose leptomen-ingeal metastases from epithelial tumors. Neuro Oncol. 2017;19(9):1248–54.
46. Kraan J, Gratama JW, Haioun C, et al. Flow cytometric immunophe-notyping of cerebrospinal fluid. Curr Protoc Cytom. 2008;Chapter 6:Unit 6.25.
47. de Jongste AH, Kraan J, van den Broek PD, et al. Use of TransFix cerebrospinal fluid storage tubes prevents cellular loss and enhances flow cytometric detection of malignant hematological cells after 18 hours of storage. Cytometry B Clin Cytom. 2014;86(4):272–9.

# Palliative Radiation Therapy for Leptomeningeal Disease

**14**

Alysa M. Fairchild

## Learning Objectives

- To review the potential roles and techniques of palliative radiotherapy in the treatment of leptomeningeal metastases.
- To review expected outcomes of palliative radiotherapy for leptomeningeal metastases including literature-reported toxicity.

## Background

Leptomeningeal metastatic disease (LM) refers to the multifocal seeding of the leptomeninges by malignant cells from a solid or hematologic tumour [1]. Once tumour cells reach the cerebrospinal fluid (CSF) via hematogenous, lymphatic spread or direct extension, they are disseminated throughout the neuraxis via dynamic flow [1]. Malignant cells within the CSF often settle through gravity on cul-de-sacs, web-like structures and stasis areas, explaining the high incidence of cranial nerve (CN) and cauda equina involvement [2, 3]. Predilection for involvement of the lower limbs reflects this gravitational effect, as well as the lengthy pathways of the cauda equina nerve roots through the subarachnoid space [4].

Two different types of LM spread have been described: free-floating non-adherent cells often difficult to discern on imaging due to the lack of discrete nodules ("diffuse, non-adherent type") and contrast-enhancing tumour nodules ("nodular type") which may have a multifocal skip pattern with intervening tumour-free areas [3, 5]. LM from solid tumours may have a propensity for the latter [6]. Even in the absence of visible nodules, microscopic infiltration may be present [7], ultimately leading to myelin loss and axonal degeneration [8].

Autopsy studies reveal that 19% of patients with cancer and neurologic signs or symptoms have meningeal involvement [9]. In a review of autopsies of patients with small cell lung cancer (SCLC) and LM, leptomeningeal involvement was considered focal in 30% and diffuse in 70% [10]. Focal LM was due to direct invasion of the leptomeninges by an underlying metastasis [10]. Diffuse involved the intracranial and/or intraspinal meninges, including the cauda equina, dorsal nerve roots, ependyma, choroid plexus and Gasserian ganglion [10].

LM is diagnosed antemortem in approximately 5–10% of patients with cancer, especially breast cancer, SCLC, non-small cell lung cancer (NSCLC), melanoma, leukaemia and lymphoma [6, 7, 10–16]. In 5–10% of those, it is the initial presentation of malignancy [3, 8], of whom 80% have a primary subsequently identified [3]. In 5% of all malignant epithelial tumours with central nervous system (CNS) involvement, LM exists in isolation, without cancer apparent elsewhere in the brain, spinal cord or peripheral nerves [17].

The CNS is a sanctuary site from water-soluble agents which are unable to penetrate the blood-brain barrier [18]. LM is being diagnosed with increasing frequency as patients live longer and as neuroimaging improves [1]. The majority of patients, 65–90%, are discovered to have LM concurrent with systemic relapse or progression [3, 10, 15]. A small proportion of those developing LM, less than 5%, recur 10 years or more after their initial diagnosis of malignancy [3]. In 2–13%, it is asymptomatic at diagnosis [3, 6, 11, 19], suggesting that LM as an incidental finding remains rare despite increased use of MRI [6]. 30–80% have concurrent parenchymal brain metastases (BM) [3, 10, 19–21], which must be considered when determining treatment options (see below). Risk factors for developing LM are summarized in Table 14.1.

A. M. Fairchild
Department of Radiation Oncology, Cross Cancer Institute,
Edmonton, AB, Canada
e-mail: alysa.fairchild@albertahealthservices.ca

© Springer International Publishing AG, part of Springer Nature 2018
E. L. Chang et al. (eds.), *Adult CNS Radiation Oncology*, https://doi.org/10.1007/978-3-319-42878-9_14

**Table 14.1** Risk factors for development of LM

| Risk factor | Example incidence | Refs |
| --- | --- | --- |
| *SCLC* | | |
| • Time since diagnosis | 0.5% at initial diagnosis vs 25% after 3 years | [10] |
| • Brain/spinal cord involvement | 54% at 3 years versus 22% in those without ($p \leq 0.02$); 35% had concurrent spinal cord compression and LM | [10] |
| • Liver metastases | 36% risk vs 21% in those without ($p \leq 0.02$) | [10] |
| • Bone metastases | 38% risk vs 17% of those without ($p \leq 0.02$) | [10] |
| • Relapse after PCI | 6–10% will recur as LM or spinal disease | [22] |
| *Breast* | | |
| • Triple negative | Increased risk (not specified) | [12] |
| *Mixed histologies* | | |
| • After resection of a BM | Seen after resection of a supratentorial BM in 3–6% vs after 16–33% of resections of a posterior fossa BM[a] | [11, 23–25] |
| • Distant in-brain failure | HR 2.0 ($p = 0.007$) for diagnosis of LM | [11] |
| • Concurrent BM | Diagnosed in 30–67% of patients with LM within 1 month of LM diagnosis | [3, 10] |
| • Adenocarcinoma | Can constitute up to 75–95% of LM cases | [4, 19, 21] |
| • Age | Younger age associated with LM (HR 0.9, $p = 0.0006$) | [11] |
| • Primary histology | Breast primary (HR 1.6, $p = 0.05$) Colorectal primary (HR 4.5, $p < 0.0001$) | [11] |

Abbreviation: *BM* brain metastasis, *HR* hazard ratio, *PCI* prophylactic cranial irradiation
[a]In part because of the large subarachnoid surface area in the posterior fossa [23]

## Diagnosis

If LM is a diagnostic consideration, patients require a contrast-enhanced neuroimaging study, preferably MRI, of the entire craniospinal axis (Table 14.2). The goals of determining extent of LM involvement are to accurately localize the cause of symptoms, to identify areas of bulky disease that may require focal therapy, to reveal concurrent brain metastases, to rule out hydrocephalus and to estimate the risk of herniation if lumbar puncture (LP) is being considered [6, 8, 14, 18]. MRI should be done before LP because pachymeningeal enhancement can be induced, especially if intracranial hypotension develops [23, 28], and may persist for weeks to months [18]. However, the risk is only ~1% in the absence of post-LP headache [29].

Fewer than 20% of patients will have a normal contrast-enhanced CT scan [14, 26]. The sensitivity of CT scan is approximately 30%, while that of MRI is ~70% [14]. In the absence of bulky disease, the false-negative rate of enhanced CT is 40%, while that of enhanced MRI is 20–30% [18, 30, 31]. In one series of 48 patients (35 with solid and 13 with hematologic primaries) who had both CSF sampling and MRI of the entire neuraxis, only 54% had concordant positive results [6]. In patients with solid tumours, the rate of positive MRI was higher, while those with hematologic tumours had a higher rate of positive CSF cytology. True sensitivity and specificity could not be calculated [6]; however, the more extensively tumour has seeded the leptomeninges, the more likely cytology is to be positive [8, 9].

If there are a high index of suspicion and no evidence of systemic cancer and CSF is inconclusive, meningeal biopsy

**Table 14.2** Clinical pearls regarding diagnosing LM

| Consider completing a diagnostic work-up for LM if: | Refs |
| --- | --- |
| The patient has neurologic dysfunction at more than one level of the neuraxis in the absence of a clear radiographic explanation | [3, 8, 26] |
| CSF cytology is positive (as this is almost never associated only with parenchymal brain metastases) | [8, 9] |
| The patient has hydrocephalus without an obstructing mass | [26] |
| Multiple small brain metastases are seen close to the cortical surface or at the base of the sulci | [18] |
| Spasm, narrowing or beading of pial vessels is seen on angiography | [3] |
| There are findings suggestive of LM on imaging of one CNS compartment | [1, 15] |
| Neurological signs on examination indicate more widespread dysfunction than neurologic symptoms | [10, 27] |
| Intramedullary spinal cord malignancy is identified (as in one series 100% had simultaneous LM) | [10, 22] |
| New-onset diabetes insipidus without a clear aetiology | [18] |

may be required [5, 26, 32]. The yield of biopsy increases if the sample is taken from a region which enhances on MRI [32]. The value of FDG-PET is still under investigation [14].

Impairment of CSF flow may occur at any level of the neuraxis as a result of tumour-related adhesions [33]. Tumour has a propensity to settle in the basal cisterns, often interfering with CSF flow or exit from the ventricular system [3]. All patients with bulky subarachnoid disease have impaired CSF flow, but some patients with normal neuroimaging also have abnormal CSF circulation [18]. During a CSF flow scan, indium-111-DTPA is administered into a ventricular catheter. Imaging is performed of the brain and spine immediately and at 4 and 24 h. CSF flow studies are abnormal in 30–75%

of patients with LM, with blocks commonly occurring at the skull base, at spinal canal and over cerebral convexities [33–35].

Both screening for and prophylaxing LM have been debated in the literature historically, commonly in the setting of SCLC, which traditionally has a high rate of leptomeningeal involvement. In a previous cooperative group study which mandated routine baseline LPs in asymptomatic patients with SCLC, all were cytologically negative [22]. Screening for LM has essentially been abandoned [15]. Additionally, because of the rarity of LM as the sole site of failure, the toxicity inherent in addressing the entire neuraxis and the low likelihood of a survival benefit, prophylactic therapy is not indicated in solid tumours [3, 15, 34].

## Multimodality Management Approach

Goals of treatment are to stabilize or improve symptoms, delay neurologic deterioration, preserve or improve quality of life (QOL) and prolong survival. Additional aims are to maintain mobility and function, prevent future complications and minimize the need for hospitalization. The optimal palliative intervention should offer a high possibility of benefit; be safe, without significant acute toxicity, with the shortest possible time investment; be minimal or non-invasive with little recovery time; and be cost-effective.

The majority of data on treatment of LM are non-randomized single-institution retrospective studies of patients with different histologies and heterogeneous prognostic features, who were not uniformly treated, and were evaluated at varying endpoints and with different response criteria [36–38]. There are no standardized diagnostic criteria, the sensitivity and specificity of current diagnostic methods are limited, conventional trial endpoints (such as RECIST) are difficult to apply, and progression is problematic to define, making cross-comparisons between trials which do exist challenging [39].

Consequently, guidance on optimal treatment strategy which can be gleaned from the literature is sparse [1, 37]. Supportive care should be offered to all (see below). Given the poor outcomes even with aggressive therapy, palliative care consultation at the diagnosis of LM should be strongly considered if that team is not already involved.

The choice of approach is largely based on performance status (PS), the trajectory of the disease to date, response to prior therapies, systemic and CNS tumour burden, age, life expectancy, current symptomatology, the probability that LM will respond to treatment, the degree of extracranial tumour control and patient wishes [1, 5, 13, 14, 18, 23, 28].

**Table 14.3** Risk stratification for treatment decision-making

| Poor risk | Refs | Good risk | Refs |
|---|---|---|---|
| • KPS <50–60<br>• Multiple, serious, fixed or major neurologic deficits<br>• Extensive systemic disease with few remaining treatment options<br>• Bulky CNS disease ± CSF flow obstruction<br>• Encephalopathy due to LM | [1, 3, 23, 28, 33, 34] | • KPS 60 or higher<br>• No major neurologic deficits<br>• Minimal systemic disease<br>• Reasonable systemic therapy options<br>• No CSF block | [1, 3, 23, 33] |

Abbreviations: *CNS* central nervous system, *CSF* cerebrospinal fluid, *KPS* Karnofsky Performance Status, *LM* leptomeningeal metastasis

Some authors advocate risk stratification (Table 14.3). Aggressive systemic and/or intrathecal (IT) therapy would be reserved for patients in the good risk group, usually in conjunction with radiotherapy (RT) [1]. Patients in the poor-risk group could be offered focal RT to symptomatic sites [1, 14]. If a marked response is observed after RT, chemotherapy may then be considered [18]. However, in practice, many patients have both good- and poor-risk characteristics, and clinical judgement dictates treatment approach [1].

The role of surgery is largely limited to placement of an Ommaya reservoir for IT chemotherapy, insertion of a ventriculoperitoneal (VP) shunt for symptomatic hydrocephalus (see below) or, rarely, resection of a large space-occupying leptomeningeal deposit or BM [5].

Prognostic and predictive factors are summarized in Table 14.4. In terms of estimation of life expectancy in breast cancer, a prognostic index (PI) has been constructed as the sum of the following: for age ≥55 years, score 1.3; for lung metastases, score 1.2; for CN involvement, score 1.5; for lumbar CSF protein 0.51–1.0 g/L, score 2; and for lumbar CSF glucose <2.5 mmol/L, score 1. A total score <1.4 predicted a median survival (MS) of 299 days; scoring 1.4–2.6 predicted a MS of 157 days; scoring 2.6–3.6 predicted a MS of 76 days; and scoring >3.6 predicted a MS of 19 days [42].

## Supportive Care

### Pharmacotherapy

Medical management should be maximized, including analgesics, antiemetics, antidepressants, and anxiolytics [24]. Prophylactic antiepileptics should not be used, since seizures are not a common occurrence and these medications require monitoring and may interact with other drugs [8, 28, 33]. 10–25% of patients eventually develop seizures and can be started on antiepileptics if necessary at that time [8].

**Table 14.4** Prognostic and predictive factors

| Poor prognostic factors | Refs | Predictive of poor survival | Refs | Predictive of improved survival | Refs |
|---|---|---|---|---|---|
| • CSF flow impairment/elevated ICP—reflects disease burden in the subarachnoid compartment | [6, 33, 35, 40] | • CSF flow impairment correlates negatively with response to treatment | [34, 35, 40] | • Delivery of IT chemotherapy | [19] |
| • Poor performance status | [12, 13, 36] | • Poor performance status | [6, 19, 20, 41] | • Use of EGFR tyrosine kinase inhibitor therapy | [19] |
| • Extent of meningeal dissemination on CT/MRI | [13] | • High CSF protein, lactate and WBC | [5, 19] | • Delivery of WBRT | [19] |
| • Age[a] | [42] | • Cranial nerve dysfunction at baseline | [43] | • VP shunt | [19] |
| • Lung metastases[a] | [42] | • Synchronous brain metastases[b] | [20] | • Correction of a CSF obstruction | [34, 35, 40] |
| • Lumbar CSF protein and glucose[a] | [42] | • Shorter interval between primary and LM diagnosis[b] | [20] | • No active systemic disease | [6] |
| • Cranial nerve involvement[a] | [42] | | | • Hematologic versus solid tumour primary | [6] |

Abbreviations: *CSF* cerebrospinal fluid, *CT* computed tomography, *EGFR* epidermal growth factor receptor, *ICP* intracranial pressure, *IT* intrathecal, *LM* leptomeningeal metastasis, *MRI* magnetic resonance image, *VP* ventriculoperitoneal, *WBC* white blood cells, *WBRT* whole brain radiotherapy
[a]Included breast patients only
[b]Included non-small cell lung patients only

Interestingly, corticosteroids have a limited role in the supportive care of LM-related symptoms because significant oedema of underlying neural tissue is uncommon [18]. However, they remain useful in treating vasogenic oedema associated with synchronous intraparenchymal BM or epidural metastases; for the symptomatic treatment of increased intracranial pressure, nausea and emesis; for prophylaxis of side effects of RT; and as an antineoplastic agent in hematologic malignancies [2, 3, 18, 20, 23, 33, 43].

## Hydrocephalus and VP Shunt Placement

Raised intracranial pressure (ICP) can occur even in the absence of an obstructive mass lesion or ventricular dilatation [3], and in those circumstances would be noted as increased opening pressure at LP [44]. This implies that subarachnoid pathways are obstructed at a microscopic level [18].

A VP shunt can significantly and immediately improve QOL and should be considered as a palliative therapy when appropriate (positional headache, persistent nausea, encephalopathy, gait apraxia, cognitive impairment, urinary incontinence), even if hydrocephalus is not clearly evident on imaging [8, 18, 23]. Approximately 10–15% of patients will require VP shunting [3, 19, 21, 45]. Peritoneal seeding is a theoretical complication although is rarely seen [11].

One drawback of VP shunt placement is that it precludes delivery of IT chemotherapy through an Ommaya reservoir [6, 18, 21]; however, increased ICP is a relative contraindication to IT chemotherapy [6]. A shunt with an on-off valve can be placed in series with a reservoir, but many patients cannot tolerate having the shunt turned off for several hours [6, 18]. Programmable values are easily opened and closed, but the valve is controlled by a magnet with which an MRI may interact [18].

Investigators from South Korea retrospectively reviewed 71 patients with BM from solid tumours (2005–2012) and LM to investigate the prognostic impact of hydrocephalus [45]. 33.8% had LM diagnosed synchronously with brain metastases and the rest metachronously (>3 months). 45/71 had lung and 14/71 had breast cancer. 63.4% had fewer than 5 BM, 14.1% had 5–10, and 22.5% greater than 10. Symptomatic hydrocephalus was seen in 18/71 patients, of whom 7 had a shunt. 25/71 had whole brain RT (WBRT) alone (median dose 30 Gy/10), 2/71 had spine RT (median 20 Gy) alone, 4/71 had both, 2/71 had IT chemotherapy, 18/71 had systemic chemotherapy and the remainder had no treatment. The MS overall was 2.1 ± 0.3 months: the MS of untreated patients was 1.4 months, and MS of those who had RT was 3.1 months. There was no statistically significant difference in MS based on hydrocephalus: patients with surgically treated hydrocephalus had a MS of 5.7 months, patients without hydrocephalus a MS of 2.3 months and those with untreated hydrocephalus a MS of 1.7 months ($p = 0.12$) [45].

# Radiation Therapy for Leptomeningeal Metastases

The optimal palliative RT regimen is one that provides prompt and effective symptom relief with minimal toxicity and patient inconvenience. In view of the fact that the intricacies of treatment planning are often outweighed by the complexities of decision-making at the end of life, Mackillop outlined ten rules to guide the prescription of palliative RT based on well-known ethical principles [46]. Among them are common-sense guidelines which serve as a reminder that "time is precious when life is short", "palliative RT should consume no more resources than necessary" and "courses should be no longer than required to achieve their therapeutic goal" [46].

## Involved-Field RT

WBRT is usually delivered to areas of cerebral involvement, especially in those with concurrent BM, with local RT delivered to areas of spinal involvement (Table 14.5) [1, 5]. Localization of the source of significant symptoms will help direct RT planning, since the intensity of LM infiltration generally corresponds [4]. Even symptoms which are not localizable to a specific location by neuroimaging, such as seizures, may benefit from WBRT [18]. RT penetrates the sulci of the brain and the Virchow-Robin spaces, areas which may not easily be reached by IT therapy [3].

Local RT restores flow in 30–35% of spinal and 50% of intracranial blockages [34, 40, 47, 48]. Restoration of normal CSF flow after RT not only relieves symptomatic hydrocephalus and potentially avoids a VP shunt but also may enable initiation of IT therapy [23]. If significant flow abnormalities remain, the patient should be treated as poor risk [1, 33].

In patients with positive CSF cytology but who are asymptomatic, with a low cerebral tumour load, without brain metastases or evidence of increased ICP, WBRT may be withheld [3, 5].

Table 14.5 Indications for involved-field radiotherapy

Symptomatic improvement, e.g. cauda equina syndrome

To address areas of CSF flow obstruction

Increased intracranial pressure even in the absence of an obstructing mass on imaging

Local shrinkage of areas of bulky disease to facilitate intrathecal chemotherapy, even if asymptomatic

Stereotactic radiosurgery (SRS) and stereotactic body RT are not considered standard of care at present [5], but appropriateness could be evaluated on a case-by-case basis [36].

If the goal of therapy is cytological CSF clearance, treatment must address the entire subarachnoid space including the ventricular system, base of the brain, cisterns and the spinal cord [18, 23]. Thus, if one is to use focal (rather than whole craniospinal) RT, additional therapy is necessary in the form of IT and/or high-dose systemic chemotherapy [3].

## Involved-Field Treatment Planning

For WBRT, opposed lateral fields with a treatment energy of 6MV photons, with appropriate immobilization and shielding, should be used [20, 43] (Fig. 14.1). Three-dimensional based planning will ensure the retroorbital area, base of skull, cerebral meninges and basal cisterns are included (Table 14.6) [5]. Radio-opaque markers placed on the lateral orbital canthi are useful [20]. Acceptable heterogeneity is 95–107% [20]. The same doses are often used for both whole brain and spinal fields [28] (Fig. 14.1). Schedules of 24 Gy/8, 30 Gy/10 and 36 Gy/12 are commonly reported [5, 10, 14, 18, 20, 28]. In patients with a predicted survival of >1 year, 40 Gy/20 could be considered to reduce late brain toxicity, while for those with a more limited prognosis 20 Gy/5 is an option [5, 20, 28]. It is unclear whether dose escalation or alternate schedules are beneficial in certain histologies [36].

## Craniospinal Irradiation (CSI)

CSI has not been used extensively since the doses needed to eradicate many solid tumours depress the bone marrow, interfering with the ability to subsequently deliver systemic chemotherapy [3, 8, 10]. Other morbidity from CSI is significant, including mucositis, pulmonary and gastrointestinal toxicity [23], especially if overlapping with previous RT fields [36]. In defined cases such as multiple circumscript plaques or nodules, or to aggressively approach radiosensitive histologies, CSI could be considered [1, 3, 28] (Fig. 14.2). Additionally, CSI may be undertaken in the rare patients who present with LM with no other CNS or systemic malignancy [17] and may also be considered in patients with leptomeningeal gliomatosis due to a primary CNS malignancy [5].

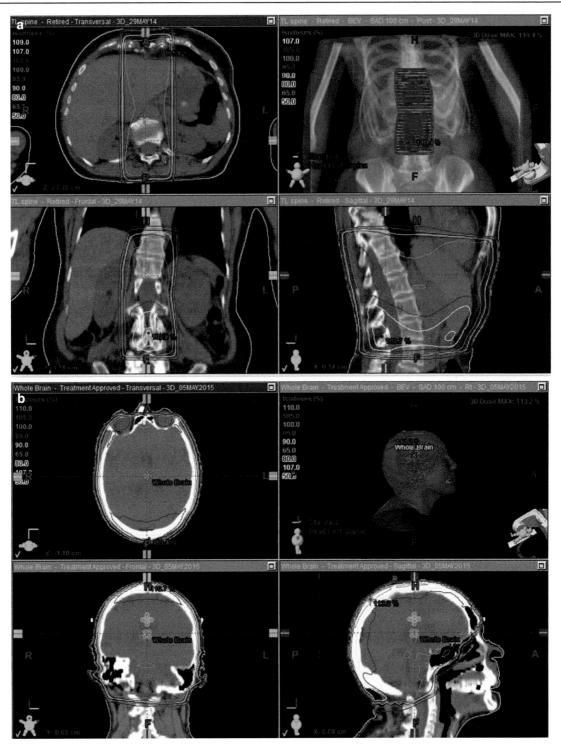

**Fig. 14.1** Example of involved-field radiotherapy for symptomatic lep-tomeningeal and intramedullary spinal metastases in a 69-year-old woman with widely metastatic breast cancer receiving palliative systemic therapy. (**a**) On initial presentation, although diffuse studding was found throughout the neuraxis, it was concentrated in the spine more than the brain, and her predominant symptom was unilateral leg weakness. Therefore, she received focal RT to T10-L4, 20 Gy/5, APPA POP fields with 15 MV photons (06/2014). While follow-up MRI 2 months later was unaltered, MRI performed almost 5 months after treatment demonstrated significant resolution along the posterior fossa, surface of the spinal cord and within the cauda equina. By 8 months after spine RT, she developed an apparent solitary focus of progression along the right cerebellar hemisphere discovered on routine imaging (asymptomatic). She was referred for consideration of stereotactic radiosurgery, which is not offered. (**b**) She consented to whole brain radiotherapy 3 months later (20 Gy/5, opposed lateral fields, 6 MV photons, [05/2015]). Follow-up MRI imaging of the brain/spine performed 3 and 6 months later was reported as stable. Nine months after WBRT, MRI revealed progressive enhancement along the anterior and posterior aspects of the spinal cord, most apparent outside of the previous spinal field, without progression in the brain. She denied lateralizing neurologic symptoms. Systemic therapy was discontinued at that time. (**c, d**) Due to the sustained response to previous focal RT and indolent disease trajectory systemically, she was offered further RT to the remaining unirradiated neuraxis. Fields encompassed C3-T10 and L4-S5, both receiving 20 Gy/5 via parallel opposed fields with 15 MV photons (03/2016). She died 8 weeks later

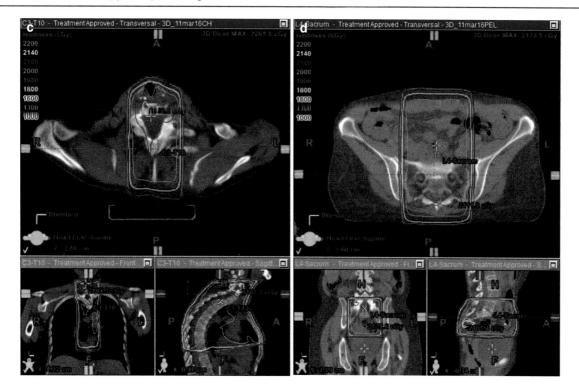

**Fig. 14.1** (continued)

**Table 14.6** Literature-derived guidance on WBRT planning

| Treatment planning | Refs |
|---|---|
| Inferior: bottom of C1 or C2 | [5, 8, |
| PTV: entire intracranial contents with a 1 cm margin around the bony skull, including the retroorbital region, base of skull and meningeal space (i.e. lamina cribrosa and basal cisterns) with sufficient margin on anterior cerebellum | 20, 28] |
| Most common dose schedule: 30 Gy/10 | |

## Radiotherapy Toxicity

Acute side effects due to increased ICP are largely prevented by administration of dexamethasone [3]. Side effects of RT to the spine are minimal, although slight leukopenia can occur [3]. Pronounced myelotoxicity is not expected even from concurrent WBRT and IT chemotherapy [5].Two patients (6.4%) in one series experienced transient subacute post-radiation L'hermitte's phenomenon [49]. There are no contemporary series reporting toxicity from CSI for solid tumours.

Approximately one third to one half of patients treated aggressively have late complications, including focal or diffuse leukoencephalopathy (LEP), diagnosed at a median of 8 months post-treatment [49, 50]. Approximately two thirds are symptomatic and one third asymptomatic [49]. Focal LEP is visualized on CT as a local hypodensity; it causes contralateral focal symptoms and/or focal seizures [49]. In diffuse LEP, CT scans demonstrate

hypodensity commonly of the periventricular white matter [49]. MRI shows cerebral atrophy, diffuse white matter signal abnormality on fluid-attenuated inversion recovery and T2-weighted images and ventricular dilatation [23]. Symptoms of diffuse LEP are cognitive change, somnolence, irritability, incontinence, neurologic deficits, seizures, ataxia, dementia and tremor [34]. It is especially likely after IT chemotherapy if patients have also received brain RT [3, 5, 18, 28] but can develop after IT chemotherapy alone [5, 50]. It is important to note that LEP is not usually seen after WBRT alone [3, 49]. LEP is irreversible and progressive [5] as a result of disseminated demyelination and axonal loss [23]. The only predictor in Siegal's series of late LEP was elevated CSF pressure at diagnosis [49].

Patients with LM secondary to breast ($N = 20$) or lung ($N = 7$) cancer who received WBRT alone (2004–2010) were retrospectively reviewed, focusing on treatment toxicity [43]. This cohort was treated with WBRT alone because of poor PS, bulky lesions, age, medical contraindications or refusal of chemotherapy. Eleven had concurrent BM, and 21/27 received 30 Gy/10. Other WBRT schedules used were 24 Gy/12, 26 Gy/13, 35 Gy/14 and 40 Gy/20. One patient required spine RT. The median time from diagnosis of LM to initiation of WBRT was 10 days (range 0–47 days). All but one patient received dexamethasone (minimum daily dose 6 mg). Treatment was completed by 21/27: three died and three pro-

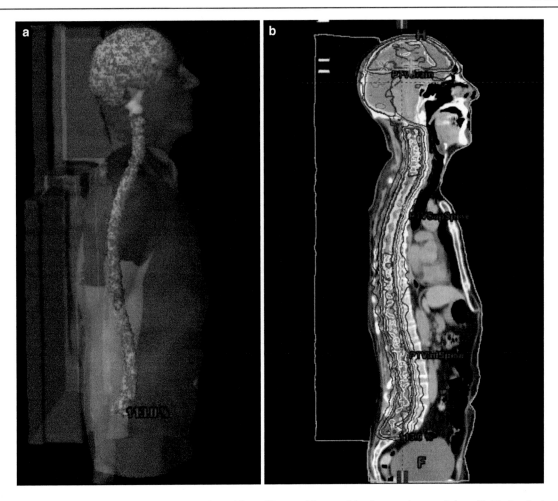

**Fig. 14.2** Example of whole craniospinal irradiation planned for a 60-year-old man with adenocarcinoma of the sella likely of minor salivary gland origin, recurrent after radical radiotherapy. He was diagnosed with leptomeningeal metastases coating the brainstem, spinal cord and cauda equina, along with disease progression in the suprasellar area. Technique: volumetric modulated arc therapy, 6 MV photons. Prescribed dose, 30 Gy/10. (**a**) Combined planning target volumes (brain, superior spinal cord and inferior spinal cord/cauda). (**b**) Dose distribution. Isodose lines: pink, 110%; yellow, 107%; purple, 105%; orange, 100%; red, 95%; light green, 90%; dark blue, 80%; dark green, 65%; light blue, 50%

gressed during RT. There was no acute grade 3–4 toxicity. 26% experienced grade 1 acute toxicity (erythema, alopecia, nausea, headache, fatigue), and three patients had grade 2 toxicity (alopecia, tinnitus, somnolence). One patient developed severe LEP at 22 months. The MS of this cohort was 8.1 weeks [43].

## Is WBRT Protective Against Subsequent Development of LM?

Data are contradictory as to whether WBRT (or prophylactic cranial irradiation [PCI]) protects against subsequent LM, especially given the potential confounding nature of intracranial BM [11]. Among 137 SCLC patients treated on two consecutive studies, 12 were eventually diagnosed with cytologically positive LM [51]. Of these 12, 7 had received 30 Gy/10 WBRT prior to the recognition of LM for brain metastases; these 7 had a median of 52 weeks to diagnosis of LM, versus 28 weeks for the 5 patients who had not had prior WBRT ($p = 0.018$). Additionally, no patient who received PCI relapsed as LM [51]. An additional

case report described a patient who received WBRT before it was recognized she had LM [8]. Eventually, she developed cauda equina syndrome and started local RT but died after one fraction. On autopsy, there was a much heavier infiltrate of tumour affecting the spinal cord versus the cranial subarachnoid space [8]. At least one other study described WBRT to be protective against (or at least delay) LM [52], while others have found no effect [11, 53, 54].

## Outcomes: Symptom Control

The natural history of LM is one of progressive neurologic dysfunction at multiple sites, often despite treatment [4, 27]. Because symptoms more often stabilize than improve once therapy is initiated, diagnosis before symptoms become devastating is essential, analogous to the situation with spinal cord compression [3, 33]. As well, symptomatic improvement (versus stabilization) is more likely to occur the earlier that treatment is started [8]. Neurologic recovery is not typi-

**Table 14.7** Symptom control outcomes

| Usually improves after RT | Refs | Usually does not improve after RT | Refs |
|---|---|---|---|
| Radicular pain | [18] | Fixed neurologic deficits such as cranial nerve palsies or paraplegia | [1, 18, 33] |
| Symptoms secondary to hydrocephalus | [3] | | |
| Symptoms relating to vascular compromise | [3] | | |
| Encephalopathy | [1] | | |
| Cognitive impairment[a] | [50] | | |

Abbreviation: *RT* radiotherapy
[a]Improved in 40%, stable in 50%

cal except in very radiosensitive tumours such as leukaemia and lymphoma [18].

20–30% of patients will be excluded from aggressive therapy at baseline due to poor condition [49]. Of those receiving therapy, an additional 10–40% will die within 1 month; consequently, evaluation of response is possible for 2/3 at best [41, 43, 49, 55]. The limited number of patients with adequate follow-up in most series makes it difficult to assess outcomes [10].

LM is associated with pain in up to 40% of patients in two main regions: headache (with or without neck stiffness) and pain in the low back/buttocks [56]. Pain tends to respond quickly to RT [18, 33], decreasing subsequent medication requirements [5] (Table 14.7). Symptoms resulting from tumour invasion—for example, into the spinal cord parenchyma—are more likely to be irreversible [3, 4, 18].

It is possible that combined IT chemotherapy and focal RT improve symptoms more effectively than IT chemotherapy alone [10]. Involved-field RT alone will not eliminate LM, nor does it likely substantially decrease the risk of future morbidity [22]. This is because the area radiated will eventually be reseeded by tumour from outside the treated volume [3, 18]. According to Chamberlain, a significant fraction of malignant cells in the CSF exist in a non-dividing state; as radiosensitivity is cell cycle-dependent, treatment failure is therefore not surprising [2].Thus, it remains unclear to what degree local RT will delay the development of further neurologic disability [3, 33]. There is minimal literature detailing QOL [57].

Elmore and colleagues described symptom outcomes after palliative RT for symptomatic LM from solid tumours diagnosed by MRI ± LP ($N = 117$) between 2008 and 2014, published thus far in abstract form only [41]. 48% had breast cancer, 19% lung, 8% melanoma and 6% prostate; median ECOG PS was 2. RT was delivered to the brain and/or spine at a dose of 30 Gy/10. Rates of improvement, stability and progression were evaluated 4 weeks after RT and were actually quite similar across different symptoms. For gait dysfunction, headache, nausea/emesis, cognitive changes and cranial neuropathies, 17–35% of patients improved, 52–56% stabilized, and 12–28% progressed. 41% died within 4 weeks of RT. Median survival was 57 days (IQR 32–158) from RT

consult (75 days for ECOG 0–1 vs 47 days for ECOG 2–4 [$p = 0.03$]). The authors suggested shorter RT schedules should be utilized, along with institution of end-of-life care planning [41].

## Outcomes: Recurrence

Relapse has been reported in 29–52% [3, 49], more commonly in solid than hematologic primaries [49]. The relapse-free interval for relapsing patients in one study ranged between 8 and 22 months, with no relationship to response attained to initial therapy [49]. 2/3 relapsed solely in the leptomeninges and 1/3 in the LM and systemically [49]. Retreatment was systemic therapy in 8/9. 5/9 had a second complete response (CR), but 4/9 deteriorated and died shortly after relapse. There has been little improvement reported after repeat WBRT for recurrent LM [8]. In general, treatment options for progressive LM are RT to symptomatic sites, systemic chemotherapy or best supportive care [1].

## Outcomes: CSF Cytology Conversion

Eradiation of tumour from the subarachnoid space with existing therapy is rare [18]. Even if it does occur, clearance of the CSF does not necessarily correlate with resolution of neurologic symptoms and signs. Neither clinical response nor survival seems dependent on cytological response [50]. In fact, outcomes seem to correlate more with symptom improvement than CSF clearing [42], and it is possible to see long patient survival in spite of persistent positive cytology [50]. Residual tumour has been found at autopsy despite treatment for LM in the majority of patients evaluated [10, 22]. For example, of 19 patients sustaining a clinical response to WBRT who ultimately underwent autopsy, tumour was found in the CSF in 17 [22]. A sustained leptomeningeal response likely also requires control of extracranial disease [49], which may not be achievable due to acquired resistance to previous systemic therapy [34].

## Outcomes: Survival

Untreated LM median survival is 4–6 weeks [4, 8, 33] (Table 14.8). It is unlikely, and probably unsurprising, that focal RT of a single CNS compartment alters survival [4, 21, 38]. Complicating the interpretation of efficacy of WBRT specifically is the potential impact of synchronous or metachronous parenchymal brain metastases [38].

In patients who receive aggressive treatment, life expectancy commonly ranges from 2 to 6 months [7, 57]. However, it is not clear if the improved survival is a result of treatment

**Table 14.8** Examples of literature-reported outcomes

| Treatment | RT dose | Years | N | Histology | Criteria for diagnosis | Outcomes | Ref |
|---|---|---|---|---|---|---|---|
| CSI | 40 Gy[a] | 1948 | 1 | Undiff carcinoma | Diagnosed on clinical findings | Symptomatic PR "almost at once" but relapses required three more RT courses; survived 28.3 m from CSI | [58] |
| RT[b] | NS | 1967–1971 | 13 | Mixed solid tumours | CSF + and/or autopsy | Breast: 37.5% improved, avg surv 5.3 m; Lymphoma: 0% improved, avg surv 3.3 m; Lung: 50% improved, avg surv 4 m | [7] |
| RT[b] + IT MTX | NS | 1967–1971 | 10 | Mixed solid tumours | CSF + and/or autopsy | Breast: 75% improved, avg surv 3.3 m; Lymphoma: 100% improved, avg surv 4.5 m; Lung: 50% improved, avg surv 3.5 m | [7] |
| WBRT | NS | Prior to 1979 | 4 | SCLC[c] | Received WBRT for BM diagnosed 1–6 months prior to LC diagnosis | Avg survival from BM diagnosis: 4.3 m; Avg survival from LC diagnosis: 44 d | [16] |
| RT[b] | 20–24 Gy/ NS | 1969–1980 | 3 | SCLC | Required cytology + CSF or autopsy | 0% cleared CSF; 0% marked symptom improvement | [10] |
| RT[b] + IT MTX | 20–24 Gy/ NS | 1969–1980 | 24 | SCLC | Required cytology + CSF or autopsy | 33.3% (8/24) cleared CSF; 8.3% (2/24) symptom CR or near CR; 20.8% (5/24) died before treatment; MS following treatment: 7 wks | [10] |
| RT[b,d] + IT MTX | 24 Gy/8 | 1975–1980 | 90 | Mixed solid tumours | Diagnosis required: typical clinical findings or CSF + or CT/ myelography + | Breast: 61% (28/46) clinical benefit, MS 7.2 m (range 1–29 m); Lung: 39% (9/23) clinical benefit, MS 4 m (range 1–10 m); Melanoma: 18% (2/11) clinical benefit, MS 3.6 m (range 1–12 m); Other: 30% (3/10) clinical benefit, MS 6.3 m (range 2–12 m); Overall: 47% (42/90) clinical benefit, MS 5.8 m (range 1–29 m) | [3] |
| WBRT + IT MTX ± spine RT[f] | 30 Gy/10 | 1981–1985 | 26 | Mixed solid tumours | BM excluded Cytology + CSF required Myelogram optional | MS overall 3.1 m (3.7 m for breast vs 1.7 mo for others; $p$ = NS); 30.8% responded: 3/8 CR, 5/8 PR; 6/26 responded and 5/26 died by 1 month after treatment start | [55] |
| RT[b] ± IT chemo ± systemic chemo | 24– 50 Gy/8–25 | 1980–1991 | 31[g] | Mixed solid tumours, primary CNS tumours and lymphoma | CSF + | NHL: 6/13 got RT; all NHL had CR; MS of NHL group not reached; Breast: 9/10 got RT; MS 21 m; Other: 8/8 got RT; MS 31 m; Overall 19/31 got WBRT ± spine RT; 79% of patients getting RT had PR; At completion of therapy, neurologic improvement in 68% and SD in 32%; overall CR 65% and PR in 35%; overall MS 23 months | [49] |
| RT[b] + IT chemo | NS | 1988–1999 | 18 | AA, GBM[b] | CSF + | 11/18 had RT: 1/11 partial brain RT, 8/11 limited spine RT, 2/11 both; 9/11 got RT for bulky disease: 8/9 SD, 1/9 PR; 3/4 who got RT for CSF obstruction re-established normal CSF flow; Avg survival post-RT: 4 m (range 2–8 m) | [2] |
| RT[b] + C ± IT chemo | 30 Gy/10 | 1991–1998 | 35 | Breast | Positive CSF cytology (97.1%) or characteristic MRI findings (2.9%) | RT + C: ¥41%; avg. survival 30.3 wks; RT + C + IT chemo: ¥33%; avg. survival 18.3 wks; COD: 42% neurologic, 28% systemic, 18% both, 6% neurotoxicity, 6% unrelated | [50] |

| Treatment | Dose | Years | N | Tumour type | Diagnosis | Outcomes | Ref. |
|---|---|---|---|---|---|---|---|
| WBRT + IT chemo | 30 Gy/10 | 1997–2005 | 85 | Mixed solid tumours | CSF +; 64% positive MRI or CT | Lung: 4/36 got IT chemo, 4/36 got WBRT alone; MS 43 d (range ≤–375 d) Breast: 19/33 got IT chemo, 5/33 got WBRT alone; MS 79 d (rang- 13–759 d) Others: 8/16 got IT chemo, 0/16 got WBRT alone; MS 30 d (range 1–523 d) 45/85 received no treatment | [13] |
| Mixed | NS | 2002–2004 | 187 | Mixed solid (N = 150) and heme (N = 37) tumours | CSF cytology (23.0%), MRI (52.9%), CSF and MRI (24.1%), or physician's clinical judgement (3.2%) | 27/150 solid and 1/37 heme received BSC alone; 67/187 had RT[b] alone; 46/187 chemo alone, 36/187 chemo and RT[b], 10/187 UNK treatment Overall MS 2.3 m for solid tumours and 4.7 m for heme ($p = 0.000$) Breast: MS 2.8 m; lung, MS 2.2 m Leukaemia, MS 5.8 m; lymphoma, 4.6 m | [6] |
| WBRT ± IT MTX | NS | 2005–2010 | 7 | Gastric[i,j] | Contrast-enhanced CT ± MRI ± CSF | 4/7 received RT, 1/4 IT MTX, 1/4 systemic chemo; 1/4 responded 3/4 have died, 1/3 of LM; average survival 88 d after RT | [59] |
| Mixed | 20–30 Gy | 2005–2012 | 71 | Mixed solid tumours, all with BM | MRI ± CSF cytology | 40.8% RPA class II, 59.2% RPA class III Histology: 45 lung, 14 breast, 12 other 25/71 WBRT, 2/71 spine RT, 4/71 WBRT + spine, 2/71 IT chemo, 18/71 systemic chemo, 33/71 no treatment Overall MS 2.1 m ± 0.3 m MS of untreated pts. 1.4 m MS of those who had RT 3.1 m | [45] |
| WBRT ± IT thiotepa | 16–30 Gy | NA | 7 | Oesophagus | CSF cytology ± imaging | 4/7 received WBRT, 1/7 IT chemo, avg. surv 6.3 wks overall (4.9 wks after WBRT); 2/4 discontinued WBRT early | [60] |

Abbreviations: *AA* anaplastic astrocytoma, *avg* average, *BM* brain metastases, *BSC* best supportive care, *C* chemotherapy (systemic), *COD* cause of death, *CR* complete response, *CSF* cerebrospinal fluid, *CSI* craniospinal irradiation, *d* days, *GBM* glioblastoma multiforme, *Gy* grey, *IT* intrathecal, *LC* leptomeningeal carcinomatosis, *m* months, *MS* median survival, *NS* not specified, *pCR* pathologic complete response, *PR* partial response, *RT* radiotherapy, *SCLC* small cell lung carcinoma, *SD* stable disease, *undiff* undifferentiated, *UNK* unknown, *WBRT* whole brain radiotherapy, *wks* weeks

[a]Deep X-ray

[b]RT to areas of bulk disease and/or most symptomatic area

[c]All relapsing after combination chemotherapy

[d]4/90 did not receive RT

[e]Clinical benefit = improved or stabilized

[f]Steroids allowed at investigator preference

[g]Minimum 6-month off-treatment follow-up data available

[h]All received 60 Gy cranial RT at initial diagnosis

[i]All with peritoneal metastases or malignant ascites

[j]All received combination chemotherapy including intraperitoneal paclitaxel

or (more likely) from patient selection [37]: only those with the best PS, least comorbidities and longest expected lifespan would be offered potentially invasive and toxic therapy [57]. Moreover, alteration of the natural history of LM with aggressive therapy may only be expected to alter survival in patients with meningeal involvement as the sole site of disease or relapse [15].

The question of survival benefit aside, some series suggest that patients receiving LM-directed treatment are less likely to die from neurologic causes and more likely to succumb to progressive systemic malignancy [3].

## Results from Landmark and Modern Series

The SWOG 8102 trial, accruing from 1981 to1985, investigated the response rate of patients with solid tumour LM after concurrent IT methotrexate (MTX) (twice weekly until CSF clearing followed by maintenance) and 30 Gy/10 WBRT [55]. Symptomatic areas of the spinal cord could also receive RT at a similar dose, but CSI was not allowed. Eligibility criteria included positive CSF cytology, absence of brain metastases and no previous WBRT. CR required CSF clearing and a normal neurologic exam, and a partial response (PR) was achievement of one of those. 26 patients (17 breast, 4 lung, 3 melanoma, 1 bladder and 1 ovary) were accrued with a median age of 54 years, and 19/26 were female. The median survival was 3.1 months overall (3.7 months for breast cancer vs 1.7 months for other histologies, $p$ = NS). Overall, 8/26 responded (3 CR, 5 PR), 6 of whom had breast cancer. By 1 month, 5/26 had died and 6/26 had responded. Excluding those who died prior to 1 month, the MS for responders was 5.7 months and for nonresponders 1.8 months ($p$ = NS). The only grade 3–4 toxicity reported was hematologic. The authors concluded that they "were unable to identify patient characteristics which would encourage [the development of] more aggressive treatment policies" [55].

Boogerd and colleagues reported their randomized trial of IT MTX concurrent with systemic therapy versus systemic therapy alone; patients in both arms had RT (30 Gy/10) delivered to "sites of clinical relevance" [50]. Only breast cancer patients with a life expectancy based on extracranial disease of at least 3 months were accrued. Patients were excluded if they had progressive or untreated BM, unless lesions were <15 mm and in continuity with the subarachnoid space. The primary endpoint was overall survival, and although the target sample size was 50 patients, the trial closed early after taking 7 years to accrue 35 participants. The median number of cycles of IT MTX delivered was 8 (range 1–21). Within 4 weeks after randomization, 6/17 of the IT group and 9/18 of the non-IT group had received RT; sites treated were not specified. MS was 18.3 weeks in the IT arm and 30.3 weeks in non-

IT arm. In the IT arm, 59% benefited (improved or stabilized), and 41% had no response; 76% ultimately progressed. The median time to progression (TTP) of initially responding patients was 43 weeks (range 25 63 weeks), and for the entire group, median TTP was 23 weeks. Six patients attained a cytological response in CSF, and their median survival was 52 weeks. In the non-IT arm, 67% benefitted and 33% had no response; 56% ultimately progressed. The median TTP of responding patients who had not received IT chemotherapy was 64 weeks (range 16 weeks to not reached), and of the entire group 24 weeks. Acute fatal LEP was seen in one patient, subacute transient LEP in one and delayed LEP in three, all in the IT group, none of whom received WBRT. One non-IT patient was diagnosed with LEP after receiving high-dose IV MTX and WBRT for LM relapse. 8/17 of IT patients had treatment-related neurologic complications versus 1/18 of the non-IT patients ($p$ = 0.007), confirming that LEP can develop in the absence of WBRT [50].

Clarke and et al. retrospectively reviewed 187 patients (2002–2004), the largest cohort in the modern era, to investigate whether MRI imaging affects diagnosis or outcomes [6]. Eligibility criteria included solid ($N$ = 150) or hematologic primary ($N$ = 37); LM diagnosed via positive CSF cytology (23.0%), suggestive MRI findings (52.9%), both (24.1%) or physician's clinical judgement (3.2%); and adequate follow-up. Breast was the most common primary (43.3%), followed by lung cancer, lymphoma, leukaemia and melanoma. Overall, 81% had metastatic disease at the time of LM diagnosis; 70% of those with solid tumours and 11% of hematologic patients had brain metastases. 42% of patients with solid tumours had previously received cranial RT for BM (97% WBRT, 3% SRS). For solid tumours, the median time from primary to LM diagnosis was 2 years, versus 11 months for hematologic tumours ($p$ = 0.004). In terms of treatment, 28 received best supportive care (BSC) alone (27 solid tumour, 1 hematologic), 67/187 had RT alone (WBRT in 40%, spine RT in 19%), 46/187 chemotherapy alone (IT ± systemic) and 36/187 both chemotherapy and RT. 10/187 had unknown treatment. MS was 2.4 months overall: 2.3 months for solid tumours and 4.7 months for hematologic ($p$ = 0.0006). MS for breast cancer was 2.8 months, lung 2.2 months, leukaemia 5.8 months and lymphoma 4.6 months. There were no statistical differences in MS within solid or hematologic groups. Patients with no active systemic disease ($N$ = 20) at the time of LM diagnosis had a MS of 3.8 months compared with 2.4 months for those with active disease ($p$ = 0.18). Twenty patients survived longer than 1 year: 10 with hematologic and 10 with solid tumours. No clear differences were found between these 20 patients and the rest of the cohort. The authors concluded the widespread availability of MRI had not significantly impacted survival [6].

Huang and colleagues at Wake Forest University retrospectively reviewed patients who received Gamma Knife SRS ± surgical resection for BM ($N$ = 795; 1999–2012) to determine risk of subsequent development of LM [11]. Those who had surgical resection before SRS received cavity-directed SRS. >90% of tumours resected were internally debulked (in a piecemeal fashion). WBRT was generally reserved for salvage of four or more BM or in the setting of short-interval distant in-brain failure. Diagnosis of LM was by MRI, CT and/or positive CSF cytology. 49/795 developed LM, all within 38 months of the first SRS. The cumulative incidence was 3.0% at 1 year, 5.5% at 2 years and 5.9% at 3 years. 13.3% were asymptomatic and diagnosed on routine imaging. Those who went on to develop LM were significantly younger, were more likely to have a breast primary, were less likely to have lung cancer and had a higher proportion of distant in-brain failure. The relative risk of developing LM after resection of an infratentorial versus supratentorial BM was 2.7 (16.4% vs 6.1%, $p = 0.024$). On MVA, colorectal primary site (HR 4.5, $p < 0.0001$), distant in-brain failure (HR 2.0, $p = 0.007$), breast primary (HR 1.6, $p = 0.05$), number of intracranial BM at the time of initial SRS (HR 1.1, $p = 0.009$) and age (HR 0.9, $p = 0.0006$) were independently associated with LM. Those who had treatment (CSI, IT chemotherapy or capecitabine) lived longer (MS 3.4 months) than those who did not undergo any intervention (MS 1.6 m; $p = 0.01$). MS of patients with breast cancer was longer than all other primary sites (MS 4 vs 1.8 months, $p = 0.03$). Death due to neurologic causes was seen in 69.6% of those with LM versus 39.7% who did not have LM ($p < 0.0001$). Median time from SRS to neurologic death was longer in the setting of LM compared to without LM (11.3 versus 7.3 months; $p = 0.12$). The authors concluded that there was no evidence that surgical resection before SRS significantly altered the risk of LM, despite the fact that the majority of tumours were removed piecemeal. They felt that LM was more likely the result of reseeding of the CNS from progressive systemic disease, given the correlation to distant in-brain failure [11].

Lee et al. reviewed 149 NSCLC patients with CSF-positive LM, 95% adenocarcinoma, from a single institution in South Korea (2001–2009) [19]. CSF sampling was done as per local clinical guidelines in those who had neurologic signs or symptoms or abnormal brain imaging; however, management decisions were at the treating physician's discretion. Median age was 58 years, 86% were ECOG 0–2, and 79.9% were stage IV disease at NSCLC diagnosis. 41.6% had previous BM treated with Gamma Knife SRS or WBRT. There was an EGFR-activating mutation found in 13/23 patients for whom this test was performed. Twenty-six (17.4%) had LM at initial diagnosis of NSCLC. IT chemotherapy was delivered to 73.2%, of whom 15/109 had cytological conversion. In addition to IT chemotherapy, 31.5% received WBRT (30 Gy/10). 18/149 received WBRT without IT chemotherapy, 3 of whom received systemic chemotherapy. 41/149 received cytotoxic chemotherapy, tyrosine kinase inhibitor (TKI) or both. 12% of patients received all three modalities and 13% supportive care only. MS overall was 14 weeks. On MVA, poor ECOG

($p = 0.026$, HR 1.36), high CSF protein level ($p = 0.027$, HR 1.69) and high CSF white blood cell count ($p = 0.015$, HR 1.69) correlated with poor survival. Delivery of IT chemotherapy ($p < 0.001$, HR 0.396), EGFR-TKI use ($p = 0.018$, HR 0.511), WBRT ($p = 0.009$, HR 0.546) and VP shunt ($p = 0.013$, HR 0.448) were associated with improved survival. Encephalopathy, cytotoxic chemotherapy and cytologic conversion were not independent predictors. Notably, the median survival of those with activating EGFR mutations was twice that of patients without [19].

Grommes et al. described a case series ($N = 9$) of EGFR-mutated NSCLC patients who received high-dose weekly erlotinib ± WBRT (5/9) for LM that developed (3/9) or worsened (6/9) following prior therapy with an EGFR TKI [61]. 5/9 had coexistent BM and 6/9 had extracranial metastases. Erlotinib monotherapy was given once weekly at a median dose of 1500 mg (range 900–1500 mg). The response rate was 6/9, with stability in 1/9 and progression in 2/9. The median time to best response was 3.3 months (range 0.8–14.5 months), and the MS was 12 months (range 2.9 m—not reached) [61]. In comparison, the MS after WBRT alone for BM without associated LM in EGFR-mutant NSCLC is 14.5 months [62]. Another published case report describes a patient with LM secondary to EGFR-mutated lung adenocarcinoma refractory to WBRT, who sustained a dramatic clinical and radiologic response to erlotinib [63]. Hata et al. suggested that a TKI should be administered even before WBRT in the EGFR-mutated population [63].

Another retrospective single-institution review focused on NSCLC with LM, without prior BM or spinal metastases [20]. Diagnosis was determined via MRI ± CSF, and all ($N = 51$) received WBRT (2007–2014). Eligibility criteria included ECOG 0–3, histologic confirmation and no previous WBRT or surgery. EGFR and ALK status were not available. WBRT dose was 30 Gy/10 (60.8%) or 20 Gy/5 (39.2%). 70.5% had concurrent BM. Median time to diagnosis of LM after lung cancer diagnosis was 13.2 months. 84.3% died of neurologic progression and 15.7% from systemic progression. MS was 3.9 months, 6-month survival was 19.6%, and 1-year survival was 5.9%. On MVA, worse PS, shorter time to LM diagnosis and concurrent BM were independent predictors of poor survival [20].

Morris and colleagues from MSKCC included 125 patients (2002–2009) with NSCLC and LM, 78% with adenocarcinoma, in a landmark analysis to try to account for the effects of selection bias [21]. This cohort was also treated before widespread testing for driver mutations and use of TKIs. Diagnosis required positive CSF cytology and/or multifocal enhancing subarachnoid nodules on MRI. However, patients were only included if they received therapy within a certain period after diagnosis, survived a predetermined time afterwards (30 days after WBRT and 45 days after IT chemotherapy) and were followed for 45 days or longer. 54/125 had received prior WBRT for BM. Median KPS was 70 (range

30–100), mean age was 59 years, and 80/125 were women. 38/125 had BSC alone, 56/125 WBRT (30–37.5 Gy/10–15), 7/125 IT chemotherapy, 20/125 systemic chemotherapy and 18/125 EGFR-directed TKI. The median survival was 3.0 months (95% CI 2–4 months). Patients receiving WBRT who were included in the landmark analysis were compared with those (N = 59) who had not received WBRT by 30 days, and no differences in OS were seen (p = 0.84). However, patients receiving IT chemotherapy and a minimum follow-up of 45 days (N = 6) survived longer than those who did not (N = 83; p = 0.001). Nine patients with EGFR mutations developed LM at a median of 12 months from primary diagnosis; their MS was 14 months (range 1–28 months). The authors concluded by questioning the routine use of WBRT given the lack of proven survival benefit but acknowledged that due to limitations of their data, improved symptoms and QOL as a result of WBRT could not be ruled out [21].

## Follow-Up

Various criteria have been used in follow-up to evaluate success of treatment, including CSF clearance, improvement in neurologic signs or symptoms, imaging changes or reversal of CSF flow obstruction [33]. QOL has rarely been reported [57]. In Boogerd's randomized trial, CSF was not routinely reexamined since conversion has not been strongly correlated with either clinical response or survival [19, 50]. While examination of MRI imaging can reveal stability or decreased contrast enhancement [20, 43], serial imaging is not yet considered standard due to the absence of data supporting correlation with symptom response [13, 20, 50]. Corticosteroid dose after therapy is also not commonly reported, probably related to a lack of evidence that LM symptomatology is responsive to steroids [2].

## Conclusions

Due to the limitations of available data in terms of heterogeneous patient populations treated largely in the absence of a standard approach, neither the relative contributions of each therapeutic modality to symptom control and survival, nor the impact of selection bias can be separated out at this time. In the spirit of MacKillop's rules for optimal palliative radiotherapy and the absence of a proven benefit from 2 weeks (10 fractions) of treatment, shorter schedules of involved-field RT should be considered if radiotherapy is to be administered. There is an absence of evidence to support whole craniospinal irradiation in solid tumours. Supportive care should be offered to all patients at the time of diagnosis, given the overwhelmingly poor prognosis most will be facing at that time in their disease trajectory. The lack of patient-reported outcomes in the literature is striking and should be considered an area for future investigation, acknowledging the challenges inherent in studying this disease entity. Finally, the potential impact of molecular biomarkers and driver mutations, such as EGFR in lung adenocarcinoma, remains to be elucidated.

## Case Presentation

A 78-year-old female never-smoker of Asian descent presented to the emergency room with a 2-week history of bifrontal headache, nausea, daily emesis, diplopia, dysphagia, decreased hearing, cough and 10 lb. weight loss. Unenhanced CT head suggested intracranial lesions compatible with malignancy, and she was admitted to hospital. MRI brain the following day confirmed multiple enhancing supra- and infratentorial intraparenchymal lesions, largest 3 cm in the left temporal lobe. There

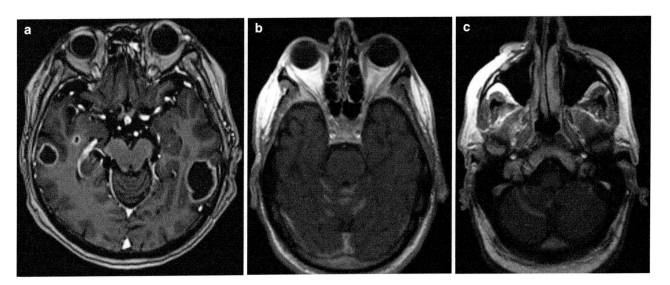

**Fig. 14.3** (a) Axial T1 MP RAGE image of parenchymal brain metastases. (b, c) Axial T1 post-gadolinium images demonstrating patchy leptomeningeal enhancement

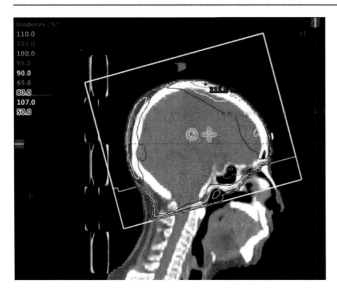

**Fig. 14.4** Digitally reconstructed radiograph of whole brain treatment volume

were also areas of patchy leptomeningeal enhancement (Fig. 14.3) without hydrocephalus, midline shift or herniation. CT chest/abdomen/pelvis revealed a 2 × 2 cm spiculated cavitating right upper lobe mass with multistation mediastinal lymphadenopathy, a small pericardial effusion and bone metastases. After bronchoscopy and CT-guided lung biopsy specimens were non-diagnostic, she underwent lumbar puncture. CSF cytology confirmed adenocarcinoma consistent with lung primary. There was no cell block available on which to perform molecular markers. Although some of her symptoms improved with institution of dexamethasone, her performance status remained poor, and she was a 1–2 person assist for transfers. She completed 20 Gy/5 palliative whole brain radiotherapy (Fig. 14.4) via daily interhospital transfer. She was subsequently admitted to hospice and passed away just over 8 weeks from diagnosis of leptomeningeal carcinomatosis.

## Summary

- Despite an increasing incidence with time, leptomeningeal metastases remain a poorly studied clinical entity, with outcomes no better now than in the 1970s.
- Stratifying patients into poor-risk and good-risk cohorts may inform treatment decision-making, although many patients will have both types of characteristics.
- Palliative radiotherapy is most commonly delivered to areas of greatest symptomatology with the intent of preserving or improving quality of life; however, there are no data supporting an extension of survival, and it is even unknown whether neurologic deterioration is delayed or prevented.

- Palliative radiotherapy to the whole brain and/or portions of the spine is planned using conventional techniques and doses, with minimal toxicity reported.
- Whole craniospinal irradiation is utilized more often for hematologic and primary CNS malignancies compared to solid tumours, however, literature supporting an improvement in outcomes is limited.

## Self-Assessment Questions

1. True or false: Local radiotherapy is more likely to reverse an intracranial versus a spinal CSF blockage.

2. True or false: The relapse-free interval is longer if the patient sustained a partial clinical response to initial therapy versus if they experienced symptom stabilization after initial therapy.

3. Which of the following is NOT both a poor prognostic and poor predictive factor?
   A. Poor performance status
   B. Lung metastases
   C. Cranial nerve dysfunction
   D. Craniospinal fluid impairment

4. A patient presents with cranial neuropathy secondary to leptomeningeal metastases from a solid tumour. Expected outcomes with involved-field (whole brain) radiotherapy are most likely:
   A. Stabilization of symptoms and increase in survival
   B. Improvement of symptoms and increase in survival
   C. Stabilization of symptoms with no impact on survival
   D. Improvement of symptoms with no impact on survival

5. Long-term survival after treatment for LM is mostly likely to correlate with:
   A. Symptom improvement
   B. Decreased contrast enhancement of the leptomeninges on MRI
   C. Decreased corticosteroid dose
   D. Conversion of CSF cytology from positive to negative

## Answers

1. True (*reverses 50% of intracranial* vs *30–35% of spinal*)
2. False ("The relapse-free interval for relapsing patients in one study ranged between 8 and 22 months, with no relationship to response attained to initial therapy [49]".)
3. B (Table 14.4)
4. C (Ref. [41]/Table 14.7)
5. A ("Outcomes seem to correlate more with symptom improvement than CSF clearing (Ref. [42])")

# References

1. National Comprehensive Cancer Network version 1.2016. Central nervous system cancers. Pgs LEPT-1 to LEPT-4, MS-29 to MS-31.
2. Chamberlain M. Combined-modality treatment of leptomeningeal gliomatosis. Neurosurgery. 2003;52(2):324–30.
3. Wasserstrom W, Glass J, Posner J. Diagnosis and treatment of leptomeningeal metastases from solid tumours: experience with 90 patients. Cancer. 1982;49:759–72.
4. Little J, Dale A, Okazaki H. Meningeal carcinomatosis. Arch Neurol. 1974;30:138–43.
5. Mack F, Baumert B, Schafer N, et al. Therapy of leptomeningeal metastasis in solid tumours. Cancer Treat Rev. 2016;43:83–91.
6. Clarke J, Perez H, Jacks L, et al. Leptomeningeal metastases in the MRI era. Neurology. 2010;74(18):1449–54.
7. Caraceni A, Martini C, Simonetti M. Neurological problems in advanced cancer. In: Doyle D, Hanks G, Cherny N, Calman K, editors. Oxford textbook of palliative medicine. 3rd ed. UK: Oxford University Press; 2005.
8. Olson M, Chernik N, Posner J. Infiltration of the leptomeninges by systemic cancer: a clinical and pathologic study. Arch Neurol. 1974;30:122–37.
9. Glass J, Melamed M, Chernik N, et al. Malignant cells in the cerebrospinal fluid: the meaning of a positive CSF cytology. Neurology. 1979;29:1369–75.
10. Rosen S, Aisner J, Makuch R, et al. Carcinomatous leptomeningitis in small cell lung cancer. Medicine. 1982;61(1):45–53.
11. Huang A, Huang K, Page B, et al. Risk factors for leptomeningeal carcinomatosis in patients with brain metastases who have previously undergone stereotactic radiosurgery. J Neurooncol. 2014;120:163–9.
12. Bartsch R, Berghoff A, Preusser M. Optimal management of brain metastases from breast cancer. CNS Drugs. 2013;27:121–34.
13. Waki F, Ando M, Takashima A, et al. Prognostic factors and clinical outcomes in patients with leptomeningeal metastasis from solid tumours. J Neurooncol. 2009;93:205–12.
14. Pavlidis N. The diagnostic and therapeutic management of leptomeningeal carcinomatosis. Ann Oncol. 2004;15(Suppl 4):iv285–91.
15. Ihde D, Glatstein E, Pass H. Small cell lung cancer. In: DeVita V, Hellman S, Rosenberg S, editors. Cancer: principles & practice of oncology. 5th ed. USA: Lippincott-Raven; 1997.
16. Aisner J, Aisner S, Ostrow S, et al. Meningeal carcinomatosis from small cell carcinoma of the lung. Acta Cytol. 1979;23(4):292–6.
17. Gonzalez-Vitale J, Garcia-Bunuel R. Meningeal carcinomatosis. Cancer. 1976;37:2906–11.
18. DeAngelis L, Boutros D. Leptomeningeal metastasis. Cancer Investig. 2005;23:145–54.
19. Lee SJ, Lee JI, Nam DH, et al. Leptomeningeal carcinomatosis in non-small cell lung cancer patients: impact on survival and correlated prognostic factors. J Thorac Oncol. 2013;8(2):185–91.
20. Ozdemir Y, Yildirim B, Topkan E. Whole brain radiotherapy in management of non-small cell carcinoma associated leptomeningeal carcinomatosis: evaluation of prognostic factors. J Neurooncol. 2016;129:329–35.
21. Morris P, Reiner A, Rosenvald Szenberg O, et al. Leptomeningeal metastasis from non-small cell lung cancer: survival and the impact of whole brain radiotherapy. J Thorac Oncol. 2012;7(2):382–5.
22. Nugent J, Bunn P, Matthews M, et al. CNS metastases in small cell bronchogenic carcinoma: increasing frequency and changing pattern with lengthening survival. Cancer. 1979;44:1885–93.
23. Clarke J. Leptomeningeal metastasis from systemic cancer. Continuum (Minneap Minn). 2012;18(2):328–42.
24. Griffo Y, Obbens E. Neurological complications. In: Walsh D, Caraceni A, Fainsinger R, Foley K, Glare P, Goh C, Lloyd-Williams M, Nunez Olarte JM, Radbruch L, editors. Palliative medicine. New York: Saunders Elsevier; 2009.
25. Van der Ree T, Dippel D, Avezaat C, et al. Leptomeningeal metastasis after surgical resection of brain metastasis. J Neurol Neurosurg Psychiatry. 1999;66(2):225–7.
26. Liaw C, Ng K, Huang J, et al. Meningeal carcinomatosis from solid tumours: clinical analysis of 42 cases. J Formos Med Assoc. 1992;91:299–303.
27. Foley KM. Acute and chronic cancer pain syndromes. In: Doyle D, Hanks G, Cherny N, Calman K, editors. Oxford textbook of palliative medicine. 3rd ed. UK: Oxford University Press; 2005.
28. Feyer P, Sautter-Bihl ML, Budach W, et al. DEGRO practical guidelines for palliative radiotherapy of breast cancer patients: brain metastases and leptomeningeal carcinomatosis. Strahlenther Onkol. 2010;186:63–9.
29. Mittl R Jr, Yousem D. Frequency of unexplained meningeal enhancement in the brain after lumbar puncture. Am J Neuroradiol. 1994;15(4):633–8.
30. Freilich R, Krol G, DeAngelis L. Neuroimaging and cerebrospinal fluid cytology in the diagnosis of leptomeningeal metastasis. Ann Neurol. 1995;38:51–7.
31. Chamberlain M. Comparative spine imaging in leptomeningeal metastases. J Neurooncol. 1995;23:233–8.
32. Cheng T, O'Neill B, Scheithauer B, et al. Chronic meningitis: the role of meningeal or cortical biopsy. Neurosurgery. 1994;34:590–5.
33. Chamberlain M. Leptomeningeal metastasis. Curr Opin Neurol. 2009;22:665–74.
34. Shapiro W, Johanson C, Boogerd W. Treatment modalities for leptomeningeal metastases. Semin Oncol. 2009;36(4 Suppl 2):S46–54.
35. Mason W, DeAngelis L, Yeh S. 111Indium-DPTA cerebrospinal fluid studies in leptomeningeal metastases predict intrathecal methotrexate distribution and outcome in patients with leptomeningeal metastases. Neurology. 1998;50:438–43.
36. Kak M, Nanda R, Ramsdale E, et al. Treatment of leptomeningeal carcinomatosis: current challenges and future opportunities. J Clin Neurosci. 2015;22:632–7.
37. Chamberlain M, Goulart B. Are prognostic factors for leptomeningeal metastases defined sufficiently to permit tailored treatment? J Thorac Oncol. 2013;8(7):E66–7.
38. Chamberlain M, Eaton K. Is there a role for whole brain radiotherapy in the treatment of leptomeningeal metastases? J Thorac Oncol. 2012;7(7):1204.
39. Chamberlain M, Soffietti R, Raizer J, et al. Leptomeningeal metastases: a response assessment in neuro-oncology critical review of endpoints and response criteria of published randomized clinical trials. Neuro Oncol. 2014;16:1176–85.
40. Glantz M, Hall W, Cole B, et al. Diagnosis, management and survival of patients with leptomeningeal cancer based on cerebrospinal fluid-flow status. Cancer. 1995;75:2919–31.
41. Elmore S, Balboni T. Symptom control and predictors of survival in leptomeningeal carcinomatosis of the neuraxis treated with radiation therapy. Int J Radiat Oncol Biol Phys. 2015;93(3 Suppl):E478–9. Abstr 3195
42. Boogerd W, Hart A, van der Sande J, et al. Meningeal carcinomatosis in breast cancer: prognostic factors and influence of treatment. Cancer. 1991;67:1685–95.
43. Gani C, Muller A, Eckert F, et al. Outcome after whole brain radiotherapy alone in intracranial leptomeningeal carcinomatosis from solid tumours. Strahlenther Onkol. 2012;188:148–53.
44. Omuro A, Lallana E, Bilsky M, et al. Ventriculoperitoneal shunt in patients with leptomeningeal metastasis. Neurology. 2005;64:1625–7.
45. Jung T, Chung W, Oh I. The prognostic significance of surgically treated hydrocephalus in leptomeningeal metastases. Clin Neurol Neurosurg. 2014;119:80–3.
46. Mackillop WJ. The principles of palliative radiotherapy: a radiation oncologist's perspective. Can J Oncol. 1996;6(Suppl 1):5–11.

47. Chamberlain M, Kormanik P. Prognostic significance of 111indium-DTPA CSF flow studies in leptomeningeal metastases. Neurology. 1996;46:1674–7.
48. Grossman S, Trump C, Chen D, et al. Cerebrospinal fluid abnormalities in patients with neoplastic meningitis. Am J Med. 1982;73:641–7.
49. Siegal T, Lossos A, Pfeffer M. Leptomeningeal metastases: analysis of 31 patients with sustained off-therapy response following combined modality therapy. Neurology. 1994;44:1463–9.
50. Boogerd W, van den Bent M, Koehler P, et al. The relevance of intraventricular chemotherapy for leptomeningeal metastasis in breast cancer: a randomized study. Eur J Cancer. 2004;40:2726–33.
51. Aisner J, Ostrow S, Govindan S, et al. Leptomeningeal carcinomatosis in small cell carcinoma of the lung. Med Pediatr Oncol. 1981;9:47–59.
52. Jo K, Lim D, Kim S, et al. Leptomeningeal seeding in patients with brain metastases treated by gamma knife radiosurgery. J Neurooncol. 2012;109:293–9.
53. Hashimoto K, Narita Y, Miyakita Y, et al. Comparison of clinical outcomes of surgery followed by local brain radiotherapy and surgery followed by whole brain radiotherapy in patients with a single brain metastasis: Single Centre retrospective analysis. Int J Radiat Oncol Biol Phys. 2011;81:E475–80.
54. Suki D, Abouassi H, Patel A, et al. Comparative risk of leptomeningeal disease after resection or stereotactic radiosurgery for solid tumour metastasis to the posterior fossa. J Neurosurg. 2008;108:248–57.
55. Sause W, Crowley J, Eyre H, et al. Whole brain irradiation and intrathecal methotrexate in the treatment of solid tumour leptomeningeal metastases – a Southwest Oncology Group study. J Neurooncol. 1988;6:107–12.
56. Victoria Hospice Society Learning Centre for Palliative Care. In: Downing GM, Wainwright W, editors. Medical care of the dying. 4th ed. Victoria: Victoria Hospice Society; 2006.
57. Dudani S, Mazzarello S, Hilton J, et al. Optimal management of leptomeningeal carcinomatosis in breast cancer patients: a systematic review. Clin Breast Cancer. 2016;16(6):456–70.
58. Heathfield K, Williams J. Carcinomatosis of the meninges: clinical and pathological aspects. Br Med J. 1956;1(4962):328–40.
59. Emoto S, Ishigami H, Yamaguchi H, et al. Frequent development of leptomeningeal carcinomatosis in patients with peritoneal dissemination of gastric cancer. Gastric Cancer. 2011;14:390–5.
60. Lukas R, Mata-Machado N, Nicholas M, et al. Leptomeningeal carcinomatosis in esophagus cancer: a case series and systematic review of the literature. Dis Esophagus. 2015;28:772–81.
61. Grommes C, Oxnard G, Kris M, et al. Pulsatile high-dose weekly erlotinib for CNS metastases from EGFR mutant non-small cell lung cancer. Neuro Oncol. 2011;13(12):1364–9.
62. Eichler A, Kahle K, Wang D, et al. EGFR mutation status and survival after diagnosis of brain metastasis in non-small cell lung cancer. Neuro Oncol. 2010;12:1193–9.
63. Hata A, Katakami N, Kaji R, et al. Erlotinib for whole brain radiotherapy refractory leptomeningeal metastases after gefitinib failure in a lung adenocarcinoma patient. J Thorac Oncol. 2012;7(4):770–1.

# Optic Pathway Gliomas

Arnold C. Paulino

## Learning Objectives

- To determine the most common histology, risk factors, and clinical presentation associated with optic pathway glioma.
- To define the roles of observation, surgery, chemotherapy, and radiotherapy in the management of optic pathway glioma.
- To describe the results of treatment, including survival, progression-free survival, and visual preservation outcomes with the different treatment modalities.
- To determine the risk of complications with the use of radiotherapy as well as tolerance doses of the surrounding normal organs in the treatment of optic pathway glioma.

## Epidemiology

Optic pathway gliomas account for about two thirds of all primary optic pathway tumors [1]. Optic pathway glioma (OPG) is a relatively rare tumor, accounting for 1% of all intracranial tumors. In children, OPG comprises about 5% of all brain tumors. These tumors usually present during the first 7 years of life, with about 90% of cases diagnosed within the first two decades of life [2]. Males and females are equally affected. In adults, OPG can be divided into two groups. The first includes patients who were diagnosed as children and followed through adulthood. The second group includes patients diagnosed with OPG during adulthood.

The optic pathway includes the retina, optic nerve, optic chiasm, optic radiations, and occipital lobe. When OPG is diagnosed, it is often classified as prechiasmatic, chiasmatic,

and postchiasmatic. Chiasmatic and postchiasmatic OPGs are more common in sporadic cases, whereas those limited to the optic nerve (prechiasmatic) are more frequently found in children with neurofibromatosis type 1 (NF1). In one study, the most common site of involvement in the NF1 patients was the optic nerve (66%), followed by the chiasm (62%). In the non-NF1 patients, the chiasm was the most common site of involvement (91%), while the optic nerves were involved in only 32% [3].

## Risk Factors

OPG is seen in about 15–20% of patients with NF1, an autosomal dominant disorder with an incidence of 1 in 2000–2500 individuals [4, 5]. The main disease manifestations of NF1 include café au lait macules, skinfold freckling (axillary and inguinal regions), Lisch nodules or iris hamartomas, OPGs, and skeletal deformities. In a study from Cincinnati, 18% of 826 NF1 individuals were identified to have OPG with a median age at detection of 3 years. Fifteen percent of OPG patients had a radiologic or clinical progression requiring therapy [6]. Conversely, in series of OPG patients, about 20–58% of patients have been reported to have NF1 [7, 8].

## Diagnosis

### Clinical Presentation

Many patients with OPG are asymptomatic, particularly those with NF1 [6]. For symptomatic patients, visual loss is the most common complaint. Patients with optic nerve gliomas typically present with unilateral, slow vision loss with a relative afferent pupillary defect, optic disk swelling or atrophy, or strabismus. Ocular pain is uncommon, but proptosis can be a presenting sign. In tumors with chiasmatic involvement, bitemporal field defects can be seen. Intracranial extension of the tumor can result in hypothalamic and endo-

A. C. Paulino
Department of Radiation Oncology, MD Anderson
Cancer Center, Houston, TX, USA
e-mail: apaulino@mdanderson.org

© Springer International Publishing AG, part of Springer Nature 2018
E. L. Chang et al. (eds.), *Adult CNS Radiation Oncology*, https://doi.org/10.1007/978-3-319-42878-9_15

crine problems. Malignant optic gliomas have been reported in adults and can present as sudden visual loss in 70–80% of patients [9].

## Diagnostic Imaging

On magnetic resonance imaging (MRI) of the brain, these lesions are T1-hypointense and T2-hyperintense with typically homogeneous gadolinium enhancement. Larger tumors may present with heterogeneous enhancement and may be associated with hydrocephalus. MRI with fat suppression can be done to visualize the entire optic pathway.

## Pathology

Most OPGs are low-grade astrocytomas, of which pilocytic astrocytomas are the predominant subtype. Malignant transformation is unusual. Optic nerve gliomas are typically expansile lesions which transgress the pia; on microscopic examination, the optic nerve is surrounded by neoplastic astrocytes with reactive elements enclosed within the dura mater. Pilomyxoid astrocytomas, fibrillary or diffuse astrocytomas, and gangliogliomas have also been reported but are not as common as pilocytic astrocytomas.

## Overall Treatment Strategy

### Tissue Diagnosis

Currently, tissue diagnosis is recommended in most tumors that look like OPG. In one study, MRI was shown to have a sensitivity of 83.3% and a specificity of 50% for diagnosing chiasmatic-hypothalamic gliomas [10]. However, most agree that radiologic diagnosis is sufficient in infants with chiasmatic-hypothalamic lesions and in children with NF1 [11].

### Observation

In general, the management of OPG can include observation, surgery, chemotherapy, and radiotherapy. Because of its indolent nature, observation of OPG has been performed, especially in children with NF1 where tumors can "wax and wane." Occasionally, OPGs may undergo spontaneous regression [12]. One of the hardest decisions is to decide when to intervene and treat the patient. Considerations for intervention include functional, typically visual, and neurologic deterioration. In patients with non-NF1 OPG, neuraxis dissemination and diencephalic syndrome may trigger intervention [13].

## Surgery

Complete resection of the tumor is recommended for the glioma confined just to the optic nerve, presenting with complete visual loss. For other tumors, a biopsy or surgical debulking have been reported. In one study of 42 children with OPG, 22 debulking procedures were performed. None of the patients had visual deterioration but six had diabetes insipidus (three permanent, three transient). One had transient hemiparesis that improved during rehabilitation. Surgery alone was found to control 13 of 17 tumors. Surgery was able to relieve mass effect and in some cases delay radiotherapy (RT). The authors conclude that surgical debulking of tumor is safe and effective for carefully selected patients [14]. Others have reported improvements in tumor control by surgical debulking while others have not [15–17].

## Chemotherapy

Chemotherapy is often used in children with OPG who have subtotal resection/biopsy to delay the use of RT. Delay in the delivery of RT can be beneficial in children with low-grade glioma as shown by better neurocognitive outcomes in older children receiving conformal RT [18]. The standard chemotherapy regimen consists of vincristine and carboplatin ("Packer regimen"). Packer et al. reported on 78 children with a mean age of 3 years who had newly diagnosed, progressive low-grade gliomas were treated with combined carboplatin and vincristine chemotherapy. Majority had diencephalic tumors, and the objective response rate was 56%. The 2- and 3-year progression-free survival (PFS) rates were 75% and 68%, respectively [19]. A phase II Pediatric Oncology Group (POG) was conducted to evaluate the activity of carboplatin in children ≤5 years with progressive optic pathway tumors (OPTs). Of the 50 children, 21 had progressive disease (15 during the course of carboplatin therapy and 6 patients progressed after) [20]. In the HIT-LGG 1996 study, 198 patients with a median age of 3.6 years had either a chiasmatic-hypothalamic ($n = 144$), chiasmatic ($n = 34$) or hypothalamic tumor ($n = 20$), and 98 of these children had severe visual impairment as their first symptom. A total of 123 children received vincristine and carboplatin at a median age of 3.7 years, of which 105 had initial complete or partial response or stable disease. The 5-year overall survival was 93% for the entire group of patients; the 5-year PFS for those receiving chemotherapy was 61%, with the 5-year radiotherapy-free survival was 83% [21]. The literature is scarce regarding the use of chemotherapy in adult patients with OPG. A Canadian study of adolescent patients with OPG suggests that chemotherapy be considered for first-line treatment rather than RT for progressive disease. In this particular report, children >10 years had PFS comparable to younger children with first-line chemotherapy, avoiding potential RT-related toxicity [22]. Many institutions, however, consider RT to be the standard treatment for progressive OPG in children greater than 10 years of age and adult patients [23].

## Indication for Irradiation

Because most of the OPG patients will survive for a long time, minimizing the sequelae of treatment is paramount in the management of this disease. As such, RT is considered to be the standard treatment for progressive OPG in adult patients, while for children <10 years old, most would consider chemotherapy to be the standard therapy. In our institution, children >10 years requiring treatment are treated with RT although there is no consensus in the literature [11, 22–25].

## Target Volume Delineation and Radiotherapy Dose Prescription

The type of OPG often dictates what imaging study to use for target delineation. In pilocytic astrocytoma, T1 enhancement is often seen and is utilized for gross tumor volume (GTV) delineation. For other low-grade gliomas, tumors are often non-enhancing, and FLAIR abnormalities are used for GTV delineation. The safety margin beyond the GTV have ranged from 0 to 10 mm for the clinical target volume (CTV). Most would use a 3 mm margin around the CTV to create the planning target volume (PTV). At St. Jude Children's Research Hospital, a 10 mm margin was added to the GTV to create the CTV, while the Children's Oncology Group ACNS0221 employed a 5 mm margin for the CTV [26]. A previous study did not find a difference between 5 or 10 mm safety margin for the CTV [27]. At the Dana-Farber Cancer Institute where stereotactic RT was used, the GTV and CTV are essentially the same, with a 2 mm expansion for the PTV [28]. Typically dose ranges from 45 to 50.4 Gy for pilocytic astrocytomas and 50.4 to 54 Gy for non-pilocytic low-grade gliomas.

For the rare malignant glioma of the optic pathway, both the contrast-enhanced T1 and FLAIR images are employed to create the GTV and CTV. In our institution the FLAIR abnormality is typically covered by the 50 Gy isodose line, while the tumor gross disease with T1 enhancement gets the higher dose, typically 54 Gy because of the tolerance of the optic nerve and chiasm.

## Organs at Risk and Tolerance Doses

Table 15.1 lists the normal tissue constraints that are used by the author for treatment of optic pathway tumors.

**Table 15.1** Normal tissue dose constraints for optic pathway glioma

| Organ | Constraints |
|---|---|
| Lens | $D_{max} \leq 6$ Gy |
| Retina | $D_{max} \leq 50.4$ Gy |
| Optic nerve | $D_{max} \leq 54$ Gy |
| Optic chiasm | $D_{max} \leq 54$ Gy |
| Hippocampus | $D_{max} \leq 16$ Gy<br>No more than 9 Gy to 100% of volume |
| Brain stem | $D_{max} \leq 54$ Gy |
| Cochleae | $D_{mean} < 37$ Gy |
| Lacrimal gland | $D_{mean} < 36$ Gy |
| Pituitary gland | $D_{max} < 45$ Gy |

$D_{max}$ = maximum dose, $D_{mean}$ = mean dose

## Radiation Toxicity: Acute and Late

The acute effects of radiation can include erythema and itching of irradiated skin, partial alopecia, fatigue, and conjunctivitis. Late effects and possible complications of radiotherapy may include cataract, cognitive dysfunction, endocrine dysfunction, Moyamoya disease, dryness of the eye, and secondary malignancy [29]. Blindness is uncommon and <5% when the $D_{max}$ or maximum dose to the optic nerves and chiasm is less than 54 Gy and retina is <50 Gy. In patients with NF1, secondary tumors and Moyamoya disease are more frequent with the use of RT [30, 31].

Protons may be able to decrease the chance of developing a secondary neoplasm as integral dose will be less [32]. It may also minimize the low-dose region in the hippocampus and hypothalamus that one gets with the use of photons. In one study, protons resulted in reduced doses to the contralateral optic nerve, optic chiasm, pituitary gland, and bilateral temporal and frontal lobes compared to photons [33].

## Radiotherapy Outcomes

### Tumor Control and Survival

Table 15.2 lists multiple single-institution studies using RT as the primary treatment for OPG. In some of the studies, about 20–40% of the patients are adolescents or adult patients. The 5- and 10-year overall survival rates range from 90% to 100% and 79% to 94%, while the 10-year PFS rates range from 69% to 100% [8, 34–38]. These results compare favorably to patients treated with primary chemotherapy where the 5-year PFS rates are in the range of 30–40% [11]. As a result many children treated with primary chemotherapy require more than one chemotherapy regimen. Despite these results, younger children <10 years old with progressive OPG are typically treated with chemotherapy first

**Table 15.2** Overall and progression-free survival and visual outcomes in patients with optic pathway gliomas treated with radiotherapy

| First author Institution Reference | Number of patients | Age | Overall survival | Progression-free survival | Visual status |
|---|---|---|---|---|---|
| Combs et al. University of Heidelberg [38] | 15 | Median, 6.9 years (8 months to 33 years) | 90% (5 years) | 92% (3 years) 72% (5 years) | Vision improved in 40% and was stable in 47% |
| Erkal et al. Ankara University [36] | 33 | Mean, 13.6 years (0.5–16.1 years) | 93% (5 years) 79% (10 years) | 82% (5 years) 77% (10 years) | Vision improved in 34% and was stable in 54% |
| Grabenbauer et al. University Hospitals of Erlangen-Nurnberg [37] | 25 | 40% were >15 years | 94% (10 years) | 69% (10 years) | Vision improved in 36% and was stable in 52% |
| Horwich et al. Royal Marsden Hospital [35] | 29 | 21% were >15 years | 100% (5 years) 93% (10 years) | 86% (10 years) | Vision improved in 43% and was stable in 48% |
| Khafaga et al. King Faisal Specialist Hospital [8] | 22 | 22% >10 years old | 79.5% (10 years) | 80% (5 years) | Vision improved in 15% and was stable in 71% |
| Tao et al. Harvard University [34] | 29 | Median, 6.6 years (1.3–19 years) | 89% (10 years) | 100% (10 years) | Vision improved in 27% and was stable in 54% |

because of the possible side effects of RT on cognition and endocrine function [39]. In NF1 patients, secondary tumors and vascular problems are heightened by the use of RT, so chemotherapy is usually the first-line treatment for progressive OPG [30, 31].

## Visual Acuity

Table 15.2 lists the visual outcomes of patients treated with RT for OPG. In general, about one third of patients had improvement in vision while another one half had stabilization [8, 34–38]. The results for visual outcome after primary chemotherapy appear to be worse compared to primary RT. In a study of 20 optic glioma patients treated with conformal RT, patients who received chemotherapy prior to RT had worse visual acuity compared to those treated with primary RT [40]. In another OPG study, older children treated with RT had better visual acuity compared to younger children treated with primary chemotherapy [41]. Published studies on childhood low-grade gliomas have not shown that chemotherapy improves vision in the majority of children with OPG [42].

## Follow-Up: Radiographic Assessment

For patients with OPG being observed for NF1, MRI of the brain is typically done every 3 months during the first year and less frequently (every 6 months then every year) thereafter. These tumors tend to wax and wane and are more indolent compared to the non-NF1 OPG.

For patients receiving RT for OPG, we typically follow these patients with a MRI of the brain and visual examina-tion every 4 months for the first 2 years and then every 6 months for the next 3 years and yearly thereafter.

## Case Presentation

The patient is a 19-year-old male who initially was diag-nosed with a hypothalamic-chiasmatic optic pathway gli-oma after a biopsy when he was 9 years old. At presentation he had right eye blindness, and he was subsequently treated with 80 weeks of vincristine and carboplatin and had stable disease until when he was 18 years old when he was noticed to have progression. Representative MRI slices are shown in Fig. 15.1a–c. The patient was treated using protons to a dose of 50.4 cobalt Gy equivalent (CGE). The CTV was 0.5 cm beyond the GTV, respecting anatomic barriers (Fig. 15.1d–f).

## Summary

Most optic pathway gliomas (OPGs) are pilocytic astrocy-tomas, but other types of low-grade and malignant gliomas have been reported. The role of surgery is to obtain tissue diagnosis or resection in the patient with glioma confined just to the optic nerve and complete visual loss. Chemotherapy consisting of carboplatin and vincristine is a popular treatment approach to delay radiotherapy (RT) in children <10 years and preserve neurocognitive function. In patients with neurofibromatosis, type 1, RT is often avoided because of the higher chance of developing Moyamoya syndrome and secondary neoplasms. RT is the mainstay of treatment for non-NF1 patients who are ≥10 years. The 10-year overall survival and progression-

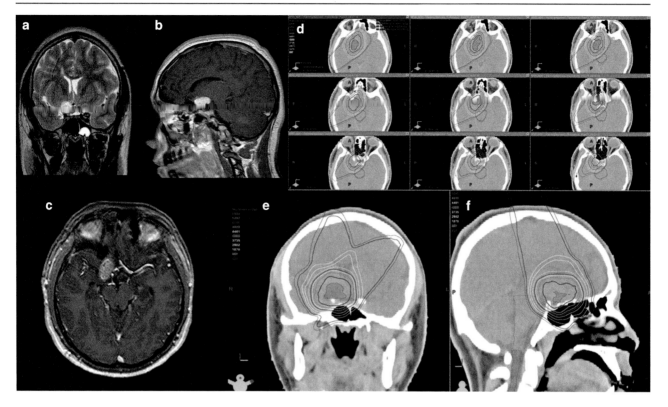

**Fig. 15.1** Proton therapy in a 19-year-old patient with optic pathway glioma. (**a–c**) Coronal, sagittal, and axial magnetic resonance imaging (MRI) slices of a patient with progressive pilocytic astrocytoma of the right hypothalamic optic pathway. (**d–f**) Axial, coronal, and sagittal slices showing treatment plan with protons. The prescribed dose was 50.4 cobalt Gy equivalent. The gross tumor volume (GTV) is outlined in maroon, while the clinical target volume (CTV) is outlined in mustard

free survival rates range from 80% to 95% and 70% to 85%, respectively, with RT. In addition, stabilization and improvement in vision have been observed in more than 70% of patients receiving RT.

## Self-Assessment Questions

1. What proportion of neurofibromatosis type 1 patients will have optic pathway glioma?
   A. <1%
   B. 15%
   C. 50%
   D. 85%

2. What is the most likely histology for an optic pathway glioma?
   A. Ganglioglioma
   B. Pleomorphic xanthoastrocytoma
   C. Pilocytic astrocytoma
   D. Subependymal giant cell astrocytoma

3. What would be the most appropriate treatment for an optic nerve glioma in an eye with complete visual loss?
   A. Stereotactic radiosurgery
   B. Carboplatin and vincristine chemotherapy

C. Intensity modulated radiation therapy
D. Surgical resection

4. At 10 years after radiotherapy, what is the expected local control for an optic pathway glioma?
   A. 20%
   B. 40%
   C. 60%
   D. 80%

5. After radiotherapy for an optic pathway glioma, what is the expected proportion of patients with stable or improved vision?
   A. 20%
   B. 40%
   C. 60%
   D. 80%

## Answers

1. B
2. C
3. D
4. D
5. C

# References

1. Dutton JJ. Gliomas of the anterior visual pathway. Surv Ophthalmol. 1994;38(5):427–52.
2. Binning MJ, Liu JK, Kestle JR, et al. Optic pathway gliomas: a review. Neurosurg Focus. 2007;23(5):E2.
3. Kornreich L, Blaser S, Schwarz M, et al. Optic pathway glioma: correlation of imaging findings with the presence of neurofibromatosis. AJNR Am J Neuroradiol. 2001;22(10):1963–9.
4. King A, Listernick R, Charrow J, et al. Optic pathway gliomas in neurofibromatosis type 1: the effect of presenting symptoms on outcome. Am J Med Genet A. 2003;122a(2):95–9.
5. Listernick R, Louis DN, Packer RJ, et al. Optic pathway gliomas in children with neurofibromatosis 1: consensus statement from the NF1 Optic Pathway Glioma Task Force. Ann Neurol. 1997;41(2):143–9.
6. Prada CE, Hufnagel RB, Hummel TR, et al. The use of magnetic resonance imaging screening for optic pathway gliomas in children with neurofibromatosis type 1. J Pediatr. 2015;167(4):851–6.e1.
7. Nicolin G, Parkin P, Mabbott D, et al. Natural history and outcome of optic pathway gliomas in children. Pediatr Blood Cancer. 2009;53(7):1231–7.
8. Khafaga Y, Hassounah M, Kandil A, et al. Optic gliomas: a retrospective analysis of 50 cases. Int J Radiat Oncol Biol Phys. 2003;56(3):807–12.
9. Hartel PH, Rosen C, Larzo C, et al. Malignant optic nerve glioma (glioblastoma multiforme): a case report and literature review. W V Med J. 2006;102(4):29–31.
10. Bommakanti K, Panigrahi M, Yarlagadda R, et al. Optic chiasmatic-hypothalamic gliomas: is tissue diagnosis essential? Neurol India. 2010;58(6):833–40.
11. Fried I, Tabori U, Tihan T, et al. Optic pathway gliomas: a review. CNS Oncol. 2013;2(2):143–59.
12. Parsa CF, Hoyt CS, Lesser RL, et al. Spontaneous regression of optic gliomas: thirteen cases documented by serial neuroimaging. Arch Ophthalmol. 2001;119(4):516–29.
13. Addy DP, Hudson FP. Diencephalic syndrome of infantile emaciation. Analysis of literature and report of further 3 cases. Arch Dis Child. 1972;47(253):338–43.
14. Goodden J, Pizer B, Pettorini B, et al. The role of surgery in optic pathway/hypothalamic gliomas in children. J Neurosurg Pediatr. 2014;13(1):1–12.
15. Hoffman HJ, Soloniuk DS, Humphreys RP, et al. Management and outcome of low-grade astrocytomas of the midline in children: a retrospective review. Neurosurgery. 1993;33(6):964–71.
16. Steinbok P, Hentschel S, Almqvist P, et al. Management of optic chiasmatic/hypothalamic astrocytomas in children. Can J Neurol Sci. 2002;29(2):132–8.
17. Wisoff JH, Abbott R, Epstein F. Surgical management of exophytic chiasmatic-hypothalamic tumors of childhood. J Neurosurg. 1990;73(5):661–7.
18. Merchant TE, Conklin HM, Wu S, et al. Late effects of conformal radiation therapy for pediatric patients with low-grade glioma: prospective evaluation of cognitive, endocrine, and hearing deficits. J Clin Oncol. 2009;27(22):3691–7.
19. Packer RJ, Ater J, Allen J, et al. Carboplatin and vincristine chemotherapy for children with newly diagnosed progressive low-grade gliomas. J Neurosurg. 1997;86(5):747–54.
20. Mahoney DH Jr, Cohen ME, Friedman HS, et al. Carboplatin is effective therapy for young children with progressive optic pathway tumors: a Pediatric Oncology Group phase II study. Neuro Oncol. 2000;2(4):213–20.
21. Gnekow AK, Kortmann RD, Pietsch T, et al. Low grade chiasmatic-hypothalamic glioma-carboplatin and vincristin chemotherapy effectively defers radiotherapy within a comprehensive treatment strategy — report from the multicenter treatment study for children and adolescents with a low grade glioma — HIT-LGG 1996 — of the Society of Pediatric Oncology and Hematology (GPOH). Klin Padiatr. 2004;216(6):331–42.
22. Chong AL, Pole JD, Scheinemann K, et al. Optic pathway gliomas in adolescence—time to challenge treatment choices? Neuro Oncol. 2013;15(3):391–400.
23. Jahraus CD, Tarbell NJ. Optic pathway gliomas. Pediatr Blood Cancer. 2006;46(5):586–96.
24. Shofty B, Mauda-Havakuk M, Weizman L, et al. The effect of chemotherapy on optic pathway gliomas and their sub-components: a volumetric MR analysis study. Pediatr Blood Cancer. 2015;62(8):1353–9.
25. Stieber VW. Radiation therapy for visual pathway tumors. J Neuroophthalmol. 2008;28(3):222–30.
26. Merchant TE, Kun LE, Wu S, et al. Phase II trial of conformal radiation therapy for pediatric low-grade glioma. J Clin Oncol. 2009;27(22):3598–604.
27. Paulino AC, Mazloom A, Terashima K, et al. Intensity-modulated radiotherapy (IMRT) in pediatric low-grade glioma. Cancer. 2013;119(14):2654–9.
28. Marcus KJ, Goumnerova L, Billett AL, et al. Stereotactic radiotherapy for localized low-grade gliomas in children: final results of a prospective trial. Int J Radiat Oncol Biol Phys. 2005;61(2):374–9.
29. Jeganathan VS, Wirth A, MacManus MP. Ocular risks from orbital and periorbital radiation therapy: a critical review. Int J Radiat Oncol Biol Phys. 2011;79(3):650–9.
30. Desai SS, Paulino AC, Mai WY, et al. Radiation-induced moyamoya syndrome. Int J Radiat Oncol Biol Phys. 2006;65(4):1222–7.
31. Sharif S, Ferner R, Birch JM, et al. Second primary tumors in neurofibromatosis 1 patients treated for optic glioma: substantial risks after radiotherapy. J Clin Oncol. 2006;24(16):2570–5.
32. Sethi RV, Shih HA, Yeap BY, et al. Second nonocular tumors among survivors of retinoblastoma treated with contemporary photon and proton radiotherapy. Cancer. 2014;120(1):126–33.
33. Fuss M, Hug EB, Schaefer RA, et al. Proton radiation therapy (PRT) for pediatric optic pathway gliomas: comparison with 3D planned conventional photons and a standard photon technique. Int J Radiat Oncol Biol Phys. 1999;45(5):1117–26.
34. Tao ML, Barnes PD, Billett AL, et al. Childhood optic chiasm gliomas: radiographic response following radiotherapy and long-term clinical outcome. Int J Radiat Oncol Biol Phys. 1997;39(3):579–87.
35. Horwich A, Bloom HJ. Optic gliomas: radiation therapy and prognosis. Int J Radiat Oncol Biol Phys. 1985;11(6):1067–79.
36. Erkal HS, Serin M, Cakmak A. Management of optic pathway and chiasmatic-hypothalamic gliomas in children with radiation therapy. Radiother Oncol. 1997;45(1):11–5.
37. Grabenbauer GG, Schuchardt U, Buchfelder M, et al. Radiation therapy of optico-hypothalamic gliomas (OHG)—radiographic response, vision and late toxicity. Radiother Oncol. 2000;54(3):239–45.

38. Combs SE, Schulz-Ertner D, Moschos D, et al. Fractionated stereotactic radiotherapy of optic pathway gliomas: tolerance and long-term outcome. Int J Radiat Oncol Biol Phys. 2005;62(3):814–9.

39. Lacaze E, Kieffer V, Streri A, et al. Neuropsychological outcome in children with optic pathway tumours when first-line treatment is chemotherapy. Br J Cancer. 2003;89(11):2038–44.

40. Awdeh RM, Kiehna EN, Drewry RD, et al. Visual outcomes in pediatric optic pathway glioma after conformal radiation therapy. Int J Radiat Oncol Biol Phys. 2012;84(1):46–51.

41. Campagna M, Opocher E, Viscardi E, et al. Optic pathway glioma: long-term visual outcome in children without neurofibromatosis type-1. Pediatr Blood Cancer. 2010;55(6):1083–8.

42. Moreno L, Bautista F, Ashley S, et al. Does chemotherapy affect the visual outcome in children with optic pathway glioma? A systematic review of the evidence. Eur J Cancer. 2010;46(12):2253–9.

# Optic Nerve Sheath Meningioma

Balamurugan A. Vellayappan, Lia M. Halasz,
Yolanda D. Tseng, and Simon S. Lo

## Learning Objectives

- To appreciate the clinical features of ONSM, including epidemiology, presenting symptoms, and radiological features.
- To understand the available treatment options—such as observation, surgery, and radiation therapy, including the benefits and drawbacks for each.
- To become familiar with the practical aspects of radiation therapy, including treatment technique, dose prescription, and organs-at-risk dose limits.

## Epidemiology

Meningiomas arise from the meningothelial cells of the arachnoid membrane and are the most common type of primary central nervous system tumors. Approximately 36% of all primary brain and spine tumors are meningiomas, with an average annual age-adjusted incidence rate of 7.86 per 100,000 persons [1]. Meningiomas show a rising incidence with age, with the peak being seen in the mid-60s [1]. Females have a predilection to develop meningiomas, with a

B. A. Vellayappan
Department of Radiation Oncology, National University Cancer Institute, National University Health System, Singapore, Singapore

L. M. Halasz · S. S. Lo (✉)
Department of Radiation Oncology, University of Washington, Seattle, WA, USA

Department of Neurological Surgery, University of Washington, Seattle, WA, USA
e-mail: simonslo@uw.edu

Y. D. Tseng
Department of Radiation Oncology, University of Washington, Seattle, WA, USA

ratio of 3:1 [1]. Meningiomas can arise anywhere in the dura and most commonly occur within the skull [2]. In contrast, ONSM is a rare condition. The estimated incidence is between 1% and 2% of all intracranial meningiomas [3]. ONSM is the second most common orbital tumor, after optic nerve gliomas [4]. ONSM can be subclassified into primary (pONSM) and secondary (sONSM). pONSM, accounting for 10% of ONSM, arise from the intra-orbital or the intra-canalicular portions of the optic nerve. The remaining 90% (sONSM) arise from the sphenoid ridge or sella and invade the orbit. Overall, 5% of cases may present with bilateral ONSM [3]. There does not seem to be a predilection for laterality among ONSM.

It is unclear if the incidence of ONSM has increased over time. However, the frequent use of imaging for evaluation of other neurological symptoms may contribute to the diagnosis of asymptomatic ONSM, which would have been undetected otherwise [5].

## Risk Factors

As with other meningiomas, ONSM is more often diagnosed in middle-aged females.

Childhood ONSM has no gender predilection and is more commonly associated with neurofibromatosis type 2 (NF2). For patients with NF2, ONSM are more commonly bilateral and may be associated with a more aggressive growth pattern [3, 6].

## Clinical Presentation

The classical triad of vision impairment, optic nerve atrophy, and optociliary shunting has been associated with ONSM since the 1970s [3, 7, 8]. However, all three signs may only be seen in a third of cases [9]. Moreover, these symptoms are not specific and have been reported with cases of glioma and sphenoid wing meningioma [7, 10].

E. L. Chang et al. (eds.), *Adult CNS Radiation Oncology*, https://doi.org/10.1007/978-3-319-42878-9_16

A majority of patients with ONSM have long-standing symptoms of painless, progressive vision loss. On average, most patients report onset of vision impairment for 3–4 years prior to diagnosis [3, 11]. Visual fields may not be affected in all cases. Dutton reported that one third of patients may have concentric or paracentric visual field defects. Proptosis (mild to moderate) does not feature prominently in cases on ONSM, unlike cases of spheno-orbital meningiomas. Upward gaze may be limited in 40–50% of patients [3, 12], although diplopia is only experienced by 4% [12]. Fundoscopic examination almost certainly reveals optic nerve pathology (disc swelling and/or optic atrophy). Most patients exhibit relative afferent pupillary defect in the ipsilateral eye [4]. Disease progression tends to be slow, and often relentless, and many patients develop blindness without treatment. A summary of clinical signs and symptoms is included in Table 16.1 [3].

**Table 16.1** Clinical signs and symptoms of optic sheath meningioma

| Symptom | Number of patients with available data | % of patients affected |
|---|---|---|
| Decreased vision | 380 | 96 |
| Decreased visual field | 135 | 83 |
| Peripheral constriction | 112 | 39 |
| Central, centro-cecal, paracentral scotoma | 112 | 29 |
| Altitudinal defect | 112 | 16 |
| Enlarged blind spot | 112 | 13 |
| Decreased color vision | 45 | 73 |
| Proptosis | 241 | 59 |
| Disc atrophy | 177 | 49 |
| Disc swelling | 208 | 48 |
| Decreased motility | 258 | 47 |
| Optociliary shunts | 238 | 30 |

## Patterns of Growth

The tumor often grows around the optic nerve without invading it. Sustained growth allows it to spread along paths of least resistance and involve the intracranial portion of the optic nerve, chiasm, and contralateral optic nerve. Occasionally, the tumor may invade the nerve through the fibrovascular septa [13, 14]. Due to the encircling nature, the tumor exerts increasing pressure on the nerve and obstructs the central retinal vein and/or artery. Further progression may cause the tumor to break through the dural sheath and invade other orbital structures. Intracanalicular ONSM usually presents with visual loss and optic atrophy earlier due to the smaller space available within the optic canal before compression occurs.

## Radiological Features

Diagnosis of ONSM is heavily reliant on imaging findings, given the precarious location and considerable morbidities associated with biopsy. High-resolution fine-cut magnetic resonance imaging (MRI) is key in establishing the diagnosis. Computed tomography (CT) plays a complementary role. Figure 16.1 illustrates the radiological findings from a patient with ONSM. Like other meningiomas, ONSM typically show homogenous and well-defined contrast enhancement and exhibit micro-/macro-calcifications which are visible on fine-cut CT. The classic description of "tramtrack" sign [15] refers to the central lucency of the optic nerve caught between the enhancing optic nerve sheath complex. However, this is not specific for ONSM and may be seen in other conditions such as lymphoma, sarcoidosis, and leptomeningeal metastasis [16]. In contrast to optic nerve gliomas, where the diameter of the nerve is enlarged, ONSM

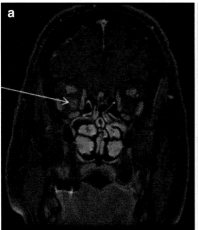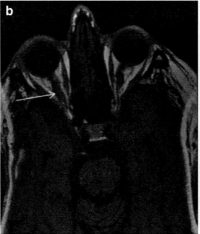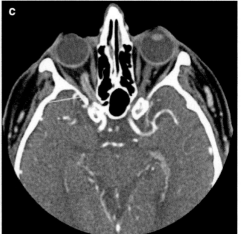

**Fig. 16.1** (**a**) Coronal T1 with contrast: yellow arrow pointing to thickened enhancement surrounding optic nerve but no enhancement of the optic nerve itself. (**b**) Axial T1 with contrast: yellow arrow pointing to "tram-track" sign. (**c**) Axial CT scan with contrast: yellow arrow pointing to "tram-track" sign

reveals an optic nerve with a reduced diameter. Radiological growth patterns have been classified by Saeed and Rootman [12] into four distinct types according to their configuration (tubular, globular, fusiform, or focal). It is suggested that tubular pattern of growth with apical extension may be associated with a poorer visual outcome.

Gadolinium-based contrast-enhanced fat-suppressed T1-weighted pulse sequences are most useful to diagnose ONSM. The tumors are isointense (T1- and T2-weighted), compared to normal optic nerve and brain tissue, but exhibit uniform and marked contrast enhancement in the post-contrast sequences [16]. Recent reports have described using functional imaging such as Ga-68-DOTA-TATE PET/CT [17] or somatostatin receptor PET/CT to aid in the diagnosis of ONSM [18].

## Pathology

ONSM share the same histological features as meningiomas that arise elsewhere in the CNS. However, literature on histology is sparse as biopsies are often not performed. ONSM are classified according to the "World Health Organization (WHO) Classification of Tumors of the Central Nervous System" [19]. This classification utilizes a three-tiered grading system that aims to predict the natural history and prognosis of meningiomas. A summary of histological criteria is presented in Table 16.2.

More than 80% of meningiomas, including ONSM, are WHO grade 1. They are slowly growing and have lower recurrence rates. In cases where histology is available, majority of ONSM are of the meningothelial or transitional variants.

NF2 is mutated in 50% of sporadic cases and in all patients with germline neurofibromatosis type 2 [20]. The

NF2 tumor suppressor gene is located on chromosome 22q, and mutations in one allele are typically associated with monosomy 22 or large deletions involving the other allele. Besides loss of heterozygosity, epigenetic mechanisms, such as hyper-methylation [21], may lead to reduced expression of NF2 gene product merlin.

## Overall Treatment Strategy

The prognosis of ONSM is excellent with no ONSM-related deaths reported in the literature [3]. As such, treatment aims are to primarily preserve and restore visual function and secondarily provide local control and halt progression. Often, these aims are interrelated.

The key question in the management of ONSM is when, and if, treatment should be initiated. The behavior of ONSM can be unpredictable [22], although most reports suggest very slow and marginal progression with loss of vision being invariable [23, 24].

As such, one must rely on strict clinical and imaging follow-up to determine progression. Treatment should be initiated before there is functional loss of vision and/or signs of clinical progression. Saeed et al. [12] have emphasized that visual acuity at the time of presentation is an important prognostic marker. Patients who had visual acuity 20/50 or better tended to retain useful vision for longer periods compared to those with a worse initial vision.

Kenerdall et al. [25] suggested to initiate treatment when visual acuity dips below 20/40 or when visual fields are constricting. This must be balanced against offering all patients treatment at diagnosis, as toxicity risks would outweigh potential benefits.

Historically, the treatment strategy has evolved from observation to invasive surgical procedures to fractionated RT. We will review these modalities, and the available evidence, below.

## Observation

Historically, due to fears of radiation-related toxicity, many patients with serviceable vision were generally treated with "watchful waiting." However, data suggests that the majority of patients will eventually experience progressive visual loss without treatment. Moreover, patients with ipsilateral visual loss are at risk of the chiasm and contralateral optic nerve being jeopardized by a slowly progressive tumor. It has been suggested that the chance of vision improvement decreases with increasing duration of visual symptoms [12]. Nevertheless, observation may be an option for patients with no discernible visual loss on careful ophthalmologic examination or in patients with a limited life expectancy where deficits from tumor progression are judged to be unlikely.

**Table 16.2** Summary of WHO grading criteria for meningioma

| | |
|---|---|
| Benign meningioma WHO grade 1 | Any histologic variant other than clear cell, choroid, papillary, or rhabdoid Lack of criteria defining atypical and anaplastic meningioma |
| Atypical meningioma WHO grade 2 (any of the three criteria) | 1. Elevated mitotic index (4–19 mitosis/10 high-power field) 2. At least three of the following five parameters: • Increased cellularity • High nuclear/cytoplasmic ratio • Large and prominent nucleoli • Uninterrupted patternless or sheetlike growth • Foci of spontaneous necrosis 3. Brain invasion |
| Anaplastic (malignant) meningioma WHO grade 3 (any of the 2 criteria) | High mitotic index (≥20/10 high-power field) Frank anaplasia (sarcoma, carcinoma, or melanoma-like histology) |

## Surgery

Unlike other intracranial meningiomas, surgery does not play a primary role in the management of pONSM. Even though the tumor can be seemingly peeled off the optic nerve [26], a majority of the cases resulted in postoperative blindness. This is due to interruption of the pial vessels and ischemic injury to the optic nerve, because the tumor and the optic nerve share the blood supply.

Surgical procedures in ONSM may be in the form of biopsy, optic nerve sheath fenestration, or surgical extirpation.

- As biopsies do carry some risk, it is often not mandated for typical cases. As mentioned above, the diagnosis is usually clinched by history, physical examination, and high-quality imaging.

Optic nerve sheath fenestration was historically performed to decompress the ON by releasing its dural sheath. However, the efficacy of this procedure was contentious with some reports of deleterious outcome resulting in massive orbital invasion necessitating exenteration [11]. Surgical extirpation was historically offered to young patients with pONSM [11]. Although a lateral orbital approach allowed access to anterior and mid-orbital tumor, apical access remained challenging. Intracranial approach (frontal craniotomy) enabled complete removal of ONSM up to the chiasm. Unfortunately, the complication rate remained high at 30%, with recurrence rates approaching 25% [3, 27]. Incomplete removal of tumor often leads to diffuse orbital invasion and intracranial spread. Improvement in visual function postsurgery has been reported, although rarely. These were likely associated with ONSM which are small, situated anteriorly, and not causing significant neural invasion [12, 27, 28].

- Although surgical intervention almost always leads to worsening visual function, surgery still has a role in the management of highly selected cases. General indications for pONSM include [29]:
  - Histological confirmation in cases with atypical clinical or radiological findings.
  - Surgical extirpation if intracranial spread threatens contralateral optic nerve and ipsilateral vision is unsalvageable.
  - Severe proptosis which is unlikely to respond to RT and/or corticosteroids.
  - Post-RT compartment syndrome of the optic nerve, causing optic nerve and macular edema, may be managed with nerve sheath surgery.

In general, complete resection is the goal of meningioma surgery. However, when there is no clear resection plane, subtotal resection has been investigated to minimize visual deficits. In these cases, adjuvant RT (as part of combined modality therapy) has been used to reduce recurrent rates. Turbin et al. [30] have published their extensive experience of patients managed with observation, surgery, radiation, or surgery with adjuvant RT. In their study, 59 patients, with visual acuity better than "no light perception," were followed for a mean of 105 months (range 51–516 m). Although visual acuity at baseline was not different between the groups, visual acuity (VA) significantly deteriorated for the observation, surgery alone, and surgery with postoperative RT groups. The radiation alone group had a nonsignificant decrease in VA. Forty-four percent of patients treated with RT alone and 31% of patients treated with surgery and postoperative RT showed sustained improvement in VA. In contrast, only 8% of patients treated without RT showed improvement in VA. Moreover, complication rates were twice as much for the surgery (66.7%) and surgery with postoperative RT groups (62.5%), compared to RT alone (33%). In addition, other studies [31] have suggested that visual improvement is reduced in patients who have undergone surgery in addition to RT, compared to RT alone. As such, subtotal resection with postoperative RT is not favored in management of pONSM.

In contrast, cases of sONSM are usually surgically managed [29]. For example, surgical removal of the intracranial component can be performed with functional vision preservation. These patients often require postoperative RT to the tumor bed and definitive RT for the intracanalicular and intra-orbital components. Meningiomas of the spheno-orbital ridge causing extrinsic compression of the ON are also managed surgically.

## Radiation Therapy

Interest in radiation therapy for treatment of ONSM was first raised by Smith et al. in 1981 [32]. RT (alone) was reported to be effective in relieving compressive symptoms with vision improving from 11/200 to 20/60. Another early report in a patient who refused surgery and was offered RT to a dose of 55 Gy documented rapid improvement in visual acuity which persisted for 2 years [33].

In the seminal review article by Dutton [3], the author reported primary RT leading to improvement in visual acuity in 75% of cases, stability in 8%, and worsening in 17%.

Similarly, the study by Turbin [30] suggested that RT alone (mixture of 2D and conformal RT 40–55 Gy over 6 weeks) had the best long-term visual function. Although the RT group had the lowest complication rate (33%), this was still considered to be high. RT-related complications included retinopathy, retinal vascular occlusion, iritis, and temporal lobe atrophy. It is likely that 2D techniques (such as lateral or wedge-pair fields), based on bony landmarks, may have led to large volumes of healthy tissue being irradiated and could have given rise to these toxicities.

However, due to lack of long-term efficacy and RT-related toxicities, the utilization of RT was still lagging. With time, more reports emerged suggesting that the risk of brain necrosis [34] and optic neuropathy [35] be <2% at doses below 54 Gy and fraction sizes of 1.8–2 Gy. Moreover, technical advancements such as CT-based planning and advanced dosimetric modeling allowed conformal radiation plans (3D conformal RT) while sparing normal brain parenchyma and other critical structures. Further improvements in imaging and delivery techniques gave rise to intensity-modulated RT and SFRT. A recent study by Saeed et al. [36] compared conventional RT with SFRT and found the visual outcomes to be similar. However, it has to be noted that visual outcomes were assessed by relatively crude means such as the Snellen eye chart. The conventional RT group had a higher complication rate (retinopathy, cataract, dry eyes). At most comprehensive cancer centers including the National University Cancer Institute of Singapore (NCIS) and University of Washington (UW), we routinely use highly conformal techniques such as SFRT, image-guided intensity-modulated RT/volumetric-modulated arc therapy or proton therapy for treatment delivery.

ONSM has a presumed low $\alpha/\beta$ [37] and therefore is sensitive to large fraction sizes. Unfortunately, ONSM is intimately associated with the optic apparatus (which are serial late-responding structures). They are also exquisitely sensitive to large fractions. Single doses of 8–12 Gy have been reported to show permanent damage to the optic apparatus [38–40]. Therefore, fractionated RT (1.8–2 Gy fractions) is still preferred over single-fraction or hypofractionated radiosurgery.

## Indications for Irradiation

In general, the indications for treatment with RT include:

- Patients diagnosed with ONSM radiologically and any visual symptom (such as decreased visual acuity/visual field/color vision, ophthalmalgia, proptosis, or orbital pain)
- Incidentally found tumors where progression of tumor is expected and patient's desire to preserve vision

## Target Volume Delineation

Patients should be simulated in a rigid relocatable thermoplastic mask. Patients are instructed to close their eyes, look forward, and keep their eyes still for the procedure. Fine-cut (1–2 mm) CT simulation images should be co-registered with contrast-enhanced T1 axial sequences. As described above, ONSM enhance on the T1-gadolinium sequence. However, the lesion can be obscured by orbital

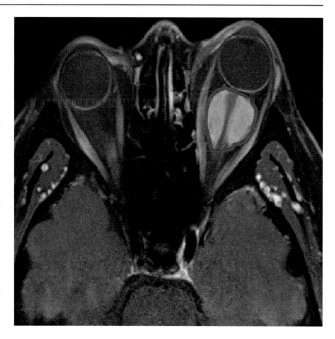

**Fig. 16.2** The gadolinium-enhanced tumor is contoured as GTV (red)

and marrow fat. Fat-suppression sequences are very useful to delineate the extent of the lesion (gross tumor volume or GTV) (Fig. 16.2). Care should be taken to trace the nerve toward the canalicular portion for at least 5 mm (longitudinal extension). Most ONSM tend to be of WHO grade 1 subtype with smooth and well-defined borders, and therefore CTV margins are not required (for microscopic spread) into the orbital fat. The PTV margin is dependent on the type of immobilization device and image-guidance used. With a stereotactic setup and daily image-guidance, a 2 mm PTV margin is usually adequate. Using a thermoplastic shell alone, without image-guidance, a 3–5 mm PTV may be required. In terms of treatment planning, multiple noncoplanar beams (or arcs) are useful to generate a conformal plan. Entry or exit through the contralateral eye should be avoided. Particular attention needs to be paid to reduce the dose to ipsilateral retina, ipsilateral lacrimal gland, optic chiasm, and contralateral eye (lens, globe, and optic nerve).

## Radiation Dose Prescription and Organ-at-Risk Tolerance

The recommended dose range for treatment of ONSM is between 50.4 and 54 Gy in 1.8 Gy fractions, which is largely determined by the tolerance of the optic nerve. This is in line with most of the studies from Table 16.1. However, there is a suggestion that lower doses may be sufficient. For example, Richards et al. [41] treated ONSM ($n = 4$) with doses ranging from 43.4 to 45 Gy in 1.67 Gy fractions and reported improvement in visual acuity and visual fields in 65% of

**Table 16.3** Suggested OAR dose limits for RT planning

| OAR | Limit (reference) | Clinical outcome |
| --- | --- | --- |
| Retina | Max dose 50 Gy [42] | Retinopathy |
| Lens | Max 7 Gy [42] | Cataract |
| Optic nerve and chiasm | Max dose [39] | Optic neuropathy risk |
| | <55 Gy | 3% or less |
| | 55–60 Gy | 3–7% |
| | >60 Gy | 7–20% |
| Pituitary | Max dose 45 Gy [43] | Pituitary dysfunction |
| Lacrimal gland | Max dose 40 Gy [44] | Xerophthalmia |

patients. However, more data is needed before adopting lower doses.

Suggested OAR dose limits are listed in Table 16.3.

At the National University Cancer Institute of Singapore and University of Washington, the optic nerve and chiasm maximum dose is limited to 54 Gy (1.8 Gy fractions). Most of our patients with ONSM are treated to 50.4 Gy (1.8 Gy fractions).

## Complication Avoidance When Treating ONSM with SFRT

- Appropriate immobilization techniques, such as a relocatable stereotactic headframe, and daily image-guidance (with stereoscopic imaging or CBCT) allow for smaller PTV margins. Patients should be instructed to look straight ahead during CT simulation and treatment.
- Accurate co-registration with high-resolution axial MRI is critical for target and organ-at-risk definition. Volumetric MRI allows reformatting into other planes. When there is doubt about the accuracy of co-registration, administering IV contrast during fine-cut CT simulation (1–2 mm) may help with target definition.
- Highly conformal RT planning techniques (such as non-coplanar volumetric arc therapy) are useful to achieve steep dose gradients. It is imperative to avoid hot spots within organs-at-risk (such as retina, optic nerve, and chiasm). It is often not possible to meet the dose limits for the lens, and patients should be counseled for radiation-induced cataracts.
- Patients will benefit from lubricating eye drops during radiation therapy treatment. Patients with symptomatic proptosis may find improvement with a low dose of dexamethasone.

## Toxicities

Acute toxicities are usually mild and well-tolerated. These include skin erythema, keratitis, and patchy alopecia (usu-

ally reversible). Because of the close proximity of ONSM to critical structures (like retina, optic apparatus, and pituitary gland), some amount of radiation exposure is unavoidable. For example, Krishnan [45] and Subramanian [46] reported radiation retinopathy in patients where the tumor was in close proximity to the globe. Other potential late toxicities include cataracts, retinal vascular occlusion, persistent iritis, temporal lobe atrophy, and pituitary dysfunction.

## Outcomes: Tumor Control and Survival

Table 16.4 summarizes the larger studies (*n* > 10) using RT in the treatment of ONSM.

Although most studies are retrospective in nature and composed of small numbers with variable follow-up, these studies enable us to draw some conclusions on the use of conformal RT. At moderately low doses between 45 and 54 Gy of fractionated RT, between 86% and 100% of patients experience stabilization and/or improvement of visual acuity. Local control, usually defined as the absence of radiological progression, of the tumor is achieved in almost all patients treated with RT. Moreover, the reported complication rates with modern conformal techniques are much lower (0–13%). In some cases, an early improvement of the visual field after SFRT is possible, as illustrated by a case from Thomas Jefferson University (Fig. 16.3). Overall survival was inconsistently reported and was 100% based on the available data. ONSM is not expected to cause disease-related mortality.

## Recommended Follow-Up Schedule

There are no guidelines with regard to frequency of follow-up. In general, most patients are followed up by ophthalmologists and radiation oncologists. At NCIS and UW, our institution, we recommend 4- to 6-monthly clinical and ophthalmologic examination. Patients are recommended to have a MR examination every 6–12 months. As late recurrences and toxicities are to be expected, patients will need lifelong follow-up.

## Case Presentation

A 43-year-old male who presented with blurred vision in the left eye for 1 year's duration. He developed proptosis in the month prior to seeking medical attention. Physical examination showed grade 3 relative afferent pupillary defect. Visual acuity was severely diminished in the left eye, with patient only being able to perceive light and hand movement. Proptosis was apparent in the left eye, with Hertel's measurement being 26 mm in the left eye, compared

**Table 16.4** Summary of studies (n > 10) where RT was used as primary treatment for ONSM

| Author (year) | Number of patients (number of lesions) | Median follow-up in months (Range) | Dose and technique | Visual outcome improved | Stable | Worse | Tumour control | Toxicity (%) | Overall survival |
|---|---|---|---|---|---|---|---|---|---|
| Tsao (1999) (abstract) [47] | 15 | 32 (11–102) | 3DCRT 50.4–54 Gy in 1.8 Gy fraction | 67% | 20% | 13% | 87% | Two patients developed radiation retinopathy (13%) | NR |
| Turbin (2002) [30] | 64 16 patients underwent surgery + RT. 18 patients RT alone | 150 (51–516) | Mixture of 2D and 3DCRT 40–55 Gy over 6 weeks. Fraction size not specified | 44% | NR | NR | 89% | 33% complication in RT alone (retinopathy, iritis, temporal lobe atrophy). 62.5% complication in surgery plus RT (retinopathy, neovascular glaucoma, cerebral infarct, CSF leak, motility defect, iritis, orbital hemorrhage) | NR |
| Andrews (2002) [48] | 30 (33) | 22 (2–71) | SFRT 51 Gy (range 50–54 Gy) | 42% | 50% | 8% | 100% | Four patients (two patients visual loss. one optic neuritis. one transient orbital pain) (13%[a]) | NR |
| Pitz (2002) [49] | 15 (16) | 37 (12–71) | SFRT 54 Gy in 1.92 Gy fractions | 40% | 60% | 0% | 100% | No severe AE reported (0%) | 100% |
| Narayan (2003) [50] | 14 | 51.3 (8.9–80.9) | 3DCRT 53–55.8 Gy in 1.8–2 Gy fraction | 36% | 50% | 14% | 100% | No severe AE reported (0%) | NR |
| Baumert (2004) [51] | 23 (23) | 20 (1–68) | SFRT 50.4 Gy (45–54) in 1.8–2 Gy fractions | 73% | 22% | 4% | 100% | One patient developed retinopathy and vitreous hemorrhage (4%[a]) | NR |
| Schroeder (2004) (abstract) [52] | 22 | 20 (2–71) | IMRT 49.3–50.4 in 1.6–2 Gy | 71% | 24% | 5% | 100% | One patient had G4 toxicity (blindness) (4%) | NR |
| Sitathanee (2006) [53] | 12 Five patients underwent surgery + RT | 34 | SFRT 55.7 Gy in 1.8 Gy fractions. one patient had 15 Gy SRS | 33% | 59% | 8% | 100% | No severe AE reported (0%) | NR |
| Arvold (2009) [54] | 25 (25) | 30 (3–168) | Conformal fractionated RT (photon, proton) 50.4 Gy (45–59.4) in 1.8 Gy fractions | 63% | 32% | 5% | 95% | Three patients retinopathy (13%) | NR |
| Milker-Zabel (2009) [55] | 32 Ten patients underwent surgery + RT | 54 (7–204) | SFRT 54.9 Gy (50.4–57.6) in 1.8 Gy | NR | 97% | 3% | 100% | No severe AE reported (0%) | NR |
| Smee (2009) [56] | 15 (16) | 86.4 (5.5–157) | SFRT 50.4 Gy (45–56 Gy) in 1.8–2 Gy fractions. Three patients SRS 20 Gy | NR | 93% (improved or stable) | 7% | 100% | No severe AE reported (0%) | NR |
| Saeed (2010) [36] | 34 | 55 (51–156) | 45 Gy to 54 Gy in 1.8 Gy fractions. 22 conventional, 12 SFRT | 41% | 50% | 9% | NR | Late toxicity[a]: dry eye (15%), cataract (9%), retinopathy (18%) | NR |
| Liu (2010) [57] | 30 Nine patients underwent surgery + RT | 56 (38–108) | SRS (Gamma-knife) 13.3 Gy (10–17 Gy) in one or two sessions | 37% | 43% | 20% | 93% | No severe AE reported (0%) | NR |

(continued)

**Table 16.4** (continued)

| Author (year) | Number of patients (number of lesions) | Median follow-up in months (Range) | Dose and technique | Visual outcome improved | Stable | Worse | Tumour control | Toxicity (%) | Overall survival |
|---|---|---|---|---|---|---|---|---|---|
| Lesser (2010) [58] | 11 | 89.6 (61–156) | Conformal fractionated (majority 3DCRT) 45–54 Gy in 1.8 Gy per fraction | NR | 91% | 9% | 100% | No severe AE reported (0%) | NR |
| Adeberg (2011) [31] | 40 (41) 21 patients underwent surgery + RT | 60 (4–228) | SFRT 54 Gy (25–66 Gy) in 1.8–5 Gy fraction | 44% | 47% | 9% | 100% | No severe AE reported (0%) | 100% |
| Marchetti (2011) [59] | 21 | 30 (11–68) | Cyberknife SFRT (hypofractionated) 25 Gy in five fractions | 35% | 65% | 0% | 100% | No severe AE reported (0%) | NR |
| Solda (2012) [60] | 45 (51) | 30 (1–156) | SFRT 50 Gy in 30–33 fractions, conformal RT | 32% | 58% | 10% | 100% | Three patients developed retinopathy. Or retinal artery embolism (6%[a]) | NR |
| Abouaf (2012) [61] | 10 | 51 (5–139) | Mixture of 2D, 3DCRT, IMRT. Majority 3DCRT, 58 Gy (50–64 Gy) in 1.8–2 Gy fractions | 80% | 10% | 10% | 100% | Two patients G3 late toxicity, (retinal) 20% | NR |
| Paulsen (2012) [62] | 109 (113) 37 pONSM | 50.5 (0.05–131.6) | SFRT 54 Gy in (50.4–54 Gy). Fraction size not specified | 13% | 75% | 12% | 98% | No severe AE reported. 5 year probability of pituitary gland function 81% | NR |
| Adams (2013) [63] | 17 (18) | 74 (11–160) | 3DCRT 46.8–55.8 Gy in 1.8 Gy fractions | NR | 89% (improved or stable) | 11% | 100% | Late toxicity[a] xeropthalmia 29%, cataract 24%, optic disc atrophy 12% | NR |
| Brower (2013) [64] | 15 | 144 (48–228) | SFRT (87%) 50.4 Gy (49.4–54.4) in 1.8 Gy fractions | 27% | 60% | 13% | 100% | Grade 4 toxicity 13% (retinopathy) | 100% |
| Moyal (2014) [65] | 15 | 22.4 (8–79) | Conformal Proton Beam 52.2 Gy in 1.8 Gy | 20% | 73% | 7% | 100% | No severe AE reported (0%) | NR |

*NR* not reported
[a]Severity not specified

| Date and SRT dose | R eye visual acuity |
|---|---|
| 6-23-05 consultation | 20/50 |
| 7-13-05 10.8 Gy | 20/200 |
| 7-20-05 19.8 Gy | 20/50 |
| 7-27-05 28.8 Gy | 20/70 |
| 8-3-05 37.8 Gy | 20/30 |
| 11-22-05 FU 3 months | 20/20 |

**Fig. 16.3** Illustrating a case where early improvement in visual acuity was demonstrated after RT. [Reprinted from Jeremic B, Werner-Wasik M, Villà S, et al. Stereotactic Radiation Therapy in Primary Optic Nerve Sheath Meningioma. In: Jeremic B, Pitz S (eds). Primary Optic Nerve Sheath Meningioma. Heidelberg Germany: Springer; 2008:105–127. With permission from Springer-Verlag]

to 21 mm in the right eye. Both CT and MRI images are shown in Fig. 16.4.

He was treated with stereotactic fractionated radiation therapy, 54 Gy in 30 fractions (1.8 Gy per fraction). The target volume definition and radiation plan are shown in Fig. 16.5.

## Summary

- ONSM is a rare tumor and can be subclassified as primary or secondary ONSM.
- ONSM usually presents with chronic visual symptoms and generally has features of optic neuropathy.
- A diagnosis can be made based on clinically and radiological features, and a biopsy is not required in most cases. A contrast-enhanced fat-suppressed T1-weighted MRI is most useful to make the diagnosis.
- Majority of ONSM are of WHO grade 1 and exhibit slow progression.
- Surgery carries a high morbidity of worsening visual function and has a limited role in the management of ONSM.
- Conformal fractionated radiation therapy (e.g. SFRT) is the mainstay in the treatment of ONSM. Doses between 50 to 54 Gy (in 1.8 to 2 Gy fractions) are recommended

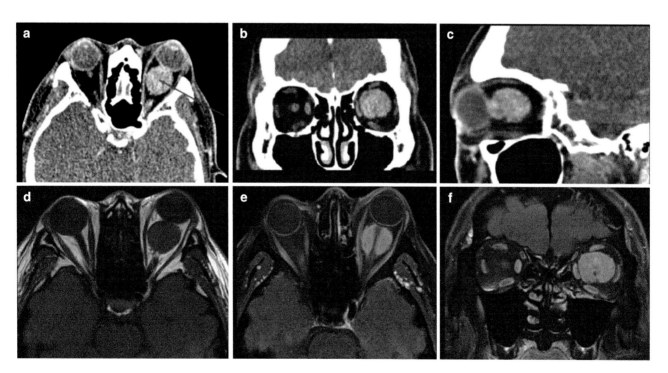

**Fig. 16.4** (a–f) Showing the pretreatment diagnostic images. (a) Axial CT, with blue arrow depicting "tram-track" sign. (b) Coronal CT. (c) Sagittal CT. (d) Axial T1 non-contrast. (e) Axial T1 with gadolinium and fat-suppression. Lobulated lesion shows avid enhancement and left eye proptosis is demonstrated. (f) Coronal T1 with gadolinium and fat-suppression

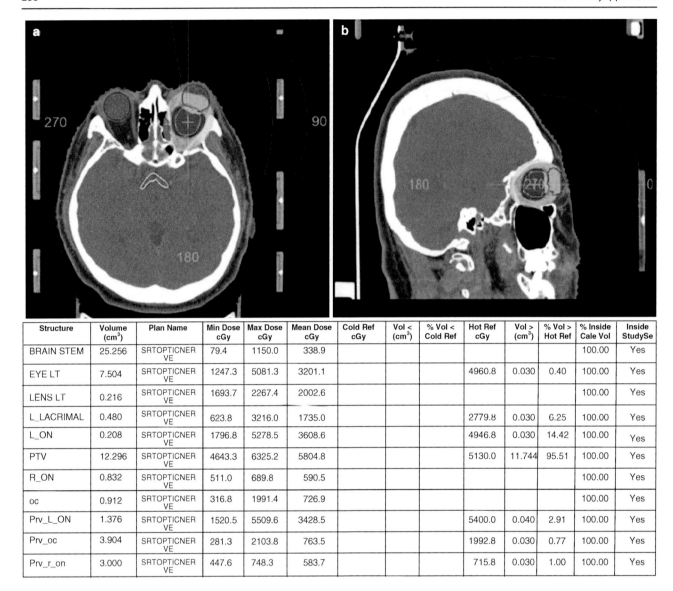

| Structure | Volume (cm³) | Plan Name | Min Dose cGy | Max Dose cGy | Mean Dose cGy | Cold Ref cGy | Vol < (cm³) | % Vol < Cold Ref | Hot Ref cGy | Vol > (cm³) | % Vol > Hot Ref | % Inside Cale Vol | Inside StudySe |
|---|---|---|---|---|---|---|---|---|---|---|---|---|---|
| BRAIN STEM | 25.256 | SRTOPTICNER VE | 79.4 | 1150.0 | 338.9 | | | | | | | 100.00 | Yes |
| EYE LT | 7.504 | SRTOPTICNER VE | 1247.3 | 5081.3 | 3201.1 | | | | 4960.8 | 0.030 | 0.40 | 100.00 | Yes |
| LENS LT | 0.216 | SRTOPTICNER VE | 1693.7 | 2267.4 | 2002.6 | | | | | | | 100.00 | Yes |
| L_LACRIMAL | 0.480 | SRTOPTICNER VE | 623.8 | 3216.0 | 1735.0 | | | | 2779.8 | 0.030 | 6.25 | 100.00 | Yes |
| L_ON | 0.208 | SRTOPTICNER VE | 1796.8 | 5278.5 | 3608.6 | | | | 4946.8 | 0.030 | 14.42 | 100.00 | Yes |
| PTV | 12.296 | SRTOPTICNER VE | 4643.3 | 6325.2 | 5804.8 | | | | 5130.0 | 11.744 | 95.51 | 100.00 | Yes |
| R_ON | 0.832 | SRTOPTICNER VE | 511.0 | 689.8 | 590.5 | | | | | | | 100.00 | Yes |
| OC | 0.912 | SRTOPTICNER VE | 316.8 | 1991.4 | 726.9 | | | | | | | 100.00 | Yes |
| Prv_L_ON | 1.376 | SRTOPTICNER VE | 1520.5 | 5509.6 | 3428.5 | | | | 5400.0 | 0.040 | 2.91 | 100.00 | Yes |
| Prv_oc | 3.904 | SRTOPTICNER VE | 281.3 | 2103.8 | 763.5 | | | | 1992.8 | 0.030 | 0.77 | 100.00 | Yes |
| Prv_r_on | 3.000 | SRTOPTICNER VE | 447.6 | 748.3 | 583.7 | | | | 715.8 | 0.030 | 1.00 | 100.00 | Yes |

**Fig. 16.5** (**a, b**) Showing the SFRT planned with three noncoplanar arcs. 54 Gy isodose wash (red) and 27 Gy isodose wash (green) are shown. Doses received by the target and organs-at-risk are shown in the table below the images

and expected to achieve uncomplicated local control and stabilization and/or improvement in visual function in majority of the patients.

## Self-Assessment Questions

1. All of the following are risk factors for development of meningioma except:
   A. Female sex
   B. Prior ionizing radiation exposure
   C. Neurofibromatosis type 2
   D. Prolonged usage of cellular devices

2. Which of the following signs or symptoms are not seen with ONSM?
   A. Decreased visual acuity
   B. Impairment of visual fields
   C. Ptosis
   D. Decreased color vision

3. "Tram-track" sign refers to central lucency of the optic nerve caught between the optic nerve sheath complexes and is specific for ONSM.
   A. True
   B. False

4. Patterns of spread of ONSM are expected to be:
   A. Radially into retro-orbital fat space
   B. Longitudinal along the optic nerve
   C. Hematogenous spread to distant organs
   D. Leptomeningeal dissemination

5. What is the most appropriate radiotherapy dose for ONSM?
   A. Single-fraction SRS 18 Gy
   B. Conformal fractionated RT 40 Gy in 1.8–2 Gy fractions
   C. Conformal fractionated RT 50–54 Gy in 1.8–2 Gy fractions
   D. Conformal fractionated RT 60 Gy in 1.8–2 Gy fractions

## Answers

1. D [66]
2. C [3]
3. B [16]
4. B [67]
5. C [62]

## References

1. Ostrom QT, Gittleman H, Fulop J, et al. CBTRUS statistical report: primary brain and central nervous system tumors diagnosed in the United States in 2008–2012. Neuro Oncol. 2015;17(Suppl 4):iv1–iv62.
2. Whittle IR, Smith C, Navoo P, et al. Meningiomas. Lancet. 2004;363(9420):1535–43.
3. Dutton JJ. Optic nerve sheath meningiomas. Surv Ophthalmol. 1992;37(3):167–83.
4. Sibony PA, Krauss HR, Kennerdell JS, et al. Optic nerve sheath meningiomas. Clinical manifestations. Ophthalmology. 1984;91(11):1313–26.
5. Vernooij MW, Ikram MA, Tanghe HL, et al. Incidental findings on brain MRI in the general population. N Engl J Med. 2007;357(18):1821–8.
6. Berman D, Miller NR. New concepts in the management of optic nerve sheath meningiomas. Ann Acad Med Singap. 2006;35(3):168–74.
7. Frisen L, Royt WF, Tengroth BM. Optociliary veins, disc pallor and visual loss. A triad of signs indicating spheno-orbital meningioma. Acta Ophthalmol. 1973;51(2):241–9.
8. Hollenhorst RW Jr, Hollenhorst RW Sr, MacCarty CS. Visual prognosis of optic nerve sheath meningiomas producing shunt vessels on the optic disk: the Hoyt-Spencer syndrome. Trans Am Ophthalmol Soc. 1977;75:141–63.
9. Carrasco JR, Penne RB. Optic nerve sheath meningiomas and advanced treatment options. Curr Opin Ophthalmol. 2004;15(5):406–10.
10. Jakobiec FA, Depot MJ, Kennerdell JS, et al. Combined clinical and computed tomographic diagnosis of orbital glioma and meningioma. Ophthalmology. 1984;91(2):137–55.
11. Wright JE, McNab AA, McDonald WI. Primary optic nerve sheath meningioma. Br J Ophthalmol. 1989;73(12):960–6.
12. Saeed P, Rootman J, Nugent RA, et al. Optic nerve sheath meningiomas. Ophthalmology. 2003;110(10):2019–30.
13. Samples JR, Robertson DM, Taylor JZ, et al. Optic nerve meningioma. Ophthalmology. 1983;90(12):1591–4.
14. Probst C, Gessaga E, Leuenberger AE. Primary meningioma of the optic nerve sheaths: case report. Ophthalmologica. 1985;190(2):83–90.
15. Kanamalla US. The optic nerve tram-track sign. Radiology. 2003;227(3):718–9.
16. Gala F, Magnetic resonance imaging of optic nerve. Indian J Radiol Imaging. 2015;25(4):421–38.
17. Klingenstein A, Haug AR, Miller C, et al. Ga-68-DOTA-TATE PET/CT for discrimination of tumors of the optic pathway. Orbit. 2015;34(1):16–22.
18. Chandra P, Purandare N, Shah S, et al. Somatostatin receptor SPECT/CT using 99mTc Labeled HYNIC-TOC aids in diagnosis of primary optic nerve sheath meningioma. Indian J Nucl Med. 2017;32(1):63–5.
19. Louis DN, Perry A, Reifenberger G, et al. The 2016 World Health Organization classification of tumors of the central nervous system: a summary. Acta Neuropathol. 2016;131(6):803–20.
20. Ragel BT, Jensen RL. Molecular genetics of meningiomas. Neurosurg Focus. 2005;19(5):E9.
21. Liu Y, Pang JC, Dong S, et al. Aberrant CpG island hypermethylation profile is associated with atypical and anaplastic meningiomas. Hum Pathol. 2005;36(4):416–25.
22. Egan RA, Lessell S. A contribution to the natural history of optic nerve sheath meningiomas. Arch Ophthalmol. 2002;120(11):1505–8.
23. Schick U, Jung C, Hassler WE. Primary optic nerve sheath meningiomas: a follow-up study. Cent Eur Neurosurg. 2010;71(3):126–33.
24. Wright JE, Call NB, Liaricos S. Primary optic nerve meningioma. Br J Ophthalmol. 1980;64(8):553–8.
25. Kennerdell JS, Maroon JC, Malton M, et al. The management of optic nerve sheath meningiomas. Am J Ophthalmol. 1988;106(4):450–7.
26. Alper MG. Management of primary optic nerve meningiomas. Current status—therapy in controversy. J Clin Neuroophthalmol. 1981;1(2):101–17.
27. Jeremic B, Pitz S. Primary optic nerve sheath meningioma: stereotactic fractionated radiation therapy as an emerging treatment of choice. Cancer. 2007;110(4):714–22.
28. Mark LE, Kennerdell JS, Maroon JC, et al. Microsurgical removal of a primary intraorbital meningioma. Am J Ophthalmol. 1978;86(5):704–9.
29. Schick U, Dott U, Hassler W. Surgical management of meningiomas involving the optic nerve sheath. J Neurosurg. 2004;101(6):951–9.
30. Turbin RE, Thompson CR, Kennerdell JS, et al. A long-term visual outcome comparison in patients with optic nerve sheath meningioma managed with observation, surgery, radiotherapy, or surgery and radiotherapy. Ophthalmology. 2002;109(5):890–9. discussion 9–900
31. Adeberg S, Welzel T, Rieken S, et al. Prior surgical intervention and tumor size impact clinical outcome after precision radiotherapy for the treatment of optic nerve sheath meningiomas (ONSM). Radiat Oncol. 2011;6:117.
32. Smith JL, Vuksanovic MM, Yates BM, et al. Radiation therapy for primary optic nerve meningiomas. J Clin Neuroophthalmol. 1981;1(2):85–99.
33. Mondon H, Hamard H, Sales J, et al. Role of radiotherapy in the treatment of meningioma of the optic nerve. Bull Soc Ophtalmol Fr. 1985;85(3):379–82.
34. Becker G, Jeremic B, Pitz S, et al. Stereotactic fractionated radiotherapy in patients with optic nerve sheath meningioma. Int J Radiat Oncol Biol Phys. 2002;54(5):1422–9.
35. Brada M, Rajan B, Traish D, et al. The long-term efficacy of conservative surgery and radiotherapy in the control of pituitary adenomas. Clin Endocrinol. 1993;38(6):571–8.
36. Saeed P, Blank L, Selva D, et al. Primary radiotherapy in progressive optic nerve sheath meningiomas: a long-term follow-up study. Br J Ophthalmol. 2010;94(5):564–8.

37. Shrieve DC, Hazard L, Boucher K, et al. Dose fractionation in stereotactic radiotherapy for parasellar meningiomas: radiobiological considerations of efficacy and optic nerve tolerance. J Neurosurg. 2004;101(Suppl 3):390–5.

38. Tishler RB, Loeffler JS, Lunsford LD, et al. Tolerance of cranial nerves of the cavernous sinus to radiosurgery. Int J Radiat Oncol Biol Phys. 1993;27(2):215–21.

39. Mayo C, Martel MK, Marks LB, et al. Radiation dose-volume effects of optic nerves and chiasm. Int J Radiat Oncol Biol Phys. 2010;76(3 Suppl):S28–35.

40. Leavitt JA, Stafford SL, Link MJ, et al. Long-term evaluation of radiation-induced optic neuropathy after single-fraction stereotactic radiosurgery. Int J Radiat Oncol Biol Phys. 2013;87(3):524–7.

41. Richards JC, Roden D, Harper CS. Management of sight-threatening optic nerve sheath meningioma with fractionated stereotactic radiotherapy. Clin Exp Ophthalmol. 2005;33(2):137–41.

42. Phase II Trial of Observation for Low-Risk Meningiomas and of Radiotherapy for Intermediate- and High-Risk Meningiomas [RTOG 0539 Protocol Information]. Available from: https://www.rtog.org/ClinicalTrials/ProtocolTable/StudyDetails.aspx?study=0539.

43. Emami B, Lyman J, Brown A, et al. Tolerance of normal tissue to therapeutic irradiation. Int J Radiat Oncol Biol Phys. 1991;21(1):109–22.

44. Parsons JT, Bova FJ, Mendenhall WM, et al. Response of the normal eye to high dose radiotherapy. Oncology (Williston Park). 1996;10(6):837–47. discussion 47–8, 51–2

45. Krishnan R, Kumar I, Kyle G, et al. Radiation retinopathy after fractionated stereotactic conformal radiotherapy for primary intraorbital optic nerve sheath meningioma. J Neuroophthalmol. 2007;27(2):143–4.

46. Subramanian PS, Bressler NM, Miller NR. Radiation retinopathy after fractionated stereotactic radiotherapy for optic nerve sheath meningioma. Ophthalmology. 2004;111(3):565–7.

47. Tsao MN, Hoyt WF, Horton J, et al. Improved visual outcome with definitive radiation therapy for optic nerve sheath meningioma. Int J Radiat Oncol Biol Phys. 1999;45(3):324–5.

48. Andrews DW, Faroozan R, Yang BP, et al. Fractionated stereotactic radiotherapy for the treatment of optic nerve sheath meningiomas: preliminary observations of 33 optic nerves in 30 patients with historical comparison to observation with or without prior surgery. Neurosurgery. 2002;51(4):890–902. discussion 3–4

49. Pitz S, Becker G, Schiefer U, et al. Stereotactic fractionated irradiation of optic nerve sheath meningioma: a new treatment alternative. Br J Ophthalmol. 2002;86(11):1265–8.

50. Narayan S, Cornblath WT, Sandler HM, et al. Preliminary visual outcomes after three-dimensional conformal radiation therapy for optic nerve sheath meningioma. Int J Radiat Oncol Biol Phys. 2003;56(2):537–43.

51. Baumert BG, Villa S, Studer G, et al. Early improvements in vision after fractionated stereotactic radiotherapy for primary optic nerve sheath meningioma. Radiother Oncol. 2004;72(2):169–74.

52. Schroeder TM, Yogeswaren ST, Augspurger ME, et al. Intensity modulated radiation therapy for optic nerve sheath meningioma. Int J Radiat Oncol Biol Phys. 2004;60(1);S315.

53. Sitathanee C, Dhanachai M, Poonyathalang A, et al. Stereotactic radiation therapy for optic nerve sheath meningioma; an experience at Ramathibodi Hospital. J Med Assoc Thail. 2006;89(10):1665–9.

54. Arvold ND, Lessell S, Bussiere M, et al. Visual outcome and tumor control after conformal radiotherapy for patients with optic nerve sheath meningioma. Int J Radiat Oncol Biol Phys. 2009;75(4):1166–72.

55. Milker-Zabel S, Huber P, Schlegel W, et al. Fractionated stereotactic radiation therapy in the management of primary optic nerve sheath meningiomas. J Neurooncol. 2009;94(3):419–24.

56. Smee RI, Schneider M, Williams JR. Optic nerve sheath meningiomas—non-surgical treatment. Clin Oncol (R Coll Radiol). 2009;21(1):8–13.

57. Liu D, Xu D, Zhang Z, et al. Long-term results of Gamma Knife surgery for optic nerve sheath meningioma. J Neurosurg. 2010;113(Suppl):28–33.

58. Lesser RL, Knisely JP, Wang SL, et al. Long-term response to fractionated radiotherapy of presumed optic nerve sheath meningioma. Br J Ophthalmol. 2010;94(5):559–63.

59. Marchetti M, Bianchi S, Milanesi I, et al. Multisession radiosurgery for optic nerve sheath meningiomas—an effective option: preliminary results of a single-center experience. Neurosurgery. 2011;69(5):1116–22. discussion 22–3

60. Solda F, Wharram B, Gunapala R, et al. Fractionated stereotactic conformal radiotherapy for optic nerve sheath meningiomas. Clin Oncol (R Coll Radiol). 2012;24(8):e106–12.

61. Abouaf L, Girard N, Lefort T, et al. Standard-fractionated radiotherapy for optic nerve sheath meningioma: visual outcome is predicted by mean eye dose. Int J Radiat Oncol Biol Phys. 2012;82(3):1268–77.

62. Paulsen F, Doerr S, Wilhelm H, et al. Fractionated stereotactic radiotherapy in patients with optic nerve sheath meningioma. Int J Radiat Oncol Biol Phys. 2012;82(2):773–8.

63. Adams G, Roos DE, Crompton JL. Radiotherapy for optic nerve sheath meningioma: a case for earlier intervention? Clin Oncol (R Coll Radiol). 2013;25(6):356–61.

64. Brower JV, Amdur RJ, Kirwan J, et al. Radiation therapy for optic nerve sheath meningioma. Pract Radiat Oncol. 2013;3(3):223–8.

65. Moyal L, Vignal-Clermont C, Boissonnet H, et al. Results of fractionated targeted proton beam therapy in the treatment of primary optic nerve sheath meningioma. J Fr Ophtalmol. 2014;37(4):288–95.

66. Lahkola A, Salminen T, Raitanen J, et al. Meningioma and mobile phone use--a collaborative case-control study in five North European countries. Int J Epidemiol. 2008;37(6):1304–13.

67. Jackson A, Patankar T, Laitt RD. Intracanalicular optic nerve meningioma: a serious diagnostic pitfall. AJNR Am J Neuroradiol. 2003;24(6):1167–70.

# Part VIII

# Ocular Oncology

# Uveal Melanoma

# 17

Richard L. S. Jennelle, Jesse L. Berry, and Jonathan W. Kim

## Learning Objectives

At the conclusion of this chapter, you should be able to:

- Discuss the different types of uveal melanoma identified by molecular profiling and the importance of each with regard to prognosis.
- Discuss the diagnostic criteria that establish the clinical diagnosis of uveal melanoma.
- Discuss the epidemiology and natural history of uveal melanoma.
- Discuss the various conservative surgical options for the treatment of uveal melanoma.
- Discuss the various types of radiotherapy that have been used to treat uveal melanoma and be able to compare and contrast the different techniques.
- Discuss the evidence that supports the eye-conserving treatment of uveal melanoma.
- Discuss the expected outcomes of conservative treatment for the different stages of uveal melanoma.
- Know the various isotopes used in brachytherapy for the treatment of uveal melanoma.
- Understand the late effects of radiotherapy used to treat uveal melanoma.
- Discuss the evolution of plaque brachytherapy with special attention to the impact of computerized treatment planning.

R. L. S. Jennelle (✉) · J. W. Kim
Children's Hospital Los Angeles, Keck School of Medicine,
Los Angeles, CA, USA
e-mail: Jennelle@usc.edu

J. L. Berry
USC Roski Eye Institute, Keck School of Medicine of USC,
Los Angeles, CA, USA

Children's Hospital Los Angeles, Keck School of Medicine,
Los Angeles, CA, USA

## Epidemiology

Primary uveal melanoma (UM) is a spectrum of disease, which encompasses intraocular tumors of the iris, ciliary body, and choroid. Uveal melanoma accounts for only 5% of melanomas in the United States [1], the remaining being predominantly skin in origin. However, mucous membranes and the conjunctiva can also harbor melanoma. It is, however, the second most common location for melanoma [2] and the most common primary intraocular malignancy in adults and the most common of all intraocular malignancies after metastatic lesions to the choroid [3]. The incidence of UM is approximately six cases per million people in the United States for an overall incidence of approximately 1500 cases per year [2]. Patients with uveal melanoma are generally 55–60 years of age, Caucasian, with light blue or green eyes and blonde or red hair [4]. Males and females are affected approximately equally [5]. Choroidal, cutaneous and iris nevi are all predisposing conditions for UM [6–8]. Ultraviolet light exposure (including via welding) [9–11] and family history [12–14] have also been correlated as risk factors. Other risk factors for the development of UM are predisposing medical conditions including dysplastic nevus syndrome [15, 16], neurofibromatosis type 1 [17–20], breast cancer-associated protein (BAP1) mutations [21, 22], and ocular melanocytosis [21–24] (GNAQ/11mutation) which significantly increases the risk of development of UM to 1/400 [25], and these individuals must be very closely monitored. Patients with choroidal nevi with known risk factors for malignant transformation must also be monitored very closely for evidence of growth, which suggests transformation. These risk factors include height >2 mm, presence of subretinal fluid, symptoms including decreased vision, flashes or floaters, presence of orange pigmentation, location adjacent the optic nerve or fovea, absence of a halo or drusen, and low internal reflectivity on B-scan ultrasonography [26–29].

## Diagnosis

Diagnosis of UM is made clinically with 99% accuracy [30]. It is based on indirect ophthalmoscopy and B-scan ultrasonography. Clinical exam generally shows an elevated, pigmented dome-shaped choroidal lesion with orange pigmentation on the surface and subretinal fluid at the base [28, 31]. There may sometimes be hemorrhage overlying the tumor; however generally there is not extensive subretinal or vitreous hemorrhage with uveal melanoma [32–34]. Amelanotic lesions are not rare but are definitely less common [35, 36]. Additionally, extensive subretinal fluid leading to a complete exudative retinal detachment can be present particularly with larger tumors [37–39].

B-scan ultrasonography classically demonstrates a choroidal tumor with dome (Fig. 17.1) or button-collar shape (Fig. 17.2) if the tumor has broken through Bruch's membrane [28, 40]. Generally B-scan is also used to measure these tumors [41]. While there are no strict measurements that determine whether or not a tumor is melanoma, in general, with the appropriate clinical features, pigmented lesions <5 mm at the base and <1 mm in height are considered choroidal nevi and lesions >10 mm at the base and >2.5 mm in height are concerning for choroidal melanoma [29]. Based on the collaborative ocular melanoma studies (COMS), small choroidal melanomas are >5 to <10 mm at the base and >1 to <2.5 mm in height and medium-sized choroidal melanomas are >10 to <15 mm at the base and >2.5 to <10 mm in height, with large-sized melanomas measuring greater than these dimensions in either the base of the height [42]. There is an indeterminate area between a choroidal nevus and a small choroidal melanoma wherein a lesion, often aptly termed an indeterminate choroidal lesion, may be a choroidal nevus with high-risk features or a small uveal melanoma. In these cases, clinical features and particularly presence or absence of growth over a short interval of monitoring are critical in the ultimate diagnosis [27]. It is also helpful to obtain a diagnostic A-scan evaluation, which for uveal melanoma classically shows a low to medium internal reflectivity lesion with descending reflectivity posteriorly after an initial high spike termed a positive angle kappa [40].

In our case presentation, the patient's tumor would be classified as a medium-sized choroidal melanoma in the COMS study based upon a tumor height measurement of 3.1 mm; however he would not have been offered brachytherapy based upon proximity to the optic disc. By AJCC criteria, the tumor would be a size category 1 (Fig. 17.3), stage T1a tumor. Table 17.1 summarizes the staging criteria for choroidal melanomas (the staging of iris melanomas differs) according to the AJCC cancer staging manual eighth edition [43]. There was no evidence of nodal or distant metastasis by imaging so the stage is T1a N0 M0 Stage IA (Table 17.1) choroidal melanoma of the right eye [43]. A biopsy is not required for diagnosis but is sometimes performed [44]. The approach to biopsy depends on the location of the tumor in the eye: biopsy may be done by fine needle aspiration (FNAB) trans-vitreally for posterior tumors and trans-sclerally for anterior tumors [45]. While biopsy is not routinely done for diagnosis, it is frequently done for prognostication regarding the risk of development of metastatic disease, with which current treatment strategies portend an extremely poor prognosis [46–48].

The differential diagnosis for choroidal melanoma includes choroidal nevus, melanocytoma, combined hamartoma of the retina and retinal pigment epithelium (RPE), congenital hypertrophy of the RPE, choroidal osteoma, choroidal hemangioma, choroidal metastases, choroidal disciform lesion, and choroidal hemorrhage [49].

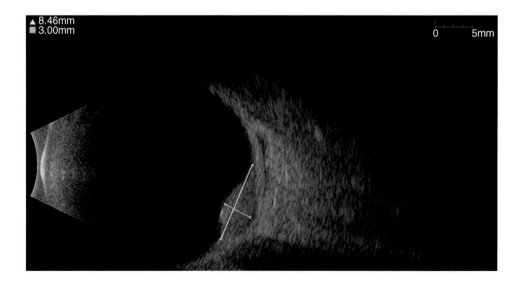

**Fig. 17.1** Ultrasound appearance of classic dome-shaped tumor

**Fig. 17.2** Ultrasound appearance of "mushroom" or "collar button" choroidal melanoma

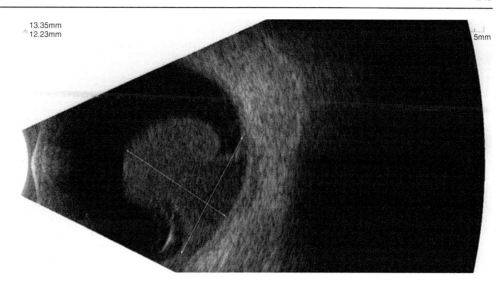

13.35mm
12.23mm

5mm

**Fig. 17.3** AJCC eighth edition size classification table. [Used with permission of the American Joint Committee on Cancer (AJCC), Chicago, IL. The original and primary source for this information is the AJCC Cancer Staging Manual, Eighth Edition (2017) published by Springer International Publishing]

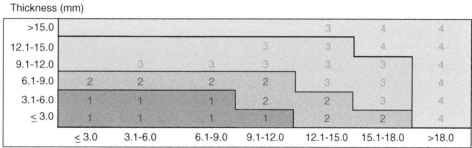

Thickness (mm)

| | | | | | | | |
|---|---|---|---|---|---|---|---|
| >15.0 | | | | | 3 | 4 | 4 |
| 12.1-15.0 | | | | 3 | 3 | 4 | 4 |
| 9.1-12.0 | | 3 | 3 | 3 | 3 | 3 | 4 |
| 6.1-9.0 | 2 | 2 | 2 | 2 | 3 | 3 | 4 |
| 3.1-6.0 | 1 | 1 | 1 | 2 | 2 | 3 | 4 |
| ≤ 3.0 | 1 | 1 | 1 | 1 | 2 | 2 | 4 |
| | ≤ 3.0 | 3.1-6.0 | 6.1-9.0 | 9.1-12.0 | 12.1-15.0 | 15.1-18.0 | >18.0 |

Largest basal diameter (mm)

**Table 17.1** Summarized AJCC eighth edition staging system for uveal melanoma

| T stage choroidal | T substage | N stage | M stage |
|---|---|---|---|
| T1 (size category 1) | a (no ciliary body involvement or extraocular extension) | N0 (no regional nodes or discrete tumor deposits in the orbit not contiguous with the eye) | M0 (no distant metastasis by clinical classification) |
| T2 (size category 2) | b (with ciliary body involvement) | N1a (regional nodal involvement) | M1a (largest diameter of largest metastasis ≤3 cm) |
| T3 (size category 3) | c (with extraocular extension ≤5 mm) | N1b (discrete tumor deposits in the orbit not contiguous with the eye) | M1b (largest diameter of largest metastasis 3.1–8 cm) |
| T4 (size category 4) | d (with both ciliary body involvement and extraocular extension ≤5 mm) | | M1c (largest diameter of largest metastasis ≥8.1 cm) |
| T4e | Any size tumor with extraocular extension >5 mm | | |
| Overall stage | TNM | | |
| I | T1aN0M0 | | |
| IIA | T1b-dN0M0 T2aN0M0 | | |
| IIB | T2bN0M0 T3aN0M0 | | |
| IIIA | T2c-dN0M0 T3b-cN0M0 T4aN0M0 | | |
| IIIB | T3dN0M0 T4b-cN0M0 | | |
| IIIC | T4d-eN0M0 | | |
| IV | Any T N1 and/or M1 | | |

Used with permission of the American Joint Committee on Cancer (AJCC), Chicago, Illinois. The original and primary source for this information is the AJCC Cancer Staging Manual, Eighth Edition (2017) published by Springer International Publishing

## Pathology

Histopathologic analysis of UM shows pigmented spindle or epithelioid-shaped melanocytes with high nuclear to cytoplasmic ratio and high mitotic and proliferation indices. Spindle cell melanomas have a better prognosis than epithelioid cell melanomas. Mixed cell type is also common and has an intermediate prognosis between the two [50, 51].

## Prognosis

Prognosis for UM depends on the risk of developing metastatic disease, which most commonly manifests in the liver (93%), the lung (24%), or the bone (16%) [52]. The risk of metastatic disease can be prognosticated based on clinical parameters such as size of the tumor, involvement of the ciliary body, and age of the patient [53, 54]. Based on COMS, the 5-year risk of tumor-specific mortality is <1% for small tumors, 10% for medium-sized tumors, and 35% for large tumors [52, 55–57]. Currently, gene expression profiling guides prognosis for metastatic disease development but does not impact choice of therapy.

Many centers now offer FNAB biopsy with various clinically available tests to evaluate cytogenetic abnormalities in chromosome 1, 3, 6, and 8 (loss of 1p, 3, and 6q and gain of 6p and 8q or 8) or gene expression profiles [58–64]. Frequent mutations have been described in the following five genes GNA11, GNAQ, BAP1, EIF1AX, and SF3B1 which are thought to be driver mutations for the development of UM [22, 65].

Gene expression profiling classifies the risk at Class 1A, 1B, and 2 with a 5-year risk of development of metastatic disease as 2%, 21%, and 72% [66]. It has never been shown that treatment modality modifies the risk of development of metastatic disease; however intraocular recurrences after treatment do occur [67, 68] and may increase this risk [69]. Our patient did not elect to have a biopsy performed, but his overall prognosis is good with an expected overall survival rate of 85% at 15 years (Fig. 17.4) [43].

## Treatment Paradigms

In this section, we will discuss treatment paradigms for uveal melanoma including trans-scleral local resection, transpupillary thermotherapy, and brachytherapy.

## Trans-Scleral Local Resection

Local trans-scleral resection of uveal melanoma is not commonly practiced in the United States and was pioneered in England for management of large tumors not amenable

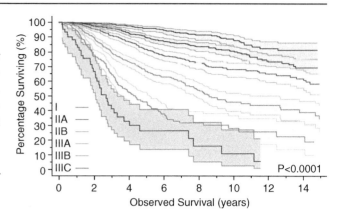

**Fig. 17.4** Survival according to AJCC eighth edition by overall stage. [Used with permission of the American Joint Committee on Cancer (AJCC), Chicago, IL. The original and primary source for this information is the AJCC Cancer Staging Manual, Eighth Edition (2017) published by Springer International Publishing]

to brachytherapy with ruthenium plaques [70]. The rates of local recurrence, systemic metastasis, and ocular complications are all higher after local resection compared to brachytherapy, but this disparity is likely associated with the larger tumors being treated with the former technique. Following local resection for large uveal melanomas, 40% of eyes were noted to have residual or recurrent tumor, with 53% of these eyes undergoing enucleation [71, 72]. The technique involves the creation of a lamellar scleral flap, which provides exposure to remove the choroidal tumor with a thin layer of attached sclera while leaving the retina undisturbed. Partial ocular decompression from a limited pars plana vitrectomy is thought to facilitate local excision by reducing retinal prolapse during the procedure and improving access to the posterior uvea. Anterior tumors are more amenable for local resection as are those tumors with overlying subretinal fluid and the absence of retinal invasion. A portion of the ciliary body can also be resected along with the choroidal component although removing more than 3 clock hours of the pars plicata can cause hypotony. Patients with large areas of extraocular extension, diffuse uveal melanomas, or optic disc involvement are poor candidates for local resection. There is no absolute size limit for local resection, but a higher rate of tumor recurrence rate has been noted with tumors greater than 15 mm in diameter [71]. For patients with uveal melanomas deemed to be too large for ruthenium plaques, local resection may be a viable alternative to enucleation for appropriate candidates.

One source of concern with surgical resection is that the majority of uveal melanomas demonstrate local invasion of the sclera, as well as the retina, which may not be completely removed with local resection. In addition, hypotensive anesthesia was thought to be necessary to decrease the chances for bleeding during the procedure and subsequent seeding of the orbit with tumor cells. The first concern has been alleviated with the common practice of using brachytherapy following local resection, treating to a tumor height of 3–5 mm post resection for any residual cells in the sclera or retina [71, 73]. The need for hypotensive anesthesia remains somewhat controversial, but it is recommended that bleeding from the procedure be carefully controlled to avoid orbital seeding. Patients should be counseled regarding the significant risk of intraocular complications such as retinal detachment, vitreous hemorrhage, and local tumor recurrence following local resection.

As mentioned, profound hypotensive anesthesia with systolic blood pressure being reduced as low as 50 mm Hg can greatly reduce the risk of intraoperative hemorrhage. The hypotensive anesthesia is typically initiated from the time the deep scleral incision is started to the moment when the scleral flap has been closed, lasting approximately 1 h. Cerebral functioning is monitored with an electroencephalogram (EEG), and an arterial line closely tracks the blood pressure. After marking the margins of the tumor, a rectangular, lamellar scleral flap is outlined 3–5 mm from the tumor borders, hinged posteriorly beyond the posterior margin of the tumor. The depth of the lamellar scleral flap is typically about 2/3 of the thickness of the sclera. Partial ocular decompression via a limited pars plana vitrectomy facilitates the rest of the procedure as it keeps the retina away from the tumor and surgical field. The deep scleral incision is made just inside the margins of the previously created scleral flap. The deep scleral incision is then extended around the tumor using corneoscleral scissors, separating the thin sclera over the base of the tumor from the surrounding sclera. The choroidal layer is then incised, and the subretinal space is entered, typically starting anteriorly and proceeding laterally and then posteriorly. Once the choroidal layer has been completely incised, the thin layer of sclera over the base of the tumor can then be used to remove the entire tumor from the eye. The retina typically peels away from the choroid, but gentle blunt dissection may be required. Once the tumor has been removed, new instruments are then used for the closure. The intraocular pressure is elevated using either a gas bubble or an intravitreal saline injection to prevent subretinal hematoma formation. The scleral flap is then closed with interrupted 8-0 nylon sutures, closing the corners first followed by the rest of the flap. Intravitreal fluid is then injected to elevate the intraocular pressure into a normal range. At this point in the procedure with the scleral flap closed and the intraocular pressure normalized, brachytherapy can be performed to prevent tumor recurrence in the retina and scleral flap. A more detailed description of the local resection procedure is beyond the scope of this chapter, but several excellent references are available in the literature [71, 73].

## Transpupillary Thermotherapy (TTT)

Using a diode laser to heat a tumor and produce cell necrosis through a transpupillary technique has been termed TTT (transpupillary thermotherapy) [74]. To perform TTT for a choroidal melanoma, an 810 nm diode laser is used either through a slit-lamp attachment or through an indirect delivery system. The technique involves treating the tumor with the diode laser at a power level which causes a visible color change (i.e., whitening) within the 45–60 s duration, which has been correlated to produce a temperature within the tumor between 45 and 60 °C. A choroidal melanoma treated with TTT has demonstrated tumor necrosis on histopathology up to a depth of 3.9 mm [75, 76].

Initial clinical series demonstrated a high rate of success in causing tumor regression for tumors less than 4 mm in thickness, and TTT was touted to be an effective primary modality for treating small posterior uveal melanomas [77, 78]. Vascular obstruction and retinal traction were observed complications [79], although overall visual results were much better than with brachytherapy [78, 80]. The margins of treatment for TTT are sharper than for brachytherapy or proton beam radiotherapy, and this factor likely explains the visual advantage for TTT. However, with longer follow-up, tumor recurrences were noted, and subsequent studies showed a 76–78% rate of long-term success for tumor control [81, 82]. Some tumor recurrences were massive and led to loss of the globe, and late recurrences many years after TTT were also noted [82]. The tumors after TTT typically demonstrate almost complete atrophy of the retina and choroid, with sharply circumscribed scars showing bare sclera. However, viable melanoma cells have been shown to invade into the sclera and emissary canals as well as the surrounding retina, and these residual cells are likely responsible for these tumor recurrences. Therefore, TTT is not thought to be curative as the sole modality for many choroidal melanomas even when treating small tumors.

Currently, TTT is utilized for choroidal melanomas in specific clinical situations. For example, TTT is an option for controlling the growth of small suspicious choroidal nevus, particularly in older patients who want to avoid brachytherapy in tumors near the optic disc. TTT is also used in combination with radiotherapy (called "sandwich" therapy), with TTT treating the apex of the tumor and brachytherapy being performed at the base [83–85]. TTT can also be used at the posterior margin of a macular tumor so that a smaller treatment zone can be used near the macula by brachytherapy to preserve vision. Finally, TTT has been used successfully to treat small edge tumor recurrences after brachytherapy [82]. Whenever TTT is used to treat a melanocytic tumor, patients require careful, long-term follow-up to monitor the patient for complications and possible local tumor recurrence.

Tumor recurrences after TTT can be treated with either brachytherapy or enucleation, depending on the level of visual acuity, size of recurrence, and metastatic status of the patient.

The technique of using TTT for melanocytic choroidal tumors has been described for both the slit-lamp application (3 mm spot size) and indirect delivery system (1.4 mm spot size). Since the spot size for the indirect system is smaller, power levels required to reach the desired temperature are also typically lower. In general, power levels should be adjusted until the desired color change (i.e., mild whitening) between 45–60 s is achieved; if the color change occurs before 45 s, then the power level is decreased. The entire surface of the tumor is treated with overlapping treatment burns, covering the margins of the tumor for 1.5 mm. Pigmented tumors are the best candidates for TTT, but even for the darkest tumors typically more than one session is required to achieve complete regression. It has been reported that the absorption of TTT may be enhanced by the intravenous infusion of ICG in amelanotic tumors [86], although we do not have experience with this technique. Treatment should be repeated for two to three sessions until the lesion has flattened significantly and very little viable tumor remains. It should be kept in mind that continued regression of the tumor can be observed for several months after the last laser session and often an atrophic scar will form at the treated site.

## Brachytherapy

Historically, the standard of care in the treatment of uveal melanoma has been enucleation. However, beginning in the early part of the twentieth century, several institutions began to evaluate brachytherapy in the management of this disease [87]. The development of plaque brachytherapy required several key elements before the modality took on its current form. Among the first plaques manufactured were those based upon the use of $^{60}$Co [87, 88]. This isotope, with a high specific activity, was naturally of interest. It could be made into an applicator that could easily be positioned in proximity to the tumor, but the highly energetic photons would require shielding that was prohibitively large when trying to spare orbital adnexal tissue. Many other isotopes were investigated as well, but it was $^{125}$I that eventually became the favored isotope for the COMS study [89] and since then has been the most common isotope for treatment in the United States. It can be incorporated into seeds with sufficiently high activity to be useful, but the relatively low energy of the emitted photons makes shielding the orbital adnexa a much easier task. The inverse square law dominates at short distances and is the key characteristic that allows for the shaping of dose to the tumor and the sparing of other nearby critical structures

in all forms of photon brachytherapy [89]. Over the years, many other isotopes with similar characteristics have been developed, but $^{125}$I (which decays by electron capture and emits a gamma photon of 35.5 keV) remains the dominant isotope largely because of the impact of the COMS study. In a similar manner, some advocate for the use of $^{103}$Pd which also decays by electron capture but with a softer gamma photon at 21 keV. The degree to which the softer gamma photon benefits the treatment or harms it is a topic of discussion within the ocular oncology community.

It is worth mentioning the use of isotopes, most commonly ruthenium, that are beta emitters. These isotopes have an even more rapid fall off of dose from the source related to the relatively short penetration range of beta particles and are typically employed for treatment of thinner tumors [90]. The main limitation of beta-emitting isotopes is excessive dose to the underlying sclera when prescribing to thicker tumors.

Although there was growing evidence, based upon multiple single institution reports, that brachytherapy could be a possible treatment for uveal melanoma, many ophthalmologists were reluctant to risk the possibility of metastatic disease in order to conserve the eye [91]. The COMS study for medium-sized melanomas was undertaken to analyze in a prospective and randomized fashion the effectiveness of plaque brachytherapy in the eye-conserving treatment of uveal melanoma. The COMS study demonstrated that, in medium-sized uveal melanomas, plaque brachytherapy could be used in place of enucleation without any impact on the rate of metastasis or overall survival [55]. A second component of the study, directed at large uveal melanomas, evaluated a short course of preoperative radiation prior to enucleation to see if this prevented metastasis from manipulation at the time of surgery. Short-course preoperative radiation did not impact the development of distant metastasis and so is no longer used [57].

Brachytherapy remains the most common eye-conserving treatment for uveal melanomas and can be used for both posterior and anterior tumors. With some adjustment in technique, brachytherapy can be used successfully for both posterior tumors near the optic nerve and anterior melanomas involving the iris and ciliary body [92–94]. The surgical technique is similar no matter which isotope is used for brachytherapy, including $^{125}$I, $^{106}$Ru, and $^{103}$Pd. However, the specific method used to localize the tumor varies significantly at different centers. Success rates appear to be high with all of the techniques described in this section. Ocular brachytherapy can be performed either under general anesthesia or under a retrobulbar block with conscious sedation. The authors' preference is general anesthesia since the local block can increase swelling and decrease surgical exposure. In addition, any patient discomfort during the procedure may require additional anesthesia and/or compromise the surgical outcome.

Before starting surgery, the surgeon performs indirect ophthalmoscopy through a dilated pupil to confirm the position of the tumor as well as any intraocular findings such as hemorrhage or subretinal fluid. After sterile prepping and draping of the marked eye, a 180 degree conjunctival peritomy is performed at the limbal location which corresponds to the center of the tumor. The Tenon's layer (i.e., capsule) is then dissected off the sclera to ensure that the scleral surface over the tumor is completely exposed. One of the rectus muscles is commonly disinserted to ensure accurate plaque placement, although this may not be necessary if the tumor is small and located in one of the oblique quadrants. The rectus muscle is isolated and imbricated in standard fashion with a double-armed 5-0 Vicryl suture and disinserted, allowing it to reflect back with the attached sutures away from the sclera. A traction suture using a 5-0 Mersilene suture is passed at the muscle insertion site or at the limbus to allow for mobilization of the globe during the procedure. The oblique muscles are thinner and typically do not have to be disinserted. We also do not recommend disturbing the vortex veins in the oblique quadrants. A small malleable retractor is used to gently retract the rectus muscle and orbital fat to visualize the entire scleral surface to ensure that no soft tissues will interfere with the positioning of the plaque on the sclera. Exposing the scleral surface is a critical part of the procedure to ensure complete plaque coverage of the tumor but also to document any areas of scleral extension. Any extra-scleral nodule less than 2 mm in thickness can be covered with the plaque and treated without a significant alteration of the treatment plan or technique.

Once the scleral surface has been exposed, attention is turned to localizing the tumor margins. At our center, three-dimensional tumor modeling is utilized to determine the plaque coordinates preoperatively (Plaque Simulator, Eye Physics LLC). The meridian and distance from the limbus are marked using a toric marker and caliper, respectively. Alternatively, the tumor margins can be determined intraoperatively using either transillumination or indirect ophthalmoscopy or a combination of the two techniques. Transillumination is most useful for pigmented, anterior tumors, and indirect ophthalmoscopy is invaluable for posterior tumors. For tumors located in the macula or near the optic nerve, it can be difficult to visualize the posterior margin, and in these cases, it may need to be estimated from the preoperative ultrasound. Transillumination is performed with a rubber adapter on a light source, with the light being directed through the pupil and the shadow of the tumor being outlined on the sclera. It should be kept in mind that highly elevated tumors can create variable shadows on the sclera depending on the angle of illumination, and amelanotic tumors may be difficult to visualize with this technique. Indirect ophthalmoscopy can be performed with scleral depression and a marking pen, or a diathermy tip. One of the

most effective devices for this technique is the diathermy-transillumination unit (MIRA 1 electrode handle) with a scleral transilluminator electrode. With the fiber-optic light marking the perimeter of the tumor (viewed with indirect ophthalmoscopy), a low intensity diathermy mark can be made on the sclera at the anterior, medial, lateral, and posterior margins. Once the surgeon has confirmed the scleral markings of the tumor margins, the dummy plaque is placed.

The dummy plaque is positioned on the sclera and partial thickness scleral passes made with two 5-0 Mersilene sutures at the position of the two eyelets. It is critical to first complete the partial thickness passes through the sclera, before passing the needle through the eyelet of the plaque. Engaging the needle through the eyelet and then sclera will lead to scleral perforation due to the angle of the needle with this technique. The passed scleral sutures are then secured to the eyelets of the dummy plaque with a temporary loop knot. The indirect ophthalmoscope is then placed on the surgeon by an assistant (maintaining sterility), and the margins of the plaque are depressed to ensure that there is complete coverage of the tumor. The depression is usually performed with a metal scleral depressor, with the assistant moving the globe with the traction suture to allow the depressor to follow the outlines of the dummy plaque. The fiber-optic light source on the MIRA unit can also be used for this indication. Ultrasound confirmation of the plaque position is becoming popular to ensure complete coverage of the tumor margins and appears to increase the accuracy of brachytherapy [95–98]. Visualizing the relationship of the plaque and scleral surface on the B-scan can also be used to assess whether posterior tilting of the plaque is occurring. However, any thin areas of tumor extension should be noted on fundoscopy and taken into account when using ultrasound confirmation. In addition, the probe of the ultrasound tip must be covered during its intraoperative use to maintain sterility.

Once its proper positioning has been confirmed, the dummy plaque is removed, and the active plaque is placed in its position; the two Mersilene sutures are tied again but this time using permanent knots. The rectus muscle is then reattached to its insertion site; the suture can be tied with a loop knot with long ends or tied with a permanent suture. The advantage of a loop, adjustable suture is that the rectus muscle does not need to be re-sutured at the time of plaque removal. However, the longer ends of the adjustable suture can cause ocular irritation if not properly tucked under the conjunctiva. If the anterior portion of the plaque covers the rectus insertion site, then the sutures are passed through the superficial sclera near the limbus; it can be properly re-sutured to the insertion site after the completion of brachytherapy. Finally, the conjunctiva is closed over the plaque using an absorbable suture.

After completion of treatment, a second operation is performed to remove the plaque (3–7 days later). The conjunctiva is gently reopened to allow for exposure of the anterior position of the plaque including the eyelets. The two Mersilene sutures are carefully lysed with Westcott scissors, being careful not to cause any traction or injury to the underlying sclera. Once the plaque is freely mobile, it is carefully removed from the scleral surface and given to the Rad Onc representative for inspection. The sclera should also be inspected for any unexpected findings such as a hematoma or dislodged seeds. The time of removal should be noted for the operative record. Again, it is critical to check the plaque for the correct number of seeds to ensure that none have become dislodged. A survey meter must also be passed over the eye and the patient to confirm complete removal of any radioactive seeds from the surgical site. If the rectus muscle had been disinserted, it is reattached to its insertion site. The conjunctiva is closed using absorbable sutures. Indirect ophthalmoscopy should also be performed at this point in the procedure to ensure that no unexpected events have occurred, such as inadvertent scleral perforation. Patients are typically seen in the first week after the removal of the plaque to ensure that healing is proceeding appropriately. The first post-brachytherapy ultrasound examination is performed at 3 months. Future follow-up exams are determined based on the clinical course.

## Surgical Complications

Inadvertent perforation of the sclera may rarely occur, and as long as appropriate steps are taken, significant complications should not be observed. If the scleral perforation with the needle occurs outside the margins of the tumor, indirect ophthalmoscopy should be performed to determine if retinal perforation has occurred. If a retinal break is noted, then laser photocoagulation should be performed around the break in an attempt to seal it. If the scleral perforation has occurred within the margins of the tumor, then no other intervention is needed as long as the scleral defect is small and immediate brachytherapy will be performed over the site of perforation. If a small amount of subretinal fluid is present around the break, then cryotherapy is recommended to seal the retinal defect.

## Brachytherapy Dose

The selection of dose is largely based upon empiric data. Based upon the pre-existing work, COMS chose a prescription dose of 100 Gy [99]. There have not been studies that systematically explore the optimal brachytherapy dose although some retrospective data supports the possibility of decreasing the dose [100]. Currently, a dose of 85 Gy is used; however this is not a decrease in prescribed dose but is related to a systematic error in the manner dose was calculated for [125]I before the mid-1990s [101]. For all intents and purposes, the 85 Gy that is currently prescribed is exactly the same as the 100 Gy used previously and should not be seen as a dose decrement.

Similarly, doses of charged particles and stereotactic radiation were chosen to mimic the dose of brachytherapy [102–104]. Accurate comparison of doses between different forms of radiation is a very difficult subject and far beyond the scope of this limited chapter. Unlike brachytherapy, studies examining dose de-escalation for proton therapy [105] and stereotactic therapy [106] are reported in the literature. These studies suggest that a substantial decrease in prescribed dose can result in similar rates of control for uveal melanoma and decreases the rate of complications.

Originally, brachytherapy use was confined to medium-sized uveal melanomas located posteriorly that spared the optic nerve. Entry in the COMS study required the tumor to be at least 2 mm from the optic nerve. This was required to ensure adequate dose to the tumor with margin. The COMS eye plaques did not have a notch or other adaptation to permit plaque placement close to the nerve. Some modern plaques have been designed with a notch so that this is no longer a restriction. Specialized brachytherapy applicators now allow for the treatment of challenging tumors with more precise techniques [107]. With experience and technical innovation, there are now few eyes that cannot be spared by using radiation. Using these more advanced techniques, we were able to use a notched plaque in our patient to adequately cover the extent of tumor with only minimal impingement on the margin (Figs. 17.5 and 17.6). In fact, it is now acceptable to treat tumors up to T4e with brachytherapy as long as there is reason to believe that the treatment will result in successful salvage of the globe without unacceptable toxicity [108]. Enucleation is now mostly reserved for eyes that have little chance for salvage irrespective of the visual acuity that may result from treatment with radiation.

Treatment planning for brachytherapy is fundamentally based upon the findings at indirect ophthalmoscopy and ultrasound examination. Using these measurements, nearly any radiation oncology service can calculate and deliver the required treatment using the COMS technique. The prescription point is typically the dimensions of the tumor with an additional margin of approximately 2 mm. Typically, it is the height of the tumor that drives the prescription as base coverage can be addressed by altering the number of sources to ensure adequate coverage. It is important to be sure that the resultant isodose line covers the base of the tumor, again with an acceptable margin. Doses are typically between 70 and 100 Gy with a typical dose rate of approximately 0.6 Gy per hour. This results in typical implant

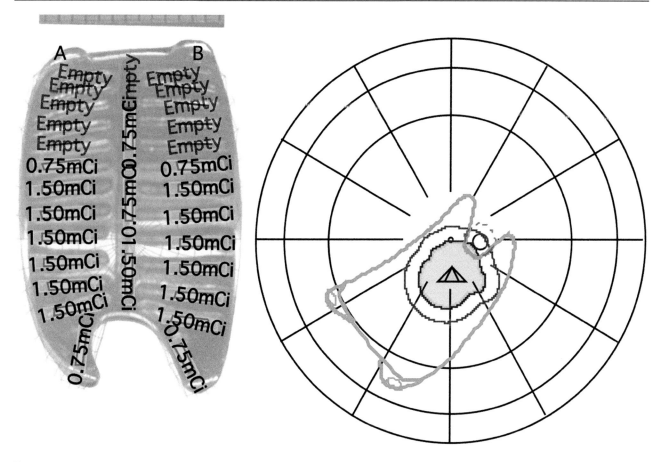

**Fig. 17.5** Plaque model, loading, and placement for case study patient

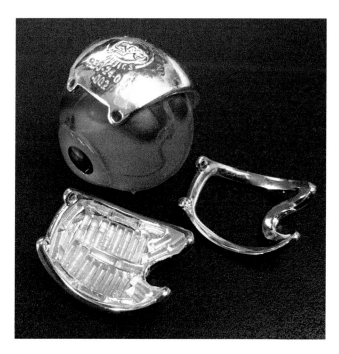

**Fig. 17.6** Eye Physics, LLC plaque for case patient placed on eye model. [Used with permission of Eye Physics, LLC]

duration of 5–7 days. Figure 17.7 shows the preplanning isodose lines superimposed on the fused imaging from our patient mentioned earlier. Figure 17.8 shows the dose area histogram of the tumor and various critical structures for our patient as well.

Treatments involving beta emitters can be a bit more variable. Since beta emitters (typically $^{106}$Ru and $^{90}$Sr) have a much longer half-life, these sources are typically reused over the course of several years. The length of time required to treat is then determined by the current activity of the source and the desired prescription. Treatment will be shorter for a new source and longer for an older one.

Since all forms of plaque brachytherapy are affixed to the globe, there is minimal difficulty ensuring adequate correction for motion. The plaque moves as a unit with the eye. However, there is great variability in the extent of treatment planning for plaque brachytherapy. Treatment planning can run from simple point source calculations on one of the standard COMS plaques to customized collimating plaques with highly accurate dose modeling supplemented by preoperative planning involving fusion of ultrasound, fundus photography, and fused CT/MRI images. The goal is to give

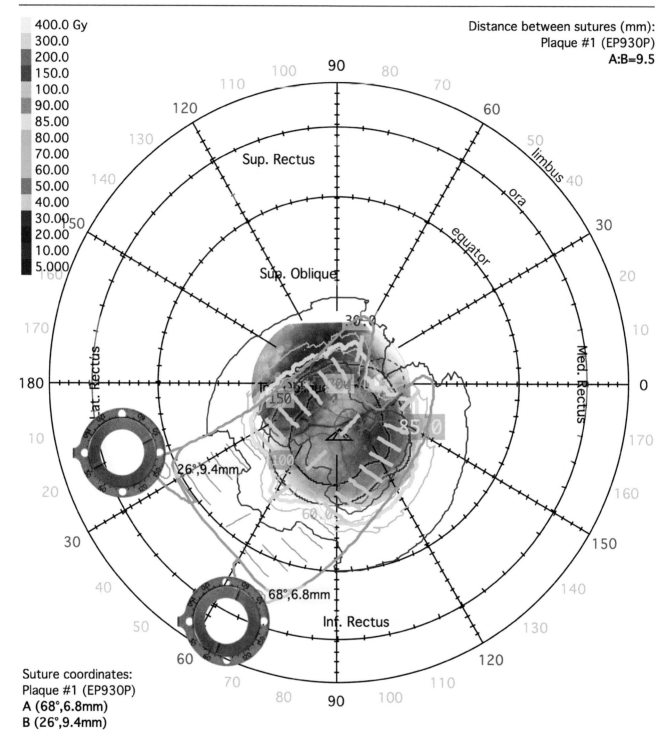

**Fig. 17.7** Tumor and normal structure contours with isodose overlay for case study patient

adequate dose to control the tumor while minimizing the dose to adjacent critical structures. The more advanced planning and treatment delivery systems allow for significant dose reduction to normal structures (Fig. 17.9) and a more streamlined procedure in the operating room, but do not allow for modification of the device during the procedure [107]. The main advantage to the advanced plaque delivery systems over traditional COMS style plaques is the increased collimation obtained by the slotted metal plaque construction (Fig. 17.10). There are no randomized trials addressing the superiority of one technique over the other, but the American Brachytherapy Society assigns level 1 importance to attempts at reducing dose to normal structures and so would favor the more advanced plaque designs [108].

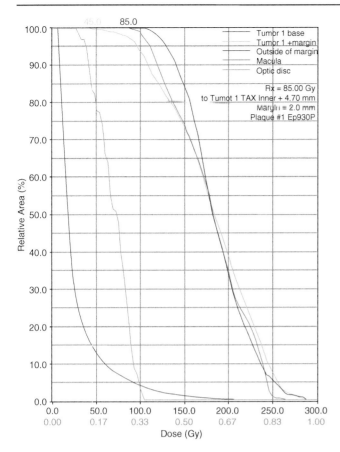

**Fig. 17.8** Dose area histograms for case study patient

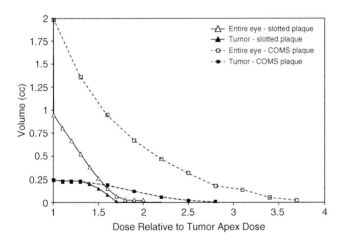

**Fig. 17.9** Dose volume histograms for COMS plaque versus advanced collimated plaque treating identical tumors. [Reprinted from Astrahan MA, Luxton G, Pu Q, Petrovich Z. Conformal episcleral plaque therapy. International Journal of Radiation Oncology Biology Physics. 1997;39:505–19. With permission from Elsevier]

## Charged Particle Radiation

At the same time that brachytherapy was beginning to be used, other institutions evaluated the use of charged particle

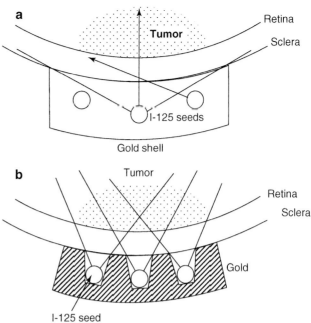

**Fig. 17.10** Effect of slotted plaque construction on collimation (**b**) of photons when compared to traditional COMS style plaque (**a**). [Reprinted from Astrahan MA, Luxton G, Pu Q, Petrovich Z. Conformal episcleral plaque therapy. International Journal of Radiation Oncology Biology Physics. 1997;39:505–19. With permission from Elsevier]

external beam irradiation in the management of uveal melanoma. Most often, this was done with proton beam radiation although helium ions have been evaluated as well [102, 109]. Charged particle radiation uses the Bragg peak to help confine the radiation to the targeted area. In short, the Bragg peak limits the effective range of the beam so that there is essentially no exit beam at any point past the physical location of the peak. The only prospective randomized trial, conducted by UCSF, compared brachytherapy with charged particle therapy in the form of helium ions. This study favored charged particle therapy for control [110]; however complication rates were significantly higher with charged particle treatment [111] especially in the anterior segment of the eye. Modern series with more advanced plaque techniques report control rates superior to COMS or the UCSF study reported above [112]. Proton beam radiation, although not supported by a study similar to COMS, nonetheless benefits from the COMS study based upon the assumption that similar rates of local control will, likewise, achieve similar rates of overall survival and distant metastasis.

## Stereotactic External Radiation

There is also a third technique, namely, stereotactic radiation. This is an outgrowth of similar work on other central nervous system tumors. In short, multiple beams can deliver conventional photon irradiation so that the dose is accurately placed at the target and demonstrates very rapid fall off in all other directions. Most forms of stereotactic radiation rigidly affix a treatment apparatus to the target and use this apparatus to guide the series of beams in a very tightly conformal manner that is highly accurate. Stereotactic radiation uses multiple beams to emulate what the Bragg peak does for charged particle therapy or what the inverse square law does for brachytherapy.

Treatment planning and prescription for external beam treatments employing charged particles or stereotactic techniques will necessarily involve the planning system for the device chosen. With charged particles, fiducial markers are typically placed to help with treatment alignment. With stereotactic techniques, some form of motion management is required. Motion management can vary from rigid fixation using various surgical apparatus to motion detection using various systems to follow visual fixation on a target [113–116]. For protons, typical doses have been in the range of 50–70 CGE (cobalt gray equivalent) usually delivered over five fractions [105]. For single faction stereotactic treatment, the range of doses is 25–50 Gy to the tumor margin [106]. As would be expected, treatment with lower doses is associated with lower rates of complication.

## Radiation Complications

Many critical structures lie close to one another within the eye, and, as a consequence, the complications experienced are not only related to dose but also related to anatomic position of the tumor with regard to these critical structures. Endpoints such as visual acuity are multifactorial in determination and can be related to damage to the nerve, macula, lens, or retina. Typical classes of complications are radiation retinopathy, glaucoma (including neovascular glaucoma), optic neuritis, keratitis, and iris neovascularization. As expected, there are wide ranges seen in reported complications both from brachytherapy and charged particle treatment [102, 117]. Table 17.2 summarizes the reported

**Table 17.2** Summarized radiotherapy complication rates by technique

| Complication | Charged particle [109] | Brachytherapy [117] |
|---|---|---|
| Glaucoma (unspecified) | 17–29% | 6–11% |
| Rubeosis | 13% | 4–23% |
| Neovascular glaucoma | 12% | 2–45% |
| Maculopathy | 67% | 13–52% |
| Cataract | 32–68% | 8–83% |
| Keratitis | 12% | 4% |
| Retinopathy | 28% | 10–63% |
| Optic neuropathy | 8% | 0–46% |

complication rates throughout the literature. Tumors that are in the anterior segment or adjacent to it also carry an increased risk of complications [118]. Depending upon beam placement, charged particle therapy may carry an increased risk of anterior chamber complications even when treating a posteriorly located tumor [111].

## Case Presentation

A 27-year-old white male was diagnosed with a retinal detachment, possibly secondary to a mass, 4 days prior and referred in for evaluation. He has no significant past medical history and no significant family history.

Physical examination reveals vision to be finger counting only in his right eye and normal visual acuity in his left. Intraocular pressures were normal bilaterally. Indirect ophthalmoscopy revealed a pigmented lesion in the right eye involving the macula and adjacent to the optic disc. The lesion was located inferotemporally extending from approximately 6 o'clock to approximately 9 o'clock (Fig. 17.11). The lesion was associated with orange pigment and subretinal fluid. B-mode ultrasound measured the lesion to be 8.4 mm by 8.5 mm with a height of 3.1 mm. He subsequently underwent thin-section computed tomography of the orbits as well as computed tomography of the chest, abdomen, and pelvis. All studies were negative for metastatic disease. He was referred for treatment with episcleral plaque

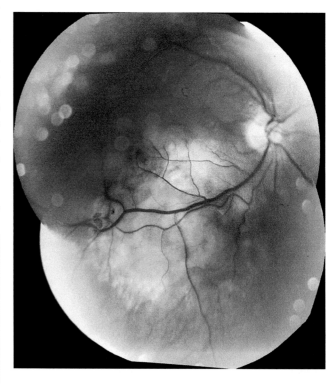

**Fig. 17.11** Fundus photo of case study patient

brachytherapy with a clinical diagnosis of choroidal melanoma of the right eye.

## Summary

UM is an uncommon disease whose management has been significantly impacted by the well-conducted COMS prospective trial. Treatment has progressed to such an extent that salvage of the eye is now a realistic possibility in all but the most advanced cases. Advances in molecular genetics have identified several subtypes of tumor with markedly different prognostic expectations but has yet to impact decisions on disease management. There are many surgical and radiotherapeutic options in the management of this disease, but episcleral plaque brachytherapy remains the mainstay of treatment at this time.

## Self-Assessment Questions

1. Which of the following is not a commonly used criterion to diagnose uveal melanoma?
   A. Appearance on indirect ophthalmoscopy
   B. Findings on B-mode ultrasound
   C. Biopsy
   D. Growth rate on serial observation

2. In the COMS study of medium-sized choroidal melanomas, patients were excluded for entry if their tumor was within 2 mm of the optic disc. Why was this an exclusion criterion?
   A. It was not possible to adequately cover the tumor volume with a COMS style plaque due to obstruction from the optic nerve.
   B. There would be unacceptable morbidity from damage to the optic nerve.
   C. There would be unacceptable toxicity from damage to the macula.
   D. Tumors in close approximation to the optic nerve are not surgically accessible.

3. All of the following radiotherapy techniques have been used to manage uveal melanoma except one. Which has not been successfully employed to manage uveal melanoma?
   A. Episcleral plaque brachytherapy
   B. IMRT
   C. Stereotactic radiotherapy
   D. Charged particle treatment

4. What is the approximate expected overall survival at 10 years for a melanoma measuring 12 × 8 mm with a height of 9 mm which does not involve the ciliary body or manifest extra-scleral extension?
   A. 95%
   B. 85%
   C. 75%
   D. 50%

5. All of the following isotopes used in the management of uveal melanoma by episcleral plaque brachytherapy are commonly used except one. Which isotope is no longer commonly used to treat uveal melanoma?
   A. $^{125}$I
   B. $^{106}$Ru
   C. $^{90}$Sr
   D. $^{60}$Co

## Answers

1. Answer: C. Biopsy is not a commonly used criterion although it can be used to help with prognostication. Both indirect ophthalmoscopy and findings on B-mode ultrasound are commonly used to diagnose uveal melanomas. Small lesions of indeterminate nature can be followed for growth on serial observation.

2. A. Tumors within 2 mm of the optic disc could not be properly covered by a COMS style plaque because of interference from the optic nerve. There were no constraints upon visual acuity toxicity in the COMS trial. There is no difficulty with surgically accessing the posterior globe.

3. B. Plaque brachytherapy, stereotactic radiation, and charged particle treatment have all been proven effective in the management of this disease. IMRT without the special immobilization and rapid fall off of the other techniques lacks the precision to treat this disease.

4. B. This tumor would stage as a T2a N0 M0 Stage IIA choroidal melanoma. The correct overall survival would be 85% at 10 years according to the AJCC staging system.

5. D. All listed isotopes have been used to treat uveal melanoma. The soft photon emitter iodine remains the most common isotope in the United States, while Europe still frequently employs ruthenium or strontium beta emitters. Although cobalt was classically used, the high energy photons proved problematic when attempting to shield the orbital adnexa, and so it is no longer used.

## References

1. Singh AD, Bergman L, Seregard S. Uveal melanoma: epidemiologic aspects. Ophthalmol Clin N Am. 2005;18(1):75–84. viii

2. Egan KM, Seddon JM, Glynn RJ, et al. Epidemiologic aspects of uveal melanoma. Surv Ophthalmol. 1988;32(4):239–51.

3. Weis E, Salopek TG, McKinnon JG, et al. Management of uveal melanoma: a consensus-based provincial clinical practice guideline. Curr Oncol. 2016;23(1):e57–64.

4. Gallagher RP, Elwood JM, Rootman J, et al. Risk factors for ocular melanoma: Western Canada Melanoma Study. J Natl Cancer Inst. 1985;74(4):775–8.

5. Zloto O, Pe'er J, Frenkel S. Gender differences in clinical presentation and prognosis of uveal melanoma. Invest Ophthalmol Vis Sci. 2013;54(1):652–6.

6. Weis E, Shah CP, Lajous M, et al. The association of cutaneous and iris nevi with uveal melanoma: a meta-analysis. Ophthalmology. 2009;116(3):536–43.e2.

7. Singh AD, Kalyani P, Topham A. Estimating the risk of malignant transformation of a choroidal nevus. Ophthalmology. 2005;112(10):1784–9.

8. Yanoff M, Zimmerman LE. Histogenesis of malignant melanomas of the uvea. II. Relationship of uveal nevi to malignant melanomas. Cancer. 1967;20(4):493–507.

9. Guenel P, Laforest L, Cyr D, et al. Occupational risk factors, ultraviolet radiation, and ocular melanoma: a case-control study in France. Cancer Causes Control. 2001;12(5):451–9.

10. Holly EA, Aston DA, Char DH, et al. Uveal melanoma in relation to ultraviolet light exposure and host factors. Cancer Res. 1990;50(18):5773–7.

11. Seddon JM, Gragoudas ES, Glynn RJ, et al. Host factors, UV radiation, and risk of uveal melanoma. A case-control study. Arch Ophthalmol. 1990;108(9):1274–80.

12. Lynch HT, Anderson DE, Krush AJ. Heredity and intraocular malignant melanoma. Study of two families and review of forty-five cases. Cancer. 1968;21(1):119–25.

13. Lynch HT, Krush AJ. Heredity and malignant melanoma: implications for early cancer detection. Can Med Assoc J. 1968;99(1):17–21.

14. Walker JP, Weiter JJ, Albert DM, et al. Uveal malignant melanoma in three generations of the same family. Am J Ophthalmol. 1979;88(4):723–6.

15. Greene MH, Sanders RJ, Chu FC, et al. The familial occurrence of cutaneous melanoma, intraocular melanoma, and the dysplastic nevus syndrome. Am J Ophthalmol. 1983;96(2):238–45.

16. Vink J, Crijns MB, Mooy CM, et al. Ocular melanoma in families with dysplastic nevus syndrome. J Am Acad Dermatol. 1990;23(5 Pt 1):858–62.

17. Singh AD, Wang MX, Donoso LA, et al. Genetic aspects of uveal melanoma: a brief review. Semin Oncol. 1996;23(6):768–72.

18. Bacin F, Kemeny JL, D'Hermies F, et al. Malignant melanoma of the choroid associated with neurofibromatosis. J Fr Ophtalmol. 1993;16(3):184–90.

19. Wiznia RA, Freedman JK, Mancini AD, et al. Malignant melanoma of the choroid in neurofibromatosis. Am J Ophthalmol. 1978;86(5):684–7.

20. Yanoff M, Zimmerman LE. Histogenesis of malignant melanomas of the uvea. 3. The relationship of congenital ocular melanocytosis and neurofibromatosis in uveal melanomas. Arch Ophthalmol. 1967;77(3):331–6.

21. Rai K, Pilarski R, Boru G, et al. Germline BAP1 alterations in familial uveal melanoma. Genes Chromosomes Cancer. 2017;56(2):168–74.

22. Decatur CL, Ong E, Garg N, et al. Driver mutations in uveal melanoma: associations with gene expression profile and patient outcomes. JAMA Ophthalmol. 2016;134(7):728–33.

23. Velazquez N, Jones IS. Ocular and oculodermal melanocytosis associated with uveal melanoma. Ophthalmology. 1983;90(12):1472–6.

24. Carreno E, Saornil MA, Garcia-Alvarez C, et al. Prevalence of ocular and oculodermal melanocytosis in Spanish population with uveal melanoma. Eye (Lond). 2012;26(1):159–62.

25. Shields CL, Kaliki S, Livesey M, et al. Association of ocular and oculodermal melanocytosis with the rate of uveal melanoma metastasis: analysis of 7872 consecutive eyes. JAMA Ophthalmol. 2013;131(8):993–1003.

26. Shields CL, Furuta M, Berman EL, et al. Choroidal nevus transformation into melanoma: analysis of 2514 consecutive cases. Arch Ophthalmol. 2009;127(8):981–7.

27. Kivela T. Diagnosis of uveal melanoma. Dev Ophthalmol. 2012;49:1–15.

28. Tarlan B, Kiratli H. Uveal melanoma: current trends in diagnosis and management. Turk J Ophthalmol. 2016;46(3):123–37.

29. Factors predictive of growth and treatment of small choroidal melanoma: COMS report no. 5. The Collaborative Ocular Melanoma Study Group. Arch Ophthalmol. 1997;115(12):1537–1544.

30. Accuracy of diagnosis of choroidal melanomas in the Collaborative Ocular Melanoma Study. COMS report no. 1. Arch Ophthalmol. 1990;108(9):1268–1273.

31. Margo CE. The accuracy of diagnosis of posterior uveal melanoma. Arch Ophthalmol. 1997;115(3):432–4.

32. Kielar RA. Choroidal melanoma appearing as vitreous hemorrhage. Ann Ophthalmol. 1982;14(5):461–4.

33. Skalka HW. Choroidal hemorrhage simulating malignant melanoma. J Clin Ultrasound. 1982;10(4):190–2.

34. Fraser DJ Jr, Font RL. Ocular inflammation and hemorrhage as initial manifestations of uveal malignant melanoma. Incidence and prognosis. Arch Ophthalmol. 1979;97(7):1311–4.

35. Giuliari GP, Connor A, Simpson ER. Amelanotic choroidal melanoma. Lancet. 2011;377(9768):848.

36. Lee DS, Anderson SF, Perez EM, et al. Amelanotic choroidal nevus and melanoma: cytology, tumor size, and pigmentation as prognostic indicators. Optom Vis Sci. 2001;78(7):483–91.

37. Gibran SK, Kapoor KG. Management of exudative retinal detachment in choroidal melanoma. Clin Exp Ophthalmol. 2009;37(7):654–9.

38. Harbour JW, Ahmad S, El-Bash M. Rate of resolution of exudative retinal detachment after plaque radiotherapy for uveal melanoma. Arch Ophthalmol. 2002;120(11):1463–9.

39. Kivela T, Eskelin S, Makitie T, et al. Exudative retinal detachment from malignant uveal melanoma: predictors and prognostic significance. Invest Ophthalmol Vis Sci. 2001;42(9):2085–93.

40. Collaborative Ocular Melanoma Study G, Boldt HC, Byrne SF, et al. Baseline echographic characteristics of tumors in eyes of patients enrolled in the Collaborative Ocular Melanoma Study: COMS report no. 29. Ophthalmology. 2008;115(8):1390–7. 7.e1–2

41. Collaborative Ocular Melanoma Study G. Comparison of clinical, echographic, and histopathological measurements from eyes with medium-sized choroidal melanoma in the collaborative ocular melanoma study: COMS report no. 21. Arch Ophthalmol. 2003;121(8):1163–71.

42. Margo CE. The collaborative ocular melanoma study: an overview. Cancer Control. 2004;11(5):304–9.

43. Amin MB, Edge SB, Cancer. AJCo. AJCC cancer staging manual 2017. 2017.

44. Augsburger JJ, Correa ZM, Schneider S, et al. Diagnostic transvitreal fine-needle aspiration biopsy of small melanocytic choroidal tumors in nevus versus melanoma category. Trans Am Ophthalmol Soc. 2002;100:225–32. discussion 32–4

45. Singh AD, Medina CA, Singh N, et al. Fine-needle aspiration biopsy of uveal melanoma: outcomes and complications. Br J Ophthalmol. 2016;100(4):456–62.

46. De Croock L, Verbraeken H. Metastatic uveal melanoma: diagnosis and treatment. A literature review. Bull Soc Belge Ophtalmol. 2002;286:59–63.

47. Kim IK, Lane AM, Gragoudas ES. Survival in patients with presymptomatic diagnosis of metastatic uveal melanoma. Arch Ophthalmol. 2010;128(7):871–5.

48. Diener-West M, Reynolds SM, Agugliaro DJ, et al. Development of metastatic disease after enrollment in the COMS trials for treatment of choroidal melanoma: Collaborative Ocular Melanoma Study Group Report No. 26. Arch Ophthalmol. 2005;123(12):1639–43.

49. Shields JA, Augsburger JJ, Brown GC, et al. The differential diagnosis of posterior uveal melanoma. Ophthalmology. 1980;87(6):518–22.

50. Histopathologic characteristics of uveal melanomas in eyes enucleated from the Collaborative Ocular Melanoma Study. COMS report no. 6. Am J Ophthalmol. 1998;125(6):745–766.

51. Coleman K, Baak JP, van Diest PJ, et al. Prognostic value of morphometric features and the Callender classification in uveal melanomas. Ophthalmology. 1996;103(10):1634–41.

52. Collaborative Ocular Melanoma Study G. Assessment of metastatic disease status at death in 435 patients with large choroidal melanoma in the Collaborative Ocular Melanoma Study (COMS): COMS report no. 15. Arch Ophthalmol. 2001;119(5):670–6.

53. McLean IW, Ainbinder DJ, Gamel JW, et al. Choroidal-ciliary body melanoma. A multivariate survival analysis of tumor location. Ophthalmology. 1995;102(7):1060–4.

54. Damato BE, Heimann H, Kalirai H, et al. Age, survival predictors, and metastatic death in patients with choroidal melanoma: tentative evidence of a therapeutic effect on survival. JAMA Ophthalmol. 2014;132(5):605–13.

55. Collaborative Ocular Melanoma Study G. The COMS randomized trial of iodine 125 brachytherapy for choroidal melanoma: V. Twelve-year mortality rates and prognostic factors: COMS report no. 28. Arch Ophthalmol. 2006;124(12):1684–93.

56. Mortality in patients with small choroidal melanoma. COMS report no. 4. The collaborative ocular melanoma study group. Arch Ophthalmol. 1997;115(7):886–893.

57. The Collaborative Ocular Melanoma Study (COMS) randomized trial of pre-enucleation radiation of large choroidal melanoma II: initial mortality findings. COMS report no. 10. Am J Ophthalmol. 1998;125(6):779–796.

58. Correa ZM. Assessing prognosis in uveal melanoma. Cancer Control. 2016;23(2):93–8.

59. Onken MD, Worley LA, Char DH, et al. Collaborative Ocular Oncology Group report number 1: prospective validation of a multi-gene prognostic assay in uveal melanoma. Ophthalmology. 2012;119(8):1596–603.

60. Dopierala J, Damato BE, Lake SL, et al. Genetic heterogeneity in uveal melanoma assessed by multiplex ligation-dependent probe amplification. Invest Ophthalmol Vis Sci. 2010;51(10):4898–905.

61. Singh AD, Donoso LA. Genetic aspects of uveal melanoma. Int Ophthalmol Clin. 1993;33(3):47–52.

62. Singh AD, Boghosian-Sell L, Wary KK, et al. Cytogenetic findings in primary uveal melanoma. Cancer Genet Cytogenet. 1994;72(2):109–15.

63. Singh AD. Prognostication of uveal melanoma: a work in progress. JAMA Ophthalmol. 2016;134(7):740–1.

64. Kilic E, van Gils W, Lodder E, et al. Clinical and cytogenetic analyses in uveal melanoma. Invest Ophthalmol Vis Sci. 2006;47(9):3703–7.

65. Field MG, Harbour JW. Recent developments in prognostic and predictive testing in uveal melanoma. Curr Opin Ophthalmol. 2014;25(3):234–9.

66. Harbour JW. A prognostic test to predict the risk of metastasis in uveal melanoma based on a 15-gene expression profile. Methods Mol Biol. 2014;1102:427–40.

67. Jampol LM, Moy CS, Murray TG, et al. The COMS randomized trial of iodine 125 brachytherapy for choroidal melanoma: IV. Local treatment failure and enucleation in the first 5 years after brachytherapy. COMS report no. 19. Ophthalmology. 2002;109(12):2197–206.

68. Marucci L, Ancukiewicz M, Lane AM, et al. Uveal melanoma recurrence after fractionated proton beam therapy: comparison of survival in patients treated with reirradiation or with enucleation. Int J Radiat Oncol Biol Phys. 2011;79(3):842–6.

69. Ophthalmic Oncology Task F. Local recurrence significantly increases the risk of metastatic uveal melanoma. Ophthalmology. 2016;123(1):86–91.

70. Foulds WS, Damato BE, Burton RL. Local resection versus enucleation in the management of choroidal melanoma. Eye. 1987;1(Pt 6):676–9.

71. Damato B, Foulds WS. Indications for trans-scleral local resection of uveal melanoma. Br J Ophthalmol. 1996;80(11):1029–30.

72. Damato BE, Paul J, Foulds WS. Risk factors for residual and recurrent uveal melanoma after trans-scleral local resection. Br J Ophthalmol. 1996;80(2):102–8.

73. Damato BE. Local resection of uveal melanoma. Dev Ophthalmol. 2012;49:66–80.

74. Oosterhuis JA, Journee-de Korver HG, Kakebeeke-Kemme HM, et al. Transpupillary thermotherapy in choroidal melanomas. Arch Ophthalmol. 1995;113(3):315–21.

75. Journee-de Korver JG, Oosterhuis JA, Kakebeeke-Kemme HM, et al. Transpupillary thermotherapy (TTT) by infrared irradiation of choroidal melanoma. Doc Ophthalmol. 1992;82(3):185–91.

76. Journee-de Korver JG, Oosterhuis JA, de Wolff-Rouendaal D, et al. Histopathological findings in human choroidal melanomas after transpupillary thermotherapy. Br J Ophthalmol. 1997;81(3):234–9.

77. Shields CL, Shields JA, DePotter P, et al. Transpupillary thermotherapy in the management of choroidal melanoma. Ophthalmology. 1996;103(10):1642–50.

78. Shields CL, Shields JA, Cater J, et al. Transpupillary thermotherapy for choroidal melanoma: tumor control and visual results in 100 consecutive cases. Ophthalmology. 1998;105(4):581–90.

79. Kashani AH, Aaberg TM Jr, Capone A Jr. Vitreomacular traction as a consequence of posterior hyaloidal contraction after transpupillary thermotherapy. Am J Ophthalmol. 2013;155(5):937–45.

80. Shields CL, Shields JA. Transpupillary thermotherapy for choroidal melanoma. Curr Opin Ophthalmol. 1999;10(3):197–203.

81. Aaberg TM Jr, Bergstrom CS, Hickner ZJ, et al. Long-term results of primary transpupillary thermal therapy for the treatment of choroidal malignant melanoma. Br J Ophthalmol. 2008;92(6):741–6.

82. Win PH, Robertson DM, Buettner H, et al. Extended follow-up of small melanocytic choroidal tumors treated with transpupillary thermotherapy. Arch Ophthalmol. 2006;124(4):503–6.

83. Shields CL, Cater J, Shields JA, et al. Combined plaque radiotherapy and transpupillary thermotherapy for choroidal melanoma: tumor control and treatment complications in 270 consecutive patients. Arch Ophthalmol. 2002;120(7):933–40.

84. Bartlema YM, Oosterhuis JA, Journee-De Korver JG, et al. Combined plaque radiotherapy and transpupillary thermotherapy in choroidal melanoma: 5 years' experience. Br J Ophthalmol. 2003;87(11):1370–3.

85. Oosterhuis JA, Journee-de Korver HG, Keunen JE. Transpupillary thermotherapy: results in 50 patients with choroidal melanoma. Arch Ophthalmol. 1998;116(2):157–62.

86. De Potter P, Jamart J. Adjuvant indocyanine green in transpupillary thermotherapy for choroidal melanoma. Ophthalmology. 2003;110(2):406–13. discussion 13–4

87. Stallard HB. Malignant melanoma of the choroid treated with radioactive applicators: Hunterian lecture delivered at the Royal College of Surgeons of England on 29th November 1960. Ann R Coll Surg Engl. 1961;29:170–82.

88. Augsburger JJ, Gamel JW, Lauritzen K, et al. Cobalt-60 plaque radiotherapy vs enucleation for posterior uveal melanoma. Am J Ophthalmol. 1990;109:585–92.

89. Earle J, Kline RW, Robertson DM. Selection of iodine 125 for the Collaborative Ocular Melanoma Study. Arch Ophthalmol. 1987;105:763–4.

90. Brualla L, Zaragoza FJ, Sauerwein W. Monte Carlo simulation of the treatment of eye tumors with (106)Ru plaques: a study on maximum tumor height and eccentric placement. Ocul Oncol Pathol. 2014;1:2–12.

91. Hawkins BS. Collaborative ocular melanoma study randomized trial of I-125 brachytherapy. Clin Trials. 2011;8:661–73.

92. Krohn J, Monge OR, Skorpen TN, et al. Posterior uveal melanoma treated with I-125 brachytherapy or primary enucleation. Eye. 2008;22:1398–403.

93. Shields CL, Naseripour M, Cater J, et al. Plaque radiotherapy for large posterior uveal melanomas (≥8-mm thick) in 354 consecutive patients 1. Ophthalmology. 2002;109:1838–49.

94. Rouberol F, Roy P, Kodjikian L, et al. Survival, anatomic, and functional long-term results in choroidal and ciliary body melanoma after ruthenium brachytherapy (15 years' experience with beta-rays). Am J Ophthalmol. 2004;137:893–900.

95. Anteby II, Pe'er J. Need for confirmation of positioning of ruthenium plaques by postoperative B-scan ultrasonography. Ophthalmic Surg Lasers. 1996;27(12):1024–9.

96. Aziz HA, Al Zahrani YA, Bena J, et al. Episcleral brachytherapy of uveal melanoma: role of intraoperative echographic confirmation. Br J Ophthalmol. 2017;101(6):747–51.

97. Chang MY, Kamrava M, Demanes DJ, et al. Intraoperative ultrasonography-guided positioning of iodine 125 plaque brachytherapy in the treatment of choroidal melanoma. Ophthalmology. 2012;119(5):1073–7.

98. Tabandeh H, Chaudhry NA, Murray TG, et al. Intraoperative echographic localization of iodine-125 episcleral plaque for brachytherapy of choroidal melanoma. Am J Ophthalmol. 2000;129(2):199–204.

99. Design and methods of a clinical trial for a rare condition: The collaborative ocular melanoma study. Control Clin Trials. 1993;14:362–391.

100. Perez BA, Mettu P, Vajzovic L, et al. Uveal melanoma treated with iodine-125 episcleral plaque: an analysis of dose on disease control and visual outcomes. Int J Radiat Oncol Biol Phys. 2014;89:127–36.

101. Nath R, Anderson LL, Luxton G, et al. Dosimetry of interstitial brachytherapy sources: recommendations of the AAPM Radiation Therapy Committee Task Group No. 43. Med Phys. 1995;22:209–34.

102. Wang Z, Nabhan M, Schild SE, et al. Charged particle radiation therapy for uveal melanoma: a systematic review and meta-analysis. Int J Radiat Oncol Biol Phys. 2013;86:18–26.

103. Dieckmann K, Georg D, Zehetmayer M, et al. LINAC based stereotactic radiotherapy of uveal melanoma: 4 years clinical experience. Radiother Oncol. 2003;67:199–206.

104. Langmann G, Pendl G, Klaus-Müllner, et al. Gamma knife radiosurgery for uveal melanomas: an 8-year experience. J Neurosurg. 2000;93:184–8.

105. Gragoudas ES, Lane AM, Regan S, et al. A randomized controlled trial of varying radiation doses in the treatment of choroidal melanoma. Arch Ophthalmol. 2000;118:773–8.

106. Langmann G, Pendl G, Müllner K, et al. High-compared with low-dose radiosurgery for uveal melanomas. J Neurosurg. 2002;97:640–3.

107. Astrahan MA, Luxton G, Pu Q, et al. Conformal episcleral plaque therapy. Int J Radiat Oncol Biol Phys. 1997;39:505–19.

108. American Brachytherapy Society – Ophthalmic Oncology Task Force. Electronic address pec, Committee AO. The American Brachytherapy Society consensus guidelines for plaque brachytherapy of uveal melanoma and retinoblastoma. Brachytherapy. 2014;13(1):1–14.

109. Verma V, Mehta MP. Clinical outcomes of proton radiotherapy for uveal melanoma. Clin Oncol. 2016;28:e17–27.

110. Mishra KK, Quivey JM, Daftari IK, et al. Long-term results of the UCSF-LBNL randomized trial: charged particle with helium ion versus iodine-125 plaque therapy for choroidal and ciliary body melanoma. Int J Radiat Oncol Biol Phys. 2015;92:376–83.

111. Char DH, Quivey JM, Castro JR, et al. Helium ions versus iodine 125 brachytherapy in the management of uveal melanoma. Ophthalmology. 1993;100:1547–54.

112. Berry JL, Dandapani SV, Stevanovic M, et al. Outcomes of choroidal melanomas treated with eye physics: a 20-year review. JAMA Ophthalmol. 2013;131:1435–42.

113. Bogner J, Petersch B, Georg D, et al. A noninvasive eye fixation and computer-aided eye monitoring system for linear accelerator-based stereotactic radiotherapy of uveal melanoma. Int J Radiat Oncol Biol Phys. 2003;56:1128–36.

114. Furdova A, Strmen P, Waczulikova I, et al. One-day session LINAC-based stereotactic radiosurgery of posterior uveal melanoma. Eur J Ophthalmol. 2011;22:226–35.

115. Petersch B, Bogner J, Dieckmann K, et al. Automatic real-time surveillance of eye position and gating for stereotactic radiotherapy of uveal melanoma. Med Phys. 2004;31:3521–7.

116. Sarici AM, Pazarli H. Gamma-knife-based stereotactic radiosurgery for medium- and large-sized posterior uveal melanoma. Graefes Arch Clin Exp Ophthalmol. 2013;251:285–94.

117. Wen JC, Oliver SC, Mccannel TA. Ocular complications following I-125 brachytherapy for choroidal melanoma. Eye. 2009;23:1254–68.

118. Puusaari I, Heikkonen J, Kivelä T. Ocular complications after iodine brachytherapy for large uveal melanomas. Ophthalmology. 2004;111:1768–77.

# Part IX

# Skull Base Tumor

# Skull Base Tumors

# 18

Ugur Selek, Frkan Topkan, and Eric L. Chang

## Learning Objectives

This chapter will enable the reader to be acquainted with olfactory neuroblastoma, chordoma, chondrosarcoma, and jugulotympanic paraganglioma which are commonly named as skull base tumors, covering common signs and symptoms of their presentations, prognostic and predictive factors, imaging findings, and multimodality management of treatment options.

## Introduction

Skull base is a challenging anatomic site for radiotherapy due to adjacent critical organs at risk (OAR) which have lower radiation dose tolerance than is required for definitive or adjuvant radiotherapy, such as lenses, eyes, optic nerves and chiasm, cochlea, and brain stem.

Evolution of radiotherapy based on image guidance of intensity-modulated radiation therapy (IMRT), volumetric modulated arc therapy (VMAT), stereotactic radiosurgery (SRS), fractionated stereotactic radiotherapy (FSRT), and proton-beam therapy has allowed improved sparing of critical organ at risks to yield safer and more effective radiation treatment of skull base tumors.

U. Selek (✉)
Koc University, School of Medicine,
Department of Radiation Oncology, Istanbul, Turkey

University of Texas, MD Anderson Cancer Center,
Radiation Oncology Department, Houston, TX, USA

E. Topkan
Baskent Department of Radiation Oncology, University Adana
Medical Faculty, Adana, Turkey

E. L. Chang
Department of Radiation Oncology, Keck School of Medicine of
University of Southern California, Los Angeles, USA

The goal is to balance the benefits and potential harms of radiation treatment to safely deliver a definitive dose to the tumor while preserving OAR by limiting the dose to the neurocritical structures such that normal tissue dose constraints are reasonably respected.

This chapter will focus mainly on olfactory neuroblastoma, chordoma, chondrosarcoma, and jugulotympanic paraganglioma which directly involve with skull base structures.

## Admission Signs, Incidence, and Prevalence

### Risk Factors

No specific environmental factors have been linked to olfactory neuroblastoma, chordoma, chondrosarcoma, and jugulotympanic paraganglioma.

### Common Signs and Symptoms

Anterior skull base involves critical structures of olfactory and optic nerves and frontal lobe, where anosmia, epistaxis, visual changes, and frontal lobe problems are expected in case of involvement. Middle central/paracentral skull base lesions can present with optic neuropathy or pituitary problems related with optic nerve, chiasm or pituitary dysfunction, or spheno-cavernous syndrome, as lateral skull base-originated tumors can denote proptosis, facial pain or dysesthesia, or trismus based on temporal or frontal lobes or trigeminal divisions of V2 and V3. Posterior skull base covers cerebellopontine angle (cranial nerves V, VII, VIII, pons, cerebellum), clivus/petrous apex (cranial nerves III–X), and jugular foramen (cranial nerves IX–XII), and lesions in this area present with mostly cranial nerve deficits such as face numbness or weakness, hearing loss, and abducens palsy that is related to the lesion location.

Orbitofrontal headaches might be related with dura invasion/stretching. Visual disturbances might be linked to optic apparatus or cavernous sinus neural involvement, including diplopia or unilateral vision loss related with lateral middle or infratemporal fossa or sphenoid wing invasion. Auditory deficits could be related to internal auditory canal or cerebellopontine angle involvement.

Several syndromes are listed based on tumor location: Olfactory syndrome as epistaxis, nasal obstruction, loss of sensation of smell, and rhinorrhea for paranasal involvement might be associated with frontal base and paranasal pressure/invasion. Frontal syndrome as seizures, increased intracranial pressure, and personality changes can be related to frontal base pressure/invasion. Hypothalamic syndrome might be seen as endocrinologic symptoms such as amenorrhea, diabetes insipidus, impotence. Pituitary apoplexy might be related to sella turcica and sphenoid sinus invasion. Dysfunction of upper cranial nerves (III, IV, V, VI) could be related to petro-clival, medial middle fossa invasion including cavernous sinus or Meckel cave. Paraneoplastic syndromes are generally related to ONB such as ectopic ACTH syndrome (EAS), syndrome of inappropriate ADH secretion (SIADH), humoral hypercalcemia of malignancy (HHM), opsoclonus-myoclonus-ataxia (OMA), hypertension due to catecholamine secretion [1].

## Physical Examination Tips

Evaluation of skull base tumors involves physical examination for cranial nerve (CN) deficits.

CN II: As visual information coming from each eye passes through to the opposite side of the optic chiasm, skull base lesions in front of optic chiasm pressing or invading eye or optic nerve cause visual deficits in one eye, though visual field deficits similar in both eyes originate due to lesions affecting optic tract, thalamus, white matter, or visual cortex.

Pupillary responses (CN II or III): If direct response is impaired when pupil illuminated, consider lesions effecting ipsilateral optic nerve or pretectal area or ipsilateral CN III parasympathetics. If consensual response is impaired when contralateral pupil illuminated, consider lesions of the *contralateral* optic nerve or pretectal area or ipsilateral CN III parasympathetics. If accommodation is impaired when looking at something moving toward the eye, consider ipsilateral optic nerve or ipsilateral CN III parasympathetics or bilateral lesions of the pathways from the optic tracts to the visual cortex. Tumors affecting pretectal area spare accommodation.

Extraocular movements (CN III, IV, VI): Eyes at rest is observed for spontaneous nystagmus or dysconjugate gaze resulting in diplopia. Double vision is also questioned with eye movements in all directions without moving the head.

Smooth pursuit is tested by having the patient visually follow a moving object with full range of horizontal/vertical eye movements. Convergence movements are tested by asking the patient to fixate vision on an object during its slow movement toward a point right between the patient's eyes.

Facial sensory and motor functions (CN V): Facial sensation is tested using a soft cotton wisp or a sharp object, and mastication muscles are tested by feeling the masseter muscles with jaw clenched.

Facial expression muscles and taste (CN VII): Asymmetry of facial shape, spontaneous facial expressions, and blinking or disproportionateness of furrows depth (e.g., nasolabial fold) are observed by asking to wrinkle brows, clench eyes tightly, smile, puff out cheeks, etc.

Hearing and vestibular sense (CN VIII): Unilateral hearing loss is consistently due to peripheral defects on neural or mechanical tracts. Skull base tumors might damage inner ear vestibular apparatus, CN VIII vestibular portion, vestibular nuclei of brain stem, or the cerebellum.

Muscles of articulation (CN V, VII, IX, X, XII): Skull base tumors which might cause injury in peripheral or central portions of CN V, VII, IX, X, or XII could result dysfunction in muscles of articulation and cause breathy, slurred, or hoarse speech, etc.

## Incidence and Prevalence

### Olfactory Neuroblastoma

Olfactory neuroblastoma (esthesioneuroblastoma, neuroendocrine carcinoma) is a rare neuroectodermal tumor originating from the olfactory epithelium in the proximal nasal septum, the superior turbinates, and the cribriform plate [2–4] which is roughly 1–5% of nasal cavity malignancies [5, 6].

Tumor site grouping International Classification of Diseases (ICD) code in Central Brain Tumor Registry of the United States (CBTRUS) is C30.0 (9522–9523) [7]. Incidence rates were lowest for olfactory tumors of the nasal cavity (0.04 per 100,000).

The incidence is highest in the 60–79 year age group, with a median age at diagnosis of 51 years [8].

Survival rate is >70% alive at 5 years after diagnosis; 5- and 10-year relative survival estimates were 72% (95% CI, 65.8–77.8%) and 62% (95% CI, 54.3–69.5%), respectively [8]. Patients <65 years old had much better survival than those ≥65 years at 10 years (P; 0.059).

There is a slight male predominance with a mean diagnosis age at 45 years [9].

Presenting symptoms are mainly nasal obstruction in addition to hyposmia, epistaxis, or nasal discharge. Major significant predictors of survival are modified Kadish stage, age, treatment modality, and nodal involvement [10]. Lymph node involvement at diagnosis is fairly common (17–47%) [11]. Though distant hematogenous metastases are not common at initial admission, metastases to the bone, lung, bone marrow, or skin were reported [6].

## Chordoma

Chordomas are slowly progressive, locally aggressive tumors arising from remnants of the notochord and constitute nearly 1% of all malignant bone tumors. Skull base chordomas mainly originate from clivus of sphenoid bone due to being the terminus of the notochord, and the skull base is the second most common site of chordomas (50%, sacrococcygeal; 35%, skull base;15%, spine) [12]. Age at diagnosis is between 30 and 50 years for skull base chordomas, younger than sacrococcygeal ones, with a slightly male predominance [12, 13].

Chordomas are defined in three pathologic subtypes, while chondroid type is the most common in skull base (incidence, classic-conventional > chondroid > dedifferentiated) [12, 14]. Chondroid and conventional chordomas seem to have a similar and a better prognosis than dedifferentiated type; dedifferentiated chordomas are mostly aneuploid with worse survival [14–16].

Brachyury appears to be a specific and sensitive immunohistochemistry biomarker of chordomas due to being a key transcription factor in development of notochord, and brachyury staining routinely distinguishes chordoma from cartilaginous tumors [17].

When whole-exome and/or whole-transcriptome sequencing are performed, skull base chordoma has recently been identified with chromosomal aberration in 1p, 7, 10, 13, and 17q. There is a high frequency of functional germ line SNP of the T gene, rs2305089, and several recurrent alterations including MUC4, NBPF1, NPIPB15 mutations and novel gene fusion of SAMD5-SASH1 [18].

Distant metastases is rare in skull base chordomas, in comparison to sacral and vertebral chordomas, and distant metastases might be intradural following surgical resection [19], or might be to lymph nodes, lungs, liver, bones, and skin [20–22].

## Chondrosarcoma

Chondrosarcomas are infrequent malignant cartilaginous neoplasms constituting 6% of all skull base and 11% of primary malignant bone tumors, mainly arising in the middle, posterior, or anterior fossa, respectively [23, 24].

World Health Organization (WHO) 2013 classification system defines chondrosarcoma in a three-step grading; as grade 1 (well-differentiated lesions without mitoses, renamed as "atypical cartilaginous tumors", ACT/CS1) [25], grade 2 (moderately differentiated chondrosarcomas, having widely scattered mitoses), and grade 3 (poorly differentiated tumors, having clearly more cellularity and nuclear pleomorphism than grade 2 tumors with prominent mitoses) [25]. High-grade mesenchymal (extraskeletal myxoid) chondrosarcoma might be rarely present at the skull base. Skull base chondrosarcomas are mostly grade 1, ACT/CS1 [26].

## Distinguishing Between Chordoma and Chondrosarcoma

The differential diagnosis is important due to significantly better prognosis of chondrosarcomas in comparison to chordomas, and differentiation should also cover myxopapillary ependymomas and adenocarcinomas. Immunohistochemistry plays a major role as cytokeratin and EMA are not positive for chondrosarcomas and myxopapillary ependymomas in addition to having no desmosomes on ultrastructural examination, despite chordomas [26–28]. Glial fibrillary acidic protein (GFAP) is only expressed in myxopapillary ependymoma, while both chondrosarcomas and chordomas do not express GFAP but S-100 protein [26, 28]. The differentiation of chordoma from adenocarcinoma might be challenging due to cytokeratin and EMA positivity in both tumors, but vimentin and S-100 protein positivity indicate diagnosis of chordoma with a small caution for interpretation that rare S-100 protein positivity can exist for adenocarcinoma [26, 28].

## Jugulotympanic Paraganglioma (JTP; Glomus Jugulare Tumor, GJ)

JTP is a paraganglioma which is a rare neuroendocrine tumor arising from the extra-adrenal autonomic paraganglia, derived from embryonic neural crest, with an approximate incidence of 1 per 1,000,000 [29, 30] while being the most common tumor of the middle ear and second to acoustic neuroma as a neurotologic tumor [31, 32].

Although paragangliomas arise both in parasympathetic and sympathetic paraganglia with similar frequency [33, 34], most paragangliomas derived from parasympathetic paraganglia are located in the skull base and neck alongside the glossopharyngeal and vagal nerves, mainly from the carotid body followed by jugulotympanic and vagal paraganglia [34, 35]. Almost 50% rise in the setting of a known genetic syndrome [36, 37]. The GJT terminology has evolved to be "jugulotympanic paraganglioma (JTP)" referring to both tumors of the jugular paraganglia (glomus jugulare) and the tympanic paraganglia (glomus tympanicum) [35, 38].

Glomus bodies might function like carotid body as chemoreceptors, reacting to variations of oxygen and carbon dioxide saturations and blood pH [39, 40]. Older terminology of chemodectoma for GJT has also been not used owing to the fact that only the carotid body paraganglia act as chemoreceptors [34]. The JTP are mainly not associated with catecholamine secretion except for the approximately 5% with symptoms related with hypersecretion [41–45].

Sporadic paragangliomas have a female predominance [46, 47] while in hereditary forms have no such predominance [48]. Typically, these tumors manifest themselves during the fifth and sixth decades of life [46].

As JTP is epicentered in the jugular bulb, symptoms might be directly related with injuries of neurovascular structures (cranial nerves VII, VIII, IX, X, XI, and XII) within the hypoglossal canal, jugular foramen, and temporal bone revealing dizziness, tinnitus, cephalgia, and an/hypo/hyperacusis.

## Diagnosis

### Imaging [49, 50]

Neuroimaging necessitates careful evaluation of the enhancement pattern, mineralized matrix, calcification, hyperostosis, flow voids, and hypervascularity, as CT and MRI might be complementary. CT is known to be superior to define calcification and minor cortical erosion. MRI is more comprehensive in soft tissue details revealing perineural tumor spread, dural involvement, intracranial invasion, neural foramina involvement, and vascular encasement.

Remodeling and/or pushing away of bony structures indicates a slow-growing process, whereas gross invasion and destruction of bone expresses a more aggressive growth. Healthy bone marrow (MRI, T1 slightly hyperintense) is mostly expected to be replaced with isointense tumor if there is invasion. Bony hyperostosis with a soft tissue mass suggests meningioma or olfactory neuroblastoma.

JTP can present as a mass originating from jugular foramen demonstrating a "moth-eaten" bony destruction pattern on CT (Fig. 18.1). JTP also has a "salt and pepper" enhancement on T1 post-contrast MR images [51].

Chordoma mostly appears with paramedian lytic clival destruction, bony fragments, and heterogeneous enhancement with a honeycomb appearance on T1 post-contrast MRI (Fig. 18.2) and T2-weighted bright signal on MRI [52–56].

Chondrosarcoma appears as a midline lesion with heterogeneous calcifications on CT in addition to a honeycomb-like heterogeneous enhancement on MRI (Fig. 18.3) [57] and a characteristic thumb sign which is indenting of the pons [52, 54, 58, 59].

Olfactory neuroblastoma (ON) presents as a homogeneous mass in the nasal vault and CT, though not characteristic, reveals moderate and uniform enhancement, involvement, and bone remodeling of cribriform plate, fovea ethmoidalis, and lamina papyracea with rare scattered speckled calcifications [60]. MRI is T1 hypointense to gray with enhancement on T1 post-contrast series (Fig. 18.4a, b) and T2 intermediate to hyperintense showing soft tissue extent

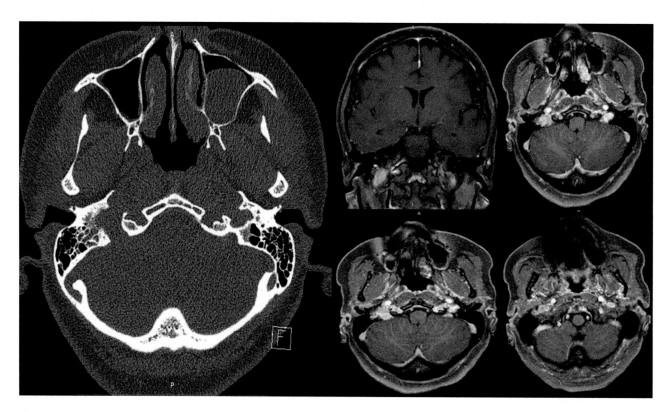

**Fig. 18.1** Globus jugulotympanicum at right jugular foramen measuring 17 × 17 × 20 mm between origin of carotid canal and level of C1, causing enlargement of jugular foramen in CT, extending to hypotympanum and mastoid

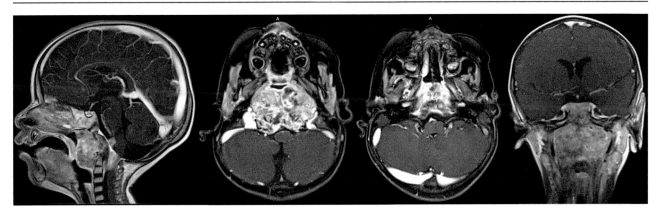

**Fig. 18.2** Large chordoma (58 × 47 × 58 mm) at the level of craniocervical junction which involves inferior part of clivus and C1 and C2 vertebral corpus causing thickening of nasopharyngeal posterior wall; the tumor is obliterating airway and compressing cervical spinal cord, while soft tissue component of tumor extends to premedullary cistern, compressing medulla oblongata and obliterating hypoglossal canals and encasing distal extracranial segments of left internal carotid artery

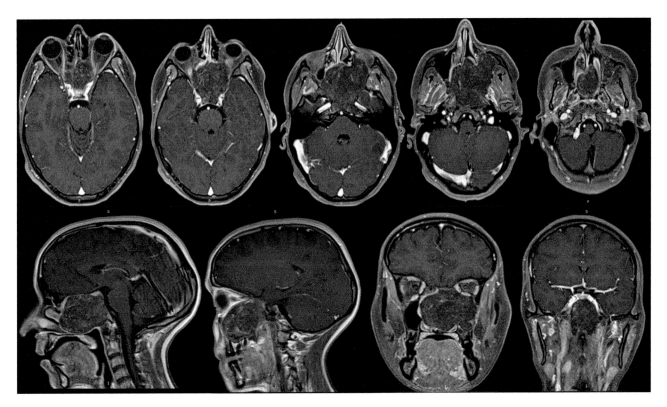

**Fig. 18.3** Chondrosarcoma, measuring 63 × 55 × 50 mm, originating from skull base, destructing clivus, filling nasal cavity and left maxillary sinus, extending to ethmoidal sinus, extending superiorly to sella without invasion of pituitary gland, causing thinning at left orbital floor and optic canal at orbital apex, pushing retro-orbital muscles superiorly

and assessment of skull base invasion, dural involvement, and perineural, orbital, and intracranial spread. 18 F-FDG PET/CT maximum standardized uptake value can help discriminating between ON and sinonasal undifferentiated carcinoma (SNUC) [61, 62].

Chondrosarcoma can be differentiated from chordoma with an off-midline growth pattern on conventional magnetic resonance imaging in the majority of patients as diffusion-weighted MR imaging (DWI) provides additional useful information [63]. Chondrosarcoma was found to be associated with the highest mean ADC value ($2051 \pm 261 \times 10^{-6}$ mm$^2$/s) with significant difference ($P < 0.001$) from classic chordoma ($1474 \pm 117 \times 10^{-6}$ mm$^2$/s) and poorly differentiated chordoma ($875 \pm 100 \times 10^{-6}$ mm$^2$/s) [64, 65].

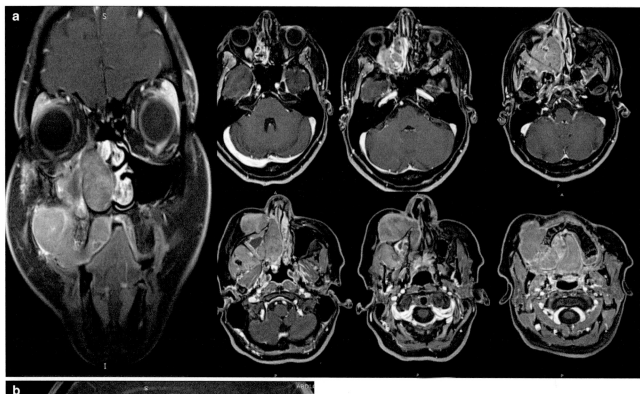

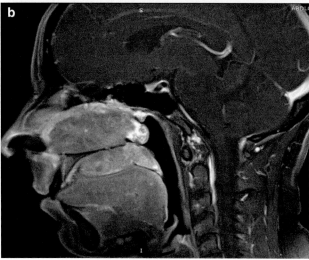

**Fig. 18.4** (**a**, **b**) Olfactory neuroblastoma, measuring 62 × 52 × 63 mm, filling the right maxillary sinus, invading right maxillary bone to the midline, filling the nasal cavity, pushing the concha, destructing anteriorly the sinus wall approximately 25 mm to anterior maxillary sinus subcutaneous fascia, filling infraorbital canal and foramen with perineural involvement, extending posteriorly filling the pterygopalatine fossa and pushing the medial pterygoid muscle with involvement of muscle insertion, protruding laterally to right masseter muscle with minimal invasion, eroding superiorly the orbital floor and inferior rec- tus muscle, invading inferiorly right maxillary and palatine bone up to oral tongue displacing it. There was no sign of foramen rotundum invasion while the lesion is adjacent to trigeminal nerve V2 branch at pterygopalatine fossa level. (**c**) January 2013, image-guided simultaneous integrated boost 9 field IMRT delivering 70 Gy (CTV70 = GTV plus 1 mm) and 63 Gy (CTV63) in 33 fractions (**d**) Olfactory neuroblastoma, status post induction chemotherapy followed by concurrent radiochemotherapy, disease-free at 5 years with initial bony destruction and teeth loss

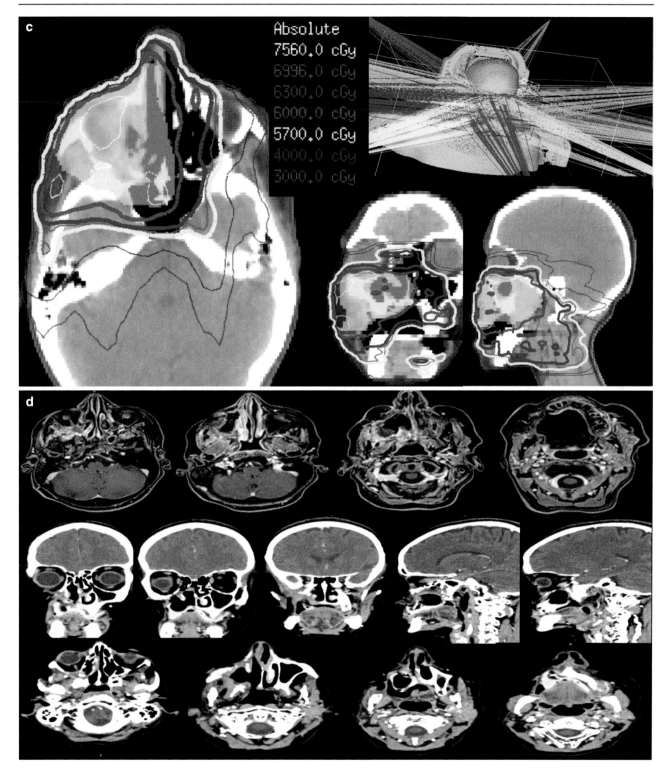

**Fig. 18.4** (continued)

## Case Study

A 10-year-old boy is admitted to the emergency service with recent fainting history in addition to increasing headaches as well as breathy and slurred speech in last month. His physical exam showed dysfunction in his muscles of articulation a mass filling the nasopharynx and continuing to the oropharynx.

MRI is thought to highlight the nature of the mass defining both bony and soft tissue extension. The MRI in Fig. 18.2

revealed a large tumor (58 × 47 × 58 mm) at the level of craniocervical junction involving inferior part of clivus and C1 and C2 vertebral body causing thickening of nasopharyngeal posterior wall and compressing the cervical spinal cord. The soft tissue component of tumor extends to premedullary cistern, compressing medulla oblongata, obliterating the hypoglossal canals, and encasing distal extracranial segments of the left internal carotid artery. Chordoma was the radiologic most possible diagnosis.

The first recommended step in management is tissue diagnosis via transoral biopsy. Though the tumor was apparently considered not possible for a surgical margin negative en bloc resection, the multidisciplinary team recommended to perform a decompressing debulking surgery which would be followed up with an adjuvant radiotherapy.

## Staging

*Olfactory neuroblastoma*: Current staging on anatomic extension of the tumor beyond the nasal cavity was first developed by Kadish et al. [66] and modified by Morita et al. [9] (Table 18.1).

*Chordoma*: Location-based classifications were clival, parasellar, and sellar [67] or basiocciput-caudal and basisphenoid-rostral [68]. Surgical approach defines the chordoma classification as superior, middle, and inferior clival [69].

*Jugulotympanic paraganglioma*: The staging systems proposed by Fisch and Glasscock/Jackson are currently the most widely used classification based on site and extent of the tumor [70, 71] (Table 18.2).

**Table 18.1** Modified Kadish staging of olfactory neuroblastoma

| Stage A | Tumors confined to nasal cavity |
| --- | --- |
| Stage B | Tumors confined to nasal cavity and paranasal sinuses |
| Stage C | Tumors extend beyond nasal cavity and paranasal sinuses, including involvement of cribriform plate, base of skull, orbit, or intracranial cavity |
| Stage D | Tumors with metastasis to cervical lymph nodes or distant sites |

**Table 18.2** Fisch classification of glomus tumors

| Type A | Tumors confined to the middle ear cleft (tympanicum) |
| --- | --- |
| Type B | Tumors limited to the tympanomastoid area with no bone destruction in the infralabyrintine compartment of the temporal bone |
| Type C | Tumors involving the infralabyrintine compartment with extension into the petrous apex |
| Type D | Tumors with intracranial extension less than 2 cm in diameter |
| Type E | Tumors with intracranial extension greater than 2 cm in diameter |

## Multimodality Management Approach

### Olfactory Neuroblastoma

Well-localized ENB is recommended to have en bloc craniofacial resection of the tumor, cribriform plate, and the attached dura [72–76]. Endoscopic surgical management approaches in years have also been adopted to craniofacial resection with comparable control rates to open approaches [77–79]. As the basic oncologic concept and surgical principles ensuring clear margins and intradural dissection, endoscopic resection correlates with similar oncologic control rates [80, 81]. Oncological surgery is the key factor, and the most significant predictor is positive surgical margins in progression and decreased overall survival rates based on common experience [82–85].

Surgery alone seems insufficient to avoid local recurrences and requires consolidation adjuvant radiotherapy to achieve adequate local control rates [73, 85–87]. Recent SEER data analysis by Villano et al. noted no survival differences between surgery alone and surgery plus adjuvant radiotherapy ($P = 0.62$), while the analysis was confounded due to combination of all stages in analysis, the majority (63%) of cases of surgery alone being stage A and adjuvant radiotherapy cases being predominantly stage C (43%) or D (20%) [8]. Therefore, as there was no stage-specific analysis for adjuvant radiotherapy, advanced cases with adjuvant radiotherapy seem to have a similar survival with early-stage cases without adjuvant radiotherapy [8].

As neck nodal metastasis is an important clinical consideration at admission or in follow-up, elective treatment of the neck primarily needs to be considered in locally advanced patients, and long-term surveillance of the neck in addition to primary site is essential [88].

Advanced ENB requires a combination of all suitable modalities such as neoadjuvant chemotherapy or radiotherapy ± concurrent chemotherapy and surgery or a maximal surgery followed by postoperative radiotherapy ± concurrent chemotherapy [89–92]. Primary definitive radiotherapy is an option only in cases surgically ineligible for an oncological resection [93].

Concurrent chemotherapy with radiotherapy generally involves cyclophosphamide, vincristine, and doxorubicin, while platinum-based chemotherapy is used for advanced, high-grade tumors. The SEER database covering 311 patients with modified Kadish staging system revealed overall and disease-specific survival rates at 10 years for stage A, B, C, and D, respectively, as 83.4% and 90%, 49% and 68.3%, 38.6% and 66.7%, and 13.3% and 35.6% [10].

We recommend aggressive, multimodality treatment as oncological radical surgery if possible with neoadjuvant or adjuvant radiochemotherapy with dose of 60–66 Gy based on respecting OAR thresholds [85, 89–91, 94–97]. Image-guided highly precise radiotherapy such as intensity-modulated RT (IMRT), volumetric modulated arc radiotherapy (VMAT), or proton therapy is the current standard to preserve the organs at risk while delivering appropriate dose to the target [98–111].

There is at present no consensus on follow-up schedule, however as late recurrence is eminent (~50% of recurrences occur after 5 years). A lifelong follow-up protocol requires clinical examination and serial scans covering both the entire intracranial compartment and neck [112, 113].

## Chordoma

Skull base chordoma requires surgical resection to obtain maximal cytoreduction of the tumor along with definitive tissue diagnosis. Skull base chordoma is associated with poor survival due to recurrences [114].

Younger age ($\leq$24 years) was found to be a favorable factor for skull base chordoma with longer progression-free survival and a good neurologic status at follow-up. Occipitocervical region location is more frequent in younger patients which tended to undergo more aggressive resection [115]. Interestingly, the tumor signal intensity in patients $\leq$24 years old was found to be higher in T2 images but lower in enhanced T1 images [116].

A nomogram by Wang et al. was generated based on independent predictors of PFS as admission visual deficits, extent of bone invasion, preoperative Karnofsky performance scale (KPS) score, pathological subtypes, and variation in perioperative KPS showed a good discriminative ability (adjusted Harrell C statistic, 0.68) to predict PFS at 3 and 5 years [114]. The nomogram applies for risk stratification of PFS and overall survival in primary cases consisting of preoperative and perioperative functional status, while marginal resection ($P = 0.018$) and adjuvant radiotherapy ($P = 0.043$) were documented to be protective factors in the recurrent group [114, 116]. Wang et al. documented their series of 238 (140 male, 98 female, mean age 38) patients with a mean follow-up of 43.7 months, revealing most common initial symptoms as headache and neck pain (33.2%) and diplopia (29%). The most common location is sphenoclival (59.2%), and the most common bone invasion type is endophytic chordoma (81.5%). Marginal resection rate is 66% (gross total 11.8%, near total 54.2%) with evident risk factors for recurrence or larger tumor volume ($\geq$40 cm$^3$) and was a major predictor for a better long-term survival. Patients with recurrent tumor or intralesional resection showed poorer long-term outcome [117]. Wang et al. also provided their single-institution data of 229 patients (183 primary, 46 recurrent) with skull base chordoma treated between 2005 and 2014. The primary group had a progression-free survival (PFS) of 51% at 5 years with a mean PFS time of 66.9 months, while the recurrent group had a post-recurrent PFS of 14% with a mean post-recurrence PFS time of 29.5 months [114].

The primary treatment of choice is maximal safe surgical resection if possible, though negative surgical margins with complete resection is rare; and positive surgical margins with microscopic or gross residual disease require adjuvant radiotherapy [118–121]. The risk of surgical seeding needs to be considered on surgical approach and therefore postoperative radiation therapy planning volume [122].

Postoperative high-dose fractionated conventional radiotherapy of 60–70 Gy provided a significantly longer recurrence-free survival in comparison to patients with residual disease who did not receive radiotherapy [123, 124].

Radiotherapy with charged particle beams was encouraged by Munzenrider et al. based on precise delivery of high-dose radiation to target area with appropriate sparing of OAR [125]. The postoperative proton radiotherapy in single-institutional retrospective studies suggested better 10-year outcomes in comparison to conventional photon radiotherapy [126, 127]. Uhl et al. published their carbon ion therapy series at the Society for Heavy Ion Research in Darmstadt, Germany, in a raster scanning technique of 155 skull base chordoma patients between 1998 and 2008, and the authors noted that carbon ion therapy (median total dose of 60 gray RBE, 3 Gy/fraction) appears to be a safe and effective treatment revealing high local control (3-, 5-, and 10-year rates: 82%, 72%, and 54%) and overall survival (3-, 5-, and 10-year rates: 95%, 85%, and 75%) rates with a median follow-up of 72 months [128]. No higher late toxicity was detected after carbon ion treatment.

McDonald et al. have recently documented their retrospective review of 39 clival chordoma patients treated with surgery and proton therapy with a median prescribed dose of 77.4 Gy (relative biological effectiveness, RBE, range 70.2–79.2 Gy) between 2004 and 2014 [121]. With a median follow-up of 51 months, local control was 69.6% and overall survival was 81.4% at 5 years. Tumor histology, GTV at radiotherapy, and prescribed radiation dose were significantly associated with local control, but only radiation dose received by 1 cm$^3$ of GTV (D1cm$^3$) was significantly associated with overall survival. The proposed treatment planning objective for D1cm$^3$ was stated to be $\geq$74.5 Gy (RBE) [121]. Weber et al. published their pencil beam scanning proton therapy series of 151 chordoma and 71 chondrosarcoma patients with a delivered mean dose of 72.5 $\pm$ 2.2 Gy RBE and a mean follow-up of 50 (range, 4–176) months [129]. The local control rate at 7 years with independent prognostic factors of optic apparatus or brain stem compression, histology, and GTV for chordoma (70.9%) was found to be significantly lower than for chondrosarcoma (93.6%) [129].

IMRT has gained acceptance in recent years to deliver precise, high-dose radiation while sparing surrounding normal structures. Sahgal et al. shared their preliminary favorable survival, local control, and adverse event outcomes of 42 skull base chordoma (24, median follow-up of 36 months) and chondrosarcoma (18, median follow-up of 67 months) patients treated with high-dose image-guided intensity-modulated radiotherapy (IG-IMRT, median 70 Gy for chondrosarcoma and 76 Gy for chordoma; 2 Gy/fraction) between August 2001 and December 2012 [130]. The overall survival and local control rates at 5 years were 85.6% and 65.3% for chordoma (8 local progression) and 87.8% and 88.1% for chondrosarcoma (2 local progression with grades 2 and 3; no failures in grade 1), respectively, mainly predicted by gross total resection and age [130]. Kim et al. reviewed their 14 consecutive clivus chordoma patients treated with postoperative intensity-modulated radiotherapy with simultaneous integrated boost (IMRT-SIB) between 2005 and 2013, achieving local control without significant morbidities with a median follow-up of 41 months [131]. The three planning target volumes were defined as gross residual/high-risk area as PTV1 (3.9 Gy/fraction to 58.5 Gy for first 2 patients in 15 fractions, 2.5 Gy/fraction to 62.5 Gy for the rest in 25 fractions), postoperative tumor bed plus a 3–5 mm as PTV2 (3.15 Gy/fraction to 47.25 Gy for first 2 patients in 15 fractions, 2.2 Gy/fraction to 55 Gy for the rest in 25 fractions), and PTV2 plus a 5–10 mm as PTV3 (2.8 Gy/fraction to 42 Gy for first 2 patients in 15 fractions, 1.8 Gy/fraction to 45 Gy for the rest in 25 fractions). The progression-free and overall survival rates at 5 years were 92.9% [131].

Jahangiri et al. suggested no additional benefit of proton radiotherapy over photon-based radiotherapy based on their retrospective review of 50 clival chordoma patients (postoperative proton beam, 19; cyberknife, 7 patients; IMRT, 6; external beam, 10; none, 4 patients) treated between 1993 and 2013, contradicting conventional presumptions [132]. They have emphasized the importance of GTR for local control and underscored the lower third of clival progression most after GTR.

Recent studies have been initiated to evaluate systemic therapies for chordoma and a number of targeted agents and their respective pathways in chordomas, such as EGFR (erlotinib, gefitinib), PDGFR (imatinib), mTOR (rapamycin), and VEGF (bevacizumab) [133].

We recommend multimodality treatment with maximal safe resection and adjuvant radiotherapy respecting OAR thresholds. Image-guided highly precise radiotherapy (IMRT, VMAT, proton or carbon ion therapy) is the current standard.

## Chondrosarcoma

Skull base chondrosarcoma requires surgical resection to obtain maximal cytoreduction of the tumor along with definitive tissue diagnosis and is known to have more than 80% tumor control rates and overall survival more than 90% at 5 years [134].

Given the difficulty of resection of skull base chondrosarcoma, complete postoperative improvements of cranial nerve deficits should not be the expectation, apart from possible additional surgical deficits [135–137]. Samii et al. noted no improvement in preoperative symptoms in 55% of their 18 patients but developing additional 25% new cranial nerve deficits [135]. Sekhar et al. also reported 41% of new cranial nerve deficits in their series of 22 patients [136]. As radical surgical procedures for chondrosarcoma are known to be highly morbid, a controversy based on the goals of surgical cure exists: aggressive initial intervention for gross total resection (complete resection rates of 50–60% [135, 137]) versus maximal safe cytoreduction and using adjunct radiotherapy [137]. If adjuvant radiotherapy has been given, the extent of resection has not been shown to offer additional benefit on local control or overall survival [26, 135, 138, 139]. The cumulative recurrence-free survival was reported as 78%, while overall survival was 88% at 5 years [134, 140, 141]. The most definitive predictor of outcome was demonstrated to be tumor histology as approximately fivefold mortality at 5 years with mesenchymal type and tumor grade among conventional types as increasing grade is associated with worse survival; fortunately mesenchymal and high-grade conventional tumors are overall less than 11%, whereas Bloch et al. reported that adjuvant radiotherapy decreased 5-year mortality from 25% to 9% [134, 140, 141].

Adjuvant conventional photon fractionated radiotherapy had an established role for skull base chondrosarcoma, with historical prescription doses of 55–65 Gy, before modern highly conformal current techniques [138, 142]; few early or late toxicities were reported with 5-year progression-free and overall survival rates of more than 80% and 90%, respectively [138, 139, 142].

Schultz-Ertner et al. documented their 54 patients with low- and intermediate-grade chondrosarcomas of the skull base carrying postoperative gross residuals, treated between 1998 and 2005, by carbon ion median total dose of 60 CGE (weekly fractionation 7 × 3.0 CGE) using the raster scan technique in Germany [143]. They declared carbon ion radiotherapy as an effective treatment, resulting with only two local recurrences in a median follow-up of 33 months, providing actuarial local control rates of 96.2% and 89.8% at 3 and 4 years, and overall survival of 98.2% at 5 years. Nikoghosyan et al. initiated a phase III study comparing experimental carbon ion radiotherapy with proton radiotherapy to reveal non-inferiority with respect to 5-year local progression-free survival in chondrosarcomas [144], with biologically isoeffective target dose to the planning target volume of 60 Gy E ± 5% in carbon ion and 70 Gy E ± 5% in proton therapy.

Martin et al. published the University of Pittsburgh initial experience of ten skull base chondrosarcoma patients receiving adjuvant stereotactic radiotherapy with a median marginal dose of 16 Gy and achieving 80% local control rate at 5 years [145]. Iyer et al. updated the series with 22 patients of which 7 were definitive primary stereotactic radiosurgery with a median marginal treatment dose of 15 Gy, revealing 22% radiation toxicity rate, 72% cumulative local control, and 70% actuarial survival rate at 5 years [146]. Kano et al. acknowledged stereotactic radiosurgery for skull base chondrosarcomas as an important adjuvant option with 46 patients (36 postoperative) from seven participating centers of the North American Gamma Knife Consortium, with a median follow-up of 75 months [147]; the actuarial overall survival was 89% at 3 years, 86% at 5 years, and 76% at 10 years with a median tumor volume of 8.0 cm$^3$ and median margin dose of 15 Gy (range 10.5–20 Gy), while progression-free survival was 88% at 3 years, 85% at 5 years, and 70% at 10 years, with improved nerve deficits (abducens nerve paralysis, 61%; oculomotor nerve paralysis, 50%; lower cranial nerve dysfunction, 50%; optic neuropathy, 43%; facial neuropathy, 38%; trochlear nerve paralysis, 33%; trigeminal neuropathy, 12%; hearing loss, 10%).

We recommend multimodality treatment with maximal safe resection and adjuvant radiotherapy respecting OAR thresholds. Image-guided highly precise radiotherapy (IMRT, VMAT, proton or carbon ion therapy) is the current standard.

## Jugulotympanic Paraganglioma

JTP management evolved in the last two decades from pure surgical approach to more individualized treatment including radiotherapy and radiosurgery. There are major concept biases: to completely remove the tumor surgically or to control the growth of the tumor by fractionated external beam radiation therapy or stereotactic single or fractionated radiosurgery to avoid progressive neurologic symptoms and deficits. As surgery carries considerable risks of morbidity and mortality [148–152], gross total resection has been shown to be performed variably (40–80%) [153–155].

Conventional external beam radiation therapy was reported to provide high local control rates (85–100%) to avoid progression of GJTs and improvement of symptoms in some patients without major complications [156–159]. Pemberton et al. documented their series of 49 GJT patients having symptoms of deafness (27 patients), tinnitus (25 patients), and cranial nerve palsies (18 patients), treated between 1965 and 1987. Patients received a median dose of 45 Gy (range, 37.5–50.0) in 15–16 fractions (over 21 days ranging between 20 and 26) following a 2D simulator-planned wedge pair basic treatment technique with a median follow-up of 7.4 years (range, 2.0–23.4) [160]. The authors noted complete clinical response in 38 patients (partial response in 4, no response in 1, and no data were available

for 6) at 6 months post-radiotherapy. The recurrence-free and cancer-specific survival at 5 and 10 years were 96% and 92%, respectively, without any radionecrosis.

Fractionated stereotactic radiosurgery has also been used as a highly effective option with less side effects, especially in different scenarios of large tumors, major morbidity, or recurrences after incomplete resections [161, 162]. Henzel et al. published their series of 17 patients with a median follow-up of 40 months and freedom from progression and overall survival at 5 years of 100% and 93.8% [161]. Wegner et al. also documented their linac-based stereotactic radiation therapy experience on 18 GJT patients (15 single, 3 bilateral; 10 primary and 8 persistent after surgery) treated with a median prescribed dose of 20 Gy in mostly 3 fractions (range, 16–25 Gy in 1–5 fx) to the 80% isodose line [162] and achieved a local control rate of 100% with a median follow-up of 22 months and no new or worsening treatment-related neurologic deficits.

Initial radiographic tumor control for jugular paragangliomas has been noted to be very similar following single- or multi-fractionated stereotactic radiosurgery [163]. Stereotactic radiosurgery has a well-known noninvasive alternative treatment option for GJT [164–169]. Ibrahim et al. documented Sheffield National Centre for Stereotactic Radiosurgery experience for long-term local control and complications of gamma knife radiosurgery for 75 patients harboring 76 GJT tumors, with a median radiological follow-up duration of 51.5 months and a clinical follow-up duration of 38.5 months [165]. The overall local control rate with the median dose to the tumor margin of 18 Gy (range 12–25 Gy) was 93.4% with low cranial nerve morbidity; only 16% had new or progressive preexisting symptoms, 20% had improvement of preexisting deficits, and no change was documented in 64%. The actuarial tumor control rates at 5 and 10 years were 92.2% and 86.3%, respectively [165]. El Majdoub et al. documented their series of 32 GJT patients treated with linear accelerator-based radiosurgery either as primary or salvage therapy [169]. With a median single dose to the tumor surface of 15 Gy (range 11–20 Gy), the actuarial overall survival rates at 5, 10, and 20 years were 100%, 95.2%, and 79.4%, respectively; a significant improvement in previous neurological complaints occurred in 10 of 27 patients, while 12 patients had no change [169].

Though there is not a randomized comparison and most patients are treated with radiotherapy having more infiltrative larger tumors with generally nerve deficits, both surgery and radiation therapy are reasonable treatments with similar long-term local control rates. Therefore, individualization is necessary along with appropriately informed consented. Surgery might be pursued in younger patients for easily resectable tumors if no significant neurologic impairment is expected. However, in any case with major neurologic sequela expected with surgery, radiotherapy should be considered.

Image-guided intensity-modulated radiotherapy or volumetric modulated arc radiotherapy is recommended for many patients with large irregularly shaped tumors in close proximity to radiosensitive normal structures with a conventional fractionated or hypofractionated dose based on dose volume histograms of OAR. Stereotactic radiosurgery for small lesions is recommended in single fraction or in fractionated approach, encompassing radiographically visible tumor alone.

## Radiotherapy

### Indications for Radiotherapy

*Olfactory neuroblastoma*: All cases diagnosed with ON require radiotherapy as a component of multimodality treatment as adjuvant following maximal safe resection or definitive approach.

*Chordoma*: En bloc R0 resection, if possible, with wide margins might avoid radiotherapy; however almost all skull base chordoma cases require radiotherapy as a component of multimodality treatment as adjuvant following maximal safe acceptable R1–R2 resection or as definitive without any resection.

*Chondrosarcoma*: Irradiation is not indicated if there is en bloc resection with wide margins which is not generally possible for skull base. Radiotherapy is considered in two clinical scenarios aside from palliative treatments: following incomplete resection and in unresectable tumors or in case the resection is not feasible with very high morbidity.

*Jugulotympanic paraganglioma*: Progressive cases in clinical and radiological follow-up who might face major neurologic sequela with radical surgery or might not be considered for gross total resection with free surgical margins are considered radiotherapy candidates.

### Target Volume Determination and Delineation Guidelines

Adequate immobilization is crucial so as not to underdose the target or overdose the organs at risk because of the tight PTV for steep dose gradients. Image-guided radiotherapy is obligatory for radiotherapy of skull base tumors. General IMRT strategy in RTOG protocols is to encompass at least 95% of the PTV and avoid delivering <93% of the prescribed dose to >1% of the PTV or >110% of the prescribed dose to >20% of the PTV.

*Gross tumor volume (GTV)*: The volume should include the gross disease at the primary site or any grossly involved lymph nodes (>1 cm or nodes with a necrotic center or PET positive) determined from CT, MRI, PET-CT, and clinical information. A thorough contouring is necessary based on the exact spreading pattern (Fig. 18.5a–d).

**Anteriorly:**
- Involvement of nasal fossa or pterygopalatine fossa (Fig. 18.6) through sphenopalatine foramen?
- Extension to foramen rotundum bearing maxillary nerve (V2) leading to intracranial fossa?
- Involvement of inferior orbital fissure which might extend into the orbital apex or of the superior orbital fissure to intracranium?

**Laterally:**
- Involvement of nasopharyngeal structures leading into nodal spread?
- Invasion of parapharyngeal space including effacement of the fat?
- Extension to retrostyloid compartment bearing the carotid space to cranial nerves IX, X, XI, and XII?
- Involvement of jugular foramen to posterior cranial fossa and IX, X, and XI cranial nerves?

**Posteriorly:**
- Involvement of the prevertebral muscles?

**Inferiorly:**
- Extension through submucosal planes to oropharynx?

**Superiorly:**
- Involvement of the foramen lacerum intact for VI nerve?
- Involvement of the foramen ovale for mandibular nerve (V3)?
- Extension to the cavernous sinus related with III, IV, ophthalmic division of V, and VI nerves?

*Clinical target volume (CTV)*: The volume would contain the GTV and a margin for subclinical disease spread which needs to be individualized and cannot be fully imaged.

**CTV1:**
- *Jugulotympanic paraganglioma*: GTV=CTV1.
- *Olfactory neuroblastoma, chordoma, chondrosarcoma*: CTV1 covering GTV with a margin of ≥5 mm–8 mm circumferentially, except being ≤1 mm adjacent to organ at risk such as brain stem or chiasm, around the GTV (Fig. 18.5a–d).
- *Postoperative*: CTV1 encompasses residual GTV and surgical bed with fusion of preoperative imaging if possible.

**CTV2:**
- *Jugulotympanic paraganglioma*: None
- *Olfactory neuroblastoma, chordoma, chondrosarcoma*: (Fig. 18.5a–d) including subclinical disease as possible

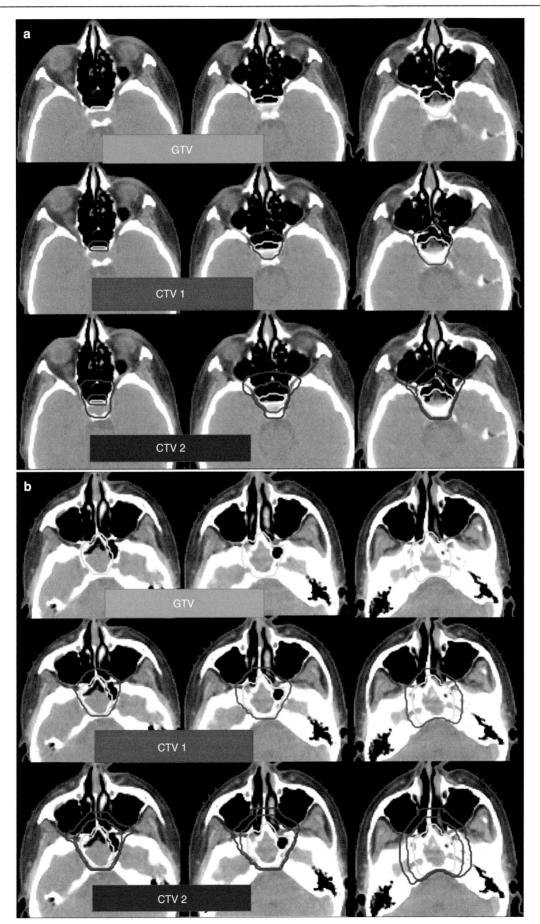

**Fig. 18.5** (a–d) Olfactory neuroblastoma, delineation of GTV, CTV1 (GTV plus 8 mm except 1 mm adjacent to brain stem and brain) and CTV2

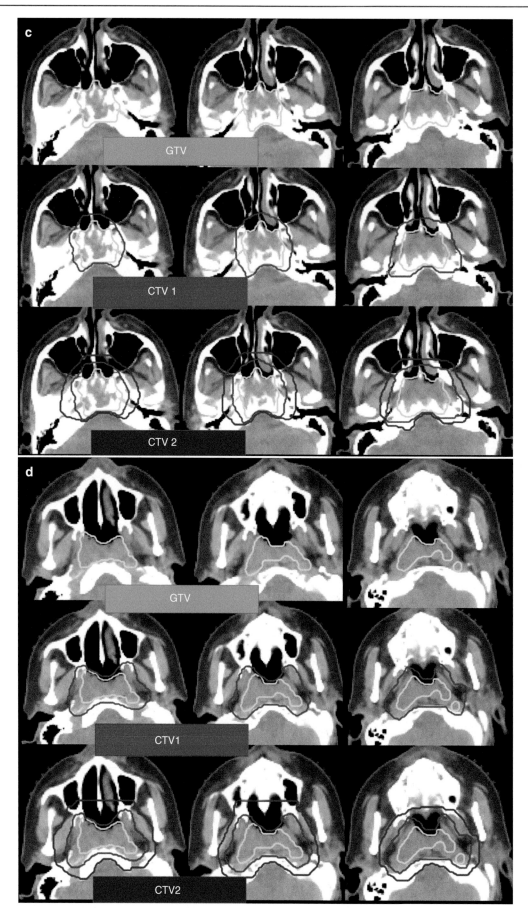

**Fig. 18.5** (continued)

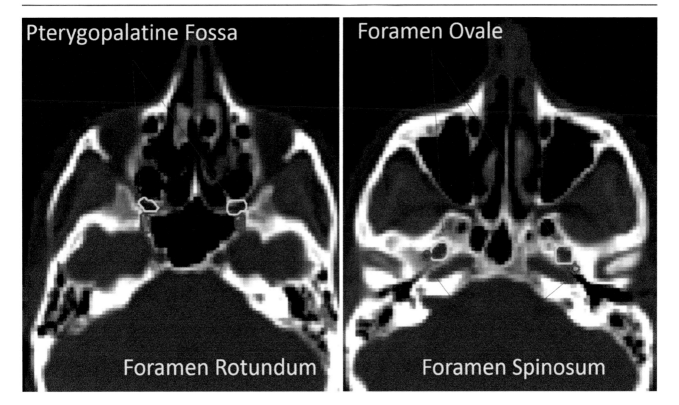

**Fig. 18.6** Pterygopalatine fossa, foramen rotundum, foramen ovale, and foramen spinosum are located cranio-caudally, respectively

microscopic disease or potential routes of spread (cavernous sinus if roof of the nasopharynx involved, entire clivus, bilaterally foramen ovale and rotundum (Fig. 18.6), pterygoid fossa, pterygopalatine fossa by inferior sphenoid sinus and posterior third of the nasal cavity and maxillary sinuses, bilateral upper deep jugular, and parapharyngeal space)

- *CTV2* requires to cover perineural track when required [170].
- *CTV2* needs to cover bilateral nodal bed if both neck is involved or ipsilateral neck if contralateral neck is free of nodal involvement.

*Planning target volume (PTV)*: The volume would contain adequate margin around the CTVs to compensate for uncertainties of setup and motion. PTV for fractionated radiotherapy is recommended to be 3–5 mm with strict daily image guidance, while each institution is encouraged to define the departmental appropriate magnitude of PTV by clinic quality assurance end-to-end tests for image guidance (Fig. 18.7a–c). PTV for stereotactic radiosurgery or fractionated radiosurgery is recommended to be typically 1–2 mm depending on the setup accuracy of the stereotactic system (Table 18.3).

**Treatment Planning Assessment Steps**

*Step 1*: Check whether the targets are adequately covered: CTV1 goal: V100% > 95%, V95% > 99%, V105% < 10%, Dmax < 120%. Although it is important to evaluate the PTV1 coverage with a tight margin on CTV1, slight underdosing of PTV1 and PTV2 could be mostly acceptable due to critical organ at risk sparing.

*Step 2*: Check for large hot spots (no more than 20% of prescription of PTV1).

*Step 3*: Check organs at risk constraints being met (Fig. 18.7).

*Step 4*: Check existence of hot/cold spots slide by slide to assure that hot spots are in the GTV and not on a nerve in the CTV.

**Normal Critical Structure Tolerance Constraints**

Major limitation in skull base definitive or adjuvant radiotherapy is the tolerance limits of various organs at risk in the field, especially the nerves and brain stem. Table 18.4 summarizes all head and neck OAR dose constraints, respectively, which need to be modified based on the fraction scheme being used based on daily fraction dose and total dose planned in order not to cause an unexpected deficit [171–174].

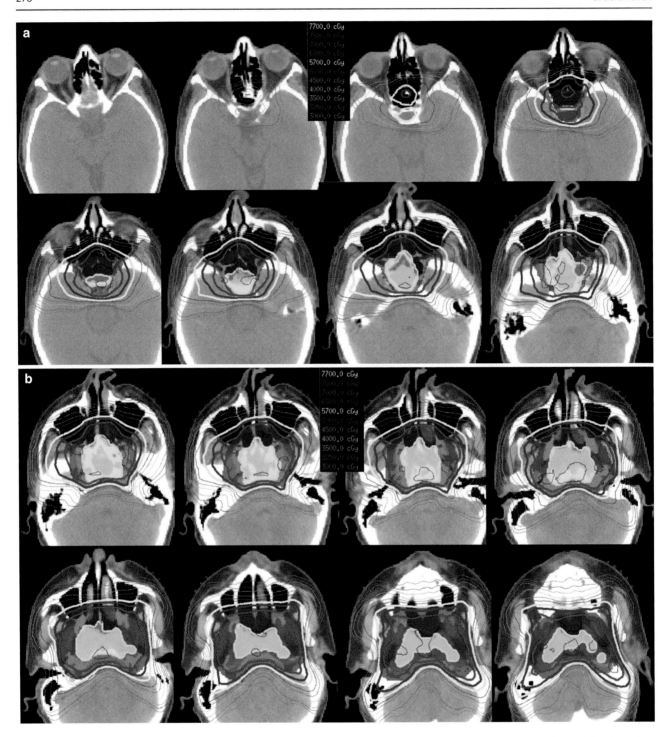

**Fig. 18.7** (a–c) Treatment delivery with IGRT, VMAT, simultaneous integrated boost 70 Gy (CTV1) and 63 Gy (CTV2) in 33 fractions, dose volume histogram details of organs at risk

## Radiation Toxicity

Skull base radiotherapy can be related to acute mucosal toxicity due to the fact that nasopharyngeal, nasal, oropharyngeal and hypopharyngeal mucosa are common adjacent structures. Strict OAR criteria to spare lacrimal, parotid, and submandibular glands would provide easier recovery in addition to dietary adjustment (avoidance of spicy and dry foods, etc.). Pain medication and hydration and oral hygiene (baking soda/salt water solutions for rinsing and gargling, etc.) are also used as supportive care.

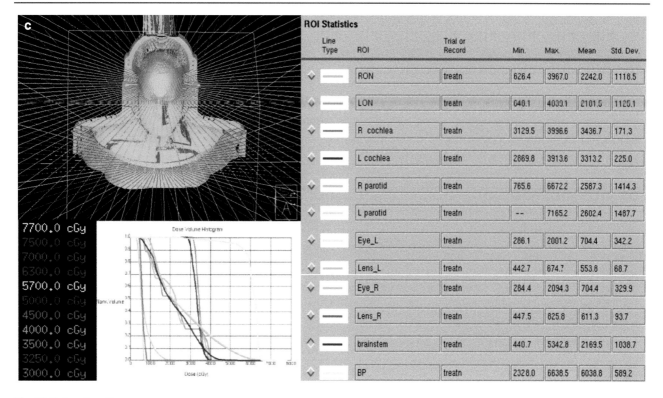

**Fig. 18.7** (continued)

**Table 18.3** Dose prescription schemes for chordoma, chondrosarcoma, olfactory neuroblastoma, and jugulotympanic paraganglioma

|  | CTV1 | CTV2 | CTV3 |
|---|---|---|---|
| Chordoma | 70 Gy | 63 Gy | 57 Gy |
| and | 2.1 Gy/fraction | 1.9 Gy/fraction | 1.72 Gy/fraction |
| Chondrosarcoma | 33 fractions | 33 fractions | 33 fractions |
| and | 66 Gy | 60 Gy | 54 Gy |
| Olfactory neuroblastoma | 2.2 Gy/fraction | 2 Gy/fraction | 1.8 Gy/fraction |
|  | 30 fractions | 30 fractions | 30 fractions |
|  | 55 Gy | 50 Gy | 45 Gy |
|  | 2.2 Gy/fraction | 2 Gy/fraction | 1.8 Gy/fraction |
|  | 25 fractions | 25 fractions | 25 fractions |
| Jugulotympanic | 12–15 Gy | NA | NA |
| paraganglioma | 1 fraction |  |  |
|  | 25 Gy | NA | NA |
|  | 5 Gy/fraction |  |  |
|  | 5 fractions |  |  |
|  | 37.5–45 Gy | NA | NA |
|  | 2.5–3 Gy |  |  |
|  | 15 fractions |  |  |
|  | 45–50 Gy | NA | NA |
|  | 1.8–2 Gy |  |  |
|  | 25 fractions |  |  |

The most late radiotherapy toxicity in skull base tumors are cranial nerve deficits related directly to the radiotherapy field with difficulty to respect OAR toxicity threshold limits in balance with delivering a sufficient dose to locally control the disease [174–176]. Therefore, patients should be well informed and consented for developing permanent deficits.

## Conclusion

In limited prospective data environment due to scarce number of patients insufficient to initiate any randomized studies, knowledge-based adaptation and optimization including consistent target coverage with respect to criti-

**Table 18.4** Institutional guidelines for organ at risk constraints for conventionally fractionated radiotherapy [174–176]

| Structure | Constraints |
|---|---|
| Brain | V30 Gy ≤ 50% |
| Brain stem | Max dose ≤54 Gy; if clinically reasonable V60 Gy ≤ 0.01 cc, V55 Gy ≤ 0.5 cc, V30 ≤ 33% |
| Spinal cord | Max dose ≤ 45 Gy V50 Gy ≤ 0.01 cc |
| Optic nerves[important] | Max dose ≤ 54 Gy; single max dose ≤ 8 Gy |
| Chiasm | Max dose ≤ 54 Gy; single max dose ≤ 8 Gy |
| Pituitary | Mean dose ≤ 36 Gy |
| Lacrimal gland | Mean dose ≤ 26 Gy |
| Hippocampus | D100% ≤ 9 Gy, max dose ≤ 16 Gy |
| Mandible (TM joint) | Max dose ≤ 69 Gy, V75Gy ≤ 1 cc |
| Brachial plexus | Max dose ≤ 66 Gy |
| Oral cavity | As low as possible, mean dose < 40 Gy |
| Submandibular glands | As low as possible |
| Parotid gland | If no neck treatment, mean dose ≤ 10 Gy Otherwise, mean dose < 26 Gy |
| | At least 20 cc of the combined volume of both parotid glands < 20 Gy |
| | At least 50% of one gland < 30 Gy (in at least one gland) |
| Esophagus, postcricoid pharynx | Mean dose < 45 Gy |
| Each cochlea | Max dose ≤ 45 Gy, mean ≤ 30 Gy |
| Each eye | Max dose ≤ 40 Gy, mean ≤ 30 Gy |
| Each lens | Max dose ≤5 Gy (as low as possible) |
| Glottic larynx | Mean dose < 36–45 Gy |

Important: Radiation dose volume effects of optic nerves and chiasm reveals a "near zero" incidence with conventionally fractionated 50 Gy, while incidence of optic neuropathy in case of conventional fractionation (1.8–2.0 Gy/fraction/day) is very unusual for a Dmax ≤ 55 Gy, but 3–7% for 55–60 Gy and 7–20% for >60 Gy [174]. Dose < 8 Gy seemed very tolerable for single-fraction stereotactic radiosurgery, and doses of 8–12 Gy might initiate risks which will increase to >10% in case of 12–15 Gy

cal OAR dose thresholds to balance the benefits and potential harms of radiation treatment is important for adjuvant, definitive, or palliative intent radiotherapy in skull base tumors, along with the best possible applicable modality of IMRT, VMAT, SRS, FSRT, and proton-beam therapy.

## Self-Assessment Questions

1. Following a severe neck pain, CT scan reveals a centrally located well-circumscribed and destructive lytic lesion in skull base with an expansile large soft tissue mass posteriorly indenting the pons. What would be the best possible radiological diagnosis?

2. Please choose the false statement below:

A. Pan-cytokeratin (panCK) and epithelial membrane antigen (EMA) are not positive for chondrosarcomas
B. Chordoma shows positivity for EMA and panCK
C. Chordoma shows positivity for Vimentin and S-100 protein
D. Chondrosarcoma does not express glial fibrillary acidic protein (GFAP)
E. Chordoma expresses GFAP

3. Brachyury appears to be a specific and sensitive immunohistochemistry biomarker of
A. Chondrosarcoma
B. Chordoma
C. Olfactory neuroblastoma
D. Jugulotympanic paraganglioma

4. What is the most significant prognostic factor below for skull base chordoma?
A. Tumor signal intensity in T2 images
B. Visual deficits
C. Extent of bony invasion
D. Extent of soft tissue mass
E. Extent of surgical resection

5. Nodal metastases are mostly expected in which tumor below?
A. Chondrosarcoma
B. Chordoma
C. Olfactory neuroblastoma
D. Jugulotympanic paraganglioma

## Answers

1. Chordoma with a "thumb sign"
2. E. Chordomas do not express glial fibrillary acidic protein
3. B. Chordoma
4. E. Extent of surgical resection
5. C Olfactory neuroblastoma

## References

1. Kunc M, Gabrych A, Czapiewski P, et al. Paraneoplastic syndromes in olfactory neuroblastoma. Contemp Oncol. 2015;19(1):6–16.
2. Taraszewska A, Czorniuk-Sliwa A, Dambska M. Olfactory neuroblastoma (esthesioneuroblastoma) and esthesioneuroepithelioma: histologic and immunohistochemical study. Folia Neuropathol. 1998;36(2):81–6.
3. Hirose T, Scheithauer BW, Lopes MB, et al. Olfactory neuroblastoma. An immunohistochemical, ultrastructural, and flow cytometric study. Cancer. 1995;76(1):4–19.
4. Shah K, Perez-Ordonez B. Neuroendocrine neoplasms of the sinonasal tract: neuroendocrine carcinomas and olfactory neuroblastoma. Head Neck Pathol. 2016;10(1):85–94.

5. Slevin NJ, Irwin CJ, Banerjee SS, et al. Olfactory neural tumours—the role of external beam radiotherapy. J Laryngol Otol. 1996;110(11):1012–6.

6. Stewart FM, Frieson HF. P.A. L: Esthesioneuroblastoma. Chichester: John Wiley; 1988.

7. Ostrom QT, Gittleman H, Liao P, et al. CBTRUS statistical report: primary brain and central nervous system tumors diagnosed in the United States in 2007–2011. Neuro Oncol. 2014;16(Suppl 4):iv1–63.

8. Villano JL, Bressler L, Propp JM, et al. Descriptive epidemiology of selected olfactory tumors. J Neurooncol. 2010;100(1):73–80.

9. Morita A, Ebersold MJ, Olsen KD, et al. Esthesioneuroblastoma: prognosis and management. Neurosurgery. 1993;32(5):706–14. discussion 714–5

10. Jethanamest D, Morris LG, Sikora AG, et al. Esthesioneuroblastoma: a population-based analysis of survival and prognostic factors. Arch Otolaryngol Head Neck Surg. 2007;133(3):276–80.

11. Davis RE, Weissler MC. Esthesioneuroblastoma and neck metastasis. Head Neck. 1992;14(6):477–82.

12. Heffelfinger MJ, Dahlin DC, MacCarty CS, et al. Chordomas and cartilaginous tumors at the skull base. Cancer. 1973;32(2):410–20.

13. O'Neill P, Bell BA, Miller JD, et al. Fifty years of experience with chordomas in southeast Scotland. Neurosurgery. 1985;16(2):166–70.

14. Mitchell A, Scheithauer BW, Unni KK, et al. Chordoma and chondroid neoplasms of the spheno-occiput. An immunohistochemical study of 41 cases with prognostic and nosologic implications. Cancer. 1993;72(10):2943–9.

15. McMaster ML, Goldstein AM, Bromley CM, et al. Chordoma: incidence and survival patterns in the United States, 1973–1995. Cancer Causes Control. 2001;12(1):1–11.

16. Hruban RH, Traganos F, Reuter VE, et al. Chordomas with malignant spindle cell components. A DNA flow cytometric and immunohistochemical study with histogenetic implications. Am J Pathol. 1990;137(2):435–47.

17. Vujovic S, Henderson S, Presneau N, et al. Brachyury, a crucial regulator of notochordal development, is a novel biomarker for chordomas. J Pathol. 2006;209(2):157–65.

18. Sa JK, Lee IH, Hong SD, et al. Genomic and transcriptomic characterization of skull base chordoma. Oncotarget. 2017;8(1):1321–8.

19. Krol G, Sze G, Arbit E, et al. Intradural metastases of chordoma. AJNR Am J Neuroradiol. 1989;10(1):193–5.

20. Chambers PW, Schwinn CP. Chordoma. A clinicopathologic study of metastasis. Am J Clin Pathol. 1979;72(5):765–76.

21. Markwalder TM, Markwalder RV, Robert JL, et al. Metastatic chordoma. Surg Neurol. 1979;12(6):473–8.

22. Volpe R, Mazabraud A. A clinicopathologic review of 25 cases of chordoma (a pleomorphic and metastasizing neoplasm). Am J Surg Pathol. 1983;7(2):161–70.

23. Adegbite AB, McQueen JD, Paine KW, et al. Primary intracranial chondrosarcoma: a report of two cases. Neurosurgery. 1985;17(3):490–4.

24. Sen CN, Sekhar LN, Schramm VL, et al. Chordoma and chondrosarcoma of the cranial base: an 8-year experience. Neurosurgery. 1989;25(6):931–40. discussion 940–1

25. Hogendoorn PCW, Bovee JM, Nielsen GP. Chondrosarcoma (grades I–III), including primary and secondary variants and periosteal chondrosarcoma. In: Hogendoorn PCW, Mertens F, editors. World Health Organization classification of tumours of soft tissue and bone, vol. 5. 4th ed. Lyon, France: IARC; 2013. p. 264.

26. Rosenberg AE, Nielsen GP, Keel SB, et al. Chondrosarcoma of the base of the skull: a clinicopathologic study of 200 cases with emphasis on its distinction from chordoma. Am J Surg Pathol. 1999;23(11):1370–8.

27. Abenoza P, Sibley RK. Chordoma: an immunohistologic study. Hum Pathol. 1986;17(7):744–7.

28. Coffin CM, Swanson PE, Wick MR, et al. An immunohistochemical comparison of chordoma with renal cell carcinoma, colorectal adenocarcinoma, and myxopapillary ependymoma: a potential diagnostic dilemma in the diminutive biopsy. Mod Pathol. 1993;6(5):531–8.

29. Thedinger BA, Glasscock ME 3rd, Cueva RA, et al. Postoperative radiographic evaluation after acoustic neuroma and glomus jugulare tumor removal. Laryngoscope. 1992;102(3):261–6.

30. Chen H, Sippel RS, O'Dorisio MS, et al. The north American neuroendocrine tumor society consensus guideline for the diagnosis and management of neuroendocrine tumors: pheochromocytoma, paraganglioma, and medullary thyroid cancer. Pancreas. 2010;39(6):775–83.

31. Spector GJ, Sobol S, Thawley SE, et al. Panel discussion: glomus jugulare tumors of the temporal bone. Patterns of invasion in the temporal bone. Laryngoscope. 1979;89(10 Pt 1):1628–39.

32. Spector GJ, Gado M, Ciralsky R, et al. Neurologic implications of glomus tumors in the head and neck. Laryngoscope. 1975;85(8):1387–95.

33. Welander J, Soderkvist P, Gimm O. Genetics and clinical characteristics of hereditary pheochromocytomas and paragangliomas. Endocr Relat Cancer. 2011;18(6):R253–76.

34. Barnes L, Tse LL, Hunt JL, et al. Tumours of the paraganglionic system: introduction. In: Barnes L, Eveson JW, Reichart P, Sidransky D, editors. World Health Organization classification of tumours pathology & genetics head and neck tumours. Lyon, France: IARC Press; 2005. p. 362.

35. Michaels L, Soucek S, Beale T, et al. Jugulotympanic paraganglioma. In: Barnes L, Eveson JW, Reichart P, Sidransky D, editors. World Health Organization classification of tumours pathology & genetics head and neck tumours. Lyon, France: IARC Press; 2005. p. 366.

36. Dannenberg H, Dinjens WN, Abbou M, et al. Frequent germ-line succinate dehydrogenase subunit D gene mutations in patients with apparently sporadic parasympathetic paraganglioma. Clin Cancer Res. 2002;8(7):2061–6.

37. Lee JA, Duh QY. Sporadic paraganglioma. World J Surg. 2008;32(5):683–7.

38. Avramovic N, Weckesser M, Velasco A, et al. Long distance endovascular growth of jugulotympanic paraganglioma evident in 68Ga-DOTATATE PET but concealed on CT. Clin Nucl Med. 2017;42(2):135–7.

39. Gulya AJ. The glomus tumor and its biology. Laryngoscope. 1993;103(11 Pt 2 Suppl 60):7–15.

40. Lawson W. The neuroendocrine nature of the glomus cells: an experimental, ultrastructural, and histochemical tissue culture study. Laryngoscope. 1980;90(1):120–44.

41. van Duinen N, Steenvoorden D, Kema IP, et al. Increased urinary excretion of 3-methoxytyramine in patients with head and neck paragangliomas. J Clin Endocrinol Metab. 2010;95(1):209–14.

42. Erickson D, Kudva YC, Ebersold MJ, et al. Benign paragangliomas: clinical presentation and treatment outcomes in 236 patients. J Clin Endocrinol Metab. 2001;86(11):5210–6.

43. Hahn S, Palmer JN, Adappa ND. A catecholamine-secreting skull base sinonasal paraganglioma presenting with labile hypertension in a patient with previously undiagnosed genetic mutation. J Neurol Surg Rep. 2012;73(1):19–24.

44. Tran Ba Huy P, Duet M, Abulizi M, et al. Skull base paraganglioma and intracranial hypertension. Arch Otolaryngol Head Neck Surg. 2010;136(1):91–4.

45. Alzahrani AS, Alshaikh O, Faiyaz-Ul-Haque M, et al. Multiple paraganglioma syndrome type 4 due to succinate dehydrogenase B mutation: diagnostic and therapeutic challenges of a skull base paraganglioma masquerading as nasopharyngeal cancer. Endocr Pract. 2010;16(3):452–8.

46. Brown JS. Glomus jugulare tumors revisited: a ten-year statistical follow-up of 231 cases. Laryngoscope. 1985;95(3):284–8.

47. Woods CI, Strasnick B, Jackson CG. Surgery for glomus tumors: the Otology Group experience. Laryngoscope. 1993;103(11 Pt 2 Suppl 60):65–70.

48. Boedeker CC, Neumann HP, Maier W, et al. Malignant head and neck paragangliomas in SDHB mutation carriers. Otolaryngol Head Neck Surg. 2007;137(1):126–9.

49. DeMonte F, Chernov M, Fuller G, et al. Skull base. In: Goepfert H, Ang KK, Clayman GL, Diaz EM, Ginsberg LE, Khuri FR, Suarez P, editors. MD Anderson Online Book: Multidisciplinary care of head and neck cancer; 2002. www.headneckcancer.org.

50. Raghavan P, Kesser BW, Wintermark M, et al. Temporal bone and skull base. In: Raghavan P, Mukherjee S, Jameson MJ, Wintermark M, editors. Manual of head and neck imaging. Berlin, Heidelberg: Springer-Verlag; 2014. p. 189–256.

51. Olsen ML, Dillon WP, Kelly WM. MR imaging of paragangliomas. AJNR Am J Neuroradiol. 1986;7:1039–42.

52. Curtin HD, Rabinov JD, Som PM. Central skull base: embryology, anatomy, and pathology, vol. 1. St. Louis, MO: Mosby; 2003.

53. Firooznia H, Pinto RS, Lin JP, et al. Chordoma: radiologic evaluation of 20 cases. Am J Roentgenol. 1976;127(5):797–805.

54. Conley LM, Phillips CD. Imaging of the central skull base. Radiol Clin N Am. 2017;55(1):53–67.

55. Meyers SP, Hirsch WL Jr, Curtin HD, et al. Chordomas of the skull base: MR features. AJNR Am J Neuroradiol. 1992;13(6):1627–36.

56. Larson TC 3rd, Houser OW, Laws ER Jr. Imaging of cranial chordomas. Mayo Clin Proc. 1987;62(10):886–93.

57. Azzopardi C, Grech R, Mizzi A. Teaching NeuroImages: chordoma. Neurology. 2014;83(10):e110–1.

58. Brown E, Hug EB, Weber AL. Chondrosarcoma of the skull base. Neuroimaging Clin N Am. 1994;4(3):529–41.

59. Oot RF, Melville GE, New PF, et al. The role of MR and CT in evaluating clival chordomas and chondrosarcomas. AJR Am J Roentgenol. 1988;151(3):567–75.

60. Dublin AB, Bobinski M. Imaging characteristics of olfactory neuroblastoma (esthesioneuroblastoma). J Neurol Surg B Skull Base. 2016;77(1):1–5.

61. Elkhatib AH, Soldatova L, Carrau RL, et al. Role of 18 F-FDG PET/CT differentiating olfactory neuroblastoma from sinonasal undifferentiated carcinoma. Laryngoscope. 2017;127(2):321–4.

62. Nguyen BD, Roarke MC, Nelson KD, et al. F-18 FDG PET/CT staging and posttherapeutic assessment of esthesioneuroblastoma. Clin Nucl Med. 2006;31(3):172–4.

63. Muller U, Kubik-Huch RA, Ares C, et al. Is there a role for conventional MRI and MR diffusion-weighted imaging for distinction of skull base chordoma and chondrosarcoma? Acta Radiol. 2016;57(2):225–32.

64. Yeom KW, Lober RM, Mobley BC, et al. Diffusion-weighted MRI: distinction of skull base chordoma from chondrosarcoma. AJNR Am J Neuroradiol. 2013;34(5):1056–61. S1051

65. Ma JP, Tian KB, Wang L, et al. Proposal and validation of a basic progression scoring system for patients with skull base chordoma. World Neurosurg. 2016;91:409–18.

66. Kadish S, Goodman M, Wang CC. Olfactory neuroblastoma. A clinical analysis of 17 cases. Cancer. 1976;37(3):1571–6.

67. Krayenbuhl H, Yasargil M. Cranial chordomas. Prog Neurol Surg. 1975;6:380–434.

68. Raffel C, Wright DC, Gutin PH, et al. Cranial chordomas: clinical presentation and results of operative and radiation therapy in twenty-six patients. Neurosurgery. 1985;17(5):703–10.

69. Sekhar LN, Sen C, Snyderman C. Anterior, anteriolateral, and lateral approaches to extradural petroclival tumors. New York: Raven Press; 1993.

70. Fisch U. Infratemporal fossa approach to tumours of the temporal bone and base of the skull. J Laryngol Otol. 1978;92(11):949–67.

71. Jackson CG, Glasscock ME 3rd, Harris PF. Glomus tumors. Diagnosis, classification, and management of large lesions. Arch Otolaryngol. 1982;108(7):401–10.

72. Resto VA, Eisele DW, Forastiere A, et al. Esthesioneuroblastoma: the Johns Hopkins experience. Head Neck. 2000;22(6):550–8.

73. Dulguerov P, Calcaterra T. Esthesioneuroblastoma: the UCLA experience 1970–1990. Laryngoscope. 1992;102(8):843–9.

74. Dulguerov P, Allal AS, Calcaterra TC. Esthesioneuroblastoma: a meta-analysis and review. Lancet Oncol. 2001;2(11):683–90.

75. Levine PA, McLean WC, Cantrell RW. Esthesioneuroblastoma: the University of Virginia experience 1960–1985. Laryngoscope. 1986;96(7):742–6.

76. Unger F, Haselsberger K, Walch C, et al. Combined endoscopic surgery and radiosurgery as treatment modality for olfactory neuroblastoma (esthesioneuroblastoma). Acta Neurochir. 2005;147(6):595–601. discussion 601–592

77. Fu TS, Monteiro E, Muhanna N, et al. Comparison of outcomes for open versus endoscopic approaches for olfactory neuroblastoma: a systematic review and individual participant data meta-analysis. Head Neck. 2016;38(Suppl 1):E2306–16.

78. Folbe A, Herzallah I, Duvvuri U, et al. Endoscopic endonasal resection of esthesioneuroblastoma: a multicenter study. Am J Rhinol Allergy. 2009;23(1):91–4.

79. Kim BJ, Kim DW, Kim SW, et al. Endoscopic versus traditional craniofacial resection for patients with sinonasal tumors involving the anterior skull base. Clin Exp Otorhinolaryngol. 2008;1(3):148–53.

80. Papacharalampous GX, Vlastarakos PV, Chrysovergis A, et al. Olfactory neuroblastoma (esthesioneuroblastoma): towards minimally invasive surgery and multi-modality treatment strategies – an updated critical review of the current literature. J BUON. 2013;18(3):557–63.

81. Devaiah AK, Andreoli MT. Treatment of esthesioneuroblastoma: a 16-year meta-analysis of 361 patients. Laryngoscope. 2009;119(7):1412–6.

82. Koka VN, Julieron M, Bourhis J, et al. Aesthesioneuroblastoma. J Laryngol Otol. 1998;112(7):628–33.

83. Eich HT, Staar S, Micke O, et al. Radiotherapy of esthesioneuroblastoma. Int J Radiat Oncol Biol Phys. 2001;49(1):155–60.

84. Eriksen JG, Bastholt L, Krogdahl AS, et al. Esthesioneuroblastoma—what is the optimal treatment? Acta Oncol. 2000;39(2):231–5.

85. Gruber G, Laedrach K, Baumert B, et al. Esthesioneuroblastoma: irradiation alone and surgery alone are not enough. Int J Radiat Oncol Biol Phys. 2002;54(2):486–91.

86. Chao KS, Kaplan C, Simpson JR, et al. Esthesioneuroblastoma: the impact of treatment modality. Head Neck. 2001;23(9):749–57.

87. Petruzzelli GJ, Howell JB, Pederson A, et al. Multidisciplinary treatment of olfactory neuroblastoma: patterns of failure and management of recurrence. Am J Otolaryngol. 2015;36(4):547–53.

88. Nalavenkata SB, Sacks R, Adappa ND, et al. Olfactory neuroblastoma: fate of the neck—a long-term multicenter retrospective study. Otolaryngol Head Neck Surg. 2016;154(2):383–9.

89. Aljumaily RM, Nystrom JS, Wein RO. Neoadjuvant chemotherapy in the setting of locally advanced olfactory neuroblastoma with intracranial extension. Rare tumors. 2011;3(1):e1.

90. Herr MW, Sethi RK, Meier JC, et al. Esthesioneuroblastoma: an update on the Massachusetts eye and ear infirmary and Massachusetts general hospital experience with craniofacial resection, proton beam radiation, and chemotherapy. J Neurol Surg B Skull Base. 2014;75(1):58–64.

91. Kim HJ, Kim CH, Lee BJ, et al. Surgical treatment versus concurrent chemoradiotherapy as an initial treatment modality in advanced olfactory neuroblastoma. Auris Nasus Larynx. 2007;34(4):493–8.

92. Rosenthal DI, Barker JL Jr, El-Naggar AK, et al. Sinonasal malignancies with neuroendocrine differentiation: patterns of failure according to histologic phenotype. Cancer. 2004;101:2567–73.

93. Benfari G, Fusconi M, Ciofalo A, et al. Radiotherapy alone for local tumour control in esthesioneuroblastoma. Acta Otorhinolaryngol Ital. 2008;28(6):292–7.

94. McElroy EA Jr, Buckner JC, Lewis JE. Chemotherapy for advanced esthesioneuroblastoma: the Mayo Clinic experience. Neurosurgery. 1998;42(5):1023–7. discussion 1027–8

95. Levine PA, Gallagher R, Cantrell RW. Esthesioneuroblastoma: reflections of a 21-year experience. Laryngoscope. 1999;109(10):1539–43.

96. Polin RS, Sheehan JP, Chenelle AG, et al. The role of preoperative adjuvant treatment in the management of esthesioneuroblastoma: the University of Virginia experience. Neurosurgery. 1998;42(5):1029–37.

97. Giridhar P, Mallick S, Laviraj MA, et al. Esthesioneuroblastoma with large intracranial extension treated with induction chemotherapy, de-bulking surgery and image guided intensity modulated radiotherapy. Eur Arch Otorhinolaryngol. 2016;273(5):1323–5.

98. Madani I, Bonte K, Vakaet L, et al. Intensity-modulated radiotherapy for sinonasal tumors: Ghent University Hospital update. Int J Radiat Oncol Biol Phys. 2009;73(2):424–32.

99. Wiegner EA, Daly ME, Murphy JD, et al. Intensity-modulated radiotherapy for tumors of the nasal cavity and paranasal sinuses: clinical outcomes and patterns of failure. Int J Radiat Oncol Biol Phys. 2010;83(1):243–51.

100. Pacholke HD, Amdur RJ, Louis DA, et al. The role of intensity modulated radiation therapy for favorable stage tumor of the nasal cavity or ethmoid sinus. Am J Clin Oncol. 2005;28(5):474–8.

101. Jensen AD, Nikoghosyan AV, Windemuth-Kieselbach C, et al. Treatment of malignant sinonasal tumours with intensity-modulated radiotherapy (IMRT) and carbon ion boost (C12). BMC Cancer. 2010;11:190.

102. Hu YW, Lin CZ, Li WY, et al. Locally advanced oncocytic carcinoma of the nasal cavity treated with surgery and intensity-modulated radiotherapy. J Chin Med Assoc. 2010;73(3):166–72.

103. Hoppe BS, Wolden SL, Zelefsky MJ, et al. Postoperative intensity-modulated radiation therapy for cancers of the paranasal sinuses, nasal cavity, and lacrimal glands: technique, early outcomes, and toxicity. Head Neck. 2008;30(7):925–32.

104. Duthoy W, Boterberg T, Claus F, et al. Postoperative intensity-modulated radiotherapy in sinonasal carcinoma: clinical results in 39 patients. Cancer. 2005;104(1):71–82.

105. Dirix P, Vanstraelen B, Jorissen M, et al. Intensity-modulated radiotherapy for sinonasal cancer: improved outcome compared to conventional radiotherapy. Int J Radiat Oncol Biol Phys. 2010;78(4):998–1004.

106. Dirix P, Nuyts S, Vanstraelen B, et al. Post-operative intensity-modulated radiotherapy for malignancies of the nasal cavity and paranasal sinuses. Radiother Oncol. 2007;85(3):385–91.

107. Chen AM, Daly ME, Bucci MK, et al. Carcinomas of the paranasal sinuses and nasal cavity treated with radiotherapy at a single institution over five decades: are we making improvement? Int J Radiat Oncol Biol Phys. 2007;69(1):141–7.

108. Buiret G, Montbarbon X, Fleury B, et al. Inverted papilloma with associated carcinoma of the nasal cavity and paranasal sinuses: treatment outcomes. Acta Otolaryngol. 2010;132(1):80–5.

109. McLean JN, Nunley SR, Klass C, et al. Combined modality therapy of esthesioneuroblastoma. Otolaryngol Head Neck Surg. 2007;136(6):998–1002.

110. Mori T, Onimaru R, Onodera S, et al. Olfactory neuroblastoma: the long-term outcome and late toxicity of multimodal therapy including radiotherapy based on treatment planning using computed tomography. Radiat Oncol. 2015;10:88.

111. Nakamura N, Zenda S, Tahara M, et al. Proton beam therapy for olfactory neuroblastoma. Radiother Oncol. 2017;122(3):368–72.

112. Rimmer J, Lund VJ, Beale T, et al. Olfactory neuroblastoma: a 35-year experience and suggested follow-up protocol. Laryngoscope. 2014;124(7):1542–9.

113. Eden BV, Debo RF, Larner JM, et al. Esthesioneuroblastoma. Long-term outcome and patterns of failure—the University of Virginia experience. Cancer. 1994;73(10):2556–62.

114. Wang L, Tian K, Wang K, et al. Factors for tumor progression in patients with skull base chordoma. Cancer Med. 2016;5(9):2368–77.

115. Tian K, Wang L, Wang K, et al. Analysis of clinical features and outcomes of skull base chordoma in different age-groups. World Neurosurg. 2016;92:407–17.

116. Tian K, Zhang H, Ma J, et al. Factors for overall survival in patients with skull base chordoma: a retrospective analysis of 225 patients. World Neurosurg. 2017;97:39–48.

117. Wang L, Wu Z, Tian K, et al. Clinical features and surgical outcomes of patients with skull base chordoma: a retrospective analysis of 238 patients. J Neurosurg. 2017;127(6):1257–67.

118. Slater JM, Slater JD, Archambeau JO. Proton therapy for cranial base tumors. J Craniofac Surg. 1995;6(1):24–6.

119. al-Mefty O, Borba LA. Skull base chordomas: a management challenge. J Neurosurg. 1997;86(2):182–9.

120. Debus J, Haberer T, Schulz-Ertner D, et al. Carbon ion irradiation of skull base tumors at GSI. First clinical results and future perspectives. Strahlenther Onkol. 2000;176(5):211–6.

121. McDonald MW, Linton OR, Moore MG, et al. Influence of residual tumor volume and radiation dose coverage in outcomes for clival chordoma. Int J Radiat Oncol Biol Phys. 2016;95(1):304–11.

122. Krengli M, Poletti A, Ferrara E, et al. Tumour seeding in the surgical pathway after resection of skull base chordoma. Rep Pract Oncol Radiother. 2016;21(4):407–11.

123. Klekamp J, Samii M. Spinal chordomas—results of treatment over a 17-year period. Acta Neurochir. 1996;138(5):514–9.

124. Romero J, Cardenes H, la Torre A, et al. Chordoma: results of radiation therapy in eighteen patients. Radiother Oncol. 1993;29(1):27–32.

125. Munzenrider JE, Liebsch NJ. Proton therapy for tumors of the skull base. Strahlenther Onkol. 1999;175(Suppl 2):57–63.

126. Amichetti M, Cianchetti M, Amelio D, et al. Proton therapy in chordoma of the base of the skull: a systematic review. Neurosurg Rev. 2009;32(4):403–16.

127. Casali PG, Stacchiotti S, Sangalli C, et al. Chordoma. Curr Opin Oncol. 2007;19(4):367–70.

128. Uhl M, Mattke M, Welzel T, et al. Highly effective treatment of skull base chordoma with carbon ion irradiation using a raster scan technique in 155 patients: first long-term results. Cancer. 2014;120(21):3410–7.

129. Weber DC, Malyapa R, Albertini F, et al. Long term outcomes of patients with skull-base low-grade chondrosarcoma and chordoma patients treated with pencil beam scanning proton therapy. Radiother Oncol. 2016;120(1):169–74.

130. Sahgal A, Chan MW, Atenafu EG, et al. Image-guided, intensity-modulated radiation therapy (IG-IMRT) for skull base chordoma and chondrosarcoma: preliminary outcomes. Neuro Oncol. 2015;17(6):889–94.

131. Kim JW, Suh CO, Hong CK, et al. Maximum surgical resection and adjuvant intensity-modulated radiotherapy with simultaneous integrated boost for skull base chordoma. Acta Neurochir. 2017;59(10):1825–34.

132. Jahangiri A, Chin AT, Wagner JR, et al. Factors predicting recurrence after resection of clival chordoma using variable surgical approaches and radiation modalities. Neurosurgery. 2015;76(2):179–85. discussion 185–176

133. Di Maio S, Yip S, Al Zhrani GA, et al. Novel targeted therapies in chordoma: an update. Ther Clin Risk Manag. 2015;11:873–83.

134. Bloch O, Parsa AT. Skull base chondrosarcoma: evidence-based treatment paradigms. *Neurosurg Clin N Am*. 2013;24(1):89–96.

135. Samii A, Gerganov V, Herold C, et al. Surgical treatment of skull base chondrosarcomas. Neurosurg Rev. 2009;32(1):67–75. discussion 75

136. Sekhar LN, Pranatartiharan R, Chanda A, et al. Chordomas and chondrosarcomas of the skull base: results and complications of surgical management. Neurosurg Focus. 2001;10(3):E2.

137. Tzortzidis F, Elahi F, Wright DC, et al. Patient outcome at long-term follow-up after aggressive microsurgical resection of cranial base chondrosarcomas. Neurosurgery. 2006;58(6):1090–8. discussion 1090–8

138. Gay E, Sekhar LN, Rubinstein E, et al. Chordomas and chondrosarcomas of the cranial base: results and follow-up of 60 patients. Neurosurgery. 1995;36(5):887–96. discussion 896–7

139. Oghalai JS, Buxbaum JL, Jackler RK, et al. Skull base chondrosarcoma originating from the petroclival junction. Otol Neurotol. 2005;26(5):1052–60.

140. Bloch OG, Jian BJ, Yang I, et al. A systematic review of intracranial chondrosarcoma and survival. J Clin Neurosci. 2009;16(12):1547–51.

141. Bloch OG, Jian BJ, Yang I, et al. Cranial chondrosarcoma and recurrence. Skull Base. 2010;20(3):149–56.

142. Cho YH, Kim JH, Khang SK, et al. Chordomas and chondrosarcomas of the skull base: comparative analysis of clinical results in 30 patients. Neurosurg Rev. 2008;31(1):35–43. discussion 43

143. Schulz-Ertner D, Nikoghosyan A, Hof H, et al. Carbon ion radiotherapy of skull base chondrosarcomas. Int J Radiat Oncol Biol Phys. 2007;67(1):171–7.

144. Nikoghosyan AV, Rauch G, Munter MW, et al. Randomised trial of proton vs. carbon ion radiation therapy in patients with low and intermediate grade chondrosarcoma of the skull base, clinical phase III study. BMC Cancer. 2010;10:606.

145. Martin JJ, Niranjan A, Kondziolka D, et al. Radiosurgery for chordomas and chondrosarcomas of the skull base. J Neurosurg. 2007;107(4):758–64.

146. Iyer A, Kano H, Kondziolka D, et al. Stereotactic radiosurgery for intracranial chondrosarcoma. J Neurooncol. 2012;108(3):535–42.

147. Kano H, Sheehan J, Sneed PK, et al. Skull base chondrosarcoma radiosurgery: report of the North American Gamma Knife Consortium. J Neurosurg. 2015;123(5):1268–75.

148. Green JD Jr, Brackmann DE, Nguyen CD, et al. Surgical management of previously untreated glomus jugulare tumors. Laryngoscope. 1994;104(8 Pt 1):917–21.

149. Patel SJ, Sekhar LN, Cass SP, et al. Combined approaches for resection of extensive glomus jugulare tumors. A review of 12 cases. J Neurosurg. 1994;80(6):1026–38.

150. Anand VK, Leonetti JP, al-Mefty O. Neurovascular considerations in surgery of glomus tumors with intracranial extensions. Laryngoscope. 1993;103(7):722–8.

151. Watkins LD, Mendoza N, Cheesman AD, et al. Glomus jugulare tumours: a review of 61 cases. Acta Neurochir. 1994;130(1–4):66–70.

152. Springate SC, Haraf D, Weichselbaum RR. Temporal bone chemodectomas--comparing surgery and radiation therapy. Oncology (Huntingt). 1991;5(4):131–7. discussion 140, 143

153. van der Mey AG, Frijns JH, Cornelisse CJ, et al. Does intervention improve the natural course of glomus tumors? A series of 108 patients seen in a 32-year period. Ann Otol Rhinol Laryngol. 1992;101(8):635–42.

154. Gstoettner W, Matula C, Hamzavi J, et al. Long-term results of different treatment modalities in 37 patients with glomus jugulare tumors. Eur Arch Otorhinolaryngol. 1999;256(7):351–5.

155. Gjuric M, Rudiger Wolf S, Wigand ME, et al. Cranial nerve and hearing function after combined-approach surgery for glomus jugulare tumors. Ann Otol Rhinol Laryngol. 1996;105(12):949–54.

156. Cole JM, Beiler D. Long-term results of treatment for glomus jugulare and glomus vagale tumors with radiotherapy. Laryngoscope. 1994;104(12):1461–5.

157. Larner JM, Hahn SS, Spaulding CA, et al. Glomus jugulare tumors. Long-term control by radiation therapy. Cancer. 1992;69(7):1813–7.

158. Schild SE, Foote RL, Buskirk SJ, et al. Results of radiotherapy for chemodectomas. Mayo Clin Proc. 1992;67(6):537–40.

159. Skolyszewski J, Korzeniowski S, Pszon J. Results of radiotherapy in chemodectoma of the temporal bone. Acta Oncol. 1991;30(7):847–9.

160. Pemberton LS, Swindell R, Sykes AJ. Radical radiotherapy alone for glomus jugulare and tympanicum tumours. Oncol Rep. 2005;14(6):1631–3.

161. Henzel M, Hamm K, Gross MW, et al. Fractionated stereotactic radiotherapy of glomus jugulare tumors. Local control, toxicity, symptomatology, and quality of life. Strahlenther Onkol. 2007;183(10):557–62.

162. Wegner RE, Rodriguez KD, Heron DE, et al. Linac-based stereotactic body radiation therapy for treatment of glomus jugulare tumors. Radiother Oncol. 2010;97(3):395–8.

163. Schuster D, Sweeney AD, Stavas MJ, et al. Initial radiographic tumor control is similar following single or multi-fractionated stereotactic radiosurgery for jugular paragangliomas. Am J Otolaryngol. 2016;37(3):255–8.

164. Winford TW, Dorton LH, Browne JD, et al. Stereotactic radiosurgical treatment of glomus jugulare tumors. Otol Neurotol. 2017;38(4):555–62.

165. Ibrahim R, Ammori MB, Yianni J, et al. Gamma Knife radiosurgery for glomus jugulare tumors: a single-center series of 75 cases. J Neurosurg. 2016;126(5):1488–97.

166. Hafez RF, Morgan MS, Fahmy OM. An intermediate term benefits and complications of gamma knife surgery in management of glomus jugulare tumor. World J Surg Oncol. 2016;14(1):36.

167. Dobberpuhl MR, Maxwell S, Feddock J, et al. Treatment outcomes for single modality management of glomus jugulare tumors with stereotactic radiosurgery. Otol Neurotol. 2016;37(9):1406–10.

168. Jacob JT, Pollock BE, Carlson ML, et al. Stereotactic radiosurgery in the management of vestibular schwannoma and glomus jugulare: indications, techniques, and results. Otolaryngol Clin N Am. 2015;48(3):515–26.

169. El Majdoub F, Hunsche S, Igressa A, et al. Stereotactic LINAC-radiosurgery for glomus jugulare tumors: a long-term follow-up of 27 patients. PLoS One. 2015;10(6):e0129057.

170. Ko HC, Gupta V, Mourad WF, et al. A contouring guide for head and neck cancers with perineural invasion. Pract Radiat Oncol. 2014;4(6):e247–58.

171. Fowler JF. 21 years of biologically effective dose. Br J Radiol. 2010;83(991):554–68.

172. Mayo C, Yorke E, Merchant TE. Radiation associated brainstem injury. Int J Radiat Oncol Biol Phys. 2010;76(3 Suppl):S36–41.

173. Lawrence YR, Li XA, el Naqa I, et al. Radiation dose-volume effects in the brain. Int J Radiat Oncol Biol Phys. 2010;76(3 Suppl):S20–7.

174. Mayo C, Martel MK, Marks LB, et al. Radiation dose-volume effects of optic nerves and chiasm. Int J Radiat Oncol Biol Phys. 2010;76(3 Suppl):S28–35.

175. Jackson A, Marks LB, Bentzen SM, et al. The lessons of QUANTEC: recommendations for reporting and gathering data on dose-volume dependencies of treatment outcome. Int J Radiat Oncol Biol Phys. 2010;76(3 Suppl):S155–60.

176. Marks LB, Yorke ED, Jackson A, et al. Use of normal tissue complication probability models in the clinic. Int J Radiat Oncol Biol Phys. 2010;76(3 Suppl):S10–9.

# Part X

# Primary Central Nervous System Lymphoma

# Primary Central Nervous System Lymphoma

**19**

Sarah A. Milgrom and Joachim Yahalom

## Learning Objectives

- Understand the appropriate evaluation of a patient with suspected primary CNS lymphoma (PCNSL).
- Know the factors associated with prognosis in PCNSL.
- Recognize the evolving role of whole-brain radiation therapy (WBRT) in the management of PCNSL.
- Appreciate the potential toxicity of WBRT in the management of PCNSL.
- Be aware of strategies to mitigate the toxicity of WBRT.
- Gain comfort with WBRT field design for PCNSL.

## Epidemiology

Primary central nervous system lymphoma (PCNSL) is an extranodal non-Hodgkin lymphoma that involves the brain, or, less commonly, the eyes, leptomeninges, or spinal cord, in the absence of systemic disease. It is estimated to represent 1% of lymphomas, 4–6% of extranodal lymphomas, and 3% of CNS tumors [1]. Its incidence in the United States is 0.47 cases per 100,000 person-years [2]. Its incidence increased in developed countries during the 1980s–1990s, in association with the acquired immune deficiency syndrome (AIDS) epidemic. Since then, the incidence has decreased in the human immunodeficiency virus (HIV)-positive population, likely due to advancements in anti-retroviral therapy. Conversely, the incidence continues to rise in elderly, immu-

nocompetent patients. Currently, this population represents the majority of affected individuals [2].

## Risk Factors

The primary risk factor for PCNSL is immunodeficiency. PCNSL is an AIDS-defining illness. As described above, its incidence in patients with AIDS increased during the 1980s–1990s, but it has decreased since that time due to advancements in controlling HIV [2]. Individuals with inherited immunodeficiency disorders, such as Wiskott-Aldrich syndrome, severe combined immunodeficiency, and X-linked immunodeficiency, are also at increased risk [3]. Likewise, immunosuppression is associated with greater rates of PCNSL; for example, it affects 1–5% of patients who have undergone solid organ transplantation [4]. Among immunocompetent patients, PCNSL is most common in the elderly population, with a peak incidence in the fifth to seventh decades of life [5].

## Diagnosis and Prognosis

Patients typically present with focal neurologic deficits, neurocognitive dysfunction, and/or signs of increased intracranial pressure [6]. Neuroimaging must be performed if the diagnosis of PCNSL is suspected. The study of choice is a brain MRI with T1-weighted gadolinium-enhanced and fluid-attenuated inversion recovery (FLAIR) sequences. MRI typically reveals one or multiple contrast-enhancing lesions, classically in the periventricular space.

The diagnosis of PCNSL requires histopathological confirmation, typically via a needle biopsy of the primary lesion. The work-up should include a lumbar puncture (if not contraindicated) and an ophthalmologic assessment with fundoscopy and slit lamp examination. Identification of lymphoma cells in the cerebrospinal or vitreous fluid may

S. A. Milgrom
Department of Radiation Oncology, MD Anderson Cancer Center, Houston, TX, USA

J. Yahalom (✉)
Department of Radiation Oncology, Memorial Sloan Kettering Cancer Center, New York, NY, USA
e-mail: yahalomj@mskcc.org

© Springer International Publishing AG, part of Springer Nature 2018
E. L. Chang et al. (eds.), *Adult CNS Radiation Oncology*, https://doi.org/10.1007/978-3-319-42878-9_19

obviate the need for a biopsy of the primary mass. Ideally, administration of steroids should be avoided until after tissue has been obtained, because it might prevent a histopathological diagnosis.

The vast majority (>95%) of lymphoma cases involving the CNS are diffuse large B-cell lymphoma (DLBCL). However, other lymphomas can affect the CNS, including T-cell lymphoma, Burkitt's lymphoma, and marginal zone lymphoma. According to the WHO classification system, the term PCNSL refers specifically to DLBCL involving the CNS [7]. Therefore, other histologies must be excluded to make the diagnosis of PCNSL. Immunohistochemical studies that are useful to diagnose DLBCL include B-cell markers, such as CD19, CD20, and CD79a. Additionally, MUM1 and BCL6 expressions are common [8].

Multiple factors have been associated with outcome in PCNSL patients. Age of greater than 60 years and poor performance status are associated with worse survival [9–12]. Other prognostic factors include elevated serum lactate dehydrogenase (LDH) level, elevated CSF protein concentration, and involvement of deep regions of the brain [13].

## Treatment Strategy

### Surgery

Given the infiltrative nature of PCNSL, it has long been accepted that surgical resection plays little role in its management. However, this belief was challenged recently by a secondary analysis of the German PCNSL Study Group-1 trial, a phase III study comprising 526 patients with PCNSL. The authors found that complete surgical resection was associated with improved progression-free survival (PFS) [14]. This finding requires validation. However, based on this report, surgical resection may be considered for well-circumscribed lesions in non-eloquent areas.

### Radiation Therapy Alone

Radiation therapy (RT) was the first treatment strategy used for PCNSL. PCNSL is often multifocal and diffusely infiltrative, so whole-brain RT (WBRT) was used, rather than focal therapy, to ensure that all disease was encompassed within the irradiated area. The Radiation Therapy Oncology Group (RTOG) 83-15 was an early, prospective, multicenter trial, in which 41 patients with newly diagnosed PCNSL were treated with WBRT to a total dose of 40 Gy, followed by a 20 Gy boost to the tumor. A subset of patients (n = 26) had posttreatment computed tomography (CT) scans performed 4 months after starting WBRT. Of these, 16 patients (62%) experienced a complete response (CR), and

an additional 5 patients (19%) had experienced "almost a CR." However, this initial response was not sustained. At 3.3 years after study completion, 27 of 41 patients (66%) experienced disease relapse, and all of these patients died of lymphoma. Most recurrences occurred in the brain (n = 25; 61%), typically within the boost field (n = 22). The median overall survival (OS) was 11.6 months. Patients who were ≥60 years of age experienced particularly poor outcomes, with a median OS of only 7.6 months [10].

A similar study, the North Central Cancer Treatment Group (NCCTG) 96-73-51, investigated the use of WBRT and high-dose steroids in patients with newly diagnosed PCNSL who were ≥70 years of age. The trial accrued 19 patients with a median age of 76 years. Patients were treated with WBRT to 41.4 Gy and a boost of 9 Gy to address gross disease, followed by high-dose steroids. Neuroimaging, typically with MRI, revealed a 42% response rate (16% CR). Based on an interim analysis, 6-month OS was 33%. Due to these poor outcomes, the trial was terminated early [15]. Thus, both RTOG 83-15 and NCCTG 96-73-51 showed that OS rates were poor after RT alone, particularly in elderly patients.

## Combined Chemotherapy and Radiation Therapy

Chemotherapy was added to WBRT in an attempt to improve upon these outcomes. Initially, the RTOG and United Kingdom Medical Research Council added cyclophosphamide, doxorubicin, vincristine, and prednisone (CHOP) or CHOP-like chemotherapy to WBRT, extrapolating from the efficacy of these agents for treating non-Hodgkin lymphomas outside of the CNS. However, the addition of CHOP-like chemotherapy did not improve survival outcomes in PCNSL when compared to those observed with WBRT alone [12, 16]. The lack of improvement was attributed to poor CNS penetration by these chemotherapeutic agents.

Conversely, the incorporation of high-dose methotrexate (HD-MTX) into management yielded a significant improvement in outcomes. In an early single-institution study, 52 patients were treated for PCNSL with HD-MTX, intrathecal (IT) MTX, procarbazine, and vincristine. Subsequently, they received WBRT to 45 Gy, followed by high-dose cytarabine. The median OS was 60 months, significantly longer than had been observed previously. Patients less than 60 years of age experienced particularly favorable outcomes: at a median follow-up time of 50 months, they had not yet reached their median overall or progression-free survival [17].

Given these impressive outcomes, this regimen was assessed further in a multi-institutional setting. In RTOG

93-10, 102 patients were treated with HD-MTX, IT-MTX, procarbazine, and vincristine, followed by WBRT. Initially the WBRT dose was 45 Gy in 25 fractions; however, in an amendment, the dose was changed to 36 Gy in 30 twice-daily fractions for patients whose disease had responded completely to induction chemotherapy. In this study, the median OS was 36.9 months and median PFS was 24 months [9]. These results confirmed the survival benefit observed when MTX-based chemotherapy was added to WBRT.

Although the combination of WBRT and MTX resulted in improved oncologic outcomes, delayed neurotoxicity emerged as a potentially devastating complication of this strategy, particularly in patients over 60 years old, as described below. Therefore, researchers have attempted to reduce the intensity of upfront therapy, with the aim of minimizing toxicity while maintaining disease control.

## Omission of WBRT

One approach that has been studied is the omission of WBRT altogether from the upfront setting. The German PCNSL Study Group reported a phase III, non-inferiority study, in which patients who achieved a CR to HD-MTX-based chemotherapy were randomized to (1) immediate consolidative WBRT (45 Gy) or (2) observation, with WBRT given only as salvage therapy if disease relapsed. Patients who did not achieve a CR to chemotherapy were treated with WBRT or high-dose cytarabine. This trial had multiple methodological limitations, including a large number of patients who dropped out or were lost to follow-up and a high proportion of serious protocol violations. In the group of patients treated per protocol, patients who received WBRT experienced improved PFS of 18.3 vs. 11.9 months ($P = 0.1$) but no improvement in OS (32.4 vs. 37.1 months, HR 1.06, 95% CI 0.80–1.40, $P = 0.7$) [18]. Importantly, the authors did not meet their prespecified non-inferiority endpoint, despite the large number of patients enrolled, because the 95% CI for OS included 0.9. Therefore, the possibility remains that omission of WBRT from the frontline setting results in a detrimental effect on survival. Nonetheless, some clinicians have proposed that WBRT should be eliminated from upfront management, based on the results of this trial.

## Altered WBRT Dose and Fractionation

Another approach that has been studied is selective WBRT dose reduction in patients whose disease responds completely to induction chemotherapy. For example, a prospective, single-institution study of chemoimmunotherapy and selectively dose-reduced WBRT yielded excellent outcomes. In this study, 52 patients with PCNSL received rituximab,

HD-MTX, procarbazine, and vincristine (R-MPV) for 5–7 cycles. Patients whose disease responded completely were treated with reduced dose WBRT (rdWBRT) to 23.4 Gy; all others received standard WBRT to 45 Gy. After WBRT, all patients received high-dose cytarabine. Two-thirds of the cohort received rdWBRT. In this subgroup, the median PFS was 7.7 years (not reached in patients <60 years old; 4.4 years in patients >60 years old), and the median OS was not reached. Twelve patients treated with rdWBRT underwent detailed neurocognitive testing during follow-up; three of these patients were ≥60 years old. There was no evidence of significant cognitive decline, with the exception of motor speed ($P < 0.05$). The authors conclude that selectively dose-reduced WBRT resulted in excellent PFS and OS, with minimal neurocognitive morbidity [19].

In addition to dose reduction, hyperfractionation has been studied. In RTOG 93-10, patients were initially treated with WBRT to a dose of 45 Gy; however, the protocol was subsequently amended so patients received 36 Gy in 30 fractions over 3 weeks. A secondary analysis assessed the cognitive function of patients who achieved a CR to chemotherapy and were treated with conventionally vs. hyperfractionated WBRT. At 8 months after treatment, MMSE scores improved in all patients. At 2 years, the decline in MMSE scores was less in patients who had received hyperfractionated vs. conventionally fractionated WBRT; however, the rates were equivalent at 4 years, suggesting that hyperfractionation delays but does not eliminate neurocognitive effects [20]. In RTOG 02-27, patients received rituximab, MTX, and temozolomide, followed by hyperfractionated WBRT (hWBRT) to 36 Gy at 1.2 Gy/fraction, given twice daily. At a median follow-up of 3.6 years, 2-year OS and PFS were 80.8% and 63.6%, respectively. All patients were evaluated by Mini-Mental Status Examination (MMSE) before treatment, at completion of hWBRT, and during follow-up. Overall, cognitive function improved or stabilized after hWBRT. A significant decline in MMSE score, defined as a reduction of >3 points, was observed in only 1 of 38 assessable patients (2.6%) at 6 months after hWBRT [21]. While these results are encouraging, longer follow-up is needed.

## Autologous Stem Cell Transplantation

Alternative consolidative approaches have been investigated as possible substitutes for WBRT. One such strategy is myeloablative high-dose chemotherapy and autologous stem cell transplantation (HDC-ASCT). For example, in one single-center phase II study, 32 patients with newly diagnosed PCNSL, who were <67 years of age, were treated with R-MPV induction followed by HDC-ASCT with thiotepa, cyclophosphamide, and busulfan. Three patients (9%)

required WBRT, due to a suboptimal response to chemotherapy. The 2-year PFS and OS rates were 79% and 81%, respectively [22]. No neurotoxicity was reported, but the follow-up time was short. These results are positive; however, it must be noted that three ASCT-related deaths occurred. Furthermore, favorable patients may have been selected for this study, because they had to be candidates for HDC-ASCT. Therefore, comparisons of these results with those of trials assessing WBRT are difficult, and randomized studies are needed.

## Intensive Polychemotherapy Alone

Another management strategy in newly diagnosed PCNSL is intensive polychemotherapy, without consolidative ASCT or WBRT. For example, the Cancer and Leukemia Group B (CALGB) reported on 44 patients treated with HD-MTX, temozolomide, and rituximab (MT-R) for four cycles, followed by consolidation with etoposide and high-dose cytarabine (EA) for patients with a CR. At a median follow-up time of 4.9 years, the 2-year PFS rate was 57%, and the median OS was not reached [23].

## Ongoing Studies

Several ongoing randomized trials will elucidate the role of WBRT in the upfront management of PCNSL. In RTOG 11-14, patients are randomized to receive R-MPV and cytarabine, with or without rdWBRT to 23.4 Gy. This trial will address whether WBRT may be avoided in the upfront setting without a detrimental effect on survival in patients receiving chemoimmunotherapy. In the International Extranodal Lymphoma Study Group-32 (IELSG-32) trial, patients <70 years of age are being randomized to one of two induction treatments and then to one of two consolidation strategies. The first randomization is to receive (1) methotrexate + cytarabine, (2) methotrexate + cytarabine + rituximab, or (3) methotrexate + cytarabine + rituximab + thiotepa. Subsequently, patients with responsive or stable disease are randomized to WBRT vs. HDC-ASCT. The results of the first randomization revealed a higher CR rate in patients receiving all four agents [24]. The final results, after the second randomization, are not yet available. A similar trial is being conducted by the Association des Neuro-Oncologues d'Expression Française/Groupe Ouest-Est d'Étude des Leucémies et Autres Maladies du Sang (ANOCEF/GOELAMS) group. Patients will be treated with rituximab, methotrexate, BCNU, etoposide, and methylprednisolone (R-MBVP) induction and then randomized to WBRT vs. HDC-ASCT. These two studies will provide a direct comparison of WBRT vs. HDC-ASCT as consolidation strategies.

## Salvage Therapy

Another potential indication for WBRT in the management of PCNSL is the treatment of relapsed or refractory disease. Two retrospective studies have been published on this topic. In one, 48 patients received salvage WBRT for PCNSL that was refractory to (50%) or relapsed after (50%) HD-MTX-based chemotherapy. The median dose was 40 Gy. After WBRT, 28 patients (58%) achieved a CR and 10 (21%) a partial response (PR). The median OS time from initiation of WBRT was 16 months, and the median PFS time was 10 months. Neurotoxicity was observed in 22% of patients [25]. In the second report, 27 patients received salvage WBRT after HD-MTX-based chemotherapy. The median dose was 36 Gy. Ten patients (37%) achieved a CR and 10 (37%) a PR. Performance status improved in 12 patients (44%) and stabilized in 6 (22%). The median OS from initiation of WBRT was 10.9 months, and median PFS was 9.7 months. Neurotoxicity was observed in 15% of patients [26].

## Indications for Irradiation

Several indications exist for WBRT in the management of PCNSL. As described above, WBRT may be used as consolidation after a CR to methotrexate-based chemotherapy. Ongoing studies will clarify the role of WBRT in this setting. Additionally, WBRT may be offered as salvage therapy in the setting of refractory or relapsed disease, definitive therapy in patients who are not eligible for chemotherapy, or palliative therapy for patients with symptomatic disease.

## Target Volume Delineation

For WBRT, equally weighted left and right opposed lateral beams should be used. The fields should be shaped with custom blocks or a multi-leaf collimator. Care should be taken in designing the fields at the skull base to avoid inadvertent shielding of the meninges in the region of the anterior temporal lobes and cribriform plate. The optic nerves and retinae are a part of the CNS and are at risk of disease involvement; therefore, the posterior aspect of the orbits must be included in the WBRT fields, even if there is no evidence of ocular disease at diagnosis (Fig. 19.1a). If ocular involvement is evident on initial slit lamp examination, the entirety of both globes should be included in the treatment volume. The inferior border can be placed at the C1–C2 or C2–C3 interspace. For patients with radiographic evidence of disease in the spine, a focal spinal field encompassing the site of involvement may be considered.

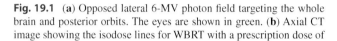
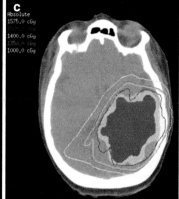

**Fig. 19.1** (**a**) Opposed lateral 6-MV photon field targeting the whole brain and posterior orbits. The eyes are shown in green. (**b**) Axial CT image showing the isodose lines for WBRT with a prescription dose of 30 Gy. (**c**) Axial CT images showing the isodose lines for the IMRT boost to the left temporal disease with a prescription dose of 15 Gy (for a total dose of 45 Gy to gross disease)

## Radiation Dose Prescription and Organ-at-Risk Tolerances

When WBRT is used for consolidation in the primary setting, after an MRI reveals a CR to methotrexate-based chemoimmunotherapy, a dose of 23.4 Gy should be used. A higher dose is needed when RT is used to treat gross disease. For less than a CR to chemotherapy, for salvage of relapsed disease, or for patients who are not candidates for chemotherapy, consideration should be given to a dose of 23.4–36 Gy for the whole brain, with a boost to the gross disease for a total dose of 45 Gy.

Typically, the tolerances of organs at risk are not exceeded with the prescription doses used for PCNSL. We recommend a dmax for the retinae and optic structures of 45 Gy and for the brainstem of 54 Gy. We recommend that the mean parotid does not exceed 26 Gy.

## Complication Avoidance

Late neurotoxicity is the most concerning complication of WBRT in the management of PCNSL. Multiple attempts have been made to reduce its incidence while maintaining disease control. One example is hyperfractionation of WBRT. As described above, in RTOG 93-10, patients were initially treated with a dose of 45 Gy, using conventional fractionation; then, the protocol was amended, so patients received 36 Gy in 30 fractions over 3 weeks. An assessment of cognitive functioning suggested that hyperfractionation delayed, but did not eliminate, the neurocognitive effects of combined modality therapy [20].

Another approach to reduce the risk of radiation-induced neurotoxicity is selective dose de-escalation in patients with chemoresponsive disease. As described above, in patients who achieve a CR to R-MPV, rdWBRT (23.4 Gy) may be used. With this regimen, researchers have observed minimal neurocognitive morbidity [19].

Pharmacologic prevention of RT-induced neurotoxicity is an area of interest. In patients receiving WBRT for brain metastases, memantine reduces the rate of decline in memory, executive function, and processing speed [27]. While the role of memantine has not been studied in PCNSL patients specifically, these findings may be extrapolated to this population, until data in PCNSL are reported.

## Radiation Toxicity

Acute, temporary treatment-related effects may include alopecia, erythema and/or dry desquamation of the scalp, and fatigue. Patients requiring treatment of the eye may experience conjunctivitis, keratitis, and xerophthalmia.

Regarding late effects, all patients, particularly those requiring treatment of the eye, are at an increased risk of cataracts. Patients requiring treatment of the eye may experience chronic dry eye. Those treated with WBRT doses >35–40 Gy may experience some degree of permanent alopecia. Sensorineural hearing loss may occur when the middle ear receives doses >45–50 Gy.

As described above, late neurocognitive decline may occur. Studies of PCNSL survivors suggest that high-dose WBRT (median 45 Gy) negatively impacts cognitive function and quality of life [28, 29]. Symptoms can range from mild effects on short-term memory to severe sequelae, such as gait disturbances, incontinence, and dementia. In patients treated on RTOG 93-10 with methotrexate-based combination chemotherapy and WBRT to 45 Gy, severe, delayed neurotoxicity was observed in 12 patients (15%), 8 of whom died. Symptoms began a median time of 504 days (range, 80–1540 days) after the start of WBRT. Patients >60 years of age were the most susceptible to this complication [9]. In another study of methotrexate-based combination chemotherapy and WBRT (45 Gy with a 10 Gy boost), five of eight surviving patients ≥60 years of age developed dementia, with associated brain atrophy and leukoencephalopathy on imaging studies, observed as early as 16 months after treatment [30].

However, prospective data suggest that the risk of neurotoxicity is significantly lower with rdWBRT. Neurocognitive testing was conducted in patients who remained progression-free after achieving a CR to R-MPV receiving rdWBRT (23.4 Gy). Twelve patients were evaluated (median age 58 years; three patients ≥60 years of age), and testing was conducted for up to 48 months after therapy. In this population, there was no evidence of cognitive decline, except for motor speed. While these results are encouraging, evaluations of larger numbers of patients with longer-term follow-up will be needed to fully characterize the incidence of neurotoxicity associated with this regimen [19].

## Outcomes

Oncologic outcomes are summarized in Table 19.1. In patients treated with WBRT alone, OS is only 48% at 1 year [10]. The addition of MTX-based chemotherapy improves OS rates to 64–80% at 2 years, in various studies [9, 17, 19]. One commonly used regimen is R-MPV, followed by rdWBRT for patients with a CR, and then high-dose cytarabine. Among

patients treated with this approach who receive rdWBRT, the reported median PFS was 7.7 years, and OS was not reached at a median follow-up time of 5.9 years. The median PFS was not reached in patients <60 years of age and was 4.4 years in patients ≥60 years. The median OS was not reached in either patients <60 years or those aged ≥60 years [19].

## Follow-Up

After the completion of therapy, patients should be followed with a brain MRI every 3 months for 2 years, then every 6 months for 3 years, and then annually for at least 5 years. Concurrent ophthalmologic evaluations are recommended. For patients with previous spinal disease, spine imaging and CSF sampling should be considered. Formal neurocognitive testing is recommended, particularly for patients treated on clinical trials.

## Case Presentation

A 62-year-old woman presented with a several week history of worsening memory deficits. A brain MRI revealed a 4 × 2 cm, enhancing lesion in the left temporal lobe (Fig. 19.2a). There was surrounding FLAIR signal abnormality, consistent with vasogenic edema (Fig. 19.2b).

**Table 19.1** Key studies assessing the use of WBRT in the management of PCNSL

| Study | n | Median age (years) | Chemotherapy | WBRT/ boost dose (Gy) | PFS | OS | Neurotoxicity |
|---|---|---|---|---|---|---|---|
| RTOG 83-15 [10] | 41 | 66 | None | 40/20 | NS | Median 12 months | NS |
| Abrey et al. [17] | 52 | 65 | MTX (IV and IT), Vin, Pro, Cyt | 45 | NS | Median 60 months | 13 |
| RTOG 93-10 [9] | 102 | 56.5 | MTX (IV and IT), Vin, Pro, Cyt | 45 or 36[a] | Median 24 months | Median 37 months | 12 cases of "severe delayed neurotoxicity," 8 deaths |
| Morris et al. [19] | 30 | 57 | RTX, HD-MTX, Pro, Vin, Cyt | 23.4 or 45[b] | Median 3.3 years | Median 6.6 years | Minimal after 23.4 Gy |
| RTOG 02-27 [21] | 53 | 57.5 | HD-MTX, TMZ, RTX | 36 | 63.6% at 2 y | 80.8% at 2 y | NS |
| G-PCNSL-SG-1 [18] | 551 (318 per protocol) | 63 | HD-MTX ± Ifos[c] | 45 vs. none[d] | Median 18.3 months (RT arm) vs. 11.9 months (no RT arm) | Median 32.4 months (RT arm) vs. 37.1 months (no RT arm) | Subset: 22/45 in RT arm (49%) vs. 9/34 (26%) in no RT arm |

*CR* complete response, *Cyt* cytarabine, *HD-MTX* high-dose methotrexate, *Ifos* ifosfamide, *IT* intrathecal, *IV* intravenous, *MTX* methotrexate, *NS* not stated, *OS* overall survival, *PFS* progression-free survival, *Pro* procarbazine, *RTX* rituximab, *Vin* vincristine, *WBRT* whole-brain radiation therapy, *y* years, *yo* years old

[a]Initially all patients received WBRT to 45 Gy with conventional fractionation, and then the trial was amended to change the dose to 36 Gy with hyperfractionation

[b]23.4 Gy for patients who responded completely to induction chemotherapy; 45 Gy for all others

[c]Initially all patients received HD-MTX alone, and then trial was amended and all patients received HD-MTX + ifosfamide

[d]Patients with a complete response to chemotherapy were randomized to 45 Gy WBRT vs. observation. Patients with persistent or relapsed disease received 45 Gy WBRT

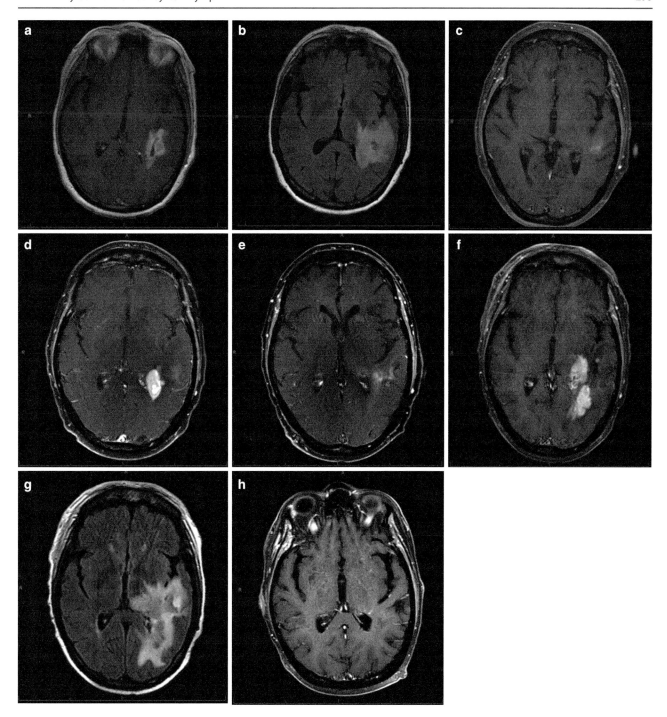

**Fig. 19.2** Brain imaging in a patient with PCNSL. (**a**) Axial T1 post-contrast image demonstrates an enhancing left temporal mass. (**b**) Axial T2 FLAIR image reveals surrounding vasogenic edema. (**c**) Axial T1 post-contrast image demonstrates a significant disease response after cycle #1 of R-MPV. (**d**) Axial T1 post-contrast image shows disease progression after cycle #2 of R-MPV. (**e**) Axial T1 post-contrast image shows a reduction in size of the mass, with a small area of residual enhancement, after three cycles of salvage etoposide, cytarabine, and rituximab. (**f**) Axial T1 post-contrast image shows interval disease progression. (**g**) Corresponding FLAIR image reveals surrounding edema. (**h**) Axial T1 post-contrast image performed 1 month after completion of radiation therapy shows no evidence of disease

A stereotactic biopsy of the mass revealed CD20-positive DLBCL with an activated B-cell (ABC) phenotype. The Ki-67 was 90%. Fluorescent in situ hybridization studies were negative for gene rearrangements in BCL2 and MYC. PET-CT imaging and a bone marrow biopsy revealed no extracranial disease. An ophthalmologic evaluation showed no evidence of intraocular lymphoma. CSF was negative for lymphomatous involvement.

The patient was initiated on R-MPV chemoimmunotherapy. After completion of the first cycle, she experienced a partial seizure. A brain MRI was repeated at that time, which revealed a significant reduction in the size of the biopsy-proven lymphoma (Fig. 19.2c). Antiepileptic therapy was initiated, and chemotherapy was continued. After the second cycle of R-MPV, she presented with acutely altered mental status. At this time, a brain MRI demonstrated interval growth of the mass to 4 × 3 cm, consistent with progressive disease (Fig. 19.2d).

She received three cycles of salvage etoposide, cytarabine, and rituximab. Subsequently, an MRI revealed a reduction in size of the left temporal mass; however, residual enhancement was appreciated (Fig. 19.2e).

Two weeks later, she presented with headaches and altered mental status. An MRI revealed marked progression of the left temporal mass, with surrounding FLAIR signal abnormality (Fig. 19.2f, g).

The patient was treated with salvage RT. The refractory disease had remained localized to the left temporal region throughout her disease course, so the decision was made to treat the whole brain to a lower dose (30 Gy) and to boost the site of refractory disease to a higher dose (45 Gy). First, she was treated with WBRT to a total dose of 30 Gy at 2 Gy per fraction, using opposed lateral fields and 6-MV photons. The posterior orbits were included within the field (Fig. 19.1a). A step-and-shoot technique was used to reduce hotspots to less than 107% (Fig. 19.1b). After completion of WBRT, she was treated with a 15 Gy boost to the site of refractory disease with six fractions of intensity-modulated RT (IMRT) for a cumulative dose of 45 Gy to the left temporal region (Fig. 19.1c). Her symptoms improved during treatment. An MRI performed 1 month after completion of RT revealed resolution of the enhancement within the left temporal lobe (Fig. 19.2h).

## Summary

- PCNSL is an aggressive form of extranodal non-Hodgkin lymphoma.
- PCNSL tends to affect elderly or immunocompromised individuals.
- The prognosis of PCNSL has improved over the past decades.
- High-dose methotrexate-based chemotherapy and WBRT to 45 Gy are associated with improved survival outcomes compared to WBRT alone; however, this approach is limited by the risk of late neurotoxicity, especially in patients over 60 years of age.
- Early data suggest that selective use of rdWBRT (23.4 Gy), in combination with chemoimmunotherapy, allows maintenance of improved survival outcomes with minimal neurotoxicity.
- Other promising consolidative strategies include ASCT and intensive polychemotherapy, which are being studied as alternatives to WBRT.

- Ongoing clinical trials will help to define the optimal consolidative approach.

## Self-Assessment Questions

1. A 58-year-old man was found to have a single 2 cm enhancing lesion in the right frontal lobe with surrounding FLAIR signal abnormality. A biopsy of the mass revealed diffuse large B-cell lymphoma. There was no evidence of intraocular or CSF involvement. He was treated with five cycles of R-MPV and achieved a complete response by MRI. You would like to use RT to consolidate this response. Which of the following describes the appropriate RT target:
   A. The site of the enhancing lesion at diagnosis with a 1.5–2 cm margin
   B. The site of the enhancing lesion and surrounding FLAIR abnormality at diagnosis with a 1.5–2 cm margin
   C. The whole brain only
   D. The whole brain, including the posterior orbits
   E. The whole brain, including the entire orbits

2. Which agent should be a part of the chemotherapy regimen used for PCNSL?
   A. Doxorubicin
   B. Methotrexate
   C. Cyclophosphamide
   D. Bleomycin
   E. Dacarbazine

3. Which of the following factors is associated with advanced age in PCNSL?
   A. A more indolent disease course
   B. Increased risk of neurotoxicity from methotrexate and whole-brain radiation therapy
   C. Equivalent disease-related mortality to younger patients
   D. Better tolerance of methotrexate than younger patients

4. Which of the following scenarios have data to support the use of whole-brain radiation therapy to a total dose of 23.4 Gy?
   A. In a patient with newly diagnosed PCNSL, who is not a candidate for chemotherapy
   B. In a patient with PCNSL that relapsed 2 months after completion of methotrexate-based chemotherapy
   C. In a patient with PNCSL who has achieved a complete response by MRI to five cycles of R-MPV chemotherapy

D. In a patient with PCNSL who has stable disease by MRI after five cycles of R-MPV chemotherapy

E. In a patient who achieved a complete response to R-MPV chemotherapy and then underwent autologous stem cell transplantation with CNS-directed high-dose chemotherapy

5. A patient presents to the emergency room with neurologic deficits. A brain MRI reveals a large enhancing mass with surrounding vasogenic edema. A diagnosis of PCNSL is suspected. Which of the following is the best sequence of events?

A. Initiate steroid therapy to reduce edema → perform a neurosurgical biopsy → perform a lumbar puncture (if safe) → perform an ophthalmologic evaluation.

B. Initiate methotrexate-based chemotherapy immediately.

C. Perform an ophthalmologic evaluation → perform a lumbar puncture (if safe) → perform a neurosurgical biopsy → initiate steroid therapy.

D. Initiate steroid therapy to reduce edema → repeat an MRI → perform a neurosurgical biopsy → perform an ophthalmologic evaluation → perform a lumbar puncture (if safe).

## Answers

1. D
2. B
3. B
4. C
5. C

## References

1. Hoang-Xuan K, Bessell E, Bromberg J, et al. Diagnosis and treatment of primary CNS lymphoma in immunocompetent patients: guidelines from the European Association for Neuro-Oncology. Lancet Oncol. 2015;16(7):e322–32. https://doi.org/10.1016/S1470-2045(15)00076-5.
2. Villano JL, Koshy M, Shaikh H, et al. Age, gender, and racial differences in incidence and survival in primary CNS lymphoma. Br J Cancer. 2011;105(9):1414–8. https://doi.org/10.1038/bjc.2011.357.
3. Hochberg FH, Miller DC. Primary central nervous system lymphoma. J Neurosurg. 1988;68(6):835–53. https://doi.org/10.3171/jns.1988.68.6.0835.
4. Schabet M. Epidemiology of primary CNS lymphoma. J Neurooncol. 1999;43(3):199–201.
5. Schlegel U. Primary CNS lymphoma. Ther Adv Neurol Disord. 2009;2(2):93–104. https://doi.org/10.1177/1756285608101222.
6. Bataille B, Delwail V, Menet E, et al. Primary intracerebral malignant lymphoma: report of 248 cases. J Neurosurg. 2000;92(2):261–6. https://doi.org/10.3171/jns.2000.92.2.0261.
7. Kluin PM, Deckert M, Ferry JA. Primary diffuse large B-cell lymphoma of the CNS. In: Swerdlow SH, Campo E, Harris NL, Jaffe

ES, Pileri SA, Stein H, Thiele J, Vardiman JW, editors. WHO classification of tumours of haematopietic and lymphoid tissues, vol. 2. 4th ed. Lyon: IARC Press; 2008. p. 240–1.
8. Giannini C, Dogan A, Salomao DR. CNS lymphoma: a practical diagnostic approach. J Neuropathol Exp Neurol. 2014;73(6):478–94. https://doi.org/10.1097/NEN.0000000000000076.
9. DeAngelis LM, Seiferheld W, Schold SC, et al. Combination chemotherapy and radiotherapy for primary central nervous system lymphoma: Radiation Therapy Oncology Group Study 93-10. J Clin Oncol. 2002;20(24):4643–8. https://doi.org/10.1200/JCO.2002.11.013.
10. Nelson DF, Martz KL, Bonner H, et al. Non-Hodgkin's lymphoma of the brain: can high dose, large volume radiation therapy improve survival? Report on a prospective trial by the Radiation Therapy Oncology Group (RTOG): RTOG 8315. Int J Radiat Oncol Biol Phys. 1992;23(1):9–17.
11. O'Neill BP, O'Fallon JR, Earle JD, et al. Primary central nervous system non-Hodgkin's lymphoma: survival advantages with combined initial therapy? Int J Radiat Oncol Biol Phys. 1995;33(3):663–73. https://doi.org/10.1016/0360-3016(95)00207-F.
12. Schultz C, Scott C, Sherman W, et al. Preirradiation chemotherapy with cyclophosphamide, doxorubicin, vincristine, and dexamethasone for primary CNS lymphomas: initial report of radiation therapy oncology group protocol 88-06. J Clin Oncol. 1996;14(2):556–64. https://doi.org/10.1200/jco.1996.14.2.556.
13. Ferreri AJ, Blay JY, Reni M, et al. Prognostic scoring system for primary CNS lymphomas: the International Extranodal Lymphoma Study Group experience. J Clin Oncol. 2003;21(2):266–72. https://doi.org/10.1200/JCO.2003.09.139.
14. Weller M, Martus P, Roth P, et al. Surgery for primary CNS lymphoma? Challenging a paradigm. Neuro Oncol. 2012;14(12):1481–4. https://doi.org/10.1093/neuonc/nos159.
15. Laack NN, Ballman KV, Brown PB, et al. Whole-brain radiotherapy and high-dose methylprednisolone for elderly patients with primary central nervous system lymphoma: Results of North Central Cancer Treatment Group (NCCTG) 96-73-51. Int J Radiat Oncol Biol Phys. 2006;65(5):1429–39. https://doi.org/10.1016/j.ijrobp.2006.03.061.
16. Mead GM, Bleehen NM, Gregor A, et al. A medical research council randomized trial in patients with primary cerebral non-Hodgkin lymphoma: cerebral radiotherapy with and without cyclophosphamide, doxorubicin, vincristine, and prednisone chemotherapy. Cancer. 2000;89(6):1359–70.
17. Abrey LE, Yahalom J, DeAngelis LM. Treatment for primary CNS lymphoma: the next step. J Clin Oncol. 2000;18(17):3144–50. https://doi.org/10.1200/jco.2000.18.17.3144.
18. Thiel E, Korfel A, Martus P, et al. High-dose methotrexate with or without whole brain radiotherapy for primary CNS lymphoma (G-PCNSL-SG-1): a phase 3, randomised, non-inferiority trial. Lancet Oncol. 2010;11(11):1036–47. https://doi.org/10.1016/S1470-2045(10)70229-1.
19. Morris PG, Correa DD, Yahalom J, et al. Rituximab, methotrexate, procarbazine, and vincristine followed by consolidation reduced-dose whole-brain radiotherapy and cytarabine in newly diagnosed primary CNS lymphoma: final results and long-term outcome. J Clin Oncol. 2013;31(31):3971–9. https://doi.org/10.1200/JCO.2013.50.4910.
20. Fisher B, Seiferheld W, Schultz C, et al. Secondary analysis of Radiation Therapy Oncology Group study (RTOG) 9310: an intergroup phase II combined modality treatment of primary central nervous system lymphoma. J Neurooncol. 2005;74(2):201–5. https://doi.org/10.1007/s11060-004-6596-9.
21. Glass J, Won M, Schultz CJ, et al. Phase I and II study of induction chemotherapy with methotrexate, rituximab, and temozolomide, followed by whole-brain radiotherapy and postirradiation temozolomide for primary CNS lymphoma: NRG oncology RTOG

0227. J Clin Oncol. 2016;34(14):1620–5. https://doi.org/10.1200/JCO.2015.64.8634.

22. Omuro A, Correa DD, DeAngelis LM, et al. R-MPV followed by high-dose chemotherapy with TBC and autologous stem-cell transplant for newly diagnosed primary CNS lymphoma. Blood. 2015;125(9):1403–10. https://doi.org/10.1182/blood-2014-10-604561.

23. Rubenstein JL, Hsi ED, Johnson JL, et al. Intensive chemotherapy and immunotherapy in patients with newly diagnosed primary CNS lymphoma: CALGB 50202 (Alliance 50202). J Clin Oncol. 2013;31(25):3061–8. https://doi.org/10.1200/JCO.2012.46.9957.

24. Ferreri AJ, Cwynarski K, Pulczynski E, et al. Chemoimmunotherapy with methotrexate, cytarabine, thiotepa, and rituximab (MATRix regimen) in patients with primary CNS lymphoma: results of the first randomisation of the International Extranodal Lymphoma Study Group-32 (IELSG32) phase 2 trial. Lancet Haematol. 2016;3(5):e217–27. https://doi.org/10.1016/S2352-3026(16)00036-3.

25. Hottinger AF, DeAngelis LM, Yahalom J, et al. Salvage whole brain radiotherapy for recurrent or refractory primary CNS lymphoma. Neurology. 2007;69(11):1178–82. https://doi.org/10.1212/01.wnl.0000276986.19602.c1.

26. Nguyen PL, Chakravarti A, Finkelstein DM, et al. Results of whole-brain radiation as salvage of methotrexate failure for immunocompetent patients with primary CNS lymphoma. J Clin Oncol. 2005;23(7):1507–13. https://doi.org/10.1200/JCO.2005.01.161.

27. Brown PD, Pugh S, Laack NN, et al. Memantine for the prevention of cognitive dysfunction in patients receiving whole-brain radiotherapy: a randomized, double-blind, placebo-controlled trial. Neuro Oncol. 2013;15(10):1429–37. https://doi.org/10.1093/neuonc/not114.

28. Doolittle ND, Korfel A, Lubow MA, et al. Long-term cognitive function, neuroimaging, and quality of life in primary CNS lymphoma. Neurology. 2013;81(1):84–92. https://doi.org/10.1212/WNL.0b013e318297eeba.

29. Correa DD, Shi W, Abrey LE, et al. Cognitive functions in primary CNS lymphoma after single or combined modality regimens. Neuro Oncol. 2012;14(1):101–8. https://doi.org/10.1093/neuonc/nor186.

30. Bessell EM, Graus F, Lopez-Guillermo A, et al. CHOD/BVAM regimen plus radiotherapy in patients with primary CNS non-Hodgkin's lymphoma. Int J Radiat Oncol Biol Phys. 2001;50(2):457–64.

# Choroid Plexus Tumors

**20**

Christina Snider, John H. Suh, and Erin S. Murphy

## Learning Objectives

- Discuss the epidemiology of choroid plexus tumors.
- Discuss prognostic and predictive factors for survival.
- Describe the histopathologic classifications, diagnostic work-up, and imaging characteristics of choroid plexus tumors.
- Describe the available treatment modalities and rationale for treatment of choroid plexus tumors based on histology and stage.
- Review appropriate radiation dose and target volume for choroid plexus tumors.

## Background Epidemiology

The choroid plexus is neuroepithelial tissue in the ventricles of the brain that produces cerebral spinal fluid (CSF). Choroid plexus tumors have very low incidence in the adult population, 0.3/1 million population/year, and are seen more frequently in children, particularly during the first 2 years of life [1]. They represent 2–4% of pediatric tumors. From a SEER review of 186 children with choroid plexus tumors, the median age at diagnosis was 4 years old for choroid plexus papilloma (CPP) and 1 year old for choroid plexus carcinoma (CPC) [2]. In adults, these tumors are most

C. Snider
Cleveland Clinic Lerner College of Medicine,
Cleveland, OH, USA

J. H. Suh · E. S. Murphy (✉)
Department of Radiation Oncology, Taussig Cancer Institute,
Cleveland Clinic, Cleveland, OH, USA

Rose Ella Burkhardt Brain Tumor and Neuro-oncology Center,
Cleveland Clinic, Cleveland, OH, USA
e-mail: murphye3@ccf.org

frequently located in the fourth ventricle and cerebellopontine angle, while lateral ventricle tumors are more commonly present in patients under the age of 20 [3–5] (Fig. 20.1).

## Risk Factors

Several rare genetic conditions have been associated with increased susceptibility to choroid plexus papilloma (CPC). Choroid plexus papilloma is a feature of Aicardi syndrome, a non-familial genetic condition linked to the X chromosome [6]. Case reports have also associated choroid plexus papilloma with hypomelanosis of Ito, a rare neurocutaneous syndrome, and with duplication of the short arm of chromosome 9 [7, 8].

While the majority of cases of CPC are sporadic, there is an association with germline *TP53* mutations/Li-Fraumeni syndrome (LFS). Multiple bodies of evidence have supported the association between CPC and *TP53* germline mutations, and pediatric cases of CPC have a high frequency of *TP53* germline mutations in association with LFS [9, 10]. As a result of this strong link between LFS and CPC, it has been recommended that patients with CPC be tested for the *TP53* germline mutations regardless of family history [9].

## Prognostic and Predictive Factors

Choroid plexus tumors are classified by 2016 World Health Organization criteria into choroid plexus papilloma (CPP, WHO Grade I), atypical choroid plexus papilloma (ACP, WHO Grade II), and choroid plexus carcinoma (CPC, WHO Grade III) [11]. CPP is most common, followed by CPC and ACP [12]. Histology is an important prognostic factor for choroid plexus tumors [2, 5].

CPP is well-differentiated, is histologically benign, and has very low or absent mitotic activity [4]. Rarely, CPP may seed cells into the CSF and result in metastasis along pathways of CSF flow [13]. A meta-analysis of choroid plexus papilloma cases reported

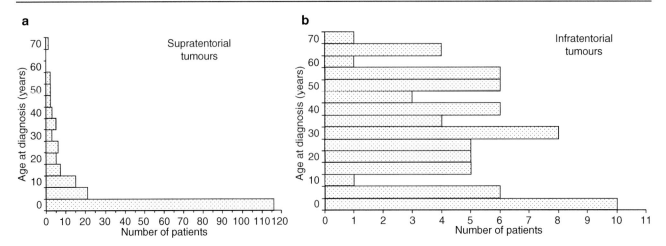

**Fig. 20.1** Distribution of (**a**) supratentorial and (**b**) infratentorial tumors by age. [Reprinted from Wolff JEA, Sajedi M, Brant R, Coppes MJ, Egeler RM. Choroid plexus tumours. Br J Cancer. 2002;87(10):1086–91. With permission from Nature Publishing Group]

1-, 5-, and 10-year projected survival rates of 90%, 81%, and 77%, respectively [5]. ACP are choroid plexus papillomas with increased mitotic activity but do not meet requirements for CPCs; they are more likely to recur than CPP [4].

CPC shows frank signs of malignancy and demonstrates at least four out of five histologic features: frequent mitoses, increased cellular density, nuclear pleomorphism, blurring of the papillary pattern with poorly structured sheets of tumor cells, and necrotic areas [4]. CPCs are highly invasive and associated with dismal prognosis, with 1-, 5-, and 10-year projected survival rates reported to be 71%, 41%, and 35%, respectively, in meta-analysis of CPC patients [5]. Over half of CPC tumors harbor somatic *TP53* mutations, and mutant *TP53* CPCs have been associated with increased genetic tumor instability and a worse prognosis [14].

Evaluation of molecular features of choroid plexus tumors has discovered that methylation profiling of choroid plexus tumors reveals three distinct subgroups (i.e., pediatric low-risk choroid plexus tumors, adult low-risk choroid plexus tumors, and pediatric high-risk choroid plexus tumors) and may provide useful prognostic information in addition to histopathology [15].

For example, this group found that for ACP of methylation cluster 3 also progressed frequently, whereas no tumor progression was observed in ACP of methylation clusters 1 and 2.

Choroid plexus carcinomas are characterized by complex chromosomal alterations related to patient age and prognosis. In one study, losses in chromosomes 9, 19p, and 22q were significantly more frequently in children <36 months, while chromosomal gains of 7 and 19 and arms 8q, 14q, and 21q were found to be significantly more frequent in older patients [16]. This study also found that loss of the 12q arm was associated

with shorter survival in addition to identifying 45 chromosomal regions that were significantly associated with survival [16].

In addition to histology, extent of surgical resection is also prognostic [2, 5, 12, 17] (Fig. 20.2). A SEER review that included 168 pediatric subjects with choroid plexus tumors found that for patients with CPC, gross total resection (GTR) was associated with a significantly lower mortality (HR = 0.21, 95% CI 0.07–0.66, $p = 0.007$) [2]. Overall survival at 5 years was 70.9% after GTR, which is significantly better than 35.9% after subtotal resection ($p = 0.012$) and 30% after no surgery ($p = 0.003$) [2]. Additionally, a meta-analysis of 102 pediatric cases of CPC found that GTR improved OS independently of patient age, gender, tumor location, and type of adjuvant therapy [17].

## Staging

Choroid plexus tumor patients often present with symptoms of intracranial pressure and therefore have a head CT and or brain MRI with and without contrast performed. After patients are stabilized, they should undergo complete staging spine MRI with and without contrast and, as long as not contraindicated, should proceed with a lumbar puncture to obtain CSF cytology.

## Imaging

On CT and MRI, CPP usually presents as an irregularly contrast-enhancing well-delineated mass within the ventricles that are isodense, hyperdense, T1-isointense, and T2-hypertense compared to the adjacent brain [3]. If dis-

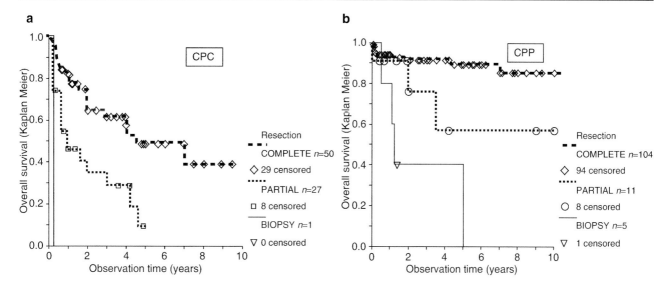

**Fig. 20.2** Extent of surgical resection is significant to survival for both (**a**) CPC and (**b**) CPP [5]. [Reprinted from Wolff JEA, Sajedi M, Brant R, Coppes MJ, Egeler RM. Choroid plexus tumours. Br J Cancer. 2002;87(10):1086–91. With permission from Nature Publishing Group]

seminated disease has occurred, tumor margins may be irregular. MRI imaging of choroid plexus carcinomas typically show large lesions within the ventricles with irregular enhancing margins, heterogenous signal on T2-weighted and T1-weighted imaging, edema in the adjacent brain parenchyma, hydrocephalus, and disseminated tumor [3]. No difference between CPC and ACP on imaging has been reported. As it may be difficult to distinguish between these tumor types, additional imaging modalities are being evaluated, and arterial spin labeling may help differentiate choroid plexus carcinomas and papillomas as demonstrated in one study [18].

## Multimodality Management Approach with Emphasis on Radiation Techniques with Guidance on Prescribed Dose and Fractionation

Owing to the rarity of these tumors, treatment for choroid plexus tumors has not been well-defined. For CPP, maximum safe resection is the typical curative approach, and tumors seldom recur after complete resection. For ACP, a curative surgical approach may be possible, but recurrence rates appear to be much higher than that of CPP; one study reported 6% recurrence for CPP and 29% recurrence for ACP [19]. The necessity of adjuvant radiotherapy and chemotherapy after gross total resection of ACP is controversial.

For CPC, treatment usually includes resection and other modalities including radiation therapy, chemotherapy [20], and second-look surgeries. Complete resection is considered

the most important predictor of survival, but due to the high vascularity of these tumors, total resection is not always possible [21–23]. A case report highlights a potential benefit to preoperative embolization but cautions the importance of understanding the anatomy of the anterior and posterior choroidal arteries to perform embolization of these tumors safely [24]. A retrospective review demonstrates that children who received neoadjuvant chemotherapy had less intraoperative blood loss and increased extent of resection compared to those who did not [25].

The survival benefit of adjuvant radiotherapy is controversial [2, 5, 17, 20, 26, 27]. Also, the most beneficial type of RT field remains controversial in treatment of CPC and has ranged from tumor/resection cavity only to whole-brain and craniospinal irradiation [27]. The role of chemotherapy in treatments of CPCs is less clear, but based on meta-analysis, it has been suggested that chemotherapy improves overall survival, particularly in patients with less than completely resected CPC [20].

In very young children, there have been efforts to avoid or delay radiotherapy. Twelve children with CPC (median age of 19.5 months) were treated on Head Start regimens which include surgical resection followed by five cycles of intensive induction followed by consolidation myeloablative chemotherapy with autologous hematopoietic stem cell rescue [28]. Seven patients progressed, five of whom ended up receiving radiotherapy. The 3- and 5-year progression-free survivals were 58% and 38% and overall survivals 83% and 62%, respectively.

There may also be a role for high-dose chemotherapy followed by stem cell rescue/transplant in the setting of recurrent disease [29, 30].

## Indications for Irradiation

Adjuvant radiation therapy is not indicated as initial treatment for CPP given the benign nature of the disease and the excellent survival outcome associated with gross total resection. In a small number of reports, Gamma Knife radiosurgery (GKRS) was used for CPP in cases of deep-seated or recurrent lesions [31]. However, the limited available data does not clarify the role of radiosurgery for these tumors. Given the worse prognosis of ACP, close monitoring after resection is warranted, and adjuvant treatment with radiation or chemotherapy may be considered in the case of local recurrence, progression, or malignant progression [32].

CPC has poor a prognosis, typically requiring aggressive multimodal therapies for treatment. Multiple studies have indicated improvement in OS and PFS for patients with CPC treated with both complete resection and RT compared to those who received complete resection only [20, 26, 27]. One retrospective study suggests that it may be possible to treat CPC with GTR only, but due to the small number of patients in the series who did not receive adjuvant therapy, a statistical comparison could not be made [22]. Further, evidence from a meta-analysis suggests that patients with CPC who received RT to the entire neuroaxis had significantly improved OS and PFS as compared to patients who received more limited RT treatment volumes, including whole-brain or involved-field RT [27]. Retrospective studies suggest that there may be a survival disadvantage for patients with CPC harboring *P53* mutations and that they should be treated with a radiation-sparing protocol due to the patients having a predilection for tumorigenesis [33].

## Treatment Field Design or Target Delineation

For CPC, craniospinal irradiation, whole brain, and tumor/tumor bed fields have been used for radiotherapy. In one retrospective analysis of 54 patients, patients with CPC treated with craniospinal irradiation improved PFS rates compared to patients with CPC treated with whole-brain and tumor/tumor bed radiotherapy (44.2% vs 15.3% 5-year PFS) [27]. Based on this analysis, craniospinal irradiation may lead to improved PFS in patients with CPC, particularly in those with disseminated disease.

Normal critical structure tolerance constraints in the context of the disease being treated. We would suggest conventional dose constraints for other diseases typically treated to the same total dose of 54–60 Gy. For example, the patients with intracranial meningiomas enrolled on the intermediate-risk arm of RTOG 0539 (NCT00895622) were treated to a total dose of 54 Gy, and the following dose constraints from that trial are very appropriate for choroid plexus tumors: The maximum point dose to a volume greater than 0.03 cc was 5 Gy for lenses, 45 Gy for retinae, 50 Gy for optic nerves, 54 Gy for optic chiasm, and 55 Gy for the brainstem.

## Radiation Dose Prescription and Organ-at-Risk Tolerances

The CPT-SIOP-2000 trial treated patients older than 3 years with radiotherapy after the second round of chemotherapy, stratifying radiation field by expected prognosis [34]. For patients with CPC nonresponsive to chemotherapy (stable disease or progressive disease) and those with metastasized CPC and APP, 35.2 Gy craniospinal irradiation was given using 1.6 Gy per fraction and a local boost up to 54 Gy. For all other choroid plexus tumor patients, local radiation with 54 Gy administered with 1.8 Gy per fraction was given. Radiation dosages of 50–60 Gy have been used to treat adults with ACP and CPC, and a total dose of 54–60 Gy for CPC patients is typically recommended [1].

In the CPT-SIOP-2000 trial, the clinical target volume (CTV) margin encompassed the visible tumor seen on T2-weighted MR plus an additional margin of 0.5 cm. The planning target volume encompassed the CTV with an additional margin depending on the precision of treatment technique. A CTV margin of 1–2 cm is reasonable for CPC and APP. When radiotherapy is necessary for CPP, smaller CTV margins can be considered.

## Complication Avoidance

Due to the rarity of choroid plexus tumors in adults, one should use strategies used for other primary brain tumors to maximize the therapeutic ratio. Organs at risk that should also be delineated include the eyes, lenses, optic nerves, optic chiasm, cochleas, brainstem, pituitary gland, brain stem, and hypothalamus. Contouring of the whole-brain volume should be done to allow evaluation of the mean brain dose. Additionally, delineation of the hippocampi may be done to estimate risk of neurocognitive decline in the patient as well as to spare these structures as much as possible using intensity-modulated radiation therapy [35].

## Radiation Toxicity, Acute and Late

Acute radiation-induced adverse effects include hair loss, skin changes, headaches, nausea, reduced appetite, and fatigue. The severity of some of these changes can be reduced with steroids. Early-delayed complications include somnolence syndrome, which is less common in adults than children but can be seen in adults in the first 2 months after radiation treatment. Corticosteroids may play preventative roles, and these symptoms usually resolve within 1–3 months [36]. Delayed complications may include focal cerebral radionecrosis, neurocognitive changes, hypopituitarism, vascular lesions, and second malignant neoplasm. The risk of radionecrosis is highest in the first 2 years of treatment. Given the challenges in discriminating radionecrosis from tumor recurrence using conventional MRI, additional images such as cerebral blood volume are often required.

## Outcomes: Tumor Control and Survival

See Figs. 20.3, 20.4, and 20.5.

## Case Study

A 64-year-old female presented with weight loss, fatigue, difficulty with ambulation, dizziness, tinnitus, numbness in the right midface and under cheek, and gait instability. She underwent imaging which demonstrated a large right cerebellopontine angle mass (Fig. 20.4). She underwent near-total resection, and pathology was consistent with choroid plexus

carcinoma, WHO grade III. Due to medical comorbidities, she was determined not to be eligible for chemotherapy. Therefore she was treated with adjuvant craniospinal irradiation (Fig. 20.5). She remains free from progression 3 years post-completion of radiotherapy but has persistent balance difficulties.

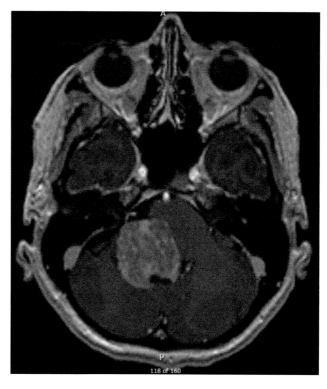

**Fig. 20.4** Axial T1 contrast-enhanced brain MRI demonstrating a right cerebellar pontine angle choroid plexus carcinoma

| Year | Author | Number of patients | Mean age | Localization | | | Pathology | | | Follow-up (mean) | Recurrence rate | V-P shunt (n) | Prognoz |
|---|---|---|---|---|---|---|---|---|---|---|---|---|---|
| | | | | LV | 3rd V | 4th V+CPA | CPP | ACPP | CPC | | | | |
| 1996 | Tacconi et al. | 33 | 30 y.o. | 14 | 1 | 18 | 32 | – | 1 | 13 years | 9 % | 6 | OS:51 %<br>Mor:27 %<br>Morb:8 % |
| 1998 | Talacchi et al. | 12 | 39.5 y.o. | – | – | 12 | 12 | – | 1 | 8.2 years | 25 % | 4 | OS:67 %<br>Mor:33 %<br>Morb:25 % |
| 2011 | Boström et al. | 14 | 46 y.o. | 1 | 1 | 12 | 12 | 2 | – | 4.8 years | 14 % | 4 | OS:100 % (CPP)<br>Mor:0<br>Morb:21 % |
| 2013 | Safaee et al. (meta analysis) | 193 | 39.9 y.o. | 18 | 7 | 158 | n.a. | | | 4.4 years | 23 % | n.a. | OS:72 %(GTR), 32 %(STR)<br>Mor:37 %<br>Morb:n.a. |
| 2014 | Turkoglu et al. | 15 | 33.7 y.o. | 4 | 2 | 9 | 9 | 4 | 2 | 5 years | 14 % | 5 | OS:100 %(CPP, ACPP), 0 % (CPC)<br>Mor:13 %<br>Morb:27 % |

ACPP: Atypical choroid plexus papilloma, CPA: Cerebellpontin angle, CPC: Choroid plexus carcinoma, CPP: Choroid plexus papilloma, GTR: Gross total resection, LV: lateral ventricle, mor: mortality, morb: morbidity, n: number, n.a.: not available, OS: Overall survival, STR: Subtotal resection, V: Ventricle, y.o.: year old

**Fig. 20.3** Review of adult series of choroid plexus tumors in the literature. [Reprinted from Turkoglu E, Kertmen H, Sanli AM, Onder E, Gunaydin A, Gurses L, et al. Clinical outcome of adult choroid plexus tumors: retrospective analysis of a single institute. Acta Neurochir (Wien). 2014 Aug 1;156(8):1461–8. With permission from Springer Verlag]

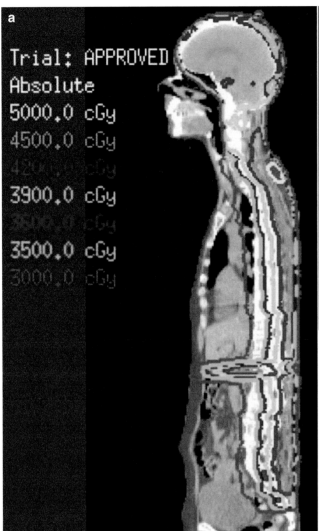

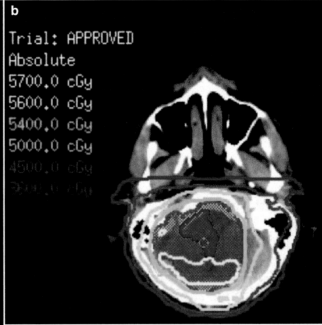

**Fig. 20.5** (**a**) Sagittal image of 36 Gy craniospinal irradiation plan for patient who underwent a near-total resection and was not eligible for chemotherapy due to medical comorbiditites and (**b**) axial image of right cerebellar pontine angle IMRT boost for total dose of 54 Gy to the resection cavity

## Summary

- Choroid plexus tumors are rare tumors, most commonly arising in young children.
- The site of choroid plexus tumors changes with age; in children, the lateral ventricles are most often affected, while the fourth ventricle is most frequently affected in adults.
- The three histopathological classifications of choroid plexus tumors from best to worse prognosis are choroid plexus papilloma, atypical choroid plexus papilloma, and choroid plexus carcinoma.
- Histology and extent of surgical resection are prognostic.
- Curative treatment for CPP and ACP is typically maximum surgical resection, but recurrence rates are higher in cases of ACP.
- CPC has the worse prognosis and often requires multiple modalities for treatment, including surgery, radiation therapy and/or chemotherapy.

## Self-Assessment Questions

1. Choroid plexus tumors arise most frequently in which age group?
   A. Young children
   B. Young adults
   C. Older adults
   D. Infants

2. Choroid plexus tumors most frequently present with:
   A. Loss of balance

B. Increased intracranial pressure

C. Seizures

D. Motor weakness

3. Which of the following histopathologic classifications is associated with worse prognosis?
   A. Choroid plexus papilloma
   B. Atypical choroid plexus papilloma
   C. Choroid plexus carcinoma

4. Curative treatment of choroid plexus papilloma is typically:
   A. Gross total resection
   B. Gross total resection with adjuvant radiotherapy
   C. Gross total resection with adjuvant chemotherapy
   D. Gross total resection with adjuvant radiotherapy and chemotherapy

5. Which of the following is NOT prognostic for choroid plexus tumors?
   A. Extent of surgical resection
   B. Histology
   C. Age of diagnosis

## Answers

1. A Young children
2. B Increased intracranial pressure
3. C Choroid plexus carcinoma
4. A Gross total resection
5. C Age of diagnosis

## References

1. Turkoglu E, Kertmen H, Sanli AM, et al. Clinical outcome of adult choroid plexus tumors: retrospective analysis of a single institute. Acta Neurochir. 2014;156(8):1461–8.
2. Lam S, Lin Y, Cherian J, et al. Choroid plexus tumors in children: a population-based study. Pediatr Neurosurg. 2013;49(6):331–8.
3. McCall T, Binning M, Blumenthal DT, et al. Variations of disseminated choroid plexus papilloma: 2 case reports and a review of the literature. Surg Neurol. 2006;66(1):62–7.
4. World Health Organization. WHO classification of tumours of the central nervous system. Revised 4th ed. In: Louis DN, Ohgaki H, Wiestler OD, Cavenee WK, editors. World Health Organization classification of tumours. Lyon: International Agency for Research on Cancer; 2016.
5. Wolff JEA, Sajedi M, Brant R, et al. Choroid plexus tumours. Br J Cancer. 2002;87(10):1086–91.
6. Aicardi J. Aicardi syndrome. Brain and Development. 2005;27(3):164–71.
7. Morigaki R, Pooh K-H, Shouno K, et al. Choroid plexus papilloma in a girl with hypomelanosis of Ito. J Neurosurg Pediatr. 2012;10(3):182–5.
8. Norman MG, Harrison KJ, Poskitt KJ, et al. Duplication of 9P and hyperplasia of the choroid plexus: a pathologic, radio-

9. logic, and molecular cytogenetics study. Pediatr Pathol Lab Med. 1995;15(1):109–20.
9. Sorrell AD, Espenschied CR, Culver JO, et al. TP53 testing and Li-Fraumeni syndrome: current status of clinical applications and future directions. Mol Diagn Ther. 2013;17(1):31–47.
10. Gozali AE, Britt B, Shane L, et al. Choroid plexus tumors; management, outcome, and association with the Li-Fraumeni syndrome: the Children's Hospital Los Angeles (CHLA) experience, 1991–2010. Pediatr Blood Cancer. 2012;58(6):905–9.
11. Louis DN, Perry A, Reifenberger G, et al. The 2016 World Health Organization classification of tumors of the central nervous system: a summary. Acta Neuropathol (Berl). 2016;131(6):803–20.
12. Cannon DM, Mohindra P, Gondi V, et al. Choroid plexus tumor epidemiology and outcomes: implications for surgical and radiotherapeutic management. J Neurooncol. 2015;121(1):151–7.
13. Irsutti M, Thorn-Kany M, Arrué P, et al. Suprasellar seeding of a benign choroid plexus papilloma of the fourth ventricle with local recurrence. Neuroradiology. 2000;42(9):657–61.
14. Tabori U, Shlien A, Baskin B, et al. TP53 alterations determine clinical subgroups and survival of patients with choroid plexus tumors. J Clin Oncol. 2010;28(12):1995–2001.
15. Thomas C, Sill M, Ruland V, et al. Methylation profiling of choroid plexus tumors reveals 3 clinically distinct subgroups. Neuro Oncol. 2016;18(6):790–6.
16. Ruland V, Hartung S, Kordes U, et al. Choroid plexus carcinomas are characterized by complex chromosomal alterations related to patient age and prognosis. Genes Chromosomes Cancer. 2014;53(5):373–80.
17. Sun MZ, Ivan ME, Clark AJ, et al. Gross total resection improves overall survival in children with choroid plexus carcinoma. J Neurooncol. 2014;116(1):179–85.
18. Dangouloff-Ros V, Grevent D, Pagès M, et al. Choroid plexus neoplasms: toward a distinction between carcinoma and papilloma using arterial spin-labeling. AJNR Am J Neuroradiol. 2015;36(9):1786–90.
19. Jeibmann A, Wrede B, Peters O, et al. Malignant progression in choroid plexus papillomas. J Neurosurg. 2007;107(3 Suppl):199–202.
20. Wrede B, Liu P, Wolff JEA. Chemotherapy improves the survival of patients with choroid plexus carcinoma: a meta-analysis of individual cases with choroid plexus tumors. J Neurooncol. 2007;85(3):345–51.
21. McEvoy AW, Harding BN, Phipps KP, et al. Management of choroid plexus tumours in children: 20 years experience at a single neurosurgical centre. Pediatr Neurosurg. 2000;32(4):192–9.
22. Fitzpatrick LK, Aronson LJ, Cohen KJ. Is there a requirement for adjuvant therapy for choroid plexus carcinoma that has been completely resected? J Neurooncol. 2002;57(2):123–6.
23. Passariello A, Tufano M, Spennato P, et al. The role of chemotherapy and surgical removal in the treatment of Choroid Plexus carcinomas and atypical papillomas. Childs Nerv Syst. 2015;31(7):1079–88.
24. Slater L-A, Hoffman C, Drake J, et al. Pre-operative embolization of a choroid plexus carcinoma: review of the vascular anatomy. Childs Nerv Syst. 2016;32(3):541–5.
25. Schneider C, Kamaly-Asl I, Ramaswamy V, et al. Neoadjuvant chemotherapy reduces blood loss during the resection of pediatric choroid plexus carcinomas. J Neurosurg Pediatr. 2015;16(2):126–33.
26. Wolff JE, Sajedi M, Coppes MJ, et al. Radiation therapy and survival in choroid plexus carcinoma. Lancet. 1999;353(9170):2126.
27. Mazloom A, Wolff JE, Paulino AC. The impact of radiotherapy fields in the treatment of patients with choroid plexus carcinoma. Int J Radiat Oncol. 2010;78(1):79–84.
28. Zaky W, Dhall G, Khatua S, et al. Choroid plexus carcinoma in children: The Head Start experience. Pediatr Blood Cancer. 2015;62(5):784–9.

29. Samuel TA, Parikh J, Sharma S, et al. Recurrent adult choroid plexus carcinoma treated with high-dose chemotherapy and syngeneic stem cell (bone marrow) transplant. J Neurol Surg A Cent Eur Neurosurg. 2013;74(Suppl 1):e149–54.

30. Mosleh O, Tabori U, Bartels U, et al. Successful treatment of a recurrent choroid plexus carcinoma with surgery followed by high-dose chemotherapy and stem cell rescue. Pediatr Hematol Oncol. 2013;30(5):386–91.

31. Kim I-Y, Niranjan A, Kondziolka D, et al. Gamma knife radiosurgery for treatment resistant choroid plexus papillomas. J Neurooncol. 2008;90(1):105–10.

32. Kamar FG, Kairouz VF, Nasser SM, et al. Atypical choroid plexus papilloma treated with single agent bevacizumab. Rare Tumors [Internet]. 2014;6(1). Available from: http://www.ncbi.nlm.nih.gov/pmc/articles/PMC3977164/. Cited 15 Jan 2017.

33. Bahar M, Kordes U, Tekautz T, et al. Radiation therapy for choroid plexus carcinoma patients with Li-Fraumeni syndrome: advantageous or detrimental? Anticancer Res. 2015;35(5):3013–7.

34. Wrede B, Hasselblatt M, Peters O, et al. Atypical choroid plexus papilloma: clinical experience in the CPT-SIOP-2000 study. J Neurooncol. 2009;95(3):383.

35. Grosu A-L, Oehlke O, Nieder C. Brain tumors. In: Grosu A-L, Nieder C, editors. Target volume definition in radiation oncology [Internet]. Berlin, Heidelberg: Springer; 2015. p. 1–21. Available from: http://link.springer.com/chapter/10.1007/978-3-662-45934-8_1. Cited 17 Jan 2017.

36. Soussain C, Ricard D, Fike JR, et al. CNS complications of radiotherapy and chemotherapy. Lancet. 2009;374(9701):1639–51.

# Hemangiopericytoma

# 21

Vincent Bernard and Amol J. Ghia

## Learning Objectives

- To describe the differential diagnosis of HPC.
- To recognize the clinical course and outcomes of HPC.
- To describe overall therapeutic and follow-up strategy for HPC.
- To describe effective approach to radiation therapy in HPC.

## Background Epidemiology

Hemangiopericytoma (HPC) is a rare mesenchymal tumor accounting for 0.4% of primary intracranial tumors and 2.5% of meningeal tumors [1]. As a whole, HPCs also arise in primary sites outside of the CNS including muscles, tendons, fat tissues, and blood vessels. These tumors are derived from the pericytes surrounding the vasculature endothelial lining. Although initially classified as a variant of meningioma due to their dural attachment, in 1993, the WHO recognized HPC as a distinct pathological entity derived from pericytes based on their aggressive behavior with tendency for extraneural metastasis, high recurrence rate, as well as distinct clinical, immunohistochemical, and molecular characteristics [2–5]. Most recently, in 2016 the WHO classification of CNS tumors re-termed both HPCs and solitary fibrous tumors (SFT) as a single entity due to their molecular similarities. Specifically, both solitary fibrous tumors and HPCs share

inversions in 12q13, resulting in *NAB2* and *STAT6* gene fusions, resulting in *STAT6* nuclear expression detectable by immunohistochemistry [6, 7].

HPCs occur equally in men and women with no racial predilection and are commonly observed in patients between 40 and 50 years old [8]. HPCs can be distributed intracranially with 70% supratentorial, 15% in the posterior fossa, and 15% in the spine, although some intraventricular lesions have been reported [9].

## Risk Factors

No risk factors have been associated with HPC.

## Diagnosis: Pathologic and Radiographic

Initial presentation of HPC is dependent on tumor location, such as in the case of supratentorial HPCs; symptoms can include peripheral neuropathy and signs and symptoms associated with increased intracranial pressure, such as headache, vertigo, nausea and vomiting, and visual disturbances. Seizures have also been reported. Duration of symptoms is typically less than a year. The prognosis of HPC warranted in its own classification in 1993 by the WHO as local recurrence and metastasis have been reported in up to 91% and 64% of patients, respectively [10, 11].

Several histologic and radiographic mimics exist for HPC and should be included in the differential diagnosis; this includes meningioma, metastatic carcinomas, mesenchymal chondrosarcomas, and hemangiomas [12–15]. CT imaging of HPCs reveals a hyperdense lesion with heterogeneous contrast enhancement. Bony erosion can at times be appreciated. MR imaging can demonstrate T1 and T2 isodensity with heterogeneous contrast enhancement. A dural tail sign or corkscrew vascular configuration can also be found. HPCs are typically detected at 4 cm of size at diagnosis (Fig. 21.1). Histological analysis confirms diagnosis, demonstrating

V. Bernard
Department of Pathology, MD Anderson Cancer Center, Houston, TX, USA

A. J. Ghia (✉)
Department of Radiation Oncology, MD Anderson Cancer Center, Houston, TX, USA
e-mail: AJGhia@mdanderson.org

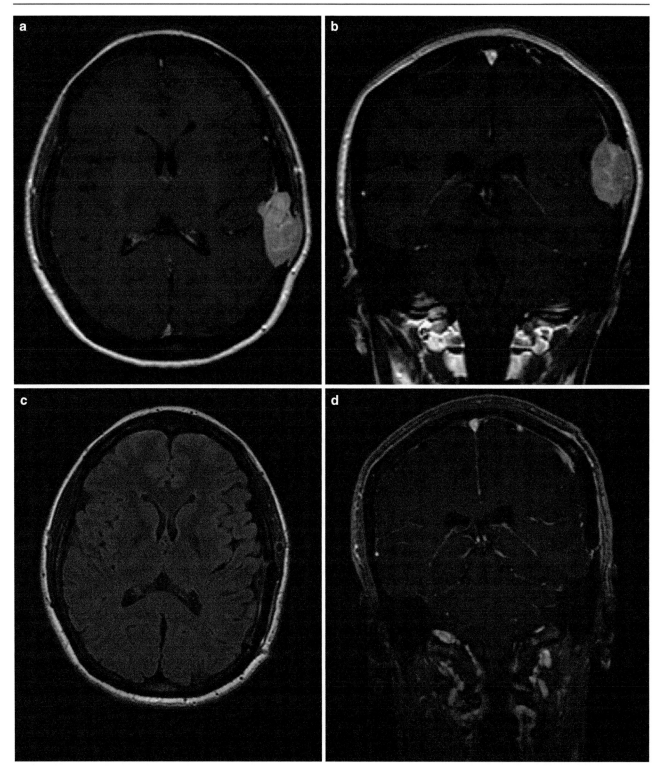

**Fig. 21.1** A 40-year-old woman, who initially noticed left scalp discomfort which evolved into a lump along her left scalp 3 months later. Initial evaluation by her primary care physician suggested a sebaceous cyst. She was referred to a surgeon, and a MRI scan was recommended revealing a 4-cm left parietal extra-axial mass extending into the skull and overlying scalp (**a**, **b**). She underwent a crani- otomy and GTR with pathology revealing a WHO Grade III anaplastic HPC. Immunohistochemistry studies showed tumor cells positive for vimentin, CD34, CD99, and BCL2, while stains for EMA, CKAE1/3, S100, and GFAP were negative. Follow-up image 1 month later shows resolution of tumor mass (**c**, **d**)

sheets of cells with uniform hypercellularity; cells have a distinct round to spindle morphology with a staghorn pattern of thin-walled vessels.

## Staging

As of 2016, the WHO has assigned three grades to the HPC/solitary fibrous tumor entity:

*Grade I*: Highly collagenous, relatively low cellularity, spindle cell lesion. Previously diagnosed as solitary fibrous tumors.

*Grade II*: More cellular, less collagenous with plump cells and staghorn appearing vascular channels. Previously diagnosed as HPC.

*Grade III*: Five or more mitoses per ten high-power fields. Previously known as anaplastic HPC and associated with poorer overall and metastatic free survival [16, 17].

## Multimodality Management Approach

HPCs are exceptionally difficult to treat with a predilection for local recurrence and distant metastasis even in a multimodality treatment setting. Treatment options for HPC include surgical resection, adjuvant radiotherapy (RT), chemotherapy, and embolization. Embolization in itself has a limited role in HPC treatment due to the ability of these tumors to avidly feed off of intracranial and extracranial collateral circulation. The role of chemotherapies also is limited with studies reporting no or marginal benefit, particularly during recurrence [18, 19].

Initial therapy of HPC typically involves complete resection when possible, resulting in immediate relief of mass effect as well as diagnostic confirmation of HPC based on histological analysis. Additionally, gross total resection (GTR) by itself is largely considered to be directly associated with increased progression free survival [11, 20]. Yet the anatomical location within the skull, dural sinus invasion, neural involvement, and its highly vascular nature make surgical intervention of HPC technically difficult. Embolization prior to surgery can sometimes help with intraoperative bleeding, but as mentioned above, the network of collateral circulation can make its utility limited. In this regard, GTR may only be possible in one-third to two-thirds of cases [21].

Due to the rarity of CNS HPCs, there is a lack of randomized prospective studies, providing consensus evidence of best practices for treatment. Thus, current therapy guidelines are typically institution dependent and derived from small-scale retrospective studies. A generally accepted approach involves initial gross tumor resection followed by postopera-

tive radiotherapy which has demonstrated effectiveness in prolonging local control and in some cases overall survival [2, 16, 18, 21–31]. Several radiation treatment modalities have been utilized in the treatment of HPC and can include conventional external radiotherapy, intensity-modulated radiotherapy (IMRT), and stereotactic radiosurgery (SRS) using a tool such as Gamma Knife radiosurgery (GKR) or Cyberknife (CK). This aggressive approach is warranted due to the propensity of HPCs to recur and metastasize. In cases of recurrence or residual tumor where further tumor resection is prohibitively invasive, radiation therapy provides a viable alternative. In addition, other novel therapeutic approaches are currently being explored, such as antiangiogenic therapies [32].

## Indications for Irradiation

RT for HPC has been widely accepted as a necessary strategy in the adjuvant setting following GTR or STR. This can be performed following GTR and STR to ablate residual tumor and improve local tumor control in the form of conventional radiotherapy, stereotactic radiosurgery, and stereotactic radiotherapy. In the case of recurrence, both repeat surgery and salvage RT are effective. Previous studies have shown that dose escalation is a prudent strategy given the aggressive nature of HPC and can provide an additional period of local tumor control and overall survival [5, 17, 20, 29]. It is important to consider the risks and benefits of repeat resection versus RT on a per patient basis as factors such as neurological status, active disease sites, timing of prior interventions or prior RT, tumor volumes, and patient wishes will influence this decision. It is also important to note that as RT is a focal therapy, it does not have a role in preventing distant metastasis, which should be aggressively monitored following initial intervention.

## Target Volume Delineation, Radiation Dose Prescription, and Organ at Risk Tolerances

A dose-response relationship has been reported in HPC with those receiving $\geq 50$ Gy and optimally beyond a threshold $\geq 60$ Gy having improved local control [23, 33, 34]. Target volumes of at least $GTV_{50}$ should be delivered with the tumor bed defined as the enhancing mass on post-contrast T1-weighted MRI. In the case of postoperative RT, GTV will consist of the tumor bed and any residual nodular enhancement if present. The $CTV_{50}$ consists of an additional 1–2 cm margin, which should encompass the dural tail if detected. Depending on setup error and reproducibility of patient positioning, $PTV_{50}$ consists of the $CTV_{50}$ plus an additional 3–5 mm. For stereotactic radiosurgery dosing, $\geq 16$ Gy in a

**Table 21.1** RT normal tissue dose constraints[a]

| Structure at risk | Recommended constraint | Maximum allowed constraint |
|---|---|---|
| Lens | <5 Gy | <7 Gy |
| Retinae | <45 Gy | <50 Gy |
| Optic nerves | <50 Gy | <55 Gy |
| Optic chiasm | <54 Gy | <56 Gy |
| | <8 Gy for SRS | <10 Gy for SRS |
| Spinal cord | <45 Gy | <50 Gy |
| Brainstem | <55 Gy | <60 Gy |
| | <12.5 Gy for SRS | |
| Cochlea | <35 Gy | <45 Gy |
| | <4 Gy for SRS | <12–14 Gy for SRS |

[a]Constraints listed are Dmax to a point

single fraction should be delivered to the GTV [35]. As with any radiotherapy to the CNS, vital structures remain at risk; recommended and maximum tolerances are described below (Table 21.1).

## Radiation Toxicity: Acute and Late

Reported up-front toxicities of RT are rare and mild when they do occur ($\leq$CTCAE Grade II). This can include skin erythema or alopecia. Possible toxicities also depend on site of therapy delivery, such as a reported case of pituitary malfunction 12 months after RT to the sellar region in one patient, but more commonly involve cases of radiation necrosis [36]. If care is not taken to avoid vital structures at risk, side effects can include cranial nerve toxicity, xerostomia, and spinal cord toxicity, among others.

## Prognostic and Predictive Factors

As previously mentioned, GTR of HPC is preferred and associated with improved overall outcomes compared with STR which is correlated to poorer local control [33, 34]. It is important to note that HPC is an aggressive tumor with a predilection for recurrence. Studies have reported recurrence rates of up to 91% of patients, occurring as late as 10 years after initial treatment [1, 19, 35]. As most studies have small patient populations, with limited follow-up intervals and incredibly heterogeneous therapeutic approaches, being able to determine consensus survival, recurrence, and metastatic rates is a challenge. Currently, overall survival rates of HPC are approximately 95%, 81%, 60%, and 23% for 1, 5, 10, and 20 years, respectively [21, 34]. Local and distant metastatic rates range from 14.3% to 63.6% and 11.1% to 55%, respectively (Table 21.2). Extraneural metastasis has been most commonly identified in the liver, lungs, and extra-axial skeleton [37]. Tumor grade has also been shown to be a predictor of overall, recurrence-free, and metastasis-free survival, with

those patients with Grade III anaplastic HPC experiencing worse prognosis [16, 17, 19, 35].

Although not all studies have found significantly improved outcomes among those patients receiving GTR + adjuvant RT, it is generally believed that this therapy combination provides the most beneficial outcomes in regard to local tumor control and overall survival (Table 21.2). Location of tumor lesion has also presented as a predictor of outcomes, with those HPCs of the posterior fossa associated with poorer overall survival versus non-posterior fossa tumors (10.75 versus 15.6 median years, respectively) [21, 34].

As poor tumor control and emergence of metastasis are intrinsic complications of HPC that led to its reclassification by the WHO, this tumor type requires aggressive follow-up.

## Follow-Up: Radiographic Assessment

Following initial therapeutic intervention, follow-up brain MRIs should be performed at 3 months, 6 months, and then every subsequent 6 months. This will allow one to assess residual tumor necessitating further adjuvant therapy, as well as tumor response and recurrence. Additionally, there should be consideration of radiograph assessment of common sites of metastasis including the lung and liver. Any change in neurological condition should be reported as this may indicate poor tumor control.

## Case Presentation

The patient is a 49-year-old male with a diagnosis of recurrent hemangiopericytoma. He was initially diagnosed 10 years ago presenting with intracranial hemorrhage. He subsequently underwent a craniotomy and subtotal resection followed by subtherapeutic external beam radiation therapy to a total dose of 35 Gy over 23 fractions. Since that time, he has been followed with serial MRIs and has had multiple recurrences at 5 and 7 years after initial surgical intervention, which were also treated with surgical resection. More recently he presented with tumor progression, with MRI of the skull base demonstrating a recurrent tumor at the right middle cranial fossa with increased invasion into the right sphenoid sinus (Fig. 21.2a).

Recurrence was managed with resection of recurrent tumor followed by radiation therapy to eliminate any residual tumor cells (Fig. 21.2b). Surgery demonstrated extensive soft tissue involvement, nerve involvement, and involvement of the eustachian tube, middle ear, ear canal, along the carotid, and sphenoid sinus. A large portion of the floor of the medial portion of the right middle fossa had been destroyed by the tumor with intracranial extension of tumor into the medial portion of the floor of the right middle fossa

**Table 21.2** Key studies on HPC

| Author year | # of patients | # of tumors | Median FU (months, range) | Median tumor volume (cm³) | Median marginal dose or mean dose (Gy, range) | Tumor control at last FU (%) | New lesions (% of patients) | Extracranial metastasis (%) | Median OS from initial diagnosis | Main findings |
|---|---|---|---|---|---|---|---|---|---|---|
| Coffey (1993) [2] | 5 | 11 | 14.8 | 7.7 | 15 (12–18) | 82 | 63.6 | 20 | N/A | Gamma knife radiosurgery resulted in tumor shrinkage of all tumors that had follow-up imaging. The authors suggest a role for radiosurgery for those tumors that have recurred after initial therapy |
| Payne (2000) [26] | 10 | 12 | 24.8 (3–56) | 7.6 | 14 (2.8–25) | 75 | 16.7 | N/A | N/A | Gamma knife radiosurgery resulted in tumor shrinkage and delayed recurrence associated with extended survival and maintenance of neurological function |
| Dufour (2001) [23] | 17 | N/A | 60 (24–259) | N/A | 50 | 48 | 29.4 | 17.6 | N/A | Surgery followed by XRT reduced risk of local recurrence. Dose greater than 50 Gy required for reducing risk of local recurrence |
| Sheehan (2002) [5] | 14 | 15 | 21 (5–76) | 5.1 | 15 (11–20) | 80 | 14.3 | 29 | N/A | Gamma knife radiosurgery achieved tumor control in 80% of lesions |
| Ecker (2003) [19] | 15 | 45 | 45.6 | 7.8 | 16 (12–21) | 93 | N/A | N/A | N/A | High-grade HPC recur earlier vs low grade (6.7 years earlier) |
| Chang and Sakamoto (2003) [38] | 8 | N/A | 44 | N/A | 20.5 (15–24) | 75 | N/A | N/A | N/A | Six out of eight patients treated with XRT at recurrence saw a decrease in tumor size |
| Kim (2003) [20] | 31 | N/A | 77 (1–216) | N/A | N/A | 61 | N/A | 13 | N/A | Complete excision followed by adjuvant radiotherapy of more than 50 Gy extended local control. Stereotactic radiosurgery suggested to be of value in the context of CNS recurrence of smaller tumors and previously irradiated fields |
| Soyuer (2004) [39] | 29 | N/A | 111.6 (2 days to 264 months) | N/A | 54 (33.4–61.2) | 39 | N/A | 55 | N/A | Although no survival advantages were found based on therapies, the authors recommend GTR followed by limited field XRT as a treatment strategy |
| Kano (2008) [40] | 20 | 29 | 46 | 4.5 | 15 (10–20) | 72.4 | N/A | 25 | 135.5 | A marginal dose of >14 Gy was associated with improved progression-free survival. The authors claim a role for adjuvant stereotactic radiosurgery, particularly for patients with residual or recurrent HPC |
| Sun (2009) [41] | 22 | 58 | 26 (5–90) | 5.4 | 13.5 (10–20) | 65 | 31.8 | 13.6 | 67.6 | Gamma knife radiosurgery is effective in postoperative management of small- to moderate-sized HPC and provides an alternative to repeat surgical resection on recurrence or residual disease |
| Iwai (2009) [42] | 8 | 13 | 61 (NA) | N/A | 15.1 (12–16) | 100 | N/A | N/A | N/A | The authors recommend using a 16 Gy marginal dose for long-term tumor growth control based on previous literature and their study group |
| Olson (2010) [29] | 21 | 28 | 68 (2–138) | 3.5 | 17 (2.8–22) | 82.4 | 33.3 | 19 | N/A | In addition to supporting the role of radiosurgery at recurrence, the authors suggest a utility in repeat radiosurgery at a higher dose in areas of recurrence and progression following initial radiation therapy |
| Kim (2010) [43] | 9 | 17 | 32 (7–82) | 1 | 20 (11–22) | 82.4 | 52.9 | 11.1 | N/A | Using gamma knife, a high marginal dose (>17 Gy) was a significant predictive factor for local control with no associated adverse events |

(continued)

**Table 21.2** (continued)

| Author year | # of patients | # of tumors | Median FU (months, range) | Median tumor volume (cm³) | Median marginal dose or mean dose (Gy, range) | Tumor control at last FU (%) | New lesions (% of patients) | Extracranial metastasis (%) | Median OS from initial diagnosis | Main findings |
|---|---|---|---|---|---|---|---|---|---|---|
| Rutkowski (2010) [34] | 277 | N/A | 78 (1 day to 399 mos) | 5.36 | N/A | 43 | N/A | 27 | 156 | GTR showed overall survival benefit. XRT demonstrated no survival benefits. Patients treated with >50 Gy has increased mortality rates than those receiving <50 Gy. Authors acknowledge this may represent a selection bias for patients with more aggressive disease and those with intrinsic poor outcomes |
| Rutkowski (2012) [31] | 35 | N/A | 2–408 | 4.4 | N/A | 46 | N/A | 20 | 194.4 | GTR and not adjuvant XRT demonstrated a statistically significant survival advantage. Although not significant, any type of surgery plus XRT showed a trend to statistical significant vs surgery alone for improved recurrence-free survival |
| Ghia (2013) [30] | 88 | N/A | N/A | N/A | N/A | N/A | N/A | N/A | 111 | Patients undergoing GTR saw an improved OS (HR, 0.28; 95% CI, 0.11–0.71; $p = 0.007$). Postoperative radiotherapy was correlated with improved OS (HR, 0.02; 95% CI, 0.00–0.31; $p = 0.005$) |
| Ghia (2013) [33] | 63 | N/A | N/A | N/A | 60 (35–66.4) | 51 | 60 | N/A | 154 | Increase in LC following postoperative RT (HR, 0.18; 95% CI, 0.04–0.82; $p = 0.027$), subtotal resection correlated with worse LC (HR, 3.06; 95% CI, 1.34–6.99, $p = 0.008$). Patients receiving >60 Gy had improved LC (HR, 0.12; 95% CI, 0.01–0.95; $p = 0.045$) |
| Sonabend (2014) [21] | 227 | N/A | 34 | 5 | N/A | N/A | N/A | N/A | N/A | Patients receiving GTR + XRT were found to have a statistically significant improved overall survival rate (HR 0.31, 95% CI 0.10–0.95; $p = 0.040$) |
| Chen (2015) [16] | 38 | N/A | 61 (15–133) | 4.6 | N/A | 66 | 34 | 13 | N/A | Low-grade tumors were associated with increased overall, recurrence-free, and metastasis-free survival. GTR followed by adjuvant RT was associated with longer overall survival and recurrence-free interval but had no impact on metastasis-free interval |
| Cohen-Inbar (2016) [35] | 90 | 133 | 59 (6–183) | 4.9 | 14 (12–16) | 55 | 27.8 | 24.4 | N/A | Margin dose of >16 Gy was a significant predictor of local tumor control. Grade III tumor was a predictor of poor tumor control |
| Kim (2017) [17] | 18 | 40 | 71.8 (3.3–153.3) | 1.2 | 20 (13–30) | 80 | 44.4 | 38.9 | 225.7 | Gamma knife radiosurgery may be used repeatedly at recurrence or progression for long-term control of intracranial lesions. Extracranial metastasis is more common in high-grade HPCs |

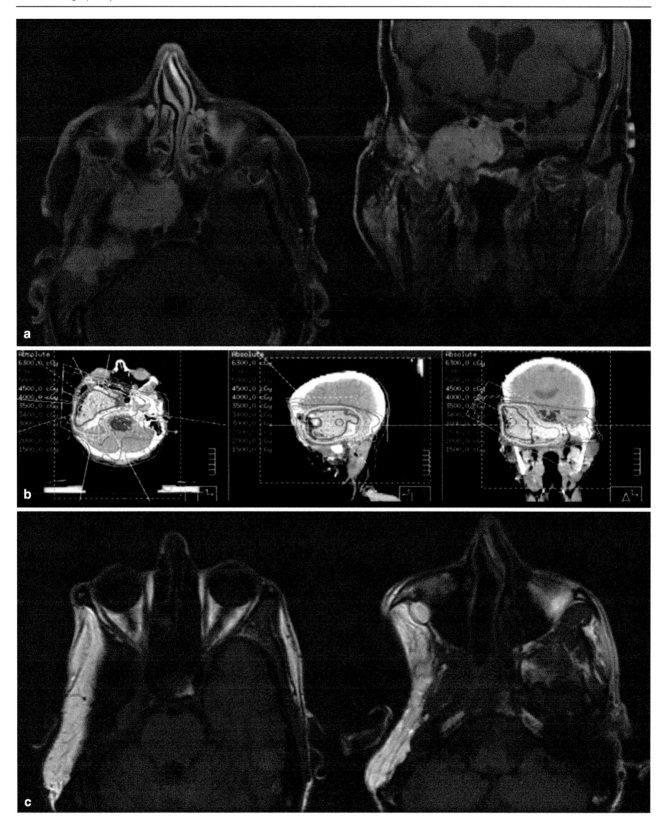

**Fig. 21.2** (**a**) Preoperative MRI showing a HPC located in the right middle cranial fossa. (**b**) Postoperative radiation therapy planning of HPC for residual tumor. (**c**) MRI at 26 months following resection and adjuvant RT showing no local recurrence

and into the right side of the sphenoid sinus. The tumor bed, especially the postoperative contrast-enhancing area on MRI including the margin, was targeted using IMRT technique treated to 60 Gy in 30 fractions (Fig. 21.2b).

Following intervention, the patient developed liver and lung metastasis at 13 months, although imaging of the treatment site remained stable even after 26 months. Complex postoperative changes are seen. Much of the patient's right lateral face and skull base have been resected and replaced by a predominately fatty graft. Some enhancement in the operated sphenoid sinus region was observed, but it did not represent progression and remained stable from previous images (Fig. 21.2c). This strategy demonstrates dose escalation to 60 Gy following tumor resection for effective local tumor control maintenance.

## Summary

- Hemangiopericytomas (HPCs) are characterized by their aggressive phenotypes with high tendencies toward recurrence and distant metastasis.
- Therapeutic intervention of HPCs should involve surgical resection followed by adjuvant radiotherapy (≥50 Gy) for increased local tumor control and overall survival.
- HPCs require close follow-up for prompt intervention of emerging recurrent or metastatic disease.

## Self-Assessment Questions

1. Which findings determine a definitive diagnosis of hemangiopericytoma?
   A. Hyperdense lesion with heterogeneous contrast enhancement on CT
   B. T1 and T2 isodensity with heterogeneous contrast enhancement on MRI
   C. Immunohistochemical analysis showing sheets of ovoid to spindle shaped cells with a staghorn pattern of thin-walled vessels
   D. Immunohistochemical positive staining for vimentin, CD34, and epithelial membrane antigen

2. What is the initial management of hemangiopericytoma to achieve optimal local tumor control?
   A. Surgical resection followed by adjuvant chemotherapy
   B. Chemotherapy followed by adjuvant radiotherapy
   C. Surgical resection followed by adjuvant radiotherapy
   D. Radiotherapy alone
   E. Chemotherapy alone

3. Which of the following mean doses delivered the tumor is most associated with a reduced risk of local recurrence in hemangiopericytoma?
   A. 20 Gy
   B. 30 Gy
   C. 40 Gy
   D. 60 Gy

4. What is an effective follow-up strategy for hemangiopericytoma following initial intervention?
   A. Follow-up head MRI every 3–6 months
   B. Follow-up head MRI every 3–6 months with radiographic assessment of metastasis to the lung and liver
   C. Follow-up head ever 1–2 years
   D. Follow-up head MRI 3 months following initial intervention and then head MRI every year

5. Which of the following is true regarding outcomes associated with radiation therapy in hemangiopericytoma?
   A. Postoperative radiotherapy has a role in improving local control.
   B. Postoperative radiotherapy leads to a decrease in distant recurrence.
   C. Postoperative radiotherapy has not demonstrated efficacy in improving local tumor control.
   D. Neoadjuvant radiotherapy is recommended prior to tumor resection for optimal local tumor control.
   E. Radiotherapy alone has demonstrated improved survival outcomes when compared to tumor resection as an initial management strategy.

## Answers

1. C
2. C
3. D
4. B
5. A

## References

1. Schiariti M, Goetz P, El-Maghraby H, et al. Hemangiopericytoma: long-term outcome revisited. Clinical article. J Neurosurg. 2011;114(3):747–55.
2. Coffey RJ, Cascino TL, Shaw EG. Radiosurgical treatment of recurrent hemangiopericytomas of the meninges: preliminary results. J Neurosurg. 1993;78(6):903–8.
3. Henn W, Wullich B, Thonnes M, et al. Recurrent t(12;19) (q13;q13.3) in intracranial and extracranial hemangiopericytoma. Cancer Genet Cytogenet. 1993;71(2):151–4.
4. Joseph JT, Lisle DK, Jacoby LB, et al. NF2 gene analysis distinguishes hemangiopericytoma from meningioma. Am J Pathol. 1995;147(5):1450–5.

5. Sheehan J, Kondziolka D, Flickinger J, et al. Radiosurgery for treatment of recurrent intracranial hemangiopericytomas. Neurosurgery. 2002;51(4):905–10. discussion 10–1

6. Schweizer L, Koelsche C, Sahm F, et al. Meningeal hemangiopericytoma and solitary fibrous tumors carry the NAB2-STAT6 fusion and can be diagnosed by nuclear expression of STAT6 protein. Acta Neuropathol. 2013;125(5):651–8.

7. Chmielecki J, Crago AM, Rosenberg M, et al. Whole-exome sequencing identifies a recurrent NAB2-STAT6 fusion in solitary fibrous tumors. Nat Genet. 2013;45(2):131–2.

8. Hall WA, Ali AN, Gullett N, et al. Comparing central nervous system (CNS) and extra-CNS hemangiopericytomas in the surveillance, epidemiology, and end results program: analysis of 655 patients and review of current literature. Cancer. 2012;118(21):5331–8.

9. Al-Brahim N, Devilliers R, Provias J. Intraventricular hemangiopericytoma. Ann Diagn Pathol. 2004;8(6):347–51.

10. Vuorinen V, Sallinen P, Haapasalo H, et al. Outcome of 31 intracranial haemangiopericytomas: poor predictive value of cell proliferation indices. Acta Neurochir. 1996;138(12):1399–408.

11. Guthrie BL, Ebersold MJ, Scheithauer BW, et al. Meningeal hemangiopericytoma: histopathological features, treatment, and long-term follow-up of 44 cases. Neurosurgery. 1989;25(4):514–22.

12. Winek RR, Scheithauer BW, Wick MR. Meningioma, meningeal hemangiopericytoma (angioblastic meningioma), peripheral hemangiopericytoma, and acoustic schwannoma. A comparative immunohistochemical study. Am J Surg Pathol. 1989;13(4):251–61.

13. Carneiro SS, Scheithauer BW, Nascimento AG, et al. Solitary fibrous tumor of the meninges: a lesion distinct from fibrous meningioma. A clinicopathologic and immunohistochemical study. Am J Clin Pathol. 1996;106(2):217–24.

14. Molnar P, Nemes Z. Hemangiopericytoma of the cerebello-pontine angle. Diagnostic pitfalls and the diagnostic value of the subunit A of factor XIII as a tumor marker. Clin Neuropathol. 1995;14(1):19–24.

15. Perry A, Scheithauer BW, Nascimento AG. The immunophenotypic spectrum of meningeal hemangiopericytoma: a comparison with fibrous meningioma and solitary fibrous tumor of meninges. Am J Surg Pathol. 1997;21(11):1354–60.

16. Chen LF, Yang Y, Yu XG, et al. Multimodal treatment and management strategies for intracranial hemangiopericytoma. J Clin Neurosci. 2015;22(4):718–25.

17. Kim BS, Kong DS, Seol HJ, et al. Gamma knife radiosurgery for residual or recurrent intracranial hemangiopericytomas. J Clin Neurosci. 2017;35:35–41.

18. Galanis E, Buckner JC, Scheithauer BW, et al. Management of recurrent meningeal hemangiopericytoma. Cancer. 1998;82(10):1915–20.

19. Ecker RD, Marsh WR, Pollock BE, et al. Hemangiopericytoma in the central nervous system: treatment, pathological features, and long-term follow up in 38 patients. J Neurosurg. 2003;98(6):1182–7.

20. Kim JH, Jung HW, Kim YS, et al. Meningeal hemangiopericytomas: long-term outcome and biological behavior. Surg Neurol. 2003;59(1):47–53. discussion –4

21. Sonabend AM, Zacharia BE, Goldstein H, et al. The role for adjuvant radiotherapy in the treatment of hemangiopericytoma: a surveillance, epidemiology, and end results analysis. J Neurosurg. 2014;120(2):300–8.

22. Bastin KT, Mehta MP. Meningeal hemangiopericytoma: defining the role for radiation therapy. J Neurooncol. 1992;14(3):277–87.

23. Dufour H, Metellus P, Fuentes S, et al. Meningeal hemangiopericytoma: a retrospective study of 21 patients with special review of post-operative external radiotherapy. Neurosurgery. 2001;48(4):756–62. discussion 62–3

24. Jaaskelainen J, Servo A, Haltia M, et al. Intracranial hemangiopericytoma: radiology, surgery, radiotherapy, and outcome in 21 patients. Surg Neurol. 1985;23(3):227–36.

25. Mena H, Ribas JL, Pezeshkpour GH, et al. Hemangiopericytoma of the central nervous system: a review of 94 cases. Hum Pathol. 1991;22(1):84–91.

26. Payne BR, Prasad D, Steiner M, et al. Gamma surgery for hemangiopericytomas. Acta Neurochir. 2000;142(5):527–36. discussion 36–7

27. Staples JJ, Robinson RA, Wen BC, et al. Hemangiopericytoma—the role of radiotherapy. Int J Radiat Oncol Biol Phys. 1990;19(2):445–51.

28. Uemura S, Kuratsu J, Hamada J, et al. Effect of radiation therapy against intracranial hemangiopericytoma. Neurol Med Chir (Tokyo). 1992;32(6):328–32.

29. Olson C, Yen CP, Schlesinger D, et al. Radiosurgery for intracranial hemangiopericytomas: outcomes after initial and repeat Gamma Knife surgery. J Neurosurg. 2010;112(1):133–9.

30. Ghia AJ, Allen PK, Mahajan A, et al. Intracranial hemangiopericytoma and the role of radiation therapy: a population based analysis. Neurosurgery. 2013;72(2):203–9.

31. Rutkowski MJ, Jian BJ, Bloch O, et al. Intracranial hemangiopericytoma: clinical experience and treatment considerations in a modern series of 40 adult patients. Cancer. 2012;118(6):1628–36.

32. Park MS, Araujo DM. New insights into the hemangiopericytoma/solitary fibrous tumor spectrum of tumors. Curr Opin Oncol. 2009;21(4):327–31.

33. Ghia AJ, Chang EL, Allen PK, et al. Intracranial hemangiopericytoma: patterns of failure and the role of radiation therapy. Neurosurgery. 2013;73(4):624–30. discussion 30–1

34. Rutkowski MJ, Sughrue ME, Kane AJ, et al. Predictors of mortality following treatment of intracranial hemangiopericytoma. J Neurosurg. 2010;113(2):333–9.

35. Cohen-Inbar O, Lee CC, Mousavi SH, et al. Stereotactic radiosurgery for intracranial hemangiopericytomas: a multicenter study. J Neurosurg. 2017;126(3):744–54.

36. Combs SE, Thilmann C, Debus J, et al. Precision radiotherapy for hemangiopericytomas of the central nervous system. Cancer. 2005;104(11):2457–65.

37. Lee EJ, Kim JH, Park ES, et al. The impact of postoperative radiation therapy on patterns of failure and survival improvement in patients with intracranial hemangiopericytoma. J Neurooncol. 2016;127(1):181–90.

38. Chang SD, Sakamoto GT. The role of radiosurgery for hemangiopericytomas. Neurosurg Focus. 2003;14(5):e14.

39. Soyuer S, Chang EL, Selek U, et al. Intracranial meningeal hemangiopericytoma: the role of radiotherapy: report of 29 cases and review of the literature. Cancer. 2004;100(7):1491–7.

40. Kano H, Niranjan A, Kondziolka D, et al. Adjuvant stereotactic radiosurgery after resection of intracranial hemangiopericytomas. Int J Radiat Oncol Biol Phys. 2008;72(5):1333–9.

41. Sun S, Liu A, Wang C. Gamma knife radiosurgery for recurrent and residual meningeal hemangiopericytomas. Stereotact Funct Neurosurg. 2009;87(2):114–9.

42. Iwai Y, Yamanaka K. Gamma knife radiosurgery for other primary intra-axial tumors. Prog Neurol Surg. 2009;22:129–41.

43. Kim JW, Kim DG, Chung HT, et al. Gamma Knife stereotactic radiosurgery for intracranial hemangiopericytomas. J Neurooncol. 2010;99(1):115–22.

# Stereotactic Radiosurgery for Hemangioblastomas

## 22

Paul Y. Windisch, Erqi L. Pollom, and Scott G. Soltys

## Learning Objectives

- Describe the epidemiology and pathologic and imaging findings of hemangioblastomas.
- Highlight the differences between sporadic and familial hemangioblastomas.
- Review the management options of observation, surgery, radiotherapy, and radiosurgery for hemangioblastomas of the brain and spine.
- Review the published literature reporting tumor control outcomes and toxicity of these management options.
- Detail stereotactic radiosurgery target delineation, dose selection, and normal organ at risk constraints.

## Background Epidemiology

Hemangioblastomas are rare, benign vascular tumors of the central nervous system that occur with an incidence of 0.17 per 100,000 person years, accounting for 0.8% of all reported brain tumors [1]. They do not have a gender predisposition or other known nongenetic risk factors. Hemangioblastomas occur sporadically or are associated with von Hippel-Lindau disease (VHL). Approximately 20% of hemangioblastomas occur in patients with VHL, and 80% of patients with VHL develop hemangioblastomas at some point in their disease course [2, 3]. While patients with sporadic hemangioblastomas are often diagnosed between 40 and 50 years of age,

P. Y. Windisch
Department of Molecular Genetics, German Cancer Research Center (DKFZ), Heidelberg, Germany

E. L. Pollom · S. G. Soltys (✉)
Department of Radiation Oncology, Stanford University, Stanford, CA, USA
e-mail: sgsoltys@stanford.edu

VHL-associated hemangioblastomas occur in younger patients, with an average age of diagnosis of 30 years [4]. Hemangioblastomas in children are extremely rare, with most cases occurring in adolescents older than 15 years [5].

## Risk Factors and Familial Syndromes

While there are no known environmental risk factors for hemangioblastoma, there is a strong association with VHL. VHL is an autosomal dominant disease, caused by a mutation in the von Hippel-Lindau tumor suppressor gene on chromosome 3, with a birth incidence estimated at 1 in 36,000 people. Twenty percent of VHL cases have no family history and are caused by a de novo mutation [6]; the remaining 80% have a known familial linkage. The VHL gene is a tumor suppressor gene that is responsible for the regulation of hypoxia-inducible factor 1 $\alpha$ (HIF1 $\alpha$). If the VHL gene is mutated, it is unable to fulfill this function, and HIF1 $\alpha$ binds to HIF1 $\beta$, leading to increased transcription of a number of genes including VEGF and several other growth factors [7]. Clinically, VHL manifests with renal cell carcinoma and renal cysts, retinal angiomas, pheochromocytomas, pancreatic lesions such as cysts, endolymphatic sac tumors, epididymal cysts, and brain and spinal hemangioblastomas [8].

Approximately 20% of patients with VHL-associated hemangioblastomas have more than one tumor. Multiple sporadic hemangioblastomas are so rare that the presence of two or more hemangioblastomas (or any other VHL-associated tumor entity) suggests a familial history of VHL [6, 9]. Therefore, a patient with a newly diagnosed hemangioblastoma should undergo genetic testing for VHL in addition to screening for the most common VHL-associated tumors such as retinal angiomas, tumors of the abdomen, and pheochromocytomas [4]. Genetic testing can consist of sequencing the VHL gene from DNA in a blood sample, which has a sensitivity and specificity of nearly 100% [9]. Although not all hemangioblastomas are associated with

VHL gene mutations, in a series of 32 sporadic hemangioblastomas, 78% of tumors showed inactivation of the VHL gene, supporting its importance in hemangioblastoma formation [10].

Although considered a benign tumor, failure to control hemangioblastomas can be life-threatening. In a series of 152 patients with VHL, 41% of patients died of progressive hemangioblastomas and 47% of renal cell carcinoma, thereby accounting for 88% of deaths [6].

## Symptoms

Symptoms caused by hemangioblastoma depend on the location of the tumor. Spinal lesions typically present with sensory disturbance, followed by pain and motor symptoms and signs [11, 12]. In the brain, cerebellar symptoms, such as ataxia or imbalance, and headaches are more common, but facial paresis, dizziness, and diplopia have been reported as well [13, 14].

## Diagnosis

Hemangioblastomas are benign tumors of vascular origin that are classified according to the World Health Organization classification system as grade 1 mesenchymal, nonmeningothelial tumors [15]. Macroscopically, hemangioblastomas appear as yellow or red, well-circumscribed tumors that can be solid or have a cystic component. Histologically, large vacuolated stromal cells are accompanied by a high number of vascular cells. Due to the high number of vessels in the tumor, intratumoral hemorrhage can be seen as well. As these characteristics may also apply to metastases formed by renal cell carcinoma, immunohistochemistry may be necessary to distinguish between the two. While epithelial markers and CD10 tend to be positive in renal cell carcinoma and negative in hemangioblastoma, the opposite is true for D2-40 and inhibin alpha.

While histopathology is required to definitively diagnose a hemangioblastoma, tumor characteristics on imaging strongly suggest the diagnosis. Hemangioblastomas are typically T1 isointense, T2 hyperintense, and often surrounded by edema, cysts, or syrinxes. Smaller tumors tend to be more homogenous than large ones. Location also helps with the diagnosis, as most tumors occur in the posterior fossa (brainstem + cerebellum) and the pial surface of the spinal cord [12]. As some hemangioblastomas show intratumoral hemorrhage, low signal intensity can be seen on gradient echo (GRE) sequences from hemosiderin deposits [16]. In addition to MRI, angiography and embolization can play a role in surgical planning [12].

## Multimodality Management Approach

Once diagnosed, management options for hemangioblastomas include observation, surgical resection, radiosurgery, or radiotherapy. As many hemangioblastomas show a biphasic growth pattern with long quiescent phases, the mere presence of an asymptomatic lesion is not an indication for treatment [17, 18]. Clinical considerations in deciding whether and how to treat a patient include the size and growth rate of the tumor, anatomic location, presence of neurological deficits, and if sporadic or VHL-associated. For example, patients with VHL-associated tumors, which are more likely to be multiple and smaller than sporadic hemangioblastomas, might benefit more from SRS as it spares them from repeated surgical procedures. Conversely, surgical resection is required to remove mass effect or edema from larger tumors or those with associated cysts. However, there are no data available on differences in growth rates between sporadic and VHL-associated hemangioblastomas as natural history studies only included patients with VHL [17, 18]. Symptoms are often not caused by the size of the tumors themselves but by tumor-associated cysts and surrounding peritumoral edema or spinal syrinx. Although the actual tumor may remain stable in size, patients may become symptomatic through enlargement of the associated cyst [17].

## Expectant Management with Observation

The incidence of cysts and cystic growth increases with the size of the tumor. In a study of the natural history of untreated VHL-associated hemangioblastomas, Wanebo et al. followed 160 patients for a median of 39 months. They found that although only 44% of tumors grew during this time, 67% of cysts enlarged. Their study was not able to provide a threshold growth rate or tumor size at which treatment should be initiated [17]. However, a study by Ammerman et al., which followed 19 patients with 143 tumors for a mean of 12.4 years suggested threshold size and growth rates which correlated with future symptomatic growth. The authors argue that prophylactic treatment of asymptomatic patients prior to the following thresholds may be considered: cerebellar tumors with a growth rate of greater than $112 \text{ mm}^3$/month or a tumor size larger than $69 \text{ mm}^3$ with a growth rate greater than $14 \text{ mm}^3$/month (100% sensitivity, 72% specificity for symptomatic progression), brainstem tumors larger than $245 \text{ mm}^3$ with growth rates greater than $0.1 \text{ mm}^3$/month (75% sensitivity, 89% specificity), and spinal tumors larger than $22 \text{ mm}^3$ (79% sensitivity, 94% specificity) [18].

Active surveillance is an option for asymptomatic hemangioblastomas, typically with MRI at 6- to 12-month intervals depending on the size of the tumor and cysts, presence of edema, and location near critical structures, with consideration of treatment prior to symptomatic or imaging progression.

## Surgical Management

Surgical resection typically provides local tumor control of over 85% if the tumor can be gross totally resected. Resection is indicated for symptomatic tumors due to mass effect or edema, to obtain histologic confirmation, or for large asymptomatic tumors or those with a cyst, as these may have decreased local control with SRS [19]. In general, surgical series report more posttreatment complications compared to reports of SRS, but the obvious selection biases inherent to such comparisons are at play, in that radiosurgical series are enriched for smaller and asymptomatic tumors compared to those requiring resection [12, 20–22].

In a surgical study of 44 patients with 71 brainstem hemangioblastomas, with a mean follow-up of 5.9 years, local control was achieved in 100%. Postoperative complications occurred in 33%, with 89% of these patients demonstrating neurologic improvement within 6 months. For surgical resection of spinal hemangioblastomas, although similarly excellent local control to intracranial tumors is reported, the risk of complications appears higher: In a study by Lonser et al., in 44 patients with 86 hemangioblastomas who underwent 55 operations, 60% of patients developed neurological deficits after surgery and 9% with permanent deficits, with only 7% improved compared to their preoperative state. Additionally, five cases of CSF leaks occurred, two patients got wound infections, one patient had aseptic meningitis, and one patient died of cardiac-related causes. The same study found that large tumor volume (>500 mm³), neurological deficits at presentation and ventral/ventrolateral location are associated with worse outcomes [22]. Although anatomically, spinal cord hemangioblastomas are at high risk of complications with any treatment intervention, the high risk of surgical complications seen in some series suggests a role for nonsurgical intervention, such as SRS, particularly for asymptomatic lesions.

## Indications for Irradiation

Resection remains the primary definitive treatment for hemangioblastomas, especially if sporadic or large and cystic. Conventionally fractionated external beam radiotherapy (EBRT) or SRS are therapeutic options as a logical extrapolation of the successful and safe treatment of other benign tumors with irradiation.

Historically, SRS was not an option for spinal hemangioblastomas given that early SRS technologies were frame-based. Therefore, non-operable patients were managed with EBRT. However, early experience with EBRT using lower dose showed poor long-term local control. As a result, the role of EBRT for hemangioblastomas was controversial until a report showed that doses greater than 50 Gy improved the disease free-interval from 67 to 129 months [23]. A more recent EBRT series of 31 brain and spinal tumors found that 50–55.8 Gy led to a 5-year disease-free survival of 80% for VHL-associated tumors. Outcomes for sporadic tumors with these doses were still comparatively poor, with a 5-year disease-free survival on only 48% [24].

Advances in image guidance and treatment planning and delivery systems have enabled non-frame-based SRS, and more data has been emerging for the use of SRS to treat hemangioblastomas (see Table 22.1). In contrast to EBRT, SRS allows the delivery of ablative doses to tumors while minimizing the amount of normal tissue irradiated through rapid dose falloff at the periphery of the target. Recent series suggest a high-rate local control (>90% after 5 years and 80% after 10 years) with a low risk of post-SRS complications [3, 26, 31]. The largest series, reported by Kano et al., reviewed the outcomes of 186 patients treated with SRS for intracranial hemangioblastomas. Local control was 89% and 79% at 5 and 10 years. Adverse radiation effects occurred in 7% of patients, including one fatality [13]. In a study by Pan et al., 28 patients with 46 spinal hemangioblastomas were treated with SRS. Local control was 92% at 5 years with no reported adverse radiation effects [31]. As patients with VHL typically have multiple tumors over time, SRS as an attractive treatment option as it can spare patients of repeated operations [31]. Similar to the EBRT experience, tumor control with SRS appears better for VHL-associated hemangioblastomas than for sporadic tumors [13, 26].

Although retrospective reports have demonstrated consistently good local control outcomes with SRS, one small prospective observational study showed worse outcomes [2]. On this study, 20 patients were treated with SRS to a mean dose of 18.9 Gy. Local control at 5, 10, and 15 years was only 83%, 61%, and 51%, respectively, and the authors concluded that SRS should only be used for lesions not surgically resectable. However, SRS was performed at multiple centers, over a long enrollment period, and dosimetric details of the plans are not reported. Contemporary series with modern imaging and dosimetry may lead to better long-term outcomes.

## Target Volume Delineation

SRS series have not consistently reported detailed GTV definitions. At the authors' institution, only the nodular tumor is delineated as the GTV when there is a large cyst that poses unfavorable dosimetry or high risk of adverse radiation

**Table 22.1** Selected literature review of local tumor control of hemangioblastomas following observation, surgery, external beam radiotherapy (EBRT), or stereotactic radiosurgery (SRS)

| Citation | Brain vs. spine (%) | Number of patients | Number of tumors | Percent of patients with VHL | Management | Total dose in Gy (range) | Median/mean tumor size in cm³ (range) | Median/mean follow-up in months (range) | Local control — Crude | 3 years | 5 years | 10 years | 15 years | Toxicity | Notes |
|---|---|---|---|---|---|---|---|---|---|---|---|---|---|---|---|
| Kano (2015) [13] | 100% brain | 186 | 517 | 43% | SRS | 17.7 Gy (VHL) and 16.1 Gy (sporadic) (8–31.4 Gy) | Median: 0.2 cm³ for VHL, 0.7 cm³ for sporadic (0.01–39.5 cm³) | Median: 115 (6–240) | | VHL: 95% Sporadic: 87% | VHL: 93% Sporadic: 81% | VHL: 82% Sporadic: 75% | | Thirteen patients (7%) developed ARE, one grade 5 | VHL has better local control than sporadic |
| Puataweepong (2014) [25] | 100% brain | 14 | 56 | 64% | SRS | Median 20 Gy in 1–5 fractions | 0.26 cm³ (range, 0.026–20.4 cm³) | Median: 24 (11–89) | | 88% (2 years) | 73% (6 years) | | | NR | |
| Hanakita (2014) [26] | 100% brain | 21 | 57 | 67% | SRS | Median 18 Gy (14–20 Gy) | Median: 0.13 cm³ (0.004–9.5 cm³) | Median: 96 (3–235) | | | VHL: 97% Sporadic: 67% | VHL: 83% Sporadic: 44% | | 14% with ARE (all reversible within 1 year) | |
| Selch (2012) [27] | 100% spine | 9 | 20 | 56% | SRS | 12–14 Gy | Median: 0.72 cm³ (0.08–14.4 cm³) | Median: 51 (14–86) | | | 90% (4 years) | | | None | |
| Daly (2011) [28] | 100% spine | 19 | 27 | 74% | SRS | 20–22 Gy in 1–3 fractions | Median: 0.16 cm³ (0.06–9.80 cm³) | Median: 33.7 (6.6–84.0) | | 86% | | | | Three patients (grade 1 in two, grade 2 in one) | |
| Sayer (2011) [29] | 100% brain | 14 | 26 | 50% | SRS | 18 Gy (10–25 Gy) | Median 1.1 cm³ (0.08–9.02 cm³) | Median: 36 (6–144) | | | 74% | 50% | | NR | |
| Karabagli (2010) [30] | 100% brain | 13 | 34 | 54% | SRS | 15.8 Gy (range: 12–25 Gy) | Median 0.22 cm³ (0.0005–0.91 cm³) | Mean: 50 (24–116) | 100% (at last study follow up) | | | | | None | |
| Asthagiri (2010) [2] | 85% brain 11% spine | 10 | 44 | 100% | SRS | 18.9 Gy (12–24 Gy) | Median: 0.03 cm³ (0.01–0.4 cm³) | Median: 96 (36–211) | | 91% (2 years) | 83% | 61% | 51% | None | Mean time to progression after SRS: 5.9 years |
| Pan (2017) [31] | 100% spine | 28 | 46 | 50% | SRS | 21.6 Gy (15–35 Gy) in 1–5 fractions | Median 0.264 cm³ (0.025–70.9 cm³) | Mean: 54.3 (3–157) | | | 92% | | | None | |
| Li (2016) [21] | 100% spine | 25 | 29 | 64% | Surgery | | NR | Median: 21.3 | 100% (at last follow-up) | | | | | 4% | |
| Mandigo (2009) [12] | 100% spine | 15 | 18 | NR | Surgery | | NR | Median: 31 (15–72) | | | | | | 20% | |

| Study | | | | | | | | | | | | |
|---|---|---|---|---|---|---|---|---|---|---|---|---|
| Lonser (2003) [22] | 100% spine | 44 | 86 | 100% | Surgery | | NR | Mean: 44 | | | 60% acute toxicity; 9% permanent toxicity | |
| Wind (2011) [32] | 100% brain | 44 | 71 | 100% | Surgery | | Median: 0.9 cm³ (0.01–7.2 cm³) | Mean: 71 (12–250) | | | 20% acute toxicity, 2% permanent toxicity | |
| Wu (2013) [20] | 100% brain | 11 | 11 | ? | Surgery | | 28.5 cm³ | Median: 41 (2–91) | 100% (at last follow-up) | | 45% | |
| Lonser (2014) [33] | 64% brain 36% spine | 225 | 1921 at beginning, 2336 at last evaluation | 100% | Observation | | Median total tumor volume per patient 0.182 (0.012–11.919) cm³ | Mean 83 (25–108) | 51% (at last follow-up) | | 49% overall grew in a salutatory (72%), linear (6%), or exponential (22%) pattern | |
| Simone (2011) [34] | NR | 7 | 84 | 100% | EBRT | 44.2 Gy (43.2–45.0 Gy) For brain; 44.1 Gy (37.5–51.6 Gy) for spine | Mean: 3.59 cm³ (0.02–22.15 cm³) | Median: 73.8 (40.3–155.6) | | | | |
| Koh (2007) [24] | 71% brain 29% spine | 18 | 31 | 28% | EBRT | 50.0–55.8 Gy | | Median: 61 (1–174) | | | 44% grade 1 | |
| Smalley (1990) [23] | 100% brain | 27 | 27 | 22% | EBRT | Either >50 Gy or <50 Gy | NR | Median: 99 | | >50 Gy: 80% <50 Gy: 30% | 4% encephalopathy | VHL outcomes better than sporadic |

effect. This approach is based on extrapolating from the surgical approach, where durable local control can be achieved with surgical resection of the mural nodule alone (rather than the entire cystic structure) [35]. Limiting the target volume in this way allows for safe dose escalation that could further improve upon SRS outcomes. For smaller, mixed solid/cystic lesions, where the inclusion of the cyst does not significantly change the treatment volume, the entire cyst in included in the target volume.

## Radiation Dose Prescription and Normal Critical Structure Tolerance Constraints

As larger or symptomatic tumors are usually surgically resected, tumor sizes in SRS series are typically small, with median size ranging from 0.03 to 1.1 cm$^3$ (see Table 22.1). Reported SRS doses vary widely, with the typical opposing considerations of local control balanced with SRS toxicity. As seen in Table 22.1, median doses range from 12 to 31 Gy in a single fraction. Hanakita et al. reported their series of 57 intracranial hemangioblastomas treated with SRS with tumor control rates of 94% and 80% at 5 and 10 years and found no significant effect on tumor control for doses >18 Gy [26]. Although a clear dose response is not seen among the series, the suboptimal local control associated with doses smaller than 50 Gy with conventional radiotherapy suggests that there is an opportunity for dose escalation [23]. As such, at the author's institution, intracranial tumors that are smaller than 1.5 cm in maximum diameter typically receive 18–22 Gy, similar to the higher doses for brain metastases as per RTOG 9005, rather than typical benign tumor doses of 13–16 Gy. Larger tumors are treated with 16 Gy or with hypofractionated SRS to a similar equivalent dose.

In the spinal cord, greater concern exists for post-SRS toxicity. Daly et al. reported the only detailed analysis of spinal cord dosimetry and outcomes from spinal SRS for hemangioblastomas [28, 36]. This review of 27 spinal hemangioblastoma treated with a median single fraction spinal SRS dose of 20 Gy showed a 3-year local control of 86%. Of note, 30% of tumors on this study had undergone previous attempt at resection and were treated for residual or recurrent disease. Despite the highest reported doses to the human spinal cord (a median maximum dose of 22.7 Gy), with maximum doses up to 30.9 Gy, the freedom from grade 2 or higher neurologic adverse effects was 96%. Doses higher than the typical spinal cord constraint of 14 Gy to a 0.03 cc volume per RTOG 0631 [37] have been routinely given to the human spinal cord for spinal metastases in other series [38].

At the authors' institution, small spinal hemangioblastomas are typically treated with 16 Gy in a single fraction, limiting the volume of cord getting greater than 10 Gy to less than 0.35 cm$^3$, as per RTOG 0631 and previously reported to be a clinically safe constraint [38]. While we don't advocate

for higher doses as retrospectively reported [36], these data highlight that the true tolerance of the human spinal cord to the partial volume dosimetry seen in SRS is unknown. Further data may reveal that human cord tolerance may be similar to animal data [39], where the 5% and 50% risk of myelopathy occur at maximum doses of 18.2 and 20.0 Gy, respectively.

## Radiation Toxicity: Stereotactic Radiosurgery Adverse Radiation Effects

Acknowledging that retrospective series are prone to underreporting of adverse effects, the risk of adverse radiation effect (ARE) following SRS for hemangioblastoma varies from 0% to 20% (see Table 22.1), within the range expected for SRS to any tumor. Most reported adverse effects were reversible. However, a grade 5 ARE following SRS [13] and radiation necrosis following EBRT [24] have been reported. Given that most spinal hemangioblastomas treated with SRS are small, the partial volume dosimetry encountered with SRS does not lend itself to formal traditional normal tissue complication probability (NTCP) modeling [36]. Additionally, smaller volumes of the spinal cord can tolerate doses exceeding the typical constraint of 14 Gy in one fraction.

## Prognostic Factors of Outcome

The prognosis after complete neurosurgical resection of a sporadic hemangioblastoma is excellent. However, patients with VHL-associated hemangioblastomas fare worse clinically, as they commonly develop new lesions [15].

Tumor control after SRS is reported as high as 90% after 5 years (see Table 22.1) and is higher for tumors that are small, solid, or VHL-associated [26, 31]. In general, female sex, young age, a high Karnofsky Performance Status, fewer tumors, and the absence of neurological symptoms correlate with increased survival [3].

## Follow-Up

Clinical and imaging follow-up recommendations depend on whether a patient has VHL or not. In most series, the first posttreatment MRI occurs 3–6 months following treatment, with subsequent imaging at 6–24 months, which depends if there are other untreated tumors or symptoms to be followed and time from treatment.

For VHL-associated hemangioblastomas, surveillance should include craniospinal MRI annually, abdominal sonography or MRI, audiometry, and screening for retinal angiomas and pheochromocytomas (fractionated metanephrines) [4, 31, 40].

## Conclusion

Given the rarity of hemangioblastomas, the reported experience with SRS in this disease has been limited to small, retrospective, single-institutional series. The heterogeneity with regard to tumor location, tumor size, SRS dosimetry, and follow-up across studies makes it challenging to compare outcomes and toxicity of this treatment modality to surgical outcomes. However, the emerging body of data thus far suggests that SRS for treatment of spinal and intracranial hemangioblastomas provides effective local control with an acceptable risk of adverse effects and may be a particularly attractive therapeutic alternative for patients with VHL who would otherwise need multiple open surgical procedures throughout their lives. Moving forward, creating a national, prospective registry for hemangioblastomas would allow standardized collection of detailed treatment and outcome data. Longer-term follow-up and better reporting of local control and ARE outcomes are needed to optimize SRS parameters and fully realize the potential of SRS in caring for patients with hemangioblastomas.

## Case Study

A representative treatment plan is shown in Fig. 22.1. A 24-year-old man with VHL had brain and spinal hemangioblastomas previously treated with four spinal surgical resections. Although a slowly progressive 5 mm left lateral L1 hemangioblastoma was not symptomatic, he pursued spinal stereotactic radiosurgery, as he desired no further open surgical interventions. Panel a and b: The L1 hemangioblastoma (red contour) was defined by post-contrast CT and MRI and treated with 16 Gy in 1 fraction to the 80% isodose line (green isodose line). Although the spinal cord (yellow contour) maximum dose was 17.5 Gy, the spinal cord volume encompassed by 10 Gy (cyan isodose line) was only 0.21 cm³, with a cord dose to 0.03 cm³ of 13.9 Gy, within the partial volume dose constraints of RTOG 0631. Follow-up imaging 7 years later (panel c) confirmed local control, without toxicity.

## Summary

- Hemangioblastomas are rare, benign vascular tumors of the posterior fossa and the spinal cord.
- Active surveillance, neurosurgical resection, and stereotactic radiosurgery are the most common management options for hemangioblastomas.
- Patients with a hemangioblastoma should receive genetic testing for VHL and screening for associated tumors.

## Self-Assessment Questions

1. In 20% of cases, hemangioblastoma is associated with which familial disease?
   A. Neurofibromatosis Type 1
   B. von Hippel-Lindau disease
   C. Li-Fraumeni syndrome
   D. MEN-2

2. Which of the following is *not* a common location of hemangioblastoma?
   A. Cerebrum
   B. Cerebellum
   C. Spinal cord
   D. Brainstem

3. Which of the following is *not* a common option for dealing with hemangioblastoma patients?
   A. Stereotactic radiosurgery
   B. Surgery
   C. Systemic chemotherapy
   D. Fractionated radiotherapy

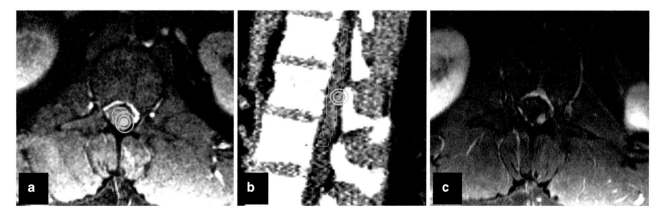

**Fig. 22.1** Representative treatment plan of a spinal hemangioblastoma from the case study

4. Which of the following statements is *false*?
   A. Female sex is associated with increased survival in hemangioblastoma patients.
   B. Adverse radiation effects after SRS for hemangioblastomas appear to be higher than for other benign tumors treated with SRS.
   C. Hemangioblastomas account for less than 5% of all brain tumors.
   D. Local tumor control 5 years after stereotactic radiosurgery is typical 80% or higher.

5. Which of the following tumors is usually *not* associated with VHL?
   A. Gastrointestinal stromal tumor
   B. Retinal angioma
   C. Pheochromocytoma
   D. Hemangioblastoma

## Answers

1. B
2. A
3. C
4. B
5. A

## References

1. Ostrom QT, Gittleman H, Xu J, et al. CBTRUS statistical report: primary brain and other central nervous system tumors diagnosed in the United States in 2009–2013. Neuro Oncol. 2016;18(Suppl 5):v1–v75.
2. Asthagiri AR, Mehta GU, Zach L, et al. Prospective evaluation of radiosurgery for hemangioblastomas in von Hippel–Lindau disease. Neuro Oncol. 2010;12(1):80–6.
3. Kano H, Niranjan A, Mongia S, et al. The role of stereotactic radiosurgery for intracranial hemangioblastomas. Neurosurgery. 2008;63(3):443–50. discussion 450–1.
4. Bamps S, Calenbergh FV, Vleeschouwer SD, et al. What the neurosurgeon should know about hemangioblastoma, both sporadic and in Von Hippel-Lindau disease: a literature review. Surg Neurol Int. 2013;4:145.
5. CBTRUS. CBTRUS statistical report: primary brain and central nervous system tumors diagnosed in the United States in 2004–2008 (March 23, 2012 revision). Source: Central Brain Tumor Registry of the United States, Hinsdale, IL; 2012. http://www.cbtrus.org/2012-NPCR-SEER/CBTRUS_Report_2004-2008_3-23-2012.pdf.
6. Maher ER, Yates JR, Harries R, et al. Clinical features and natural history of von Hippel-Lindau disease. Q J Med. 1990;77(283):1151–63.
7. Bader HL, Hsu T. Systemic VHL gene functions and the VHL disease. FEBS Lett. 2012;586(11):1562–9.
8. Maher ER, Neumann HP, Richard S. von Hippel-Lindau disease: a clinical and scientific review. Eur J Hum Genet. 2011;19(6):617–23.
9. Decker J, Neuhaus C, Macdonald F, et al. Clinical utility gene card for: von Hippel–Lindau (VHL). Eur J Hum Genet. 2013;22(4). https://doi.org/10.1038/ejhg.2013.180.
10. Shankar GM, Taylor-Weiner A, Lelic N, et al. Sporadic hemangioblastomas are characterized by cryptic VHL inactivation. Acta Neuropathol Commun. 2014;2:167.
11. Na JH, Kim HS, Eoh W, et al. Spinal cord hemangioblastoma: diagnosis and clinical outcome after surgical treatment. J Korean Neurosurg Soc. 2007;42(6):436–40.
12. Mandigo CE, Ogden AT, Angevine PD, et al. Operative management of spinal hemangioblastoma. Neurosurgery. 2009;65(6):1166–77.
13. Kano H, Shuto T, Iwai Y, et al. Stereotactic radiosurgery for intracranial hemangioblastomas: a retrospective international outcome study. J Neurosurg. 2015;122(6):1469–78.
14. Dwarakanath S, Suri A, Sharma BS, et al. Intracranial hemangioblastomas: an institutional experience. Neurol India. 2006;54(3):276–8.
15. International Agency for Research on Cancer. WHO classification of tumours of the central nervous system. Geneva: World Health Organization; 2016.
16. Ho VB, Smirniotopoulos JG, Murphy FM, et al. Radiologic-pathologic correlation: hemangioblastoma. AJNR Am J Neuroradiol. 1992;13(5):1343–52.
17. Wanebo JE, Lonser RR, Glenn GM. The natural history of hemangioblastomas of the central nervous system in patients with von Hippel–Lindau disease. J Neurosurg. 2003;98:82–94.
18. Ammerman JM, Lonser RR, Dambrosia J, et al. Long-term natural history of hemangioblastomas in patients with von Hippel–Lindau disease: implications for treatment. J Neurosurg. 2006;105(2):248–55.
19. Matsunaga S, Shuto T, Inomori S, et al. Gamma knife radiosurgery for intracranial haemangioblastomas. Acta Neurochir. 2007;149(10):1007–13. discussion 1013
20. Wu P, Liang C, Wang Y, et al. Microneurosurgery in combination with endovascular embolisation in the treatment of solid haemangioblastoma in the dorsal medulla oblongata. Clin Neurol Neurosurg. 2013;115(6):651–7.
21. Li X, Wang J, Niu J, et al. Diagnosis and microsurgical treatment of spinal hemangioblastoma. Neurol Sci. 2016;37(6):899–906.
22. Lonser RR, Weil RJ, Wanebo JE. Surgical management of spinal cord hemangioblastomas in patients with von Hippel–Lindau disease. J Neurosurg. 2003;98:106–16.
23. Smalley SR, Schomberg PJ, Earle JD, et al. Radiotherapeutic considerations in the treatment of hemangioblastomas of the central nervous system. Int J Radiat Oncol Biol Phys. 1990;18(5):1165–71.
24. Koh E-S, Nichol A, Millar B-A, et al. Role of fractionated external beam radiotherapy in hemangioblastoma of the central nervous system. Int J Radiat Oncol Biol Phys. 2007;69(5):1521–6.
25. Puataweepong P, Dhanachai M, Hansasuta A, et al. The clinical outcome of intracranial hemangioblastomas treated with linac-based stereotactic radiosurgery and radiotherapy. J Radiat Res. 2014;55(4):761–8.
26. Hanakita S, Koga T, Shin M, et al. The long-term outcomes of radiosurgery for intracranial hemangioblastomas. Neuro Oncol. 2014;16(3):429–33.
27. Selch MT, Tenn S, Agazaryan N, et al. Image-guided linear accelerator-based spinal radiosurgery for hemangioblastoma. Surg Neurol Int. 2012;3:73.
28. Daly ME, Choi CYH, Gibbs IC, et al. Tolerance of the spinal cord to stereotactic radiosurgery: insights from hemangioblastomas. Int J Radiat Oncol Biol Phys. 2011;80(1):213–20.
29. Sayer FT, Nguyen J, Starke RM, et al. Gamma knife radiosurgery for intracranial hemangioblastomas—outcome at 3 years. World Neurosurg. 2011;75(1):99–105. discussion 45–8

30. Karabagli H, Genc A, Karabagli P, et al. Outcomes of gamma knife treatment for solid intracranial hemangioblastomas. J Clin Neurosci. 2010;17(6):706–10.

31. Pan J, Ho AL, D'Astous M, et al. Image-guided stereotactic radiosurgery for treatment of spinal hemangioblastoma. Neurosurg Focus. 2017;42(1):E12.

32. Wind JJ, Bakhtian KD, Sweet JA, et al. Long-term outcome after resection of brainstem hemangioblastomas in von Hippel-Lindau disease. J Neurosurg. 2011;114(5):1312–8.

33. Lonser RR, Butman JA, Huntoon K, et al. Prospective natural history study of central nervous system hemangioblastomas in von Hippel-Lindau disease. J Neurosurg. 2014;120(5):1055–62.

34. Simone CB 2nd, Lonser RR, Ondos J, et al. Infratentorial craniospinal irradiation for von Hippel-Lindau: a retrospective study supporting a new treatment for patients with CNS hemangioblastomas. Neuro Oncol. 2011;13(9):1030–6.

35. Jeffreys R. Clinical and surgical aspects of posterior fossa haemangioblastomata. J Neurol Neurosurg Psychiatry. 1975;38(2):105–11.

36. Daly ME, Luxton G, Choi CYH, et al. Normal tissue complication probability estimation by the Lyman-Kutcher-Burman method does not accurately predict spinal cord tolerance to stereotactic radiosurgery. Int J Radiat Oncol Biol Phys. 2012;82(5):2025–32.

37. Ryu S, Pugh SL, Gerszten PC, et al. RTOG 0631 phase 2/3 study of image guided stereotactic radiosurgery for localized (1-3) spine metastases: phase 2 results. Pract Radiat Oncol. 2014;4(2):76–81.

38. Schipani S, Wen W, Jin JY, et al. Spine radiosurgery: a dosimetric analysis in 124 patients who received 18 Gy. Int J Radiat Oncol Biol Phys. 2012;84(5):e571–6.

39. Medin PM, Foster RD, van der Kogel AJ, et al. Spinal cord tolerance to single-fraction partial-volume irradiation: a swine model. Int J Radiat Oncol Biol Phys. 2011;79(1):226–32.

40. VHL Surveillance guidelines. VHL Alliance. http://vhl.org/wp-content/uploads/2016/05/Surveillance-guidelines.pdf. Published 2016. Accessed 24 Jan 2017.

# NF2-Related Tumors and Malignant Peripheral Nerve Sheath Tumors

# 23

Timothy D. Struve, Luke E. Pater, and John Breneman

## Learning Objectives

- Identify the genetic factors associated with NF2.
- List the CNS tumors which have an increased incidence in patients with NF2.
- Describe the differences in epidemiology of CNS tumors in patients with and without NF2.
- Discuss the differences in therapeutic decision-making for treatment of CNS tumors in NF2 and non-NF2 patients.
- Describe the differences in prognosis and treatment outcomes of CNS tumors in NF2 and non-NF2 patients.
- Describe the work-up and prognosis of malignant peripheral nerve sheath tumor (MPNST).
- Discuss the role of radiotherapy in the treatment of MPNST.

## Background

Neurofibromatosis type 2 (NF2) is a multiple neoplasia syndrome caused by a mutation in the *NF2* gene on chromosome 22 [1]. The condition was first described in 1822 in a deaf patient with tumors of the skull, dura mater, and brain [2]. Initially thought to be linked to neurofibromatosis type 1 (NF1), it was not until 1987 that the two conditions were formally separated after they were localized to different chromosomes [3, 4]. NF2 patients are prone to develop vestibular schwannomas (the bilateral form being pathognomonic of the condition), non-vestibular schwannomas, meningiomas, spinal ependymomas and astrocytomas, and neurofibromas, as well as non-tumor conditions such as juvenile cataracts, epiretinal membranes, retinal hamartomas,

and cutaneous lesions [1]. These patients pose a particular challenge to radiation oncologists as they often present at a young age and form tumors in eloquent locations.

## Epidemiology

The birth incidence for NF2 is 1 in 25,000 live births. As many as 7% of patients with vestibular schwannoma may have NF2 and that risk increases as the age of the patient decreases [1, 5]. NF2 shows a wide phenotypic variability and nearly 100% penetrance by 60 years of age [6].

## Risk Factors and Genetics

NF2 is an autosomal-dominant mutation in the *NF2* tumor suppressor gene on chromosome 22q12. The mutation affects the 69 kDa protein product called merlin (moesin-ezrin-radixin-like protein), also known as schwannomin. Merlin acts through several intermediary steps and ultimately regulates the phosphoinositide-3 kinase (PI3K) and the mitogen-activated protein kinase (MAPK) signaling pathways. These pathways are known to promote cell growth, protein translation, and cellular proliferation [1].

Approximately half of patients inherit one affected allele from a parent in an autosomal-dominant manner, and the other half acquires a de novo mutation in *NF2*. Tumor formation is a result of the loss of function in the wild-type *NF2* allele in susceptible target organs, i.e., the "two-hit hypothesis." Patients who develop NF2 through a de novo mutation will exhibit somatic mosaicism, and the later the mutation is acquired, generally the milder the disease phenotype will be [1]. If NF2-related tumors are predominantly on one side of the body, mosaicism may be particularly likely [5].

While there is phenotypic heterogeneity of the disease within the general population, the phenotypic expression

T. D. Struve · L. E. Pater · J. Breneman (✉)
Department of Radiation Oncology, University of Cincinnati, Cincinnati, OH, USA
e-mail: john.breneman@uc.edu

© Springer International Publishing AG, part of Springer Nature 2018
E. L. Chang et al. (eds.), *Adult CNS Radiation Oncology*, https://doi.org/10.1007/978-3-319-42878-9_23

of NF2 within a family is often similar [1]. This interfamilial phenotypic heterogeneity is related to different mutations within the *NF2* gene itself. *NF2* nonsense or frameshift mutations lead to truncated proteins and are associated with severe disease, whereas missense mutations and in-frame or large deletions are associated with mild disease [1, 7, 8].

## Clinical Presentation

NF2 typically presents in the third decade of life in the form of hearing loss from vestibular schwannoma. Children with NF2 more frequently present with non-vestibular schwannomas and symptoms such as visual and skin manifestations, spinal tumors, or other intracranial, non-vestibular tumors [1].

## Diagnosis and Screening

The diagnosis of NF2 is based on clinical criteria, and constitutional *NF2* mutation is not part of the present diagnostic requirement. The most recent and widely used diagnostic criteria are the Manchester criteria (Table 23.1).

Screening of NF2 patients, or children of NF2-affected parents, for NF2-related tumors should begin at an early age. Magnetic resonance imaging (MRI) of the head and spine starts at age 10–12 years or even earlier in severely affected families. MRI screening should occur every 2 years for patients less than 20 years old and every 3 years for older patients. Once tumors are identified on screening MRI, annual follow-up scans should be obtained until the growth rate is determined [1, 9]. MRI screening is supplemented with yearly ophthalmologic, neurologic, and audiology exams which these patients should have beginning in infancy.

**Table 23.1** Manchester criteria for the diagnosis of NF2. Patients must have the primary finding plus one or more of the associated additional findings

| Primary finding | Additional findings needed for diagnosis |
|---|---|
| Bilateral vestibular schwannomas | • None |
| Family history of NF2 | • Unilateral vestibular schwannoma or two NF2-associated lesions (meningioma, glioma, neurofibroma, schwannoma, or cataract) |
| Unilateral vestibular schwannoma | • Two additional NF2-associated lesions (meningioma, glioma, neurofibroma, schwannoma, or cataract) |
| Multiple meningiomas | • Unilateral vestibular schwannoma or two other NF2-associated lesions (glioma, neurofibroma, schwannoma, or cataract) |

Based on data from Refs. [1, 9]

## NF2-Related Tumors

While many of the tumors that NF2 patients are prone to develop also occur in the sporadic population, it is important for the radiation oncologist to know the distinguishing features of these tumors in NF2 and the different management approach utilized when these tumors develop as part of the NF2 syndrome.

## Vestibular Schwannoma

### Epidemiology

Bilateral VS are a distinguishing feature of this syndrome with 90–95% of NF2 patients being affected [1]. NF2-related VS exhibit several differing clinical characteristics compared to their sporadic counterparts. Sporadic VS tends to originate in the inferior vestibular portion of the vestibulocochlear nerve, whereas in NF2, there is predilection for the superior branch [5, 10–12]. NF2-associated VS tumors are diagnosed at a younger age than non-NF2 VS. They often exhibit a more lobular growth pattern and are more adherent to adjacent cranial nerves [13].

Reported growth rates of NF2-related VS are highly variable in the literature, but there appears to be a trend toward higher growth rate in younger patients [14]. Investigators from the House Ear Institute reported on the natural history of 84 NF2-related VS. They found a mostly linear growth rate with a mean growth of 1.3–1.9 mm/year [15]. Dirks et al., on the other hand, found that approximately half of patients will exhibit a saltatory pattern characterized by patterns of growth and intervening quiescence. Over a mean follow-up period of 9.5 years, they observed the overall growth rate to be approximately 0.6 cm$^3$ per year [16]. While larger tumors appear to be associated with worse hearing, the rate of hearing loss does not appear to be associated with tumor growth [17–19].

### Diagnosis

Vestibular schwannomas have a characteristic appearance on MRI which is iso- to slightly hypointense on T1-weighted images, and they enhance brightly with contrast administration. They are typically solid and nodular though there may be associated cystic components, especially in larger tumors. Most have an intracanalicular component, and many extend into the cerebellopontine angle. The primary differential diagnosis is between VS and meningioma, the latter often distinguished by its dural tail. Occasionally metastases will present with a similar appearance.

The radiographic appearance of VS is usually diagnostic, so the great majority of patients do not undergo biopsy prior to treatment. Histologically, neoplastic Schwann cells form two basic patterns; Antoni A pattern has compact, elongated cells, while Antoni B pattern is less cellular with loosely textured cells with indistinct processes.

## Overall Treatment Strategy for NF2-Related Vestibular Schwannoma

The management of non-NF2-related vestibular schwannoma (VS) is described in Chap. 4. Here, we discuss the management of these tumors in this special population. Management of these tumors is challenging and is best done at a high-volume center with a multidisciplinary approach. The focus of treatment should be on quality of life including hearing and facial nerve preservation. Initial observation should be considered for small tumors in patients with good serviceable hearing.

### Surgery

For patients with small, bilateral VS and intact hearing, an attempt at hearing preserving surgery on one side should be considered. If successful, resection of the contralateral tumor can be performed subsequently. However, even in expert hands, hearing preservation rates are less than 50% with this approach. Surgical morbidity associated with these tumors is related to the fact that NF2-related VS are often multifocal and intimately associated with the facial nerve [9]. Large tumors in non-hearing ears which show progression on serial imaging should also be considered for resection, especially if they are associated with mass effect. Outcomes for resection of NF2-associated VS are given in Table 23.2.

### Systemic Therapy

Interest in systemic therapy has increased in recent years. It is important to note that while the majority of data regarding systemic therapy for NF2-related tumors focuses on VS, results may be applicable to other NF2-related tumors given that the underlying genetic driver is the same.

The focus of systemic therapies has been inhibition of the merlin signaling pathways. VEGF inhibitors such as bevaci-zumab have shown early promise. Plotkin et al. have published the largest series of patients treated with bevacizumab for NF2-associated VS to date. In their analysis of 31 patients, 87% and 54% of patients had either decreased tumor size or stable disease at 1 and 3 years, respectively [20]. Other smaller series have shown similar promising results [21]. Additional agents such as lapatinib, nilotinib, and mTOR inhibitors are also being investigated and show promise in preclinical studies and small patient series [21].

## Indications for Irradiation

There has been some reluctance to consider radiotherapy for NF2-related VS. The principle concerns are limited data regarding long-term control, especially in this young patient population, and concerns over secondary malignancy. Nonetheless, radiotherapy, especially radiosurgery, is increasingly being used in the management of NF2-related VS. Radiosurgery is an attractive option as it is noninvasive, is associated with low risks of facial nerve dysfunction, and results in relatively good local control [22–28]. Radiotherapy is generally indicated when there is evidence of growth of a VS and there is functional hearing in the affected ear. Preservation of any existing hearing in NF2 patients is especially important since virtually all have bilateral tumors putting them at risk for complete hearing loss. In general, long-term control rates are between 80% and 90% with hearing preserved in 30–50% of patients who had serviceable hearing prior to treatment. The rates of facial nerve complications are less than 10% when using modern radiosurgery techniques and dosing (Table 23.3).

## Radiation Technique

The radiation techniques for NF2-related VS are similar to non-NF2 tumors and are described in Chap. 4. There are, however, additional considerations in this special population. These patients are generally younger, and there are theoretical concerns of increased secondary malignancy risks in these patients. Therefore, every attempt to limit integral dose should be made.

**Table 23.2** Results for surgical resection of acoustic schwannoma in patients with NF2

| Author | Pub year | N | Surgery | Follow-up (mo) | Local control | Hearing preserved | Facial nerve injury |
|---|---|---|---|---|---|---|---|
| Samii et al. | 1997 | 120 | Suboccipital | n/a | n/a | 36% | 33% |
| Doyle and Shelton | 1993 | 13 | Middle fossa | Up to 240 | 77% | 39% | 20% |
| Slattery et al. | 1998 | 23 | Middle fossa | n/a | n/a | 48% | 0% |
| Moffat et al. | 2003 | 15 | Translabyrinthine/retrosigmoid | n/a | 100% | 0% | 45% |
| Slattery et al. | 2007 | 47 | Middle fossa | 34 | n/a | 55% | 19% |
| Friedman et al. | 2011 | 55 | Middle fossa | 24 mo | 40% | 50% | 25% |

**Table 23.3** Results for single-fraction stereotactic radiosurgery for acoustic schwannoma in patients with NF2

| Author | Pub year | N | Follow-up (mo) | Dose (Gy) | Local control | Hearing preserved | Facial nerve injury |
|---|---|---|---|---|---|---|---|
| Roche et al. | 2000 | 35 | 32 | 13 | 74% | 57% | 9% |
| Kida et al. | 2000 | 20 | 34 | 13 | 100% | 33.30% | 10% |
| Rowe et al. | 2003 | 122 | 96 | 13–25 | 50% | 40% | 5% |
| Linskey et al. | 1992 | 19 | 30 | 18 | 89.50% | 33% | 30.80% |
| Subach et al. | 1999 | 45 | 36 | 15 | 98% | 43% | 19% |
| Mathieu et al. | 2007 | 74 | 53 | 14 | 83% (81% actuarial control at 15 years) | 48% | 8% |
| Wentworth et al. | 2009 | 12 | 60 | 12 | 75% | 50% | 33% |

## Target Delineation

Vestibular schwannomas are best defined on contrast-enhanced T1 MRI. It is recommended that a gadolinium-enhanced MRI be obtained in the axial and coronal plane with a slice thickness of 1 mm. Additionally, a high-resolution T2-weighted gradient echo sequence can assist with definition of adjacent critical structures such as cranial nerves and the cochlea. The GTV target is the enhancing tumor and no CTV or PTV is used when utilizing radiosurgery. For fractionated cases, an institutionally defined PTV can be used.

## Radiation Dose Prescription

Single-fraction radiosurgery is appropriate for most tumors <3 cm in size unless there is a significant degree of abutment to the brainstem. A marginal dose of 12.5–13 Gy is typically used. Patients not suitable for single-fraction radiosurgery are offered fractionated radiotherapy using 46.8–50.4 Gy in 1.8 Gy fractions. In this setting, proton therapy can be considered if available as it may reduce integral dose to normal, uninvolved tissues. There are, however, few reports utilizing proton therapy for VS in the literature, and these mostly utilize outdated techniques with none specific to NF2 patients [29–32].

## Toxicity and Normal Tissue Constraints

The toxicity and normal tissue constraints, namely, to the cochlea and brainstem, are identical to non-NF2 patients and described in Chap. 4. Hearing preservation rates appear to be lower in this population than the sporadic VS population. Hearing preservation rates as high as 77% have been reported in sporadic VS following radiosurgery [33]. However, hearing preservation rates in NF2-associated VS are approximately 50% (Table 23.3). This discrepancy is likely related to differences in tumor biology rather than toxicity attributable to therapy. Facial nerve complication rates are low with modern radiosurgery techniques (Table 23.3).

It is widely quoted that NF2 patients have an increased risk of malignant transformation or secondary malignan-

cies following radiotherapy. This concern stems from the fact that NF2 patients already have a mutated tumor suppressor pathway, and radiotherapy could provide the mutagen for the "two-hit" hypothesis [25]. This fear has been heightened after the reporting of several case reports and a publication that indicated a tenfold increase in the incidence of malignant peripheral nerve sheath tumor (MPNST) following radiotherapy [34–37]. Using a survey of North American and European centers, Baser et al. collected data on 1348 NF2 patients. A total of five patients underwent malignant transformation of their tumor or development of a secondary cancer in the high-dose area following treatment with radiosurgery. Nine patients in the non-radiosurgery group also had malignant transformation of their tumors. By extrapolating from other experiences where utilization rates of radiosurgery for NF2-related tumors are known to be approximately 8%, they concluded that 106 of the 1348 patients received radiosurgery. Thus, they postulated that the rate of secondary malignancy was 5 out of 106 patients which was ten times higher than the sporadic malignant tumor rate in NF2 patients, i.e., 9 of 1242 [35]. Whether or not this is a valid conclusion could be questioned.

In addition to the survey-derived data, there are several case reports in the literature linking malignant transformation of VS to prior radiosurgery [34, 36–38]. It has been pointed out that in only one case was the benign histology confirmed prior to radiosurgery [25]. Therefore, while an association between radiosurgery and malignant transformation may exist, there is no conclusive evidence of this phenomenon to date.

## Outcomes

The University of Pittsburgh has one of the largest published series of NF2 patients treated with radiosurgery for VS [25]. Seventy four NF2-related VS in 62 patients were treated from 1987 to 2005. The median patient age was 33 years old. Prior to 1992, marginal doses of up to 20 Gy were used, but after this date, marginal dose did not exceed 14 Gy. The actuarial rate of local control was 81% at 15 years. No cases of malignant transformation or secondary malignancy were noted in their cohort of patients.

The Mayo Clinic has also published long-term radiosurgery results for 26 NF2 patients with 32 treated VS [24]. The median age of the patients was 37 years, and the median margin dose was 14 Gy (range, 12–20 Gy). At a median follow-up of 7.6 years, 84% of the tumors were either stable or decreased in size. The Kaplan-Meier estimates for 5- and 10-year progression-free survival were 85% and 80%, respectively. Their data also suggest a dose-response relationship with a median marginal dose of 15.5 Gy associated with radiographic decrease in tumor size, whereas the median marginal dose for tumors that enlarged was 13 Gy. The hazard ratio for this dose response was 0.49 (95% CI 0.17–0.92; $p = 0.02$).

Reported outcomes are not universally favorable, however. The National Centre for Stereotactic Radiosurgery in the United Kingdom reported on 122 VS treated with radiosurgery in 96 NF2 patients [27]. Treatment was conducted in an earlier era (1986–2000), and over an 8-year follow-up period, only approximately 50% of tumors were controlled as defined by need for subsequent treatment or imaging changes. It is unclear why these results are inferior to other studies. It is possible that target localization was less precise in the earlier era. Also, the majority of tumors treated in their study were treated due to growth noted on surveillance scans which may have led to a selection bias in favor of more aggressive lesions.

## Follow-Up and Radiographic Assessment

Clinical follow-up is recommended at 3–6-month intervals for the first year after therapy and can be extended to 6–12-month intervals in the setting of clinical stability. Audiology examination should be performed at 6 months post-SRS (for those with hearing prior to treatment) and then yearly thereafter if stable. Patients should undergo contrast-enhanced MRI scans at 6-month intervals following therapy until tumor size stability is observed. Subsequently, yearly contrast-enhanced MRI scans should be obtained until 10 years, at which point, a 2-year interval is reasonable.

## Meningioma

### Epidemiology

Meningioma is the second most common tumor in NF2 patients [1]. Approximately 50% of patients will have intracranial meningiomas at the time of initial presentation, and another 20% will have intradural, extramedullary spinal tumors. Nearly all patients will develop meningiomas over their lifetime [1, 39–43]. These tumors often present as an asymptomatic finding on imaging [43]. Similar to NF2-related VS, NF2-related meningioma tend to develop at a younger age. Children who present with what appears to be sporadic meningioma should be screened for NF2 as up to 20% of these patients will harbor the mutation [1, 44]. Children that present with optic nerve sheath meningiomas have an even higher incidence of NF2 at 28% [45, 46].

NF2-related meningiomas tend to behave more aggressively and are frequently higher grade than their sporadic counterparts [1, 42]. Approximately a third of patients will experience more than 20% growth of their meningioma over the course of 1 year, and approximately half will require surgery for meningioma-related symptoms over a 9-year period [47]. The presence of meningiomas in NF2 patients carries a relative risk of mortality two-and-a-half-fold higher than NF2 patients without meningiomas [48]. When meningiomas develop in addition to vestibular schwannoma in NF2 patients, as is often seen, there appears to be a synergistic effect of increased growth rate of the schwannoma and meningioma beyond that expected of these tumors in the sporadic setting [43]. The transitional and fibroblastic histologies appear to be overrepresented in NF2-related meningioma although all histologies are reported [42]. NF2-related meningiomas occur most commonly in the parasagittal and convexity locations as in sporadic tumors. However, there is also a predilection for the spinal cord, intraventricular locations, and the optic nerve sheaths [45, 47, 49]. The intraventricular meningiomas often occur in the lateral ventricles in close association with the choroid plexus.

The incidence of optic nerve sheath meningiomas (ONSM) is approximately 7% in NF2 patients. Bosch et al. published a series of 30 consecutive NF2 patients presenting to an ophthalmology clinic over 12 years. Imaging of the brain with MRI revealed eight (27%) cases of ONSM, two of which had bilateral tumors. Half of the patients had no prior diagnosis of ONSM. Of the ten total tumors, six were classified as primary or probably primary ONSM meaning that they had originated from the optic nerve sheath itself and were not a result of extension from an intracranial meningioma [46].

A rare entity known as meningioangiomatosis can occur in association with NF2. In fact, up to 25% of meningioangiomatosis are associated with NF2. This condition is characterized by a plaque-like, cerebral hemispheric mass, most often involving the temporal and frontal lobes. Histologically, these tumors consist of an intracortical and leptomeningeal collection of small blood vessels with perivascular spindle cells. They should be considered in the differential diagnosis of cortical lesions in NF2 patients [47].

### Diagnosis

As in meningiomas not associated with NF2, MRI imaging is often diagnostic. Tumors arise from the dura, are typically isointense to brain on T1 and T2 sequences, and enhance

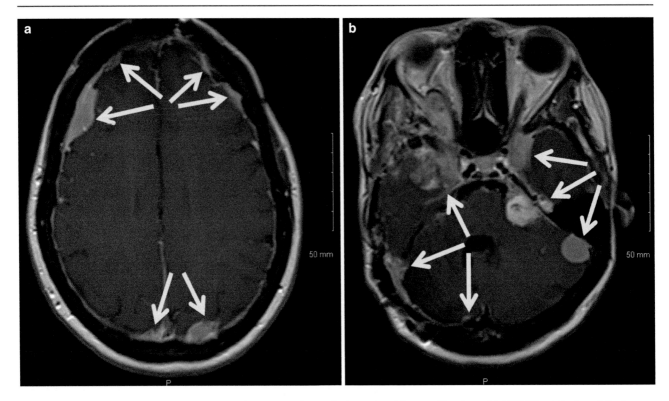

**Fig. 23.1** Multiple convexity (panel **a**) and base of skull (panel **b**) meningiomas in a 35-year-old patient with NF2. The right sigmoid lesion was surgically debulked with the remainder of the tumors managed by a combination of observation and stereotactic radiosurgery

brightly after administration of contrast (Fig. 23.1). A "dural tail" may be present and can help differentiate them from acoustic schwannoma for tumors in the region of the cerebellopontine angle. Calcifications are often seen on CT imaging. As in non-NF2-related meningiomas, a wide variety of histologic appearances are seen, and these are described in Chap. 1.

## Overall Treatment Strategy

Similar to sporadic meningioma, asymptomatic tumors are often managed with observation. Surgery and radiotherapy should be reserved for growing lesions or those causing symptoms.

Surgery is the primary treatment for symptomatic NF2-associated meningioma if the lesion is in an operable location. However, in patients with numerous intracranial meningiomas, many practitioners avoid surgery for asymptomatic tumors, even when they exhibit growth, in an attempt to limit the morbidity associated with multiple craniotomies. For optic nerve sheath meningiomas, surgery is reserved for tumors with intracranial extension, disfiguring proptosis, and rapid visual deterioration, with radiotherapy favored for all other scenarios [50]. Spinal meningiomas, on the other hand, are nearly always resectable, and radiotherapy plays a relatively small role for these tumors.

## Indications for Irradiation

Radiotherapy is indicated for progressing or symptomatic tumors that are not amenable to surgical resection. In a few instances, "pre-emptive" radiotherapy may be indicated for a tumor that is in a particularly eloquent location where even minimal growth could cause significant morbidity – i.e., optic nerve sheath meningiomas. Both radiosurgery and fractionated radiotherapy are used, depending upon the size and location of the tumor.

## Radiotherapy Technique

NF2-associated meningiomas are treated similarly to sporadic meningiomas. Fully fractionated or hypofractionated radiotherapy and single-fraction radiosurgery are all commonly used, depending on the size and location of the tumor. Target delineation, radiation dose prescription, and normal tissue constraints are identical to sporadic meningiomas as described in Chap. 1.

## Outcomes

Data regarding radiotherapy for NF2-related meningiomas is relatively sparse. Historically, it had been thought that

NF2-associated meningiomas had unfavorable outcomes following radiosurgery compared to sporadic tumors. Santacroce et al. published results of 4564 patients treated with radiosurgery for intracranial meningioma. Of those patients, 60 had a confirmed diagnosis of NF2. The 10-year progression-free survival rate for NF2-associated tumors was 77.6% vs. 89.9% for sporadic tumors [51]. Kondziolka et al. reported on six NF2 patients treated with radiosurgery for convexity meningiomas in a larger series of 125 patients. The NF2-associated tumors were found to have poorer overall survival compared to their sporadic counterparts [52]. Wentworth et al. treated 49 meningiomas associated with NF2, mostly with radiosurgery delivering 12–14 Gy to the 50% isodose line. They reported a 5-year progression-free survival rate of 86% [53].

More recent series appear to show favorable outcomes. The Mayo Clinic group published results of 15 NF2 patients with 62 intracranial meningiomas treated with radiosurgery. The median prescription dose was 16 Gy (range 13–20). At a median follow-up of approximately 9 years, the 5- and 10-year local control rates were both 96% [54]. Liu et al. reported on 12 NF2 patients with 87 tumors treated with radiosurgery. Using a marginal dose between 12 and 15 Gy, the 5-year local control rate was 92% [55].

## Follow-Up and Radiographic Assessment

For WHO grade I and II meningiomas following radiosurgery, clinical and radiographic follow-up with contrast-enhanced MRI should be obtained at 3, 6, and 12 months posttreatment. If stable, surveillance can be extended to every 6–12 months for 5 years and then every 1–2 years. Shorter follow-up intervals are appropriate for patients with malignant lesions, numerous lesions, or lesions near critical structures.

## Malignant Peripheral Nerve Sheath Tumor

Malignant peripheral nerve sheath tumors (MPNSTs) are rare, high-grade sarcomas of nerve sheath differentiation comprising approximately 5–10% of soft tissue sarcomas [56, 57]. They most commonly arise from a peripheral nerve, a pre-existing neurofibroma, or in extra-neural soft tissue. While uncommon in the general population, their incidence may approach ~10% in patients diagnosed with NF1. They are less commonly reported in NF2, but have been observed. Peak incidence is at 30–40 years of age in patients with NF1 compared to 70–80 years of age for sporadic tumors [58]. They have also been described arising as a secondary malignancy following prior radiotherapy [59, 60].

## Diagnosis and Prognosis

The 2016 WHO classification recognizes two subtypes of MPNST—epithelioid MPNST and MPNST with perineural differentiation [57]. The epithelioid variant is only rarely associated with neurofibromatosis; MPNST with perineural differentiation make up the vast majority of cases. Histologically, tumors have a heterogenous appearance, frequently showing tightly packed spindle cells in a herringbone pattern, and many have a pseudocapsule. MRI findings typically show tumors to be hyperintense on STIR- and T2-weighted images. They are isointense to muscle on T1 images and enhance with contrast administration (Fig. 23.2).

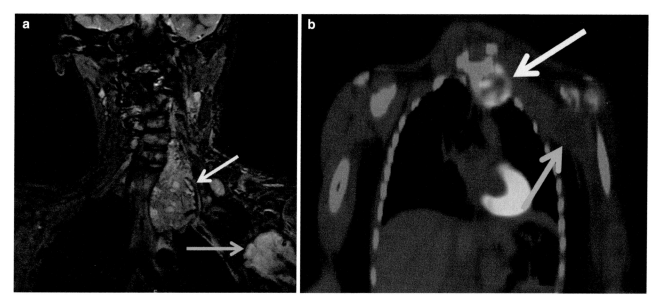

**Fig. 23.2** (a) Post-contrast MRI of a left cervical MPNST (yellow arrow) and a benign left axillary neurofibroma (green arrow). (b) PET/CT of the same patient showing an SUV of 9.7 in the MPNST (yellow arrow) and SUV of 2.5 in the left axillary neurofibroma (green arrow)

## Overall Treatment Strategy for Malignant Peripheral Nerve Sheath Tumors

Treatment of MPNSTs is guided by the same principles as those applied to other high-grade sarcomas. Both surgery and radiotherapy are required to optimize local control. There is limited data to support the use of chemotherapy.

### Surgery

Incisional biopsy or core biopsy is preferred for pathologic confirmation. This biopsy should be performed in a manner to allow for subsequent en bloc definitive removal if feasible. Several studies have shown that gross total resection is associated with improved local control and perhaps survival [61]. Amputation may be necessary in advanced cases or for unfavorable locations; however, this has not been associated with improved survival if wide excision is possible, and local control is only improved if negative margins are not feasible with more limited resections [62]. Lymph node sampling is recommended only in patients with clinical concern for lymphadenopathy via exam or imaging and is typically not performed electively.

### Systemic Therapy

Cytotoxic chemotherapy has shown minimal benefit in the treatment of MPNST [63]. More recent emphasis has been placed on utilizing targeted therapies such as tyrosine kinase inhibitors and vascular endothelial growth factor inhibitors in addition to radiotherapy and surgery. The Children's Oncology Group and the NRG cooperative group are currently conducting a trial to assess the use of pazopanib for these tumors.

## Indications for Irradiation

Current standard of care for treatment of high-grade sarcomas with radiotherapy is applied to MPNST, meaning that essentially all patients require the use of radiotherapy either adjuvantly with surgery or as the sole local control modality for those patients with inoperable tumors.

## Radiation Technique

Radiotherapy is preferentially given prior to definitive surgical resection. Compared to postoperative radiotherapy, preoperative radiotherapy treatment volumes are usually smaller, resulting in less radiation exposure to normal tissue. Additionally, a lower radiation dose is typically used when radiation is given preoperatively, and it has been postulated that preoperative radiotherapy decreases the risk of disseminating viable tumor at the time of resection. Specific approach and technique are largely dependent on lesion location as these tumors may originate in a variety of body sites. Intracranial lesions and lesions of the base of skull are typically treated with IMRT or proton therapy if available due to necessity of limiting exposure to critical structures that may lie in close approximation to the targeted tumor. Brachytherapy may play a role as a boost in selected tumors, though its use is not as prevalent as is seen in other soft tissue sarcomas.

## Target Delineation

MPNSTs frequently have irregular enhancement on T1 contrast-enhanced MRI and tumor borders can be indistinct. In addition, MPNST arising within a background of neurofibroma may be difficult to differentiate from the benign component. Positron emission tomography (PET/CT) may be specific for this distinction when an SUV cutoff of 3.5 is applied [64].

The GTV consists of all palpable or visible disease on imaging at presentation. For patients treated postoperatively, the GTV should include all surgically exposed tissue including drain sites and surgical incisions. CTV expansions vary in the longitudinal plane from 2 to 5 cm and radially 1–3 cm with the smaller margins typically used in children who have not achieved complete growth of adjacent normal tissue (Fig. 23.3). CTV expansions for boosts are typically limited to 1 cm. PTV expansions vary depending on the immobilization technique used for the respective disease site and considerations for any physiologic motion that may occur.

## Radiation Dose Prescription

When delivered preoperatively, 45–50 Gy is given in 1.8–2.0 Gy fractions. Patients with positive margins after surgery may be considered for a postoperative boost of 16–20 Gy in 2 Gy fractions for microscopic and macroscopic margins, respectively. When only postoperative radiotherapy is used, a dose of 60 Gy in 2.0 Gy fractions is given for microscopic residual tumor, with a boost to 66–70 Gy for gross residual. Brachytherapy may also be used and is most commonly applied as a boost in conjunction with external beam radiotherapy.

## Toxicity and Normal Tissue Constraints

Normal tissue dose constraints vary based on the tumor location. Given the relatively high dose required for disease control, standard CNS dose constraints should be respected. Standard fractionation dose limit to the spinal cord is conservatively recommended as 45 Gy. Brachial plexus dose constraints are 60–63 Gy.

Toxicity of therapy is related to lesion location. Spinal cord myelopathy and brachial plexopathy are chief considerations. Extremity lesion treatment risks joint arthropathy so

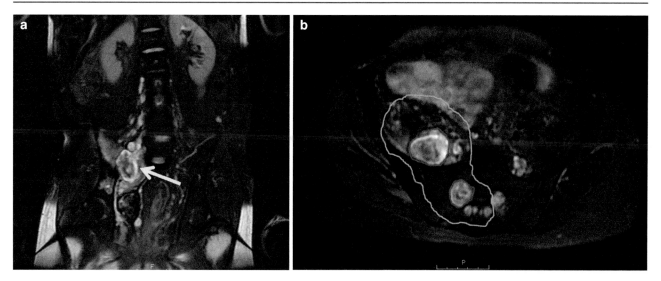

**Fig. 23.3** (**a**) MPNST (yellow arrow) arising in a pre-existing neurofibroma in a 22-year-old patient with NF1. (**b**) The patient was treated with 50 Gy pre-op radiotherapy followed by resection. The GTV is indicated by the red contour with the CTV indicated in green. Note that the CTV has been partially constrained by the sacral canal and iliac wing as there was no evidence of bone invasion on imaging

radiotherapy fields crossing the joint are avoided when possible. In addition, lymphedema risk is high when a <2 cm strip of normal tissue can be spared. Normal structure constraints are applied for bowel, lung, and cardiac doses when appropriate. Secondary malignancy risk may be greater given the coexistence of the NF1 mutation, though, in practice, this is not a significant consideration given the guarded prognosis of MPNST and the essential role that radiotherapy plays in its treatment.

## Outcomes

Current outcomes for patients diagnosed with MPNSTs remains poor. Five-year disease-free survival is typically in the range of 40%, and 5-year overall survival is approximately 60% [65]. Poor prognostic factors include tumor location in the trunk or head and neck region, deep-seated tumors, tumors >10 cm in size, locally invasive lesions, positive surgical margins, and omission of adjuvant radiotherapy [65, 66]. In addition, some reports have associated a poorer prognosis for patients with NF1 compared to those whose tumors arise spontaneously [65, 67].

## Follow-Up and Radiographic Assessment

Follow-up for patients with MPNST includes physical exam and imaging of the affected site every 3 months for the first 2–3 years, given the high risk of recurrence in this timeframe. Patients are typically then followed every 6 months for 5 years and annually thereafter. Follow-up should also include CT of the chest given the risk of lung metastases.

## Challenging Case Study

A 24-year-old female patient with no family history of neurofibromatosis was diagnosed with NF2 when bilateral vestibular schwannomas were found on MRI performed to evaluate left-sided hearing loss and severe headaches. Due to progressive growth of the left vestibular schwannoma with loss of functional hearing in that ear, she underwent a left translabyrinthine tumor resection at the age of 26. She was subsequently followed with imaging and audiograms for 5 years. At the age of 31, growth of her right-sided lesion was noted with associated decrease in her word recognition score on audiogram. Bevacizumab was started and she completed eight cycles of this drug. Her hearing improved and remained stable for 2 years with no active therapy. At age 33, she reported recurrent right-sided hearing deficit and a word recognition score was 40%. Bevacizumab was again initiated. She completed 15 cycles of this drug with initial improvement of hearing, but subsequent progressive decline in spite of radiographic stability (Fig. 23.4).

At the time of radiation oncology consultation, the patient was 33 years of age with a chief concern of regaining/retaining functional hearing. Though she could communicate well and had excellent lip reading skills, she had two young children and wanted to be able to hear them at all times and communicate more fully. The patient underwent single-fraction stereotactic radiosurgery to the right acoustic schwannoma, receiving 13 Gy (Fig. 23.5). Follow-up imaging showed

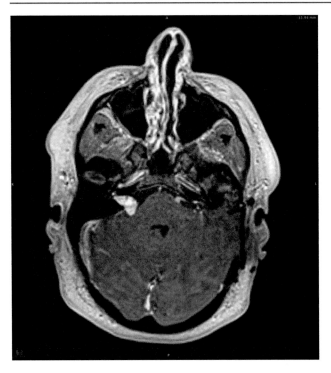

**Fig. 23.4** Appearance of the right acoustic schwannoma at the time radiosurgery. Note that the left acoustic schwannoma had been resected

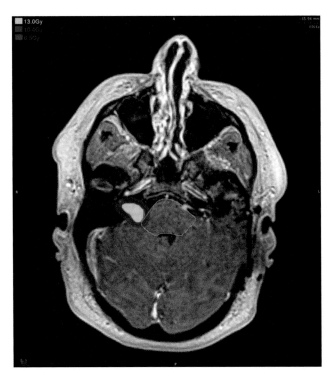

**Fig. 23.5** Radiosurgery color wash isodoses

stable tumor size and speech recognition score was also stable at 30%. Two years later, the patient underwent elective placement of a cochlear implant and is currently receiving ongoing auditory rehabilitation with some improvement in her functional hearing.

## Summary

- NF2 is a phacomatosis with an autosomal-dominant inheritance pattern.
- Bilateral acoustic schwannomas are a hallmark of NF2.
- Management of acoustic schwannomas in patients with NF2 utilizes both surgery and radiotherapy with an emphasis on preservation of function.
- Patients with NF2 are at risk for developing multiple meningiomas.
- Management of meningiomas in patients with NF2 parallels that used for non-NF2 patients, though local control is not as favorable in the NF2 patient population.
- MPNST is a highly malignant sarcoma occurring primarily in patients with NF1.
- Optimal treatment for MPNST consists of preoperative radiotherapy followed by gross total resection. The role of chemotherapy and targeted agents is currently being investigated.

## Self-Assessment Questions

1. What is the hereditary pattern of type 2 neurofibromatosis (NF2)?
   A. Autosomal dominant
   B. Autosomal recessive
   C. X-linked dominant
   D. X-linked recessive

2. What is the most common presenting symptom of type 2 neurofibromatosis (NF2)?
   A. Headache
   B. Seizure
   C. Hearing loss
   D. Vision loss

3. A 32-year-old male with type 2 neurofibromatosis (NF2) is found to have a 1.5 cm right acoustic schwannoma and a 1.8 cm left acoustic schwannoma. Speech discrimination is 90% bilaterally. What is the most appropriate management for these tumors?
   A. Resection of the larger, left-sided tumor and radiosurgery of the right-sided tumor
   B. Radiosurgery for both tumors
   C. Systemic bevacizumab q2 weeks for six cycles
   D. Repeat audiogram and imaging in 6 months

4. A patient with type 2 neurofibromatosis (NF2) has a 3 cm falcine meningioma. Compared to a patient with a similar tumor but without NF2, what is the prognosis of the patient with NF2?
   A. Better
   B. The same
   C. Worse

5. What is the preferred radiotherapy technique for treatment of malignant peripheral nerve sheath tumors?
   A. Preoperative radiotherapy using 45 Gy in 1.8 Gy fractions
   B. Postoperative radiotherapy using 60 Gy in 2.0 Gy fractions
   C. Interstitial HDR brachytherapy delivering 30 Gy in six fractions
   D. SBRT delivering 24 Gy in three fractions

## Answers

1. A
2. C
3. D
4. C
5. A

## References

1. Asthagiri AR, Parry DM, Butman JA, et al. Neurofibromatosis type 2. Lancet. 2009;373(9679):1974–86.
2. Wishart JH. Case of tumours in the skull, dura mater and brain. Edinburgh Med Surg J. 1822;18:393–7.
3. Rouleau GA, Wertelecki W, Haines JL, et al. Genetic linkage of bilateral acoustic neurofibromatosis to a DNA marker on chromosome 22. Nature. 1987;329(6136):246–8.
4. Seizinger BR, Rouleau GA, Ozelius LJ, et al. Genetic linkage of von Recklinghausen neurofibromatosis to the nerve growth factor receptor gene. Cell. 1987;49(5):589–94.
5. Evans DG, Moran A, King A, et al. Incidence of vestibular schwannoma and neurofibromatosis 2 in the North West of England over a 10-year period: higher incidence than previously thought. Otol Neurotol. 2005;26(1):93–7.
6. Evans DG, Huson SM, Donnai D, et al. A genetic study of type 2 neurofibromatosis in the United Kingdom. I. Prevalence, mutation rate, fitness, and confirmation of maternal transmission effect on severity. J Med Genet. 1992;29(12):841–6.
7. Evans DG, Trueman L, Wallace A, et al. Genotype/phenotype correlations in type 2 neurofibromatosis (NF2): evidence for more severe disease associated with truncating mutations. J Med Genet. 1998;35(6):450–5.
8. Parry DM, MacCollin MM, Kaiser-Kupfer MI, et al. Germ-line mutations in the neurofibromatosis 2 gene: correlations with disease severity and retinal abnormalities. Am J Hum Genet. 1996;59(3):529–39.
9. Evans DG, Baser ME, O'Reilly B, et al. Management of the patient and family with neurofibromatosis 2: a consensus conference statement. Br J Neurosurg. 2005;19(1):5–12.
10. Brackmann DE, Fayad JN, Slattery WH 3rd, et al. Early proactive management of vestibular schwannomas in neurofibromatosis type 2. Neurosurgery. 2001;49(2):274–80. discussion 80–3
11. Khrais T, Romano G, Sanna M. Nerve origin of vestibular schwannoma: a prospective study. J Laryngol Otol. 2008;122(2):128–31.
12. Slattery WH 3rd, Brackmann DE, Hitselberger W. Hearing preservation in neurofibromatosis type 2. Am J Otol. 1998;19(5):638–43.
13. Jaaskelainen J, Paetau A, Pyykko I, et al. Interface between the facial nerve and large acoustic neurinomas. Immunohistochemical study of the cleavage plane in NF2 and non-NF2 cases. J Neurosurg. 1994;80(3):541–7.
14. Baser ME, Makariou EV, Parry DM. Predictors of vestibular schwannoma growth in patients with neurofibromatosis Type 2. J Neurosurg. 2002;96(2):217–22.
15. Slattery WH 3rd, Fisher LM, Iqbal Z, et al. Vestibular schwannoma growth rates in neurofibromatosis type 2 natural history consortium subjects. Otol Neurotol. 2004;25(5):811–7.
16. Dirks MS, Butman JA, Kim HJ, et al. Long-term natural history of neurofibromatosis Type 2-associated intracranial tumors. J Neurosurg. 2012;117(1):109–17.
17. Fisher LM, Doherty JK, Lev MH, et al. Concordance of bilateral vestibular schwannoma growth and hearing changes in neurofibromatosis 2: neurofibromatosis 2 natural history consortium. Otol Neurotol. 2009;30(6):835–41.
18. Masuda A, Fisher LM, Oppenheimer ML, et al. Hearing changes after diagnosis in neurofibromatosis type 2. Otol Neurotol. 2004;25(2):150–4.
19. Plotkin SR, Merker VL, Muzikansky A, et al. Natural history of vestibular schwannoma growth and hearing decline in newly diagnosed neurofibromatosis type 2 patients. Otol Neurotol. 2014;35(1):e50–6.
20. Plotkin SR, Merker VL, Halpin C, et al. Bevacizumab for progressive vestibular schwannoma in neurofibromatosis type 2: a retrospective review of 31 patients. Otol Neurotol. 2012;33(6):1046–52.
21. Ruggieri M, Pratico AD, Evans DG. Diagnosis, management, and new therapeutic options in childhood neurofibromatosis type 2 and related forms. Semin Pediatr Neurol. 2015;22(4):240–58.
22. Kida Y, Kobayashi T, Tanaka T, et al. Radiosurgery for bilateral neurinomas associated with neurofibromatosis type 2. Surg Neurol. 2000;53(4):383–9. discussion 9–90
23. Linskey ME, Lunsford LD, Flickinger JC. Tumor control after stereotactic radiosurgery in neurofibromatosis patients with bilateral acoustic tumors. Neurosurgery. 1992;31(5):829–38. discussion 38–9
24. Mallory GW, Pollock BE, Foote RL, et al. Neurosurgery. 2014;74(3):292–300. discussion −1
25. Mathieu D, Kondziolka D, Flickinger JC, et al. Stereotactic radiosurgery for vestibular schwannomas in patients with neurofibromatosis type 2: an analysis of tumor control, complications, and hearing preservation rates. Neurosurgery. 2007;60(3):460–8. discussion 8–70
26. Roche PH, Regis J, Pellet W, et al. Neurofibromatosis type 2. Preliminary results of gamma knife radiosurgery of vestibular schwannomas. Neurochirurgie. 2000;46(4):339–53. discussion 54
27. Rowe JG, Radatz MW, Walton L, et al. Clinical experience with gamma knife stereotactic radiosurgery in the management of vestibular schwannomas secondary to type 2 neurofibromatosis. J Neurol Neurosurg Psychiatry. 2003;74(9):1288–93.
28. Subach BR, Kondziolka D, Lunsford LD, et al. Stereotactic radiosurgery in the management of acoustic neuromas associated with neurofibromatosis Type 2. J Neurosurg. 1999;90(5):815–22.
29. Bush DA, McAllister CJ, Loredo LN, et al. Fractionated proton beam radiotherapy for acoustic neuroma. Neurosurgery. 2002;50(2):270–3. discussion 3–5
30. Harsh GR, Thornton AF, Chapman PH, et al. Proton beam stereotactic radiosurgery of vestibular schwannomas. Int J Radiat Oncol Biol Phys. 2002;54(1):35–44.
31. Vernimmen FJ, Mohamed Z, Slabbert JP, et al. Long-term results of stereotactic proton beam radiotherapy for acoustic neuromas. Radiother Oncol. 2009;90(2):208–12.
32. Weber DC, Chan AW, Bussiere MR, et al. Proton beam radiosurgery for vestibular schwannoma: tumor control and cranial nerve toxicity. Neurosurgery. 2003;53(3):577–86. discussion 86–8
33. Lunsford LD, Niranjan A, Flickinger JC, et al. Radiosurgery of vestibular schwannomas: summary of experience in 829 cases. J Neurosurg. 2005;102(Suppl):195–9.

34. Bari ME, Forster DM, Kemeny AA, et al. Malignancy in a vestibular schwannoma. Report of a case with central neurofibromatosis, treated by both stereotactic radiosurgery and surgical excision, with a review of the literature. Br J Neurosurg. 2002;16(3):284–9.

35. Baser ME, Evans DG, Jackler RK, et al. Neurofibromatosis 2, radiosurgery and malignant nervous system tumours. Br J Cancer. 2000;82(4):998.

36. Noren G. Long-term complications following gamma knife radiosurgery of vestibular schwannomas. Stereotact Funct Neurosurg. 1998;70(Suppl 1):65–73.

37. Thomsen J, Mirz F, Wetke R, et al. Intracranial sarcoma in a patient with neurofibromatosis type 2 treated with gamma knife radiosurgery for vestibular schwannoma. Am J Otol. 2000;21(3):364–70.

38. Comey CH, McLaughlin MR, Jho HD, et al. Death from a malignant cerebellopontine angle triton tumor despite stereotactic radiosurgery. Case report. J Neurosurg. 1998;89(4):653–8.

39. Evans DG, Huson SM, Donnai D, et al. A clinical study of type 2 neurofibromatosis. Q J Med. 1992;84(304):603–18.

40. Mautner VF, Lindenau M, Baser ME, et al. The neuroimaging and clinical spectrum of neurofibromatosis 2. Neurosurgery. 1996;38(5):880–5. discussion 5–6

41. Patronas NJ, Courcoutsakis N, Bromley CM, et al. Intramedullary and spinal canal tumors in patients with neurofibromatosis 2: MR imaging findings and correlation with genotype. Radiology. 2001;218(2):434–42.

42. Perry A, Giannini C, Raghavan R, et al. Aggressive phenotypic and genotypic features in pediatric and NF2-associated meningiomas: a clinicopathologic study of 53 cases. J Neuropathol Exp Neurol. 2001;60(10):994–1003.

43. Slattery WH. Neurofibromatosis type 2. Otolaryngol Clin N Am. 2015;48(3):443–60.

44. Evans DG, Birch JM, Ramsden RT. Paediatric presentation of type 2 neurofibromatosis. Arch Dis Child. 1999;81(6):496–9.

45. Ardern-Holmes S, Fisher G, North K. Neurofibromatosis type 2: presentation, major complications, and management, with a focus on the pediatric age group. J Child Neurol. 2017;32(1):9–22

46. Bosch MM, Wichmann WW, Boltshauser E, et al. Optic nerve sheath meningiomas in patients with neurofibromatosis type 2. Arch Ophthalmol. 2006;124(3):379–85.

47. Goutagny S, Kalamarides M. Meningiomas and neurofibromatosis. J Neurooncol. 2010;99(3):341–7.

48. Baser ME, Friedman JM, Aeschliman D, et al. Predictors of the risk of mortality in neurofibromatosis 2. Am J Hum Genet. 2002;71(4):715–23.

49. Evans DG, Sainio M, Baser ME. Neurofibromatosis type 2. J Med Genet. 2000;37(12):897–904.

50. Roser F, Nakamura M, Martini-Thomas R, et al. The role of surgery in meningiomas involving the optic nerve sheath. Clin Neurol Neurosurg. 2006;108(5):470–6.

51. Santacroce A, Walier M, Regis J, et al. Long-term tumor control of benign intracranial meningiomas after radiosurgery in a series of 4565 patients. Neurosurgery. 2012;70(1):32–9. discussion 9

52. Kondziolka D, Madhok R, Lunsford LD, et al. Stereotactic radiosurgery for convexity meningiomas. J Neurosurg. 2009;111(3):458–63.

53. Wentworth S, Pinn M, Bourland JD, et al. Clinical experience with radiation therapy in the management of neurofibromatosis-associated central nervous system tumors. Int J Radiat Oncol Biol Phys. 2009;73(1):208–13.

54. Birckhead B, Sio TT, Pollock BE, et al. Gamma Knife radiosurgery for neurofibromatosis type 2-associated meningiomas: a 22-year patient series. J Neuro-Oncol. 2016;130(3):553–60.

55. Liu A, Kuhn EN, Lucas JT Jr, et al. Gamma Knife radiosurgery for meningiomas in patients with neurofibromatosis Type 2. J Neurosurg. 2015;122(3):536–42.

56. Huang JH, Zhang J, Zager EL. Diagnosis and treatment options for nerve sheath tumors. Expert Rev Neurother. 2005;5(4):515–23.

57. Louis DN, Ohgaki H, Wiestler OD, et al. WHO classification of tumours of the central nervous system. Lyon, France: International Agency for Research on Cancer; 2016.

58. Evans DG, Baser ME, McGaughran J, et al. Malignant peripheral nerve sheath tumours in neurofibromatosis 1. J Med Genet. 2002;39(5):311–4.

59. LaFemina J, Qin LX, Moraco NH, et al. Oncologic outcomes of sporadic, neurofibromatosis-associated, and radiation-induced malignant peripheral nerve sheath tumors. Ann Surg Oncol. 2013;20(1):66–72.

60. Seferis C, Torrens M, Paraskevopoulou C, et al. Malignant transformation in vestibular schwannoma: report of a single case, literature search, and debate. J Neurosurg. 2014;121(Suppl):160–6.

61. Byerly S, Chopra S, Nassif NA, et al. The role of margins in extremity soft tissue sarcoma. J Surg Oncol. 2016;113(3):333–8.

62. Rosenberg SA, Tepper J, Glatstein E, et al. The treatment of soft-tissue sarcomas of the extremities: prospective randomized evaluations of (1) limb-sparing surgery plus radiation therapy compared with amputation and (2) the role of adjuvant chemotherapy. Ann Surg. 1982;196(3):305–15.

63. Ferrari A, Bisogno G, Carli M. Management of childhood malignant peripheral nerve sheath tumor. Paeditr Drugs. 2007;9:239–48.

64. Derlin T, Tornquist K, Munster S, et al. Comparative effectiveness of 18F-FDG PET/CT versus whole-body MRI for detection of malignant peripheral nerve sheath tumors in neurofibromatosis type 1. Clin Nucl Med. 2013;38(1):e19–25.

65. Valentin T, Le Cesne A, Ray-Coquard I, et al. Management and prognosis of malignant peripheral nerve sheath tumors: the experience of the French Sarcoma Group (GSF-GETO). Eur J Cancer. 2016;56:77–84.

66. Zou C, Smith KD, Liu J, et al. Clinical, pathological, and molecular variables predictive of malignant peripheral nerve sheath tumor outcome. Ann Surg. 2009;249(6):1014–22.

67. Kolberg M, Holand M, Agesen TH, et al. Survival meta-analyses for >1800 malignant peripheral nerve sheath tumor patients with and without neurofibromatosis type 1. Neurooncology. 2013;15(2):135–47.

# Germ Cell Tumors

# 24

Kenneth Wong, Chenue Abongwa, Eric L. Chang, and Girish Dhall

## Learning Objectives

- Understand the incidence, prevalence, and risk factors of intracranial germ cell tumors.
- Understand the clinical and radiological presentation of intracranial germ cell tumors.
- Identify key prognostic factors, and understand genetic and molecular changes associated with these tumors.
- Understand the overall treatment strategy and the role of surgery, chemotherapy, and radiation therapy in treatment.
- Understand the evidence supporting radiation therapy, and apply these principles in planning therapy for patients with intracranial germ cell tumors.
- Identify key treatment-related late effects associated with therapy for intracranial germs cell tumors.

K. Wong (✉)
Department of Radiation Oncology, Keck School of Medicine of USC, Los Angeles, CA, USA

Radiation Oncology Program, Children's Center for Cancer and Blood Diseases, Children's Hospital Los Angeles, Los Angeles, CA, USA
e-mail: KeWong@chla.usc.edu

C. Abongwa
Department of Pediatrics, Loma Linda University School of Medicine, Loma Linda, CA, USA

E. L. Chang
Department of Radiation Oncology, Keck School of Medicine of USC, Los Angeles, CA, USA

Radiation Oncology Program, Children's Center for Cancer and Blood Diseases, Children's Hospital Los Angeles, Los Angeles, CA, USA

Department of Radiation Oncology, University of Texas MD Anderson Cancer Center, Houston, TX, USA

G. Dhall
Neuro-Oncology Program, Children's Center for Cancer and Blood Diseases, Children's Hospital Los Angeles, Los Angeles, CA, USA

Department of Pediatrics, Keck School of Medicine of USC, Los Angeles, CA, USA

## Epidemiology

### Incidence and Prevalence

Overall, intracranial germ cell tumors (IGCTs) are rare, with only 120–200 new cases per year in the United States (US). These cases comprise about 3–5% of all primary childhood central nervous system (CNS) tumors. In adults, IGCTs make up about 0.3–0.5% of all primary CNS tumors with a reported incidence of about 0.10 per 100,000 person-years in the United States and Canada [1].

Germ cell tumors are classified into two main clinicopathologic groups, germinomas and non-germinomatous germ cell tumors (NGGCTs), which are a heterogeneous group comprising embryonal carcinoma, yolk sac or endodermal sinus tumor, choriocarcinoma, mixed germ cell tumor, mature or immature teratoma, and teratoma with malignant transformation.

The peak incidence of IGCTs occurs around early puberty or in the second decade of life, with a median age of about 10 years. More than 90% of cases occur in patients younger than 20 years of age, and few patients develop tumors after the age of 30 years. There is also a striking sex predilection, with males more likely to develop IGCTs. The male predilection is even higher for pineal tumors [2]. These tumors typically occur in the pineal and suprasellar regions in the brain and rarely in other subcortical structures such as the basal ganglia, ventricles, thalamus, cerebral hemispheres, and cerebellum. About 5–10% of patients with CNS germ cell tumors have bifocal lesions involving both the pineal and suprasellar regions. Although this phenomenon is typically seen with pure germinomas, there have been reports in patients with NGGCTs [3].

Much of what is known about IGCTs was described by Jennings et al. in one of the largest early series of 389 cases. Most IGCTs are germinomas (65%) with the other histologic subgroups represented as follows: teratomas (18%), embryonal carcinomas (5%), endodermal sinus tumors (7%), and choriocarcinomas (5%). The majority of germinomas (57%)

arise in the suprasellar cistern, while most NGGCTs (68%) preferentially involve the pineal gland. NGGCTs demonstrate an earlier age of onset than do germinomas. Prolonged symptomatic intervals prior to diagnosis are common in suprasellar germinomas and among females. Suprasellar germinomas commonly present with diabetes insipidus, visual field defects, and hypothalamic-pituitary failure. NGGCTs present as posterior third ventricular masses with hydrocephalus and midbrain compression. Tumors may infiltrate the hypothalamus (11%), third ventricle (22%), or spinal cord (10%) and are associated with a poorer prognosis [4].

The incidence of IGCTs based upon older studies had been considered to be higher in East Asia than in the United States. Pineal region masses represent about 1–3% of all the intracranial masses in the United States, but this proportion was higher in Asia where they make up to 9% of all intracranial tumors [4–6].

## Standard Mortality Ratio CBTRUS (Central Brain Tumor Registry of the United States)

A more recent study of pooled data did not find significant differences in incidence rates or distribution by location or gender in the United States or Japan. McCarthy et al. estimated the incidence of IGCTs in Japan and the United States utilizing data from four databases, the Japan Cancer Surveillance Research Group (JCSRG; 2004–2006); Surveillance, Epidemiology, and End Results (SEER; 2004–2008); Brain Tumor Registry of Japan (BTRJ; 1984–2000); and the US National Cancer Database (NCDB; 1990–2003). The incidence between Japan (males = 0.143, females = 0.046) and the United States (males = 0.118, females = 0.030) was not statistically different, and there was the same gender-based pattern by location [1].

The exact incidence of pineal germ cell tumors was largely unknown, and Villano et al. reported the largest study using data from Surveillance, Epidemiology, and End Results (SEER 1973–2001), the Central Brain Tumor Registry of the United States (CBTRUS; 1997–2001), and National Cancer Database (NCDB; 1985–2003). The peak number of cases occurred in the 10- to 14-year age group in the CBTRUS data and in the 15- to 19-year age group in the SEER and NCDB data. The majority of tumors were germinomas, which had the highest survival rate (>79% at 5 years). All three databases showed a male predominance for pineal IGCTs and 72% of patients were Caucasian. Patients that received radiation therapy in the treatment plan either with surgery or alone survived the longest [7].

The same investigators examined the epidemiology of non-pineal IGCTs and used data from CBTRUS from 2000 to 2004 and SEER from 1992 to 2005. Males had a greater frequency (59.7%) than females (40.3%). However, by age group, the male-to-female rate ratio was about 1:1 for children and adults, but there was a 2:1 male predilection in young adults (15–29 years). For children and young adults, most tumors were malignant (86.8% and 89.0%, respectively), whereas for adults, more than half were nonmalignant (56.8%). Germinoma was the most frequent diagnosis (61.5%). In SEER, the frequency of malignant IGCTs (2.5%) was greater than that in the mediastinum (2.1%). Of 408 malignant IGCTs, 216 (52.9%) were non-pineal. The male-to-female IRR was 1.5. Overall relative survival for non-pineal IGCTs was 85.3% at 2 years, 77.3% at 5 years, and 67.6% at 10 years. Previous studies of IGCTs that have not stratified by site have suggested greater gender disparity. Non-pineal IGCTs show no significant gender preference yet have outcomes similar to pineal IGCTs [8].

Surawicz et al. analyzed 5 years of incidence data from the CBTRUS (1990–1994) from 11 collaborating state cancer registries. IGCTs were more common in men than in women and more common in Whites than in Blacks. The incidence rate was highest in the 0–19-year-old age group, then fell by half in the 20–34-year-old age group, and decreased again in half throughout adulthood [9].

## Risk Factors

Patients with Klinefelter syndrome [10] and Down's syndrome [11] appear to be predisposed to the development of both intracranial and gonadal germ cell tumors. Patients with trisomy 21 may develop tumors in atypical locations. There does not appear to be an association of IGCTs with radiation exposure. Familial clusters have not been reported for IGCTs as opposed to gonadal germ cell tumors [12].

## Familial Syndromes

Although there are case reports of testicular germ cell tumors with neurofibromatosis type 1, there are few case reports of IGCTs [13]. There does not appear to be an association of IGCTs with familial cancer syndromes, such as von Hippel-Lindau, Cowden, Turcot, Gorlin, or Li-Fraumeni syndrome.

## Non-suprasellar or Pineal Location

The majority of IGCTs occur in suprasellar or pineal regions, but uncommon locations involving the basal ganglia, thalamus, cerebral hemispheres, cerebellum, and optic chiasm have been reported [14]. Of the atypical locations, the basal ganglia are the most common and well documented and are associated with cerebral and/or brain stem atrophy in about a third of cases.

Phi et al. retrospectively reviewed 17 patients and described four different MRI features characterized by degree of contrast enhancement, size, and presence or absence of subependymal seeding. Subtle lesions with faint or no enhancement had a significantly longer time from initial MRI to diagnosis. Radiation therapy fields without whole ventricular coverage were significantly associated with tumor progression. Motor deficits at diagnosis were associated with deterioration in motor function after tumor remission. The actuarial progression-free survival (PFS) and overall survival (OS) 5 years after diagnosis were 66% and 77%, respectively. High clinical suspicion and active diagnostic procedures were recommended, and for optimal radiation therapy, whole ventricular fields were recommended by Phi et al. even if subependymal seeding was not detected [15]. Twelve patients with basal ganglia lesions were reviewed by Tian et al., and five had histopathologic confirmation of germinoma after a median duration of symptoms of 18 months [16]. Ozelame et al. described four males with basal ganglia germinoma, three of whom had cognitive decline, psychosis, and slowly progressive hemiparesis. CT findings showed a hyperdense or calcified lesion on pre-contrast scans, and additional imaging showed ipsilateral cerebral and/or brain stem hemiatrophy [17].

## Diagnosis and Prognosis

The clinical presentation of IGCTs varies by the location and the extent of the tumor. Pineal tumors, because of their close location to the tectum, typically present with signs and symptoms of raised intracranial pressure due to obstructive hydrocephalus. These patients typically have a shorter prodromal period from the onset of symptoms to diagnosis and typically present with headaches, vomiting, visual signs and symptoms, pyramidal signs, and altered mental status [4]. Parinaud's syndrome, which is upward gaze palsy with eyelid retraction, may be seen in some cases due to raised intracranial pressure [18]. Suprasellar tumors tend to present with endocrinopathies due to hypothalamic/pituitary dysfunction and ophthalmological abnormalities due to involvement of the optic chiasm and visual pathways. Diabetes insipidus, growth failure, secondary hypothyroidism, and, in children, precocious puberty or delayed sexual development have been described, and time to diagnosis may be prolonged [4, 18, 19]. Some unusual presentations include psychosis and behavioral problems, and patients will ultimately develop panhypopituitarism, hypothyroidism, or central adrenal insufficiency [20]. Following a diagnosis of IGCT, full endocrinological and ophthalmological evaluations are recommended to fully identify endocrinopathies and visual disorders. Tumors in the basal ganglia may present with motor dysfunction such as hemiparesis, dystonia, chorea, and neuropsychiatric

disturbances such as abnormal behavior and poor school performance [15].

IGCTs may secrete detectable levels of proteins into the blood and/or cerebrospinal fluid (CSF), and these proteins can be used for diagnostic purposes or to monitor tumor recurrence (Table 24.1). Marked elevations of alpha-fetoprotein (AFP) and beta-human chorionic gonadotropin (ß-hCG) in serum and/or CSF may serve as surrogate diagnostic markers for NGGCTs, but it is less clear for germinomas. Allen et al. reported on 58 newly diagnosed histologically confirmed patients with germinoma gathered from two prospective clinical trials, which required that patients have normal AFP and ß-hCG ≤ 50 mIU/mL in serum and lumbar CSF [21]. There were four categories of ß-hCG profiles: normal serum and lumbar CSF ß-hCG (60%), normal serum and elevated CSF ß-hCG (34.5%), elevated serum and CSF ß-hCG (3.5%), and elevated serum and normal CSF ß-hCG (2%). The lumbar CSF value was higher than the serum value in 87% of patients with ß-hCG elevations. Allen et al. concluded that lumbar CSF was a more informative screen for ß-hCG than serum. The majority of patients had normal ß-hCG values at diagnosis, thus histologic confirmation remains the standard of care.

In most American and European trials, germinoma trials are limited to patients with ß-hCG ≤ 50 mIU/mL in serum and lumbar CSF. There are patients with germinomas with higher levels of ß-hCG, but as levels rise, a small component of choriocarcinoma cannot be completely excluded. There are, however, confirmed secretory germinomas that have ß-hCG levels of up to 200 mIU/mL without adverse impact on survival [22, 23]. Complete diagnostic staging is mandatory, and relapses have been correlated with incomplete diag-

**Table 24.1** Classification of germ cell tumors using tumor markers

| Tumor types | Tumor markers | | | | |
|---|---|---|---|---|---|
|  | β-HCG | AFP | PLAP | OCT4 | c-Kit |
| *Germinoma variants* | | | | | |
| Germinoma | – | – | +/– | + | + |
| Germinoma, syncytiotrophoblastic type | + | – | +/– | + | + |
| *Non-germinomatous germ cell tumors* | | | | | |
| Endodermal sinus (yolk sac) tumor | – | + | +/– | – | – |
| Choriocarcinoma | ++ | – | +/– | – | – |
| Embryonal carcinoma | – | – | + | +/– | – |
| Mixed germ cell tumors | +/– | +/– | +/– | +/– | +/– |
| *Teratoma variants* | | | | | |
| Mature teratoma | – | – | – | +/– | – |
| Immature teratoma | +/– | +/– | – | +/– | +/– |

Abbreviations: *AFP* alpha-fetoprotein, *β-HCG* β-human chorionic gonadotropin, *PLAP* placental alkaline phosphatase

Adapted from Louis DN, Ohgaki H, Wiestler O et al., eds. WHO Classification of Tumours of the Central Nervous System, Third Edition. Albany, NY: WHO Publication Center, 2007:203

nostic work-up [24, 25]. Disseminated disease may occur in about a quarter to a third of patients at diagnosis.

## Pathologic or Radiographic

Imaging by itself cannot differentiate IGCTs from the other CNS tumors and cannot differentiate germinomas reliably from NGGCTs. For this reason, a combination of clinical presentation, tumor markers, MRI and CT imaging, CSF cytology, and histology is used for diagnosis. In cases with normal tumor markers in the serum and CSF, histologic confirmation remains the standard of care [24]. The surgical morbidity and mortality for pineal region tumors have been significant prior to the implementation of minimally invasive procedures such as neuroendoscopy and improvements in neurointensive care [26]. In the future, with the use of highly sensitive methods, low ß-hCG levels may be detected in all germinomas [27]. Several new candidate tumor markers, detectable in CSF or by immunohistochemical staining, include c-kit (CD117), OCT4, NANOG, and SALL4 [28–31].

Germinomas typically are slightly hyperdense on CT when compared to normal brain parenchyma. The tumor border is clearly defined where the tumor interfaces with CSF and more obscure where it merges into the brain parenchyma [32, 33]. Germinomas enhance homogeneously and may have intratumoral cysts and calcifications [18, 34]. On T1 MRI sequences, they appear as well-demarcated lesions which can be isointense or hypointense to the gray matter. On T2 sequences, they are isointense to slightly hyperintense to the gray matter [35]. Teratomas generally appear heterogeneous, are well demarcated on CT, and contain multiple small and large cysts and some calcifications. The entire tumor or parts of it may be enhancing based on the amount of soft tissue content. Mature or malignant teratomas have similar patterns to malignant teratomas, but the cystic component and calcifications may be smaller. Both germinomas and the soft tissue components of teratomas restrict diffusion on advanced MRI sequences [35]. Choriocarcinomas may be accompanied by intracranial hemorrhage and yolk sac tumors tend to be irregular in shape and, unlike germinomas, may be isodense or hypodense on non-contrast enhanced CT [33].

Following initial diagnosis, the neuroaxis is generally staged using imaging with spinal MRI and lumbar CSF cytology [24]. Neuroaxial dissemination is classified based on the medulloblastoma staging system described by Chang et al. [36].

### World Health Organization Pathologic Criteria (2016 Edition)

In most centers, CNS germ cell tumors are classified according to the World Health Organization (WHO) classification system, which is based on histology, the expression of tumor markers in tumor cells and the associated protein markers secreted in both the serum and the CSF [24]. The WHO classification was updated in 2016, and for the first time, the classification uses molecular parameters in addition to histology to define many tumor entities [37]. The classification presents major restructuring of gliomas, medulloblastomas, and other embryonal tumors. However, for germ cell tumors, entities remain unchanged with germinoma, embryonal carcinoma, yolk sac tumor, choriocarcinoma, teratoma (mature and immature), teratoma with malignant transformation, and mixed germ cell tumor (Table 24.2).

A second classification system, which is based on the elevation of serum and/or CSF markers, has been used in some European studies. Based on this system, IGCTs are classified into secreting and non-secreting tumors. Elevated levels of CSF AFP $\geq$ 10 ng/mL and/or CSF ß-hCG > 50 IU/L or either greater than the institutional normal range are considered secretory tumors [2].

A third system is used by the Japanese group and stratifies tumors into risk groups based on the histological subtype and responsiveness to therapy. These risk groups include the good, intermediate, and poor prognostic groups based on the classification described by Matsutani et al. (Table 24.3) [22, 38].

### Prognostic Factors and Molecular Subtypes

Complex chromosomal anomalies have been described in IGCTs including gains of chromosomes 12p, 8q, 1q, and X, as well as losses of 11q, 13, and 18q [39]. Two studies using molecular analysis suggest that activation of the KIT/RAS and AKT pathways may be involved in oncogenesis in the majority of germinomas.

Wang et al. reported an analysis of 62 cases by next-generation sequencing, single nucleotide polymorphism array, and expression array. They found the KIT/RAS signaling pathway was frequently mutated in more than 50% of IGCTs, including novel recurrent somatic mutations in KIT, its downstream mediators KRAS and NRAS, and its negative regulator CBL. There were also novel somatic alterations in

**Table 24.2** World Health Organization classification of intracranial germ cell tumors 2016

| Intracranial germ cell tumors | Notes |
| --- | --- |
| Germinoma | |
| Embryonal carcinoma | |
| Yolk sac tumor | Also known as endodermal sinus tumor |
| Choriocarcinoma | Often associated with markedly elevated β-HCG |
| Teratoma | May be mature or immature |
| Teratoma with malignant transformation | |
| Mixed germ cell tumor | Comprised of a mix of the above histological types |

Adapted from Louis DN, Ohgaki H, Wiestler OD, Cavenee WK: WHO classification of tumours of the central nervous system, ed. 4 Lyon, IARC Press, 2016

**Table 24.3** Japanese classification of intracranial germ cell tumors by histologic subtype and prognosis

| Most aggressive | Choriocarcinoma |
|---|---|
| | Yolk sac tumor |
| | Embryonal carcinoma |
| | Mixed tumors (comprised mainly of choriocarcinoma, yolk sac tumor, or embryonal tumor) |
| Intermediate | Germinoma with elevated levels of β-HCG |
| | Extensive or multifocal germinoma |
| | Immature teratoma |
| | Teratoma with malignant transformation |
| | Mixed tumors (comprised mainly of germinoma or teratoma) |
| Favorable prognosis | Pure germinoma |
| | Mature teratoma |

Intracranial germ cell tumors may be divided by response to therapy into good, intermediate, and poor prognosis groups. Pure germinomas and mature teratomas have the best prognosis, followed by germinomas with elevated levels of β-HCG, extensive or multifocal germinoma, immature teratoma, teratoma with malignant transformation, and mixed tumors composed mainly of germinoma or teratoma. The most aggressive histologic subtypes include choriocarcinoma, yolk sac tumor, embryonal carcinoma, and mixed tumors comprised mainly of choriocarcinoma, yolk sac tumor, or embryonal carcinoma

Abbreviations: *β-HCG* β-human chorionic gonadotropin

Adapted from Matsutani M, Sano K, Takakura K, Fujimaki T, Nakamura O, Funata N, Seto T. Primary intracranial germ cell tumors: a clinical analysis of 153 histologically verified cases. J Neurosurg. 1997 Mar;86 (3):446–55

the AKT/mTOR pathway in 19% of patients with upregulation of AKT1 expression. Less frequently, there were loss-of-function mutations in BCORL1 and mutations in JMJD1C, which is a coactivator of the androgen receptor [40].

Schulte et al. performed genome-wide analysis of genomic copy number alterations in 49 germinomas by molecular inversion profiling. Mutational analysis was performed by resequencing of candidate genes, including KIT and RAS family members. Ras/Erk and Akt pathway activation was analyzed by immunostaining with antibodies against phospho-Erk, phosho-Akt, phospho-mTOR, and phospho-S6. All germinomas coexpressed Oct4 and Kit and showed extensive global DNA demethylation compared to other tumors and normal tissues. Co-activation of Ras/Erk and Akt pathways was present in 83% of germinomas [41].

## Overall Treatment Strategy

Due to the predominance in the younger age group, most of the data and recommendations for young adults are extrapolated from studies in children. There are a few small published series of adult patients (Table 24.4) [42–45]. Currently, the Dutch Society of Neuro-Oncology is conducting a trial for patients 18 years or older with IGCTs.

**Table 24.4** Publications with adult patients

| Author Pub year Institution | Number Histology Characteristics | Median Follow-up | Chemotherapy | Radiation therapy | Notes |
|---|---|---|---|---|---|
| Foote 2010 Toronto | *N* = 10 males Germinoma Median age 24 From 1990–2007 | 130 months | None | CSI 25 Gy with simultaneous boost to 40 Gy | All were alive without relapsed disease. Seven of ten had hypopituitarism prior to radiation therapy and hormonal function was not affected in those with an intact pituitary axis. No reported cognitive decline in the treated cohort |
| Cho 2009 Seoul | *N* = 81 (*N* = 23 age ≥ 20) Germinoma From 1971–2002 | 120 months | None | Focal, WB, but all had CSI after 1982 | Doses reduced from 34.2 to 19.5 Gy with boost to 39.3 to 59 Gy. All failures occurred in focal (4/13) or whole brain (1/8) |
| Calugaru 2007 Paris | *N* = 10 males Germinoma Median age 27 From 1997 to 2005 | 46 months | CDDP, VP16 × 3–4 | 24–30 Gy focal RT, *n* = 5 20 Gy CSI, *n* = 5 | All were alive and free of disease with median follow-up of 46 months. Two patients had memory deficits |
| Silvani 2005 Milan | *N* = 18 Germinoma Median age 21 | 55 months | CDDP, VBL, BLM × 3 | Local, WV, or CSI | All were alive without evidence of recurrence. No decline in neurocognitive function was seen |
| Dutch Society for Neuro-oncology | Adults > 18 years | | Germinoma: None | Germinoma: WVI (M0) or CSI (M+) 24 Gy followed by boost to 40 Gy | Prospective trial |
| | | | Non-germinoma: CDDP, VP16, IF × 4 | Non-germinoma: Focal tumor bed (M0) to 54 Gy CSI (M+) 30 Gy followed by boosts to 54 Gy (50.8 Gy spinal metastases) | |

Abbreviations: *CSI* craniospinal irradiation, *WB* whole brain, *WV* whole ventricular irradiation, *CDDP* cisplatin, *VP16* etoposide, *VBL* vinblastine, *BLM* bleomycin, *IF* ifosfamide

The management for IGCTs is still being refined to maintain high cure rates while potentially reducing morbidity from late effects of treatment. Surgery plays an important role in the management of these tumors. At diagnosis, most pineal tumors will present with obstructive hydrocephalus which will need a CSF diversion procedure. When endoscopic third ventriculostomy is performed, biopsy is generally attempted in this initial stage via the aqueduct if the tumor is accessible to achieve a histological diagnosis. Given the heterogeneity of these tumors, however, sampling may not actually reflect the full range of elements these tumors contain [26]. Since the extent of tumor resection is also associated with improved survival rates [46], some authors advocate radical removal for precise histologic characterization and in cases when chemotherapy is not feasible. In Europe and America, delayed surgery after chemotherapy is generally preferred, while in Japan upfront aggressive surgery is preferred for treatment and prognostic reasons [22, 47–49]. Increasingly in the recent pediatric studies, the role of second-look surgery is being recognized [22, 50, 51].

Germinomas have long been known to be highly curable with radiation therapy alone with cure rates greater than 85% with 30–36 Gy CSI followed by boost to 45–50 Gy to primary tumor [42, 43, 52, 53]. However, the late effects of whole brain or craniospinal irradiation (CSI) have been well documented, with adverse impacts on hearing, endocrine regulation, neurocognitive function, risk of stroke, and secondary malignancies. To mitigate these risks, strategies have been developed to reduce the dose and volume of radiation therapy, often in combination with chemotherapy.

This strategy is increasingly being adopted in adult centers and has led to a reduction in the irradiation dose to about 21–24 Gy in most centers from the previously used 30–40 Gy and a reduction in radiation fields from CSI to whole ventricular irradiation (WVI) with an additional boost to 40–45 Gy to the primary tumor. Fields less than WVI are not recommended due to the increased risk for recurrence in the periventricular region [43, 54–57]. The use chemotherapy with radiation therapy has allowed a reduction in the radiation dose and field volumes. Chemotherapy is able to convert macroscopic to microscopic disease, with response rates of 91% for germinomas and 55% for NGGCT, permitting WVI and CSI dose reductions to 21 Gy and cumulative doses to 30 Gy with 3–5-year estimated event-free survivals (EFS) of 89–93% [22, 58–61]. Further dose reductions to 18 Gy are currently being studied in the COG ACNS1123 trial. There are reports of treatment with WVI treatment alone without boost. Chemotherapy alone cannot replace radiation therapy [62–64]. New treatment technologies such as intensity-modulated radiation therapy or proton therapy permit a dose reduction to nontarget brain [65, 66]. It is unclear as of now whether this reduction in radiation dose is meaningful in avoiding late effects as large studies on outcomes following these recent advances have not yet been carried out. Germinomas in the basal ganglia may still require whole brain irradiation due to the concern that they invade deeply into the brain tissue and relapse can occur in the extraventricular area [38, 67]. CSI alone or combined with chemotherapy has been used for patients with dissemination at diagnosis [25, 68].

In contrast, for NGGCTs, radiation therapy as a single modality is curative for only a small percentage of tumors. Calaminus et al. reviewed the data from several European intracranial NGGCT studies and found that 9 of 11 patients treated with chemotherapy alone died of disease, while 20 of 27 treated with chemotherapy and radiation were disease-free 4 years after diagnosis [69]. In another study, nearly 40% of NGGCT patients who obtained a complete response to multi-agent chemotherapy without radiation went on to relapse with very poor salvage rates with subsequent radiation therapy [62]. These results suggest that radiation therapy, although rarely curative alone, is a required component of the treatment approach. Taken together, these results suggest that NGGCTs respond poorly to radiation therapy alone with only about 30–40% survival rates, and results are improved to about 60% with combined modality therapy with local tumor control using surgery, chemotherapy, and radiation therapy [70]. In general, NGGCTs require higher doses and more extensive fields when compared to germinomas with CSI at doses of 30–36 Gy and local boosts to the tumor site of 50–54 Gy. For metastatic disease, CSI should be given [24]. For localized disease, there is some controversy, as some have reported good results with focal therapy. However, in the NYU study in which patients received CSI ($n = 5$) or involved field RT ($n = 13$), there were four of six patients who had isolated recurrences outside the involved radiation field [71]. Also, Balmaceda et al. found almost a 50% rate of ventricular relapses among patients who achieved complete response with chemotherapy and did not receive radiation therapy [62]. Calaminus et al. reported 80% progression-free survival for patients treated with chemotherapy and CSI [69]. This supports CSI as a conservative strategy for maximizing local control for all patients with NGGCTs. The Children's Oncology Group (COG) phase II trial of induction chemotherapy with or without second-look surgery for newly diagnosed NGGCTs, ACNS0122, reported high response rates and excellent survival outcomes (5-year EFS 84% and OS 93%) [72]. The current COG study, ACNS1123, is evaluating whether the use of pre-irradiation chemotherapy can permit a reduction in the field of irradiation by eliminating spinal irradiation in those patients who respond well to chemotherapy. This arm of the study was recently closed suggesting that there may have been an increased incidence of relapse in this group.

Mature teratomas are generally thought to be less sensitive to chemotherapy and are treated with surgical resection only [24]. Teratomas with immature elements are generally treated using multimodality therapy with chemotherapy and surgical resection, followed by radiation therapy.

Outcomes following multimodality therapy have improved, but morbidity still remains significant due to complications of the tumor itself, surgical resection, and late effects from chemotherapy and/or radiation therapy. Chemotherapy is most commonly associated with otoxocity and nephrotoxicity. The change to carboplatin, which is generally less ototoxic and nephrotoxic than cisplatin, will hopefully lead to less toxicity while maintaining comparative efficacy [72]. The alkylating agents ifosfamide and cyclophosphamide cause hemorrhagic cystitis, which can be prevented with the use of hyperhydration, but the accompanying fluid and electrolyte problems can be difficult to manage in patients with suprasellar tumors who have diabetes insipidus. Secondary therapy-related leukemias can occur with alkylating agents, such as ifosfamide or epipodophyllotoxins, usually between 5–7 years and 3–5 years after treatment, respectively. Bleomycin can also lead to pulmonary toxicities. These complications, although rare, can pose a significant problem in the few patients who have them. Radiation therapy can be associated with multiple complications including a risk for stroke, vascular changes in the circle of Willis, and neurocognitive deficiency and secondary brain tumors including glioblastoma multiforme [73].

## Chemotherapy Only

Chemotherapy was initially used for IGCTs after it was recognized that some of the agents used in the treatment of testicular germ cell tumors also had good CNS penetration [74]. The most common active agents include alkylating agents and platinum compounds, such as cisplatin, carboplatin, ifosfamide, cyclophosphamide, bleomycin, and etoposide. However, the use of chemotherapy alone strategies to avoid radiation therapy did not led to encouraging results [62–64, 75]. Kellie et al. explored treatment of patients with CNS germinoma with the primary objective to determine whether intensive cisplatin- and cyclophosphamide-based combination chemotherapy was effective without radiotherapy. Nineteen patients were enrolled. With a median follow-up of 6.5 years, only 8 of 19 patients remained in complete remission, with a 5-year OS rate of 68% [64]. Kellie et al. also explored a similar approach for patients with NGGCTs and enrolled 20 patients. The authors concluded that intensive chemotherapy was effective in one-third of patients in this study. Salvage therapy, including irradiation, was feasible in patients with recurrent disease [63]. In a third study, da Silva et al. reported on 25 patients treated with 1 of 2 risk-tailored chemotherapy regimens. Eleven patients relapsed at a mean of 30.8 months; eight of them subsequently received radiation therapy. The 6-year EFS and OS for the 25 patients were 45.6% and 75.3%, respectively. These intensive chemotherapy regimens proved less effective than irradiation-containing regimens [75].

## The Role of High-Dose Chemotherapy

High-dose chemotherapy (HDC) has been used in the treatment of germ cell tumors in pediatrics [76]. The rationale for using HDC in these tumors is that most chemotherapeutic agents only achieve a fraction of their concentration in the CSF when administered intravenously. By delivering a high dose, the concentration achieved in the CSF is increased, and since most tumors demonstrate a dose-dependent response to treatment, outcomes can be improved [77]. High-dose carboplatin and thiotepa have been used in the setting of relapse for IGCTs [78]. The current consensus is that patients with NGGCTs can generally not be salvaged without the use of HDC as these tumors are generally not radiosensitive and most of the agents which are typically used to salvage these patients are agents which may have been used in upfront therapy already [24]. The role of HDC for upfront management of IGCTs is unclear.

## COG Trials

Wara et al. reported the survey results of the Brain Tumor Committee of Children's Cancer Study Group. A total of 140 patients were seen during the period from 1960 to 1975, and 118 patients had adequate treatment records to be evaluable. The majority (86%) were younger than 30 years of age with a 2:1 male predominance. Thirty-six of the 57 biopsied patients (63%) were found to have germinomas. The survival of patients in the germinoma group (72%) was comparable to that of the patients without biopsy (71%). The OS rate for all patients (biopsied and unbiopsied) was 65% with follow-up times ranging from 2 to 15 years. Nine patients developed spinal cord metastases (8%), two of whom also had simultaneous primary recurrence; none of these patients had received adjunctive spinal irradiation [79].

Goldman et al. reported the results of COG ACNS0122, a phase II trial evaluating the effect of neoadjuvant chemotherapy with or without second-look surgery before CSI, for 102 children with NGGCTs. Induction chemotherapy consisted of six cycles of carboplatin/etoposide alternating with ifosfamide/etoposide. Patients who had less than complete response after induction chemotherapy were encouraged to undergo second-look surgery. Patients who did not achieve complete response or partial response after chemotherapy with or without second-look surgery proceeded to HDC with thiotepa and etoposide and autologous transplant before CSI. During the median follow-up of 5.1 years, 16 patients recurred or progressed, with seven deaths after relapse. No deaths were attributed to therapy-related toxicity. Relapse occurred at the site of primary disease in ten patients, at a distant site in three patients, or both in one patient. Neoadjuvant chemotherapy achieved high response rates and contributed to excellent survival outcomes in children with newly diagnosed NGGCTs [72]. This regimen is used as the backbone for ACNS1123, the current COG study.

## Indications for Irradiation

### Newly Diagnosed IGCT

All patients with newly diagnosed IGCT should be considered for radiation therapy with or without chemotherapy based on the unsatisfactory results of the chemotherapy alone trials discussed above.

### Recurrent Tumors

There are no standard approaches for patients with recurrent germ cell tumors. Curative options are limited by prior treatment. For patients with pure germinomas treated initially with either radiation therapy or with chemotherapy alone, high salvage rates are achieved. However, for patients with prior chemoradiation or those with relapsed NGGCTs, sustained responses to commonly used salvage chemotherapy regimens are difficult to achieve. To date, cure rates of about 50% have been achieved using a salvage paradigm with surgical resection and intensive chemotherapy to achieve minimal residual tumor, followed by HDC with autologous stem cell rescue [76, 78]. Though compared to germinomas, relapsed NGGCTs patients have a worse prognosis with two-thirds progressing within 18 months of treatment. When re-irradiating recurrent IGCTs, cumulative doses to the optic apparatus or brain stem will often be an issue since these tumors tend to occur in the suprasellar cistern or pineal gland [80].

## Target Volume Delineation

For newly diagnosed metastatic NGGCTs, the best outcomes have been reported with multimodality therapy, incorporating chemotherapy, surgery, and CSI to 30–36 Gy with boosts to 54 Gy (45 Gy to spinal metastases) [24, 70, 72, 81]. For localized NGGCTs, there is some controversy, with some evidence supporting focal irradiation [82], though others demonstrated that recurrences can occur beyond focal irradiation fields [62, 71]. COG ACNS1123 is testing induction chemotherapy and WVI to 30.6 Gy plus boost; however, this arm has been closed to accrual. For adult patients, the Dutch Society of Neuro-Oncology is testing a strategy of induction chemotherapy with focal irradiation for patients with localized disease and CSI for patients with dissemination. The remainder of this section will focus on treatment recommendations for germinomas.

Germinomas are radiosensitive, and there are high cure rates with a variety of varying treatment volumes and dose prescriptions. Traditionally, craniospinal irradiation was followed by a boost to the tumor site. While no longer recommended in histologically unverified cases, radiation therapy was historically used empirically with presumptive evidence of an IGCT based on rapid response. The selection of treatment can be controversial, but the treatment to following protocol guidelines is probably associated with a superior outcome [25]. In this section, CSI, whole brain, WVI, and focal irradiation are discussed. When combined with chemotherapy, volume and dose reductions are effective.

Most contemporary reviews report high survival rates regardless of the volume or dose of radiation therapy [2, 25, 38]. Traditionally, CSI has ranged from 30 to 36 Gy with boost doses to 45–50 Gy. Whole brain or whole ventricular fields with a boost have used doses from 24 to 30 Gy [83]. Proponents of CSI and whole brain argue that these approaches assure the highest cure rates. However, there remains concern that these larger treatment volumes can result in long-term cumulative toxicity. A consensus strategy favors WVI and a focal boost to the suprasellar and/or pineal regions when radiation therapy is used as a single modality for both M0 and occult multifocal disease [24]. The treatment paradigm for COG ACNS0232 for localized or occult multifocal disease was WVI to 24 Gy with boosts to 45 Gy without chemotherapy. The current COG ACNS1123 study has reduced doses to 18 Gy with boosts to 30 Gy for complete responders after chemotherapy and 24 Gy with boost to 36 Gy for partial responders.

## CSI

The most robust data for CSI alone were generated in two prospective European studies. Calaminus et al. reported the results of a nonrandomized international study for intracranial germinoma that compared chemotherapy followed by local radiotherapy to reduced-dose CSI alone. Patients with localized germinoma received either CSI or two courses of chemotherapy followed by local radiotherapy. Metastatic patients received CSI with focal boosts to primary tumor and metastatic sites, with the option to be preceded with chemotherapy. Patients with localized germinoma ($n = 190$) received either CSI alone ($n = 125$) or combined therapy ($n = 65$), demonstrating no differences in 5-year EFS or OS. Seven of 65 patients receiving combined treatment experienced relapse (6 of 7 with ventricular recurrence outside the radiotherapy field), and only 4 of 125 patients treated with CSI alone experienced relapse (all at the primary tumor site). Metastatic patients (n = 45) had 98 ± 2.3% EFS and OS. Localized germinoma can be treated with reduced-dose CSI alone or with chemotherapy and reduced-field radiotherapy. The pattern of relapse suggests inclusion of ventricles in the radiation field. Reduced-dose craniospinal radiation alone is effective in metastatic disease [56]. Bamberg et al. reported the results of 60 patients enrolled between 1983 and 1993 with histologically (n = 58) or cytologically (n = 2) confirmed germinoma enrolled onto a multicenter prospective study (MAKEI 83/86/89). Patients received radiotherapy alone (craniospinal axis/local boost). In the MAKEI 83/86 study (involving 11 patients), the dose to the craniospinal axis was 36 Gy and the dose to the tumor region was 14 Gy. In the MAKEI 89 study (involving 49 patients), doses were 30 and 15 Gy, respectively. Complete remission was achieved in all patients. The estimated (Kaplan-Meier) 5-year relapse-free survival rate was 91.0% at a mean follow-up of 59.5 months with the estimated OS rate was 93.7% [53].

## Whole Brain or WVI

The omission of spinal irradiation with radiation therapy alone has long been debated, with spinal recurrence rates estimated at 6% [84]. Rogers et al. analyzed 278 cases in which whole brain or WVI only was given. The recurrence rate after whole brain or whole ventricular radiotherapy plus boost was 7.6% compared with 3.8% after craniospinal radiotherapy, with no predilection for isolated spinal relapses (2.9% versus 1.2%) [54]. Even with bifocal disease, spinal irradiation may be omitted provided staging is complete [85].

The further volume reduction to WVI has been based on observations that extraventricular intracranial relapses are rare [54, 55, 86]. There can be considerable variability with contouring the whole ventricular volume. In a survey, most respondents were in favor of including the third ventricle, fourth ventricle, and suprasellar and pineal cisterns. Including the prepontine cistern should be considered when patients have had an endoscopic third ventriculostomy. The consensus contouring atlas [87] for COG ACNS1123 is available online [88]. An example of the whole ventricular volume is shown in Fig. 24.1. Of note, for basal ganglia germinomas,

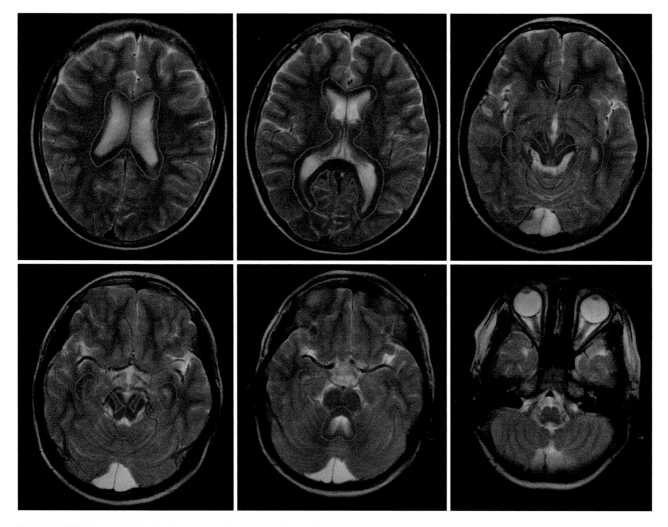

**Fig. 24.1** Whole ventricular planning target volume overlaid on T2-weighted MRI brain. The prepontine cistern was not included in this patient who did not have an endoscopic third ventriculostomy

some advocate whole brain irradiation rather than WVI [38, 67], but further studies are needed.

## Focal or Radiosurgery

Multiple studies using focal irradiation limited to the tumor bed have demonstrated reduced PFS rates, and in one cohort, 36% of patients treated with focal irradiation had intraventricular relapses outside the primary radiation field [52, 54, 89]. Alapetite et al. reviewed the data for all germinoma patients registered in the French protocol from 1990 to 1999, and 10 of 60 patients developed a recurrence. In eight patients, the site of recurrence was in the periventricular area suggesting that recurrences could have been avoided with WVI [57]. Radiosurgery is another focal radiation therapy modality, and cannot be recommended without extended radiation fields [90, 91], but may have a role at disease recurrence.

## Radiation Dose Prescription and Organ-at-Risk Tolerances

Radiation dose prescriptions have been discussed in the section for target volume delineation. The doses used for IGCTs are usually associated with a low risk of radiation necrosis [80], but late effects of treatment have prompted strategies incorporating chemotherapy to allow further dose reduc-

tions or advanced radiation therapy techniques discussed in the following section.

## Complication Avoidance

### IMRT

With intensity-modulated radiation therapy (IMRT) or volumetric-modulated arc therapy (VMAT), cerebral hemisphere sparing with WVI can be improved compared to conformal radiation therapy. IMRT can achieve more conformal plans with absolute percentage reductions of irradiated brain of about 10–15% [65, 92, 93]. An example of the whole ventricular dose distribution is shown in Fig. 24.2, and IMRT plans may use a variable number of beams, coplanar or noncoplanar beam arrangements, or multiple VMAT arcs (Fig. 24.3).

### Proton

Additional dosimetric improvement over IMRT may be achieved with proton beam therapy, whether conformal or intensity-modulated with pencil beam scanning [66, 94]. An example of a non-coplanar IMRT plan compared to a proton plan is shown in Fig. 24.4 and demonstrates that the proton plan can reduce the volume of normal brain outside the target volumes receiving radiation dose.

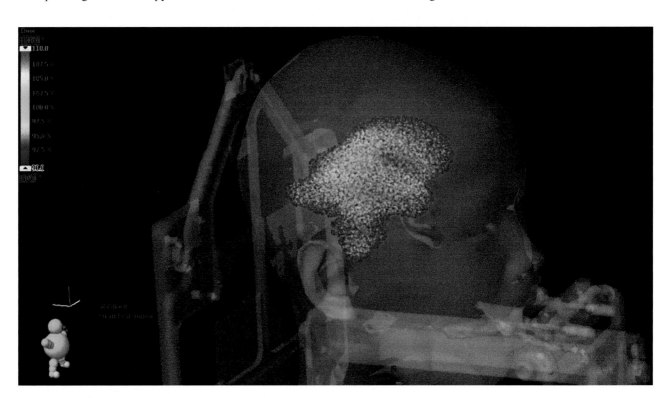

**Fig. 24.2** Dose color wash for whole ventricular irradiation from 90% to 110%

| Ten beam coplanar IMRT plan | Ten beam non-coplanar IMRT plan | Three arc non-coplanar VMAT plan |
|---|---|---|

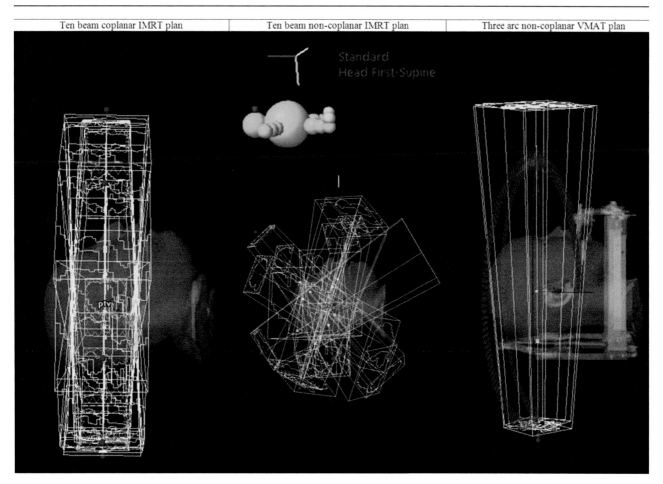

**Fig. 24.3**   Examples of three different beam arrangements for IMRT plans

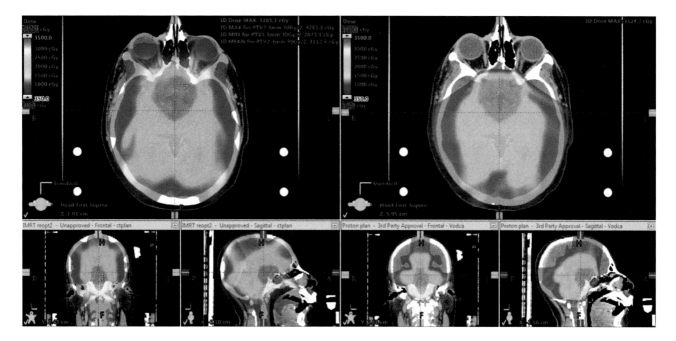

**Fig. 24.4**   Axial, coronal, and sagittal view of non-coplanar IMRT plan compared to proton plan (right) with dose color wash from 3.5 to 35 Gy

## Radiation Toxicity, Acute and Late

The late effects of whole brain or craniospinal irradiation (CSI) have been well documented, with adverse impacts on hearing, endocrine regulation, neurocognitive function, risk of stroke, and secondary malignancies. However, it may be difficult to separate radiation therapy-associated effects from late effects related to the tumor itself, associated hydrocephalus, surgery, and/or chemotherapy. Numerous retrospective series report conflicting results, and reliable prospective data are not yet available. O'Neil et al. evaluated neurocognitive outcomes after chemoradiation in a cohort of 20 patients treated for germinoma from 2003 to 2009 and found that the group performed in the average range on all neurocognitive measures administered and did not decline over time [95].

## Outcomes: Tumor Control and Survival

Outcomes for germinomas are quite favorable; however, recurrence still occurs. There are no standard approaches for patients with recurrent IGCTs, but cure rates of about 50% have been achieved using a salvage paradigm with surgical resection and intensive chemotherapy followed by HDC with autologous stem cell rescue [76, 78]. Re-irradiation has been shown to be effective, although patients may be at increased risk of hormonal or neurocognitive dysfunction [96, 97].

## Follow-Up: Radiographic Assessment

Patients should be monitored during treatment and during follow-up with serum tumor markers for IGCTs, even if initially negative [24]. However, patients may have evidence of tumor recurrence or development of secondary malignancy on imaging, so serum biomarkers alone are insufficient [98, 99]. Dynamic contrast-enhanced MRI may play a role in predicting tumor response to radiation therapy [100].

## Case Presentation

The patient is an 8-year-old Asian boy who presented with a shift in height from the 15th to the 25th percentile and an increase in weight from the 13th to the 63rd percentile over 6 months. He was seen by a pediatric endocrinologist, and initial biochemical and radiological evaluations showed a bone age of 10 years, normal AFP, elevated serum ß-hCG 43 mIU/mL, and testosterone 927 ng/dL. He had imaging studies, including a testicular ultrasound; CT scan of the chest, abdomen, and pelvis; PET scan; and MRI brain, which did not reveal any unusual masses. A repeat serum ß-hCG

1 month later was 29 mIU/mL. After consultation with a pediatric hematologist-oncologist, a lumbar puncture was performed and CSF ß-hCG was 121 mIU/mL. The CSF AFP, protein, and cytology were within normal limits. Two months later, repeat MRI brain and spine showed a prominent pineal gland measuring 6 mm, within the normal limits of size, but contrast enhancement was slightly more prominent than normal. A second lumbar puncture revealed an elevated ß-hCG of 43 mIU/mL and a negative AFP of <0.9 ng/mL. A biopsy was not performed. He was enrolled on COG study ACNS1123 with four cycles of neoadjuvant carboplatin and etoposide with normalization of serum ß-hCG and interval decrease in size of the pineal gland. The patient then received radiation therapy.

## Summary

- Intracranial germ cell tumors are rare and are most common in childhood and early puberty.
- These tumors most often occur in the pineal gland or suprasellar region.
- Overall, there is a male predominance, which is more pronounced for pineal gland tumors.
- There are two groups, germinomas and non-germinomatous germ cell tumors. Histological subtype is an important factor for stratification of prognosis and treatment.
- Germinomas are more common and can be cured with radiation therapy alone. For localized disease, fields have decreased from craniospinal irradiation to whole brain or whole ventricular fields. Further reduction to focal irradiation fields have resulted in an increase of intraventricular failure. Combination of irradiation with chemotherapy has permitted further decreases in dose. Chemotherapy only strategies that omit irradiation have not been proven to be satisfactory.
- Non-germinomatous germ cell tumors have a poorer prognosis, and best results have been achieved with chemotherapy and craniospinal irradiation.
- The most recent Children's Oncology Group trial has been studying smaller volumes and lower doses for those patients who respond well to neoadjuvant chemotherapy.
- Long-term survivors may have changes in quality of life, neurocognition, and endocrine function. These may be reduced with modern radiation therapy techniques such as intensity-modulated radiation therapy or proton beam therapy.
- There is not a standard of care for recurrent germ cell tumors though high-dose chemotherapy and re-irradiation may play a role.

## Self-Assessment Questions

1. This 8-year boy was diagnosed with a pure CNS germinoma with elevated serum and CSF ß-hCG and normal AFP levels. After complete tumor marker response and radiographic response to chemotherapy, which of the following treatment recommendations would be most appropriate?
   A. Craniospinal irradiation with a boost to the primary site
   B. Focal radiation therapy to the pineal gland
   C. Whole ventricular irradiation with a boost to the primary site
   D. Radiation therapy is not necessary after four cycles of chemotherapy
   E. Stereotactic radiosurgery

2. A response to induction chemotherapy may allow a lower radiation dose and smaller irradiation volume for which of the following tumor types?
   A. Anaplastic astrocytoma
   B. CNS germinoma involving suprasellar region and pineal gland
   C. Medulloblastoma
   D. CNS lymphoma
   E. Myxopapillary ependymoma

3. Which of the following diagnoses is most likely for a 17-year-old male who has Parinaud's syndrome and an elevated serum AFP level and a normal ß-hCG level?
   A. Hepatoblastoma
   B. Primary pineal parenchymal tumor
   C. Hypothalamic germinoma
   D. Yolk sac tumor
   E. Pilocytic astrocytoma

4. Which of the following tumor types is least likely to be treated with chemotherapy and craniospinal irradiation?
   A. Non-germinomatous germ cell tumor
   B. Medulloblastoma
   C. Pure germinoma
   D. Pineoblastoma

5. Which of the following complications most commonly occurs in patients receiving fractionated radiation therapy for suprasellar non-germinomatous germ cell tumor?
   A. Radiation necrosis
   B. Optic neuropathy
   C. Diabetes insipidus
   D. Growth hormone deficiency
   E. Meningioma

## Answers

1. C
   Rationale: Chemotherapy alone and focal radiation strategies are regarded as inadequate therapy for focal CNS germinoma with higher rates of local and intraventricular recurrences. Rogers et al. demonstrated that whole brain or whole ventricular irradiation followed by a boost yielded identical rates of local/neuraxis control and survival compared to craniospinal irradiation followed by a boost in adequately staged patients. In patients with complete response to induction chemotherapy, the COG trial is investigating reduced-dose 18 Gy whole ventricular irradiation followed by a boost to 30 Gy.

2. B
   Rationale: Bifocal CNS germ cell tumors that respond to induction chemotherapy may be treated with whole ventricular irradiation followed by a boost. This was the treatment schema on COG ACNS0232, and the rationale for treatment as localized disease is supported by the Canadian data by Lafay-Cousin et al.

3. D
   Rationale: Parinaud's syndrome is an upward gaze palsy that can be caused by a pineal gland tumor. An elevated AFP is suggestive of a NGGCT.

4. C

5. D
   Rationale: Growth hormone is the most radiosensitive hormone followed by TSH and FSH. Patients with suprasellar germ cell tumors may present with diabetes insipidus, but is uncommon to develop following radiation therapy.

## References

1. McCarthy BJ, Shibui S, Kayama T, et al. Primary CNS germ cell tumors in Japan and the United States: an analysis of 4 tumor registries. Neuro Oncol. 2012;14(9):1194–200.
2. Echevarría ME, Fangusaro J, Goldman S. Pediatric central nervous system germ cell tumors: a review. Oncologist. 2008;13(6):690–9.
3. Aizer AA, Sethi RV, Hedley-Whyte ET, et al. Bifocal intracranial tumors of nongerminomatous germ cell etiology: diagnostic and therapeutic implications. Neuro Oncol. 2013;15(7):955–60.
4. Jennings MT, Gelman R, Hochberg F. Intracranial germ-cell tumors: natural history and pathogenesis. J Neurosurg. 1985;63(2):155–67.
5. Rickert CH, Paulus W. Epidemiology of central nervous system tumors in childhood and adolescence based on the new WHO classification. Childs Nerv Syst. 2001;17(9):503–11.
6. Nomura K. Epidemiology of germ cell tumors in Asia of pineal region tumor. J Neurooncol. 2001;54(3):211–7.

7. Villano JL, Propp JM, Porter KR, et al. Malignant pineal germ-cell tumors: an analysis of cases from three tumor registries. Neuro Oncol. 2008;10(2):121–30.

8. Villano JL, Virk IY, Ramirez V, et al. Descriptive epidemiology of central nervous system germ cell tumors: nonpineal analysis. Neuro Oncol. 2010;12(3):257–64.

9. Surawicz TS, McCarthy BJ, Kupelian V, et al. Descriptive epidemiology of primary brain and CNS tumors: results from the Central Brain Tumor Registry of the United States, 1990–1994. Neuro Oncol. 1999;1(1):14–25.

10. Queipo G, Aguirre D, Nieto K, et al. Intracranial germ cell tumors: association with Klinefelter syndrome and sex chromosome aneuploidies. Cytogenet Genome Res. 2008;121(3–4):211–4.

11. Chik K, Li C, Shing MM, et al. Intracranial germ cell tumors in children with and without Down syndrome. J Pediatr Hematol Oncol. 1999;21(2):149–51.

12. Giambartolomei C, Mueller CM, Greene MH, et al. A mini-review of familial ovarian germ cell tumors: an additional manifestation of the familial testicular germ cell tumor syndrome. Cancer Epidemiol. 2009;33(1):31–6.

13. Wong TT, Ho DM, Chang TK, et al. Familial neurofibromatosis 1 with germinoma involving the basal ganglion and thalamus. Childs Nerv Syst. 1995;11(8):456–8.

14. Wei X-H, Shen H-C, Tang S-X, et al. Radiologic features of primary intracranial ectopic germinomas: case reports and literature review. Medicine (Baltimore). 2016;95(52):e5543.

15. Phi JH, Cho B-K, Kim S-K, et al. Germinomas in the basal ganglia: magnetic resonance imaging classification and the prognosis. J Neurooncol. 2010;99(2):227–36.

16. Tian C, Pu C, Wu W, et al. Is biopsy needed to guide management for all patients with presumed intracranial ectopic germinomas. J Neurooncol. 2009;92(1):37–44.

17. Ozelame RV, Shroff M, Wood B, et al. Basal ganglia germinoma in children with associated ipsilateral cerebral and brain stem hemiatrophy. Pediatr Radiol. 2006;36(4):325–30.

18. Packer RJ, Cohen BH, Cooney K, et al. Intracranial germ cell tumors. Oncologist. 2000;5(4):312–20.

19. Legido A, Packer RJ, Sutton LN, et al. Suprasellar germinomas in childhood. A reappraisal. Cancer. 1989 15;63(2):340–4.

20. Malbari F, Gershon TR, Garvin JH, et al. Psychiatric manifestations as initial presentation for pediatric CNS germ cell tumors, a case series. Childs Nerv Syst. 2016;32(8):1359–62.

21. Allen J, Chacko J, Donahue B, et al. Diagnostic sensitivity of serum and lumbar CSF bHCG in newly diagnosed CNS germinoma. Pediatr Blood Cancer. 2012;59(7):1180–2.

22. Matsutani M, Japanese Pediatric Brain Tumor Study Group. Combined chemotherapy and radiation therapy for CNS germ cell tumors—the Japanese experience. J Neurooncol. 2001;54(3):311–6.

23. Finlay J, da Silva NS, Lavey R, et al. The management of patients with primary central nervous system (CNS) germinoma: current controversies requiring resolution. Pediatr Blood Cancer. 2008;51(2):313–6.

24. Murray MJ, Bartels U, Nishikawa R, et al. Consensus on the management of intracranial germ-cell tumours. Lancet Oncol. 2015;16(9):e470–7.

25. Kortmann R-D. Current concepts and future strategies in the management of intracranial germinoma. Expert Rev Anticancer Ther. 2014;14(1):105–19.

26. Souweidane MM, Krieger MD, Weiner HL, et al. Surgical management of primary central nervous system germ cell tumors: proceedings from the second international symposium on central nervous system germ cell tumors. J Neurosurg Pediatr. 2010;6(2):125–30.

27. Fukuoka K, Yanagisawa T, Suzuki T, et al. Human chorionic gonadotropin detection in cerebrospinal fluid of patients with a germinoma and its prognostic significance: assessment by using a highly sensitive enzyme immunoassay. J Neurosurg Pediatr. 2016;18(5):573–7.

28. Miyanohara O, Takeshima H, Kaji M, et al. Diagnostic significance of soluble c-kit in the cerebrospinal fluid of patients with germ cell tumors. J Neurosurg. 2002;97(1):177–83.

29. Ngan K-W, Jung S-M, Lee L-Y, et al. Immunohistochemical expression of OCT4 in primary central nervous system germ cell tumours. J Clin Neurosci. 2008;15(2):149–52.

30. Santagata S, Hornick JL, Ligon KL. Comparative analysis of germ cell transcription factors in CNS germinoma reveals diagnostic utility of NANOG. Am J Surg Pathol. 2006;30(12):1613–8.

31. Mei K, Liu A, Allan RW, et al. Diagnostic utility of SALL4 in primary germ cell tumors of the central nervous system: a study of 77 cases. Mod Pathol. 2009;22(12):1628–36.

32. Chang T, Teng MM, Guo WY, et al. CT of pineal tumors and intracranial germ-cell tumors. AJR Am J Roentgenol. 1989;153(6):1269–74.

33. Fujimaki T, Matsutani M, Funada N, et al. CT and MRI features of intracranial germ cell tumors. J Neurooncol. 1994;19(3):217–26.

34. Smirniotopoulos JG, Rushing EJ, Mena H. Pineal region masses: differential diagnosis. Radiographics. 1992;12(3):577–96.

35. Borja MJ, Plaza MJ, Altman N, et al. Conventional and advanced MRI features of pediatric intracranial tumors: supratentorial tumors. AJR Am J Roentgenol. 2013;200(5):W483–503.

36. Chang CH, Housepian EM, Herbert C. An operative staging system and a megavoltage radiotherapeutic technic for cerebellar medulloblastomas. Radiology. 1969;93(6):1351–9.

37. Louis DN, Perry A, Reifenberger G, et al. The 2016 World Health Organization classification of tumors of the central nervous system: a summary. Acta Neuropathol (Berl). 2016;131(6):803–20.

38. Kamoshima Y, Sawamura Y. Update on current standard treatments in central nervous system germ cell tumors. Curr Opin Neurol. 2010;23(6):571–5.

39. Schneider DT, Zahn S, Sievers S, et al. Molecular genetic analysis of central nervous system germ cell tumors with comparative genomic hybridization. Mod Pathol. 2006;19(6):864–73.

40. Wang L, Yamaguchi S, Burstein MD, et al. Novel somatic and germline mutations in intracranial germ cell tumours. Nature. 2014 10;511(7508):241–5.

41. Schulte SL, Waha A, Steiger B, et al. CNS germinomas are characterized by global demethylation, chromosomal instability and mutational activation of the Kit-, Ras/Raf/Erk- and Akt-pathways. Oncotarget. 2016;7(34):55026–42.

42. Foote M, Millar B-A, Sahgal A, et al. Clinical outcomes of adult patients with primary intracranial germinomas treated with low-dose craniospinal radiotherapy and local boost. J Neurooncol. 2010;100(3):459–63.

43. Cho J, Choi J-U, Kim D-S, et al. Low-dose craniospinal irradiation as a definitive treatment for intracranial germinoma. Radiother Oncol. 2009;91(1):75–9.

44. Calugaru V, Taillibert S, Lang P, et al. Neoadjuvant chemotherapy followed by radiotherapy adapted to the tumor response in the primary germinoma of the central nervous system: experience of the Pitié-Salpêtrière Hospital and review of literature. Cancer Radiother. 2007;11(3):122–8.

45. Silvani A, Eoli M, Salmaggi A, et al. Combined chemotherapy and radiotherapy for intracranial germinomas in adult patients: a single-institution study. J Neurooncol. 2005;71(3):271–6.

46. Schild SE, Scheithauer BW, Haddock MG, et al. Histologically confirmed pineal tumors and other germ cell tumors of the brain. Cancer. 1996;78(12):2564–71.

47. Calaminus G, Bamberg M, Jürgens H, et al. Impact of surgery, chemotherapy and irradiation on long term outcome of intracranial malignant non-germinomatous germ cell tumors: results of the German Cooperative Trial MAKEI 89. Klin Padiatr. 2004;216(3):141–9.

48. Sawamura Y, de Tribolet N, Ishii N, et al. Management of primary intracranial germinomas: diagnostic surgery or radical resection? J Neurosurg. 1997;87(2):262–6.

49. Sawamura Y, Ikeda J, Shirato H, et al. Germ cell tumours of the central nervous system: treatment consideration based on 111 cases and their long-term clinical outcomes. Eur J Cancer. 1998;34(1):104–10.

50. Ogiwara H, Kiyotani C, Terashima K, et al. Second-look surgery for intracranial germ cell tumors. Neurosurgery. 2015;76(6):658–61. discussion 661–2

51. Weiner HL, Finlay JL. Surgery in the management of primary intracranial germ cell tumors. Childs Nerv Syst. 1999;15(11–12):770–3.

52. Nguyen Q-N, Chang EL, Allen PK, et al. Focal and craniospinal irradiation for patients with intracranial germinoma and patterns of failure. Cancer. 2006;107(9):2228–36.

53. Bamberg M, Kortmann RD, Calaminus G, et al. Radiation therapy for intracranial germinoma: results of the German cooperative prospective trials MAKEI 83/86/89. J Clin Oncol. 1999;17(8):2585–92.

54. Rogers SJ, Mosleh-Shirazi MA, Saran FH. Radiotherapy of localised intracranial germinoma: time to sever historical ties? Lancet Oncol. 2005;6(7):509–19.

55. Aoyama H. Radiation therapy for intracranial germ cell tumors. Prog Neurol Surg. 2009;23:96–105.

56. Calaminus G, Kortmann R, Worch J, et al. SIOP CNS GCT 96: final report of outcome of a prospective, multinational nonrandomized trial for children and adults with intracranial germinoma, comparing craniospinal irradiation alone with chemotherapy followed by focal primary site irradiation for patients with localized disease. Neuro Oncol. 2013;15(6):788–96.

57. Alapetite C, Brisse H, Patte C, et al. Pattern of relapse and outcome of non-metastatic germinoma patients treated with chemotherapy and limited field radiation: the SFOP experience. Neuro Oncol. 2010;12(12):1318–25.

58. Buckner JC, Peethambaram PP, Smithson WA, et al. Phase II trial of primary chemotherapy followed by reduced-dose radiation for CNS germ cell tumors. J Clin Oncol. 1999;17(3):933–40.

59. Khatua S, Dhall G, O'Neil S, et al. Treatment of primary CNS germinomatous germ cell tumors with chemotherapy prior to reduced dose whole ventricular and local boost irradiation. Pediatr Blood Cancer. 2010;55(1):42–6.

60. Kretschmar C, Kleinberg L, Greenberg M, et al. Pre-radiation chemotherapy with response-based radiation therapy in children with central nervous system germ cell tumors: a report from the Children's Oncology Group. Pediatr Blood Cancer. 2007;48(3):285–91.

61. Eom K-Y, Kim IH, Park CI, et al. Upfront chemotherapy and involved-field radiotherapy results in more relapses than extended radiotherapy for intracranial germinomas: modification in radiotherapy volume might be needed. Int J Radiat Oncol Biol Phys. 2008;71(3):667–71.

62. Balmaceda C, Heller G, Rosenblum M, et al. Chemotherapy without irradiation—a novel approach for newly diagnosed CNS germ cell tumors: results of an international cooperative trial. The first international central nervous system germ cell tumor study. J Clin Oncol. 1996;14(11):2908–15.

63. Kellie SJ, Boyce H, Dunkel IJ, et al. Primary chemotherapy for intracranial nongerminomatous germ cell tumors: results of the second international CNS germ cell study group protocol. J Clin Oncol. 2004;22(5):846–53.

64. Kellie SJ, Boyce H, Dunkel IJ, et al. Intensive cisplatin and cyclophosphamide-based chemotherapy without radiotherapy for intracranial germinomas: failure of a primary chemotherapy approach. Pediatr Blood Cancer. 2004;43(2):126–33.

65. Chen MJ, Santos A da S, Sakuraba RK, et al. Intensity-modulated and 3D-conformal radiotherapy for whole-ventricular irradiation as compared with conventional whole-brain irradiation in the management of localized central nervous system germ cell tumors. Int J Radiat Oncol Biol Phys. 2010;76(2):608–14.

66. MacDonald SM, Trofimov A, Safai S, et al. Proton radiotherapy for pediatric central nervous system germ cell tumors: early clinical outcomes. Int J Radiat Oncol Biol Phys. 2011;79(1):121–9.

67. Sonoda Y, Kumabe T, Sugiyama S-I, et al. Germ cell tumors in the basal ganglia: problems of early diagnosis and treatment. J Neurosurg Pediatr. 2008;2(2):118–24.

68. Jackson C, Jallo G, Lim M. Clinical outcomes after treatment of germ cell tumors. Neurosurg Clin N Am. 2011;22(3):385–94. viii

69. Calaminus G, Bamberg M, Baranzelli MC, et al. Intracranial germ cell tumors: a comprehensive update of the European data. Neuropediatrics. 1994;25(1):26–32.

70. Robertson PL, Jakacki R, Hukin J, et al. Multimodality therapy for CNS mixed malignant germ cell tumors (MMGCT): results of a phase II multi-institutional study. J Neurooncol. 2014;118(1):93–100.

71. Robertson PL, DaRosso RC, Allen JC. Improved prognosis of intracranial non-germinoma germ cell tumors with multimodality therapy. J Neurooncol. 1997;32(1):71–80.

72. Goldman S, Bouffet E, Fisher PG, et al. Phase II trial assessing the ability of neoadjuvant chemotherapy with or without second-look surgery to eliminate measurable disease for nongerminomatous germ cell tumors: a Children's Oncology Group Study. J Clin Oncol Off J Am Soc Clin Oncol. 2015;33(22):2464–71.

73. Acharya S, DeWees T, Shinohara ET, et al. Long-term outcomes and late effects for childhood and young adulthood intracranial germinomas. Neuro Oncol. 2015;17(5):741–6.

74. Matsukado Y, Abe H, Tanaka R, et al. Cisplatin, vinblastine and bleomycin (PVB) combination chemotherapy in the treatment of intracranial malignant germ cell tumors—a preliminary report of a phase II study—The Japanese Intracranial Germ Cell Tumor Study Group. Gan No Rinsho Jpn J Cancer Clin. 1986;32(11):1387–93.

75. da Silva NS, Cappellano AM, Diez B, et al. Primary chemotherapy for intracranial germ cell tumors: results of the third international CNS germ cell tumor study. Pediatr Blood Cancer. 2010;54(3):377–83.

76. Bouffet E. The role of myeloablative chemotherapy with autologous hematopoietic cell rescue in central nervous system germ cell tumors. Pediatr Blood Cancer. 2010;54(4):644–6.

77. Butturini A, Frappaz D. The challenges of high-dose chemotherapy in CNS tumors. Pediatr Blood Cancer. 2010;54(4):652–3.

78. Modak S, Gardner S, Dunkel IJ, et al. Thiotepa-based high-dose chemotherapy with autologous stem-cell rescue in patients with recurrent or progressive CNS germ cell tumors. J Clin Oncol. 2004;22(10):1934–43.

79. Wara WM, Jenkin RD, Evans A, et al. Tumors of the pineal and suprasellar region: Childrens Cancer Study Group treatment results 1960–1975: a report from Childrens Cancer Study Group. Cancer. 1979;43(2):698–701.

80. Marks LB, Yorke ED, Jackson A, et al. Use of normal tissue complication probability models in the clinic. Int J Radiat Oncol Biol Phys. 2010;76(3 Suppl):S10–9.

81. Calaminus G, Bamberg M, Harms D, et al. AFP/beta-HCG secreting CNS germ cell tumors: long-term outcome with respect to initial symptoms and primary tumor resection. Results of the cooperative trial MAKEI 89. Neuropediatrics. 2005;36(2):71–7.

82. Baranzelli MC, Patte C, Bouffet E, et al. Nonmetastatic intracranial germinoma: the experience of the French Society of Pediatric Oncology. Cancer. 1997;80(9):1792–7.

83. Dattoli MJ, Newall J. Radiation therapy for intracranial germinoma: the case for limited volume treatment. Int J Radiat Oncol Biol Phys. 1990;19(2):429–33.

84. Shikama N, Ogawa K, Tanaka S, et al. Lack of benefit of spinal irradiation in the primary treatment of intracranial germinoma: a multiinstitutional, retrospective review of 180 patients. Cancer. 2005;104(1):126–34.

85. Lafay-Cousin L, Millar B-A, Mabbott D, et al. Limited-field radiation for bifocal germinoma. Int J Radiat Oncol Biol Phys. 2006;65(2):486–92.

86. Shirato H, Aoyama H, Ikeda J, et al. Impact of margin for target volume in low-dose involved field radiotherapy after induction chemotherapy for intracranial germinoma. Int J Radiat Oncol Biol Phys. 2004;60(1):214–7.

87. Mailhot R, Rotondo R, Murphy E, et al. A consensus atlas for whole ventricular irradiation for pediatric germ cell tumors: survey results and guidelines. Int J Radiat Oncol Biol Phys. 2012;84(3):S65.

88. ACNS1123_Atlas [Internet]. Available from: http://www.qarc.org/cog/ACNS1123_Atlas.pdf.

89. Haas-Kogan DA, Missett BT, Wara WM, et al. Radiation therapy for intracranial germ cell tumors. Int J Radiat Oncol Biol Phys. 2003;56(2):511–8.

90. Zissiadis Y, Dutton S, Kieran M, et al. Stereotactic radiotherapy for pediatric intracranial germ cell tumors. Int J Radiat Oncol Biol Phys. 2001;51(1):108–12.

91. Hasegawa T, Kondziolka D, Hadjipanayis CG, et al. Stereotactic radiosurgery for CNS nongerminomatous germ cell tumors. Report of four cases. Pediatr Neurosurg. 2003;38(6):329–33.

92. Yang JC, Terezakis SA, Dunkel IJ, et al. Intensity-modulated radiation therapy with dose painting: a brain-sparing technique for intracranial germ cell tumors. Pediatr Blood Cancer. 2016;63(4):646–51.

93. Sakanaka K, Mizowaki T, Hiraoka M. Dosimetric advantage of intensity-modulated radiotherapy for whole ventricles in the treatment of localized intracranial germinoma. Int J Radiat Oncol Biol Phys. 2012;82(2):e273–80.

94. Park J, Park Y, Lee SU, et al. Differential dosimetric benefit of proton beam therapy over intensity modulated radiotherapy for a variety of targets in patients with intracranial germ cell tumors. Radiat Oncol. 2015;10:135.

95. O'Neil S, Ji L, Buranahirun C, et al. Neurocognitive outcomes in pediatric and adolescent patients with central nervous system germinoma treated with a strategy of chemotherapy followed by reduced-dose and volume irradiation. Pediatr Blood Cancer. 2011;57(4):669–73.

96. Merchant TE, Davis BJ, Sheldon JM, et al. Radiation therapy for relapsed CNS germinoma after primary chemotherapy. J Clin Oncol Off J Am Soc Clin Oncol. 1998;16(1):204–9.

97. Hu Y-W, Huang P-I, Wong T-T, et al. Salvage treatment for recurrent intracranial germinoma after reduced-volume radiotherapy: a single-institution experience and review of the literature. Int J Radiat Oncol Biol Phys. 2012;84(3):639–47.

98. Cheung V, Segal D, Gardner SL, et al. Utility of MRI versus tumor markers for post-treatment surveillance of marker-positive CNS germ cell tumors. J Neurooncol. 2016;129(3):541–4.

99. Martinez S, Khakoo Y, Gilheeney S, et al. Marker (+) CNS germ cell tumors in remission: are surveillance MRI scans necessary? Pediatr Blood Cancer. 2014;61(5):853–4.

100. Feng C, Gao P, Qiu X, et al. Prediction of radiosensitivity in primary central nervous system germ cell tumors using dynamic contrast-enhanced magnetic resonance imaging. Chin J Cancer Res. 2015;27(3):231–8.

# Pineal Region Tumors

Nicholas Trakul and Jason Ye

## Learning Objectives

- Discuss the epidemiology, histologic variants, and oncologic behavior of pineal parenchymal tumors (PPTs).
- List the most common presenting clinical signs and symptoms and discuss standard workup and staging.
- Outline the overall treatment strategy for PPTs, including the roles for chemotherapy, radiation, and surgery.
- Outline basic principles of radiation treatment planning.
- Review the current evidence for treatment and outcomes.
- Discuss guidelines for follow-up, surveillance, and possible treatment-related toxicity.

The pineal gland is the endocrine organ in humans, located at the center of the posterior and habenular commissures of the brain. It measures 5–8 mm in humans and gets its name from its resemblance to a pine cone (Latin: pineas) [1]. Its function is to produce melatonin, a hormone responsible for modulating sleep patterns in both circadian rhythm and seasonal cycles. The "pineal region" is generally defined as an area bounded by the splenium of the corpus callosum and tela choroidea dorsally (superior), the tectum and quadrigeminal plate ventrally (inferior), the posterior third ventricle rostrally (anterior), and the cerebellar vermis caudally (posterior) [2]. In addition to those arising from pineal gland tissue, multiple other cell types can cause tumors in the pineal region. These include germ cell tumors (GCTs), glio-

mas, meningiomas, ependymomas, lymphomas, and metastases and are discussed in their respective chapters accordingly. This chapter focuses its discussion on tumors arising from the pineal gland, also known as pineal parenchymal tumors (PPTs), which account for approximately 27% of pineal region tumors [3].

## Epidemiology

The three histologic tumors that account for most neoplasms arising within the pineal gland are GCTs, PPTs, and gliomas. In a series of 633 cases from the SEER database, these comprised 59%, 30%, and 5% of patients, respectively [4]. Germ cell tumors, the most frequent tumor type found in the pineal region, are discussed elsewhere (Chap. 24).

Tumors involving the pineal gland or body are uncommon, accounting for less than 1% of all adult CNS tumors in Europe and North America [4]. Pineal tumors are more common in children aged 1–12 years where these constitute about 3% of brain tumors [5].

The 2016 WHO classification of CNS tumors divides pineal gland tumors into four subgroups [3]:

- Pineocytoma (grade I) (20% of PPT).
- Pineal parenchymal tumors of intermediate differentiation (grade II or III) (45% of PPT).
- Papillary tumor of the pineal region (grade II or III) (<1% of PPT).
- Pineoblastoma (grade IV) (35% of PPT).

Papillary tumor of the pineal region (PTPR) is a newly recognized rare entity of PPT added to the WHO pineal region tumor classification system in 2007. To date, only 181 cases have been reported in the literature in both adults and children.

N. Trakul (✉)
Department of Radiation Oncology, Stanford University, Stanford, CA, USA
e-mail: ntrakul@stanford.edu

J. Ye
Department of Radiation Oncology, Keck School of Medicine of USC, Los Angeles, CA, USA

© Springer International Publishing AG, part of Springer Nature 2018
E. L. Chang et al. (eds.), *Adult CNS Radiation Oncology*, https://doi.org/10.1007/978-3-319-42878-9_25

## Presentation and Symptoms

Pineal tumors most commonly cause neurologic dysfunction by compressing and direct invading surrounding structures [2]. Up to 75% of patients with pineal tumors can have impairment of oculomotor function such as Parinaud's syndrome, impaired upward gaze resulting from pressure on the pretectal region (the dorsal aspect of the upper midbrain, which contains the rostral interstitial nucleus of medial longitudinal fasciculus (riMLF)) [6].

Alternatively, they can also obstruct cerebrospinal fluid (CSF) flow by exerting mass effect on the third (most common) and fourth ventricles, as well as the aqueduct of Sylvius, which connects the two. Hydrocephalus is common at presentation, manifested by headaches, lethargy, and other signs of increased intracranial pressure.

Progressive local tumor growth may result in cranial neuropathies or hypothalamic dysfunction. Malignant tumors of the pineal gland can destroy the gland and lead to decreased levels of melatonin, which may cause sleep irregularities [7]. While extracranial metastases are rare, symptoms can develop in cases of leptomeningeal dissemination, which is present at diagnosis in up to 19% of pineoblastomas [8].

The rate of tumor growth determines the rapidity of symptom onset and is an important prognostic factor. In a review of over 200 patients with pineal region tumors, average duration between the onset of symptoms to presentations was 11 months, with range of 1 month to 11 years [6] (Table 25.1).

Age at presentation and sex of the patient can assist in forming differential diagnoses. Pineoblastomas tend to occur in young children under the age of 10 (40% of cases), with mean age at presentation of 18, while PPTID and pineocytoma tend to be in older adults in the 40s–60s (mean 41–43) [3]. This is in contrast to germ cell tumors, which tend to occur in the teens and 20s.

Pineocytomas, PPTID, and pineoblastomas all have a female predominance, with a male-to-female ratio of 0.6:1, 0.8:1, and 0.7:1, respectively [3].

**Table 25.1** Signs and symptoms of pineal tumors

| |
| --- |
| *Symptoms* |
| Headaches (73%) |
| Vision abnormalities (47%) |
| Nausea and vomiting (40%) |
| Impaired ambulation (37%) |
| *Signs* |
| Papilledema (60%) |
| Ataxia (50%) |
| Loss of upward gaze (30%) |
| Tremor (20%) |
| Altered pupillary reflexes (17%) |
| Hyperactive deep tendon reflexes (13%) |

Based on data from Ref. [9]

## Diagnosis

The diagnosis and staging workup for suspected pineal tumors include a contrast-enhanced magnetic resonance imaging (MRI) of the entire neural axis. If a lumbar puncture can be safely performed, the CSF should be examined cytologically for leptomeningeal spread. If CSF cannot be obtained by lumbar puncture, it should be obtained at the time of surgery. Whenever possible and felt to be safe, tissue sample should always be obtained in order to definitively establish a diagnosis.

Since germ cell tumor is the most common histology of tumors in the pineal region, serum and CSF levels of alpha-fetoprotein and beta-human chorionic gonadotropin (beta-hCG) need to be obtained to help with the diagnosis. Once tissue is obtained, immunohistochemistry can also be obtained for these markers or placental alkaline phosphatase. There is no serum marker used for diagnosing PPTs at this time.

Measurement of daily variation in serum melatonin levels does not have an established role but remains an area of interest for patients with tumors of the pineal region. In a series of 29 patients with a histologically well-defined pineal tumor and 24-h melatonin profile determination before and/or after surgery, melatonin rhythm was dramatically reduced for undifferentiated or invasive tumors [10]. An abnormal melatonin profile following surgery could be a reflection of either residual tumor or surgical damage to the pineal gland.

## Imaging

MRI is the most useful initial study to identify the tumor and delineate its relationship to adjacent structures.

In some cases, the imaging findings may suggest certain tumor types. While germ cell tumors and malignant gliomas characteristically "invade" through the wall of the third ventricle, expansive compression is more common with pineal parenchymal tumors, low-grade astrocytomas, and meningiomas [11].

The characteristic appearance of each of the PPTs is summarized below:

## Pineocytomas

- Usually present as globular, well-delineated masses <3 cm in diameter.
- Cysts and calcifications are present in up to one-half of cases.
- Peripheral calcifications are more suggestive of pineocytoma than germinoma (due to preexisting pineal calcifications dispersing to the periphery of the lesions) [12–14].
- Typically isodense on CT.

- MRI: hypointense on T1-weighted images and hyperintense on T2-weighted images [15].
- Strongly and homogeneously enhance with contrast.

## PPTIDs

- Usually present as bulky masses with local invasion.
- More rarely circumscribed than pineocytomas.
- May show occasional peripheral "exploded calcifications" on CT.
- MRI: heterogeneous and mostly hypointense on T1-weighted images and hyperintense on T2.
- Postcontrast enhancement is usually marked and heterogeneous.

## Pineoblastomas

- Usually present as large, multilobulated masses in the pineal region and show frequent invasion of surrounding structures, including the tectum, thalamus, and splenium corpus callosum.
- Often have associated hydrocephalus.
- Hyperdense and rarely have associated calcifications on CT [11].
- MRI: poorly demarcated, hypointense to isointense on T1, and isointense to mildly hyperintense on T2-weighted images [16].
- Enhance heterogeneously with contrast in both CT and MRI.

## Papillary Tumors of the Pineal Region

- Well-circumscribed heterogeneous masses composed of cystic and solid portions.
- Frequently associated with aqueductal obstruction with hydrocephalus.
- MRI: T1 hyperintensity (may be related to secretory material with high protein and glycoprotein content).
- Postcontrast enhancement is usually heterogeneous.

However, imaging alone is generally not reliable enough to establish a histologic diagnosis.

## Histology and Prognosis

A tissue diagnosis is generally needed prior to therapy, since treatment is histology-dependent.

Accessing pineal tumors can be challenging because of the gland's deep location and its vicinity to important vascular and neural structures.

Due to concerns about injury to the deep cerebral veins, a direct, visually guided biopsy of the mass with open or neuro-endoscopic surgery has been the preferred approach. An open procedure also allows collection of CSF for tumor marker studies, visualization of the third ventricle for staging purposes, and, if needed, third ventriculostomy for CSF diversion [17].

Despite these potential advantages of an open procedure, contemporary series suggest that stereotactic biopsy is also a safe and well-tolerated alternative, provided a low frontal approach is used to access the tumor below the level of the internal cerebral veins [18]. With this approach, CSF sampling is also possible from the lateral ventricle, which is usually adjacent to the biopsy track. Diagnostic sample can be obtained in 94–100% of the cases with multiple targeted biopsies. Morbidity related to stereotactic biopsy is generally limited to transient worsening of ocular symptoms, although fatal complications have been reported [18]. If the biopsy is nondiagnostic, equivocal, or suggests a benign tumor such as mature teratoma or meningioma, surgery is recommended to establish a definitive diagnosis or to identify focal areas of malignant disease.

Histologic diagnosis of pineal gland tumor is based on the most recent World Health Organization pathologic criteria, 2016 edition.

Pinealocytes are thought to arise from photoreceptor cells, similar to the retina, modified to gain secretory function. Clinical evidence of shared histogenesis is the occurrence of trilateral retinoblastoma syndrome, which consists of bilateral familial retinoblastoma with pineoblastoma. PPTs share morphologic and immunohistochemical features of cells from both the developing human pineal gland and the retina. Pinealocytes are positive for neuron-specific enolase (NSE) and synaptophysin, supporting their neuroendocrine nature. Both pineocytomas and pineoblastomas stain for NSE, and IHC may be used to distinguish PPT from astrocytic tumors.

Pineocytoma—Pineocytoma is a rare neoplasm. It accounts for about 20% of all pineal parenchymal tumors. Pineocytomas are classified as grade I on the World Health Organization (WHO) grading scale for brain tumors (WHO, are well circumscribed, and generally do not seed the CSF [19, 20].

Microscopically, pineocytomas are well-differentiated, moderately cellular neoplasm composed of relatively small, uniform, mature cells resembling pinealocytes. They are composed of sheets of mature-appearing cells arranged in lobules, with rare or absent mitotic figures, and no pleomorphism, hyperchromatic nuclei, or necrosis. They can be associated with rosettes arranged around eosinophilic central areas. While normal pineal gland does not have pineocytomatous rosettes, the absence of rosettes (i.e., lack of neuronal differentiation) in pineocytomas carries poorer prognosis [19, 20].

Pineoblastoma—Pineoblastomas correspond to WHO grade IV tumors with poor prognosis. They are considered by some to be a variant of supratentorial primitive neuroectodermal tumors (PNETs). Like supratentorial PNETs, pineoblastomas are poorly differentiated, infiltrative, and have a significant potential for leptomeningeal and extracranial dissemination.

Pineoblastomas are seen as densely packed small cells with irregular or round nuclei and high mitotic activity ("small blue round cell" tumors). They are commonly associated with necrosis. Pineoblastomas do not express pineocytomatous rosettes, but can have Homer-Wright or Flexner-Wintersteiner rosettes, which are indicative of retinoblastic differentiation [19, 20].

PPTs of intermediate differentiation (PPTID)—Pineal parenchymal tumors (PPTs) of intermediate differentiation are classified as grade II–III according to the WHO classification. They are characterized by moderately high cellularity, round nuclei with mild atypia and "salt and pepper" chromatin, occasional mitoses, and lack pineocytomatous rosettes [3, 21].

Papillary tumor of the pineal region (PTPR) is a rare neuroepithelial tumor that was added to the 2007 WHO classification of CNS tumors. They are classified as WHO grade II or III.

Histologically, PTPRs are epithelial-looking tumors characterized by a papillary architecture, positive for cytokeratin and glial fibrillary acidic protein (GFAP) on immunohistochemistry. The nuclei are round to oval, with stippled chromatin; pleomorphic nuclei may be present. Precise histologic criteria have not been defined [22]. Although microscopically indistinguishable from pineocytoma, the histology is incompatible with a pineal parenchymal tumor.

Prognosis—The main prognostic indicators for pineal region tumors are disease extent and histologic subtype. Tumors with leptomeningeal or spinal metastases have a poor prognosis regardless of treatment.

Pineocytomas have the best prognosis, followed by PPTs of intermediate differentiation, and then pineoblastomas. Pineocytomas are characterized by an indolent clinical course, with long interval (4 years in one series) between the onset of symptoms and surgery. No strictly classified pineocytomas have been known to metastasize. The reported 5-year survival rate of patients with pineocytoma ranges from 86% to 91%. However, a small subset of pineocytomas can take an aggressive form, with multiple recurrences despite aggressive therapy. Extent of surgery is considered to be the major prognostic factor for pineocytoma [23].

PPTIDs have the increased propensity to spread in the neural axis, with approximately 10% of the cases having craniospinal dissemination at diagnosis. They can also recur locally (22%) and have craniospinal dissemination (15%) after therapy. However, they have better prognosis compared to pineoblastomas, with a median overall survival of 165 months (vs. 77 months for pineoblastoma) and a median progression-free survival of 93 months (vs. 46 months for pineoblastoma). Increased mitotic bodies (< or ≥6 per 10 HPF), lack of neuronal differentiation (NFP negative tumor by IHC), and increased Ki-67 proliferation index have been shown to be predictive of poor survival [24, 25].

Pineoblastoma is the most aggressive of the pineal parenchymal tumors, with high incidence of craniospinal seeding and even rare instances of extracranial metastasis [24, 26–28]. Overall survival rates are low, with older studies reporting median survival in the range of 1.3–2.5 years [24, 29, 30] and more recent studies showing improved median overall survival times reaching 4.1–8.7 years [31, 32]. Disseminated disease at diagnosis, young age, and incomplete resection are poor prognostic factors. Radiation therapy has been shown to improve the prognosis in this group of patients [28, 31, 33].

PTPRs is an extremely rare entity, for which there is limited data to guide prognosis. The only prognostic factor currently identified in the literature is whether or not surgical resection was complete. In an updated retrospective series of 44 patients, only gross total resection and younger patient age were associated with improved overall survival. However, in a small series of patients in four published reports, 15 of 21 patients experienced recurrences even after total resection [34]. Radiation therapy and chemotherapy have not shown a significant impact on survival [35]. Increased mitotic and proliferative activity has also been associated with a worse prognosis and may prove to be useful in identifying patients at increased risk for recurrence [36].

## Overall Treatment Strategy

Pineal parenchymal tumors (PPTs) are rare, and there are no large, randomized trials to inform their management. Most data regarding the management of these tumors comes from retrospective case series, and there is no consensus management algorithm.

It is often difficult to distinguish PPTs from other tumors arising from the pineal region (e.g., germ cell tumors) by imaging alone. Establishing a histologic diagnosis is critical to determining the need for metastatic workup, choice of adjuvant systemic therapy, and prognosis. Standard staging workup prior to surgery includes neuroaxis imaging by MRI and CSF analysis. It is increasingly common to obtain an endoscopic biopsy along with third ventriculostomy, if needed, prior to surgery in order to obtain a histologic diagnosis and relieve hydrocephalus if present.

Surgery plays an important role in both diagnosis and treatment of pineal region tumors. The goals of surgery are (1) to confirm histologic diagnosis and (2) relieve hydrocephalus if present and (3) cytoreduction. Complete surgical removal is often difficult, due to the deep location and proximity of critical vascular structures. Pineal region tumors are commonly resected using either an infratentorial suprasellar approach [37] or an occipital transtentorial approach (OTA) [38]. The goal of surgery is maximal tumor resection. For pineoblastoma, there is some controversy regarding whether maximal resection impacts outcome, with some studies reporting that >50% reduction of tumor mass is correlated with increased survival [39]. Other studies have suggested no link between completeness of resection and survival [40]. Reported gross total resection rates for PPTs are 40–50% [38, 41]. Surgery has associated morbidity, with reported rates of mortality ranging from 0% to 11%, major morbidity 3–6.8% and minor morbidity rates of 3–28% [42].

Adjuvant treatment is determined by the completeness of resection and the WHO grade of the tumor (see next section).

## Indications for Irradiation

The role of adjuvant radiation for PPTs is dependent on the histology of the primary tumor. Pineocytomas can often be cured by a gross total resection (GTR), with radiation commonly utilized in the setting of subtotal resection (STR) or biopsy, although recurrence rates in this setting appear to be inferior to that achieved with GTR [41]. Pineoblastomas, due to their propensity to spread throughout the CSF, are often treated similarly to medulloblastomas, with irradiation of the complete craniospinal axis. This can be done with concurrent or adjuvant chemotherapy. Adjuvant radiation is often recommended for PPTIDs and papillary tumors, although its role is less well defined and is still being explored. This has led to a high degree of heterogeneity in regard to use and extent of adjuvant radiation for these tumors. For example, a review of published literature on the treatment of these tumors found that 30.4% of patients received CSI with 32.6% local radiation only. Additionally, 22.8% of patients received chemotherapy, illustrating the wide variety of treatment paths available for this intermediate group [43]. PPTIDs can disseminate throughout the spinal axis, like pineoblastoma, but this occurs at a much lower rate. It is an open question as to whether patients with PPTIDs may benefit from prophylactic CSI, as some limited series have shown little benefit to the practice of these tumors [44].

Unlike germ cell tumors, well-differentiated pineal parenchymal tumors are thought to be relatively radioresistant. This has led to the investigation of stereotactic radiosurgery (SRS) as possible treatment modality, either as a primary treatment for unresectable or subtotally resected tumors or for recurrent disease. While still investigational, early results have been promising, with reported local tumor control rates ranging from 67% to 100% [45–49].

## Target Volume Delineation

### Fractionated Radiation

A thin slice (at least 2 mm through area of interest) MRI with gadolinium contrast should be obtained for treatment planning. If possible, preoperative MRI should be fused with treatment planning imaging set in order to better delineate at-risk areas for coverage in treatment planning. Treatment planning CT is obtained using a thermoplastic mask for immobilization. GTV is typically defined as all visible gross disease on postoperative imaging. CTV is typically delineated as a combination of gross disease and at-risk resection cavity with an expansion to account for microscopic disease spread. For non-infiltrative tumors, such as pineocytoma, a 5 mm CTV expansion is typically used. For the more infiltrative pineoblastoma, a 10–20 mm expansion is utilized. PTV expansion is typically 3–5 mm depending on the availability of image-guided radiotherapy (IGRT) and cone beam CT (CBCT).

Intensity-modulated radiation therapy (IMRT) is preferred at our institution in order to provide maximal sparing of nearby critical structures. Typically, static field or volumetric-modulated arc therapy (VMAT) is utilized. Treatment plans seek to maximize PTV coverage (typically 90% or greater covered by the prescription dose) while sparing critical structures (see next section).

The techniques for CSI are discussed in detail in Chap. 43. The local boost to the tumor bed is typically given in a sequential fashion upon completion of CSI, until the desired total dose is achieved.

For radiosurgery, GTV is usually contoured as the enhancing and non-enhancing tumor as delineated by MRI without CTV or PTV expansion. Typically, SRS is done using Gamma Knife [45] or, if fractionated treatment is desired, with CyberKnife or some other platform which supports fractionated stereotactic radiation therapy [47].

## Radiation Dose Prescription and Organ-at-Risk Tolerances

A radiation dose of greater than 50 Gy is suggested to the tumor and/or resection bed, based on an early report where a high percentage of local failures were seen in patients receiving less than 50 Gy [28]. Typical prescription doses used at our institution are 50.4–54 Gy in 1.8 Gy per fraction covering the PTV, as described previously.

Radiosurgical prescription doses vary, but most series report doses of 12–16 Gy prescribed the tumor margin for single-fraction treatments [45] and 30–36 Gy in five fractions for multifraction treatments [47]. Doses are typically prescribed to the 50–80% isodose line.

Doses to at-risk organs should be constrained using standard treatment planning constraints for CNS structures, for both fractionated and radiosurgery (see Chap. 45).

## Complication Avoidance

Improvements in radiation delivery technique, such as IMRT, VMAT, and IGRT, allow greater conformality and accuracy of delivery of radiation. However, complications can arise when irradiating deep brain structures. As mentioned previously, obstructive hydrocephalus is a common presenting sign for tumors located in this region. This is usually relieved by surgery, but surgery is not done in all cases. Even if pressure is relieved by partial resection, tumor swelling during radiotherapy can lead to recurrence of hydrocephalus, especially if a shunt has not been placed. A series from China examining Gamma Knife SRS in pineal region tumors noted three cases of severe elevation of intracranial pressure requiring ICU admission and one death due to brain herniation [46]. Close monitoring, with quick intervention in the form of corticosteroids and mannitol and intraventricular shunt placement, should be performed when signs of increased intracranial pressure are noted.

## Radiation Toxicity, Acute and Late

Commonly reported radiation-induced acute toxicities in patients undergoing radiation to the pineal region include alopecia and mild to moderate nausea. Long-term toxicities include cognitive decline, hearing loss, and seizure disorder [31]. Endocrine dysfunction has also been reported in the adolescent/adult population [50].

## Outcomes: Tumor Control and Survival

Pineal tumors are rare in adults, and outcomes data are limited to single or multiple institution case series consisting of small numbers of patients. Several literature reviews have also been performed compiling relevant reports into analyses, but are limited by the heterogeneity and limited numbers of the source material. In general, it has been noted that for both pineocytoma and pineoblastoma, adult outcomes are much better than pediatric, suggesting that these tumors behave more aggressively when presenting in children [51].

In adults, outcomes for pineocytomas are generally excellent, and high cure rates achieved with surgery alone. Clark et al. reported a literature review comprising 64 relevant reports on outcomes for pineocytoma, which demonstrated progress-free survival (PFS) rates of 89% at 5 years for patients undergoing surgery, including 100% PFS for patients undergoing GTR. This was superior to that of patients undergoing biopsy alone which has a 5-year PFS of 75%. In this study, radiation did not improve outcomes in patients with STR [41] (Table 25.2).

Stereotactic radiosurgery has been investigated as an alternative to surgery for pineocytoma. Wilson et al. reported on a series of three adults treated at the Barrow Neurological Institute in Phoenix with subtotally resected pineocytoma, none of which demonstrated recurrence at median follow-up of 6 years [48]. A report from the University of Pittsburgh likewise demonstrated 100% control of local disease in 13 patients with pineocytoma treated with SRS [45]. Park et al. looked at SRS using both Gamma Knife (single fraction) and CyberKnife (five fractions) as an upfront treatment, finding 100% tumor control at a mean follow-up of 78 months [47]. These reports suggest that SRS may be a viable alternative for patients unwilling or unable to undergo surgery.

At the opposite end of the spectrum, pineoblastoma outcomes are much poorer when compared to lower-grade tumors, although, as mentioned previously, outcomes for adults are generally superior to pediatric tumors. In a pooled, retrospective analysis, Lutterbach et al. reported a 5-year survival of 51% for a group of adults with primarily pineoblastoma. Increasing age and lower amount of residual disease after primary treatment were found to be positively associated with survival [39]. A smaller combined analysis from Indiana University and the Mayo Clinic likewise noted median survival rates of 118 months with 42% of adult patients alive past 5 years [40]. This is in stark contrast to the pediatric population, especially patients younger than 4 years old, where 5-year survival rates are about 12%. Interestingly, patients older than 4 display survival closer to adults, with 5-year OS rates of 66% [52]. One attempt was made using a population registry database to examine outcomes for pineoblastoma in adults.

Selvanathan et al. were able to identify 95 patients in the Surveillance, Epidemiology and End Results (SEER) database diagnosed between 1990 and 2007. Median survival was 176 months in this cohort and 5-year overall survival was 62.8% [53].

There are few studies that focus solely on PPTIDs, and many older studies may have included patients with this pathology in their analysis, incorrectly classified as higher- or lower-grade tumors. Mallick et al., identifying and analyzing published series of PPTIDs, performed a comprehensive literature review. They were able to identify 29 studies with

**Table 25.2** Published outcomes for pineal tumors in adults

| References | Type | Number | Histology | Surgery | Radiation | PFS | OS |
|---|---|---|---|---|---|---|---|
| Clark et al. (2010) [41] | Literature review | 166 | PC | Biopsy 21%<br>STR 38%<br>GTR 42% | Local 28% | GTR 94% (5 years)<br>STR + XRT 84%<br>(5 years) | NR |
| Wilson et al. (2012) [48] | Single institution | 14 | PC | GTR 36%<br>STR 64% | SRS 35% | 100% with<br>STR + SRS | NR |
| Park et al. (2015) [47] | Single institution | 9 | PC 33%<br>PPTID 67% | Biopsy 100% | SRS 100% | 100% local control<br>1 case spinal metastasis | NR |
| Kano et al. (2009) [45] | Single Institution | 20 | PC 65%<br>PB 25% | Biopsy 75% | SRS 100% | PC 100% (5 years)<br>PB 67% (3 years) | PC 92.3%<br>PB 28.6% |
| Mallick et al. (2016) [43] | Literature review | 127 | PPTID | Biopsy 31.7%<br>STR 31.9%<br>GTR 25.2% | CSI 30.5%<br>Local 32.6% | 52.2% (5 years) | 84.1% (5 years) |
| Das et al. (2016) [44] | Single institution | 5 | PPTID | Biopsy 20%<br>STR 80% | Local 100% | 100% (21 months) | 100% (21 months) |
| Gener et al. (2015) [40] | 2 institution pooled | 12 | PB | Biopsy 50%<br>STR 25%<br>GTR 25% | 75% | 42% (7 years) | 68% (7 years) |
| Lutterbach et al. (2002) [39] | Multicenter | 101 | PPTID 37%<br>PB 63% | Biopsy 44%<br>Surgery 56% | CSI 60%<br>Local 38% | PPTID 93 months (median)<br>PB 46 months (median | PPTID 165 months (median)<br>PB 77 months (median) |
| Selvanathan et al. (2012) [53] | SEER | 95 | PB | Biopsy 15%<br>STR 21%<br>GTR 16%<br>Unknown 48% | Any 47% | NR | 62.8% (5 years) |

Abbreviations: *PC* pineocytoma, *PPTID* pineal parenchymal tumor of intermediate differentiation, *PB* pineoblastoma, *GTR* gross total resection, *STR* subtotal resection, *CSI* craniospinal irradiation, *SRS* stereotactic radiosurgery, *PFS* progress-free survival, *OS* overall survival, *NR* not reported

127 patients. As expected, survival rates for PPTID were superior to pineoblastoma, with median overall survival of 14 years and a 5-year OS rate of 84.1%. Twenty-four patients had recurrence of disease, and of these recurrences, 15 (62.5%) occurred within the spine/leptomeninges and 9 (37.5%) were local recurrences. This study also illustrates the wide variety of adjuvant approaches used in these tumors. Adjuvant radiation was used in only 36% of cases, ranging from CSI (15 cases) to SRS (4 cases) [43]. Das et al. reported a smaller series of five patients using a uniform technique of adjuvant local fractionated radiation to 54 Gy. They reported that no patients suffered failure either locally or within the spine and all were alive at a median follow-up of 21.4 months. The authors suggest that spinal/leptomeningeal failure may not occur commonly enough to warrant CSI in this population [44].

## Follow-Up: Radiographic Assessment

Standard follow-up includes MRI of the brain and spine (for PPTID and pineoblastoma) at regular intervals with clinical exam. Routine monitoring of pituitary axis should also be done, with referral to endocrinology as indicated. Routine clinical exam should be performed with emphasis on cranial nerve function and neurocognitive assessment as warranted.

## Case Study

Patient is a 37-year-old female that initially presented with hearing loss that developed over 5 months. She was eventually worked up with MRI brain, which identified a 3.9 × 3.9 × 3.4 cm (APxTVxCC) contrast enhancing pineal mass (Fig. 25.1). She was referred to neurosurgeon, who identified a slight right cranial nerve IV palsy and gait ataxia on physical exam. She underwent suboccipital craniotomy with subtotal resection. Post-op MRI demonstrated surgical changes and blood products with 1.5 × 2.1 ×1.2 cm residual tumor in the right lateral edge of the resection cavity (Fig. 25.2). Final pathology identified a pineal parenchymal tumor of intermediate differentiation with mitotic index of 9.8% suggestive of WHO grade III.

CSF sampling on that day was negative for malignancy. She was subsequently discharged to physical therapy with residual right eye lateral gaze palsy and gait ataxia. Patient was evaluated by radiation oncology, and whole spine MRI done approximately 4 weeks post-op confirmed the absence of spinal metastases. Thus, patient was recommended to undergo post-operative radiation therapy with IMRT to a dose of 54 Gy in 30 fractions to the residual disease with a margin. Had she had disease in the spine, treatment recommendation would have changed to CSI 36 Gy in 20 fractions followed by a boost to the residual disease to total dose of 54 Gy.

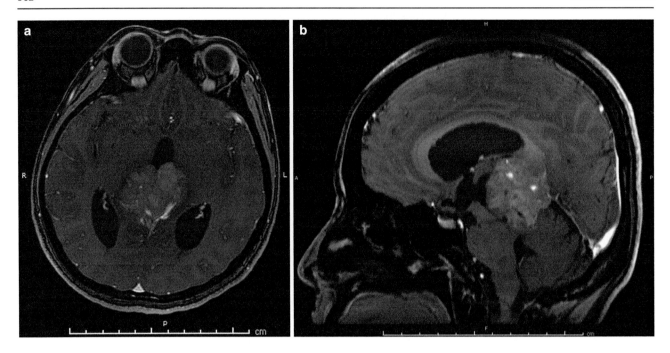

**Fig. 25.1** Axial (**a**) and sagittal (**b**) views of MRI with IV contrast demonstrating a large pineal mass causing mass effect on the midbrain and hydrocephalus

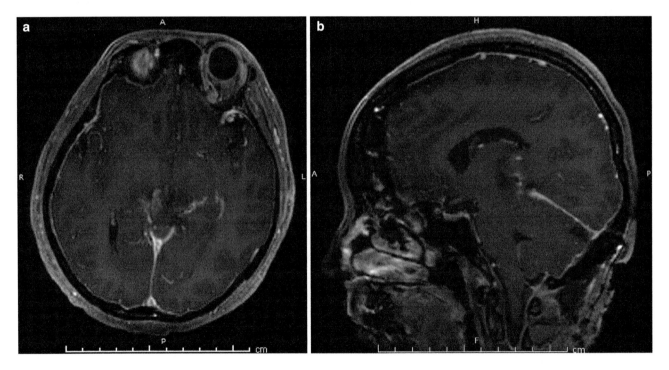

**Fig. 25.2** Post-operative axial (**a**) and sagittal (**b**) views of MRI with IV contrast showing resolution of hydrocephalus and a small enhancing residual tumor in the surgical cavity

## Summary

- Pineal parenchymal tumors (PPTs) comprise 27% of pineal region tumors.
- PPTs are rare in adults, comprising <1% of all diagnosed brain tumors.
- WHO grade has important implications in terms of risk of craniospinal axis spread and prognosis.
- PPTs are behaving less aggressively in the adult population when compared to the pediatric experience.
- Adjuvant treatment is usually indicated for higher-grade tumors and subtotal resections.
- Craniospinal irradiation is indicated for tumors that have the capability of leptomeningeal and spinal dissemination.

## Self-Assessment Questions

1. Which WHO grade corresponds to pineoblastoma?
   A. WHO grade I
   B. WHO grade II
   C. WHO grade III
   D. WHO grade IV

2. Which adult pineal region tumor can be cured using surgery alone?
   A. Pineocytoma
   B. Germ cell tumor
   C. Pineoblastoma
   D. Glioma

3. In which pineal parenchymal tumor is the risk of spinal dissemination the highest?
   A. Pineocytoma
   B. Pineoblastoma
   C. Pineal parenchymal tumor of intermediate differentiation (PPTID)
   D. Pineal papillary tumor (PPT)

## Answers

1. D
2. A
3. B

## References

1. Brastianos HC, Brastianos PK, Blakeley J. Pineal region tumors. In: Norden AD, Reardon DA, Wen PCY, editors. Primary central nervous system tumors. Totowa, NJ: Humana Press; 2011. p. 435–55.
2. Chin LS, Regine WF. Principles and practice of stereotactic radiosurgery. New York: Springer; 2015.
3. Louis DN, Perry A, Reifenberger G, et al. The 2016 World Health Organization classification of tumors of the central nervous system: a summary. Acta Neuropathol. 2016;131:803–20.
4. Al-Hussaini M, Sultan I, Abuirmileh N, et al. Pineal gland tumors: experience from the SEER database. J Neurooncol. 2009;94:351–8.
5. Ostrom QT, Gittleman H, Fulop J, et al. CBTRUS statistical report: primary brain and central nervous system tumors diagnosed in the United States in 2008–2012. Neuro Oncol. 2015;17(Suppl 4):iv1–iv62.
6. Konovalov AN, Pitskhelauri DI. Principles of treatment of the pineal region tumors. Surg Neurol. 2003;59:250–68.
7. Norden AD, Reardon DA, Wen PY. Primary central nervous system tumors: pathogenesis and therapy. New York: Springer; 2011.
8. Luther N, Stetler WR, Dunkel IJ, et al. Subarachnoid dissemination of intraventricular tumors following simultaneous endoscopic biopsy and third ventriculostomy. J Neurosurg Pediatr. 2010;5:61–7.
9. Chang CG, Kageyama N, Kobayashi T, et al. Pineal tumors: clinical diagnosis, with special emphasis on the significance of pineal calcification. Neurosurgery. 1981;8:656–68.
10. Leston J, Mottolese C, Champier J, et al. Contribution of the daily melatonin profile to diagnosis of tumors of the pineal region. J Neurooncol. 2009;93:387–94.
11. Chiechi MV, Smirniotopoulos JG, Mena H. Pineal parenchymal tumors: CT and MR features. J Comput Assist Tomogr. 1995;19:509–17.
12. Awa R, Campos F, Arita K, et al. Neuroimaging diagnosis of pineal region tumors-quest for pathognomonic finding of germinoma. Neuroradiology. 2014;56:525–34.
13. Ganti SR, Hilal SK, Stein BM, et al. CT of pineal region tumors. AJR Am J Roentgenol. 1986;146:451–8.
14. Vaquero J, Ramiro J, Martínez R, et al. Clinicopathological experience with pineocytomas: report of five surgically treated cases. Neurosurgery. 1990;27:612–8. discussion 618–9
15. Korogi Y, Takahashi M, Ushio Y. MRI of pineal region tumors. J Neurooncol. 2001;54:251–61.
16. Nakamura M, Saeki N, Iwadate Y, et al. Neuroradiological characteristics of pineocytoma and pineoblastoma. Neuroradiology. 2000;42:509–14.
17. Reddy AT, Wellons JC, Allen JC, et al. Refining the staging evaluation of pineal region germinoma using neuroendoscopy and the presence of preoperative diabetes insipidus. Neuro Oncol. 2004;6:127–33.
18. Regis J, Bouillot P, Rouby-Volot F, et al. Pineal region tumors and the role of stereotactic biopsy: review of the mortality, morbidity, and diagnostic rates in 370 cases. Neurosurgery. 1996;39:907–12. discussion 912–4
19. Borit A, Blackwood W, Mair WG. The separation of pineocytoma from pineoblastoma. Cancer. 1980;45:1408–18.
20. Jouvet A, Saint-Pierre G, Fauchon F, et al. Pineal parenchymal tumors: a correlation of histological features with prognosis in 66 cases. Brain Pathol. 2000;10:49–60.
21. Cohan JN, Moliterno JA, Mok CL, et al. Pineal parenchymal tumor of intermediate differentiation with papillary features: a continuum of primary pineal tumors? J Neurooncol. 2011;101:301–6.
22. Louis DN, Ohgaki H, Wiestler OD, et al. The 2007 WHO classification of tumours of the central nervous system. Acta Neuropathol. 2007;114:97–109.
23. Deshmukh VR, Smith KA, Rekate HL, et al. Diagnosis and management of pineocytomas. Neurosurgery. 2004;55:349–55. discussion 355–7
24. Fauchon F, Jouvet A, Paquis P, et al. Parenchymal pineal tumors: a clinicopathological study of 76 cases. Int J Radiat Oncol Biol Phys. 2000;46:959–68.
25. Fèvre-Montange M, Vasiljevic A, Frappaz D, et al. Utility of Ki67 immunostaining in the grading of pineal parenchymal tumours: a multicentre study. Neuropathol Appl Neurobiol. 2012;38:87–94.
26. Herrick MK, Rubinstein LJ. The cytological differentiating potential of pineal parenchymal neoplasms (true pinealomas). A clinicopathological study of 28 tumours. Brain. 1979;102:289–320.
27. Jacobs JJ, Rosenberg AE. Extracranial skeletal metastasis from a pinealoblastoma. A case report and review of the literature. Clin Orthop Relat Res. 1989;(247):256–60.
28. Schild SE, Scheithauer BW, Schomberg PJ, et al. Pineal parenchymal tumors. Clinical, pathologic, and therapeutic aspects. Cancer. 1993;72:870–80.
29. Chang SM, Lillis-Hearne PK, Larson DA, et al. Pineoblastoma in adults. Neurosurgery. 1995;37:383–90. discussion 390–1
30. Mena H, Ribas JL, Enzinger FM, et al. Primary angiosarcoma of the central nervous system. Study of eight cases and review of the literature. J Neurosurg. 1991;75:73–6.
31. Farnia B, Allen PK, Brown PD, et al. Clinical outcomes and patterns of failure in pineoblastoma: a 30-year, single-institution retrospective review. World Neurosurg. 2014;82:1232–41.
32. Jakacki RI, Burger PC, Kocak M, et al. Outcome and prognostic factors for children with supratentorial primitive neuroectodermal tumors treated with carboplatin during radiotherapy: a report

from the Children's Oncology Group. Pediatr Blood Cancer. 2015;62:776–83.

33. Lee JYK, Wakabayashi T, Yoshida J. Management and survival of pineoblastoma: an analysis of 34 adults from the brain tumor registry of Japan. Neurol Med Chir (Tokyo). 2005;45:132–41. discussion 141–2

34. Fèvre-Montange M, Hasselblatt M, Figarella-Branger D, et al. Prognosis and histopathologic features in papillary tumors of the pineal region: a retrospective multicenter study of 31 cases. J Neuropathol Exp Neurol. 2006;65:1004–11.

35. Fauchon F, Hasselblatt M, Jouvet A, et al. Role of surgery, radiotherapy and chemotherapy in papillary tumors of the pineal region: a multicenter study. J Neurooncol. 2013;112:223–31.

36. Heim S, Beschorner R, Mittelbronn M, et al. Increased mitotic and proliferative activity are associated with worse prognosis in papillary tumors of the pineal region. Am J Surg Pathol. 2014;38:106–10.

37. Hernesniemi J, Romani R, Albayrak BS, et al. Microsurgical management of pineal region lesions: personal experience with 119 patients. Surg Neurol. 2008;70:576–83.

38. Tsumanuma I, Tanaka R, Fujii Y. Occipital transtentorial approach and combined treatments for pineal parenchymal tumors. Prog Neurol Surg. 2009;23:26–43.

39. Lutterbach J, Fauchon F, Schild SE, et al. Malignant pineal parenchymal tumors in adult patients: patterns of care and prognostic factors. Neurosurgery. 2002;51:44–55. discussion 55–6

40. Gener MA, Conger AR, Van Gompel J, et al. Clinical, pathological, and surgical outcomes for adult pineoblastomas. World Neurosurg. 2015;84:1816–24.

41. Clark AJ, Ivan ME, Sughrue ME, et al. Tumor control after surgery and radiotherapy for pineocytoma. J Neurosurg. 2010;113:319–24.

42. Bruce JN, Ogden AT. Surgical strategies for treating patients with pineal region tumors. J Neurooncol. 2004;69:221–36.

43. Mallick S, Benson R, Rath GK. Patterns of care and survival outcomes in patients with pineal parenchymal tumor of intermediate differentiation: an individual patient data analysis. Radiother Oncol J Eur Soc Ther Radiol Oncol. 2016;121:204–8.

44. Das P, Mckinstry S, Devadass A, et al. Are we over treating Pineal Parenchymal tumour with intermediate differentiation? Assessing the role of localised radiation therapy and literature review. Springerplus. 2016;5:26.

45. Kano H, Niranjan A, Kondziolka D, et al. Role of stereotactic radiosurgery in the management of pineal parenchymal tumors. Prog Neurol Surg. 2009;23:44–58.

46. Li W, Zhang B, Kang W, et al. Gamma knife radiosurgery (GKRS) for pineal region tumors: a study of 147 cases. World J Surg Oncol. 2015;13:304.

47. Park JH, Kim JH, Kwon DH, et al. Upfront stereotactic radiosurgery for pineal parenchymal tumors in adults. J Korean Neurosurg Soc. 2015;58:334–40.

48. Wilson DA, Awad A-W, Brachman D, et al. Long-term radiosurgical control of subtotally resected adult pineocytomas. J Neurosurg. 2012;117:212–7.

49. Yianni J, Rowe J, Khandanpour N, et al. Stereotactic radiosurgery for pineal tumours. Br J Neurosurg. 2012;26:361–6.

50. Stoiber EM, Schaible B, Herfarth K, et al. Long term outcome of adolescent and adult patients with pineal parenchymal tumors treated with fractionated radiotherapy between 1982 and 2003—a single institution's experience. Radiat Oncol. 2010;5:122.

51. Sonabend AM, Bruce JN. Management paradigms along a histologic spectrum of pineal cell tumors. World Neurosurg. 2014;81:685–7.

52. Mynarek M, Pizer B, Dufour C, et al. Evaluation of age-dependent treatment strategies for children and young adults with pineoblastoma: analysis of pooled European Society for Paediatric Oncology (SIOP-E) and US Head Start data. Neuro Oncol. 2017;19(4):576–85.

53. Selvanathan SK, Hammouche S, Smethurst W, et al. Outcome and prognostic features in adult pineoblastomas: analysis of cases from the SEER database. Acta Neurochir (Wien). 2012;154:863–9.

# Glomus Tumors

# 26

Jenny Yan and Kristin Janson Redmond

## Abbreviations

| | |
|---|---|
| 3DCRT | Three-dimensional conformal radiation therapy |
| GK | Gamma Knife |
| GTR | Gross total resection |
| HSRT | Hypofractionated stereotactic radiation therapy |
| IMRT | Intensity-modulated radiation therapy |
| LINAC | Linear accelerator |
| MEN2B | Multiple endocrine neoplasia type 2 |
| MIBG | Meta-iodobenzylguanidine |
| NF1 | Neurofibromatosis type 1 |
| PET | Positron-emission tomography |
| RT | Radiation therapy |
| SRS | Stereotactic radiosurgery |
| STR | Subtotal resection |
| VHL | Von Hippel-Lindau |

## Learning Objectives

- Understand the epidemiology, diagnosis, and prognosis of different types of paragangliomas.
- Understand past and current treatment methods of paragangliomas.
- Understand indications for radiation therapy as well as potential dose fractionation schedules.
- Understand side effects and outcomes of radiation therapy.

## Introduction

Glomus tumors, or paragangliomas, are neuroendocrine tumors that are from neural crest-derived cells (chromaffin cells) of the extra-adrenal autonomic paraganglia. These tumors may come from either sympathetic or parasympathetic paraganglia and can have catecholamine-secreting functions [1, 2]. Sympathetic-derived paragangliomas account for most of the catecholamine-secreting tumors (86% in a study of 236 patients), typically with high levels of norepinephrine in biochemical screening tests [3]. Almost all secreting paragangliomas are from the sympathetic chain along the thorax (10%), abdomen (75%), bladder, and prostate (10%) [1, 4]. Parasympathetic-derived tumors are usually benign, non-catecholamine-secreting tumors most commonly found in the skull and neck bases near cranial nerves. There are three main sites for these latter head and neck tumors: carotid body, jugulotympanic, and vagal paraganglia. Depending on the location of the tumor, head and neck paragangliomas often have various presentations, complications, and therapeutic options that differ from paragangliomas below the neck [1, 5]. The focus of this chapter will be on the epidemiology, diagnosis, prognosis, and treatment of head and neck paragangliomas.

## Background/Epidemiology

Paragangliomas of the head and neck are the most common tumor of the middle ear and second most common of the temporal bone [5]. The annual incidence is about one case per 1.3 million patients in the USA. Sporadic cases are more commonly found in females than males (3:1), mostly in the fifth decade of life [5, 6]. Tumors in nonhereditary cases generally present as single (multiple tumors in 1.2% of cases), unilateral, and are often found on the left side for unknown mechanisms [5].

J. Yan · K. J. Redmond (✉)
Department of Radiation Oncology and Molecular Radiation Services, Johns Hopkins University, Baltimore, MD, USA
e-mail: kjanson3@jhmi.edu

© Springer International Publishing AG, part of Springer Nature 2018
E. L. Chang et al. (eds.), *Adult CNS Radiation Oncology*, https://doi.org/10.1007/978-3-319-42878-9_26

Approximately one-third of paragangliomas are hereditary and are more likely to present with multiple tumors at an earlier age than sporadic types [7]. Hereditary forms are commonly associated with neurofibromatosis type 1 (NF1), von Hippel-Lindau (VHL), Carney-Stratakis dyad, and some rare cases of multiple endocrine neoplasia type 2 (MEN2B) [5, 8]. Mutations of the familial form are often from defective B, C, and D subunits of succinate dehydrogenase (SDH), an enzyme important in the citric acid cycle and electron transport chain of the mitochondria. Screenings for mutations in *SDHD*, *SDHC*, *SDHAF2*, and *SDHB* are recommended for all patients with paraganglioma [8].

Most head and neck paragangliomas are benign, but about 20% may become malignant over time. Diagnosis of malignancy is complicated since imaging and histology may not always reveal evidence of tumor invasion and metastasis [1]. Malignancy rates differ for various locations of paragangliomas with 10–19% for vagal tumors, 4–6% for carotid body tumors, and 2–4% for jugulotympanic tumors [9]. Spread of tumor cells is more likely to be regional (69% of cases) than distant metastases and tends to have better survival outcomes with regional disease (77%) than distant disease (12%), but the rates of survival outcomes vary greatly between different study reports between reports of 35% to 100% [10].

## Diagnosis and Prognosis

### Pathologic or Radiographic

Diagnosis of both catecholamine-secreting and non-catecholamine-secreting paragangliomas typically starts with biochemical testing of urinary and/or plasma fractionated metanephrine and catecholamine levels [11]. Although head and neck paragangliomas rarely secrete catecholamines (3.6%), biochemical screening is still an essential diagnostic tool to avoid complications of catecholamine crises during surgical and radiation treatments [5].

Patients suspected of head and neck paragangliomas usually present with symptoms of pulsatile tinnitus with or without conductive hearing loss and/or non-tender masses in the lateral neck area [12]. For these patients, ultrasound, CT, and MRI imaging are the gold standards for diagnoses. Ultrasound is usually better for patients with suspected carotid body paragangliomas, while MRI and CT are often used for jugulotympanic or vagal paragangliomas [13]. CT scans are commonly used to look for invasion of surrounding osseous structures and displacement of major blood vessels [4]. Before administering contrast for CT scans, patients must show negative biochemical results for catecholamine hypersecretion or be given an alpha-blockade therapy due to possible complications of a catecholamine crisis.

To further characterize vascular involvement of the tumor, gadolinium-enhancing MRI is usually performed. MRI may also help to detect tumor spread to the dura mater and is the test of choice for children and pregnant women. T2 images show classic signal patterns of "salt and pepper" appearance from areas of hemorrhage or slow flow (salt) and high vascularity with flow voids (pepper) in majority of lesions larger than 2 cm (Fig. 26.1) [14, 15].

Definitive diagnosis of paragangliomas requires a tissue histopathology at the time of resection. Typical histological features show nesting (Zellballen) or trabecular patterns of cells with prominent vascular networks highlighted with reticulin [16]. Nests are made up of round/oval cells with giant cells and granular eosinophilic cytoplasms, intracytoplasmic hyaline globules, and abundant stroma.

Despite the usefulness of biopsies, they are often difficult to obtain because aspiration or incision may cause severe hemorrhage or hypertension from a catecholamine crisis. Patients undergoing resection or biopsy must first have a negative biochemical test or receive alpha-adrenergic blockade therapy. Even with biopsies, head and neck paraganglioma samples are often mistaken for other types of cancers such as neurofibroma, neurofibrosarcoma, malignant mela-

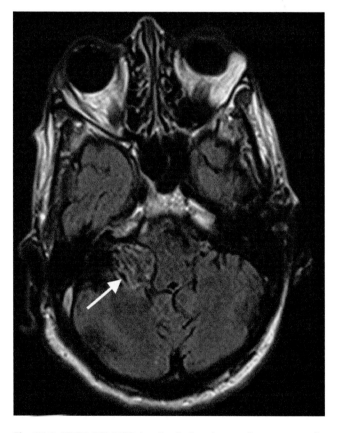

**Fig. 26.1** T2 FLAIR MRI showing "salt and pepper" appearance of a right-sided paraganglioma pushing on the right lateral brainstem at the pontomedullary junction, as shown by arrow

noma, thyroid cancer, or metastases from other cancers [17]. Thus, the combination of radiographic localization, signaling patterns, and physical examination are usually the main determinants for diagnosis. In situations where surgical resection is deemed unsafe, other imaging techniques can be used to differentiate paragangliomas from more common head and neck tumors including meningiomas and schwannomas. Noninvasive somatostatin receptor scintigraphy has been proposed as the next diagnostic step following CT and MRI due to the high expression of somatostatinergic receptors in paragangliomas and meningiomas compared to other head and neck tumors such as schwannomas [18]. Invasive arteriography can further separate meningiomas from paragangliomas due to greater vascular involvement of paragangliomas. DynaCT angiograms are an emerging test of choice for better vascular visualization and clarifying vessel relationships to the surrounding anatomy (Fig. 26.2) [19].

Metastatic disease is often screened using radioisotope imaging such as metaiodobenzylguanidine (MIBG) scanning, somatostatin receptor scintigraphy, or positron-emission tomography (PET) scans. MIBG is a compound that resembles norepinephrine and is taken up by adrenergic tissue. 123I-MIBG scans can detect tumors that are negative on CT or MRI scans, but have high false-negative rates especially for patients with SDH-mutated paragangliomas [20, 21]. FDG-PET has been shown to be more specific than MIBG and CT/MRI for detecting metastatic disease. In a study of 216 patients, detection of metastasis was greater for PET/CT (89%) than CT/MRI (74%) and 123I-MIBG (50%). For patients with SDH mutations, PET/CT had a sensitivity of 92% compared to 45% in 123I-MIBG scans [13]. For metastases in unexpected foci of disease, somatostatin receptor scintigraphy has been shown to have benefits due to high sensitivity in detecting the high density of somatostatin type 2 receptors expressed in paragangliomas [18]. Screening for metastases is thus indicated in all patients with SDHB germline mutation tumors using PET/CT scans [11].

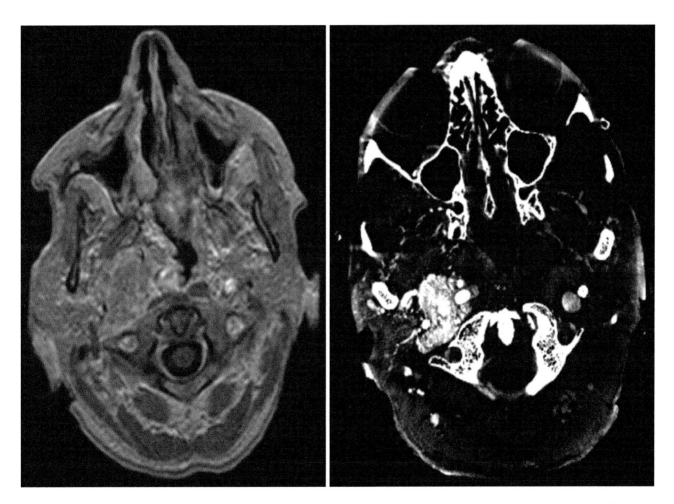

**Fig. 26.2** Seventy-five-year-old woman with right-sided paraganglioma. MRI (left) and DynaCT angiogram (right) in same axial slice. Enhanced region reveals the improved vascular visualization using the DynaCT angiogram technique

## Prognostic Factors and Molecular Subtypes

Classification of paragangliomas depends on tumor size, location, and infiltrative areas. Carotid body (paraganglioma) tumors (CBTs) use the Shamblin classification system where class I CBTs are localized tumors with little attachment to carotid vessels, class II CBTs partially surround carotid vessels, and class III CBTs completely surround the carotid [14, 22] (Table 26.1).

Jugulotympanic paragangliomas follow the Fisch classification rule. Class A tumors are only in the promontory and mesotympanum; Class B surround the ossicles; Class C are divided into C1–C4 depending on extent of osseous erosion around the carotid foramen, carotid canal, and foramen lacerum; and Class D have intracranial extension that may or may not involve the dura mater [23, 24]. Class D classification must always accompany Class C classification to clarify location of osseous destruction (Table 26.2).

Most paragangliomas are benign and carry a very good prognosis. Treatment of jugular paragangliomas and vagal paragangliomas with radiotherapy showed disease control of 89.1% and 93.7%, respectively [25]. Prognosis of malignant paragangliomas is more variable. In a report of 86 malignant head and neck paraganglioma cases, the 5-year survival rate was 82% for regional metastases and 41% for distant metastases [26]. Another report of 19 patients showed a 5-year sur-

vival rate of 84%, with 14 of 19 patients having distant metastases [27]. A report from the National Cancer Database of 59 malignant head and neck paragangliomas cases showed a 77% 5-year survival rate for regional metastases and 12% for distant metastases [9]. The high discrepancies between the survival rates of regional and local metastatic tumors could be due to varying definitions of malignancies, location of the metastases, tumor burden, and other systemic complications.

## Overall Treatment Strategy

Treatment for skull base and neck paragangliomas differ depending on symptoms, size, location, and vascularization. For small (<3 cm), asymptomatic, non-secreting paragangliomas, initial observation can be a viable approach. Patients with larger tumors have two main therapeutic options—surgery or radiation therapy.

Historically, resection has been considered the gold standard, especially for symptomatic, catecholamine-secreting paragangliomas. Prior to therapy, patients are given combined alpha- and beta-adrenergic blockade, calcium channel blockers, and metyrosine to prevent hypertensive crises. Additionally, preoperative arterial embolization may be given 2 days before surgery to reduce complications of bleeding and tumor size since head and neck paragangliomas tend to be highly vascular. However, embolization is a risky procedure associated with complications such as skin necrosis, blindness, cranial nerve deficits, and more; thus, there are no clear indications for use of embolization prior to resection [28–30]. Some criteria for use include patients with class C and D jugular paragangliomas [28]. Resection of head and neck paragangliomas have cure rates of 89–100% and a report of 93% long-term disease control in a systematic review of 211 cases of vagal paragangliomas. Despite high control rates, rates of surgical morbidity are high. The aforementioned review reported 147 cases of cranial nerve damage in the 211 patients and preservation of vagal nerve function in only 11 patients [31].

**Table 26.1** Shamblin classification of carotid body paraganglioma tumors

| Class | Tumor characteristics | Resection prognostics |
|---|---|---|
| I | Little attachment to carotid vessels | Complete resection has low morbidity |
| II | Partially surrounds internal + external carotid | Complete resection more challenging |
| III | Completely surrounds carotid vessels | Resection requires major vessel reconstruction |

Based on data from Ref. [14]

**Table 26.2** Fisch classification of jugulotympanic paragangliomas

| Class | Location and extension of paraganglioma |
|---|---|
| A | Along tympanic plexus on promontory |
| B | Invasion of hypotympanon; cortical bone over jugular bulb intact |
| C1 | Erosion of carotid foramen |
| C2 | Destruction of vertical carotid canal |
| C3 | Involvement of horizontal portion of carotid canal; foramen lacerum intact |
| C4 | Invasion of foramen lacerum and cavernous sinus |
| De (1/2) | Intracranial but extradural extension; displacement of the dura: De1 < 2 cm, De2 > 2 cm |
| Di (1/2/3) | Intracranial and intradural extension; depth of invasion into posterior cranial fossa: Di1 < 2 cm, Di2 2–4 cm; Di3 > 4 cm |

Based on data from Ref. [23]

## Indications for Radiation Therapy

Radiation therapy (RT) management of paragangliomas is mostly used for treating non-catecholamine-secreting benign paragangliomas in the skull base and neck where tumor progression may be associated with progressive cranial nerve deficits, as surgery is associated with the adverse side effects including hemorrhage and cranial nerve damage [11]. RT is most commonly delivered using conventionally fractionated RT at 1.8–2 Gy daily for 5 days per week to a total dose of 45–50.4 Gy, stereotactic radiosurgery (SRS) at a single-fraction dose of 12–15 Gy, or hypofractionated stereotactic radiation therapy (HSRT) at 25 Gy in five fractions. Conventionally fractionated RT is normally given using three-dimensional conformal radiation therapy (3DCRT) or intensity-modulated radiation therapy (IMRT). SRS can be done with Gamma Knife (GK), robotic radiosurgery platform (CyberKnife, Accuray, Inc.), or linear accelerator (LINAC)-based systems [32, 33]. Regardless of the treatment device used, the long-term disease control rates are reported to be 80–90% [34]. Advantages of SRS include convenience (fewer fractions), increased sparing of healthy tissues, and feasibility of re-irradiation after failure of conventionally fractionated RT. However, historically, single-fraction treatment has been limited to small tumors that are <3 cm. Hypofractionated approaches of 2–5 fractions may allow more conformal and convenient treatment of lesions greater than 3 cm, but the data is limited.

Historically, radiation therapy has been reserved for surgically unresectable tumors or for recurrent/progressive tumors following surgery. However, recent data suggest that excellent local control can be achieved with low rates of morbidity, and this has led to an increase in utilization of SRS or conventionally fractionated stereotactic radiation therapy (FSR) as a primary treatment modality. Details of outcomes from key studies using SRS from 1999 to 2016 are outlined in Table 26.3, which is updated from comprehensive meta-analysis by Guss et al. [60]. Emerging data suggest excellent local control, with lower morbidity than invasive surgical approaches. However, long-term follow-up data is lacking, and the rates of local control decades after treatment remain uncertain. In addition, there are concerns regarding the long-term risk of secondary malignancy following RT which remains unclear. Based on the pediatric literature, it may be as high as 13.9% [61].

**Table 26.3** Selected studies showing outcomes using stereotactic radiosurgery from 1999 to 2016

| Study | Year | Patients | Modality | Mean margin dose (Gy) | Follow-up (mo) | Tumor control | Symptom control |
|---|---|---|---|---|---|---|---|
| Dobberpuhl [34] | 2016 | 12 | GK | 15.5 | 27.6 | 100% | 80% |
| Ibrahim [35] | 2016 | 75 | GK | 18 | 51.5 | 93.4% | 84% |
| Scheick [36] | 2016 | 11 | LINAC | 15 | 63 | 81% | 82% |
| Hafez [37] | 2016 | 22 | GK | 14.7 | 56 | 95.5% | 86% |
| Martin [38] | 2016 | 39 | LINAC | 18 | 71 | 94.8% | 83% |
| El Majdoub [39] | 2015 | 27 | LINAC | 15 | 132 | 95.2% | 82% |
| Liscak [40] | 2014 | 46 | GK | 20 | 118 | 98% | 96% |
| Sager [41] | 2014 | 21 | LINAC | 15 | 49 | 100% | 100% |
| Chun [42] | 2014 | 31 | GK | 25 | 26.3 | 100% | 94% |
| de Andrade [43] | 2013 | 15 | LINAC | 14 | 27 | 100% | 80% |
| Hurmuz [44] | 2013 | 14 | GK | 25 | 39 | 100% | 93% |
| Wegner [2] | 2010 | 18 | LINAC | 20 | 22 | 100% | 100% |
| Navarro [14] | 2010 | 10 | GK | 14 | 10 | 100% | 100% |
| Genc [45] | 2010 | 18 | GK | 15.6 | 53 | 94% | 94% |
| Miller [46] | 2009 | 5 | GK | 15 | 34 | 100% | 100% |
| Ganz [47] | 2009 | 14 | GK | 13.6 | 28 | 100% | 100% |
| Sharma [48] | 2008 | 24 | GK | 16.4 | 26 | 100% | 100% |
| Lim [49] | 2007 | 18 | LINAC | 20.4 | 60 | 100% | 100% |
| Henzel [50] | 2007 | 17 | LINAC | a | 40 | 100% | 100% |
| Gerosa [45] | 2006 | 20 | GK | 17.5 | 50 | 100% | 90% |
| Varma [25] | 2006 | 17 | GK | 15 | 48 | 76% | 88% |
| Poznanovic [51] | 2006 | 8 | LINAC | 15.1 | 16 | 100% | 100% |
| Bitaraf [52] | 2006 | 16 | GK | 18 | 19 | 100% | 100% |
| Feigl [53] | 2006 | 12 | GK | 17 | 33 | 100% | 92% |
| Sheehan [54] | 2005 | 8 | GK | 15 | 28 | 100% | 100% |
| Pollock [55] | 2004 | 42 | GK | 14.9 | 44 | 97% | N/A |
| Maarouf [56] | 2003 | 14 | LINAC | 15 | 48 | 100% | 92% |
| Feigenberg [53] | 2002 | 5 | GK | 15 | 27 | 80% | 80% |
| Saringer [57] | 2001 | 13 | GK | 12 | 50 | 100% | 100% |
| Jordan [58] | 2000 | 8 | GK | 16.3 | 27 | 100% | 100% |
| Liscak [59] | 1999 | 66 | GK | 16.5 | 24 | 100% | 96% |

*GK* Gamma Knife, *LINAC* linear accelerator, *N/A* not available
Summary of data adapted from Guss et al. systematic review [60]
[a]Fractionated

## General Principles of Simulation and Target Delineation

- CT stimulation with thermoplastic mask for immobilization.
- 1 mm thick volumetric slice MRI T1 pre- and post-gadolinium, T2 + FLAIR for target delineation.
- In postoperative cases, fusion of both the preoperative and postoperative T2/FLAIR and post-gadolinium MRIs help delineate target volume.
- In patients without pathologic confirmation of the diagnosis, CT angiography with DynaCT angiogram may be beneficial to confirm the diagnosis and assist with accurate target delineation.
- SRS, HSRT, IMRT, 3DCRT, or proton therapy may be utilized.

## Treatment Planning Techniques

For SRS, HSRT, IMRT, and 3DCRT, the gross tumor volume (GTV) is delineated based on CT angiogram, T2/FLAIR, and T1 post-gadolinium diagnostic images of the gross tumor. The clinical target volume (CTV) expansion is variable and is dependent upon whether the case is a de novo or a postoperative case. In postoperative setting, reference to preoperative imaging is necessary to map out regions at risk. CTV margins may be reduced to as low as 1 mm when GTV close to brainstem, spinal cord, or middle/inner ear structures [62]. The planning target volume (PTV) expansion is also variable, dependent upon the immobilization technique and the treatment device used. It is typically 0.3–0.5 cm for 3DCRT and IMRT to account for uncertainties in patient positioning and systematic errors, but there is data supporting no significant difference using 0.3 cm expansion margins compared to 0.5 [45]. SRS and HSRT PTV is typically much smaller ranging from 0 to 2 mm. For definitive radiation therapy, GTV, CTV, and PTV were on average 1 mm less than postoperative RT in retrospective studies [63]. All tumor volume descriptions are outlined in Table 26.4.

Suggested dose prescriptions of RT vary depending on the method used (SRS, HSRT, or IMRT/3DCRT) and do not have any prospective data to provide evidence-based outcomes. A table of commonly used prescriptions for each RT technique is outlined in Table 26.5. Structures most at risk from RT for head and neck paragangliomas include the brainstem, spinal cord, vascular structures (carotid artery, internal jugular vein), ipsilateral inner ear structures (vestibule, semicircular canals, cochlea), and ipsilateral parotid gland. Guidelines based on clinical experience are outlined for SRS, HSRT, and IMRT/3DCRT in Table 26.6, although these are not intended to be definitive and should not be used for clinical decision-making without a comprehensive review of the most recently published literature. Case example for contouring and dose determinations are demonstrated in Figs. 26.3 and 26.4.

RT-related toxicities are generally classified as acute or long-term. Most common acute symptoms include skin irritation and redness, darkened skin and dryness, sore throat, transient hearing loss, transient hoarseness, otalgia, dysphagia, tinnitus, low-grade nausea, vertigo, and headaches. Higher rates of permanent nerve damage were reported in

**Table 26.4** Suggested target volumes for RT

| Target volumes | Definition and description |
|---|---|
| GTV | Gross tumor extent based on CT angiogram, T2/FLAIR, and T1 post-gadolinium images |
| CTV | GTV + regions believed to be at risk based on preoperative imaging + a radial expansion of up to 0.5–1 cm for 3DCRT and IMRT; 0–0.1 cm for SRS and HSRT[a]. May be reduced down to as low as 1 mm if close to the brainstem or spinal cord. CTV expansion should respect anatomic boundaries such as the bone and dura |
| PTV | CTV + 0.3–0.5 cm for 3DCRT and IMRT; 0–0.2 cm for SRS and HSRT[a] |

[a]CTV and PTV are not always used for Gamma Knife techniques

**Table 26.5** Suggested dose prescription for RT

| Technique | Dose |
|---|---|
| Stereotactic radiosurgery (SRS) | 13–16 Gy in one fraction |
| Fractionated stereotactic radiosurgery (FSR) | 25 Gy in five fractions |
| Three-dimensional conformal radiation therapy (3DCRT) and intensity-modulated radiation therapy (IMRT) | 1.8 Gy/fraction for total 45–50.4 Gy 1.8–2Gy/fraction for total 45–50.4 Gy |

There is no prospective data to guide the prescription dose. Above are reasonable prescriptions from past clinical experiences [63, 64]

**Table 26.6** Organ-at-risk dose constraints (volume max)

| Organ | One fraction (Gy) | Five fractions (Gy) | Conventional fractionation (Gy) |
|---|---|---|---|
| Brainstem | 12 | 25 | 54 |
| Cochlea | 9 | 25 | 45 |
| Inner ear (cochlea + vestibular organ) | N/A | 25 | 45 |
| Internal auditory canal | N/A | 25 | 50 |
| Oral cavity | N/A | 30–40 | 60 |
| Parotid | 14 | 20–30 | 40 |
| Spinal cord | 12 | 25 | 45 |

Note that these represent guidelines based on clinician experience. They are not data driven and must be validated in future studies. The most appropriate doses are dependent upon the unique patient and clinical scenario Abbreviations: *N/A* not available. Source: [39, 60, 62, 65, 66]

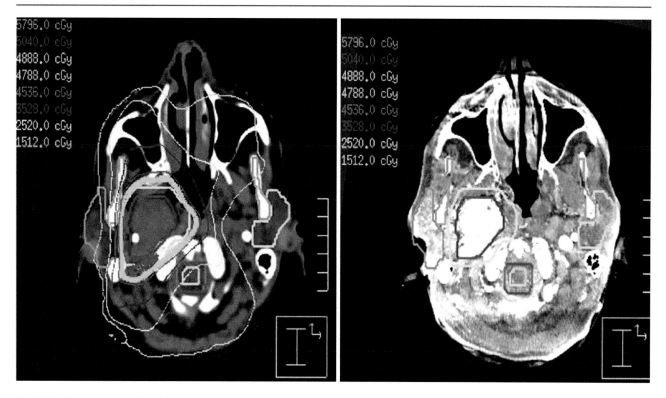

**Fig. 26.3** Treatment plan for a 75-year-old female with right-sided jugular paraganglioma depicting isodose lines on conventional CT (left) and contours on DynaCT angiogram (right)

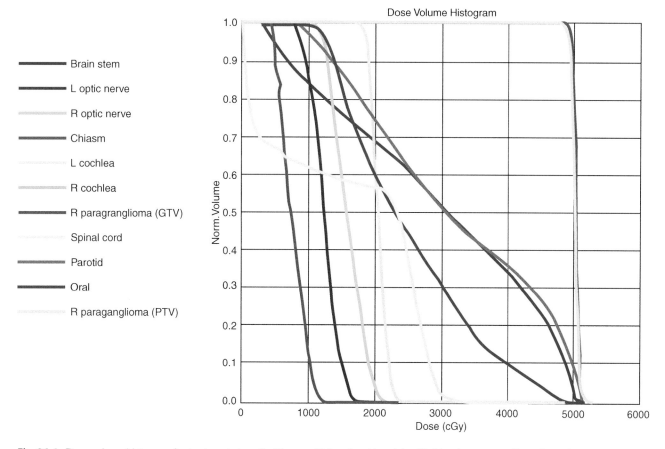

**Fig. 26.4** Dose volume histogram for treatment plan of a 75-year-old female with a right-sided jugular paraganglioma for various organs

surgical patients, while more patients recovered from transient nerve paralysis after radiotherapy [39, 42, 50, 60].

Long-term complications include xerostomia with dysphagia, otitis media, otitis externa, stenosis of external auditory canal, hearing loss, hoarseness, vocal cord paresis, and osteonecrosis which are uncommon and more associated with older 2D conventional radiotherapy techniques [62, 64]. Possible permanent injury to cranial nerves IX, X, XI, and XII is more common in SRS techniques. Other rare but serious problems include radiation-induced tumors, paralysis of upper and lower limbs, and brain necrosis but are very uncommon effects [64] (Table 26.7).

## Outcomes: Tumor Control and Survival

Results from multiple studies have shown high local control rates following radiation treatment of paragangliomas. Tumor control rates range typically around 90% at 5 years posttreatment for IMRT/3DCRT and around 95% with mean follow-up of 3 years for SRS and HSRT techniques [36, 60]. In addition to high tumor control, patients also report 90–100% control of pretreatment symptoms such as tinnitus, headache, CN damage, and facial palsy. In a review of 1084 patients, surgical resection of class C and D jugulotympanic paragangliomas showed in tumor control in 85% of cases [31] but also created 965 new cranial nerve deficits. Another review of 461 patients showed radiation therapy had local control rates of 89–98%, a decrease of cranial neuropathies from 242 prior to treatment to 232 after RT. Comparison of stereotactic radiosurgery (SRS) v. gross total resection (GTR) and subtotal resection (STR) over 109 reports with a total of 869 patients showed control rates of 86%, 69%, 71%, and 95% for GTR, STR, STR and SRS, and SRS alone, respectively. Cranial nerve damage for GTR and SRS in CN IX, X, and XI was 38 vs. 9.7%, 26 vs. 9.7%, and 40 vs. 12%, respectively [64, 67, 68]. A full list of studies analyzing SRS outcomes from 1999 to 2016 is outlined in Table 26.3.

**Table 26.7** Radiation toxicity, acute and long-term

| Acute | Skin redness and irritation in treated area, darkened skin and dryness in treated area, sore throat, transient facial palsy/spasm, tinnitus, otalgia, dysphagia, transient hoarseness, reddening or irritation of mucous membrane, low-grade nausea, vertigo, and headache |
|---|---|
| Long term | Xerostomia with dysphagia, otitis media, otitis externa, stenosis of external auditory canal, hearing loss, hoarseness, vocal cord paresis, and osteonecrosis. Possible permanent injury to cranial nerves IX, X, XI, and XII |
| Uncommon or rare risks | Low risk of radiation-induced tumor, paralysis of upper and lower limbs, and brain necrosis |

## Follow-Up: Radiographic Assessment

Post-treatment surveillance of paragangliomas include lifelong follow-up with magnetic resonance imaging due to the long disease course and possibility for late recurrences or development of metachronous primary tumors. A reasonable approach for monitoring is a complete physical exam and biochemical marker (if appropriate) monitoring every 6–12 months for the first 3 years, and lifelong annual biochemical tests and images. Patients with non-catecholamine-secreting paragangliomas may have longer times between follow-up visits. Somatostatin receptor scintigraphy is another emerging method of posttreatment assessment of residual tumor [18].

## Case Study

A 66-year-old male was diagnosed with a right-sided glomus jugulare after presenting with rightward tongue deviation and thinning of the right side of the tongue with wrinkling and fasciculation. The patient first had symptoms of tongue deviation 2 years prior to consultation. MRI scans showed an abnormality proximal to the right hypoglossal canal, but an initial biopsy of the mass was nondiagnostic. No treatment was initiated and the patient opted for serial observations. Patient continued to notice symptoms of diminished taste, tongue atrophy, rightward tongue deviation with some numbness on the right side of the tongue, and occasional episodes of dizziness with right arm pain.

Latest MRI showed a tumor in the posterior medial aspect of the ascending segment of the petrous portion of the right internal carotid artery, measuring 1.5 × 1.4 × 2.4 cm, with no evidence of extra-axial fluid collection, intracranial hemorrhage, or hydrocephalus. The trigeminal nerves were normal without evidence of mass effect and no significant distortion of sinuses or arteries noted (Fig. 26.5).

Given the location of the lesion, stereotactic radiosurgery could not be performed, and the patient was started on conventionally fractionated image-guided IMRT using stereotactic techniques which delivered 45 Gy over 25 fractions (1.8 Gy/fraction). Patient was followed every 6 months after treatment with repeat MRI. Six years after completion of treatment, MRI showed stable findings and clinical examination showed stable tongue atrophy and deviation, and there were no other symptoms or complaints.

## Summary

- Paragangliomas are rare tumors that often arise in the head and neck in the carotid body, jugulotympanic and vagal paraganglia.

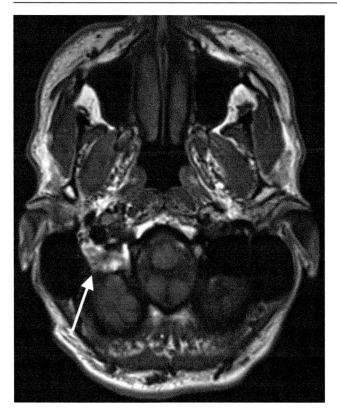

**Fig. 26.5** MRI of a 66-year-old male with right-sided paraganglioma, as shown by arrow

- Parasympathetic-derived tumors are often benign, non-catecholamine secreting but can be malignant.
- Diagnosis of paragangliomas are through biochemical screening of catecholamine levels, MRI, angiogram, and definitive histology showing Zellballen nesting patterns.
- Metastatic disease is visualized with 123I-MIBG, MRI, and PET-CT scans.
- Historical treatment has been surgical removal but, recent studies reveal high tumor control rates using stereotactic radiosurgery (SRS).
- Dosing for various techniques are the following: stereotactic radiosurgery (SRS) at 13–16 Gy in one fraction, hypofractionated stereotactic radiosurgery (HSRT) at a total 25 Gy in five fractions, and 3D conformal radiotherapy and intensity-modulated radiotherapy (IMRT) at 1.8 Gy/fraction for total 45–50.4 Gy, but no prospective data on prescription dose is currently available [63, 64].
- Tumor and symptom control rates are 80–100% for SRS studies between 1999 and 2016.
- Important organs at risk from RT include the brainstem, spinal cord, vascular structures, ipsilateral inner/middle ear structures, and ipsilateral parotid gland.
- Follow-up includes annual lifelong surveillance with imaging and biochemical tests in some patients.

## Self-Assessment Questions

1. Which of the following would NOT be considered an indication for radiation therapy consultation in patients with a paraganglioma?
   A. Tumor smaller than 3 cm
   B. Catecholamine-secreting tumor greater than 7 cm
   C. Recurrent tumor after resection
   D. Symptomatic tumor affecting hearing and balance
   E. Tumor below the neck that is highly vascularized near important anatomic organs

2. Where is the best way to visualize metastatic sites for patients with SDH (succinate dehydrogenase)-mutated paragangliomas?
   A. CT/MRI
   B. 123I-MIBG
   C. SRS
   D. PET/CT
   E. DynaCT

3. Which of the following statements regarding the toxicities of radiation therapy for paraganglioma is CORRECT?
   A. Brain necrosis and paralysis of upper and lower limbs are severe and common risks of therapy.
   B. Vertigo, skin irritation, facial spasms, and loss of cranial nerve function are often long-term effects of radiation therapy.
   C. Acute effects from therapy may include tinnitus, hearing loss, skin redness, and irritation.
   D. Patients often experience loss of visual and auditory function for many years following treatment.
   E. Radiation-induced tumors occur in majority of treated patients.

4. What is the preferred radiation technique used for paragangliomas <3 cm and suggested dose?
   A. Stereotactic radiosurgery of single-fraction 50 Gy dose
   B. Stereotactic radiosurgery of single-fraction 13–16 Gy dose
   C. Stereotactic radiosurgery of single-fraction 5 Gy dose
   D. Stereotactic radiosurgery of single-fraction 30 Gy dose
   E. Stereotactic radiosurgery of single-fraction 25 Gy

5. Which of the following is NOT a main structure to monitor dose constraints in paraganglioma radiation treatment planning?
   A. Parotid glands
   B. Thyroid
   C. Cochlea
   D. Vestibular organ
   E. Carotid

## Answers

1. B.

   Surgical consultation should be considered in patients with catecholamine-secreting tumors that are large if it is anatomically feasible to remove the source of excess catecholamine in the body [11].

2. D

   Detection of metastasis was greater for PET/CT (89%) than CT/MRI (74% and 123I-MIBG (50%). For patients with SDH mutations, PET/CT had a sensitivity of 92% compared to 45% in 123I-MIBG scans [31]. Screening for metastases is indicated in all patients with SDHB germline mutation paragangliomas using FDG-PET/CT scans [11].

3. C

   Toxicities associated with radiation therapy are usually acute including skin redness and irritation, transient facial palsy/spasm, tinnitus, hearing loss, dysphagia, etc. Radiation-induced tumors, limb paralysis, and brain necrosis are very rare complications [12].

4. B

   Small tumors <3 cm have best response to stereotactic radiosurgery of a single fraction (13–16 Gy dose), with benefits of sparing healthy tissue, convenience of one treatment, and high efficacy after tumor recurrence [34]

5. B

   Important structures to contour during treatment planning include brainstem, spinal cord, vascular structures, ipsilateral inner ear structures, and ipsilateral parotid gland [64]. The thyroid is typically lower in the neck and not immediately adjacent to the tumor.

## References

1. Lee JH, Barich F, Karnell LH, et al. National Cancer Data Base report on malignant paragangliomas of the head and neck. Cancer. 2002;94(3):730–7.
2. Wegner RE, Rodriguez KD, Heron DE, et al. Linac-based stereotactic body radiation therapy for treatment of glomus jugulare tumors. Radiother Oncol. 2010;97(3):395–8.
3. Erickson D, Kudva YC, Ebersold MJ, et al. Benign paragangliomas: clinical presentation and treatment outcomes in 236 patients. J Clin Endocrinol Metab. 2001;86(11):5210–6.
4. Ramlawi B, David EA, Kim MP, et al. Contemporary surgical management of cardiac paragangliomas. Ann Thorac Surg. 2012;93(6):1972–6.
5. Young WF Jr. Paragangliomas: clinical overview. Ann N Y Acad Sci. 2006;1073:21–9.
6. Boedeker CC, Neumann HP, Maier W, et al. Malignant head and neck paragangliomas in SDHB mutation carriers. Otolaryngol Head Neck Surg. 2007;137(1):126–9.
7. Fishbein L, Merrill S, Fraker DL, et al. Inherited mutations in pheochromocytoma and paraganglioma: why all patients should be offered genetic testing. Ann Surg Oncol. 2013;20(5):1444–50.
8. Burnichon N, Briere JJ, Libe R, et al. SDHA is a tumor suppressor gene causing paraganglioma. Hum Mol Genet. 2010;19(15):3011–20.
9. Lee JA, Duh QY. Sporadic paraganglioma. World J Surg. 2008;32(5):683–7.
10. Fliedner SM, Lehnert H, Pacak K. Metastatic paraganglioma. Semin Oncol. 2010;37(6):627–37.
11. Lenders JW, Duh QY, Eisenhofer G, et al. Pheochromocytoma and paraganglioma: an endocrine society clinical practice guideline. J Clin Endocrinol Metab. 2014;99(6):1915–42.
12. Fayad JN, Keles B, Brackmann DE. Jugular foramen tumors: clinical characteristics and treatment outcomes. Otol Neurotol. 2010;31(2):299–305.
13. Stoeckli SJ, Schuknecht B, Alkadhi H, et al. Evaluation of paragangliomas presenting as a cervical mass on color-coded Doppler sonography. Laryngoscope. 2002;112(1):143–6.
14. Navarro Martin A, Maitz A, Grills IS, et al. Successful treatment of glomus jugulare tumours with gamma knife radiosurgery: clinical and physical aspects of management and review of the literature. Clin Transl Oncol. 2010;12(1):55–62.
15. Olsen WL, Dillon WP, Kelly WM, et al. MR imaging of paragangliomas. AJR Am J Roentgenol. 1987;148(1):201–4.
16. Rao AB, Koeller KK, Adair CF. From the archives of the AFIP. Paragangliomas of the head and neck: radiologic-pathologic correlation. Armed Forces Institute of Pathology. Radiographics. 1999;19(6):1605–32.
17. Monabati A, Hodjati H, Kumar PV. Cytologic findings in carotid body tumors. Acta Cytol. 2002;46(6):1101–4.
18. Duet M, Sauvaget E, Petelle B, et al. Clinical impact of somatostatin receptor scintigraphy in the management of paragangliomas of the head and neck. J Nucl Med. 2003;44(11):1768–74.
19. Namba K, Niimi Y, Song J, et al. Use of Dyna-CT angiography in neuroendovascular decision-making: a case report. Interv Neuroradiol. 2009;15(1):68–72.
20. Intenzo CM, Jabbour S, Lin HC, et al. Scintigraphic imaging of body neuroendocrine tumors. Radiographics. 2007;27(5):1355–69.
21. Timmers HJ, Chen CC, Carrasquillo JA, et al. Staging and functional characterization of pheochromocytoma and paraganglioma by 18F-fluorodeoxyglucose (18F-FDG) positron emission tomography. J Natl Cancer Inst. 2012;104(9):700–8.
22. Dorobisz K, Dorobisz T, Temporale H, et al. Diagnostic and therapeutic difficulties in carotid body paragangliomas, based on clinical experience and a review of the literature. Adv Clin Exp Med. 2016;25(6):1173–7.
23. Offergeld C, Brase C, Yaremchuk S, et al. Head and neck paragangliomas: clinical and molecular genetic classification. Clinics (Sao Paulo). 2012;68(Suppl 1):19–28.
24. Schuster D, Sweeney AD, Stavas MJ, et al. Initial radiographic tumor control is similar following single or multi-fractionated stereotactic radiosurgery for jugular paragangliomas. Am J Otolaryngol. 2016;37(3):255–8.
25. Varma A, Nathoo N, Neyman G, et al. Gamma knife radiosurgery for glomus jugulare tumors: volumetric analysis in 17 patients. Neurosurgery. 2006;59(5):1030–6. discussion 1036
26. Sethi RV, Sethi RK, Herr MW, et al. Malignant head and neck paragangliomas: treatment efficacy and prognostic indicators. Am J Otolaryngol. 2013;34(5):431–8.
27. Moskovic DJ, Smolarz JR, Stanley D, et al. Malignant head and neck paragangliomas: is there an optimal treatment strategy? Head Neck Oncol. 2010;2:23.
28. Green JD Jr, Brackmann DE, Nguyen CD, et al. Surgical management of previously untreated glomus jugulare tumors. Laryngoscope. 1994;104(8 Pt 1):917–21.
29. Litle VR, Reilly LM, Ramos TK. Preoperative embolization of carotid body tumors: when is it appropriate? Ann Vasc Surg. 1996;10(5):464–8.
30. Valavanis A. Preoperative embolization of the head and neck: indications, patient selection, goals, and precautions. AJNR Am J Neuroradiol. 1986;7(5):943–52.

31. Suarez C, Rodrigo JP, Bodeker CC, et al. Jugular and vagal paragangliomas: systematic study of management with surgery and radiotherapy. Head Neck. 2013;35(8):1195–204.
32. Feigl GC, Horstmann GA. Intracranial glomus jugulare tumors: volume reduction with Gamma Knife surgery. J Neurosurg. 2006;105(Suppl):161–8.
33. Gerosa M, Visca A, Rizzo P, et al. Glomus jugulare tumors: the option of gamma knife radiosurgery. Neurosurgery. 2006;59(3):561–9. discussion 561–9
34. Dobberpuhl MR, Maxwell S, Feddock J, et al. Treatment outcomes for single modality management of glomus jugulare tumors with stereotactic radiosurgery. Otol Neurotol. 2016;37(9):1406–10.
35. Ibrahim R, Ammori MB, Yianni J, et al. Gamma Knife radiosurgery for glomus jugulare tumors: a single-center series of 75 cases. J Neurosurg. 2016;8:1–10.
36. Scheick SM, Morris CG, Amdur RJ, et al. Long-term outcomes after radiosurgery for temporal bone paragangliomas. Am J Clin Oncol. 2018;41(3):223–6.
37. Hafez RF, Morgan MS, Fahmy OM. An intermediate term benefits and complications of gamma knife surgery in management of glomus jugulare tumor. World J Surg Oncol. 2016;14(1):36.
38. Martin IT, Avila Rdel M, Herrera MZ, et al. Role of radiosurgery in the management of glomus tumors. Head Neck. 2016;38(Suppl 1):E798–804.
39. El Majdoub F, Hunsche S, Igressa A, et al. Stereotactic LINAC-radiosurgery for glomus jugulare tumors: a long-term follow-up of 27 patients. PLoS One. 2015;10(6):e0129057.
40. Liscak R, Urgosik D, Chytka T, et al. Leksell Gamma Knife radiosurgery of the jugulotympanic glomus tumor: long-term results. J Neurosurg. 2014;121(Suppl):198–202.
41. Sager O, Beyzadeoglu M, Dincoglan F, et al. Evaluation of linear accelerator-based stereotactic radiosurgery in the management of glomus jugulare tumors. Tumori. 2014;100(2):184–8.
42. Chun SG, Nedzi LA, Choe KS, et al. A retrospective analysis of tumor volumetric responses to five-fraction stereotactic radiotherapy for paragangliomas of the head and neck (glomus tumors). Stereotact Funct Neurosurg. 2014;92(3):153–9.
43. de Andrade EM, Brito J, Mario SD, et al. Stereotactic radiosurgery for the treatment of glomus jugulare tumors. Surg Neurol Int. 2013;4(Suppl 6):S429–35.
44. Hurmuz P, Cengiz M, Ozyigit G, et al. Robotic stereotactic radiosurgery in patients with unresectable glomus jugulare tumors. Technol Cancer Res Treat. 2013;12(2):109–13.
45. Genc A, Bicer A, Abacioglu U, et al. Gamma knife radiosurgery for the treatment of glomus jugulare tumors. J Neuro-Oncol. 2010;97(1):101–8.
46. Miller JP, Semaan M, Einstein D, et al. Staged Gamma Knife radiosurgery after tailored surgical resection: a novel treatment paradigm for glomus jugulare tumors. Stereotact Funct Neurosurg. 2009;87(1):31–6.
47. Ganz JC, Abdelkarim K. Glomus jugulare tumours: certain clinical and radiological aspects observed following gamma knife radiosurgery. Acta Neurochir. 2009;151(5):423–6.
48. Sharma MS, Gupta A, Kale SS, et al. Gamma knife radiosurgery for glomus jugulare tumors: therapeutic advantages of minimalism in the skull base. Neurol India. 2008;56(1):57–61.
49. Lim M, Bower R, Nangiana JS, et al. Radiosurgery for glomus jugulare tumors. Technol Cancer Res Treat. 2007;6(5):419–23.
50. Henzel M, Hamm K, Gross MW, et al. Fractionated stereotactic radiotherapy of glomus jugulare tumors. Local control, toxicity, symptomatology, and quality of life. Strahlenther Onkol. 2007;183(10):557–62.
51. Poznanovic SA, Cass SP, Kavanagh BD. Short-term tumor control and acute toxicity after stereotactic radiosurgery for glomus jugulare tumors. Otolaryngol Head Neck Surg. 2006;134(3):437–42.
52. Bitaraf MA, Alikhani M, Tahsili-Fahadan P, et al. Radiosurgery for glomus jugulare tumors: experience treating 16 patients in Iran. J Neurosurg. 2006;105(Suppl):168–74.
53. Feigenberg SJ, Mendenhall WM, Hinerman RW, et al. Radiosurgery for paraganglioma of the temporal bone. Head Neck. 2002;24(4):384–9.
54. Sheehan J, Kondziolka D, Flickinger J, et al. Gamma knife surgery for glomus jugulare tumors: an intermediate report on efficacy and safety. J Neurosurg. 2005;102(Suppl):241–6.
55. Pollock BE. Stereotactic radiosurgery in patients with glomus jugulare tumors. Neurosurg Focus. 2004;17(2):E10.
56. Maarouf M, Voges J, Landwehr P, et al. Stereotactic linear accelerater-based radiosurgery for the treatment of patients with glomus jugulare tumors. Cancer. 2003;97(4):1093–8.
57. Saringer W, Khayal H, Ertl A, et al. Efficiency of gamma knife radiosurgery in the treatment of glomus jugulare tumors. Minim Invasive Neurosurg. 2001;44(3):141–6.
58. Jordan JA, Roland PS, McManus C, et al. Stereotastic radiosurgery for glomus jugulare tumors. Laryngoscope. 2000;110(1):35–8.
59. Liscak R, Vladyka V, Wowra B, et al. Gamma Knife radiosurgery of the glomus jugulare tumour – early multicentre experience. Acta Neurochir. 1999;141(11):1141–6.
60. Guss ZD, Batra S, Limb CJ, et al. Radiosurgery of glomus jugulare tumors: a meta-analysis. Int J Radiat Oncol Biol Phys. 2011;81(4):e497–502.
61. Lee JS, DuBois SG, Coccia PF, et al. Increased risk of second malignant neoplasms in adolescents and young adults with cancer. Cancer. 2016;122(1):116–23.
62. Chen AM, Farwell DG, Luu Q, et al. Evaluation of the planning target volume in the treatment of head and neck cancer with intensity-modulated radiotherapy: what is the appropriate expansion margin in the setting of daily image guidance? Int J Radiat Oncol Biol Phys. 2011;81(4):943–9.
63. Dupin C, Lang P, Dessard-Diana B, et al. Treatment of head and neck paragangliomas with external beam radiation therapy. Int J Radiat Oncol Biol Phys. 2014;89(2):353–9.
64. Hinerman RW, Amdur RJ, Morris CG, et al. Definitive radiotherapy in the management of paragangliomas arising in the head and neck: a 35-year experience. Head Neck. 2008;30(11):1431–8.
65. Rogers L, Zhang P, Vogelbaum MA, et al. Intermediate-risk meningioma: initial outcomes from NRG oncology/RTOG-0539. Int J Radiat Oncol Biol Phys. 2017;93(3):S139–40.
66. Truong MT, Zhang Q, Rosenthal DI, et al. Quality of life and performance status from a substudy conducted within a prospective phase 3 randomized trial of concurrent accelerated radiation plus cisplatin with or without cetuximab for locally advanced head and neck carcinoma: NRG oncology radiation therapy oncology group 0522. Int J Radiat Oncol Biol Phys. 2017;97:687–99.
67. Chino JP, Sampson JH, Tucci DL, et al. Paraganglioma of the head and neck: long-term local control with radiotherapy. Am J Clin Oncol. 2009;32(3):304–7.
68. Gittleman HR, Lim D, Kattan M, et al. An independently validated nomogram for individualized estimation of survival among patients with newly diagnosed glioblastoma: NRG Oncology/RTOG 0525 and 0825. Int J Radiat Oncol Biol Phys. 2017;96(2):S92.

# Adult Medulloblastoma

# 27

Anthony Pham, Kenneth Wong, and Eric L. Chang

## Learning Objectives

- Describe the molecular pathways involved in the pathogenesis of medulloblastoma.
- Differentiate between molecular subtypes according to the WHO 2016 classification.
- Be familiar with the staging and multidisciplinary management of adult medulloblastoma.
- Gain competency in contouring target volumes and critical structures.
- Summarize the outcomes and prognostic factors of key studies investigating adult medulloblastoma.
- Describe acute and late toxicity associated with craniospinal irradiation.

## Epidemiology

Medulloblastoma is a highly cellular malignant embryonal neoplasm defined as a malignant, invasive embryonal tumor of the cerebellum with preferential manifestation in children [1]. Though more common in the pediatric population, these tumors do occur in the adult population as well. By defini-

A. Pham (✉)
Department of Radiation Oncology, Keck School of Medicine of USC, Los Angeles, CA, USA
e-mail: anthony.pham@med.usc.edu

K. Wong
Department of Radiation Oncology, Keck School of Medicine of USC, Norris Cancer Hospital, Los Angeles, CA, USA

Department of Radiation Oncology, Children's Center for Cancer and Blood Diseases, Children's Hospital Los Angeles, Los Angeles, CA, USA

E. L. Chang
Department of Radiation Oncology, Keck School of Medicine of USC, Norris Cancer Hospital, Los Angeles, CA, USA

Department of Radiation Oncology, UT MD Anderson Cancer Center, Houston, TX, USA

tion, medulloblastomas arise in the posterior fossa, usually from the cerebellar vermis in the roof of the fourth ventricle. Medulloblastomas have a marked propensity to seed within the cerebrospinal fluid (CSF) pathways, with evidence of metastatic spread occurring in up to 35% of cases at diagnosis. Though previously classified under the historical category of primitive neuroectodermal tumor (PNET) due to similar histological, radiological, and clinical characteristics, medulloblastomas are now distinct entity after use of molecular markers has led to the reclassification of these tumors.

## Incidence and Prevalence

Medulloblastoma is the most common malignant brain neoplasm in childhood, accounting for 15–25% of all childhood primary central nervous system (CNS) neoplasms, with about 70% of all cases diagnosed in patients less than 15 years of age [2]. Average age of presentation is children aged 3–6 years, with only 25% of patients being between 15 and 44 years of age [3]. There is a slight increase in incidence between the ages of 20 to 24 years, but the disease is rare after the fourth decade [2]. The Central Brain Tumor Registry of the United States (CBTRUS) obtained data on all newly diagnosed primary brain and CNS tumors from multiple national databases diagnosed between 2006 and 2010. This study found that the incidence of medulloblastoma was 1.5 cases per million in the general population, children being ten times more likely to develop the disease than adults [4]. The incidence of medulloblastoma in patients older than 19 was 0.6 per million adults. Similar to the US data, the European annual incidence is about 1.1 per million in the male and 0.8 per million in the female adult population [5]. Males are 1.58 times more likely than females to be diagnosed with medulloblastoma during childhood, but this difference is not maintained in adulthood [2].

E. L. Chang et al. (eds.), *Adult CNS Radiation Oncology*, https://doi.org/10.1007/978-3-319-42878-9_27

## Standard Mortality Ratio CBTRUS (Central Brain Tumor Registry of United States)

Using Surveillance, Epidemiology, and End Results (SEER) data from 2006–2010, the CBTRUS reported the mortality and relative survival rates for 1573 cases of medulloblastoma [4]. The 1-, 2-, 5-, and 10 year relative survival rates for patients with medulloblastoma were 88.2%, 81.7%, 71.1%, and 62.8% respectively. Age-stratified survival was reported for patients with embryonal tumors (including medulloblastoma). The 1-, 2-, 5-, and 10-year relative survival rates for these patients were 84.3%, 75.7%, 58.9%, and 49.6%. Five-year relative survival decreased with age from 64% in the youngest (20–44 years) age group to 31.8% in the older group of patients (45 years and over). No age-stratified survival was reported separately for medulloblastoma.

Similar to the CBTRUS, population-based cancer registries of about 20 European countries in the EUROCARE study reported survival data for patients with PNET [3]. The analysis included 867 adults with PNET of the brain diagnosed during the period 1995–2002 and with follow-up until 2003. Relative survival was 78% at 1 year, 61% at 3 years, and 52% at 5 years, with no differences between genders. Five-year relative survival decreased with age from 56% in the youngest (15–44 years) age group to 9% in the older group of patients (45 years and over).

## Risk Factors:

## Radiation and Heritable

There are few clear environmental risk factors for medulloblastoma. Exposure to ionizing radiation has been established as a cause of various brain tumors in patients with prior therapeutic radiation therapy and among atomic bomb survivors. Effective treatment of primary brain tumors, acute leukemia, and other tumors has allowed patients to survive for extended periods, thereby placing them at risk for secondary malignancies [6, 7]. Patients treated with low-dose irradiation for benign conditions such as tinea capitis and skin disorders as children have an increased risk of CNS tumors well into adulthood [8]. Armstrong et al. found that the latency period between irradiation and the development of brain tumors may be as short as 5 years or as long as many decades. High-grade gliomas and meningiomas are the two most common subsequent CNS neoplasms, although medulloblastoma/(PNETs), schwannomas, and low-grade gliomas have also been reported at much lower rates in some studies. Other environmental risk factors for CNS tumors including medulloblastoma are unclear. Workers in vinyl chloride, petrochemical, agricultural, and rubber industries have been found to have an increased risk of brain tumors in retrospective cohorts studied. However, there is no consistent evidence implicating any particular chemical exposure as a risk factor for CNS tumors.

## Familial Syndromes

Approximately 2–5% of medulloblastomas occur in association with inherited genetic syndromes. Both nevoid basal cell carcinoma syndrome (NBCCS, also called Gorlin syndrome), caused by germline mutations in the patched-1 (PTCH1) gene, and familial adenomatous polyposis (FAP), caused by inactivating mutations in the adenomatous polyposis coli (APC) gene, are associated with an increased risk for medulloblastoma [9]. In both syndromes, mutations occur in pathways that are related to the pathogenesis of medulloblastoma.

NBCCS is the most common genetic syndrome associated with medulloblastoma. It is a hereditary condition characterized by multiple basal cell skin cancers with other common findings including jaw cysts, pits on the palms of the hands or soles of the feet, calcium deposits in the brain, developmental disability, and skeletal bone changes. Medulloblastoma develops in 3–5% of patients with NBCCS and typically presents in patients before the age of three [10]. It is inherited in an autosomal dominant manner due to mutations in the sonic hedgehog (SHH) pathway, most commonly occurring in the PTCH1 gene on chromosome 9 [11]. Less commonly, NBCCS may be due to mutations in suppressor of fused homologue (SUFU) gene. During normal cerebellar development, SHH is produced by Purkinje neurons and stimulates growth and migration of granule neuron precursor (GNP) cells. Overactive SHH signaling plays a key role in the pathogenesis of a subset of sporadic medulloblastomas as well as those associated with NBCCS.

Turcot syndrome is a historical term that originally described an association between brain tumors (primarily medulloblastomas and gliomas) and two different forms of inherited colonic polyposis, FAP and hereditary nonpolyposis colorectal cancer (HNPCC) [12]. It is now clear that medulloblastomas are associated with FAP and not HNPCC. FAP is an autosomal dominant condition caused by inactivating mutations in the APC gene on chromosome 5 [13]. Medulloblastoma develops in less than 1% of patients with FAP, and the risk may not be uniform in patients with FAP, with those mutations in segment 2 of the APC gene at the highest risk. A germline mutation in one APC allele plus a "second hit" deletion of the other allele results in loss of function of the APC protein. This protein complex plays a role in the wingless (WNT) signaling pathway, which is a network of proteins that controls cell proliferation and differentiation during development and healing. Loss of APC, as occurs in FAP, ultimately leads to excessive intranuclear accumulation of β-catenin, an intracellular protein involved in the eventual pathogenesis of medulloblastoma [14].

## Diagnosis and Prognosis

Patients with medulloblastoma demonstrate a combination of signs and symptoms caused by increased intracranial pressure and cerebellar dysfunction that evolve over a period of weeks to a few months. The predominant clinical symptom of medulloblastoma is increased intracranial pressure, especially when the tumor is obstructing the flow of CSF causing hydrocephalus. Most patients present with a history of nocturnal or morning headaches caused by increased intracranial pressure. Nausea and vomiting occurring upon waking is also a common symptom. Changes in mental status may also be seen. Prolonged elevation of intracranial pressure can lead to papilledema and complete or partial loss of vision.

Specific neurologic exam findings depend upon the location of the tumor. Tumors in the midline may cause gait ataxia or truncal instability, manifested by a broad-based gait or difficulty with heel-to-toe walking, whereas tumors in the lateral cerebellar hemispheres are more likely to cause limb clumsiness or incoordination. This may manifest as dysmetria on finger-to-nose testing, intention tremor, and difficulty with heel-to-shin testing upon examination. Medulloblastoma in adults occurs more commonly in the lateral cerebellum, unlike in children, where medulloblastoma occurs medially more commonly [15].

Though uncommon, signs and symptoms related to the compression of cranial nerves may arise. This may occur when there is infiltration of the floor of the fourth ventricle by the tumor or by spinal metastases. Diplopia, nystagmus, and abnormalities of extraocular movements caused by impairment of cranial nerves IV or VI can be observed. Other focal neurologic deficits, such as hearing loss and cranial nerve VII palsies, can occur but are rare. If there is metastatic spread to the spine, upper motor neuron signs may be present.

## Radiographic Characteristic

The classic computed tomography (CT) finding is a hyperdense mass within the posterior fossa on an unenhanced study that markedly enhances after the injection of IV contrast medium [16]. However, many medulloblastomas may be missed on CT scan. On magnetic resonance imaging (MRI), medulloblastoma typically appears usually iso- to hypointense on T1-weighted images, with contrast enhancement. The T2 signal varies, ranging from hyperintense to hypointense. Other typical features are increased signals on diffusion-weighted images (DWI) and a decreased apparent diffusion coefficient (ADC), which is a marker of high cellularity and may help in differentiating from other posterior fossa tumors, such as pilocytic astrocytoma and ependy-moma [17]. In addition, the desmoplastic/nodular variant, which is more common in adults, may lack uniform contrast enhancement. In cases of spinal involvement, MRI typically shows linear or nodule enhancement along the pial surface of the spinal cord and/or drop metastases within the cauda equina. Enhancing nodules or more linear patterns of enhancement may be evident in the ventricles, over the surface of the brain, or in the spinal canal and are indicative of leptomeningeal dissemination.

The differential diagnosis of a posterior fossa mass includes other tumors with a predisposition for the cerebellum, including pilocytic astrocytoma, ependymoma, high-grade glioma and atypical teratoid/rhabdoid tumors (ATRT). In an adult with a posterior fossa mass lesion, the differential diagnosis also includes metastatic tumors, which are rare in childhood. Certain imaging findings can help to differentiate these posterior fossa tumors. Pilocytic astrocytomas are typically cystic with a mural nodule or centrally necrotic with a thick rim of enhancing tissue. Ependymomas grow to fill the fourth ventricle and extend inferiorly through the foramen of Magendie or laterally through the foramen of Luschka, but usually do not invade through the ventricles like medulloblastomas. ATRT are much rarer than medulloblastomas but can have a similar appearance on MRI. Compared with medulloblastoma, ATRT are more likely to involve the lateral hemispheres or cerebellopontine angle and contain intratumoral hemorrhage [18]. In addition, decreased ADC values are characteristic of medulloblastoma and ATRT but not ependymoma or pilocytic astrocytoma.

## Staging Work-Up

Standard staging procedures include the diagnostic imaging with MRI that should be performed before surgery to clearly delineate the tumor. Because these tumors have a propensity to spread through the CSF to distant CNS sites, patients should ideally have MRI of the entire brain and spine preoperatively. CT and myelography can be performed for staging purposes if there is no access to MRI or if the patient's condition does not allow MRI. Postoperative MRI of the brain should be performed within 24–48 h to determine the extent of resection since enhancement after this time period may not represent residual disease. On the other hand, interpretation of a spinal MRI obtained too soon after surgery may be difficult to interpret due to the challenge of distinguishing between subdural blood products and drop metastases. Therefore, a postoperative spinal MRI should be delayed for 2 weeks if performed.

In addition, cytological evaluation of CSF is suggested to detect medulloblastomas that have metastasized throughout the CNS. Fouladi et al. studied 106 consecutive patients, in which 17% of leptomeningeal spread would have been missed if no CSF was collected and analyzed [19]. Elevated protein and a mild pleocytosis are often seen in association with a positive cytology, but these findings are nonspecific. A positive CSF cytology either pre- or postoperatively predicts for an increased rate of relapse and poor outcome. However, lumbar puncture should be delayed until after surgery if there is evidence of increased intracranial pressure and/or obstructive hydrocephalus to avoid possible brain herniation. If collected after surgery, CSF cytology should be performed after waiting 2–3 weeks to avoid potential contamination of the specimen with surgical debris.

Medulloblastomas rarely metastasize outside of the nervous system at diagnosis, and therefore systemic staging with CT of the chest, abdomen, and pelvis, positron emission tomography, or bone scan are not required at the time of diagnosis. Complete surgical information and imaging data allow staging to be carried out according to the Chang staging system, which helps guide the appropriate treatment for average- and high-risk patients.

## World Health Organization Pathologic Diagnostic Criteria 2016

Regardless of histological or genetic characterization, medulloblastoma is a malignant invasive tumor classified as WHO grade 4, with a predominantly neuronal differentiation and inherent tendency to metastasize via CSF. Microscopically, they are highly cellular tumors with abundant dark staining, round or oval nuclei, and little cytoplasmic differentiation. Homer Wright rosettes are a prototypical histopathological characteristic of medulloblastoma. Immunohistochemical studies most often demonstrate nodules of neural differentiation, staining for synaptophysin as well as markers of primitive neuroepithelial cells, including neuron-specific enolase and nestin. This is consistent with their presumed origin from neuronal progenitor cells from the ventricular zone (VZ), which differentiate into Purkinje cells, basket cells, and other glial and neuronal cells of the cerebellum. Other medulloblastoma subtypes express markers specific for cerebellar granule cells and are thought to arise from distinctly different cells in the external germinal layer (EGL) that produces cerebellar granule cells [20]. These cell groups are related to different molecular subtypes of medulloblastoma with VZ cells giving origin to the WNT subtype, while SHH medulloblastomas are derived from EGL cells.

Several histologic variants of medulloblastoma have been described with a spectrum of histopathological appearances ranging from tumors with extensive nodularity to those with large-cell/anaplastic features. Previous WHO classification of tumors of the CNS characterized medulloblastoma into classic medulloblastoma and several variants: desmoplastic/nodular, anaplastic, and large-cell medulloblastomas. These

subtypes are described in adults as well as children, but with a different frequency in adults compared to the pediatric age group.

Classical ("undifferentiated") medulloblastomas are tumors composed of densely packed cells with round nuclei surrounded by scant cytoplasm. Neuroblastic rosettes, ganglion cells, necrosis, calcifications, intratumoral hemorrhage, and infiltrative behavior can be found. Most childhood cases are classic medulloblastoma (80%).

Desmoplastic/nodular medulloblastomas are more frequent in adults than in children (25–40% versus 15–20%, respectively) and are more often located in the cerebellar hemispheres. These tumors tend to be firm and more circumscribed with small foci of necrosis can be grossly evident, but extensive necrosis is rare. Histologically, these tumors are characterized by the presence of reticulin-free nodules ("pale islands") with decreased cellularity and more prominent neuronal differentiation of the tumor cells within these islands. These are often correlated with the neurotrophin receptor p75NTR, which is rarely observed in classical childhood medulloblastoma, which supports that the desmoplastic/nodular variant is a different tumor type. Loss of heterozygosity in chromosome 9q associated with PTCH1 has been found as well. While there is evidence that these tumors are biologically less aggressive, the prognostic significance of the desmoplastic/nodular phenotype is not yet clear [21–24].

Large-cell/anaplastic medulloblastomas carry a relatively poor prognosis and represent 2–4% of the medulloblastomas in children, but are rare in adults [25–27]. Though focal anaplastic change is a very frequent feature in almost all medulloblastomas, large-cell and anaplastic medulloblastomas are characterized histologically by pronounced and widespread large-cell or anaplastic features. These features include relatively large, partly vesicular nuclei with prominent nucleoli and a variable amount of eosinophilic cytoplasm in large-cell, while anaplastic features include markedly pleomorphic tumor cell nuclei with nuclear molding, cell-cell wrapping, and high mitotic activity. This variant has a higher propensity for CSF dissemination and a more aggressive clinical course. The large-cell/anaplastic variant is most commonly associated with the group 3 molecular subtype in children and with group 4 tumors in adults.

More recently, multiple molecular/genetic abnormalities have been discovered by using routine immunohistochemistry (IHC) in medulloblastomas and have been used to stratify medulloblastoma molecular subtypes [28–30]. The most common abnormalities include isochromosome 17q (present in 30–40% of tumors), MYC/MYC-N amplification, and abnormalities in the SHH-PTCH and Wnt/WG pathways [31]. The Hedgehog signaling pathway plays an important role in the pathogenesis of medulloblastoma. This pathway controls the development of cerebellar granular progenitor cells in the external granular layer. PTCH, a tumor suppressor gene on chromosome 9, encodes PTCH1, which inhibits the Hedgehog pathway by binding to Patched. Secreted by Purkinje cells, SHH is an inhibitory ligand for the PTCH1. Thus SHH overexpression prevents the inhibition of downstream expression of smoothened (SMO), which leads to the transcription of specific target genes including MYC-N which cause increased proliferation of these cells and thus contributes to the pathogenesis of medulloblastoma.

Alterations in the SHH pathway are present in approximately 30% of medulloblastomas, though more common in infants and adults and underrepresented in children. Abnormalities in the multiple genes involved in this pathway are found, mainly in the desmoplastic/nodular subtype of medulloblastomas [32, 33]. Activation of the SHH pathway can occur in the absence of germline or somatic mutations to PTCH1 in patients with medulloblastoma. These include truncating mutations of PTCH2, a homologue of PTCH1 that is localized to the short arm of chromosome 1. In some cases, SHH signaling is enhanced by loss of function of the tumor suppressor gene GNAS, which encodes the G protein alpha subunit (Gαs) which suppresses SHH signaling through cAMP-dependent pathway regulation. Other alterations include both somatic and germline mutations in the SUFU, another gene involved in the SHH pathway that is localized to chromosome 10q as well as mutations in GLI3, a downstream component of the SHH pathway, located on chromosome 7p.

The WNT pathway involves the APC gene. WNT binds to its receptor, Frizzled, which destabilizes a multi-protein complex that includes the APC protein. This complex initiates a sequence of events that leads to the accumulation of β-catenin that can activate various transcription factors, which are important in the pathogenesis of medulloblastoma. Nuclear β-catenin staining is present in most WNT pathway tumors. Activation or inactivation of the factors involved in this pathway by genetic mutations is reported in especially the classic subtype of medulloblastomas. Loss of chromosome 6 and somatic mutations of catenin beta 1 gene (CTNNB1) that promote stabilization and nuclear localization of β-catenin are present in the vast majority of WNT pathway tumors. The interaction of CTNNB1 with TCF/LEF family proteins to form a transcription factor complex increases the expression of MYC.

MYC/MYC-N have multiple effects in the cell cycle and appear to be necessary for progenitor cells to exit the cell cycle. MYC, MYCN, and MYCL expression in the developing posterior fossa appears to be cell context dependent. GNPs express MYCN, but not MYC, in their proliferative phase in response to SHH. Neuronal progenitors in the Purkinje cell layer and in the ventricular zone express MYCL but not MYCN or MYC. In addition, amplification of MYC and MYCN occurs in 5–10% of medulloblastomas [34]. Some authors have found the overexpression of MYC/MYCN mRNA to be a significant predictor of worse out-

come [35]. Although promoting proliferation in medulloblastoma, the MYC genes play different roles in each subtype.

## Molecular Subtypes

The WHO now classifies medulloblastomas into four groups: WNT-activated, SHH-activated and TP53-mutant, SHH-activated and TP53-wild-type, and non-WNT/non-SHH (groups 3 and 4) (Table 27.1). SHH subgroup is the most predominant subtype in adult patients, consisting of 60% of patients [36]. Al-Halabi et al. found SHH-driven tumorigenesis in more than 80% of adult medulloblastoma [37]. Northcott et al. performed a gene expression profiling study which included an independent cohort of 14 adult medulloblastoma and indicated that these tumors were allocated to SHH (72%), CDK6/MYC (21%), and WNT (7%) subtypes [30]. A similar study found a greater number of SHH-activated tumors (50%) compared to CDK6/MYC-activated (29%) and WNT-activated tumors (21%) [36].

The SHH subgroup may have the greatest clinical implications in the future, as SHH pathway inhibitors (specifically Smo inhibitors) have been proven to be effective in preliminary studies and are currently being evaluated in phase III

Table 27.1 World Health Organization (WHO) classification of medulloblastoma

| Medulloblastomas, genetically defined | |
|---|---|
| Medulloblastoma, WNT-activated | Least common, associated with Turcot syndrome, metastasis infrequent, 5y OS >95% |
| Medulloblastoma, SHH-activated and TP53-wild-type | Often desmoplastic, associated with Gorlin syndrome |
| Medulloblastoma, SHH-activated and TP53-mutant | Chromosome instability, peak in adolescence, worse OS than TP53-wt |
| Medulloblastoma, non-WNT/non-SHH | |
| Medulloblastoma, group 3 | Amplification of MYC, rare in adults, frequently metastatic, 5y OS ~50% |
| Medulloblastoma, group 4 | Amplification of MYCN and CDK6, large-cell/anaplastic histology in adults, male predominance, 5y OS ~50% |
| Medulloblastomas, histologically defined | |
| Medulloblastoma, classic | Sheets of small round blue cells with neuroblastic or neuronal differentiation, as demonstrated by immunoreactivity for synaptophysin |
| Desmoplastic/nodular medulloblastoma | Nodular areas of densely packed reticulin-rich cells, with features of neuronal differentiation |
| Medulloblastoma with extensive nodularity | Expanded reticulin-free lobular architecture with neutrophil-like tissue nodular grape-like appearance on MRI |
| Large-cell/anaplastic medulloblastoma | Prominent and pleomorphic nuclei with large areas of necrosis and high mitotic rate |

trials. The most commonly found genetic mutations in the SHH subgroup are PTCH1 (28%) or SUFU, in addition to other frequently mutated genes [30]. A recent study demonstrated that the presence of TP53 mutations, which occurs in 13% of SHH medulloblastomas, allows for further prognostic stratification, as this mutation being associated with a poorer survival [38]. TP53 mutant SHH tumors have a peak incidence in adolescence, while SHH tumors with wild-type TP53 are overrepresented in infants and adults with medulloblastoma [28]. Patients with TP53 wild-type SHH tumors have an intermediate prognosis, with overall survival (OS) rates of approximately 80%. Comparatively, patients with TP53-mutant SHH tumors have much worse survival, with a five-year OS of approximately 40%. TP53 can also be mutated in WNT tumors, but in this subgroup it does not seem to be of prognostic significance.

The least common subtype of medulloblastomas, WNT-activated tumors account for 10% of all medulloblastomas (15% in adults) [36]. Typically, they occur in children over 3 years of age and are rarely found in adults with medulloblastoma. These tumors occur equally as often between males and females. WNT-activation is associated with the classical medulloblastoma histology as well as a low propensity for metastasis. Their prognosis is best in children, with 5-year OS rates of >95%, compared to 80% in adults. This subgroup is characterized by enhanced WNT-beta catenin pathway activation. A mutation in CTNNB1 is the most common genetic alteration in this subgroup (present in 90% of the cases), which leads to an enhanced activation of MYC and MYC-N oncogenes, with a subsequent increase in cellular proliferation [39]. Given its better prognosis, de-escalated therapeutic protocols are being investigated in the pediatric population of this subgroup in order to minimize any long-term adverse events.

Group 3, which has the worst prognosis with 5-year OS rates of 40 to 50%, makes up 25% of the diagnoses, the condition occurring in children and infants, with a predominance in males (2:1). It has rarely been described in adults (<2%) [28]. The tendency to metastasize is high (45%), and the most commonly found genetic alteration is proto-oncogene MYC mutation/amplification (16.7%). This group is characterized by an elevated genomic instability with frequent chromosome 1p gains, 10q and 5q loss, and the presence of isochromosome 17 [40].

Group 4 is the largest subgroup of all, accounting for 35% of all medulloblastomas [40]. Almost all cases have classic or large-cell histology. The incidence in males is three times higher than in female. The condition occurs in adults (20–25% of all adult medulloblastomas) and children (35%), the latter having better prognosis than adults. Overall, the prognosis is intermediate, with an OS rate of 75%. Metastases occur in 35–40% of cases. MYCN and CDK6 amplifications are the most commonly found genetic alterations in this group.

## Prognosis

In most studies, adults with medulloblastoma have a similar prognosis compared with children with no reported significant differences in survival [22, 41, 42], although some found a worse survival in infants compared to adults and children due to early recurrences without therapeutic options [43]. In a population-based study using the SEER database that included 454 adults treated between 1970 and 2004, 5- and 10-year survival rates were 65% and 52%, respectively [44]. The prognostic factors associated with worse prognosis include disseminated or metastatic disease at the time of diagnosis, residual disease after resection, and large-cell and anaplastic histology. Among adults, localized disease at presentation has been associated with a better outcome [45, 46]. Female sex has been associated with increased survival in some retrospective studies [45, 46], but not in others [47]. Poor postoperative performance status has been also shown to impact survival [24]. Other factors such as age and location of tumor in the cerebellum have not been shown to impact survival and recurrence of the disease [48]. However, in a large retrospective series, Padovani et al. analyzed 253 patients showing that brain stem and fourth ventricle involvement and dose <50 Gy to the posterior cranial fossa were negative prognostic factors in a multivariate analysis, with most relapses occurring in the posterior fossa [49].

Based on the knowledge of favorable and adverse prognostic factors, medulloblastoma is staged using the Chang staging system (Table 27.2) [50]. Treatment in children is tailored to risk factors with a division into average-risk and high-risk categories. Average-risk patients are defined as

**Table 27.2** Modified Chang staging system

| | |
|---|---|
| *Tumor extent* | |
| T1 | Tumor less than 3 cm in diameter |
| T2 | Tumor greater than 3 cm in diameter |
| T3a | Tumor greater than 3 cm in diameter with extension into the aqueduct of Sylvius and/or the foramen of Luschka |
| T3b | Tumor greater than 3 cm in diameter with unequivocal extension into the brain stem |
| T4 | Tumor greater than 3 cm in diameter with extension up past the aqueduct of Sylvius and/or down past the foramen magnum |
| No consideration is given to the number of structures invaded or the presence of hydrocephalus | |
| T3b can be defined by intraoperative demonstration of tumor extension into the brain stem in the absence of radiographic evidence | |
| *Metastasis* | |
| M0 | No evidence of gross subarachnoid or hematogenous metastasis |
| M1 | Microscopic tumor cells found in the cerebrospinal fluid |
| M2 | Gross nodular seeding demonstrated in the cerebellar/cerebral subarachnoid space or in the third or lateral ventricles |
| M3 | Gross nodular seeding in the spinal subarachnoid space |
| M4 | Metastasis outside the cerebrospinal axis |

total or near-total resection at the time of surgery and no evidence of disseminated disease by brain and spine MRI and CSF analysis. High-risk patients are defined as the presence of $\geq 1.5$ cm$^2$ of residual tumor after surgery and/or evidence of disseminated or metastatic disease. Since data on these prognostic factors are scarce in adult medulloblastoma, the risk profile has been extrapolated mainly from data on childhood medulloblastoma. Like children, adults are typically stratified into risk groups based on the extent of surgical resection and the presence or absence of disseminated or metastatic disease. However, there is increasing understanding that histopathological and molecular classification of the tumor affects prognosis and is being integrated into new clinical trials.

It has been thought that the degree of tumor resection is related to outcome of medulloblastoma, where 5-year progression-free survival (PFS) in patients more than 3 years of age was 78% in children with tumor residual <1.5 cm$^2$ and 53% in patients with larger tumor residual. In adults, the data supporting the prognostic relevance of postoperative residual disease is conflicting. The advantage of gross total resection has also been shown in a cohort of 454 patients analyzed within the SEER database [51]. Carrie et al. analyzed 156 patients without showing an impact of residual tumor on OS, but found that complete resection resulted in severely reduced postoperative performance status only without any benefit in OS [23]. The 5-year PFS rate was 59% in 109 patients without residual disease, compared with 64% in 50 patients with residual tumor. By contrast, Chan observed a 5-year PFS rate of 86% for 17 patients without residual tumor vs. 27% for patients with residual tumor [52]. Data from the updated analysis performed by Brandes et al. showed that postoperative residual disease did not significantly impact the 5-year PFS, while T stage showed a borderline correlation with 5-year PFS, being 82% in patients with T1–T3a disease and 44% in patients with T3b–T4 disease ($p = 0.06$) [53]. Atalar et al. found that residual volume less than 1.5 cm$^2$ after surgery correlated with better disease-free survival, though this did not hold on multivariate analyses. The impact of residual disease after surgery may be mitigated by adjuvant chemotherapy and radiotherapy, which can salvage and improve outcomes for this group of patients.

Medulloblastoma has a propensity to spread through CSF to seed the craniospinal axis. The relevance of leptomeningeal spread of medulloblastoma detected in the CSF or by MRI is reported in several studies in children [50, 54]. The study of 86 pediatric patients of Miralbell et al. found differences in 5- and 10-year OS by stage of 76/54% for M0, 36/25% for M1, and 22/22% for M2–3 disease [55]. Zeltzer et al. studied 203 patients with medulloblastoma, and the difference in 5-year PFS in M0, M1, and M2+ was 70%, 57%, and 40% respectively [56]. The prognostic relevance of macroscopic metastatic disease has been confirmed in the analy-

sis of 454 patients reported by Lai et al. and 251 patients reported by Padovani et al. [49, 51].

On the other hand, the tendency for metastatic spread is much lower in adults than in children (8% and 13%, respectively, in two series of adult patients), and the influence of metastatic disease is less clear [57]. For example, in one French series, positive CSF was found in 8% of cases [49]. Positive CSF did appear to be of prognostic significance, with a 10-year OS of 49% compared to 60% in CSF negative patients. Spinal involvement had an important prognostic influence as well. The 10-year OS was 24% in patients with spinal metastases, compared to 58% in patients without metastatic deposits. Frost et al. reported a 5-year PFS of 42% in patients without metastatic disease, whereas none of the patients with metastases survived [57]. In the series reported by Chan et al., the 5-year PFS was 47% as compared to 59% in patients without tumor dissemination [52]. Although early data in the prospective series of Brandes et al. suggested that patients without metastases showed a significantly better outcome than those with metastatic spread (PFS at 5 years of 75% vs. 45%, respectively, $p = 0.01$), more recent data on the same population, after a median follow-up of 7.6 years, showed that this difference was not significant, with PFS at 5 years 61% and 78% in metastatic and nonmetastatic patients, respectively [53, 54]. This data is consistent with those reported by Carrie et al., which could not detect an impact of metastatic disease on prognosis [23]. In their study, the 5-year OS rates were 51% for patients with metastases and 58% for metastases-free patients, which was a statistically insignificant difference.

Histologic grading of medulloblastoma has been recently proposed as an important prognostic factor. In a large series of pediatric medulloblastomas from the Pediatric Oncology Group (POG), moderate and severe anaplasia was identified on histopathological examination in 14% and 10% of cases, respectively, and was associated with poor prognosis [58]. The prognostic significance of severe anaplasia on survival has been confirmed in a more recent study from patients enrolled in the International Society of Paediatric Oncology (SIOP) II clinical trial. Mild, moderate, and severe anaplasia was present in 7%, 59%, and 34%, respectively, of cases in this cohort, severe anaplasia predicted a significantly worse outcome. In the study by Lamont et al. in pediatric medulloblastoma, severe anaplasia/large-cell morphology was found in 20% of cases and was independent prognostic indicator for worse outcomes [59]. Similarly, large-cell/anaplastic subtype is an unfavorable prognostic pathologic factor in adults [43, 51].

Other histological subtypes have been shown to impact prognosis in adults. In a study of 30 adult patients presenting with medulloblastoma, only histological type had a statistically significant influence on survival and recurrence after multivariate analysis, with patients presenting classic medulloblastoma demonstrating a long PFS and OS [48]. The desmoplastic/nodular type often has been found to be more common in adults and to be correlated with a better outcome in pediatrics with several studies have reported similar findings in adults [23, 48, 60]. However, other studies have not demonstrated that the desmoplastic/nodular histological subtype predicts a better outcome [57, 61, 62].

Important prognostic molecular markers reported in children include nuclear accumulation of β-catenin as a marker for favorable prognosis, while p53 and EGFR overexpression and MYC amplification are unfavorable. In the future, pediatric protocols risk group stratification will also be based on β-catenin and MYC amplification. However, MYC/MYCN amplifications were rarely observed in adult tumors [63]. In addition, adult medulloblastomas with 6q deletion and nuclear β-catenin activation did not share the excellent prognosis with their pediatric counterparts. In adults, MDM2 overexpression has been reported as a marker for unfavorable prognosis [26, 32, 64, 65]. Other poor prognostic factors in adult medulloblastoma include CDK6 amplification, 10q loss, and 17q gain [63].

## Multi-Modality Management Approach

In the past, adult patients with medulloblastoma were frequently treated according to various pediatric protocols, under the assumption that the tumors display the same properties in adults as in children (Table 27.3). Previously, prospective controlled trials were lacking and current experience

**Table 27.3** Studies investigating adjuvant radiation with or without chemotherapy

| Study | No. of patients | Treatment | 5-year OS |
|---|---|---|---|
| Bloom 1990 | 47 | RT<br>RT → CT (in 1971–1981) | 1952–1963: 38%<br>1964–1981: 59%<br>1971–1981: 76% |
| Prados 1995 | 47 | RT → CT (in 32 pts) | AR: 81%<br>HR: 54% |
| Frost 1995 | 48 | RT (only 1 pt. treated with CT) | 62% |
| Chan 2000 | 32 | RT → CT (in 24 pts) | 83% |
| Greenberg 2000 | 17 | CRT → CT | 24.3% |
| Louis 2002 | 24 | RT → CT (in 6 pts) | 82% |
| Padovani 2007 | 253 | CRT (in 142 pts) | 72% |
| Brandes 2003 and 2007 | 10AR<br>26 HR | RT<br>CT → RT → CT | AR: 80%<br>HR: 73% |
| Friedrich 2012 | 70 (nonmetastatic) | RT → CT | 4-Year OS: 89% |
| Beier 2017 | 30 (50% M0) | CRT → CT | 3-Year OS: 70% |

was based exclusively on retrospective studies. These studies comprised small patient numbers and have utilized varying treatments spanning decades during which time diagnostic procedures, neurosurgical skills, and radiation therapy techniques have changed considerably. Given the paucity and heterogeneity of data, the recent German NOA-07 prospectively investigated the use of chemoradiation followed by adjuvant chemotherapy in adult patients with medulloblastoma in order to define a standard treatment regimen.

Based on experience in children, craniospinal irradiation (CSI) is followed by a boost to the posterior fossa. Appropriate conventional doses based on the prognostic factors as used in the pediatric population may be used in adults although dose de-escalation is of lesser importance in adults than the developing child. In children, adjuvant chemotherapy has been used to lower doses of radiation to minimize the long-term toxicity to children. However, the toxicity of chemotherapy is higher in adults especially in those with poor performance status or multiple medical comorbidities, and there is less need to reduce the total radiation dose in an adult patient. For average-risk patients, surgery followed by radiotherapy (CSI followed by a boost to the posterior fossa) using conventional doses (without dose reductions) with or without concurrent and adjuvant chemotherapy is a reasonable option. On the other hand, many practitioners have adopted the paradigm of average-risk pediatric protocols using lower doses of CSI and smaller boost fields to the posterior fossa surgical bed with margin.

For high-risk patients, it is difficult to establish detailed treatment recommendations due to the rarity of this disease in adults. It may be reasonable to treat high-risk adult patients with conventional dose CSI followed by posterior fossa boost followed by chemotherapy. However, as in children, conventional treatment schedules are associated with a poorer outcome, and consequently novel approaches are being investigated. It is therefore recommended that individualized treatment decisions in adults should involve a multidisciplinary team including medical or neuro-oncologist, radiation oncologist, and/or pediatric oncologist to weigh the potential yet unproven benefits of chemotherapy on long-term survival against the risks of toxicity in adult patients.

## Surgery

Maximal safe resection is a key component of the treatment of all patients with medulloblastoma. Resection confirms the diagnosis, relieves increased intracranial pressure, and helps establish local control. Surgery is used to remove as much of the tumor as possible without causing serious neurologic sequelae, such as persistent ataxia, cranial nerve deficits and posterior fossa syndrome which entails swallowing difficulties, mutism, truncal ataxia, and emotional instability. Because of the potential for neurologic complications, total or radical resection is not always possible, and overly aggressive attempts to achieve complete resection should be avoided. Today, with modern surgical techniques and imaging guidance in the operating room, gross total or near-total resection is achieved in a majority of patients and peri- or postoperative complications and neurological deficits resulting from surgery have become rare event [34]. In the presence of hydrocephalus, it might be necessary to relieve intracranial pressure with ventriculoperitoneal shunt or third ventriculostomy before proceeding with the surgical tumor resection. Ventriculostomy is often undertaken prior to resection in order to spare the patient ventriculoperitoneal shunt placement.

## Chemotherapy

The necessity and timing of chemotherapy in adults (before or after radiotherapy) is still a matter of debate. In young children, efforts have been made to reduce irradiation dose whenever possible using chemotherapy to minimize the impact on neurological and intellectual development caused by radiotherapy. Packer et al. reported positive results from the Children's Oncology Group (COG) study where children older than 3 with nonmetastatic medulloblastoma were treated with postoperative, reduced-dose CSI (23.4 Gy in 13 fractions) plus a boost to the posterior fossa (32.4 Gy in 17 fractions) with concomitant vincristine and adjuvant lomustine, vincristine, and cisplatin. In this study, the PFS rate was 86% at 3 years and 79% at 5 years, which was comparable to historical controls treated with full-dose radiotherapy. In an update, EFS and OS at 10 years were 81% and 86%, respectively [66, 67]. Following these results, this approach using concomitant vincristine with radiation followed by maintenance chemotherapy has become widely used in various institutions for the treatment of average-risk children.

Because of the differences in terms of long-term toxicities between adult and pediatric patients, the use of chemotherapy is challenging in adult patients, and some adult patients with average-risk medulloblastoma may be treated with postoperative radiation therapy alone. Retrospective series of adolescents and adults with medulloblastoma suggest poor tolerance of chemotherapy after CSI [68, 69]. Chemotherapy after surgery but before radiotherapy has the advantage of increased tolerance because of uncompromised bone marrow reserve and increased delivery due to the decreased blood-brain barrier after surgery. This comes at the expense of an inevitable delay in the initiation of radiotherapy. In children, randomized studies showed a disadvantage for pre-radiation chemotherapy, or when radiotherapy was postponed for more than 20 weeks after surgery [56, 70]. Hematological toxicities due to chemotherapy in adult patients can be higher than pediatric patients, possibly causing treatment delays [68, 69]. In addition, increased and irreversible vincristine-induced neuropathies have been documented in adults at doses that are common in pediatric protocols. There are several small retrospective studies and one prospective trial that suggest the use of chemotherapy in average-risk adults is feasible as well, though at the expense of increased toxicity [49, 54]. In Germany, 49 out of 70 adult patients without metastatic disease received additional chemotherapy according to the German HIT'91 protocol, which used concurrent vincristine during radiation followed by maintenance of lomustine, vincristine, and cisplatin [71]. This same regimen was used in the German NOA-07 trial, and 70% of enrolled patients were able to complete at least four cycles of adjuvant chemotherapy with 49.7% of patients able to complete all eight cycles as intended per protocol [72]. Based on these more recent studies, the use of chemotherapy in average-risk adult patients with medulloblastoma may be possible with proper toxicity management.

Chemotherapy is part of the treatment for high-risk pediatric patients, but there is no consensus on regimens, doses, and timing of the chemotherapy in either pediatric or adult settings to date. In children, different schedules have been used in clinical trials and the optimal treatment in unknown. A reasonable multiagent chemotherapy regimen consists of carboplatin and vincristine administered concurrently with radiation therapy, followed by six maintenance cycles of cyclophosphamide and vincristine with or without cisplatin [73]. A similar regimen that incorporates chemotherapy before radiation can be used in adults, which is based on the results of the prospective study by Brandes et al. [74]. In this trial, all patients received two courses of pre-radiation chemotherapy with carboplatin-etoposide, followed by radiotherapy with vincristine, followed by four maintenance courses of chemotherapy with carboplatin, vincristine, and cyclophosphamide (DEC). Data from this high-risk trial suggested this regimen provides long-term outcomes similar to that obtained with radiotherapy alone in average-risk patients. However, a recent small phase II prospective study by the ECOG-ACRIN Cancer Research Group reports that 11 adult patients with high-risk medulloblastoma treated with three cycles of postoperative cisplatin, etoposide, cyclophosphamide, and vincristine prior to CSI experience much lower than expected outcomes with 5-year PFS and OS of 27% and 55% [75]. Therefore, the feasibility of various chemotherapy regimens in the high-risk group has not been firmly established.

## Indication for Irradiation

Radiation therapy (RT) is an integral component of the initial management of patients with medulloblastoma, both to control residual posterior fossa disease and to treat any disease that has spread along the craniospinal axis. Prior to use of radiation, no children survived with surgical resection alone. In adults, surgery alone is associated with a high relapse rate and requires adjuvant radiation therapy. Hubbard et al. reported six spinal recurrences in eight patients undergoing surgery alone [62]. Starting in 1930, RT was incorporated to reduce the rate of local recurrence in the surgical bed and along the craniospinal axis [76]. Two large series of adult medulloblastoma treated patients over a 30-year period from the 1950s to the 1980s. The 5-year OS was about 50–60% and 10-year OS was about 40% [57, 61]. Ferrante et al. analyzed 32 patients and showed that radiation therapy increased OS from 6.5 months to 6.6 years [15, 46]. Since there, there has been progressive improvement in the delivery and quality of CSI, resulting in the current long-term OS rate of 60–70% in children and adults. Because of the propensity of medulloblastomas to disseminate within the CSF, postoperative radiotherapy should be given to the entire craniospinal axis with a boost to both the primary tumor site and focal CNS metastatic sites [24, 69, 77, 78]. Dosage to the craniospinal axis appears to be critical as well. According to the Children's Cancer Study Group experience, dose reductions from 36 to 23.4 Gy were associated with a significantly increased risk of recurrences outside the posterior fossa [79]. However, these dose reductions appear to be feasible when combined with chemotherapy with a 5-year PFS rate of 79% [66, 67]. For adults, the only available data from Bloom et al. demonstrated an increased relapse rate after dose reductions from 32 to 35 Gy down to 15–25 Gy [61]. The dose to the spinal axis depends on the presence or absence of microscopic or macroscopic metastases.

The rationale for additional radiation to the tumor bed is based upon the observation that 50–70% of recurrences occur in the posterior fossa. The radiation dose to the posterior fossa should be at least 54 Gy as a dose–response relationship for treatment of tumors located within the posterior fossa has clearly been documented [24, 80–82]. Berry et al. noted a 10-year PFS of 77% if the dose to the posterior fossa exceeded 52 Gy [83]. Lower doses were associated with a 5-year PFS rate of 47%. In adults, Hazuka et al. noted a tumor control of 75% in the posterior fossa after 55 Gy or more, compared to 40% tumor control if doses less than 50 Gy where given [84]. Abacioglu et al. confirmed these observations finding that the 5-year local control rates being 33% after doses of less than 54 Gy, as compared to 91% in patients receiving higher doses [82].

Radiotherapy should start within 4 weeks of the operation. In case of combined modality treatment, the concurrent chemotherapy should be initiated at the same time. It has been demonstrated that delay beyond 47 days is associated with worse local control and an impaired prognosis [15, 24]. Herrlinger et al. reported that the interval between surgery and the start of radiotherapy influenced survival [77]. Furthermore, time to completion of RT has been demon-

strated to be important in terms of prognosis, as delays and interruptions may have a negative impact on PFS [53]. The expected duration of radiotherapy is approximately 6 weeks. Studies have shown a correlation between improved posterior fossa control and shorter periods for the completion of radiotherapy [52, 85]. An overall treatment time of less than or equal to 45–48 days has therefore been proposed [86, 87]. Concerning time intervals, another study found a significant better survival if the time interval between surgery and start of radiotherapy was kept below 25 days [82].

## Treatment Field Design and Target Delineation

For accurate dose delivery and reproducibility, an individual immobilization system is made for simulation and treatment. The patient can be in prone or supine position, depending on the radiation technique, but the supine technique is growing in popularity due to patient comfort and easier airway access for children needing anesthesia. A CT simulation scan encompassing the entire cranium to below the thecal sac is obtained. The caudal termination of the thecal sac is best identified on a sagittal T2-weighted spine MRI. This planning CT scan should be fused using image registration with the postoperative cranial MRI scan or with the preoperative MRI scan.

For CSI, the CTV is defined as the entire craniospinal axis encompassing the whole brain and thecal sac. Extra attention should be taken to include the cribriform plate, which is the inferior border of the anterior fossa and frontal sinus and can be identified by following the anterior clinoids anteriorly and locating the superior orbital plate. Planning target volume (PTV) can be defined as the CTV plus 0.3–0.5 cm margin for setup inaccuracies. For conventional CSI technique, the brain and spine are treated with separate but abutting RT fields (Fig. 27.1). The patient is treated in the prone or supine position such that two opposed lateral 6 MV photon beams should cover the head and cervical spine to about C5/C6. The inferior border of these fields should geometrically match with the superior border of the spinal irradiation field. Placement of the junction between these two fields must be done precisely. Feathering the field junction the cranial and spine fields every five fractions during the course of CSI is routinely done to minimize the potential of overlapping dose to the spinal cord. Due to the length of the adult spinal cord, the spinal irradiation field is often split into designated upper and lower spine fields or alternatively treated at extended skin to surface distance (SSD).

After CSI, the patient should be treated supine to deliver the boost to the posterior fossa and any spine metastases. Traditionally, boost volume includes the entire posterior fossa. However, posterior fossa failures occur primarily in the tumor bed, and the COG ACNS0331 trial has shown in a

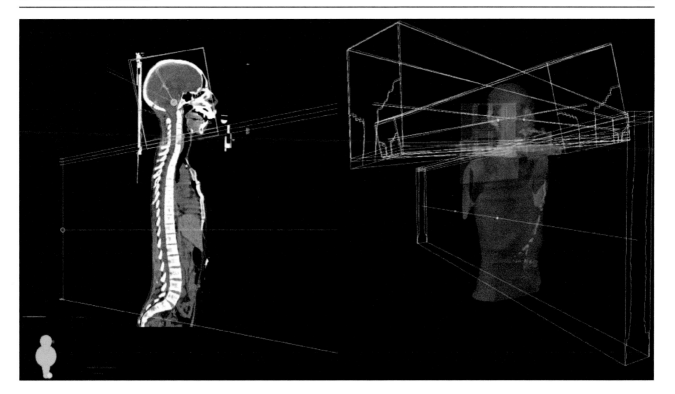

**Fig. 27.1** CSI beam arrangement. A supine patient is treated with two lateral opposed cranial fields matched to a single posterior spine field. The field junction was moved 0.5 cm twice during CSI, after the seventh and fourteenth fractions

randomized setting that the use of reduced volume posterior fossa boost is non-inferior to entire posterior fossa boost [88]. When delineating the target volumes, the gross tumor volume (GTV) is contrast-enhancing lesion on MRI scan, including the primary tumor plus the walls of the resection cavity. In light of the outcomes in the pediatric population, the clinical target volume (CTV) should be the GTV plus entire surgical bed with a 1.5 cm expansion anatomically constrained by the posterior fossa excluding extension beyond barriers such as the bone and tentorium. The PTV is the CTV plus a 0.3–0.5 cm margin. Cranial and spinal metastases GTV can be boosted with a 0.5–1 cm margin to create a PTV.

For all average-risk patients or high-risk patients treated with combined modality, the craniospinal PTV should receive 36 Gy in 20 fractions followed by a posterior fossa boost of 18–19.8 Gy in 10–11 fractions for a total dose of 54 to 55.8 Gy. For high-risk patients with M+ disease treated with radiotherapy only, the craniospinal PTV should receive 39.6 Gy in 22 fractions followed by a posterior fossa boost of 16.2 Gy for a total of 55.8 Gy.

## Normal Critical Structure Tolerance and Constraints

Whenever possible, without compromising CTV, attempts should be made to limit the dose to the optic chiasm and optic nerves to a point dose less than 54 Gy, while the retina (eye) should receive a point dose less than 45 Gy. The brain stem should be limited to a point dose less than 54 Gy, while normal spinal cord should be limited to 45 Gy. The cochlea to a median dose should be less than 37 Gy with platinum-based chemotherapy or 45 Gy without chemotherapy. The lens dose should be minimized by avoiding direct fields and should not be higher than 5 Gy. The pituitary and hypothalamus should receive less than 45 Gy. Direct irradiation of the thyroid by vertex fields should be avoided and dose to the thyroid should be minimized.

## Complication Avoidance

With the advent of conformal radiation planning and delivery, reducing the target volume for RT has been the primary aim of many clinical investigators in order to minimize side effects from the treatment. Given that the distribution of radiation dose to an organ-at-risk correlates with its functional outcome, the expectation is that newer methods of RT will decrease side effects without affecting the rate of local control or the pattern of failure. With these goals in mind, recent technical advances such as intensity-modulated radiotherapy (IMRT) can be used for both the irradiation of the spine and posterior fossa boost. Image-guided RT (IGRT) allows for the adjustment and positional correction of the patient or treatment fields based on daily low-dose kilovoltage imaging to account for the daily setup variability allowing the use of small PTV margins.

Volumetric modulated arc therapy (VMAT) and helical tomotherapy have been evaluated and described in the literature to deliver highly conformal doses while minimizing doses to OAR [89, 90]. Compared to conventional IMRT, these techniques are delivered continuously while varying the gantry rotational speed, multileaf collimator leaf position, and dose rate simultaneously during treatment delivery, therefore reducing treatment times while delivering an extremely conformal radiation dose [91–93]. Tomotherapy and VMAT seem to be favorable in terms of target volume coverage, dose homogeneity, and reduction of dose to nontarget tissues, but concerns have been raised regarding longer radiation beam-on times that could lead to higher whole-body isodoses compared to conventional techniques.

Proton beam therapy exploits the favorable physical characteristics of charged particle beams to deliver less radiation dose to normal tissues compared to external beam photon radiotherapy [94]. Proton therapy allows the delivery of high therapeutic dose within the target area, with lower nontarget tissue irradiation than for standard and three-dimensional conformational therapy. For example, in the study by St. Clair et al., the dose to 90% of the cochlea was reduced from 101.2% of the prescribed dose with conventional X-rays to 2.4% with protons. Similarly, the dose to 50% of the heart volume was reduced from 72.2% with conventional X-rays to 0.5% with protons [80]. In their study, Merchant et al. created models to compare the effects of proton therapy versus photon therapy in medulloblastoma and other brain tumors and found that proton therapy could lead to a reduction in hearing impairment and reduced doses to the hypothalamic–pituitary axis [81]. These dosimetric advantages have been borne out in the clinical setting with a retrospective study comparing proton CSI to photon CSI demonstrating significantly decreased rates of GI toxicity and hematologic toxicity using proton therapy [95].

## Radiation Toxicity, Acute and Late Toxicity

Although RT is an effective adjuvant therapy, the side effects of RT limit the therapeutic benefit of many treatment regimens. The main drawback of radiation therapy is its acute and late toxicity. Acute side effects include fatigue, skin changes, hair loss, nausea, vomiting, headache, weight loss, taste alteration, hearing loss, and transient radiation myelopathy (Lhermitte's phenomena). CSI can cause depressed hematologic counts (thrombocytomenia, lymphopenia, neutropenia) since the radiation fields encompass large volumes of bone marrow in the vertebral bodies, which is extremely radiosensitive [96, 97]. This hematological toxicity can lead to increased rates of infections, bleeding, and transfusions,

and possibly decreased tolerance of chemotherapy. Gastrointestinal toxicity can occur commonly during CSI due to exit doses and can include complaints such as mucositis, nausea, dysphagia, odynophagia, esophagitis, abdominal pain, cramping, and diarrhea. Proton CSI can limit exit dose that occurs with photon CSI, thus minimizing toxicity. Patients treated using proton therapy experience less significant weight loss (16% vs. 64%; $P = 0.004$), grade 2+ nausea and vomiting (26% vs. 71%; $P = 0.004$), esophagitis (5% vs. 57%, $P < 0.001$), and hematologic toxicity (white blood cells 46% vs. 55%, $P = 0.04$; hemoglobin 88% vs. 97%, $P = 0.009$; platelets 48% vs. 65%, $P = 0.05$) [95].

Late toxicity can include hypopituitarism, chronic myleopathic neuropathy, neurocognitive impairment (concentration, memory, and behavior), benign tumors (meningioma), second malignancies (skin, thyroid, CNS), and hearing impairment. Neurocognitive and psychological symptoms were among the most frequently observed sequelae in brain tumor survivors [98]. The dose-dependent and volume-dependent neurotoxicity of RT to the supratentorial brain, the temporal lobes, and the hippocampus is implicated in cognitive dysfunction [99]. It has been theorized that the thinning of white matter in the cerebral cortex or hippocampus impacts attention and learning [100]. The hypothesized mechanism of injury includes damage of endothelial cell with consequent microvascular damage, direct injury to neurons and oligodendrocytes and direct oxidative stress on the myelin membrane [101].

Other complications, such as hearing impairment, hypothalamic and pituitary endocrinopathies, and visual impairment, may occur depending on the field of radiation [102]. Hearing loss is a significant risk in medulloblastoma survivors given the doses of RT used in medulloblastoma protocols and as well as synergistic toxicity between RT and cisplatin chemotherapy. Enhanced utilization of IMRT or proton techniques with attention to avoidance of auditory structures may diminish the incidence of this side effect. Endocrine abnormalities are very common following RT for medulloblastoma [103]. Higher RT doses to the hypothalamus and pituitary are associated with an increased risk of multiple endocrinopathies. Irradiation of the pituitary hypothalamic axis can result in growth hormone (GH), adrenocorticotrophic hormone (ACTH), and thyroid-stimulation hormone (TSH) deficiencies [103–105]. In addition, irradiation of the thyroid can cause primary hypothyroidism.

Patients who have received spinal radiation may also experience direct RT toxicity on vertebral bodies. Skeletal complications of radiation therapy include alterations in bone growth, radiation osteopenia with secondary stress fractures, and radiation-induced sarcoma [106]. Growth arrest is less of a concern for patients who have reached their adult height, unlike children, who experience dose-dependent decline in sitting height due to the direct RT effect on the spine [107]. In addition, osteopenia is common in survivors, though it is reversible and the severity is dose dependent [105]. Weakening of the bone can cause insufficiency fractures to occur after radiation therapy. Alteration in signal intensity of the vertebral bodies after radiation changes secondary to replacement of marrow by fatty tissue can be seen up to 10 years after radiation and may present poor hematopoietic reserve [108, 109].

The incidence of second malignancies is increased following RT and/or chemotherapy for primary central nervous system malignancies [110]. Increased whole-body doses could increase the risk of radiation-induced tumors, especially in younger patients. Radiation-associated malignancies included soft tissue sarcomas, thyroid cancer, acute and chronic myelogenous leukemia, breast cancer, and lung cancer. Radiation-induced leukemia generally occurs within 3–5 years of radiation exposure; solid tumors usually start to be diagnosed a minimum of 10–15 years after exposure and often do not appear much later in life [67]. However, estimates of rates of radiation-associated malignancy require a large population size that is usually required to evaluate the risk of cancer, because cancer is a rare outcome, especially in children. Large cohort studies from Japanese atomic bomb survivors and children treated with radiation for benign conditions demonstrate the risk of secondary cancers is dose dependent [111]. Proton therapy has been used to attempt to minimize total dose to the patient and thus reduce the rate of secondary malignancy [112].

## Outcomes: Tumor Control and Survival

Adults with average-risk medulloblastoma have generally good outcomes even with radiation alone, with 5-year PFS ranging from 55% to 80% [24, 42, 113]. In children with medulloblastoma, chemotherapy has been used for years in order to improve outcome for poor prognosis patients or to decrease radiotherapy dose in standard prognosis patients. Similarly, investigators have attempted to demonstrate the efficacy of chemotherapy in adult patients (Table 27.3). In the series by Chan et al., additional chemotherapy yielded a 5-year PFS rate of 47% [52]. Prados et al. achieved a 5-year PFS rate of 38% when additional chemotherapy was given [42]. The Brandes group retrospectively analyzed the results of average-risk patients who were treated with postoperative radiation with or without chemotherapy. They demonstrated that OS was 100% at 15 years when chemotherapy was added [114].

In a large French retrospective analysis and its subsequent update, there was improved 5-year PFS with combined therapy compared to radiotherapy alone (74.2% versus 59.8%), but no difference was observed regarding overall survival (73% versus 71%) [23, 49]. The investigators hypothesized that the heterogeneity of chemotherapy regimens used at multiple centers treating patients over a long period may have obscured a chemotherapy benefit. At the same time, radiation therapy at reduced doses (<34 Gy) in conjunction with chemotherapy yielded identical results as compared with standard dose radiotherapy alone [49]. These promising results suggest that dose de-escalation combined with chemotherapy may also be possible in adults with average-risk disease.

More recently, in a large multicenter retrospective study of 204 adult patients treated between 1976 and 2014, Atalar et al. found that the addition of adjuvant chemotherapy using vincristine- and cisplatin-based regimens improved local control (74% vs. 50%, $P = 0.03$) and subsequently overall survival (73% vs. 55%, $P = 0.03$) [24]. Only performance status and use of CSI was similarly related to oncologic outcomes on multivariate analysis. A recent meta-analysis by Kocakaya et al. showed that patients receiving chemotherapy first-line survived significantly longer than patients treated with radiotherapy alone (median OS 108 months versus 57 months) [115]. Efforts have been made to pursue prospective studies in adult patients with medulloblastoma in order to standardize chemotherapy regimens. Brandes et al. conducted a study in which 36 adult patients with average or high-risk medulloblastoma were treated prospectively with the DEC regimen followed by standard dose radiotherapy. The median PFS was 81 months and the 5-year EFS and OS rates were 65.4% and 75.3%, respectively [54]. By treating adult patients without metastatic disease according to the German HIT'91 protocol, Friedrich et al. followed the majority of which received additional chemotherapy achieved 4-year EFS and OS of 68% and 89%, respectively [71]. In a similar prospective study using the same HIT'91 protocol, 3-year EFS, PFS, and OS rates were 66.6%, 66.6%, and 70.0%, respectively [72].

Adult patients with metastatic medulloblastoma appear to benefit from combination therapy, though the data are limited. In the HIT'91 study, the 3-year PFS for patients with M2/M3 disease after radiotherapy followed by maintenance chemotherapy was 30%, compared to 83% for patients without metastatic disease [116]. In the early CCSG trial published by Evans et al., the overall outcome for patients with M1–M3 disease was 5-year EFS of 36% compared to 59% for patients with M0 disease [117]. This study also demonstrated that the addition of maintenance chemotherapy improved 5-year EFS to 46% compared to 0% for patients treated with radiotherapy alone. Brandes et al. demonstrated in their phase II study that high-risk patients treated with both pre-radiation and maintenance chemotherapy after radiotherapy had an exceptionally good prognosis, comparable to that in children with acceptable rates of toxicity [53, 54]. After a median follow-up of 7.6 years, updated data showed that the risk of recurrence appeared to increase markedly after 7 years of follow-up in low-risk patients. Nevertheless, medulloblastoma patients with residual or metastatic disease are at higher risk for recurrence and death, even despite intensive chemotherapy and radiation with an expected 5-year survival of approximately 50% [24]. Future studies are limited by the fact that metastatic disease, as described by Chang's classification, seems to be a rare condition in adults as opposed to the situation in children [50]. Because of the heterogeneity of patients and protocols, no recommendations can be made yet with respect to a preferred regimen, though existing pediatric protocols may be reasonable. Further studies to determine the correct sequence and combination of chemotherapy are under investigation for children with high-risk medulloblastoma. In the meantime, treatment decisions in adults should be individualized, taking into account higher risks of toxicity in adult patients, performance status, or medical comorbidities.

Lastly, the quality and timing of radiation therapy has an impact on tumor control and survival. The development of modern technologies and the introduction of quality assurance programs have highlighted the necessity for precise and reproducible irradiation schedules in medulloblastoma. Grabenbauer et al. noted an increase in survival during the last decades and concluded that the use of modern techniques in recent years has allowed better overall radiotherapeutic management [118]. Miralbell et al. analyzed the precision of treatment techniques and the impact on survival [119]. They detected that inadequate field alignment in whole-brain irradiation was associated with a significantly worse survival. Carrie et al. performed a detailed analysis of treatment techniques with special attention to coverage of clinical target volume in SFOP protocols [41]. They noted an increased risk of relapses with increasing frequency of protocol violations. In the German HIT'91 study, detailed radiotherapeutic guidelines were given in the protocol with a high degree of adherence to the guidelines and the actual treatment delivered. It was concluded that the high quality of treatment was a major contributing factor to the overall outcome [70, 116]. Image-guided radiation therapy can help ensure precise field alignment during treatment.

## Follow-Up: Radiographic Assessment

Following completion of therapy, patients should be routinely monitored for treatment complications and disease recurrence. Patients should be seen every 3 months for the first 1–2 years and then every 6–12 months thereafter. At these visits, a history and physical examination should be performed and obtain brain and spine MRIs to monitor for recurrence.

Imaging will be performed every 3 months in the first year and every 4 months in the second year starting 3 months after radiotherapy [120]. Late relapses are common with a report by Frost et al. showing that OS decreased from 62% to 41% after 10 years [57]. Similarly, Chan et al. observed a 5-year OS of 83% which had decreased to 45% by 8 years [52].

The utility of routine screening spine MRIs has been questioned in patients without a history of disseminated disease. In an observational study that included 89 patients with medulloblastoma followed with screening brain and spine MRIs, 990 brain MRIs and 758 spine MRIs were obtained over a median follow-up of 52 months [121]. An isolated spine recurrence was detected on five spine MRIs, with a detection rate of 7/1000. Therefore, cranial MRI alone may be considered for surveillance unless other localizing signs are present initially and unless new symptoms prompt additional or more extensive imaging.

## Case Illustration

A 21-year-old man presents with progressive dizziness over 1 year, particularly when standing or walking, exhibiting an ataxic gait. The patient reported nausea, vomiting, and diaphoresis, which was worse upon wakening. This was also accompanied with intermittent headaches.

The physical examination revealed horizontal nystagmus and a positive Romberg's sign. The remaining cranial nerve, motor, and sensory examinations were normal.

Magnetic resonance imaging (MRI) of the brain was conducted that showed a right-sided posterior fossa mass, which had an iso-hypointense appearance on T1-weighted images, an inhomogenously enhanced appearance in T1-weighted contrast images, and iso-hyperintense in T2-weighted images. MRI spine did not demonstrate dissemination of disease elsewhere.

The patient underwent a suboccipital craniotomy, which revealed a grayish solid mass, with undefined border, which was totally excised. Frozen section revealed malignant small round cells. Histopathological analysis showed nodules of small round cells with occasional neurocytic differentiation and surrounding collagen-rich tissue suggestive of desmoplastic medulloblastoma. In addition, immunohistochemical stains were also conducted, with the tumor staining positive for glial fibrillary acidic protein (GFAP), synaptophysin, and neuron-specific enolase and negative for cytokeratin, desmin, and epithelial membrane antigen (EMA). The patient was discharged with slight balance disturbance, and no significant postoperative complication was observed. However, his postoperative CSF cytology was persistently positive suggestive of disseminated disease.

Following his surgery, the patient was treated with radiotherapy of the whole-brain and spinal cord dose to 36 Gy, with posterior cranial fossa boost to 55.8 Gy with concurrent vincristine (Fig. 27.2). The planning target volume (PTV) included the whole brain plus a 0.3 cm uniform margin together with a spine clinical target volume to the bottom of the thecal sac as identified on MRI plus margins of between 0.5 and 1 cm. The larger margin for the spine was considered due to less rigid body immobilization and higher variability with spine setup. The RapidArc VMAT plan was created using three isocenters, with two partial arcs encompassing the brain and cervical spine, a partial arc for the mid spine and a partial arc for the lower spine (Fig. 27.3). The plans were optimized with high weightings for PTV coverage while sparing the maximal amount of OARs without sacrificing coverage of the PTV (Fig. 27.4).

The patient was treated on a Varian TrueBeam linear accelerator with the 120 Leaf Millennium MLC. He positioned in his immobilization devices with skin marks. Then optical surface imaging used to finely adjust the patient's longitudinal position, roll, and pitch prior to daily kilovoltage cone beam CT (CBCT) image verification of his position prior to treatment. His position would be re-setup for rotational shift errors greater than 0.5 cm, while smaller translational shifts were adjusted with the treatment couch. To ensure delivery as planned with overlapping VMAT arcs, rotational errors were ignored, and when translational shifts were applied, equal shifts were applied to each isocenter. When different translational shifts were needed for each isocenter, the lower spine isocenter was allowed up to a 5 mm residual error while the brain and upper spine isocenter was limited to a 2 mm residual error. The planned separation of the isocenters was always preserved.

He completed his radiation treatment as planned. This was followed by maintenance chemotherapy with cisplatin and vincristine for six cycles. He has done well for 3 years with no evidence of recurrence on follow-up MRI scans of the brain and spine.

## Summary

- Medulloblastoma is a highly cellular malignant, invasive embryonal neoplasm of the cerebellum that is more common in children but does occur in adults.
- Patients with medulloblastoma demonstrate a combination of signs and symptoms caused by increased intracranial pressure and cerebellar dysfunction that evolve over a period of weeks to a few months.

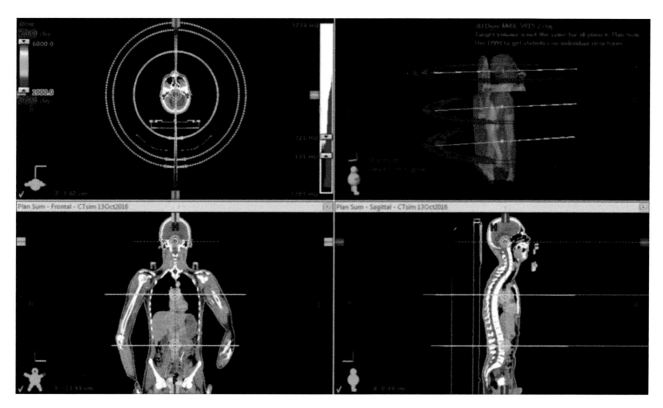

**Fig. 27.2** Treatment simulation was performed with immobilization using an abutted custom head and body fixation system consisting of a vacuum-assisted mouthpiece connected to the couch by a carbon fiber frame, while a vacuum bag system was used for immobilization below the neck. He was immobilized in the supine position with his arms at his side. Simulation included a 2 mm slice width computed tomography (CT) scan of the brain and spine in the treatment position, and the PTV and OARs were delineated for treatment planning

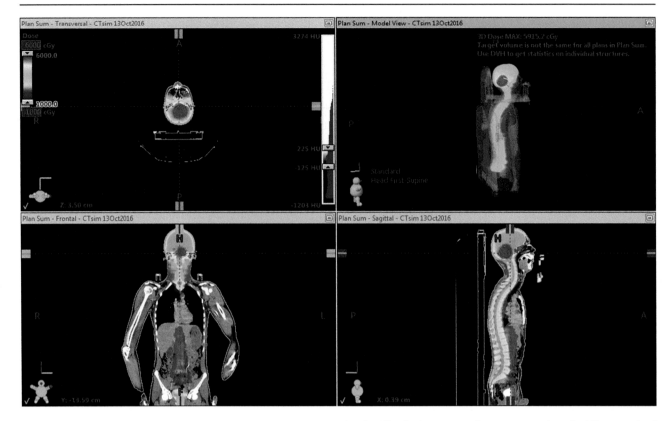

**Fig. 27.3** The RapidArc VMAT plan was created using three isocenters, with two partial arcs encompassing the brain and cervical spine, a partial arc for the mid spine and a partial arc for the lower spine. For the brain and upper spine, approximately 80° was omitted anteriorly to avoid the face, oral cavity, lenses, and solid carbon fiber mouthpiece bracket. For the lower two spine arcs, approximately 40° was omitted bilaterally to avoid entry through the arms. Junctions between arcs overlapped by about 2–3 cm and the dose in that region was automatically feathered by the planning system. No junction shifts were executed. The collimator was rotated 10–15° to minimize interleaf leakage

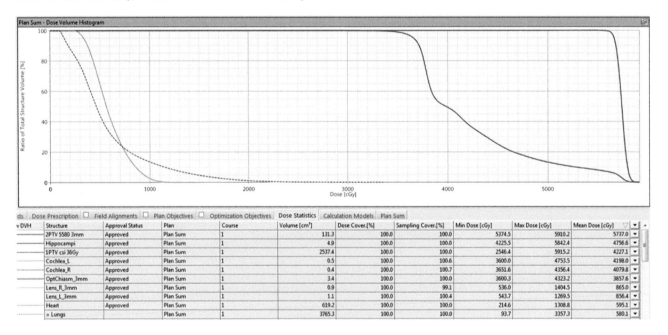

ds | Dose Prescription ☐ Field Alignments ☐ Plan Objectives ☐ Optimization Objectives | Dose Statistics | Calculation Models | Plan Sum

| Structure | Approval Status | Plan | Course | Volume [cm³] | Dose Cover.[%] | Sampling Cover.[%] | Min Dose [cGy] | Max Dose [cGy] | Mean Dose [cGy] |
|---|---|---|---|---|---|---|---|---|---|
| 2PTV 5580 3mm | Approved | Plan Sum | 1 | 131.3 | 100.0 | 100.0 | 5374.5 | 5910.2 | 5737.0 |
| Hippocampi | Approved | Plan Sum | 1 | 4.9 | 100.0 | 100.0 | 4225.5 | 5842.4 | 4756.6 |
| 1PTV csi 36Gy | Approved | Plan Sum | 1 | 2537.4 | 100.0 | 100.0 | 2546.4 | 5915.2 | 4227.1 |
| Cochlea_L | Approved | Plan Sum | 1 | 0.5 | 100.0 | 100.6 | 3600.0 | 4753.5 | 4198.0 |
| Cochlea_R | Approved | Plan Sum | 1 | 0.4 | 100.0 | 100.7 | 3651.6 | 4356.4 | 4079.8 |
| OptChiasm_3mm | Approved | Plan Sum | 1 | 3.4 | 100.0 | 100.0 | 3600.3 | 4323.2 | 3857.6 |
| Lens_R_3mm | Approved | Plan Sum | 1 | 0.9 | 100.0 | 99.1 | 536.0 | 1404.5 | 865.0 |
| Lens_L_3mm | Approved | Plan Sum | 1 | 1.1 | 100.0 | 100.4 | 543.7 | 1269.5 | 856.4 |
| Heart | Approved | Plan Sum | 1 | 619.2 | 100.0 | 100.0 | 214.6 | 1308.8 | 595.1 |
| = Lungs | | Plan Sum | 1 | 3765.3 | 100.0 | 100.0 | 93.7 | 3357.3 | 580.1 |

**Fig. 27.4** Dose volume histogram for the CSI and posterior fossa treatment volumes as well as heart and lung. All plans were optimized with high weightings for PTV coverage and homogeneity (V95% = 95% and V107% < 10%). OAR weighting was increased until PTV dose coverage began to be compromised

- Standard staging procedures include the diagnostic imaging with that should be performed before surgery and after surgery as well as CSF fluid cytology.
- Previous WHO classification of tumors of the CNS characterized medulloblastoma histologically into classic, desmoplastic/nodular, anaplastic, and large-cell medulloblastomas.
- The latest WHO classification of tumors of the CNS (2016) has incorporated molecular characteristics to stratify medulloblastoma into four subtypes by using routine immunohistochemistry (IHC): WNT-activated, SHH-activated and TP53-mutant, SHH-activated and TP53-wild-type, and non-WNT/non-SHH (groups 3 and 4).
- Medulloblastomas are staged by the Chang staging system into average-risk patients with total or near-total resection (<1.5 cc residual disease) at the time of surgery and no evidence of disseminated disease by brain and spine magnetic resonance imaging (MRI) and CSF analysis or high-risk patients who have ≥1.5 cc of residual tumor after surgery and/or evidence of disseminated or metastatic disease.
- Adult patients with medulloblastoma were frequently treated according to various pediatric protocols, as the data for treating adult medulloblastoma is limited to studies with small patient numbers.
- For standard-risk patients, the standard recommendation is surgery followed by radiotherapy (CSI to 36 Gy followed by a boost to the posterior fossa to 54–55.8 Gy). Average-risk pediatric protocols using chemotherapy, lower doses of CSI radiation, and tumor bed boost should be considered given the excellent outcomes of this group. Proton CSI radiotherapy has been shown to have less toxicity than photon CSI radiation.
- Adult patients with a high-risk medulloblastoma appear to benefit from combination therapy in prospective studies by Brandes et al. and Beier et al. demonstrating that high-risk patients treated with both pre-irradiation chemotherapy and maintenance chemotherapy had an good prognosis with acceptable toxicity.
- Following completion of therapy, patients should be seen every 3 months for the first 1–2 years and then every 6–12 months thereafter, with brain and spine MRI to be evaluated for treatment complications and disease recurrence.

## Self-Assessment Questions

1. What is the appropriate staging work up for suspected medulloblastoma?
   A. Pre- and postoperative MRI brain/spine only
   B. Postoperative MRI brain/spine, CSF cytology
   C. Preoperative MRI brain/spine, postoperative MRI brain, CSF cytology
   D. Pre- and postoperative MRI brain/spine, CSF cytology
   E. Pre- and postoperative MRI brain/spine, CSF cytology, CT of the chest, abdomen, and pelvis

2. The Hedgehog signaling pathway plays an important role in the pathogenesis of medulloblastoma. The following are true about this signaling pathway except?
   A. The majority of adult medulloblastomas have SHH mutations.
   B. Patients with FAP have mutations in the Wnt pathway.
   C. SHH is an inhibitory ligand for the PTCH1, which is a tumor suppressor gene.
   D. SHH-mutated medulloblastomas may respond to SMO inhibitors.
   E. SHH is produced by Purkinje neurons.

3. The most common histological subtype of medulloblastoma that occurs in adults is?
   A. Classic medulloblastoma
   B. Desmoplastic/nodular
   C. Anaplastic
   D. Large-cell medulloblastomas.

4. What is the incidence of medulloblastoma in patients older than 19 in the United States?
   A. 0.1 per million
   B. 0.6 per million
   C. 1.2 per million
   D. 2.0 per million

5. The following are poor prognostic factors for adult medulloblastoma except:
   A. Residual disease
   B. Disseminated disease
   C. Desmoplastic/nodular subtype
   D. TP53-mutant SHH tumors
   E. Overexpression of MYC

6. Which of the following is not an anticipated late side effect of craniospinal radiation in adults?
   A. Hypopituitarism
   B. Neurocognitive impairment
   C. Second malignancy
   D. Growth arrest
   E. Ototoxicity

7. What is the appropriate dose for CSI in a high-risk patient receiving concurrent chemotherapy?
   A. 23.4 Gy
   B. 36.0 Gy
   C. 39.6 Gy
   D. 55.8 Gy

8. What was the maintenance chemotherapy regimen in the prospective German NOA-07 trial?
   A. Cisplatin, etoposide, and cyclophosphamide
   B. Lomustine, vincristine, and cisplatin
   C. Carboplatin, vincristine, and cyclophosphamide
   D. Cisplatin and etoposide

9. Following completion of therapy and restaging, how often should patients be routinely monitored with MRI?
   A. Three months for the first 1 to 2 years and then every 6 to 12 months
   B. Four to six months for the first year and then every 6 to 12 months
   C. Six months for the first 1 to 2 years and then yearly
   D. Every 3 months until progression

## Answers

1. D
2. B
3. B
4. B
5. C
6. D
7. B
8. B
9. A

## References

1. Louis DN, Perry A, Reifenberger G, et al. The 2016 World Health Organization classification of tumors of the central nervous system: a summary. Acta Neuropathol. 2016;131(6):803–20. https://doi.org/10.1007/s00401-016-1545-1.
2. Smoll NR, Drummond KJ. The incidence of medulloblastomas and primitive neurectodermal tumours in adults and children. J Clin Neurosci. 2012;19(11):1541–4. https://doi.org/10.1016/j.jocn.2012.04.009.
3. Verdecchia A, Francisci S, Brenner H, et al. Recent cancer survival in Europe: a 2000–02 period analysis of EUROCARE-4 data. Lancet Oncol. 2007;8(9):784–96. https://doi.org/10.1016/S1470-2045(07)70246-2.
4. Ostrom QT, Gittleman H, Farah P, et al. CBTRUS statistical report: primary brain and central nervous system tumors diagnosed in the United States in 2006–2010. Neuro Oncol. 2013;15(Suppl 2):ii1–ii56. https://doi.org/10.1093/NEUONC/NOT151.
5. Peris-Bonet R, Martínez-García C, Lacour B, et al. Childhood central nervous system tumours – incidence and survival in Europe (1978–1997): report from Automated Childhood Cancer Information System project. Eur J Cancer. 2006;42(13):2064–80. https://doi.org/10.1016/j.ejca.2006.05.009.
6. Shore RE, Moseson M, Harley N, et al. Tumors and other diseases following childhood X-ray treatment for ringworm of the scalp (Tinea capitis). Health Phys. 2003;85(4):404–8. http://www.ncbi.nlm.nih.gov/pubmed/13678280. Accessed 27 Aug 2016.
7. Armstrong GT, Liu Q, Yasui Y, et al. Long-term outcomes among adult survivors of childhood central nervous system malignancies in the Childhood Cancer Survivor Study. J Natl Cancer Inst. 2009;101(13):946–58. https://doi.org/10.1093/jnci/djp148.
8. Taylor AJ, Little MP, Winter DL, et al. Population-based risks of CNS tumors in survivors of childhood cancer: the British childhood cancer survivor study. J Clin Oncol. 2010;28(36):5287–93. https://doi.org/10.1200/JCO.2009.27.0090.
9. Ellison DW, Clifford SC, Gajjar A, et al. What's new in neuro-oncology? Recent advances in medulloblastoma. Eur J Paediatr Neurol. 2003;7(2):53–66. http://www.ncbi.nlm.nih.gov/pubmed/12697428. Accessed 26 Nov 2016
10. Amlashi SFA, Riffaud L, Brassier G, et al. Nevoid basal cell carcinoma syndrome: relation with desmoplastic medulloblastoma in infancy. A population-based study and review of the literature. Cancer. 2003;98(3):618–24. https://doi.org/10.1002/cncr.11537.
11. Smith MJ, Beetz C, Williams SG, et al. Germline mutations in SUFU cause Gorlin syndrome-associated childhood medulloblastoma and redefine the risk associated with PTCH1 mutations. J Clin Oncol. 2014;32(36):4155–61. https://doi.org/10.1200/JCO.2014.58.2569.
12. Hamilton SR, Liu B, Parsons RE, et al. The molecular basis of Turcot's syndrome. N Engl J Med. 1995;332(13):839–47. https://doi.org/10.1056/NEJM199503303321302.
13. Vasen HFA, Möslein G, Alonso A, et al. Guidelines for the clinical management of familial adenomatous polyposis (FAP). Gut. 2008;57(5):704–13. https://doi.org/10.1136/gut.2007.136127.
14. Attard TM, Giglio P, Koppula S, et al. Brain tumors in individuals with familial adenomatous polyposis: a cancer registry experience and pooled case report analysis. Cancer. 2007;109(4):761–6. https://doi.org/10.1002/cncr.22475.
15. Brandes AA, Franceschi E, Tosoni A, et al. Adult neuroectodermal tumors of posterior fossa (medulloblastoma) and of supratentorial sites (stPNET). Crit Rev Oncol Hematol. 2009;71(2):165–79. https://doi.org/10.1016/j.critrevonc.2009.02.002.
16. Bourgouin PM, Tampieri D, Grahovac SZ, et al. CT and MR imaging findings in adults with cerebellar medulloblastoma: comparison with findings in children. AJR Am J Roentgenol. 1992;159(3):609–12. https://doi.org/10.2214/ajr.159.3.1503035.
17. Eran A, Ozturk A, Aygun N, et al. Medulloblastoma: atypical CT and MRI findings in children. Pediatr Radiol. 2010;40(7):1254–62. https://doi.org/10.1007/s00247-009-1429-9.
18. Koral K, Gargan L, Bowers DC, et al. Imaging characteristics of atypical teratoid-rhabdoid tumor in children compared with medulloblastoma. AJR Am J Roentgenol. 2008;190(3):809–14. https://doi.org/10.2214/AJR.07.3069.
19. Fouladi M, Gajjar A, Boyett JM, et al. Comparison of CSF cytology and spinal magnetic resonance imaging in the detection of leptomeningeal disease in pediatric medulloblastoma or primitive neuroectodermal tumor. J Clin Oncol. 1999;17(10):3234–7. https://doi.org/10.1200/jco.1999.17.10.3234.
20. Fan X, Eberhart CG. Medulloblastoma stem cells. J Clin Oncol. 2008;26(17):2821–7. https://doi.org/10.1200/JCO.2007.15.2264.
21. Sarkar C, Pramanik P, Karak AK, et al. Are childhood and adult medulloblastomas different? A comparative study of clinicopathological features, proliferation index and apoptotic index. J Neurooncol. 2002;59(1):49–61. https://doi.org/10.1023/A:1016357731363.
22. Giordana MT, Cavalla P, Dutto A, et al. Is medulloblastoma the same tumor in children and adults? J Neurooncol. 1997;35(2):169–76. http://www.ncbi.nlm.nih.gov/pubmed/9266455. Accessed 13 Aug 2016
23. Carrie C, Lasset C, Alapetite C, et al. Multivariate analysis of prognostic factors in adult patients with medulloblastoma. Retrospective study of 156 patients. Cancer. 1994;74(8):2352–60.

24. Atalar B, Ozsahin M, Call J, et al. Treatment outcome and prognostic factors for adult patients with medulloblastoma: the Rare Cancer Network (RCN) experience. Radiother Oncol. 2018;127(1):96–102. https://doi.org/10.1016/j.radonc.2017.12.028.

25. Giordana MT, D'Agostino C, Pollo B, et al. Anaplasia is rare and does not influence prognosis in adult medulloblastoma. J Neuropathol Exp Neurol. 2005;64(10):869–74.

26. Gajjar A, Hernan R, Kocak M, et al. Clinical, histopathologic, and molecular markers of prognosis: toward a new disease risk stratification system for medulloblastoma. J Clin Oncol. 2004;22(6):984–93. https://doi.org/10.1200/JCO.2004.06.032.

27. Lai R. Survival of patients with adult medulloblastoma: a population-based study. Cancer. 2008;112(7):1568–74. https://doi.org/10.1002/cncr.23329.

28. Kool M, Koster J, Bunt J, et al. Integrated genomics identifies five medulloblastoma subtypes with distinct genetic profiles, pathway signatures and clinicopathological features. PLoS One. 2008;3(8):e3088. https://doi.org/10.1371/journal.pone.0003088.

29. Thompson MC. Genomics identifies medulloblastoma subgroups that are enriched for specific genetic alterations. J Clin Oncol. 2006;24(12):1924–31. https://doi.org/10.1200/JCO.2005.04.4974.

30. Northcott PA, Korshunov A, Witt H, et al. Medulloblastoma comprises four distinct molecular variants. J Clin Oncol. 2009;28. https://doi.org/10.1200/JCO.2009.27.4324.

31. Louis DN, Ohgaki H, Wiestler OD, et al. The 2007 WHO classification of tumours of the central nervous system. Acta Neuropathol. 2007;114(2):97–109. https://doi.org/10.1007/s00401-007-0243-4.

32. Pomeroy SL, Tamayo P, Gaasenbeek M, et al. Prediction of central nervous system embryonal tumour outcome based on gene expression. Nature. 2002;415(6870):436–42. https://doi.org/10.1038/415436a.

33. Fernandez-Teijeiro A, Betensky RA, Sturla LM, et al. Combining gene expression profiles and clinical parameters for risk stratification in medulloblastomas. J Clin Oncol. 2004;22(6):994–8. https://doi.org/10.1200/JCO.2004.03.036.

34. Shih DJH, Northcott PA, Remke M, et al. Cytogenetic prognostication within medulloblastoma subgroups. J Clin Oncol. 2014;32(9):886–96. https://doi.org/10.1200/JCO.2013.50.9539.

35. Ryan SL, Schwalbe EC, Cole M, et al. MYC family amplification and clinical risk-factors interact to predict an extremely poor prognosis in childhood medulloblastoma. Acta Neuropathol. 2012;123(4):501–13. https://doi.org/10.1007/s00401-011-0923-y.

36. Remke M, Hielscher T, Northcott PA, et al. Adult medulloblastoma comprises three major molecular variants. J Clin Oncol. 2011;29(19):2717–23. https://doi.org/10.1200/JCO.2011.34.9373.

37. Al-Halabi H, Nantel A, Klekner A, et al. Preponderance of sonic hedgehog pathway activation characterizes adult medulloblastoma. Acta Neuropathol. 2011;121(2):229–39. https://doi.org/10.1007/s00401-010-0780-0.

38. Zhukova N, Ramaswamy V, Remke M, et al. Subgroup-specific prognostic implications of TP53 mutation in medulloblastoma. J Clin Oncol. 2013;31(23):2927–35. https://doi.org/10.1200/JCO.2012.48.5052.

39. Ramaswamy V, Northcott PA, Taylor MD. FISH and chips: the recipe for improved prognostication and outcomes for children with medulloblastoma. Cancer Genet. 2011;204(11):577–88. https://doi.org/10.1016/j.cancergen.2011.11.001.

40. Kool M, Korshunov A, Remke M, et al. Molecular subgroups of medulloblastoma: an international meta-analysis of transcriptome, genetic aberrations, and clinical data of WNT, SHH, Group 3, and Group 4 medulloblastomas. Acta Neuropathol. 2012;123(4):473–84. https://doi.org/10.1007/s00401-012-0958-8.

41. Carrie C, Hoffstetter S, Gomez F, et al. Impact of targeting deviations on outcome in medulloblastoma: study of the French

Society of Pediatric Oncology (SFOP). Int J Radiat Oncol Biol Phys. 1999;45(2):435–9. http://www.ncbi.nlm.nih.gov/pubmed/10487567. Accessed 9 Apr 2016

42. Prados MD, Warnick RE, Wara WM, et al. Medulloblastoma in adults. Int J Radiat Oncol Biol Phys. 1995;32(4):1145–52. http://www.ncbi.nlm.nih.gov/pubmed/7607936. Accessed 28 Aug 2016

43. Brandes AA, Palmisano V, Monfardini S. Medulloblastoma in adults: clinical characteristics and treatment. Cancer Treat Rev. 1999;25(1):3–12. https://doi.org/10.1053/ctrv.1998.0096.

44. Curran EK, Le GM, Sainani KL, et al. Do children and adults differ in survival from medulloblastoma? A study from the SEER registry. J Neurooncol. 2009;95(1):81–5. https://doi.org/10.1007/s11060-009-9894-4.

45. Le QT, Weil MD, Wara WM, et al. Adult medulloblastoma: an analysis of survival and prognostic factors. Cancer J Sci Am. 1997;3(4):238–45. http://www.ncbi.nlm.nih.gov/pubmed/9263630. Accessed 13 Aug 2016

46. Ferrante L, Mastronardi L, Celli P, et al. Medulloblastoma in adulthood. J Neurosurg Sci. 1991;35(1):23–30. http://www.ncbi.nlm.nih.gov/pubmed/1890457. Accessed 7 Nov 2016

47. Coulbois S, Civit T, Grignon Y, et al. Adult medulloblastoma. Review of 22 patients. Neurochirurgie. 2001;47(1):6–12. http://www.ncbi.nlm.nih.gov/pubmed/11283450. Accessed 7 Nov 2016

48. Aragonés MP, Magallón R, Piqueras C, et al. Medulloblastoma in adulthood: prognostic factors influencing survival and recurrence. Acta Neurochir. 1994;127(1–2):65–8. http://www.ncbi.nlm.nih.gov/pubmed/7942185. Accessed 9 Nov 2016

49. Padovani L, Sunyach MP, Perol D, et al. Common strategy for adult and pediatric medulloblastoma: a multicenter series of 253 adults. Int J Radiat Oncol Biol Phys. 2007;68(2):433–40. https://doi.org/10.1016/j.ijrobp.2006.12.030.

50. Chang CH, Housepian EM, Herbert C. An operative staging system and a megavoltage radiotherapeutic technic for cerebellar medulloblastomas. Radiology. 1969;93(6):1351–9. https://doi.org/10.1148/93.6.1351.

51. Lai SF, Wang CW, Chen YH, et al. Medulloblastoma in adults: treatment outcome, relapse patterns, and prognostic factors. Strahlenther Onkol. 2012;188(10):878–86. https://doi.org/10.1007/s00066-012-0168-2.

52. Chan AW, Tarbell NJ, Black PM, et al. Adult medulloblastoma: prognostic factors and patterns of relapse. Neurosurgery. 2000;47(3):623–32.

53. Brandes AA, Franceschi E, Tosoni A, et al. Long-term results of a prospective study on the treatment of medulloblastoma in adults. Cancer. 2007;110(9):2035–41. https://doi.org/10.1002/cncr.23003.

54. Brandes AA, Ermani M, Amista P, et al. The treatment of adults with medulloblastoma: a prospective study. Int J Radiat Oncol Biol Phys. 2003;57(3):755–61. https://doi.org/10.1016/S0360-3016(03)00643-6.

55. Miralbell R, Bieri S, Huguenin P, et al. Prognostic value of cerebrospinal fluid cytology in pediatric medulloblastoma. Swiss Pediatric Oncology Group. Ann Oncol. 1999;10(2):239–41. http://www.ncbi.nlm.nih.gov/pubmed/10093696. Accessed 28 Nov 2016

56. Zeltzer PM, Boyett JM, Finlay JL, et al. Metastasis stage, adjuvant treatment, and residual tumor are prognostic factors for medulloblastoma in children: conclusions from the Children's Cancer Group 921 randomized phase III study. J Clin Oncol. 1999;17(3):832–45. https://doi.org/10.1200/jco.1999.17.3.832.

57. Frost PJ, Laperriere NJ, Wong CS, et al. Medulloblastoma in adults. Int J Radiat Oncol Biol Phys. 1995;32(4):951–7.

58. Eberhart CG, Kepner JL, Goldthwaite PT, et al. Histopathologic grading of medulloblastomas. Cancer. 2002;94(2):552–60. https://doi.org/10.1002/cncr.10189.

59. Lamont JM, McManamy CS, Pearson AD, et al. Combined histopathological and molecular cytogenetic stratification of medullo-

blastoma patients. Clin Cancer Res. 2004;10(16):5482–93. https://doi.org/10.1158/1078-0432.CCR-03-0721.

60. Hartsell WF, Montag AG, Lydon J, et al. Treatment of medulloblastoma in adults. Am J Clin Oncol. 1992;15(3):207–11. http://www.ncbi.nlm.nih.gov/pubmed/1590272. Accessed 14 Aug 2016

61. Bloom HJG, Bessell EM, Between T. Medulloblastoma in adults: a review of 47 patients treated between 1952 and 1981. Int J Radiat Oncol. 1990;18(4):763–72. https://doi.org/10.1016/0360-3016(90)90395-Z.

62. Hubbard JL, Scheithauer BW, Kispert DB, et al. Adult cerebellar medulloblastomas: the pathological, radiographic, and clinical disease spectrum. J Neurosurg. 1989;70(4):536–44. https://doi.org/10.3171/jns.1989.70.4.0536.

63. Korshunov A, Remke M, Werft W, et al. Adult and pediatric medulloblastomas are genetically distinct and require different algorithms for molecular risk stratification. J Clin Oncol. 2010;28(18):3054–60. https://doi.org/10.1200/JCO.2009.25.7121.

64. Giordana MT, Duo D, Gasverde S, et al. MDM2 overexpression is associated with short survival in adults with medulloblastoma. Neuro Oncol. 2002;4(2):115–22. https://doi.org/10.1093/neuonc/4.2.115.

65. Ray A, Ho M, Ma J, et al. A clinicobiological model predicting survival in medulloblastoma. Clin Cancer Res. 2004;10(22):7613–20. https://doi.org/10.1158/1078-0432.CCR-04-0499.

66. Packer RJ, Gajjar A, Vezina G, et al. Phase III study of craniospinal radiation therapy followed by adjuvant chemotherapy for newly diagnosed average-risk medulloblastoma. J Clin Oncol. 2006;24(25):4202–8. https://doi.org/10.1200/JCO.2006.06.4980.

67. Packer RJ, Zhou T, Holmes E, et al. Survival and secondary tumors in children with medulloblastoma receiving radiotherapy and adjuvant chemotherapy: results of Children's Oncology Group trial A9961. Neuro Oncol. 2013;15(1):97–103. https://doi.org/10.1093/neuonc/nos267.

68. Greenberg HS, Chamberlain MC, Glantz MJ, et al. Adult medulloblastoma: multiagent chemotherapy. Neuro Oncol. 2001;3(1):29–34. https://doi.org/10.1093/neuonc/3.1.29.

69. Tabori U, Sung L, Hukin J, et al. Medulloblastoma in the second decade of life: a specific group with respect to toxicity and management: a Canadian Pediatric Brain Tumor Consortium Study. Cancer. 2005;103(9):1874–80. https://doi.org/10.1002/cncr.21003.

70. Kortmann RD, Kühl J, Timmermann B, et al. Postoperative neoadjuvant chemotherapy before radiotherapy as compared to immediate radiotherapy followed by maintenance chemotherapy in the treatment of medulloblastoma in childhood: results of the German prospective randomized trial HIT '91. Int J Radiat Oncol Biol Phys. 2000;46(2):269–79. http://www.ncbi.nlm.nih.gov/pubmed/10661332. Accessed 11 Nov 2016

71. Friedrich C, von Bueren AO, von Hoff K, et al. Treatment of adult nonmetastatic medulloblastoma patients according to the paediatric HIT 2000 protocol: a prospective observational multicentre study. Eur J Cancer. 2013;49(4):893–903. https://doi.org/10.1016/j.ejca.2012.10.006.

72. Beier D, Proescholdt M, Reinert C, et al. Multicenter pilot study of radiochemotherapy as first-line treatment for adults with medulloblastoma (NOA-07). Neuro Oncol. 2018;20(3):400–10. https://doi.org/10.1093/neuonc/nox155.

73. Jakacki RI, Burger PC, Zhou T, et al. Outcome of children with metastatic medulloblastoma treated with carboplatin during craniospinal radiotherapy: a Children's Oncology Group Phase I/II study. J Clin Oncol. 2012;30(21):2648–53. https://doi.org/10.1200/JCO.2011.40.2792.

74. Brandes AA, Bartolotti M, Marucci G, et al. New perspectives in the treatment of adult medulloblastoma in the era of molecular oncology. Crit Rev Oncol Hematol. 2015;94(3):348–59. https://doi.org/10.1016/j.critrevonc.2014.12.016.

75. Moots PL, O'neill A, Londer H, et al. Preradiation chemotherapy for adult high-risk medulloblastoma: a trial of the ECOG-ACRIN Cancer Research Group (E4397). Am J Clin Oncol. 2016. https://doi.org/10.1097/coc.0000000000000326.

76. Paterson E, Farr RF. Cerebellar medulloblastoma: treatment by irradiation of the whole central nervous system. Acta Radiol. 1953;39(4):323–36. http://www.ncbi.nlm.nih.gov/pubmed/13057640. Accessed 11 Nov 2016

77. Herrlinger U, Steinbrecher A, Rieger J, et al. Adult medulloblastoma: prognostic factors and response to therapy at diagnosis and at relapse. J Neurol. 2005;252(3):291–9. https://doi.org/10.1007/s00415-005-0560-2.

78. Taylor MD, Mainprize TG, Rutka JT. Molecular insight into medulloblastoma and central nervous system primitive neuroectodermal tumor biology from hereditary syndromes: a review. Neurosurgery. 2000;47(4):888–901. http://www.ncbi.nlm.nih.gov/pubmed/11014429. Accessed 30 Nov 2016

79. Thomas PR, Deutsch M, Kepner JL, et al. Low-stage medulloblastoma: final analysis of trial comparing standard-dose with reduced-dose neuraxis irradiation. J Clin Oncol. 2000;18(16):3004–11. https://doi.org/10.1200/jco.2000.18.16.3004.

80. St Clair WH, Adams JA, Bues M, et al. Advantage of protons compared to conventional X-ray or IMRT in the treatment of a pediatric patient with medulloblastoma. Int J Radiat Oncol Biol Phys. 2004;58(3):727–34. https://doi.org/10.1016/S0360-3016(03)01574-8.

81. Merchant TE, Hua C, Shukla H, et al. Proton versus photon radiotherapy for common pediatric brain tumors: comparison of models of dose characteristics and their relationship to cognitive function. Pediatr Blood Cancer. 2008;51(1):110–7. https://doi.org/10.1002/pbc.21530.

82. Abacioglu U, Uzel O, Sengoz M, et al. Medulloblastoma in adults: treatment results and prognostic factors. Int J Radiat Oncol Biol Phys. 2002;54(3):855–60. https://doi.org/10.1016/S0360-3016(02)02986-3.

83. Berry MP, Jenkin RDT, Keen CW, et al. Radiation treatment for medulloblastoma. J Neurosurg. 1981;55(1):43–51. https://doi.org/10.3171/jns.1981.55.1.0043.

84. Hazuka MB, DeBiose DA, Henderson RH, et al. Survival results in adult patients treated for medulloblastoma. Cancer. 1992;69(8):2143–8. http://www.ncbi.nlm.nih.gov/pubmed/1544120. Accessed 11 Nov 2016

85. Skołyszewski J, Gliński B. Results of postoperative irradiation of medulloblastoma in adults. Int J Radiat Oncol Biol Phys. 1989;16(2):479–82. http://www.ncbi.nlm.nih.gov/pubmed/2921151. Accessed 30 Nov 2016

86. del Charco JO, Bolek TW, Mark McCollough W, et al. 15 Medulloblastoma: time-dose relationship based on a 30-year review. Int J Radiat Oncol. 1996;36(1):166. https://doi.org/10.1016/S0360-3016(97)85357-6.

87. Brandes AA, Paris MK. Review of the prognostic factors in medulloblastoma of children and adults. Crit Rev Oncol Hematol. 2004;50(2):121–8. https://doi.org/10.1016/j.critrevonc.2003.08.005.

88. Michalski JM, Janss A. Results of COG ACNS0331: a Phase III Trial of Involved-Field Radiotherapy (IFRT) and Low Dose Craniospinal Irradiation (LD-CSI) with chemotherapy in average-risk medulloblastoma: a report from the children's oncology group. In: ASTRO 2016 Abstract, vol. 96. Amsterdam: Elsevier; 2017. p. 937–8. https://doi.org/10.1016/j.ijrobp.2016.09.046.

89. Otto K. Volumetric modulated arc therapy: IMRT in a single gantry arc. Med Phys. 2008;35(1):310. https://doi.org/10.1118/1.2818738.

90. Bedford JL, Warrington AP. Commissioning of Volumetric Modulated Arc Therapy (VMAT). Int J Radiat Oncol. 2009;73(2):537–45. https://doi.org/10.1016/j.ijrobp.2008.08.055.

91. Lee YK, Brooks CJ, Bedford JL, et al. Development and evaluation of multiple isocentric volumetric modulated arc therapy technique for craniospinal axis radiotherapy planning. Int J Radiat

Oncol Biol Phys. 2012;82(2):1006–12. https://doi.org/10.1016/j.ijrobp.2010.12.033.

92. Lopez Guerra JL, Marrone I, Jaen J, et al. Outcome and toxicity using helical tomotherapy for craniospinal irradiation in pediatric medulloblastoma. Clin Transl Oncol. 2014;16(1):96–101. https://doi.org/10.1007/s12094-013-1048-7.

93. Myers P, Stathakis S, Mavroidis P, et al. Evaluation of localization errors for craniospinal axis irradiation delivery using volume modulated arc therapy and proposal of a technique to minimize such errors. Radiother Oncol. 2013;108(1):107–13. https://doi.org/10.1016/j.radonc.2013.05.026.

94. Yock TI, Tarbell NJ. Technology insight: proton beam radiotherapy for treatment in pediatric brain tumors. Nat Clin Pract Oncol. 2004;1(2):97–103.; quiz 1 p following 111. https://doi.org/10.1038/ncponc0090.

95. Brown AP, Barney CL, Grosshans DR, et al. Proton beam craniospinal irradiation reduces acute toxicity for adults with medulloblastoma. Int J Radiat Oncol Biol Phys. 2013;86(2):277–84. https://doi.org/10.1016/j.ijrobp.2013.01.014.

96. Chang EL, Allen P, Wu C, et al. Acute toxicity and treatment interruption related to electron and photon craniospinal irradiation in pediatric patients treated at the University of Texas M. D. Anderson Cancer Center. Int J Radiat Oncol. 2002;52(4):1008–16. https://doi.org/10.1016/S0360-3016(01)02717-1.

97. Jefferies S, Rajan B, Ashley S, et al. Haematological toxicity of cranio-spinal irradiation. Radiother Oncol. 1998;48(1):23–7. https://doi.org/10.1016/S0167-8140(98)00024-3.

98. Mulhern RK, Merchant TE, Gajjar A, et al. Late neurocognitive sequelae in survivors of brain tumours in childhood. Lancet Oncol. 2004;5(7):399–408. https://doi.org/10.1016/S1470-2045(04)01507-4.

99. Abayomi OK. Pathogenesis of irradiation-induced cognitive dysfunction. Acta Oncol. 1996;35(6):659–63. http://www.ncbi.nlm.nih.gov/pubmed/8938210. Accessed 28 Oct 2015

100. Schultheiss TE, Kun LE, Ang KK, et al. Radiation response of the central nervous system. Int J Radiat Oncol Biol Phys. 1995;31(5):1093–112. https://doi.org/10.1016/0360-3016(94)00655-5.

101. Belka C, Budach W, Kortmann RD, et al. Radiation induced CNS toxicity – molecular and cellular mechanisms. Br J Cancer. 2001;85(9):1233–9. https://doi.org/10.1054/bjoc.2001.2100.

102. Mulhern RK, Butler RW. Neurocognitive sequelae of childhood cancers and their treatment. Pediatr Rehabil. 2014;7(1):1–14 discussion 15–6. https://doi.org/10.1080/13638490310001655528.

103. Eaton BR, Esiashvili N, Kim S, et al. Endocrine outcomes with proton and photon radiotherapy for standard risk medulloblastoma. Neuro Oncol. 2016;18(6):881–7. https://doi.org/10.1093/neuonc/nov302.

104. Paulino AC. Hypothyroidism in children with medulloblastoma: a comparison of 3600 and 2340 cGy craniospinal radiotherapy. Int J Radiat Oncol Biol Phys. 2002;53(3):543–7. http://www.ncbi.nlm.nih.gov/pubmed/12062595. Accessed 30 Mar 2016

105. Gurney JG, Kadan-Lottick NS, Packer RJ, et al. Endocrine and cardiovascular late effects among adult survivors of childhood brain tumors: Childhood Cancer Survivor Study. Cancer. 2003;97(3):663–73. https://doi.org/10.1002/cncr.11095.

106. Bluemke DA, Fishman EK, Scott WW Jr. Skeletal complications of radiation therapy. Radiographics. 1994;14(1):111–21. https://doi.org/10.1148/RADIOGRAPHICS.14.1.8128043.

107. Xu W, Janss A, Moshang T. Adult height and adult sitting height in childhood medulloblastoma survivors. J Clin Endocrinol Metab. 2003;88(10):4677–81. https://doi.org/10.1210/jc.2003-030619.

108. Ramsey RG, Zacharias CE. MR imaging of the spine after radiation therapy: easily recognizable effects. Am J Neuroradiol. 1985;6(2):247–51.

109. Yankelevitz DF, Henschke CI, Knapp PH, et al. Effect of radiation therapy on thoracic and lumbar bone marrow: evaluation with MR imaging. AJR Am J Roentgenol. 1991;157(1):87–92. https://doi.org/10.2214/ajr.157.1.1904679.

110. Meadows AT, Friedman DL, Neglia JP, et al. Second neoplasms in survivors of childhood cancer: findings from the Childhood Cancer Survivor Study cohort. J Clin Oncol. 2009;27(14):2356–62. https://doi.org/10.1200/JCO.2008.21.1920.

111. Preston DL, Ron E, Tokuoka S, et al. Solid cancer incidence in atomic bomb survivors: 1958–1998. Radiat Res. 2007;168(1):1–64. https://doi.org/10.1667/RR0763.1.

112. Chung CS, Yock TI, Nelson K, et al. Incidence of second malignancies among patients treated with proton versus photon radiation. Int J Radiat Oncol. 2013;87(1):46–52. https://doi.org/10.1016/j.ijrobp.2013.04.030.

113. Tabori U, Sung L, Hukin J, et al. Distinctive clinical course and pattern of relapse in adolescents with medulloblastoma. Int J Radiat Oncol Biol Phys. 2006;64(2):402–7. https://doi.org/10.1016/j.ijrobp.2005.07.962.

114. Franceschi E, Bartolotti M, Paccapelo A, et al. Adjuvant chemotherapy in adult medulloblastoma: is it an option for average-risk patients? J Neurooncol. 2016;128(2):235–40. https://doi.org/10.1007/s11060-016-2097-x.

115. Kocakaya S, Beier CP, Beier D. Chemotherapy increases long-term survival in patients with adult medulloblastoma – a literature-based meta-analysis. Neuro Oncol. 2016;18(3):408–16. https://doi.org/10.1093/neuonc/nov185.

116. Kortmann RD, Timmermann B, Kühl J, et al. HIT '91 (prospective, co-operative study for the treatment of malignant brain tumors in childhood): accuracy and acute toxicity of the irradiation of the craniospinal axis. Results of the quality assurance program. Strahlenther Onkol. 1999;175(4):162–9. http://www.ncbi.nlm.nih.gov/pubmed/10230458. Accessed 9 Apr 2016

117. Evans AE, Jenkin RD, Sposto R, et al. The treatment of medulloblastoma. Results of a prospective randomized trial of radiation therapy with and without CCNU, vincristine, and prednisone. J Neurosurg. 1990;72(4):572–82. https://doi.org/10.3171/jns.1990.72.4.0572.

118. Grabenbauer GG, Beck JD, Erhardt J, et al. Postoperative radiotherapy of medulloblastoma. Impact of radiation quality on treatment outcome. Am J Clin Oncol. 1996;19(1):73–7. http://www.ncbi.nlm.nih.gov/pubmed/8554041. Accessed 12 Nov 2016

119. Miralbell R, Fitzgerald TJ, Laurie F, et al. Radiotherapy in pediatric medulloblastoma: quality assessment of Pediatric Oncology Group Trial 9031. Int J Radiat Oncol Biol Phys. 2006;64(5):1325–30. https://doi.org/10.1016/j.ijrobp.2005.11.002.

120. Kramer ED, Vezina LG, Packer RJ, et al. Staging and surveillance of children with central nervous system neoplasms: recommendations of the Neurology and Tumor Imaging Committees of the Children's Cancer Group. Pediatr Neurosurg. 1994;20(4):254–62. discussion 3. http://www.ncbi.nlm.nih.gov/pubmed/8043464. Accessed 9 Feb 2017

121. Bartels U, Shroff M, Sung L, et al. Role of spinal MRI in the follow-up of children treated for medulloblastoma. Cancer. 2006;107(6):1340–7. https://doi.org/10.1002/cncr.22129.

# Intracranial Ependymoma

## Intracranial Ependymoma

# 28

Jaipreet S. Suri, Paul Youn, and Michael T. Milano

## Learning Objectives

- Explain classification of ependymomas.
- Describe clinical presentation and work-up of ependymomas.
- Outline prognostic factors.
- Describe current management guidelines.
- Outline role of radiation therapy in management of ependymomas.

## Introduction/Epidemiology

Ependymomas are uncommon tumors arising from the ependymal cells lining the ventricles, central canal, filum terminale, or choroid plexus [1]. The origin of these cancers, possibly neuroectodermal, remains controversial; recently a possible glial origin has been speculated [1–3]. Ependymal tumors constitute approximately 1.8% of primary brain and central nervous system tumors diagnosed in the United States between 2009 and 2013 with 1420 estimated new cases in 2017 as per the Central Brain Tumor Registry of the United States (CBTRUS) Statistical Report [4]. Historically, they were first described by Percival Bailey in 1924 as an independent histopathological entity [5]. They are usually childhood tumors and relatively less common in adults with a bimodal peak distribution at ages 5 and 35 years [6]. Ependymal tumors in adults are most common in the spinal canal, comprising the majority of patients in most reports [3,

J. S. Suri · P. Youn
Department of Radiation Oncology,
University of Rochester Medical Center/James P. Wilmot
Cancer Center, Rochester, NY, USA

M. T. Milano (✉)
Department of Radiation Oncology, University
of Rochester Medical Center, Rochester, NY, USA
e-mail: Michael_milano@urmc.rochester.edu

**Table 28.1** Clinical presentation of ependymoma

| Location | Clinical symptoms | Pathophysiology |
|---|---|---|
| Supratentorial | Confusion, lethargy, seizures, focal neurological deficits | Mass effect |
| Intraventricular | Headaches, nausea, vomiting, papilledema, ataxia, vertigo, CN deficits | Increase in intracranial pressure |
| Infratentorial | Visual disturbances, ataxia, dizziness, neck pain/stiffness, CN palsies, hemiparesis (rare) | Compression of posterior fossa structures (posterior fossa syndrome) |

7, 8]. Among intracranial ependymomas, 50–60% are supratentorial [7]. The clinical presentation depends on the tumor location and size/mass effect [1, 9] as detailed in the Table 28.1.

## Diagnosis and Prognosis

The work-up for patients with adult intracranial ependymoma should include a detailed history, physical examination, contrast-enhanced magnetic resonance imaging (or computerized tomography if MRI is contraindicated) of the brain and entire neuraxis, biopsy (if applicable), and cerebrospinal fluid (CSF) cytology (at least 2 weeks after surgery). Heterogeneous enhancement (more pronounced with higher grade) is usually appreciated on MRI and could be considered diagnostic if there is characteristic involvement through the foramen of Luschka [1, 9, 10]. CSF evaluation is critical with incidence of spinal seeding ranging from 1.6% for supratentorial tumors and 2–4.5% for low-grade lesions to 9.7% for infratentorial lesions and 8.4–20% for high-grade tumors [1, 11, 12].

As per the recently updated 2016 World Health Organization (WHO) pathologic classification, adult ependymal tumors can be classified as grade I (subependymoma

**Table 28.2** World Health Organization (WHO) pathologic classification of ependymoma

| Classification | Tumor cell | Mitotic activity | Key histological features |
|---|---|---|---|
| WHO grade I [myxopapillary] | Cuboidal | Absent/very low | Mucoid matrix with GFAP expression and lack of cytokeratin expression |
| WHO grade I [subependymoma] | Isomorphic | Absent/very low | Dense fibrillary matrix with frequent microcysts |
| WHO grade II [ependymoma (papillary, clear cell, tanycytic subtypes)] | Monomorphic | Rare/absent | Perivascular pseudorosettes and ependymal rosettes |
| WHO grade III [anaplastic] | Cellular/nuclear pleomorphism | High | Perivascular rosettes, pseudopalisading necrosis, endothelial proliferation |

or myxopapillary), grade II [ependymoma (with papillary, clear cell, tanycytic subtypes)], or grade III (anaplastic) as summarized in the Table 28.2 [1, 13]. However, as acknowledged in the updated 2016 classification, current WHO criteria is difficult to apply and of questionable clinical utility [13]. Hence, a more prognostic and reproducible classification/grading scheme is warranted.

## Prognostic Factors

All of the published data on prognostic factors are derived from retrospective analyses extending over several decades. The prognostic factors reported in the literature include extent of resection, tumor grade, age at time of diagnosis, Karnofsky performance status (KPS), tumor location, and adjuvant radiation therapy [14]. Low-grade histology ($p = 0.052$) was found to be a significant prognostic factor for progression-free survival (PFS) in a study of 31 patients with age at diagnosis ranging from 1 to 56 years (median 9 years) [15]. Grade III (anaplastic) histology ($p < 0.01$), supratentorial location ($p < 0.01$), and subtotal resection (STR) ($p < 0.01$) were found to be significant adverse prognostic factors on multivariate Cox proportional hazard model analysis of the Collaborative Ependymoma Research Network (CERN Foundation) data from 19 institutions that included 282 adult ependymoma patients (46% spine, 35% infratentorial, 19% supratentorial) [16]. Rooney et al. retrospectively analyzed 42 adult patients (>18 years; median age, 36.8 years; 26/42 patients with grade II and 14/42 with grade III histology) with supratentorial ependymoma diagnosed between 1969 and 2008 from the Mayo Clinic tumor registry; they found that extent of resection ($p = 0.009$), lack of recurrence ($p = 0.02$), and age ≤ 40 years ($p = 0.05$) were significantly favorable factors for improved overall survival (OS) [17]. Metellus et al. analyzed 114 adult patients (mean age 48 years, range 18–82 years) with intracranial WHO grade II ependymomas from 32 French neurosurgical centers diagnosed between 1990 and 2004. With multivariate analyses, they demonstrated that improved OS rates were associated with higher preoperative KPS score ($p = 0.027$), greater extent of surgery ($p = 0.008$), and infratentorial vs. supraten-

torial tumor location ($p = 0.012$) [18]. Supratentorial tumors are usually of higher grade, and it is more difficult to achieve gross total resection (GTR) [8]. Among patients who underwent STR, adjuvant radiation therapy was correlated with a significant improvement in both overall ($p = 0.005$) and PFS ($p = 0.002$) [18]. Gender and age group (<55 and ≥55) were not significant [18]. Extent of resection and tumor grade were found to be significant prognostic factors for PFS and OS in a study of 109 adult supratentorial hemispheric ependymomas patients (clinical information for 101 patients was collected from literature review, and the remaining eight patients were retrospectively accrued from the University of Michigan) [14].

## Management

The management of intracranial ependymoma in adults remains controversial due to the rarity of the disease and lack of prospective clinical trials. As per the National Comprehensive Cancer Network (NCCN) guidelines, the standard of care remains maximum safe resection as the first-line treatment [8]. Not only is extent of resection important prognostic factor; it also provides tissue for pathologic diagnosis, opportunity for GTR/debulking, and possible alleviation of cerebral spinal fluid (CSF) obstruction [1]. If maximum resection is not feasible, then stereotactic/open biopsy is recommended with consideration of second-look surgery to complete the resection. Postoperative contrast-enhanced MRI of the brain and spine should be obtained along with CSF cytology. Adjuvant radiation therapy is recommended for WHO grade II tumors after incomplete resection and for all WHO grade III tumors. Supratentorial WHO grade I/II ependymoma after GTR could be observed; alternatively, adjuvant fractionated external beam radiation therapy could also be considered. These recommendations are consistent with a population-based analysis by Ghia et al. of 92 patients [median age 17.5 years (range 1–83 years); 75% Caucasian; 58% female] with non-anaplastic supratentorial ependymoma; there was not a significant difference in 5- and 10-year cause-specific survival (CSS) and estimated overall survival between patients who underwent GTR alone vs.

GTR followed by adjuvant radiotherapy (50% of patients; radiotherapy mean/median dose unknown) [5]. Rogers et al. evaluated 37 adult patients (age ≥ 18 years; median age 44; 23 male) with nondisseminated intracranial ependymomas (33/37 infratentorial; 32/37 low grade) treated between 1975 and 2001 with GTR alone (20/37), GTR + radiotherapy (8/37), STR + radiotherapy (8/37), or STR alone (1/37); adjuvant radiotherapy (mean posterior fossa dose 54 Gy in 30 fractions) was associated with an improvement in 10-year local control from 51% (GTR alone) to 100% (GTR + radiotherapy) for infratentorial ($p = 0.07$) and 56% (GTR alone) to 88% (GTR + radiotherapy) for all intracranial ependymoma patients ($p = 0.15$) [19]. However, for patients with posterior fossa ependymomas, adjuvant postoperative radiation therapy does significantly improve local control and is recommended for patients with GTR and STR [20]. In an analysis of 45 patients with posterior fossa ependymomas, adjuvant radiation therapy was delivered to 13 patients after GTR and 12 patients after STR. The 10-year actuarial local control rates for patients with GTR + radiotherapy, GTR alone, and STR + radiotherapy were 100%, 50%, and 36%, respectively, with significant differences between GTR + radiotherapy and GTR alone cohorts ($p = 0.018$) and GTR + radiotherapy and STR + radiotherapy cohorts ($p = 0.003$) [20]. Management for patients with evidence of metastatic disease within the CSF and/or brain and spinal canal includes craniospinal axis irradiation (CSI), but is not covered in this chapter [8]. Currently, there is no well-defined role of chemotherapy in adjuvant setting either [8].

## Radiation Dose, Target Volume Delineation, Tumor Control, and Survival

Based upon the prescribed doses that were utilized in published studies, generally 54–60 Gy in 1.8–2 Gy fractions is prescribed to the tumor bed with 1–2 cm circumferential margins. One can choose to generate a volume expanded (1–2 cm) clinical target volume (CTV), appropriately modified to exclude regions unlikely to harbor disease, and then add an additional PTV margin to account for setup uncertainty (which would be treatment machine and institution dependent) [8, 21]. The predominant site of recurrence for both low-grade and high-grade ependymomas is local recurrence [1]. A predominance of local (vs. spinal) recurrence is consistent with data from Paulino et al. who analyzed 28 patients [18 male; median age 12 years (range, 2–81 years)] with posterior fossa ependymoma treated between 1984 and 1998 with median follow-up of 127 months [22]. In this small series, 3 of 11 patients who received craniospinal or whole brain radiotherapy developed recurrences, of which one was a local recurrence and another posterior fossa outside of tumor bed + spine recurrence. Among nine patients who had

tumor bed radiotherapy alone and six who did not receive radiotherapy, there were three relapses, all within the tumor bed. In another study, 31 patients with age at diagnosis ranging from 1 to 56 years (median 9 years), 19 of whom had anaplastic tumors were analyzed, and all 16 relapses were at the primary intracranial sites with no spinal failures [15]. Additionally, this study also analyzed prescribed dose; patients treated to a dose greater than or equal to 50 Gy experienced improved long-term PFS ($p = 0.04$), although this was not significant on multivariate analysis [15]. The only treatment variable found to be significant for PFS was volume of cranial irradiation favoring local fields ($p = 0.002$) [15].

A recent population-based National Cancer Database (NCDB) study identified 2507 adult patients with intracranial WHO grades I–III ependymoma treated between 1998 and 2012 and failed to demonstrate significant overall survival with adjuvant radiation therapy [23]. Forty-five percent of patients underwent radiotherapy with a median dose of 54 Gy (<54 Gy = 20.5%, 54–59.3 Gy = 50.3%, ≥ 59.4 Gy = 29.2%). With median follow-up of 49 months, the unadjusted 5-year overall survival was 73% (95% CI of 70–76%) in irradiated patients versus 75.8% (95% CI of 73.2–78.4%) who underwent observation [23]. Subset analysis of tumor grade, extent of resection (GTR vs. STR), size, and location (supratentorial vs. infratentorial) also did not show significant overall survival improvement with radiotherapy [23]. Presently, this data is only published in an abstract form, and a careful review of manuscript is needed.

Though treatment with radiotherapy was not associated with improved outcomes in the NCDB and other studies, this may reflect a bias in that patients who received radiotherapy were perhaps more likely to have had adverse risk factors. Given the retrospective nature of these studies, specific recommendations about which situations warrant radiotherapy cannot be readily ascertained, though higher-grade disease, STR, and tumor location warrant more serious consideration of adjuvant radiation therapy. The 10-year overall survival ranges approximately from 50% to 72.5% as summarized in the Table 28.3.

**Table 28.3** Published survival outcomes of adult ependymoma patients

| Study | OS (10 year) | Comment |
| --- | --- | --- |
| Schwartz et al. [24] | 72.5% | Adults with supratentorial ependymoma |
| Stuben et al. [25] | 58% | Heterogeneous study population (age > 16 years) |
| Reni et al. [26] | 50% | Multi-institutional experience with adult intracranial ependymomas (age > 17 years; 70 patients) |

## Acute- and Late-Term Sequelae of Radiation Toxicity

Acute side effects from radiation therapy depend on the tumor location and generally include fatigue, headache, nausea, vomiting, radiation dermatitis, and alopecia. Long-term side effects include memory loss, apathy, concentration difficulties, personality changes, and delayed leukoencephalopathy with cognitive dysfunction, sometimes even in patients with Karnofsky performance status ≥90% [1]. Long-term cognitive impairment has also been correlated with volume of supratentorial brain in the radiation field and fraction size ≥2 Gy [1, 5]. Occasionally, cranial nerve dysfunction and endocrine dysfunction (even for tumors away from hypothalamus-pituitary axis) are also reported [1]. There is also a risk of radionecrosis dependent on radiation dose and volume, usually at median of 1–2 years post-radiotherapy and with an estimated risk of 5% with biologically effective dose (BED) of 120 Gy and 10% with BED of 150 Gy, for conventional fractionated radiation therapy (<2.5 Gy fraction size) [27].

## Follow-Up

NCCN guidelines recommend follow-up with serial MRIs every 3–4 months for the first year, then 4–6 months for the second year, and then every 6–12 months for at least 12 years [8].

## Case Presentation: Highlight Radiation Therapy Management with Neuroimaging and Thought Process

A 23-year-old man presented with a 3-month history of daily headaches and four episodes of associated expressive aphasia. His past medical history was significant for childhood acute lymphoblastic leukemia (ALL) status post chemotherapy (vincristine, mercaptopurine, and methotrexate) and whole brain radiation therapy (WBRT) to 18 Gy with twice-daily radiotherapy in March 1990 at age 2½ on a prospective protocol in which he was randomized to receive WBRT. MRI of the brain during work-up of his headache showed a mass centered in the left thalamus measuring 3.7 × 3.6 cm with compression of the third ventricle and extension into the left lateral ventricle. MRI of the cervical-thoracic-lumbar spine did not demonstrate any evidence of metastatic disease. He underwent GTR, and final pathology results demonstrated WHO grade III ependymoma with Ki67 15%. Postoperative MRI did not reveal any residual tumor, and the CSF was negative. We recommended adjuvant radiation therapy to the tumor bed, and he received total dose of 58 Gy in 29 once-daily fractions to clinical target volume (CTV) and 52.2 Gy in 29 once-daily fractions to planning target volume (PTV) using intensity-modulated radiation therapy (IMRT) as illustrated in Figs. 28.1, 28.2, 28.3, and 28.4. He tolerated treatment very well with-

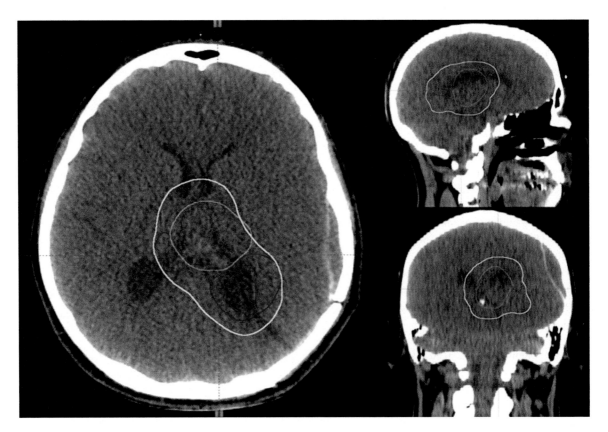

**Fig. 28.1** Planning CT treatment volumes: pre-op tumor (green), pre-op cyst (blue), CTV (pink), and PTV (yellow)

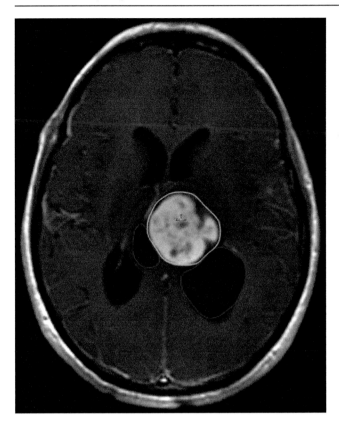

**Fig. 28.2** Delineation of the treatment volumes on diagnostic pre-op MRI: pre-op tumor (green) and pre-op cyst (blue)

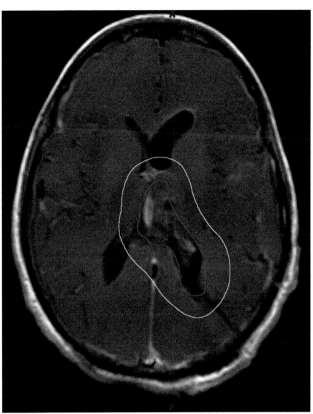

**Fig. 28.3** Delineation of the treatment volumes on diagnostic post-op MRI: CTV (pink) and PTV (yellow)

out any significant side effects. He continues to do very well with no evidence of disease recurrence, now >6 years since completion of radiation therapy. His only long-term toxicity seems to be concentration difficulties being managed with methylphenidate.

## Summary

- Ependymomas are uncommon tumors arising from the ependymal cells lining the ventricles, central canal, filum terminale, or choroid plexus.
- Clinical presentation depends on the tumor location.
- As per WHO 2016 pathologic classification, ependymal tumors can be classified as grade I (subependymoma or myxopapillary), grade II [ependymoma (with papillary, clear cell, tanycytic subtypes)], or grade III (anaplastic).
- Prognostic factors include extent of resection, tumor grade, age at time of diagnosis, Karnofsky performance status (KPS), tumor location, and adjuvant radiation therapy, with arguably extent of resection being the most significant factor.
- Predominant pattern of recurrence is local.
- Management of adult intracranial ependymoma remains controversial, and multi-institutional prospective trials are needed.

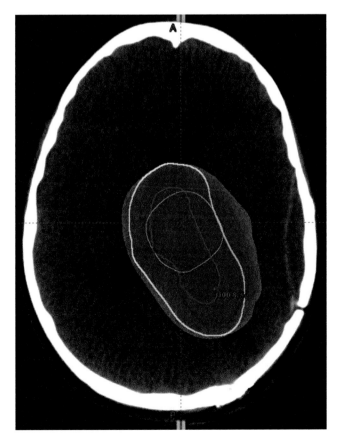

**Fig. 28.4** IMRT plan with treatment volumes [pre-op tumor (green), pre-op cyst (blue), CTV (pink), and PTV (yellow)] and dose color wash

## Self-Assessment Questions

1. Which of the histologic subtypes of ependymoma is associated with the worst prognosis?
   A. Myxopapillary
   B. Subependymoma
   C. Classical
   D. Anaplastic

2. Compared to pediatric ependymoma, adult ependymoma predominantly occurs in?
   A. Frontal lobe
   B. Spinal cord
   C. Cerebellum
   D. Brain stem

3. What seems to be the most important prognostic factor in adult intracranial ependymoma?
   A. Radiation therapy dose
   B. Supratentorial location
   C. Extent of resection
   D. Age at diagnosis

4. Which of the following statements about adult intracranial ependymoma is true?
   A. Adjuvant radiation therapy dose is around 50.4 Gy.
   B. Predominant pattern of recurrence is local.
   C. Gross total resection is more common for supratentorial location.
   D. Adjuvant chemotherapy is always recommended for anaplastic histology.

5. Observation would be an acceptable management option for which of the following?
   A. Supratentorial WHO grade I ependymoma after GTR
   B. Infratentorial WHO grade II ependymoma after GTR
   C. Supratentorial WHO grade III ependymoma after GTR
   D. Infratentorial WHO grade III ependymoma after GTR

## Answers

1. D
   (Please refer to "Prognostic Factors" section for explanation)
2. B
   (Please refer to "Introduction/Epidemiology" section for explanation)
3. C
   (Please refer to "Prognostic Factors" section for explanation)

4. B
   (Please refer to "Radiation Dose, Target Volume Delineation, Tumor Control, and Survival" section for explanation)
5. A
   (Please refer to "Management" section for explanation)

## References

1. Reni M, Gatta G, Mazza E, et al. Ependymoma. Crit Rev Oncol Hematol. 2007;63(1):81–9.
2. Asaid M, Preece P, Rosenthal M, et al. Ependymoma in adults: local experience with an uncommon tumour. J Clin Neurosci. 2015;22(9):1392–6.
3. Gilbert M, Ruda R, Soffietti R. Ependymomas in adults. Curr Neurol Neurosci Rep. 2010;10(3):240–7.
4. Ostrom Q, Gittleman H, Fulop J, et al. CBTRUS statistical report: primary brain and central nervous system tumors diagnosed in the United States in 2008–2012. Neurooncology. 2015;17(Suppl 4):iv1–iv62.
5. Ghia A, Mahajan A, Allen P, et al. Supratentorial gross-totally resected non-anaplastic ependymoma: population based patterns of care and outcomes analysis. J Neurooncol. 2013;115(3):513–20.
6. Thompson Y, Ramaswamy V, Diamandis P, et al. Posterior fossa ependymoma: current insights. Childs Nerv Syst. 2015;31(10):1699–706.
7. Chamberlain M. Ependymomas. Curr Neurol Neurosci Rep. 2003;3(3):193–9.
8. National Comprehensive Cancer Network. Central Nervous System Cancers (version 1.2016). https://www.nccn.org/professionals/physician_gls/pdf/cns.pdf. Accessed 12 Apr 2017.
9. Halperin E, Brady L, Perez C. Perez & Brady's principles and practice of radiation oncology. 6th ed. Philadelphia: Wolters Kluwer; 2015.
10. Constine LS, Tarbell NJ, Halperin EC. Pediatric radiation oncology, LWW. 6th ed. Philadelphia: Wolters Kluwer; 2016.
11. Schild S, Nisi K, Scheithauer B, et al. The results of radiotherapy for ependymomas: the mayo clinic experience. Int J Radiat Oncol Biol Phys. 1998;42(5):953–8.
12. Vanuytsel L, Brada M. The role of prophylactic spinal irradiation in localized intracranial ependymoma intracranial ependymoma. Int J Radiat Oncol Biol Phys. 1991;21(3):825–30.
13. Louis D, Perry A, Reifenberger G, et al. The 2016 World Health Organization classification of tumors of the central nervous system: a summary. Acta Neuropathol. 2016;131(6):803–20.
14. Hollon T, Nguyen V, Smith B, et al. Supratentorial hemispheric ependymomas: an analysis of 109 adults for survival and prognostic factors. J Neurosurg. 2016;125(2):410–8.
15. Kovalic J, Flaris N, Grigsby P, et al. Intracranial ependymoma long term outcome, patterns of failure. J Neurooncol. 1993;15(2):125–31.
16. Vera-Bolanos E, Aldape K, Yuan Y, et al. Clinical course and progression-free survival of adult intracranial and spinal ependymoma patients. Neurooncology. 2015;17(3):440–7.
17. Rooney J, Stauder M, Laack N. Adult supratentorial ependymoma: the Mayo Clinic experience. Int J Radiat Oncol Biol Phys. 2011;81((2):S299–300.
18. Metellus P, Guyotat J, Chinot O, et al. Adult intracranial WHO grade II ependymomas: long-term outcome and prognostic factor analysis in a series of 114 patients. Neurooncology. 2010;12(9):976–84.
19. Rogers L, Pueschel J, Spetzler R, et al. Intracranial ependymomas in the adult patient: the barrow neurological institute experience. Int J Radiat Oncol Biol Phys. 2003;57(2):S371.

20. Rogers L, Pueschel J, Spetzler R, et al. Is gross-total resection sufficient treatment for posterior fossa ependymomas? J Neurosurg. 2005;102(4):629–36.

21. Donahue B, Steinfeld A. Intracranial ependymoma in the adult patient: successful treatment with surgery and radiotherapy. J Neurooncol. 1998;37(2):131–3.

22. Paulino A. The local field in infratentorial ependymoma: does the entire posterior fossa need to be treated? Int J Radiat Oncol Biol Phys. 2001;49(3):757–61.

23. Kalash R, Glaser S, Balasubramani G, et al. Adult ependymoma (AE) patients: practice patterns and overall survival. Int J Radiat Oncol Biol Phys. 2016;96(2):E90.

24. Schwartz T, Kim S, Glick R, et al. Supratentorial ependymomas in adult patients. Neurosurgery. 1999;44(4):721–31.

25. Stüben G, Stuschke M, Kroll M, et al. Postoperative radiotherapy of spinal and intracranial ependymomas: analysis of prognostic factors. Radiother Oncol. 1997;45(1):3–10.

26. Reni M, Brandes A, Vavassori V, et al. A multicenter study of the prognosis and treatment of adult brain ependymal tumors. Cancer. 2004;100(6):1221–9.

27. Lawrence Y, Li X, el Naqa I, et al. Radiation dose–volume effects in the brain. Int J Radiat Oncol Biol Phys. 2010;76(3):S20–7.

# Central Neurocytoma

Shireen Parsai, Senthilkumar Gandhidasan, and John H. Suh

## Learning Objectives

- To understand the clinical presentation of central neurocytoma.
- To identify key radiologic and pathologic features of central neurocytoma.
- To understand indications for conventional radiation therapy and stereotactic radiosurgery.

## Background/Epidemiology

Central neurocytoma (CNC) was first recognized by Hassoun et al. in 1982 when they identified two patients with intraventricular tumors with neuronal features [1]. The term central neurocytoma was derived from the tumor's neuronal origin and midline location [2, 3]. Since the 1980s, CNC has been further defined as a subset of benign tumors which are composed of cells undergoing neuronal differentiation typically located in the supratentorial ventricular system.

CNC is rare and comprises approximately 0.1–0.5% of all primary brain tumors [4]. The tumors generally affect young adults with the highest incidence occurring in the third decade and with equal prevalence among males and females and across all races [4, 5].

S. Parsai · J. H. Suh (✉)
Department of Radiation Oncology, Taussig Cancer Institute,
Cleveland Clinic,
Cleveland, OH, USA
e-mail: suhj@ccf.org

S. Gandhidasan
Department of Radiation Oncology, Illawarra Cancer Care Centre,
Wollongong, NSW, Australia

## Diagnosis and Prognosis

### Clinical Presentation

Classically, CNC presents with a gradual onset of symptoms associated with increased intracranial pressure caused by the lesion obstructing the interventricular foramina and leading to obstructive hydrocephalus [3–5]. Signs and symptoms of increased intracranial pressure are often generalized and may include headache, dizziness, visual disturbances, nausea, vomiting, ataxia, and papilledema. There are no pathognomonic symptoms to diagnose CNC. Incidental identification on neuroimaging may also lead to diagnosis in asymptomatic patients early in the disease process [4, 5].

### Radiologic Findings

Typical appearance of CNC on imaging is a well-demarcated, lobulated mass located in the supratentorial ventricular system. The majority of all CNC occur within the anterior half of the lateral ventricles, although it may also be observed in the third or fourth ventricles [4, 6]. Tumors are frequently attached to the superior and lateral walls of the ventricles and septum pellucidum distorting its appearance on imaging [3–5]. Analyses of angiographic findings of CNC have led to the hypothesis that the tumors originate from neuronal cells of the subependymal zone (SEZ) located on the floor of the lateral ventricle around the interventricular foramina, rather than the septum pellucidum. The size of CNC can be variable, ranging from subcentimeter lesions, which are identified incidentally, to larger biventricular lesions. The average size at diagnosis is approximately 4–5 cm in maximum dimension [7].

Non-contrasted computed tomography (CT) scans usually reveal a mixed density mass. The tumor mass itself is isodense but may exhibit hypodense areas which represent cystic degeneration. About one-fourth to one-half of all CNC also demonstrate hyperdense calcification. Contrast-enhanced

© Springer International Publishing AG, part of Springer Nature 2018
E. L. Chang et al. (eds.), *Adult CNS Radiation Oncology*, https://doi.org/10.1007/978-3-319-42878-9_29

CT is not necessarily helpful in the diagnosis of CN as it has a variable pattern of enhancement with contrast [3–5, 7].

Magnetic resonance imaging (MRI) is the preferred imaging modality in evaluating CNC. T1-weighted images reveal solid, isointense components with hypointense areas corresponding to areas of cystic degeneration (see Fig. 29.1). Heterogeneous enhancement may be seen after administration of gadolinium. T2-weighted images demonstrate "soap-bubble" multicystic masses with hyperintense fluid and isointense solid components. Peritumoral edema on FLAIR or T2 sequences are generally not observed (see Fig. 29.2) [3–5, 7].

## Pathologic Characteristics

Historically, CNC commonly has been misdiagnosed as intraventricular oligodendroglioma or ependymoma due to similar histopathologic appearance. Therefore, immunohis-

tochemistry and electron microscopy (EM) play a pivotal role in establishing the correct diagnosis. EM demonstrates ultrastructural features of neuronal differentiation. Similar to oligodendrogliomas, CNC may demonstrate the classic "fried egg" and "chicken wire" appearance. This results from small uniform cells with round to oval nuclei containing granular chromatin, scant cytoplasm, perinuclear halos with plexiform capillary microvascular architecture and often associated microcalcification (see Fig. 29.3). Resembling ependymomas, CNC cells may be arranged in straight lines or as perivascular rosettes. Although synaptophysin has been proven to be the most reliable immunohistochemical marker, neuron-specific enolase (NSE) and neuronal nuclear antigen (NeuN) are also markers for neuronal origin (see Fig. 29.3). Glial fibrillary acidic protein (GFAP) positivity is not necessary for diagnosis but suggests bipotential properties of true CNC cells [2–5, 8, 9].

CNC was first established as a distinct entity in the 1993 World Health Organization (WHO) classification. Although

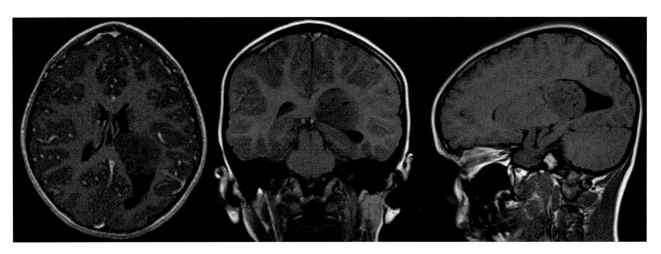

**Fig. 29.1** Axial, coronal, and sagittal views (*left to right*) of a T1-weighted post-contrast MRI demonstrates well-demarcated non-enhancing lesion (*arrow*) in the atrium of the left lateral ventricle, mea-

suring 3.9 cm in maximum dimension in a 7-year-old girl diagnosed with central neurocytoma

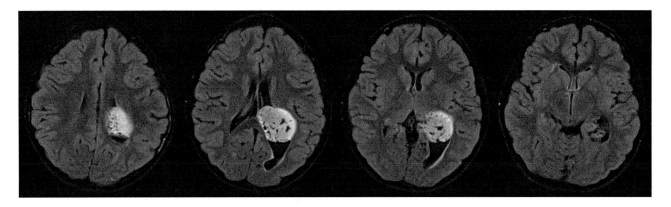

**Fig. 29.2** Axial T2-weighted FLAIR MRI demonstrates a hyperintense lesion occupying and dilating the atrium and posterior horn of the left lateral ventricle. Multiple small internal cystic spaces are noted in the lesion

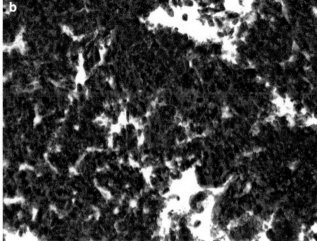

**Fig. 29.3** (**a**) Central neurocytoma marked by a proliferation of monomorphic appearing cells with rounded nuclei and a "salt and pepper" chromatin pattern (hematoxylin and eosin, original magnification 200×). (**b**) The tumor demonstrates diffuse cytoplasmic immunoreactivity with antibody to synaptophysin, consistent with neurocytic differentiation (original magnification 200×)

>75% CNC are deemed as a histologically benign tumor, CNC is designated as WHO grade II, owing in part to subsets of CNC demonstrating increased mitosis, microvascular proliferation, and focal necrosis which are associated with more aggressive clinical behavior. This subset is termed "atypical" CNC and can be designated based on the proliferation index of ≥2% (via MIB-1 labeling index). Clinically, atypical neurocytomas have been associated with increased risk of local recurrence and worse overall survival as compared to typical neurocytomas which exhibit more indolent histologies. A meta-analyses of 129 patients treated for central neurocytoma demonstrated that MIB-1 labeling index >3% was associated with an increased risk of local failure (45% vs 12%) and death (25% vs 3%) as compared to MIB labeling index ≤3% [10]. Extraventricular neurocytomas (EVN) exist as a separate entity in the 2007 and 2016 WHO classifications as they demonstrate a much wider morphologic spectrum. Discussion regarding EVN is beyond the scope of this chapter [2, 11–13].

## Overall Treatment Strategy

Primary treatment is maximal safe surgical resection with neurologic preservation, but this is variably achieved due to the highly vascular nature of central neurocytoma and its adherence to local critical structures. Surgical resection relieves obstruction and allows for tissue diagnosis [14–16]. Radiotherapy may be used in the upfront setting for inoperable patients or adjuvantly when indicated as discussed below. Chemotherapy is generally reserved as a last resort, often in cases with extracranial or leptomeningeal spread and in cases of recurrent neurocytoma after surgery or radiotherapy.

## Indications for Irradiation

The decision to proceed with radiotherapy is best made in a multidisciplinary setting. Clinicians may recommend close observation for lesions exhibiting an indolent natural history. Adjuvant radiotherapy should be considered for atypical histologies (i.e., elevated MIB-1 labeling index), residual, and recurrent disease. Following gross total resection, 5-year local control rates are estimated at 85% as compared to 46% with subtotal resection. When considering atypical CNC, the 5-year local control rates are lower: 57% after GTR as compared to 31% after STR [17–20]. Studies have demonstrated that adjuvant radiotherapy significantly increases local control in both typical and atypical histologies following subtotal resection [21, 22]. Adjuvant radiotherapy may be administered using conventionally fractionated schedules or stereotactic radiosurgery. Over time, more institutions have adopted SRS for adjuvant therapy or salvage of small recurrences given the theoretical benefit of smaller treatment volumes and potentially less neurotoxicity [21, 23].

## Target Volume Delineation

The target volume is delineated on a simulation CT with the aid of a fusion with both preoperative and postoperative MRIs. For definitive conventional radiotherapy, the gross tumor volume (GTV) is defined by the area of disease as evident on CT and MRI. For adjuvant cases, the GTV is defined as the tumor bed on postoperative CT and MRI. Tumor expansions may be extrapolated from the meningioma experience. The clinical target volume (CTV) is created by a 1 cm expansion of the GTV while carving out of the bone and other natural barriers to disease spread. Rades et al. recommend a 1.5–2.0 cm GTV to CTV expansion for incompletely resected atypical neurocytomas [24]. The planning target volume (PTV) is an additional margin of 3–5 mm to account for variabilities in treatment setup. Organs at risk (OAR) must be delineated as well as planning risk volume (PRV) for each OAR. For radiosurgery cases, the GTV is defined similarly to the definitive conventionally fractionated cases without further CTV or PTV expansions.

## Radiation Dose Prescription and Organ at Risk Tolerances

No published guidelines exist on radiation dosing and normal tissue constraints in treating CNC. Conventionally fractionated doses generally range from 45 to 54 Gy in 1.8–2.0 Gy per fraction (refer to Table 29.1). A dose-effect relationship should be considered in treating atypical neurocytomas which have been incompletely resected. Radiation doses >54 Gy are associated with better local control compared to doses ≤54 Gy. Per Rades et al., a total dose of 54–60 Gy at 2 Gy per fraction is recommended for incompletely resected atypical neurocytomas, except in the treatment of young children in which the risk of radiation-induced toxicity must be respected [24]. Dose constraints for normal tissues in conventionally fractionated cases may be borrowed from protocols for other intracranial tumors treated to similar total doses at 1.8–2.0 Gy per day. For example, dose constraints used to treat intracranial meningiomas are appropriate.

**Table 29.1** Compilation of studies of treating central neurocytoma with conventionally fractionated radiation therapy

| Study (year published) | No. of patients | Median dose Gy (range) | Median follow-up, months (range) | Local control |
|---|---|---|---|---|
| Louis et al. (1990) [25] | 4 | 54 to tumor; 30 to axis | 40 (11–78) | 100% |
| Fujimaki et al. (1997) [26] | 10 | 55.8 (50–60) | 72 (23–160) | 90% |
| Sharma et al. (1999) [27] | 15 | Not reported (40–60) | 36 (6–72) | 100% |
| Ashkan et al. (2000) [28] | 4 | 55 (not reported) | 6 (3–40) | 100% |
| Lenzi et al. (2006) [29] | 5 | 45 (not reported) | 84 (36–240) | 40% |
| Leenstra et al. (2007) [30] | 18 | 54.5 (48.6–61.2) | 19 (19–281) | 78% |
| Paek et al. (2008) [31] | 6 | 54 (50.4–55.8) | 171 (128–229) | 100% |
| Chen et al. (2008) [32] | 5 | 44.18 (20.5–54.0) | 29 (15–33) | Not reported |

**Table 29.2** Maximum point (defined as volume greater than 0.03 cc) doses permissible to critical structures per RTOG 0539 protocol

| Critical structure | Maximum point dose |
|---|---|
| Lenses | 5 Gy |
| Retinae | 45 Gy |
| Optic nerves | 50 Gy |
| Optic chiasm | 54 Gy |
| Brainstem | 55 Gy |

Constraints per RTOG 0539 for lesions treated to 54 Gy (NCT00895622) are shown in Table 29.2. In addition to the constraints as below, less than 0.03 cc volume of spinal cord may exceed 50 Gy.

Experiences delivering single-session stereotactic radiosurgery have delivered a mean marginal dose ranging from 10.5 to 20 Gy (refer to Table 29.3). Larger lesions have been treated with hypofractionated radiation schedules of 30 Gy in five fractions [17]. Normal tissue constraints are as follows; less than 1 cc volume of brainstem may exceed 12 Gy; maximum point dose to a volume greater than 0.03 cc should not exceed 8 Gy to the optic chiasm and 12.5 Gy to the brainstem. The volume of the spinal cord receiving 10 Gy should be limited to less than 10%. See Fig. 29.4 for an SRS plan involving recurrent atypical neurocytoma treated with Gamma Knife radiosurgery (Elekta; Stockholm, Sweden).

## Complication Avoidance

Strict adherence to normal tissue constraints allows for complication avoidance. Radiation-induced toxicities may be divided into acute toxicities which occur within 6 weeks of completing radiotherapy and late toxicities which occur greater than 6 weeks after completing radiotherapy. Acute toxicities may include fatigue, alopecia, skin erythema, and symptoms of cerebral edema (secondary to BBB disruption) such as nausea, vomiting, headaches, and seizures. Tinnitus, sensation of aural fullness, hearing impairment, xerostomia, and dysgeusia are less common. Late toxicities may include leukoencephalopathy, endocrine dysfunction, radiation necrosis, neurocognitive decline, and secondary malignancy. Permanent hearing impairment, visual changes, and cataract development are less common [45, 46]. In a reported experience by Karlsson et al. treating 42 patients treated with Gamma Knife radiosurgery, 45% of the patients developed ventricular enlargement following radiotherapy, and six of these patients required surgical intervention. The cause of ventricular enlargement remains unclear but confirms the importance of long-term follow-up of patients after completion of therapy to identify unanticipated toxicities which may require surgical or medical intervention [42].

**Table 29.3** Compilation of select studies of treating central neurocytoma with stereotactic radiosurgery

| Study (year published) | No. of patients | Mean marginal dose, Gy (range) | Prescription isodose line, % (mean) | Median follow-up, months (range) | Local control |
|---|---|---|---|---|---|
| Pollock et al. (2001) [33] | 1 | 18 (NA) | Not reported | 34 (NA) | 100% |
| Bertalanffy et al. (2001) [34] | 3 | Not reported (9.6–19) | 30–60 (not reported) | 24 (12–60) | 100% |
| Anderson et al. (2001) [35] | 4 | 17.0 (16–20) | Not reported | 13 (12–28) | 100% |
| Cobery et al. (2001) [15] | 4 | 10.5 (9–13) | 30–50 (42.5) | 32.5 (12–99) | 100% |
| Martin et al. (2003) [36] | 4 | 16.5 (16–18) | 89–110 (94.8) | 33 (3–54) | 100% |
| Hara et al. (2003) [37] | 1 | 20 (NA) | 50 (NA) | 12 (NA) | 100% |
| Kim et al. (2007) [38] | 7 | 15.7 (15–18) | 50 (50) | 61 (26–77) | 71% |
| Yen et al. (2007) [39] | 6 | 15.1 (9–20) | 30–60 (32.5) | 72 (6–123) | 100% |
| Matsunaga et al. (2010) [40] | 7 | 13.9 (12–18) | 50–75 (55.6) | 63.6 (15–136) | 88% |
| Genc et al. (2011) [41] | 18 | 16.7 (9–20) | 50 (50) | 31 (6–110) | 93% |
| Karlsson et al. (2012) [42] | 35 | 14 (11–25) | Not reported | 30 (1.4–14.1) | 83% |
| Monaco et al. (2015) [43] | 8 | 14.6 (12–20) | 50 (50) | 63.3 (12.9–139.1) | 88% |
| Yamanaka et al. (2016) [44] | 36 | 15 (10–20) | 50 (40–55) | 54.5 (3–180) | 94% |

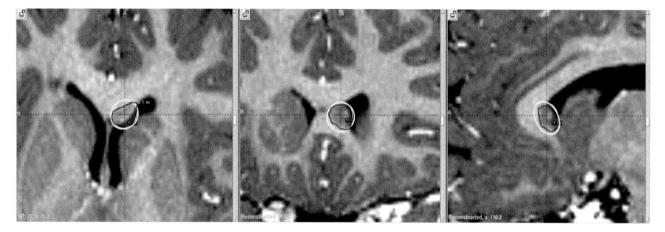

**Fig. 29.4** Gamma Knife radiosurgery plan for recurrent atypical neurocytoma with aggressive pathologic features including Ki-67 index of 20–25% involving the left frontal horn of the lateral ventricle, 6 months after surgical resection (*left to right*: axial, coronal, sagittal representations). Lesion contour represented in blue. Prescription isodose line (16 Gy) represented in yellow

## Outcomes: Tumor Control

Local control is generally favorable for CNC. Outcomes after conventionally fractionated radiation therapy and SRS are summarized in Tables 29.1 and 29.3, respectively. Barani et al. published a review of radiotherapy experiences including conventionally fractionated RT and SRS with a total of 158 cases. Overall control rate was 91% (93% and 88% for SRS and conventional radiotherapy, respectively). There was a trend toward increased local control in the SRS group; however this was not statistically significant. Furthermore, histologic atypia was found to correlate to the risk of local recurrence after radiotherapy [47]. Park et al. conducted a systematic review of five retrospective case series with a total of 64 cases treated with SRS (median marginal dose ranged from 12.1 to 16.0 Gy), reporting local control rates of 91.1% with a mean of 59.3 months of follow-up [23]. The decision to treat patients adjuvantly with conventionally fractionated radiation therapy or stereotactic radiosurgery is at the discretion of the treating physician given the comparable local control rates. In patients with incompletely resected CNC, there is no significant difference in 5-year local control rates when treated with conventionally fractionated RT as compared to SRS [21].

Although surgical resection remains the main therapy as previously discussed, SRS may be used as definitive therapy when patients are deemed medically inoperable. Kim et al. reviewed 20 patients treated with SRS, and of these, half did not have prior surgical resection. Results demonstrated a trend toward improved tumor control with definitive SRS compared to adjuvant SRS, although this was not found to be statistically significant [48].

## Follow-Up: Radiographic Assessment

No published guidelines exist on appropriate follow-up imaging. Physician discretion should be used to schedule routine follow-up visits with serial MRI brain with and without contrast to examine tumor response to therapy and continued surveillance for disease recurrence. For benign neurocytomas, our institution recommends follow-up with imaging every 6 months for 3 years from completing therapy, then yearly for at least 10 years. For atypical neurocytomas, our institution follows these patients every 3 months for 3 years from completing therapy, then at least yearly for a minimum of 10 years.

## Case Presentation

A 49-year-old male with past medical history of attention deficit/hyperactivity disorder and hypertension first presented to a neurologist with a 1-week history of intermittent nausea and vomiting, vertigo, and a sense of dysequilibrium following a recent barotrauma after jumping in a pool. He also described progressive bitemporal headaches and tinnitus. An MRI brain demonstrated a 4.4 cm infiltrating mass lesion centered at the left inferomedial cerebellum resulting in severe narrowing of the fourth ventricle at the level of the lower posterior fossa (see Fig. 29.5). No overt hydrocephalus was identified though the degree of effacement of the fourth ventricle raised concern for impending hydrocephalus. The patient was admitted for further evaluation and management. Systemic imaging with CT chest, abdomen, and pelvis was unrevealing for an extracranial site of primary disease. Surgical resection was completed via a suboccipital craniotomy with implementation of neuronavigation and electrophysiologic monitoring as well as placement of an external ventricular drain. Intraoperative frozen section was suggestive of ependymoma vs grade 3 astrocytoma. Gross total resection was achieved. Postoperative pathology demonstrated a fairly monomorphic proliferation of cells with generally round to oval nuclei and salt and pep-

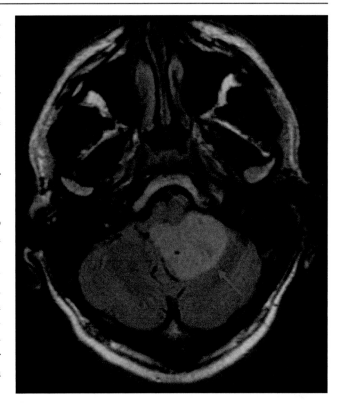

**Fig. 29.5** Axial T2-weighted FLAIR MRI demonstrates an infiltrating mass lesion (*red arrow*), measuring 4.4 cm in maximum dimension, centered at the left inferomedial cerebellum contributing to rightward displacement and severe narrowing of the fourth ventricle at the level of the lower posterior fossa

per chromatin pattern. The tumor demonstrated diffuse and strong immunoreactivity with antibodies to NeuN and synaptophysin. Occasional S-100 positive staining cells were noted along with background staining with antibody to GFAP, Ki-67 reported as 3%. Diagnosis was established as atypical central neurocytoma, favor WHO grade II. A repeat MRI brain with and without contrast was obtained within 24 h after surgical resection. After surgery, symptoms of nausea, vomiting, and dizziness resolved. Balance continued to improve with physical therapy. He was seen by the radiation oncologist postoperatively to discuss the role of adjuvant radiation therapy.

He was recommended adjuvant radiation therapy given the risk of recurrence in the setting of high Ki-67 index. CT simulation scan without contrast was obtained 3 weeks postoperatively for planning purposes, and he began radiotherapy within 4 weeks after surgical resection. The surgical bed was contoured as the GTV on the planning CT with guidance from postoperative MRI fusion. The GTV included the region of the fourth ventricle previously involved by tumor on preoperative imaging. A CTV

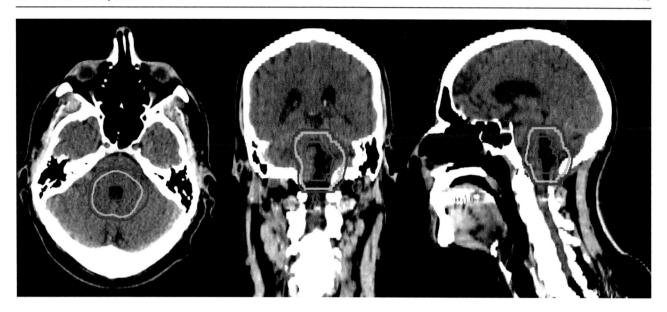

**Fig. 29.6** Axial, coronal, and sagittal (*left to right*) CT brain images representing delineated tumor volumes: GTV shown in red, CTV shown in green, and PTV shown in blue

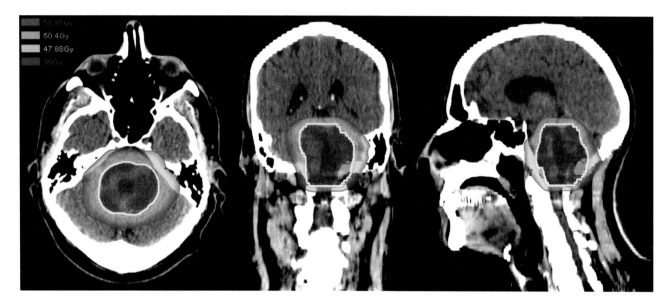

**Fig. 29.7** Axial, coronal, and sagittal slices (*left to right*) representing radiation dose distribution. Yellow line represents PTV

was created by 1.0 cm expansion on the GTV, carving out of bone. A 3 mm expansion on the CTV was used to define the PTV (see Fig. 29.6). A radiation dose of 5040 cGy in 28 fractions was prescribed to the PTV. Intensity-modulated radiation therapy (IMRT) planning was performed with volumetric-modulated arc therapy (VMAT) technique using 6 MV photons prescribed to the 97.8% isodose line (see Fig. 29.7). The plan was delivered with two VMAT arcs. Normal tissue constraints were respected (see Fig. 29.8). Image guidance was performed with daily cone beam CT (CBCT).

He completed therapy over 37 days and tolerated treatment well. On the last day of treatment, he was noted to have grade 2 fatigue, grade 1 alopecia, grade 1 nausea, and grade 1 headache per CTCAE criteria. He was also noted to have mild numbness in his left hand and left foot. He required a prolonged steroid taper due to ongoing nausea and headaches which recurred with radiotherapy. He has been followed for 1 year to date, at which time nausea and headaches have resolved, steroids have been successfully tapered, and the two follow-up MRIs obtained at 6-month intervals have been without evidence of disease progression.

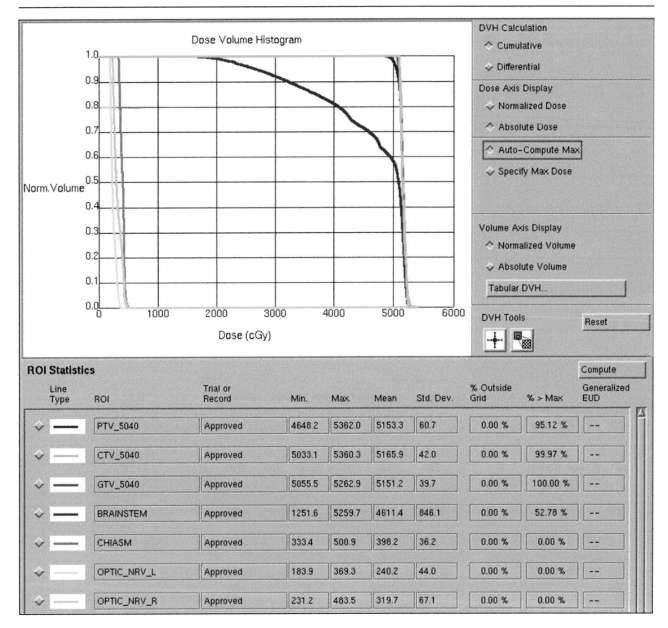

**Fig. 29.8** Representative images of dose-volume histograms (DVH) for the radiation plan, plotting dose delivered to the target volume and normal tissue volumes

## Summary

- Central neurocytoma is a rare brain tumor which occurs most commonly in young adults and arises in the supratentorial ventricular system.
- The clinical presentation of CNC is usually secondary to intracranial pressure with nausea, vomiting, headaches, and dizziness.
- Diagnosis is established based on characteristic pathologic findings consistent with neuronal differentiation including immunoreactivity with antibody to synaptophysin.
- Treatment paradigms include maximal safe surgical resection ± adjuvant radiotherapy or definitive radiotherapy.
- After surgical resection, adjuvant radiotherapy is recommended in cases of subtotal resection, recurrent disease, or atypical features.
- In general, radiation therapy may be prescribed as conventionally fractionated radiotherapy to doses of 45–54 Gy at 1.8–2.0 Gy/fraction for benign neurocytomas or 54–60 Gy in 2.0 Gy/fraction for atypical neurocytomas. Stereotactic radiosurgery series have used mean marginal doses ranging from 10.5 to 20 Gy, though the

majority was treated with mean marginal doses of 14–18 Gy in a single session.

- After completing radiotherapy, patients should be followed in the long term to evaluate for potential recurrences and radiation-induced late toxicities.

## Self-Assessment Questions

1. What is the most common region neurocytoma arises?
   A. Lateral ventricle
   B. Third ventricle
   C. Fourth ventricle
   D. Skull base

2. What is the specific pathologic marker for neurocytoma?
   A. Neuron-specific enolase (NSE)
   B. Neuronal nuclear antigen (NeuN)
   C. Synaptophysin
   D. Glial fibrillary acidic protein (GFAP) positivity

3. What defines an atypical neurocytoma?
   A. Number of mitotic figures per high-power field
   B. Microvascular proliferation
   C. Focal necrosis
   D. Proliferation index $\geq 2\%$

4. All of the following are indications for adjuvant radiation therapy except:
   A. MIB-1 labeling index >2%
   B. Subtotal resection
   C. Recurrent disease
   D. Tumor >5 cm

5. What is an appropriate dose for conventionally fractionated radiotherapy used to treat a benign neurocytoma?
   A. 30 Gy
   B. 40 Gy
   C. 50 Gy
   D. 60 Gy

## Answers

1. A
2. C
3. D
4. D
5. C

## References

1. Hassoun J, Gambarelli D, Grisoli F, et al. Central neurocytoma. An electron-microscopic study of two cases. Acta Neuropathol. 1982;56(2):151–6.
2. Kim DG, Park CK. Central neurocytoma: establishment of the disease entity. Neurosurg Clin N Am. 2015;26(1):1–4.
3. Schmidt MH, Gottfried ON, von Koch CS, et al. Central neurocytoma: a review. J Neurooncol. 2004;66(3):377–84.
4. Patel DM, Schmidt RF, Liu JK. Update on the diagnosis, pathogenesis, and treatment strategies for central neurocytoma. J Clin Neurosci. 2013;20(9):1193–9.
5. Yang I, Ung N, Chung LK, et al. Clinical manifestations of central neurocytoma. Neurosurg Clin N Am. 2015;26(1):5–10.
6. Wong J, Teo C, Kwok B. Central neurocytoma in third and fourth ventricles with aqueductal involvement. Br J Neurosurg. 2006;20(1):57–62.
7. Donoho D, Zada G. Imaging of central neurocytomas. Neurosurg Clin N Am. 2015;26(1):11–9.
8. Choudhari KA, Kaliaperumal C, Jain A, et al. Central neurocytoma: a multi-disciplinary review. Br J Neurosurg. 2009;23(6):585–95.
9. Paek SH, Kim JE, Kim DG, et al. Angiographic characteristics of central neurocytoma suggest the origin of tumor. J Korean Med Sci. 2003;18(4):573–80.
10. Rades D, Schild SE, Fehlauer F. Prognostic value of the MIB-1 labeling index for central neurocytomas. Neurology. 2004;62(6):987–9.
11. Louis DN, Ohgaki H, Wiestler OD, et al. The 2007 WHO classification of tumours of the central nervous system. Acta Neuropathol. 2007;114(2):97–109.
12. Louis DN, Perry A, Reifenberger G, et al. The 2016 World Health Organization classification of tumors of the central nervous system: a summary. Acta Neuropathol. 2016;131(6):803–20.
13. Soylemezoglu F, Scheithauer BW, Esteve J, et al. Atypical central neurocytoma. J Neuropathol Exp Neurol. 1997;56(5):551–6.
14. Sgouros S, Carey M, Aluwihare N, et al. Central neurocytoma: a correlative clinicopathologic and radiologic analysis. Surg Neurol. 1998;49(2):197–204.
15. Cobery ST, Noren G, Friehs GM, et al. Gamma knife surgery for treatment of central neurocytomas. Report of four cases. J Neurosurg. 2001;94(2):327–30.
16. Qian H, Lin S, Zhang M, et al. Surgical management of intraventricular central neurocytoma: 92 cases. Acta Neurochir. 2012;154(11):1951–60.
17. Imber BS, Braunstein SE, Wu FY, et al. Clinical outcome and prognostic factors for central neurocytoma: twenty year institutional experience. J Neurooncol. 2016;126(1):193–200.
18. Rades D, Fehlauer F. Treatment options for central neurocytoma. Neurology. 2002;59(8):1268–70.
19. Rades D, Fehlauer F, Schild SE. Treatment of atypical neurocytomas. Cancer. 2004;100(4):814–7.
20. Rades D, Fehlauer F, Lamszus K, et al. Well-differentiated neurocytoma: what is the best available treatment? Neuro Oncol. 2005;7(1):77–83.
21. Rades D, Schild SE. Value of postoperative stereotactic radiosurgery and conventional radiotherapy for incompletely resected typical neurocytomas. Cancer. 2006;106(5):1140–3.
22. Kim DG, Paek SH, Kim IH, et al. Central neurocytoma: the role of radiation therapy and long term outcome. Cancer. 1997;79(10):1995–2002.

23. Park HK, Steven DC. Stereotactic radiosurgery for central neurocytoma: a quantitative systematic review. J Neurooncol. 2012;108(1):115–21.

24. Rades D, Fehlauer F, Ikezaki K, et al. Dose-effect relationship for radiotherapy after incomplete resection of atypical neurocytomas. Radiother Oncol. 2005;74(1):67–9.

25. Louis DN, Swearingen B, Linggood RM, et al. Central nervous system neurocytoma and neuroblastoma in adults—report of eight cases. J Neurooncol. 1990;9(3):231–8.

26. Fujimaki T, Matsuno A, Sasaki T, et al. Proliferative activity of central neurocytoma: measurement of tumor volume doubling time, MIB-1 staining index and bromodeoxyuridine labeling index. J Neurooncol. 1997;32(2):103–9.

27. Sharma MC, Sarkar C, Karak AK, et al. Intraventricular neurocytoma: a clinicopathological study of 20 cases with review of the literature. J Clin Neurosci. 1999;6(4):319–23.

28. Ashkan K, Casey AT, D'Arrigo C, et al. Benign central neurocytoma. Cancer. 2000;89(5):1111–20.

29. Lenzi J, Salvati M, Raco A, et al. Central neurocytoma: a novel appraisal of a polymorphic pathology. Our experience and a review of the literature. Neurosurg Rev. 2006;29(4):286–92. discussion 292

30. Leenstra JL, Rodriguez FJ, Frechette CM, et al. Central neurocytoma: management recommendations based on a 35-year experience. Int J Radiat Oncol Biol Phys. 2007;67(4):1145–54.

31. Paek SH, Han JH, Kim JW, et al. Long-term outcome of conventional radiation therapy for central neurocytoma. J Neurooncol. 2008;90(1):25–30.

32. Chen CM, Chen KH, Jung SM, et al. Central neurocytoma: 9 case series and review. Surg Neurol. 2008;70(2):204–9.

33. Pollock BE, Stafford SL. Stereotactic radiosurgery for recurrent central neurocytoma: case report. Neurosurgery. 2001;48(2):441–3.

34. Bertalanffy A, Roessler K, Dietrich W, et al. Gamma knife radiosurgery of recurrent central neurocytomas: a preliminary report. J Neurol Neurosurg Psychiatry. 2001;70(4):489–93.

35. Anderson RC, Elder JB, Parsa AT, et al. Radiosurgery for the treatment of recurrent central neurocytomas. Neurosurgery. 2001;48(6):1231–7. discussion 1237–8

36. Martin JM, Katati M, Lopez E, et al. Linear accelerator radiosurgery in treatment of central neurocytomas. Acta Neurochir. 2003;145(9):749–54. discussion 754

37. Hara M, Aoyagi M, Yamamoto M, et al. Rapid shrinkage of remnant central neurocytoma after gamma knife radiosurgery: a case report. J Neurooncol. 2003;62(3):269–73.

38. Kim CY, Paek SH, Jeong SS, et al. Gamma knife radiosurgery for central neurocytoma: primary and secondary treatment. Cancer. 2007;110(10):2276–84.

39. Yen CP, Sheehan J, Patterson G, et al. Gamma knife surgery for neurocytoma. J Neurosurg. 2007;107(1):7–12.

40. Matsunaga S, Shuto T, Suenaga J, et al. Gamma knife radiosurgery for central neurocytomas. Neurol Med Chir. 2010;50(2):107–12. disucussion 112–3

41. Genc A, Bozkurt SU, Karabagli P, et al. Gamma knife radiosurgery for cranial neurocytomas. J Neurooncol. 2011;105(3):647–57.

42. Karlsson B, Guo WY, Kejia T, et al. Gamma knife surgery for central neurocytomas. J Neurosurg. 2012;117(Suppl):96–101.

43. Monaco EA 3rd, Niranjan A, Lunsford LD. The management of central neurocytoma: radiosurgery. Neurosurg Clin N Am. 2015;26(1):37–44.

44. Yamanaka K, Iwai Y, Shuto T, et al. Treatment results of gamma knife radiosurgery for central neurocytoma: report of a Japanese multi-institutional cooperative study. World Neurosurg. 2016;90:300–5.

45. Lawrence YR, Li XA, el Naqa I, et al. Radiation dose-volume effects in the brain. Int J Radiat Oncol Biol Phys. 2010;76(3 Suppl):S20–7.

46. Douw L, Klein M, Fagel SS, et al. Cognitive and radiological effects of radiotherapy in patients with low-grade glioma: long-term follow-up. Lancet Neurol. 2009;8(9):810–8.

47. Barani IJ, Raleigh DR, Larson D. The management of central neurocytoma: radiotherapy. Neurosurg Clin N Am. 2015;26(1):45–56.

48. Kim JW, Kim DG, Kim IK, et al. Central neurocytoma: long-term outcomes of multimodal treatments and management strategies based on 30 years' experience in a single institute. Neurosurgery. 2013;72(3):407–13. discussion 413–4

# Prognostic Classification Systems for Brain Metastases

# 30

Paul W. Sperduto

## Learning Objectives

- To understand how prognosis varies by diagnosis.
- To understand the diagnosis-specific prognostic factors for each of the most common cancers associated with brain metastases.
- To understand how to calculate the Graded Prognostic Assessment (GPA) for each diagnosis.
- To understand how the prognosis should influence clinical judgment regarding whether and what treatment is appropriate.

## Introduction

Brain metastases are a common and complex conundrum for cancer care. An estimated 300,000 patients are diagnosed each year with brain metastases in the United States [1], and that incidence is growing due to advances in treatment that result in patients living longer and thus at risk for brain metastases [2]. It is a complex problem because of the marked heterogeneity of this patient population: brain metastases may arise from a wide variety of tumor types and subtypes. Furthermore, these patients may have already received a plethora of different treatments for their cancer or may present with brain metastases at the time of initial diagnosis. This heterogeneity has long plagued interpretation of clinical trials involving this patient population because it was essentially impossible to sufficiently stratify studies to verify similar groups of patients were being compared [3]. Interpretation of clinical trials and efforts to estimate prognosis are further complicated by the plethora of possible combinations of currently available treatment options [surgery, stereotactic

radiosurgery (SRS), whole-brain radiation therapy (WBRT), chemotherapy, targeted drug therapies, and immunotherapies]. Furthermore, four prospective randomized trials have shown WBRT adds no survival benefit over SRS alone in SRS-eligible patients [4–7], and, on the other end of the prognostic spectrum, in poor prognosis patients, there is evidence that supportive care may be as effective as WBRT [8]. Accordingly, WBRT is used less commonly than in the past.

## Classification Systems

These concerns led to efforts to better understand prognosis. The purpose of a prognostic index is to predict outcome before, not after, treatment. It is important to distinguish prognostic from predictive factors. A prognostic factor identifies good vs. bad outcome irrespective of treatment used, whereas a predictive factor identifies good versus bad outcome for a specific treatment. Gaspar et al. published the Radiation Therapy Oncology Group (RTOG) Recursive Partitioning Analysis for brain metastases (Table 30.1) in 1997 [9]. This prognostic index consisted of three classes: I (age < 65, Karnofsky Performance Status (KPS) ≥ 70, controlled primary tumor, no extracranial metastases), II (all patients not in class I or III), and III (KPS < 70) which correlated with median survival of 7.1, 4.2, and 2.3 months, respectively, at that time. Weltman et al. published the Score Index for Radiosurgery (SIR) (Table 30.2) in 2000 [10]. This

**Table 30.1** Radiation Therapy Oncology Group (RTOG) Recursive Partitioning Analysis (RPA) for patients with brain metastases

| Class | Criteria | Median survival |
|---|---|---|
| Class I: | Age < 65 years and | 7.1 months |
| | KPS ≥ 70 and | |
| | controlled primary tumor and | |
| | no extracranial metastases | |
| Class II: | All patients not in class I or III | 4.2 months |
| Class III: | KPS < 70 | 2.3 months |

*KPS* Karnofsky Performance Status
Based on data from Ref. [9]

P. W. Sperduto
Minneapolis Radiation Oncology and Gamma Knife Center,
University of Minnesota Medical Center, Minneapolis, MN, USA
e-mail: psperduto@mropa.com

© Springer International Publishing AG, part of Springer Nature 2018
E. L. Chang et al. (eds.), *Adult CNS Radiation Oncology*, https://doi.org/10.1007/978-3-319-42878-9_30

**Table 30.2** Score Index for Radiosurgery (SIR)

|  | Score | | |
|---|---|---|---|
|  | 0 | 1 | 2 |
| Age (years) | ≥60 | 51–59 | ≤50 |
| KPS | ≤50 | 60–70 | 80–100 |
| Systemic disease | Progressive | Stable | CR or NED |
| Number of lesions | ≥3 | 2 | 1 |
| Vol. largest lesion (ml) | >13 | 5–13 | <5 |

*KPS* Karnofsky Performance Status, *CR* complete response, *NED* no evidence of disease
Median survival (MS) by SIR score: SIR 1–3 (MS 2.91 months), SIR 4–7 (MS 7.00 months), SIR 8–10 (MS 31.38 months)
Based on data from Ref. [10]

**Table 30.3** Basic Score for Brain Metastases (BSBM)

|  | Score | |
|---|---|---|
|  | 0 | 1 |
| KPS | 50–70 | 80–100 |
| Control of primary tumor | No | Yes |
| Extracranial metastases | Yes | No |

*KPS* Karnofsky Performance Status
Median survival (MS) by BSBM: BSBM 3 (MS >32 months), BSBM 2 (MS 13.1 months), BSBM 1 (MS 3.3 months), BSBM 0 (MS 1.9 months)
Based on data from Ref. [11]

index used the sum of scores (0–2) for each of five prognostic factors (age, KPS, status of systemic disease, number of brain metastases, and the volume of the largest metastasis). Lorenzoni et al. published the Basic Score for Brain Metastases (BSBM) (Table 30.3) in 2004 [11]. This index is based on the sum of scores (0–1) for three prognostic factors (KPS, control of primary tumor, and extracranial metastases). Sloan-Barnholtz published a nomogram (Fig. 30.1) in an effort to further individualize prognosis [12]. Kondziolka published an interesting survey study in which experts in the field were asked to estimate survival for a series of patients given all relevant clinical parameters. This study showed even experts cannot predict outcomes with certainty for all patients [13]. All prognostic indices have limitations but can provide guidance for clinical decision-making and are essential for stratification of clinical trials so that those trials are comparing comparable patients, thus making the results of those trials worthwhile, relevant, and interpretable.

Our group published the Graded Prognostic Assessment (GPA) in 2008 [14] based on 1960 patients from five randomized Radiation Therapy Oncology Group (RTOG) trials (7916, 8528, 8905, 9104, and 9508). Analysis showed four prognostic factors (age, KPS, extracranial metastases, and number of brain metastases) were significant for survival. Those prognostic factors were weighted in proportion to their regression coefficients and scaled such that patients with the best/worst prognosis would have a GPA of 4.0/0.0, respectively. In 2010, we refined the GPA based on an analy-

sis of a retrospective multi-institutional database of 4259 patients. That study found survival varies by diagnosis and diagnosis-specific prognostic factors [15]. The breast-GPA was then further refined using tumor subtype [16], and a summary report was published [17]. More recently, the GPA indices for lung cancer and melanoma were updated using new data from patients (2186 lung cancer and 823 melanoma patients) diagnosed since 2005 including molecular factors. The lung-molGPA incorporates EGFR and ALK gene status [18, 19], and similarly the melanoma-molGPA incorporates *BRAF* status [20, 21]. The original melanoma-GPA found only two factors were significant (KPS and the number of brain metastases), whereas in the updated melanoma-molGPA, other clinical factors (age and extracranial metastases) were found to be significant, in addition to *BRAF* status.

Table 30.4 shows the median survival time for patients with brain metastases by diagnosis-specific GPA. Table 30.5 shows a user-friendly worksheet to facilitate calculation of the Graded Prognostic Assessment by diagnosis and estimate survival for patients with brain metastases. A free online/smartphone application is available at brainmetgpa.com which further simplifies calculation of the GPA. Table 30.6 shows a multivariate analysis of risk of death and median survival by treatment (excluding drug therapies) and diagnosis. It is important to understand these data are retrospective in nature with the selection bias inherent in all retrospective studies so one should not conclude that one treatment is better than another based on these data. Fig. 30.2 shows Kaplan-Meier curves for survival for six diagnoses by GPA, demonstrating excellent separation between groups.

The diagnosis-specific GPA indices presented here hold several implications for clinical management and research involving patients with brain metastases:

1. There is marked heterogeneity in outcomes for patients with brain metastases, and these outcomes vary not only by diagnosis but also by diagnosis-specific prognostic factors, as detailed herein. Because of this heterogeneity, we should not treat all patients with brain metastases the same way; treatment should be individualized, and the past philosophy of fatalistic futility should be abandoned.

2. On the other hand, as shown in Table 30.4, if a patient has a GPA of 0–1.0, regardless of diagnosis, their expected survival is poor. For these patients, supportive care, as suggested by the QUARTZ trial [8], may be the best option.

3. For patients with GPA scores above 1.0, the median survival time (Table 30.4) varies more by diagnosis, and more aggressive treatment strategies may be appropriate, but these retrospective data do not provide a basis for assuming that longer survival is a consequence of

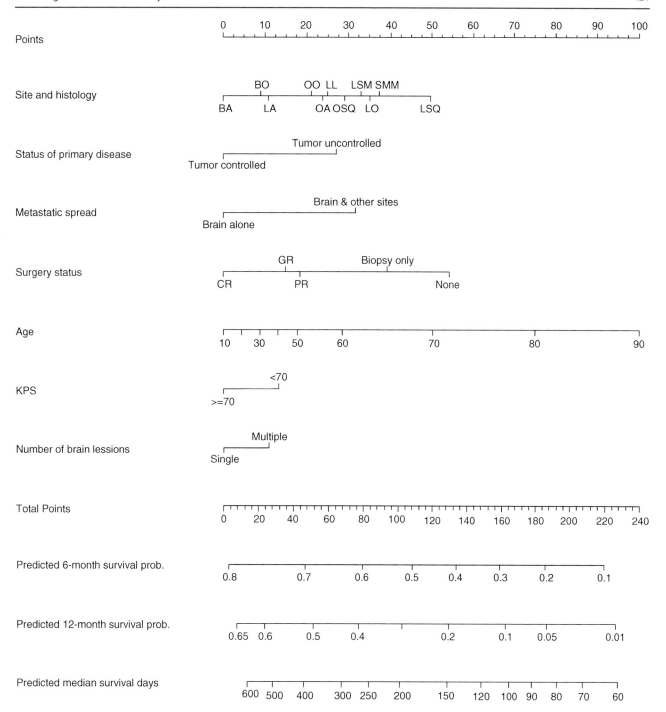

**Fig. 30.1** Nomogram for 6- and 12-month survival probability and median survival prediction for RTOG brain metastases patients. Abbreviations for site and histology: *BA* breast and adenocarcinoma, *BO* breast and other, *LA* lung and adenocarcinoma, *LL* lung and large cell, *LO* lung and other, *LSM* lung and small cell, *LSQ* lung and squamous cell, *OA* other and adenocarcinoma, *OSQ* other and squamous cell, *SMM* skin melanoma, *OO* other and other. Surgery: *PR* partial resection, *CR* complete resection, *GR* gross resection. [Reprinted from Sloan-Barnholtz-Sloan JS, Yu C, Sloan AE, et al. A nomogram for individualized estimation of survival among patients with brain metastasis. Neuro Oncol 2012;14:910–918. With permission from Oxford University Press]

more aggressive treatment. Indeed, the survival by treatment data shown in Table 30.6 is certainly fraught with selection bias and should not be blindly applied or expected. Nonetheless, these data reflect patterns of care for patients with brain metastases.

4. Performance status is prognostic in every diagnosis. Clinicians should take the time to accurately assess and document their patients' performance status.
5. Table 30.5 shows the number of brain metastases is a significant prognostic factor for lung cancer, melanoma,

**Table 30.4** Median survival time for patients with brain metastases by diagnosis-specific Graded Prognostic Assessment score

| | | DS-GPA | | | | |
|---|---|---|---|---|---|---|
| Diagnosis | Overall MST (95% CI) N | 0–1.0 MST (95% CI) n (%) | 1.5–2.0 MST (95% CI) n (%) | 2.5–3.0 MST (95% CI) n (%) | 3.5–4.0 MST (95% CI) n (%) | p (log-rank) |
| NSCLC | 15,23 (14.17–16.53) 1521 | 6.90 (5.73–8.70) 337 (22%) | 13.67 (11.97–15.33) 664 (44%) | 26.47 (23.40–30.63) 455 (30%) | 46.77 (36.87–NE) 65 (4%) | <0.001 |
| SCLC | 4.90 (4.30–6.20) 281 | 2.79 (1.83–3.12) 65 (23%) | 4.90 (4.04–6.51) 119 (42%) | 7.67 (6.27–9.13) 84 (30%) | 17.05 (4.70–27.43) 13 (5%) | <0.001 |
| Melanoma | 9.80 (9.08–10.59) 823 | 4.92 (3.67–6.92) 136 (17%) | 8.30 (7.34–9.28) 386 (47%) | 15.77 (13.12–18.82) 256 (31%) | 34.07 (23.61–50.46) 45 (5%) | <0.001 |
| RCC | 9.63 (7.66–10.91) 286 | 3.27 (2.04–5.10) 43 (15%) | 7.29 (3.73–10.91) 76 (27%) | 11.27 (8.80–14.80) 104 (36%) | 14.77 (9.73–19.79) 63 (22%) | <0.001 |
| Breast cancer | 13.80 (11.53–15.87) 400 | 3.35 (3.13–3.78) 23 (6%) | 7.70 (5.62–8.74) 104 (26%) | 15.07 (12.94–15.87) 140 (35%) | 25.30 (23.10–26.51) 133 (33%) | <0.001 |
| GI cancer | 5.36 (4.30–6.30) 209 | 3.13 (2.37–4.57) 76 (36%) | 4.40 (3.37–6.53) 65 (31%) | 6.87 (4.86–11.63) 50 (24%) | 13.54 (9.76–27.12) 18 (9%) | <0.001 |
| Others | 6.37 (5.22–7.49) 450 | – | – | – | – | – |

The top row in each cell is the median survival time (MST) in months and its associated 95% CI. The bottom row is the frequency and percentage of patients with the corresponding DS-GPA category for a given diagnosis. Abbreviations: *DS-GPA* Diagnosis-Specific Graded Prognostic Assessment, *NSCLC* non-small cell lung cancer (adenocarcinoma), *SCLC* small cell lung cancer, *RCC* renal cell carcinoma, *GI* gastrointestinal, *NE* not estimable
Based on data from Refs. [17, 19, 21]

and renal cell carcinoma, but not for breast or gastrointestinal cancers. Patients should not be denied treatment because of the number of brain metastases.

6. Extracranial metastases are only prognostic in lung cancer and melanoma but not in breast cancer, renal cell carcinoma, or gastrointestinal cancers. The implication here is that those patients with non-lung, non-melanoma malignancies should not be denied aggressive treatment for their brain metastases because they have extracranial metastases.

7. Age is strongly prognostic in lung cancer and weakly prognostic in breast cancer and melanoma but not prognostic in renal cell carcinoma or gastrointestinal cancers. Thus, age should not be used as a rationale to withhold aggressive treatment for non-lung malignancies.

8. Because lung cancer and brain metastases from lung cancer are so common, those patients have masked our understanding of the distinct course for patients with

non-lung malignancies and brain metastases, as demonstrated by points 5, 6, and 7.

9. Tumor subtype in breast cancer is of paramount importance and prognostic significance, but it is not as prognostic as the breast-GPA index.

10. A disproportionate number of patients with gastrointestinal cancers present with GPA of 0–1.0. Whether this is due to lack of screening MRI in these patients versus other biological reasons remains unclear, but the finding should serve as a reminder that brain metastases are not uncommon in GI cancer patients. Ongoing research will better elucidate prognosis for these patients, and the GI-GPA will be updated accordingly.

11. Clinicians may use the worksheet in Table 30.5 to calculate their patient's GPA score and estimate survival.

12. The GPA may be used for purposes of stratification in clinical trials dealing with patients with brain metastases.

**Table 30.5** GPA worksheet to estimate survival from brain metastases by diagnosis

| Non-small cell/small cell lung cancer | | | | |
|---|---|---|---|---|
| | GPA scoring criteria | | Patient | |
| | 0 | 0.5 | 1.0 | Score |
| Age | ≥70 | <70 | n/a | ____ |
| KPS | ≤70 | 80 | 90–100 | ____ |
| ECM | Present | | Absent | ____ |
| #BM | >4 | 1–4 | n/a | ____ |
| Gene status | EGFR neg/unk and ALK neg/unk | n/a | EGFR pos or ALK pos | ____ |
| | | | Sum total | ____ |

Adenocarcinoma MS by GPA: GPA 0–1.0 = 6.9; 1.5–2.0 = 13.7; 2.5–3.0 = 26.5; 3.5–4.0 = 46.8
Non-adenocarcinoma MS by GPA: GPA 0–1.0 = 5.3; 1.5–2.0 = 9.8; 2.5–3.0 = 12.8

| Melanoma | | | | |
|---|---|---|---|---|
| | 0 | 0.5 | 1.0 | Score |
| Age | ≥70 | <70 | n/a | ____ |
| KPS | <70 | 80 | 90–100 | ____ |
| ECM | Present | n/a | Absent | ____ |
| #BM | >4 | 2–4 | 1 | ____ |
| Gene status | BRAF neg/unk | BRAF pos | n/a | ____ |
| | | | Sum total = | ____ |

MS (months) by GPA: GPA 0–1.0 = 4.9; 1.5–2.0 = 8.3; 2.5–3.0 = 15.8; 3.5–4.0 = 34.1

| Breast cancer | | | | | | |
|---|---|---|---|---|---|---|
| | 0 | 0.5 | 1.0 | 1.5 | 2.0 | Score |
| KPS | ≤50 | 60 | 70–80 | 90–100 | n/a | ____ |
| Subtype | Basal | n/a | LumA | HER2 | LumB | ____ |
| Age | ≥60 | <60 | n/a | n/a | n/a | ____ |
| | | | | | Sum total = | ____ |

Subtype:
Basal, triple negative (ER/PR/HER2-neg)
LumA, luminal A (ER/PR-pos, HER2-neg)
LumB, luminal B (triple positive, ER/PR/HER2-pos)
HER2, HER2-pos, ER/PR-neg

MS (months) by GPA: GPA 0–1.0 = 3.4; 1.5–2.0 = 7.7; 2.5–3.0 = 15.1; 3.5–4.0 = 25.3

| Renal cell carcinoma | | | | |
|---|---|---|---|---|
| | 0 | 1.0 | 2.0 | Score |
| KPS | <70 | 70–80 | 90–100 | ____ |
| #BM | >3 | 2–3 | 1 | ____ |
| | | | Sum total = | ____ |

MS (months) by GPA: GPA 0–1.0 = 3.3; 1.5–2.0 = 7.3; 2.5–3.0 = 11.3; 3.5–4.0 = 14.8

| GI cancers | | | | | | |
|---|---|---|---|---|---|---|
| | 0 | 1 | 2 | 3 | 4 | Score |
| KPS | <70 | 70 | 80 | 90 | 100 | ____ |

MS (months) by GPA: GPA 0–1.0 = 3.1; 2.0 = 4.4; 3.0 = 6.9; 4.0 = 13.5

Abbreviations: *GPA* Graded Prognostic Assessment, *KPS* Karnofsky Performance Status, *ECM* extracranial metastases, *#BM* number of brain metastases, *ER* estrogen receptor, *PR* progesterone receptor, *HER2* human epidermal growth factor receptor 2, *MS* median survival in months, *neg/unk* negative or unknown
Based on data from Refs. [17, 19, 21]

**Table 30.6** Multivariable analysis of risk of death and median survival[a] by treatment and diagnosis

| Diagnosis | Statistics | Treatment | | | | | |
|---|---|---|---|---|---|---|---|
| | | WBRT | SRS | WBRT + SRS | S + SRS | S + WBRT | S + WBRT+SRS |
| NSCLC | Risk of death (HR) | 1.0 | 1.08 | 1.20 | 0.66[b] | 0.78 | 0.79 |
| n = 1521 | 95% CI | | 0.92–1.27 | 0.94–1.54 | 0.50–0.88 | 0.58–1.06 | 0.40–1.58 |
| | p-Value | | 0.35 | 0.15 | <0.01 | 0.11 | 0.51 |
| | Median survival[a] | 13 | 14 | 10 | 32 | 20 | 20 |
| | n (%) | 342 (22%) | 767 (50%) | 139 (9%) | 114 (7%) | 76 (5%) | 13 (1%) |
| SCLC | Risk of death (HR) | 1.0 | 0.97 | 0.24[b] | 0.00 | 0.42[b] | 0.00 |
| n = 281 | 95% CI | | 0.41–2.26 | 0.10–0.59 | NA | 0.25–0.73 | NA |
| | p-Value | | 0.94 | 0.002 | 0.99 | 0.002 | 0.98 |
| | Median survival[a] | 4 | 7 | 15 | 12 | 15 | 15 |
| | n (%) | 229 (81%) | 13 (5%) | 21 (7%) | 1 (0.4%) | 16 (6%) | 1 (0.4%) |
| Melanoma | Risk of death (HR) | 1.0 | 0.69[b] | 0.62[b] | 0.50[b] | 0.54[b] | 0.70 |
| n = 823 | 95% CI | | 0.54–0.89 | 0.45–0.86 | 0.36–0.69 | 0.35–0.84 | 0.36–1.36 |
| | p-Value | | <0.01 | <0.01 | <0.01 | <0.01 | 0.29 |
| | Median survival[a] | 6 | 10 | 9 | 13 | 11 | 11 |
| | n (%) | 91 (11%) | 464 (56%) | 73 (9%) | 95 (12%) | 34 (4%) | 12 (1%) |
| Renal cell | Risk of death (HR) | 1.0 | 0.83 | 0.70 | 0.87 | 0.66 | 0.68 |
| n = 286 | 95% CI | | 0.56–1.21 | 0.43–1.14 | 0.42–1.83 | 0.37–1.17 | 0.09–5.01 |
| | p-Value | | 0.33 | 0.15 | 0.71 | 0.16 | 0.70 |
| | Median survival[a] | 5 | 11 | 12 | 13 | 16 | 9 |
| | n (%) | 78 (27%) | 131 (46%) | 46 (16%) | 11 (4%) | 18 (6%) | 2 (1%) |
| Breast cancer | Risk of death (HR) | 1.0 | 1.07 | 0.74 | 0.59 | 0.72 | 0.47[b] |
| n = 400 | 95% CI | | 0.66–1.73 | 0.47–1.16 | 0.28–1.23 | 0.43–1.21 | 0.23–0.96 |
| | p-Value | | 0.80 | 0.18 | 0.16 | 0.72 | 0.04 |
| | Median survival[a] | 7 | 13 | 15 | 24 | 18 | 30 |
| | n (%) | 131 (33%) | 115 (29%) | 86 (22%) | 19 (5%) | 28 (7%) | 20 (5%) |
| GI cancer | Risk of death (HR) | 1.0 | 0.72 | 0.69 | 2.30 | 0.33[b] | 0.39[b] |
| n = 209 | 95% CI | | 0.40–1.28 | 0.39–1.22 | 0.43–12.4 | 0.19–0.56 | 0.17–0.90 |
| | p-Value | | 0.26 | 0.21 | 0.33 | <0.001 | 0.03 |
| | Median survival[a] | 3 | 7 | 7 | 9 | 10 | 8 |
| | n (%) | 95 (45%) | 35 (17%) | 35 (17%) | 2 (1%) | 34 (16%) | 8 (4%) |

Diagnoses: *NSCLC* non-small cell lung cancer (adenocarcinoma), *SCLC* small cell lung cancer, *GI* gastrointestinal

Treatments: *S* surgery, *WBRT* whole-brain radiation therapy, *SRS* stereotactic radiosurgery

Statistics: Risk of death: hazard ratio (HR) normalized to patients treated with whole-brain radiation therapy alone (HR = 1.0) and calculated by multivariable Cox regression, adjusted for DS-GPA and stratified by institution

Based on data from Refs. [17, 19, 21]

[a]Median survival in months based on one-sample Kaplan-Meier method

[b]Statistically significantly better than WBRT alone; 95% confidence interval

## Case Study

A 36-year-old [22] white female marathon runner presented in August 2005 with a right neck mass. Fine needle aspiration initially confirmed a malignancy, later confirmed as a malignant melanoma by excisional biopsy of a posterior scalp lesion on 9-15-05. This malignant melanoma was histopathologically staged as Clark's Level IV, Breslow depth at least 6 mm, with angiolymphatic invasion, and positive deep and peripheral margins. Brain MRI for initial radiologic staging on September 27, 2005, showed multiple scalp lesions but no evidence of parenchymal brain metastases. PET scan September 27, 2005, showed hypermetabolic activity only in the left neck. On October 11, 2005, she underwent a left modified radical neck dissection and wide local excision of the scalp lesion. Pathology confirmed meta-

static melanoma in 3 of 28 lymph nodes with extension into the adjacent soft tissues in two areas. Pathology from the scalp excision showed a maximum tumor depth of 1.9 cm, and the deep margin remained positive. She underwent two additional scalp excisions, and the deep margin remained positive. Her stage was T4bN2bM0, stage IIIC. She received 64 Gy radiation therapy to the left neck and scalp, completed 1-20-06. She then received three cycles of cisplatinum, interferon, and vinblastine followed by interleukin-2, completed in March 2006. She did well without evidence of recurrence until November 2006 when she underwent a debridement of necrotic tissue in the scalp lesion. PET scan on December 05, 2006, showed a 0.7 cm hypermetabolic nodule in the retroperitoneum consistent with metastatic recurrence. Brain MRI on December 06, 2006, showed three brain metastases (2.5 cm right caudate, 1.1 cm left parieto-occipital, and

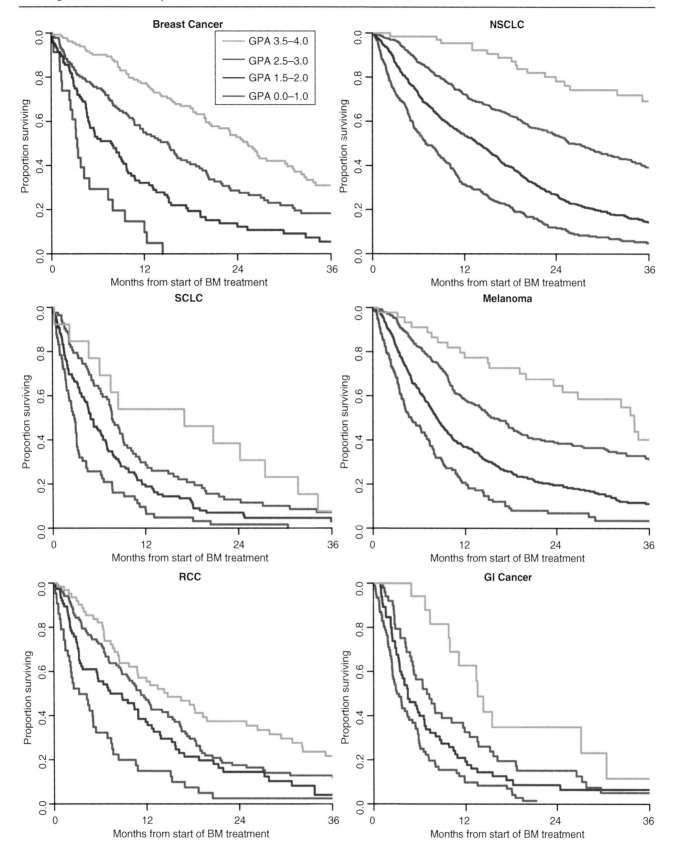

**Fig. 30.2** Kaplan-Meier curves for survival by GPA for six diagnoses: breast cancer, non-small cell lung cancer, small cell lung cancer, melanoma, renal cell carcinoma, gastrointestinal cancers

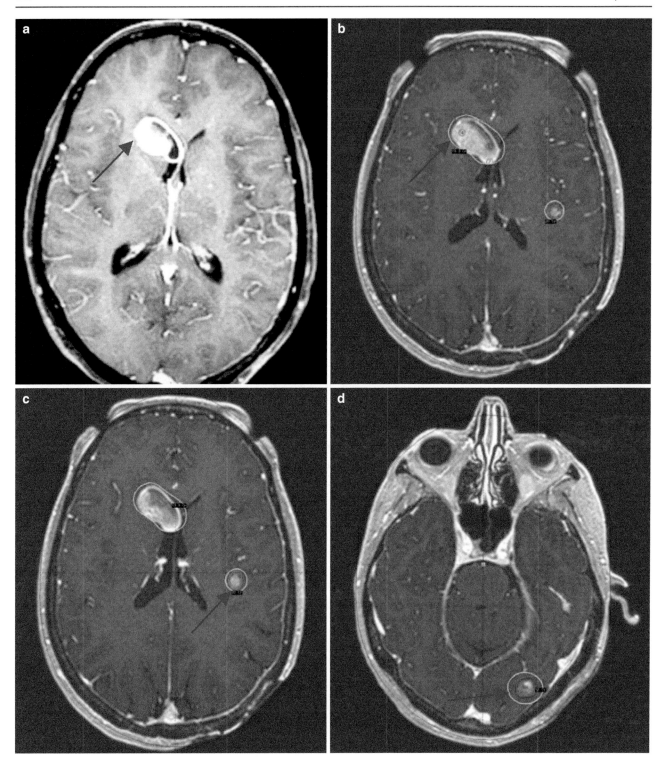

**Fig. 30.3** Serial brain MRI images of case study. (**a**) Initial MRI shows largest of three brain metastases, December 06, 2006. (**b**) Gamma Knife plan for right frontal brain metastasis, December 13, 2006. (**c**) Gamma Knife plan for left frontal brain metastasis, December 13, 2006. (**d**) Gamma Knife plan for left occipital brain metastasis, December 13, 2006. (**e**) MRI 9 months after GK shows marked radiation necrosis and edema, September 26, 2007. (**f**) MRI 18 months after GK shows resolving radiation necrosis, May 23, 2008. (**g**) MRI 21 months after GK shows minimal residual enhancement, October 23, 2008. (**h**) MRI 10.7 years after GK shows no evidence of disease, August 02, 2017

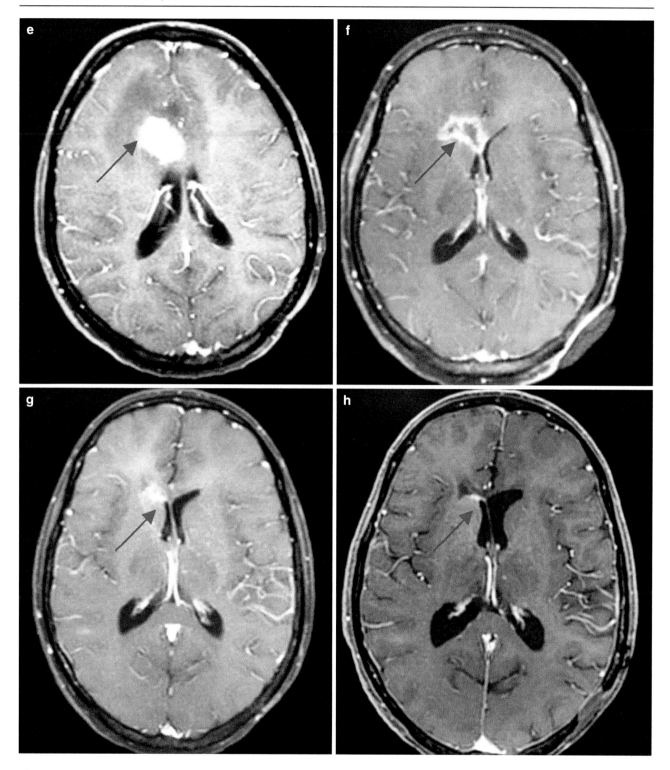

**Fig. 30.3** (continued)

0.7 cm left posterior frontal) (Fig. 30.3a), which were not present on the prior scan of June 22, 2006.

Whole-brain radiation therapy was not given (and has not been given) due to the prior scalp radiation. She underwent SRS (Gamma Knife) on December 13, 2006, to all three lesions: right caudate, 20 Gy to a volume of 8.4 cc (Fig. 30.3b); left posterior frontal, 24 Gy to a volume of 0.47 cc (Fig. 30.3c); and left parieto-occipital, 24 Gy to a volume of 1.6 cc (Fig. 30.3d). She underwent SABR to the pelvic soft tissue metastasis (25 Gy in five fractions over 2 weeks, completed on February 23, 2007). Between March and June 2007, she received four cycles of carboplatin, paclitaxel, and temozolomide treatment. In September 2007, she developed headaches, nausea, vomiting, and confusion. MRI on September 26, 2007, showed a marked increase in enhancement and edema in the right frontal lobe consistent with radiation necrosis (Fig. 30.3e). Due to increased headaches and possible radiation necrosis, the temozolomide was discontinued. She has received no treatment since September 2007. The edema was treated with steroids, which were gradually tapered off over 4 months. Brain MRI on May 23, 2008, showed improvement with central necrosis of the previously solid-appearing lesion (Fig. 30.3f). Brain MRI on October 23, 2008, showed further resolution of the enhancement/necrosis with minimal residual enhancement (Fig. 30.3g). Serial imaging since that time has shown no evidence of recurrent tumor or necrosis.

She remains clinically and radiographically free of disease 11 years after the diagnosis of multiple brain metastases and more than 10 years after completion of treatment. Brain MRI on August 02, 2017, showed no change in the minimal residual enhancement/scar tissue (Fig. 30.3h), and PET scan on August 02, 2017, showed no evidence of disease. She has remained asymptomatic for over a decade and continues to run marathons, as recently as October 14, 2017. In November 2017, she completed the FACT-Brain questionnaire, a patient-reported QOL tool to reassess brain cognition. Her FACT-BR score was perfect (200 on a scale of 200), 11 years after diagnosis of her brain metastases. Notably, this patient never underwent craniotomy or whole-brain radiation therapy and thus avoided the related long-term neurocognitive toxicity of these interventions.

To fully appreciate this patient's remarkable outcome, it is appropriate to review how her outcome compares to the best available evidence of survival for melanoma patients with brain metastases. We recently updated and published the melanoma-molGPA [7] based on a multi-institutional retrospective study of 483 melanoma patients with brain metastases diagnosed between January 01, 2006, and December 31, 2015. Notably, the patient presented here was diagnosed in 2006, so she is a contemporary of the patients in the melanoma-molGPA update study. The study showed five prognostic factors significant for survival. Table 30.5 shows

a worksheet with which to calculate the melanoma-molGPA. To further simplify calculation of the melanoma-molGPA, a free user-friendly app is available at brainmetgpa.com. Overall median survival has improved from 6 to 10 months since the 1980s, and the median survival by melanoma-molGPA groups for GPA of 0–1.0, 1.5–2.0, 2.5–3.0, and 3.5–4.0 was 4.9, 8.3, 15.8, and 34.1 months, respectively. The patient presented here had a melanoma-GPA of 3.0 on a 4.0 scale on both the original and updated GPA index, correlating with an estimated survival of 8.8 and 15.8 months, respectively. This patient is disease-free and asymptomatic with a perfect FACT-Brain QOL score 11 years after the diagnosis of multiple brain metastases. Clearly, prognostic indices are imperfect but nonetheless provide our best estimate of survival for these patients.

## Summary

Patients with brain metastases are a heterogeneous population and outcomes vary widely by diagnosis and diagnosis-specific prognostic factors. Because of this heterogeneity and the plethora of available treatment options, it is difficult to estimate survival. These problems have complicated clinical decision-making as well as interpretation of clinical trials. The Graded Prognostic Assessment (GPA) is a diagnosis-specific prognostic index which has been updated to reflect the current treatment era by incorporating diagnosis-specific prognostic factors including molecular factors such as tumor subtype and gene status. The GPA is useful for clinical decision-making as physicians determine whether and what treatment is appropriate for these patients. It can also be useful to stratify clinical trials to ensure those trials are comparing comparable patients, which is especially important in such a heterogeneous patient population. Without accurate stratification, the results of clinical trials are uninterpretable and a waste of resources.

## Self-Assessment Questions

1. According to the updated Diagnosis-Specific Graded Prognostic Assessment (DS-GPA) for lung cancer (lung-molGPA), the significant prognostic factors for patients with lung cancer and brain metastases are which of the following?
   A. Age, KPS, number of brain metastases
   B. Age, KPS, presence of extracranial metastases
   C. Age, KPS, EGFR status, presence of extracranial metastases
   D. Age, KPS, EGFR and ALK status, presence of extracranial metastases, number of brain metastases

2. According to the updated Diagnosis-Specific Graded Prognostic Assessment (DS-GPA) for breast cancer (breast-GPA), the significant prognostic factors for patients with breast cancer and brain metastases are which of the following?
   A. Age, KPS, number of brain metastases
   B. Age, KPS, presence of extracranial metastases
   C. Age, KPS, estrogen, and progesterone receptor status
   D. Age, KPS, tumor subtype

3. According to the updated Diagnosis-Specific Graded Prognostic Assessment (DS-GPA) for melanoma (melanoma-molGPA), the significant prognostic factors for patients with melanoma and brain metastases are which of the following?
   A. Age, KPS, BRAF status, number of brain metastases
   B. Age, KPS, presence of extracranial metastases, number of brain metastases
   C. Age, KPS, BRAF status, presence of extracranial metastases
   D. Age, KPS, BRAF status, presence of extracranial metastases, number of brain metastases

4. The two prognostic indices, the Radiation Therapy Oncology Group Recursive Partitioning Analysis (RTOG RPA) and the Diagnosis-Specific Graded Prognostic Assessment (DS-GPA) for patients with brain metastases differ in which of the following ways?
   A. Both consider control of the primary tumor.
   B. They use the same factors but the DS-GPA is based on larger, more current data.
   C. The DS-GPA considers the molecular profile of the tumor.
   D. The estimated survival for the best prognostic group for each index is about the same.

5. What is the GPA and estimated survival for a 69-year-old patient with ALK-positive lung adenocarcinoma, KPS 90, no extracranial metastases, and four brain metastases?
   A. GPA 4.0, estimated survival 47 months
   B. GPA 3.0, estimated survival 26.5 months
   C. GPA 2.0, estimated survival 13.7 months
   D. GPA 3.5, estimated survival 12 months

## Answers

1. D
2. D
3. D
4. C
5. A

**Acknowledgments** This work has been a collaborative multi-institutional effort. The faculty and residents of the following institutions have selflessly contributed time and energy to one or more of the studies on the Graded Prognostic Assessment: MD Anderson; Memorial Sloan Kettering Cancer Center; Mayo Clinic; University of California, San Francisco; Massachusetts General Hospital; Dana-Farber Cancer Institute; Duke University; Yale University; University of Colorado Denver; Cleveland Clinic; University of Wisconsin-Madison; McGill University; Centre Hospitalier de l' Université de Montreal; University of Maryland; University of Alabama at Birmingham; and the University of Minnesota. This work would not have been possible without the tireless work of these dedicated colleagues. Special recognition is appropriate for Ryan Shanley who has provided his statistical wisdom for nearly a decade.

## References

1. Gavrilovic IT, Posner JB. Brain metastases: epidemiology and pathophysiology. J Neurooncol. 2005;75(1):5–14.
2. Park DM, Posner JB. Management of intracranial metastases: history. In: Sawaya R, editor. Intracranial metastases: current management strategies. Oxford, England: Blackwell Publishing Ltd; 2004. p. 3–19.
3. Yamamoto M, Serizawa T, Shuto T, et al. Stereotactic radiosurgery for patients with multiple brain metastases (JLGK0901): a multi-institutional prospective observational study. Lancet Oncol. 2014;15(4):387–95.
4. Aoyama H, Shirato H, Tago M, et al. Stereotactic radiosurgery plus whole-brain radiation therapy vs stereotactic radiosurgery alone for treatment of brain metastases, a randomized controlled trial. JAMA. 2006;295:2483–91.
5. Chang EL, Wefel JS, Hess KR, et al. Neurocognition in patients with brain metastases treated with radiosurgery or radiosurgery plus whole-brain irradiation: a randomized controlled trial. Lancet Oncol. 2009;10:1037–44.
6. Kocher M, Soffietti R, Abacioglu U, et al. Adjuvant whole-brain radiotherapy versus observation after radiosurgery or surgical resection of one to three cerebral metastases: results of the EORTC 22952–26001 Study. J Clin Oncol. 2011;29:134–41.
7. Brown PD, Jaeckle K, Ballman KV, et al. Effect of radiosurgery alone vs radiosurgery with whole brain radiation therapy on cognitive function in patients with 1 to 3 brain metastases. JAMA. 2016;4:401–9.
8. Mulvenna P, Nankivell M, Barton R, et al. Dexamethasone and supportive care with or without whole brain radiotherapy in treating patients with non-small cell lung cancer with brain metastases unsuitable for resection or stereotactic radiotherapy (QUARTZ): results from a phase 3, non-inferiority, randomized trial. Lancet. 2016;388:2004–14.
9. Gaspar LE, Scott C, Rotman M, et al. Recursive partitioning analysis (RPA) of prognostic factors in three Radiation Therapy Oncology Group (RTOG) brain metastases trials. Int J Radiat Oncol Biol Phys. 1997;37:745–51.
10. Weltman E, Salvajoli JV, Brandt RA, et al. Radiosurgery for brain metastases: a score index for predicting prognosis. Int J Radiat Oncol Biol Phys. 2000;46:1155–61.
11. Lorenzoni J, Devriendt D, Massager N, et al. Radiosurgery for treatment of brain metastases: estimation of patient eligibility using three stratification systems. Int J Radiat Oncol Biol Phys. 2004;60:218–24.
12. Sloan-Barnholtz-Sloan JS, Yu C, Sloan AE, et al. A nomogram for individualized estimation of survival among patients with brain metastasis. Neuro Oncol. 2012;14:910–8.

13. Kondziolka D, Parry PV, Lunsford DL, et al. The accuracy of predicting survival in individual patients with cancer. J Neurosurg. 2014;120:24–30.
14. Sperduto PW, Berkey B, Gaspar LE, et al. A new prognostic index and comparison to three other indices for patients with brain metastases: an analysis of 1960 patients in the RTOG database. Int J Radiat Oncol Biol Phys. 2008;70:510–4.
15. Sperduto PW, Chao ST, Sneed PK, et al. Diagnosis-specific prognostic factors, indexes, and treatment outcomes for patients with newly diagnosed brain metastases: a multi-institutional analysis of 4,259 patients. Int J Radiat Oncol Biol Phys. 2010;77:655–61.
16. Sperduto PW, Kased N, Roberge D, et al. The effect of tumor subtype on survival and the Graded Prognostic Assessment (GPA) for patients with breast cancer and brain metastases. Int J Radiat Oncol Biol Phys. 2011. https://doi.org/10.1016/j.ijrobp.2011.02.027.
17. Sperduto PW, Kased N, Roberge D, et al. Summary report on the graded prognostic assessment: an accurate and facile diagnosis-specific tool to estimate survival for patients with brain metastases. J Clin Oncol. 2011;30:419–25.
18. Sperduto PW, Yang TJ, Beal K, et al. The effect of gene alterations and tyrosine kinase inhibition on survival and cause of death in patients with adenocarcinoma of the lung and brain metastases. Int J Radiat Oncol Biol Phys. 2016;96(2):406–13.
19. Sperduto PW, Yang TJ, Beal K, et al. Improved survival and prognostic ability in lung cancer patients with brain metastases: an update of the graded prognostic assessment for lung cancer using molecular markers (lung-molGPA). JAMA Oncol. 2016;3:827–31. https://doi.org/10.1001/jamaoncol.2016.3834.
20. Sperduto PW, Jiang W, Brown PD, et al. The prognostic value of BRAF, cKIT and NRAS mutations in melanoma patients with brain metastases. Int J Radiat Oncol Biol Phys. 2017;98(5):1069–77.
21. Sperduto PW, Jiang W, Brown PD, et al. Estimating survival in melanoma patients with brain metastases: an update of the graded prognostic assessment for melanoma using molecular markers (melanoma-molGPA). Int J Radiat Oncol Biol Phys. 2017;99(4):812–6.
22. Sperduto WA, King D, Watanabe Y, et al. Case report of extended survival and quality of life in a melanoma patient with multiple brain metastases and review of literature. Cureus. 2017;9(12):e1947. https://doi.org/10.7759/cureus.1947.

# Neurosurgical Management of Single Brain Metastases

# 31

Sherise D. Ferguson, Richard G. Everson, Kathryn M. Wagner, Debra Nana Yeboa, Ian E. McCutcheon, and Raymond Sawaya

## Learning Objectives

- To understand the surgical indications for brain metastasis.
- To describe the RPA classification and its impact on patient selection for surgical resection.
- To understand the indication for radiosurgery in the management of brain metastasis.
- To describe surgical adjuncts available for resection of metastasis located in eloquent cortex.

## Introduction

Brain metastases are the most common brain tumors in adults and will be diagnosed in ~200,000 patients in the United States alone this year, outnumbering primary brain tumors by more than 5:1 [1–3]. Overall, approximately 8–10% of patients with systemic cancer will develop symptomatic brain metastases [4–6]. Lung cancer, breast cancer, and melanoma are the most common solid tumors to spread to the central nervous system (CNS) [4]. The frequency of brain metastases in melanoma is the highest of all major cancers, with 40–60%

of all patients with melanoma developing brain metastases [7]. Approximately 37–50% of patients with solid tumors present with single brain metastases, but 50–63% have multiple metastases at initial presentation [8, 9]. Of all the patients diagnosed with brain metastases, half will die within 3–27 months after the initial diagnosis [4–6].

These issues are pressing, as the incidence of brain metastasis may be increasing due to newer therapies (targeted inhibitors and immunotherapy) that lengthen the survival of patients with systemic cancer [6, 10]. Care of patients with brain metastases is best performed by multispecialty teams consisting of medical oncologists, neurosurgeons, and radiation oncologists. Members of the interdisciplinary team must understand the nuances of available treatment modalities in order to provide optimal, individualized care for patients. In this chapter, we will focus on the neurosurgical management of single brain metastasis with an emphasis on patient selection, surgical technique, and treatment outcome. As evidence from well-designed randomized controlled trials continues to accumulate and factors beyond oncologic control are increasingly being included as endpoints, members of the neuro-oncology community are utilizing individualized and disease-specific approaches. The treatment of brain metastasis has become tailored, and treatment paradigms vary depending on the individual patient. Surgery remains the cornerstone in brain metastasis treatment, and this review will outline its role and the role of radiosurgery in the treatment of single brain metastases.

S. D. Ferguson (✉) · I. E. McCutcheon · R. Sawaya
Department of Neurosurgery, The University of Texas MD Anderson Cancer Center, Houston, TX, USA
e-mail: sdferguson@mdanderson.org

R. G. Everson
Department of Neurosurgery, UCLA Medical Center, Los Angeles, CA, USA

K. M. Wagner
Department of Neurosurgery, Baylor College of Medicine, Houston, TX, USA

D. N. Yeboa
Department of Radiation Oncology, The University of Texas MD Anderson Cancer Center, Houston, TX, USA

## Single Brain Metastases

### Surgery

A solitary brain metastasis is one brain lesion without evidence of extracranial metastasis, whereas a single brain metastasis is defined as one lesion in the brain with at least one other site of extracranial disease or uncontrolled primary cancer. The essential role of surgical resection in the treatment of single brain metastases is firmly established. The positive impact of surgery was solidified after the completion of two landmark, randomized clinical trials. The first was conducted by Patchell and colleagues, who randomized patients with a single brain metastasis to receive tumor resection followed by whole-brain radiation therapy (WBRT) ($n = 25$) or WBRT alone ($n = 23$) and subsequently reported the indispensable advantages of surgical resection. First, patients in the surgical resection group survived significantly longer than patients treated with WBRT alone (median survival of 40 weeks versus 15 weeks, respectively). Surgery was also associated with a lower risk of local recurrence (20%) relative to WBRT alone (52%). Finally, surgical patients maintained functional independence (defined by a Karnofsky Performance Scale [KPS] score of >70) significantly longer (median, 38 weeks) relative to patients treated with only WBRT (median, 8 weeks) [11]. Vecht et al. conducted another prospective randomized trial that included 63 patients, which similarly confirmed the benefits of surgical resection. Patients undergoing surgery improved in functional status more quickly than those exclusively treated with radiation. Surgical patients also benefited from significantly longer survival and had prolonged functional independence compared with patients undergoing WBRT alone [12].

In addition to the evidence presented above, tumor resection has several other practical clinical advantages. This is particularly the case with large (>3 cm in maximal diameter), symptomatic lesions. When patients present urgently with significant neurological symptoms or impending herniation, surgical resection is the only way to promptly reduce intracranial pressure and address compressive mass effect. In their analysis of 206 brain metastasis patients (~58% of patients had solitary or single metastases), Schödel et al. reported improved neurological function in 56.8% of all patients, most notably in patients with increased intracranial pressure and hemiparesis [13]. Moreover, large metastases involving the posterior fossa (cerebellum) or ventricular system can obstruct the flow of cerebrospinal fluid (CSF), causing hydrocephalus, which can pose a life-threatening emergency. Surgical removal of the mass can quickly restore CSF pathways and rapidly reverse associated symptoms and neurological deficits. Brain metastases may also cause cortical irritation and seizures in a subset of patients, and surgery may help in attaining seizure control when medical management fails. It is important to note that there is no firm evidence that prophylactic administration of antiepileptic drugs in patients with brain metastases is beneficial in patients who have never had a seizure [14–16]. Brain metastases are also

commonly associated with vasogenic cerebral edema, which can be mild or substantial, causing neurological sequelae. Edema can often be managed with the administration of steroids (i.e., dexamethasone), but in the circumstance of refractory symptomatic edema, tumor resection is beneficial [17] (Fig. 31.1).

In the setting of known systemic cancer, a newly discovered brain lesion is often correctly assumed to be a brain metastasis. However, in a patient with an unknown primary cancer, multiple primaries, or imaging characteristics concerning for an alternative pathology (e.g., lymphoma, glioma), surgical intervention (i.e., biopsy/resection) may be required to confirm diagnosis and formulate an appropriate treatment plan. This scenario is not rare, as 11% of patients with a primary cancer outside the CNS may have a nonmetastatic lesion [11] (Figs. 31.2 and 31.3).

When possible, the goal of surgery is gross-total resection (GTR), as it is well accepted that complete resection significantly improves patient outcome [18, 19]. A single-institution study evaluated the outcome of 271 patients with single brain metastases and specifically focused on predictors of patient outcome. These authors reported that GTR of the metastasis was associated with a median patient survival time of 10.6 months versus subtotal resection (STR), which led to a median survival time of 8.7 months. This result did not quite reach statistical significance ($p = 0.07$), but it should be noted that the patients in this study were treated from 1984 to 2004, and surgical techniques and their adjuncts have advanced since then [18]. In a more recent study, Lee et al. conducted a retrospective study (1995–2011) detailing the surgical outcome of 157 patients with brain metastases. Approximately 60% of patients had a single brain metastasis ($n = 96$), and their median overall survival post resection was 19.3 months. The authors reported that extent of surgical resection significantly correlated with survival. Specifically, patients who had a STR had a median survival time of 15.1 months compared with 20.4 months in patients where GTR was achieved [19]. Even though the cancer patient population can be a challenging one (i.e., typically it includes many older patients, those with medical comorbidities, and most are undergoing systemic chemotherapy), surgical resection is generally well tolerated in these carefully selected patients. A retrospective study evaluating the surgical outcome of 69 patients undergoing resection of single brain metastases reported clinical improvement of neurological symptoms in 90% of patients and no major complications occurring within 30 days of surgery [20]. A large retrospective review of 208 patients undergoing resection for brain metastases (191 with single lesions) reported an overall operative mortality of

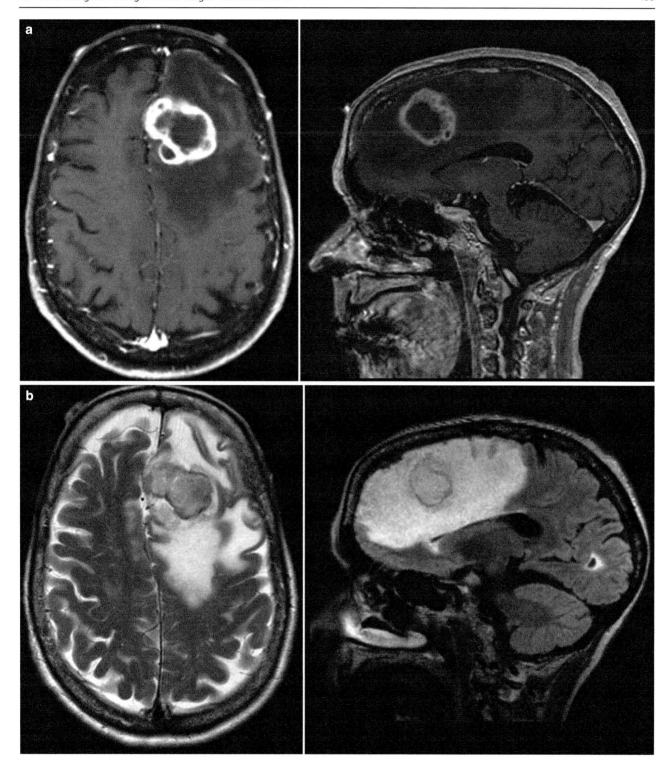

**Fig. 31.1** (**a**) A 56-year-old female with a history of lung adenocarcinoma who presented with worsening headaches. T1 contrast-enhanced MRI in the axial (left) and sagittal (right) planes shows a 3.3 cm in diameter heterogeneously enhancing lesion in the left frontal lobe. (**b**) T2/FLAIR-weighted MR images (axial and sagittal) show the signifi- cant edema surrounding the lesion. (**c**) Left panel: T1-weighted con- trast-enhanced MRI (sagittal plane) immediately post resection showing gross-total resection. Right panel: T2-weighted MRI obtained 30 days postoperatively showing improvement of surrounding edema

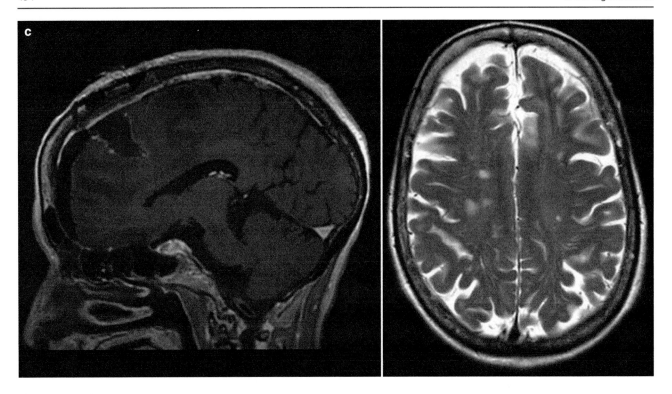

**Fig. 31.1** (continued)

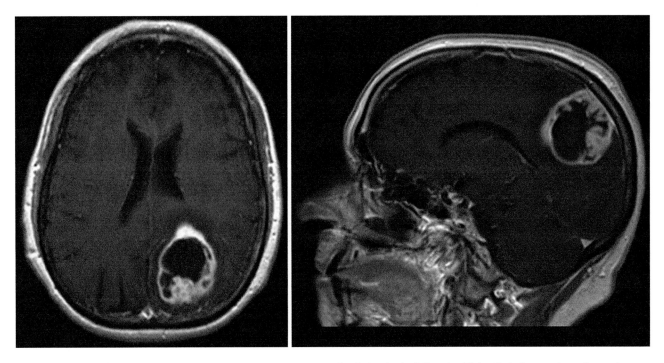

**Fig. 31.2** A 64-year-old female with a history of endometrial stromal sarcoma who presented with headaches and dizziness. MRI [axial (left) and sagittal (right)] showed a 4 cm in diameter heterogeneously enhanc- ing lesion in the left parietal lobe. Pathology at time of resection was consistent with glioblastoma

1.9% [21]. Another study analyzed a cohort of 206 patients with brain metastases treated with surgical resection, with the majority of patients having a single or solitary metastasis (~58%). The authors reported similarly low complication rates, with mortality and morbidity rates of 0% and 10.3%, respectively [13]. However, despite the many advantages of surgery, its use must be tempered by the overall clinical picture.

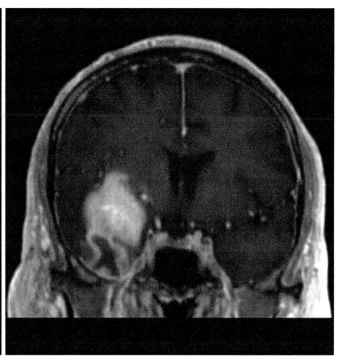

**Fig. 31.3** A 79-year-old male with a history of melanoma. Routine staging post-contrast MRI [axial (left) and coronal (right) plane] showed a complex heterogeneously enhancing lesion in the right anterior tempo- ral lobe and a second lesion in the medial posterior temporal lobe. Pathology findings at time of resection of the larger lesion were consis- tent with glioblastoma (the smaller secondary lesion was not biopsied)

Achieving the full benefit of surgical resection requires good patient selection. To that end, prognostic scales have been generated in order to optimize treatment algorithms and more accurately predict surgical outcomes for brain metastasis. Surgery is most suited for patients with con- trolled systemic disease and high functional performance status. A recent study reviewed the outcome of 264 patients with brain metastasis undergoing resection and analyzed the clinical factors associated with early postoperative death (defined as death within 6 months). Multivariate analysis demonstrated that a lower KPS score (<70), uncontrolled systemic disease, and lack of postoperative systemic ther- apy were all associated with early death after resection [22]. Focusing on these salient factors, the Radiation Therapy Oncology Group (RTOG) developed the recursive partition- ing analysis [RPA] classification system based on patient age, control of systemic disease, KPS score, and status of extracranial disease. RPA class I is associated with the best anticipated outcome, whereas RPA class III patients have the worst prognosis. Tendulkar et al. [18] analyzed the sur- gical outcome of 271 patients undergoing resection of a single brain metastasis. They reported a significant correla- tion between patient survival and RPA class; post resection, the mean survival times of RPA class I, II, and II patients were 21.4 months, 9 months, and 8.9 months, respectively. Since this landmark study, the predictive impact of RPA class has been validated in multiple surgical series [19, 21, 23, 24]. Overall in RPA class I patients, surgery carries a

favorable prognosis, making this patient population most suitable for surgical resection. The Graded Prognostic Assessment (GPA) is a newer prognostic index for patients with brain metastases. The GPA score is based on age, KPS score, number of intracranial lesions, and status of systemic disease. Median overall survival times based on GPA score are 2.6 months for 0–1 points, 3.8 months for 1.5–2.5 points, 6.9 months for 3 points, and 11 months for 3.5–4 points. This prognostic index was generated from a database of 1960 patients accrued to four RTOG protocols for patients with brain metastasis [25, 26]. This index has been shown to be equally accurate as the RPA score in predicting survival, but it is inherently more quantitative and potentially more clinical relevant [27]. Moreover, the diagnosis-specific GPA accounts for tumor histology, and the unique characteristics of each primary tumor are taken into account, making this grading system pertinent to clinical practice. These histol- ogy-specific prognostic indices are based on multi-institu- tional analysis of 4259 patients with brain metastases from breast carcinoma, small-cell and non-small cell lung carci- noma, GI cancers, melanoma, and renal cell carcinoma [26, 28, 29]. Overall, these prognostic scales emphasize the impact of systemic disease status. Moreover, recent data suggest that systemic disease and a patient's individual responsiveness to systemic therapy may be more likely to impact mortality than the presence of brain metastases [30].

In regard to surgery, the value of GTR is undisputed. A number of recent studies contend that the method of surgical resection is also a key component in determining patient outcome. Historically, tumor resection has involved internal debulking of the lesion followed by dissection of the tumor capsule from the surrounding brain parenchyma. Resection in this piecemeal fashion can successfully achieve GTR, but from an oncological prospective, it may be suboptimal because violation of the tumor capsule potentially exposes the surrounding cortex to malignant cells. In order to avoid this and to prevent the increased bleeding that can be encountered when directly entering the lesion, multiple studies now advocate an en bloc resection technique. En bloc resection entails circumferential dissection of the tumor along the brain tumor interface without violating the tumor capsule; hence it avoids spillage of tumor contents. Additionally, this method is technically feasible for metastatic lesions in particular as they have macroscopically sharp borders, are surrounded by a gliotic pseudocapsule, and usually infiltrate the surrounding cortex to a limited distance (<5 mm) [31–33]. Moreover, confining dissection to the typically hypovascular brain margin reduces intraoperative bleeding and allows surgical boundaries to be more clear. Recent data support the en bloc technique as both feasible and safe. An analysis of 1033 surgical patients, 62% of which underwent en bloc resection, demonstrated that an en bloc technique was not associated with increased complication rates compared with piecemeal resection, even when tumors were located in eloquent (functional) cortex [34].

En bloc resection has several other clinical benefits. First, it has been associated with a lower risk of local recurrence relative to traditional piecemeal resection. One notable study analyzed the predictors of local recurrence in 570 surgical patients who underwent GTR of a single brain metastasis (without postoperative WBRT). In this patient cohort, the overall incidence of local recurrence was 15%. It showed that patients who underwent piecemeal resection were 1.7 times more likely to develop local recurrence than those with tumors resected in an en bloc fashion [35]. Patients undergoing en bloc resection have also been shown to have a lower risk of developing leptomeningeal disease (LMD), a devastating sequela of CNS metastases with a very poor prognosis. Ahn et al. retrospectively analyzed 242 patients who underwent surgical resection for brain metastases (68% of whom had a single lesion) to determine the predictors of LMD. An en bloc technique was utilized in 36% of cases, while the remaining cases were resected in a piecemeal fashion. Overall, 10% of patients subsequently developed LMD. Multivariate analysis showed that piecemeal resection carried ~3× the risk for subsequent LMD development as en bloc resection (HR 3.67) did. Of note, direct contact of the tumor with the CSF space (the surface of the tumor contacting the pia mater or the ventricle wall without intervening brain parenchyma) or involvement of the CSF space (observing pial or ependymal contrast enhancement on magnetic resonance [MR] imaging) also significantly increased the risk of LMD (HRs of 6.3 and 9, respectively) [36].

Metastases in the posterior fossa are of particular concern due to the proximity of CSF spaces that may predispose patients to the development of LMD. As such, the University of Texas MD Anderson Cancer Center (MD Anderson) reported the impact of tumor resection method on 260 surgically treated posterior fossa metastases, with 123 of these surgeries being performed in an en bloc fashion. Overall, GTR was achieved in 96% of patients, and 10% of patients developed LMD ($n = 26/260$). Piecemeal resection was significantly associated with an increased risk of LMD, with 13.9% of such patients developing subsequent LMD compared with only 5.7% of en bloc resection patients [37].

The principle of en bloc resection has recently been expanded, and the concept of supramarginal resection has emerged in recent literature. Unlike primary brain tumors, which are diffusely infiltrating, brain metastases are classically considered to have distinct borders. However, even though at gross inspection the borders of metastases may appear distinctive, recent pathological studies suggest that microscopic tumor infiltration of adjacent brain may be present in a subset of these lesions. In a prospective study, biopsies were taken from the edge of the surgical resection cavity of 39 patients after GTR and underwent pathological analysis. The authors reported that 64% of patients had infiltrative tumor cells extending beyond the glial tumor pseudocapsule [38]. Autopsy studies have supported this clinical observation. An autopsy study of 57 brain metastases reported that a majority (51%) of brain metastases displayed clear demarcation from the surrounding parenchyma. However, one-third of cases were diffusely infiltrating, and a small proportion (18%) demonstrated perivascular protrusion of tumor cells into the surrounding cortex [39]. Another autopsy study involving immunohistochemical analysis of 76 brain metastases reported that only 37% of brain metastases showed sharp demarcation from the surrounding cortex, whereas 63% displayed evidence of infiltration of adjacent brain parenchyma [31]. In light of these findings, recent surgical series have investigated the feasibility of supramarginal resection. A recent surgical series described the clinical outcome using this technique. Specifically, the authors compared the outcomes of 94 patients undergoing standard GTR with those of patients receiving "microscopic total resection" (MTR). The authors described MTR as resection of the lesion followed by removal of an additional 5 mm of surrounding cortex (supramarginal). All lesions in this study were confined to non-eloquent cortex. Surgical margins were confirmed with subsequent biopsies of the resulting resection cavity [33]. The mean patient follow-up time was 12.8 months; 51 and 23 patients received GTR and MTR, respectively. The authors reported that MTR significantly decreased the risk of local recurrence relative to GTR alone

(23% versus 43%). Multivariate analysis showed that MTR was associated with a statistically significant decrease in the risk of local recurrence compared with GTR (23% versus 43%) [33]. Supramarginal resection has also been deemed feasible for lesions located in eloquent cortex [32, 40]. A recent series analyzed the outcome of 34 surgical patients who underwent supramarginal resection of lesions located in eloquent cortex. The mean follow-up interval was 16 months, and the authors reported that 15% of patients experienced temporary new or worsening neurological deficits; however, these deficits were resolved by the time of follow-up [40].

Once a patient has been deemed a good candidate for resection, consideration must be given to reaching this goal with limited morbidity. The benefit of aggressive surgical resection is reduced if it creates new crippling neurological deficits postoperatively, which can reduce patient functional status, predispose to medical complications, and negatively impact quality of life. Moreover, if surgical complications result in a significant drop in KPS score, patients may no longer be eligible for clinical trials or be able to tolerate aggressive adjuvant therapy. With this in mind, the use of surgical mapping adjuncts has proven to be vital in making surgical resection effective and safe. For brain metastases located in functional (eloquent) cortex (speech, motor areas), an additional careful preoperative evaluation is necessary to document existing deficits. At MD Anderson we often obtain neurocognitive testing preoperatively in patients whose lesions involve or sit adjacent to language areas. Additionally, predicting the exact location of eloquent cortex with standard anatomical imaging can be difficult, and at times such imaging is insufficient due to several factors including redistribution of functional cortex around the lesion and individual tumor-induced plasticity. With this in mind, functional neuroimaging plays an increasingly important role. Preoperative localization of eloquent brain regions is invaluable for visualizing the spatial relationship between the lesion and surrounding eloquent cortex, planning a resection strategy, calculation of risk, and counseling the patient on postoperative expectations. Diffusion tensor imaging (DTI) tractography, functional MR imaging, and transcranial magnetic stimulation (TMS) are examples of advanced imaging modalities for eloquent regions. These noninvasive tests are useful for localization of functional cortex in order to optimize surgical planning, accurately assess surgical risk, and adequately counsel the patient regarding postoperative recovery and expectations [41–43].

It is important to realize that even with these significant advancements in neuroimaging, the gold standard for surgery within eloquent cortex remains the use of intraoperative mapping for real-time information regarding proximity to critical structures, particularly motor and speech areas. For lesions located close to or involving the posterior frontal lobe/precentral gyrus (motor cortex) or the deep subcortical

motor tracts (corticospinal tract), intraoperative localization is critical. Intraoperatively, the precise location of the motor cortex can be confirmed by placement of a grid electrode on the cortical surface. Subcortical motor fibers can be localized using direct stimulation with a monopolar or bipolar electrode. Once the location of the motor fibers is confirmed, resection can be alternated with direct motor stimulation in order to continuously monitor these critical fiber tracts. The benefit of intraoperative motor mapping has been reported for the resection of brain metastases. A 33-patient surgical series, focusing on lesions in proximity to the motor cortex, described favorable outcomes using mapping techniques. In this report, GTR was achieved in 94% of patients (31/33). Postoperatively, six patients (18%) experienced worsening neurological symptoms, but all patients had recovered by their 3-month follow-up visit [44]. Kellogg and Munoz reported the 3-month neurological outcome of 17 patients after resection of brain metastases in the precentral gyrus. All patients were symptomatic preoperatively. Postoperatively, the authors reported favorable surgical outcomes with stable or improved symptoms in 94% of patients [45] (Figs. 31.4 and 31.5).

Unlike motor mapping, which can be performed with the patient under general anesthesia, intraoperative language mapping is done with the patient awake. After surgical exposure of the cortex in proximity to or involving the tumor, a current-generating bipolar electrode is used to

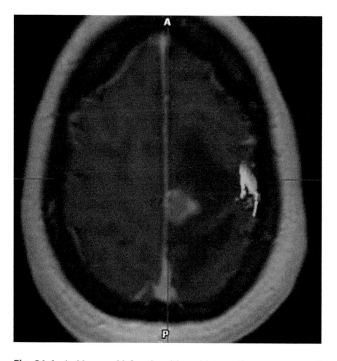

**Fig. 31.4** A 46-year-old female with no history of cancer presented with right leg weakness. MRI showed a 2 cm in diameter lesion adjacent to the precentral gyrus. DTI tractography showed the displaced motor fibers (blue and green fibers)

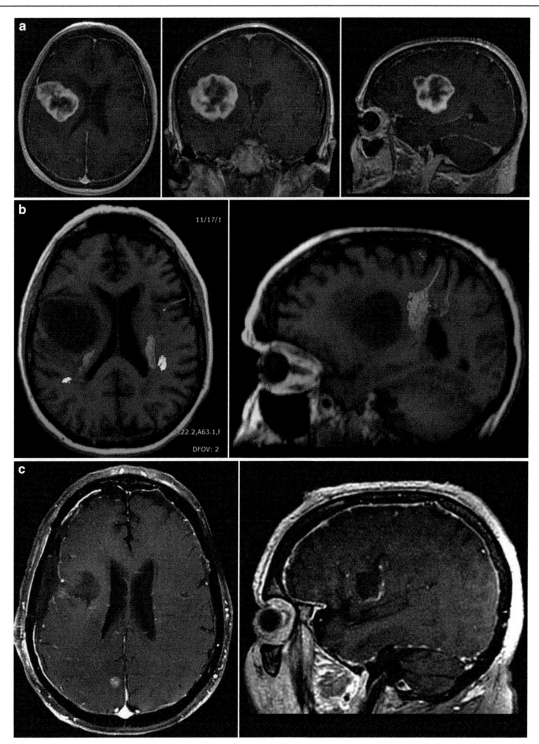

**Fig. 31.5** (**a**) An 80-year-old male with a history of esophageal cancer who presented with altered mental status. Post-contrast MRI [axial (left), coronal (middle), and sagittal (right) images] showed a 5 cm in diameter heterogeneously enhancing mass in the right inferior frontal lobe extending into the basal ganglia. (**b**) DTI tractography showed the corticospinal tract fibers (blue) in proximity to the lesion. (**c**) Patient underwent right frontal craniotomy for tumor resection with the aid of subcortical motor mapping. Postoperative MRI showed GTR. Patient had no postoperative motor deficits following resection

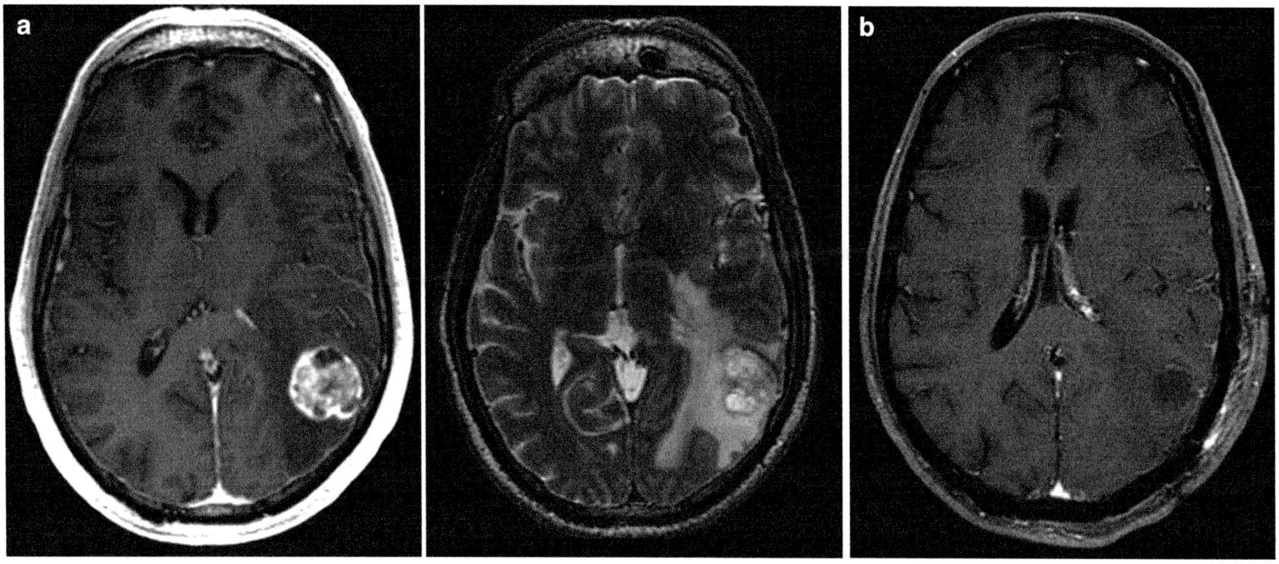

**Fig. 31.6** (**a**) A 58-year-old male with a history of esophageal cancer who presented with word-finding difficulty. MRI [T1 with contrast (left) and T2-weighted (right)] showed a 3.1 cm in diameter enhancing lesion in the posterior left temporal lobe with surrounding vasogenic edema. (**b**) Patient underwent an awake craniotomy for tumor resection. Postoperative MRI showed GTR. Patient had no postoperative speech deficits

stimulate the cortical region of interest. Language mapping is performed, while the patient is asked to complete a variety of verbal tasks using multiple picture cards for naming. The cortex is stimulated during these tasks, and areas on the cortex that produce semantic errors, paraphasias, or speech arrest are noted and avoided during resection (Fig. 31.6). Kamp et al. [32] retrospectively analyzed the outcome of 19 patients who underwent awake craniotomy for resection for metastases in eloquent cortex. In this series, 16% of patients experienced transient deficits after surgery, but none had permanent deficits. Overall, the benefit of intraoperative mapping is clear and has shown improved neurological outcome in patients with brain metastases in difficult to access locations.

Ideally, surgical resection is followed by adjuvant radiotherapy, traditionally WBRT. This treatment paradigm is the result of a multicenter randomized trial that compared the outcome of patients with a single brain metastasis undergoing complete resection followed by postoperative WBRT ($n = 49$) or observation alone ($n = 46$). This study demonstrated that postoperative irradiation significantly reduced the rate of tumor recurrence (18% versus 70%, respectively) and neurological death (14% versus 44%, respectively) relative to the observation group [46]. Neider et al. also demonstrated the significant impact of postoperative irradiation in a pooled analysis of multiple studies focused on surgical resection of single brain metastases. Data were collected on 643 patients from ten studies and analyzed. The authors reported local recurrence in 40% and 12% of patients treated with surgery alone and surgery followed by postoperative WBRT, respectively [47]. Of note, recent studies have sug-

gested potentially negative effects of WBRT on patient cognition and quality of life [48, 49]. Growing concern regarding the neurotoxicity associated with WBRT has resulted in the use of alternative forms of adjuvant radiation methods such as stereotactic radiosurgery (SRS). This will be discussed in the "Radiosurgery" section below.

## Radiosurgery

Over the past two decades, SRS has emerged as a common treatment option for patients with a limited number of brain metastases. SRS consists of a targeted dose of radiation delivered to one or more intracranial lesions with high accuracy. SRS allows the delivered radiation to tightly conform to the target volume and spare the surrounding normal tissue as much as possible. Depending on the system used for delivery, radiosurgery can be administered in single or multiple fractions. Often it provides ablative treatment in a single treatment session. The most commonly used delivery devices are the Gamma Knife (multisource cobalt-60 unit), specially modified linear accelerators (LINACs), or charged-particle (e.g., proton beam) irradiators [50]. Multiple studies have confirmed the efficacy of SRS as a sole modality, showing excellent local tumor control, particularly for the treatment of smaller lesions [51].

Several series have shown that the most reliable predictor of local tumor control with SRS alone is tumor volume [52–54]. Baschnagel and colleagues performed a retrospective analysis of a single-institution experience of 548 metastases treated with SRS in 250 patients [52]. They showed that both local control and overall survival were inversely associated with tumor volume. Local control at 1 year for tumors sized at <2 cm³ was 97% compared with only 75% for tumors ≥2 cm³. Another study reviewed the outcomes of 172 patients with brain metastases managed with SRS alone. Univariate and multivariate analyses confirmed that tumor volume was the only significant predictor of local control in this patient cohort. Specifically, in lesions with tumor volumes of <4 cm³, local control rates were 84% and 77% at 1 and 2 years, respectively. However, in metastases of ≥4 cm³, the local control rate was 49% at 1 and 2 years [55]. The impact of tumor volume on local control was also demonstrated in a retrospective analysis of 103 melanoma patients who underwent LINAC-based SRS. Among the patients treated with SRS alone, the 1-year local control rates for patients with tumors ≤2 cm³ and >2 cm³ were 75% and 42%, respectively [56]. In addition to the matter of decreased local control, larger lesions also carry an increased risk of radiation necrosis with single-fraction radiosurgery [57–59]. Of note, even though SRS has been used traditionally for brain metastases <3 cm in maximal diameter, recent studies have advocated the utility of multi-session SRS for larger brain metastases [60–62].

In addition to being effective for appropriately sized lesions, SRS has the advantage of being minimally invasive, which makes it ideal for patients with multiple medical morbidities or coagulopathy. This therapy can also be used in lesions that are less surgically accessible or are inaccessible [63–65]. For example, a single-institution study of 161 patients with brainstem metastases (*n* = 189) evaluated the safety and efficacy of SRS in this highly eloquent region. The authors reported a local control rate of 87% and a survival time of 5.5 months after treatment, and notably the severe toxicity rate was only 1.8% [63]. A larger study by Triffletti et al. retrospectively analyzed the outcome of a total of 596 brainstem lesions (547 patients). Less than 10% of patients experienced severe toxicity as a result of SRS. This toxicity risk increased with increasing tumor volume and treatment margins. However, local control rates were quite high (82%), indicating a favorable outcome with SRS treatment of these difficult lesions [64]. This matter had been examined prospectively in a 2016 study of 51 brainstem lesions in 48 patients with a median follow-up time of ~5 months and a median tumor volume of 0.12 cm³ (maximum volume 3.7 cm³). These authors also reported a favorable outcome with a 12-month local control rate of 89% and with only 4% of patients experiencing grade 3 toxicity. Moreover, the majority of patients (69%) had improvement or resolution of clinical symptoms after treatment [66] (Fig. 31.7). Manipulation of the motor cortex also produces higher surgical risk (Fig. 31.8). Park et al. retrospectively reviewed the clinical features of 60 brain metastases in the motor cortex, with 51% of the patients having preexisting

motor deficits. The mean target volume of this cohort was 3.2 cm³ (max 14 cm³), and the median follow-up interval was 12.3 months. One-third of patients (35%) experienced new or worsening deficits. The development of deficits was associated with increasing treatment dose (>20 Gy) in multivariate analysis. Fifty percent of patients experienced neurological improvement. This study indicated that SRS involving the motor strip is feasible, with favorable local control rates of 90% and 77% at 6 and 12 months, respectively. However, neurological comprise is not uncommon [67].

Other analyses also suggest that SRS is a very cost-effective treatment. A recent study compared the cost of SRS (using the Gamma Knife) and surgical resection among multiple intracranial pathologies, including brain metastases. Patients were accrued over a 3-year period with a minimum follow-up period of 12 months. The average costs of treating brain metastases with surgery and SRS were approximately $55K and $23K, respectively; these sums demonstrate that SRS is a cost-effective treatment option for brain metastases [68]. SRS can be performed on an outpatient basis, and multiple lesions can be treated simultaneously. Lastly, because it is minimally invasive, SRS typically does not significantly disrupt systemic therapy, giving it an advantage over open surgical resection in this regard.

## Post-resection SRS

As discussed earlier, after surgical resection, it is well established that adjuvant radiation is necessary to reduce the risk of local recurrence. Traditionally, the radiation modality has been WBRT, but several studies have associated this treatment with irreversible cognitive dysfunction and a negative impact on quality of life. Moreover, this neurotoxicity may be amplified by systemic chemotherapy [48, 69–73]. To avoid potential toxicities and to leverage the strong evidence for local control after SRS, multiple groups have investigated the utility of administering SRS to the post-resection cavity, with encouraging results [74–79]. A retrospective study analyzed the outcome of 106 patients who underwent resection of brain metastases followed by treatment of the resection bed with SRS (112 cavities). Most patients had a GTR (96%), and the median time from surgery to SRS was 24 days. The median overall survival time was 10.9 months, and the local control rate was 80%. Multivariate analysis demonstrated that lesions >3 cm in maximal diameter were at higher risk of local treatment failure. Specifically, these patients had a 13.6 times increased risk of treatment failure compared with patients who had lesions that were ≤3 cm [76]. Brennan et al. published the first prospective study of post-resection SRS (39 patients; median follow-up of 1 year) and again showed

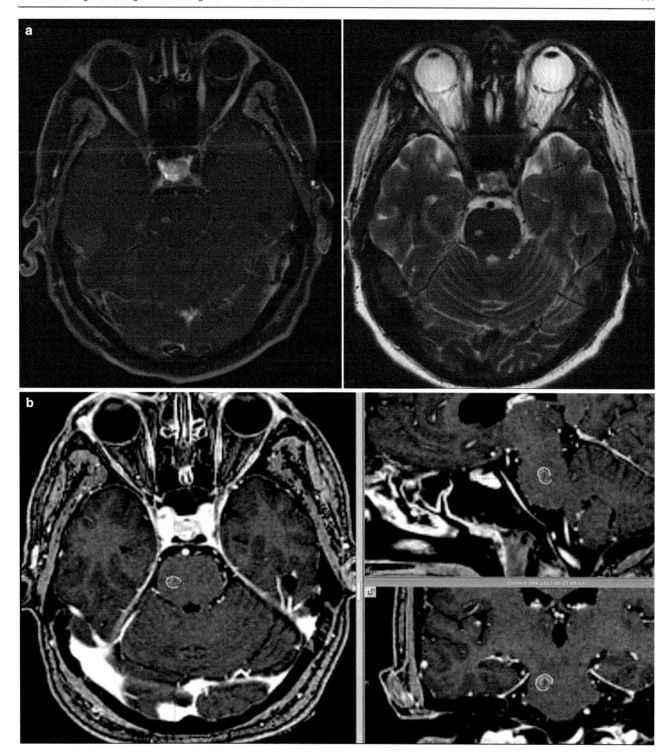

**Fig. 31.7** (**a**) A 70-year-old male with metastatic lung non-small cell lung cancer discovered to have a 6 mm in diameter asymptomatic pontine lesion on staging workup. T1 with contrast and T2-weighted MRI images are shown. (**b**) Patient was treated with frame-based SRS (Gamma Knife) with 16 Gy to 50% isodose line

good local control. Additionally, they also reported that tumors ≥3 cm in maximal diameter with superficial dural/pial involvement had an increased risk of local failure [80]. Robbins et al. reviewed 85 patients over 11 years in whom surgical resection cavities were treated with SRS alone,

adding a 2–3 mm margin to the cavity when planning the treatment volume. Local control was 81% at 1 year, and approximately one-third (35%) of these patients needed salvage WBRT treatment [78]. These authors also reported larger tumor size and dural involvement as risk factors for

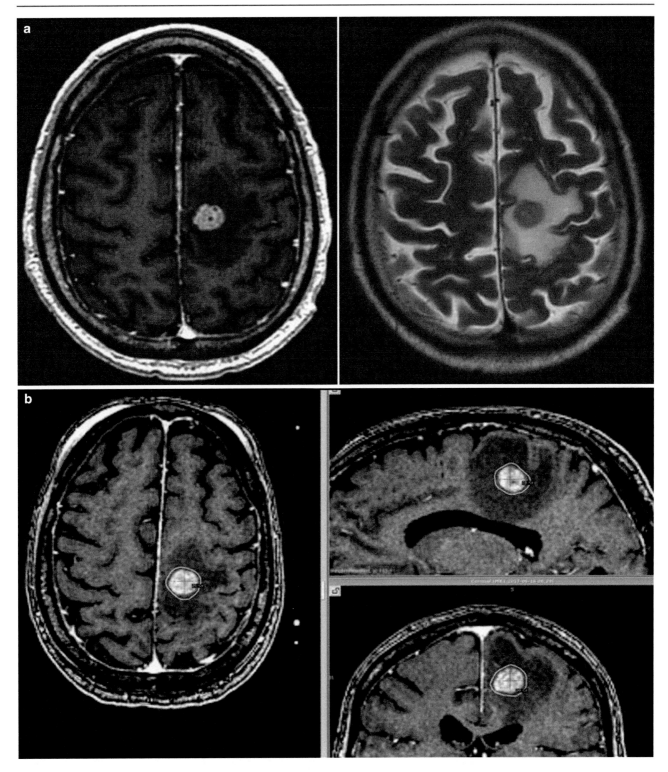

**Fig. 31.8** (a) A 66-year-old male with metastatic lung non-small cell lung cancer discovered to have a 2 cm in diameter enhancing lesion in the precentral gyrus. T1 with contrast and T2-weighted MRI images are shown. (b) Patient was treated with frame-based SRS (Gamma Knife) with 20 Gy delivered to 50% isodose line

local control failure. The impact of tumor size on the risk of local recurrence has also been demonstrated in additional studies [81]. The timing of post-resection SRS can also affect the rate of local recurrence: SRS administered more than 3 weeks after surgery is associated with higher rates of local recurrence [82].

Two recent randomized phase 3 clinical trials have evaluated the outcome of resection cavity SRS. The prospective,

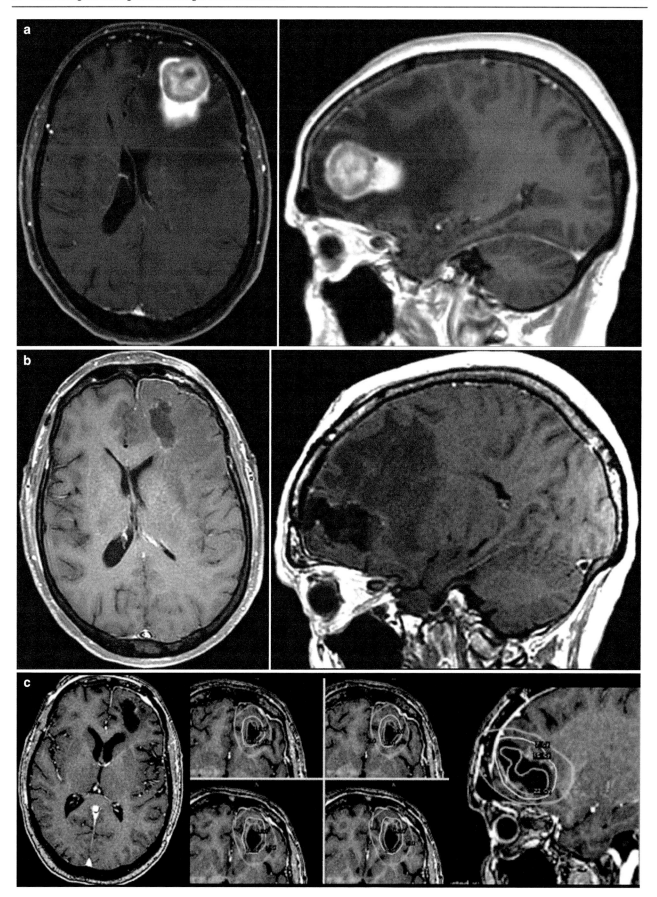

**Fig. 31.9** (**a**) A 65-year-old female with metastatic breast cancer discovered to have a 3.1 cm in diameter enhancing lesion in the left frontal lobe. T1 with contrast MRI images (axial and sagittal) are shown. (**b**) Patient underwent left frontal craniotomy for tumor resection. Postoperative MRI showing GTR. (**c**) Patient was treated with post-resection Gamma Knife irradiation of the cavity with 15 Gy to the 50% isodose line

randomized trial completed at MD Anderson compared the efficacy of cavity SRS with observation alone for completely resected brain metastases. To be included, patients had to have undergone complete resection of one to three brain metastases. This study included 132 patients, 68 patients in the observation group and 64 in the SRS group. The primary outcome measure was time to recurrence in the surgical cavity, with a median follow-up time of 11.1 months. The 12-month freedom from local recurrence percentages were 72% and 43% for the SRS and observation groups, respectively [83]. A second randomized phase 3 trial compared the effect of SRS treatment of the resection cavity with that of WBRT on patient survival and cognitive outcome. This study was multi-institutional, and a total of 194 patients were enrolled (with 98 randomized to cavity SRS and 96 receiving WBRT), and the median follow-up time was 11.1 months. The authors reported no statistically significant difference in survival between the two treatment groups and that patients undergoing SRS experienced significantly less cognitive decline than those receiving WBRT [84]. With this degree of evidence, post-resection SRS treatment of the cavity is quickly becoming the standard of care (Fig. 31.9).

## Pre-resection SRS

The novel concept of pre-resection SRS has recently been introduced as an alternative treatment strategy. This approach has the technical advantage of delivering radiation prior to surgical anatomical distortion, allowing for clear target definition and allowing treatment of a target with an intact blood supply, which is thought to confer a therapeutic advantage [85]. Additionally, presurgical radiation may potentially limit tumor dissemination by preoperative sterilization of the operative field [86]. Additionally, it is hypothesized that tumors may be more radioresponsive because the target is not a hypoxic tumor bed. Asher et al. [85] presented the first series employing the use of SRS prior to surgical resection. They reported this technique to be safe and effective, with rates of local control at 12 and 24 months of 86% and 72%, respectively. Local control was also high even with lesions >3 cm in maximal diameter, for which there had previously consistently been shown to be worse outcomes after SRS. Patel et al. compared the outcomes of pre-resection SRS and post-resection SRS. This study included 180 patients at two institutions; 66 had pre-resection SRS (within 48 h of resection), and 114 had post-resection SRS. Similar rates of local control, distal recurrence, and overall survival occurred between the two treatment arms. Interestingly, preoperative SRS was associated with significantly lower rates of symptomatic radiation necrosis and LMD [86]. Another study by Patel and colleagues compared clinical outcomes and toxicities for presurgery SRS and postoperative WBRT

for resectable brain metastases. In that study, the authors retrospectively reviewed 102 patients who underwent resection at two institutions. Overall, 66 patients with 71 lesions received presurgery SRS, whereas 36 patients (with 42 resection cavities) received postoperative WBRT. The authors found no statistically significant difference in local tumor recurrence rate, distant tumor recurrence rate, or the development of LMD between the two treatment groups [87].

### Conclusion

In the contemporary management of metastatic cancer, brain metastasis is a challenging issue and carries a poor prognosis. Despite these factors, concepts in the management of this devastating clinical problem are advancing, and tailored multimodal therapy has become the standard of care. The role of surgery in managing brain metastases is well accepted, particularly for single metastases, and it is likely to continue as a cornerstone of therapy.

## Self-Assessment Questions

1. What are the three most common solid tumors to metastasize to the brain?
   A. Melanoma, renal cell carcinoma, and colon cancer
   B. Lung cancer, breast cancer, and melanoma
   C. Breast cancer, thyroid cancer, and lung cancer
   D. Lung cancer, colon cancer, and breast cancer
   E. Melanoma, lung cancer, and renal cell carcinoma

2. What is the goal of surgical resection for brain metastasis?
   A. Gross-total resection
   B. Confirmation of diagnosis
   C. Address neurological symptoms
   D. Reduce intracranial pressure
   E. All of the above

3. Which RPA class is associated with the best surgical outcome?
   A. I
   B. II
   C. III

4. Which of the following are potential benefits of SRS?
   1. Minimally invasive
   2. Ideal to address large (>4 cm) symptomatic lesions
   3. Can be performed on an outpatient basis
      A. 2 only
      B. 2 and 3
      C. 1 and 3
      D. 1 and 2
      E. All of the above

5. True or False? Recent phase 3 clinical trials have established the role and efficacy of pre-resection SRS.
   A. True
   B. False

## Answer Key

1. B
2. E
3. A
4. C
5. B

**Acknowledgments** We thank David M. Wildrick, PhD, for editorial assistance.
**Conflict of Interest** The authors declare that they have no conflicts of interest.

## References

1. Sul J, Posner JB. Brain metastases: epidemiology and pathophysiology. Cancer Treat Res. 2007;136:1–21.
2. Jemal A, Siegel R, Ward E, et al. Cancer statistics, 2008. CA Cancer J Clin. 2008;58(2):71–96.
3. Fox BD, Cheung VJ, Patel AJ, et al. Epidemiology of metastatic brain tumors. Neurosurg Clin N Am. 2011;22(1):1–6, v.
4. Nayak L, Lee EQ, Wen PY. Epidemiology of brain metastases. Curr Oncol Rep. 2012;14(1):48–54.
5. Brastianos PK, Curry WT, Oh KS. Clinical discussion and review of the management of brain metastases. J Natl Compr Cancer Netw. 2013;11(9):1153–64.
6. Eichler AF, Chung E, Kodack DP, et al. The biology of brain metastases-translation to new therapies. Nat Rev Clin Oncol. 2011;8(6):344–56.
7. Kibbi N, Kluger H. The treatment of melanoma brain metastases. Curr Oncol Rep. 2016;18(12):73.
8. Delattre JY, Krol G, Thaler HT, et al. Distribution of brain metastases. Arch Neurol. 1988;45(7):741–4.
9. Gavrilovic IT, Posner JB. Brain metastases: epidemiology and pathophysiology. J Neurooncol. 2005;75(1):5–14.
10. Rostami R, Mittal S, Rostami P, et al. Brain metastasis in breast cancer: a comprehensive literature review. J Neurooncol. 2016;127(3):407–14.
11. Patchell RA, Tibbs PA, Walsh JW, et al. A randomized trial of surgery in the treatment of single metastases to the brain. N Engl J Med. 1990;322(8):494–500.
12. Vecht CJ, Haaxma-Reiche H, Noordijk EM, et al. Treatment of single brain metastasis: radiotherapy alone or combined with neurosurgery. Ann Neurol. 1993;33(6):583–90.
13. Schödel P, Schebesch KM, Brawanski A, et al. Surgical resection of brain metastases-impact on neurological outcome. Int J Mol Sci. 2013;14(5):8708–18.
14. Forsyth PA, Weaver S, Fulton D, et al. Prophylactic anticonvulsants in patients with brain tumour. Can J Neurol Sci. 2003;30(2):106–12.
15. Franceschetti S, Binelli S, Casazza M, et al. Influence of surgery and antiepileptic drugs on seizures symptomatic of cerebral tumours. Acta Neurochir. 1990;103(1–2):47–51.
16. Glantz MJ, Cole BF, Friedberg MH, et al. A randomized, blinded, placebo-controlled trial of divalproex sodium prophylaxis in adults with newly diagnosed brain tumors. Neurology. 1996;46(4):985–91.
17. Ryken TC, McDermott M, Robinson PD, et al. The role of steroids in the management of brain metastases: a systematic review and evidence-based clinical practice guideline. J Neurooncol. 2010;96(1):103–14.
18. Tendulkar RD, Liu SW, Barnett GH, et al. RPA classification has prognostic significance for surgically resected single brain metastasis. Int J Radiat Oncol Biol Phys. 2006;66(3):810–7.
19. Lee CH, Kim DG, Kim JW, et al. The role of surgical resection in the management of brain metastasis: a 17-year longitudinal study. Acta Neurochir. 2013,155(3):389–97.
20. Pessina F, Navarria P, Cozzi L, et al. Role of surgical resection in patients with single large brain metastases: feasibility, morbidity, and local control evaluation. World Neurosurg. 2016;94:6–12.
21. Paek SH, Audu PB, Sperling MR, et al. Reevaluation of surgery for the treatment of brain metastases: review of 208 patients with single or multiple brain metastases treated at one institution with modern neurosurgical techniques. Neurosurgery. 2005;56(5):1021–34.
22. Arita H, Narita Y, Miyakita Y, et al. Risk factors for early death after surgery in patients with brain metastasis: reevaluation of the indications for and role of surgery. J Neurooncol. 2014;116(1):145–52.
23. Obermueller T, Schaeffner M, Gerhardt J, et al. Risks of postoperative paresis in motor eloquently and non-eloquently located brain metastases. BMC Cancer. 2014;14:21.
24. Schackert G, Schmiedel K, Lindner C, et al. Surgery of recurrent brain metastases: retrospective analysis of 67 patients. Acta Neurochir. 2013;155(10):1823–32.
25. Sperduto CM, Watanabe Y, Mullan J, et al. A validation study of a new prognostic index for patients with brain metastases: the graded prognostic assessment. J Neurosurg. 2008;109(Suppl):87–9.
26. Sperduto PW, Berkey B, Gaspar LE, et al. A new prognostic index and comparison to three other indices for patients with brain metastases: an analysis of 1,960 patients in the RTOG database. Int J Radiat Oncol Biol Phys. 2008;70(2):510–4.
27. Estabrook NC, Lutz ST, Johnson CS, et al. Does graded prognostic assessment outperform recursive partitioning analysis in patients with moderate prognosis brain metastases? CNS Oncol. 2016;5(2):69–76.
28. Sperduto PW, Chao ST, Sneed PK, et al. Diagnosis-specific prognostic factors, indexes, and treatment outcomes for patients with newly diagnosed brain metastases: a multi-institutional analysis of 4,259 patients. Int J Radiat Oncol Biol Phys. 2010;77(3):655–61.
29. Antoni D, Clavier JB, Pop M, et al. Institutional, retrospective analysis of 777 patients with brain metastases: treatment outcomes and diagnosis-specific prognostic factors. Int J Radiat Oncol Biol Phys. 2013;86(4):630–7.
30. Yamamoto M, Serizawa T, Shuto T, et al. Stereotactic radiosurgery for patients with multiple brain metastases (JLGK0901): a multi-institutional prospective observational study. Lancet Oncol. 2014;15(4):387–95.
31. Baumert BG, Rutten I, Dehing-Oberije C, et al. A pathology-based substrate for target definition in radiosurgery of brain metastases. Int J Radiat Oncol Biol Phys. 2006;66(1):187–94.
32. Kamp MA, Dibue M, Niemann L, et al. Proof of principle: supramarginal resection of cerebral metastases in eloquent brain areas. Acta Neurochir. 2012;154(11):1981–6.
33. Yoo H, Kim YZ, Nam BH, et al. Reduced local recurrence of a single brain metastasis through microscopic total resection. J Neurosurg. 2009;110(4):730–6.
34. Patel AJ, Suki D, Hatiboglu MA, et al. Impact of surgical methodology on the complication rate and functional outcome of patients with a single brain metastasis. J Neurosurg. 2015;122(5):1132–43.
35. Patel AJ, Suki D, Hatiboglu MA, et al. Factors influencing the risk of local recurrence after resection of a single brain metastasis. J Neurosurg. 2010;113(2):181–9.
36. Ahn JH, Lee SH, Kim S, et al. Risk for leptomeningeal seeding after resection for brain metastases: implication of tumor location with mode of resection. J Neurosurg. 2012;116(5):984–93.

37. Suki D, Abouassi H, Patel AJ, et al. Comparative risk of lepto-meningeal disease after resection or stereotactic radiosurgery for solid tumor metastasis to the posterior fossa. J Neurosurg. 2008;108(2):248–57.

38. Siam L, Bleckmann A, Chaung HN, et al. The metastatic infiltration at the metastasis/brain parenchyma-interface is very heterogeneous and has a significant impact on survival in a prospective study. Oncotarget 2015;6(30):29254 67.

39. Berghoff AS, Rajky O, Winkler F, et al. Invasion patterns in brain metastases of solid cancers. Neuro Oncol. 2013;15(12):1664–72.

40. Kamp MA, Rapp M, Slotty PJ, et al. Incidence of local in-brain progression after supramarginal resection of cerebral metastases. Acta Neurochir. 2015;157(6):905–10; discussion 10-1.

41. Hendrix P, Senger S, Griessenauer CJ, et al. Preoperative navigated transcranial magnetic stimulation in patients with motor eloquent lesions with emphasis on metastasis. Clin Anat. 2016;29(7):925–31.

42. Huberfeld G, Trebuchon A, Capelle L, et al. Preoperative and intra-operative neurophysiological investigations for surgical resections in functional areas. Neurochirurgie. 2017;63(3):142–9.

43. Sollmann N, Wildschuetz N, Kelm A, et al. Associations between clinical outcome and navigated transcranial magnetic stimulation characteristics in patients with motor-eloquent brain lesions: a com-bined navigated transcranial magnetic stimulation-diffusion tensor imaging fiber tracking approach. J Neurosurg. 2018;128:800–10.

44. Sanmillan JL, Fernandez-Coello A, Fernandez-Conejero I, et al. Functional approach using intraoperative brain mapping and neurophysiological monitoring for the surgical treatment of brain metastases in the central region. J Neurosurg. 2017;126:698–707.

45. Kellogg RG, Munoz LF. Selective excision of cerebral metastases from the precentral gyrus. Surg Neurol Int. 2013;4:66.

46. Patchell RA, Tibbs PA, Regine WF, et al. Postoperative radiother-apy in the treatment of single metastases to the brain: a randomized trial. JAMA. 1998;280(17):1485–9.

47. Nieder C, Astner ST, Grosu AL, et al. The role of postoperative radiotherapy after resection of a single brain metastasis. Combined analysis of 643 patients. Strahlenther Onkol. 2007;183(10):576–80.

48. Aoyama H, Tago M, Kato N, et al. Neurocognitive function of patients with brain metastasis who received either whole brain radiotherapy plus stereotactic radiosurgery or radiosurgery alone. Int J Radiat Oncol Biol Phys. 2007;68(5):1388–95.

49. Tallet AV, Azria D, Barlesi F, et al. Neurocognitive function impair-ment after whole brain radiotherapy for brain metastases: actual assessment. Radiat Oncol. 2012;7(1):77.

50. Mehta MP, Tsao MN, Whelan TJ, et al. The American Society for Therapeutic Radiology and Oncology (ASTRO) evidence-based review of the role of radiosurgery for brain metastases. Int J Radiat Oncol Biol Phys. 2005;63(1):37–46.

51. Auchter RM, Lamond JP, Alexander E, et al. A multiinstitu-tional outcome and prognostic factor analysis of radiosurgery for resectable single brain metastasis. Int J Radiat Oncol Biol Phys. 1996;35(1):27–35.

52. Baschnagel AM, Meyer KD, Chen PY, et al. Tumor volume as a predictor of survival and local control in patients with brain metastases treated with Gamma Knife surgery. J Neurosurg. 2013;119(5):1139–44.

53. Ebner D, Rava P, Gorovets D, et al. Stereotactic radiosurgery for large brain metastases. J Clin Neurosci. 2015;22(10):1650–4.

54. Molenaar R, Wiggenraad R, Verbeek-de Kanter A, et al. Relationship between volume, dose and local control in stereotactic radiosurgery of brain metastasis. Br J Neurosurg. 2009;23(2):170–8.

55. Hasegawa T, Kondziolka D, Flickinger JC, et al. Brain metastases treated with radiosurgery alone: an alternative to whole brain radio-therapy? Neurosurgery. 2003;52(6):1318–26.

56. Selek U, Chang EL, Hassenbusch SJ III, et al. Stereotactic radiosur-gical treatment in 103 patients for 153 cerebral melanoma metasta-ses. Int J Radiat Oncol Biol Phys. 2004;59(4):1097–106.

57. Blonigen BJ, Steinmetz RD, Levin L, et al. Irradiated volume as a predictor of brain radionecrosis after linear accelerator stereotactic radiosurgery. Int J Radiat Oncol Biol Phys. 2010;77(4):996–1001.

58. Minniti G, Clarke E, Lanzetta G, et al. Stereotactic radiosurgery for brain metastases: analysis of outcome and risk of brain radionecro-sis. Radiat Oncol. 2011;6:48.

59. Sneed PK, Mendez J, Vemer-van den Hoek JG, et al. Adverse radiation effect after stereotactic radiosurgery for brain metas-tases: incidence, time course, and risk factors. J Neurosurg. 2015;123(2):373–86.

60. Hasegawa T, Kato T, Yamamoto T, et al. Multisession gamma knife surgery for large brain metastases. J Neurooncol. 2017;131(3):517–24.

61. Minniti G, Scaringi C, Paolini S, et al. Single-fraction versus mul-tifraction (3 x 9 Gy) stereotactic radiosurgery for large (>2 cm) brain metastases: a comparative analysis of local control and risk of radiation-induced brain necrosis. Int J Radiat Oncol Biol Phys. 2016;95(4):1142–8.

62. Yomo S, Hayashi M, Nicholson C. A prospective pilot study of two-session Gamma Knife surgery for large metastatic brain tumors. J Neurooncol. 2012;109(1):159–65.

63. Trifiletti DM, Lee CC, Winardi W, et al. Brainstem metastases treated with stereotactic radiosurgery: safety, efficacy, and dose response. J Neurooncol. 2015;125(2):385–92.

64. Trifiletti DM, Lee CC, Kano H, et al. Stereotactic radiosurgery for brainstem metastases: an international cooperative study to define response and toxicity. Int J Radiat Oncol Biol Phys. 2016;96(2):280–8.

65. Gans JH, Raper DM, Shah AH, et al. The role of radiosurgery to the tumor bed after resection of brain metastases. Neurosurgery. 2013;72(3):317–25; discussion 25–6.

66. Joshi R, Johnson MD, Maitz A, et al. Utility of graded prog-nostic assessment in evaluation of patients with brainstem metastases treated with radiosurgery. Clin Neurol Neurosurg. 2016;147:30–3.

67. Park CY, Choi HY, Lee SR, et al. Neurological change after gamma knife radiosurgery for brain metastases involving the motor cortex. Brain Tumor Res Treat. 2016;4(2):111–5.

68. Caruso JP, Moosa S, Fezeu F, et al. A cost comparative study of Gamma Knife radiosurgery versus open surgery for intracranial pathology. J Clin Neurosci. 2015;22(1):184–8.

69. Chang EL, Wefel JS, Hess KR, et al. Neurocognition in patients with brain metastases treated with radiosurgery or radiosurgery plus whole-brain irradiation: a randomised controlled trial. Lancet Oncol. 2009;10(11):1037–44.

70. Chow E, Davis L, Holden L, et al. Prospective assessment of patient-rated symptoms following whole brain radiotherapy for brain metastases. J Pain Symptom Manag. 2005;30(1):18–23.

71. McDuff SG, Taich ZJ, Lawson JD, et al. Neurocognitive assess-ment following whole brain radiation therapy and radiosurgery for patients with cerebral metastases. J Neurol Neurosurg Psychiatry. 2013;84(12):1384–91.

72. Pulenzas N, Khan L, Tsao M, et al. Fatigue scores in patients with brain metastases receiving whole brain radiotherapy. Support Care Cancer. 2014;22(7):1757–63.

73. Taillibert S, Le Rhun E, Chamberlain MC. Chemotherapy-related neurotoxicity. Curr Neurol Neurosci Rep. 2016;16(9):81.

74. Mathieu D, Kondziolka D, Flickinger JC, et al. Tumor bed radio-surgery after resection of cerebral metastases. Neurosurgery. 2008;62(4):817–23; discussion 23–4.

75. Jagannathan J, Yen CP, Ray DK, et al. Gamma Knife radiosurgery to the surgical cavity following resection of brain metastases. J Neurosurg. 2009;111(3):431–8.

76. Jensen CA, Chan MD, McCoy TP, et al. Cavity-directed radio-surgery as adjuvant therapy after resection of a brain metastasis. J Neurosurg. 2011;114(6):1585–91.

77. Choi CY, Chang SD, Gibbs IC, et al. Stereotactic radiosurgery of the postoperative resection cavity for brain metastases: prospective evaluation of target margin on tumor control. Int J Radiat Oncol Biol Phys. 2012;84(2):336–42.

78. Robbins JR, Ryu S, Kalkanis S, et al. Radiosurgery to the surgical cavity as adjuvant therapy for resected brain metastasis. Neurosurgery. 2012,71(5):1037–43.

79. Atalar B, Modlin LA, Choi CY, et al. Risk of leptomeningeal disease in patients treated with stereotactic radiosurgery targeting the postoperative resection cavity for brain metastases. Int J Radiat Oncol Biol Phys. 2013;87(4):713–8.

80. Brennan C, Yang TJ, Hilden P, et al. A phase 2 trial of stereotactic radiosurgery boost after surgical resection for brain metastases. Int J Radiat Oncol Biol Phys. 2014;88(1):130–6.

81. Ojerholm E, Lee JY, Thawani JP, et al. Stereotactic radiosurgery to the resection bed for intracranial metastases and risk of leptomeningeal carcinomatosis. J Neurosurg. 2014;121(Suppl):75–83.

82. Iorio-Morin C, Masson-Cote L, Ezahr Y, et al. Early Gamma Knife stereotactic radiosurgery to the tumor bed of resected brain metastasis for improved local control. J Neurosurg. 2014;121(Suppl):69–74.

83. Mahajan A, Ahmed S, McAleer MF, et al. Post-operative stereotactic radiosurgery versus observation for completely resected brain metastases: a single-Centre, randomised, controlled, phase 3 trial. Lancet Oncol. 2017;18(8):1040–8.

84. Brown PD, Ballman KV, Cerhan JH, et al. Postoperative stereotactic radiosurgery compared with whole brain radiotherapy for resected metastatic brain disease (NCCTG N107C/CEC.3): a multicentre, randomised, controlled, phase 3 trial. Lancet Oncol. 2017;18(8):1049–60.

85. Asher AL, Burri SH, Wiggins WF, et al. A new treatment paradigm: neoadjuvant radiosurgery before surgical resection of brain metastases with analysis of local tumor recurrence. Int J Radiat Oncol Biol Phys. 2014;88(4):899–906.

86. Patel KR, Burri SH, Asher AL, et al. Comparing preoperative with postoperative stereotactic radiosurgery for resectable brain metastases: a multi-institutional analysis. Neurosurgery. 2016;79(2):279–85.

87. Patel KR, Burri SH, Boselli D, et al. Comparing pre-operative stereotactic radiosurgery (SRS) to post-operative whole brain radiation therapy (WBRT) for resectable brain metastases: a multi-institutional analysis. J Neurooncol. 2017;131(3):611–8.

# Multiple Brain Metastases

# 32

Isabella Zhang, Masaaki Yamamoto, and Jonathan P. S. Knisely

## Abbreviations

| | |
|---|---|
| DRIVL | Delayed radiation-induced vasculitic leukoencephalopathy |
| fSRS | Fractionated SRS |
| KPS | Karnofsky performance status |
| OSC | Optimal supportive care |
| QALY | Quality-adjusted life year |
| QOL | Quality of life |
| SRS | Stereotactic radiosurgery |
| WBRT | Whole brain radiation therapy |

## Learning Objectives

- To describe the epidemiology and presentation of brain metastases.
- To discuss the treatment options of multiple brain metastases with surgery, radiation, and systemic therapy.
- To discuss the risks and benefits of combined stereotactic radiosurgery (SRS) and whole brain radiation therapy (WBRT) versus SRS alone.
- To discuss the toxicities of radiation treatment for brain metastases.
- To highlight the neurocognitive sequelae of radiation treatment.

I. Zhang
Department of Radiation Medicine, Northwell Health, Lake Success, NY, USA

M. Yamamoto
Department of Neurosurgery, Katsuta Hospital Mito GammaHouse, Hitachi-naka, Ibaraki, Japan

J. P. S. Knisely (✉)
Department of Radiation Oncology, Weill Cornell School of Medicine, New York Presbyterian Hospital, New York, NY, USA
e-mail: jok9121@med.cornell.edu

## Background/Epidemiology/Risk Factors

Brain metastases are the most common intracranial malignancy, occurring at a frequency of ten times that of primary brain tumors. An estimated 97,800–170,000 patients will be diagnosed with brain metastases in the United States every year, and this number is rising as a result of increased survival from systemic treatments and the increasing availability and use of imaging [1].

The most common primary tumor from which brain metastases arise is lung cancer, followed by breast and gastrointestinal cancer. Over their lifetimes, 20–40% of patients with cancer will develop brain metastases. The likelihood of developing brain metastases depends on the primary tumor type—the risk appears to be highest in lung cancer, followed by renal cell carcinoma, melanoma, breast cancer, and colorectal cancer [2].

## Presentation/Imaging Findings

Patients' presenting symptoms may include headaches, nausea and vomiting, focal weakness, visual field defects, cognitive or speech disturbances, gait or limb ataxia, and/or seizures. However, with the increased use of high-performance CT and MR imaging of the central nervous system (CNS) for staging and follow-up of advanced malignancies, metastases are often diagnosed in asymptomatic patients. The vast majority of patients with intracranial metastases present with more than one brain metastasis, with 50% of patients presenting with three or more metastases [3]. Over 80% of brain metastases are found in the cerebral hemispheres, while 15% are in the cerebellum and less than 5% are found in the brainstem [4]. Hematogenous metastases are often found in the watershed areas of the brain or at the gray-white junction, where embolic tumor cells lodge and extravasate into the brain parenchyma. Metastases enhance on MRI after contrast administration because of diffusion of the paramagnetic gadolinium contrast agent

© Springer International Publishing AG, part of Springer Nature 2018
E. L. Chang et al. (eds.), *Adult CNS Radiation Oncology*, https://doi.org/10.1007/978-3-319-42878-9_32

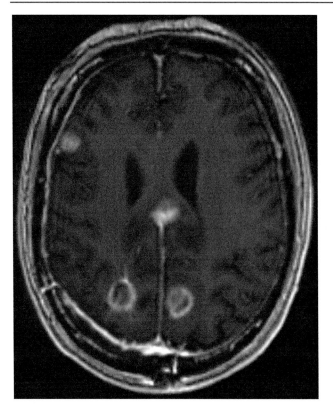

**Fig. 32.1** Multiple brain metastases demonstrating ring enhancement on a T1-weighted contrast-enhanced MRI

through neovasculature that lacks a blood-brain barrier (Fig. 32.1). Larger lesions may be "ring-enhancing," and the differential diagnosis for CNS ring-enhancing lesions includes high-grade gliomas, CNS lymphoma in the setting of immunosuppression, toxoplasmosis, or abscesses. Hemorrhagic metastases are more commonly seen with certain histologies, including renal cell carcinoma, melanoma, and choriocarcinoma.

Intracranial metastases can also present as leptomeningeal carcinomatosis, where tumor cells spread along the surface of the CNS, including perivascular Virchow-Robin spaces. Clinically, patients can present with the same symptoms as above—headache, nausea and vomiting, mental status changes, and seizures—or with focal cranial nerve deficits or neurologic deficits including compromised control of urination or defecation arising from compression of the spinal cord or lumbosacral nerve roots. On imaging of the brain, this can be seen as diffuse enhancement along the gyri and sulci, with or without focal areas of nodularity (Fig. 32.2). In the setting of a questionable radiographic diagnosis, a definitive diagnosis of leptomeningeal carcinomatosis can be made with a lumbar puncture demonstrating tumor cells in the cerebrospinal fluid (CSF). Leptomeningeal disease is most commonly seen with breast cancer but is also found frequently in small-cell lung cancer and melanoma [5]. Generally, treatment options are more limited, and patient survival is worse with leptomeningeal carcinomato-

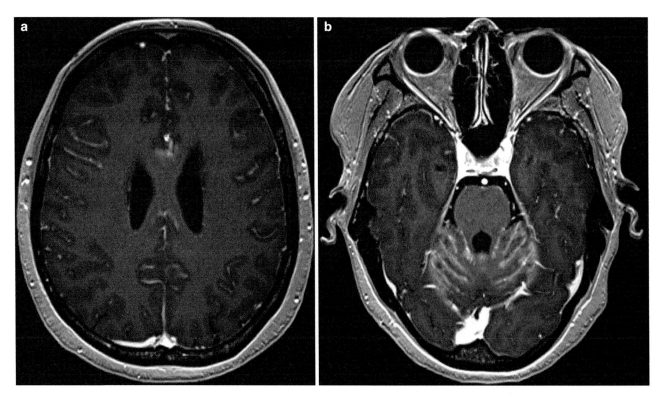

**Fig. 32.2** Diffuse leptomeningeal disease. Contrast enhancement is seen throughout the sulci of the cerebrum (**a**) and the folia of the cerebellum (**b**)

sis, and the management of leptomeningeal carcinomatosis is discussed later in this chapter.

Patients with a known history of metastatic cancer and MRI findings suggestive of intracranial disease may proceed with treatment—either with surgery or radiation—without the need for a histopathological confirmation, if the risks of a biopsy outweigh the benefits. Surgical resection will identify patients with CNS lesions not caused by metastatic disease or is metastatic from a previously undiagnosed primary tumor and will provide additional tissue for histopathologic evaluation, which can be invaluable in cases where there may have been a change in the histopathological nature of the metastatic disease [6]. In patients with no known history of malignancy, a systemic workup to locate the primary tumor should be performed with a CT of the chest, abdomen, and pelvis and other appropriate diagnostic testing. If extracranial disease is found and can be safely biopsied, then that is the preferred approach; however, if no other evidence of disease is seen, then a biopsy or resection of a brain lesion should be performed to establish a diagnosis. Patients with a dominant, symptomatic CNS metastasis will benefit from surgical relief of mass effect if resection can be accomplished safely.

## Prognostic and Predictive Factors

Historically, the median survival of patients with brain metastases who receive supportive care only was 1 month [7]. This historical benchmark predated the routine use of cross-sectional imaging, where more patients likely were diagnosed with symptomatic disease than most patients presenting today. For example, contemporary data on lung cancer patients who were deemed ineligible for surgery or radiosurgery for brain metastases showed a survival with optimal supportive care to be approximately 8–9 weeks in the recently published QUARTZ trial [8].

Within the cohort of patients with multiple brain metastases, the median survival can range from only several months to many years. Multiple prognostication systems have been proposed and validated and are helpful for clinicians in the discussion of appropriate treatments. Historically, a recursive partitioning analysis (RPA) was created based on patients enrolled in multiple Radiation Therapy Oncology Group (RTOG) studies and found that performance status, age, control of the primary tumor, and extracranial disease control could stratify patients treated with WBRT into three groups with median survivals of 2.3–7.1 months [9]. A graded prognostic assessment (GPA) index was later created using a more granular stratification system for age, performance status, and extracranial metastases that incorporated the number of brain metastases [10]. Further improvements in prognostication with that approach were achieved by

including information about histopathological features of the primary site and information about important driver mutations. With this approach, median survival ranges were found to vary from 2.8 months for poor performers with small-cell lung cancer to 25.4 months for the best subgroup of patients with breast cancer and 46.8 months for lung cancer patients with EGFR mutations or ALK translocations and other good prognostic features [11, 12]. These and other prognostic systems are described in greater detail in Chap. 30.

Improved survival in patients with one brain metastasis compared with those with multiple brain metastases has been demonstrated in multiple studies. In the GPA, patients with 2–3 metastases appeared to have better survival than those with greater than 3; however, the prognostic value of the number of brain metastases has come into question. In a recently published study by Yamamoto and Serizawa et al. of patients treated with Gamma Knife stereotactic radiosurgery, patients with a single brain metastasis had the best survival (median 13.8 months), while those with 2–4 and 5–10 brain metastases had equal survival rates (median 10.8 months in both groups) [13]. The total volume of brain metastases has been demonstrated to be a better prognostic factor than the total number of metastases and has been associated with overall survival, distant brain failure, and local tumor control [14, 15].

## Overall Treatment Strategy

Patients who present with symptomatic disease should be started on steroids to reduce tumor-related edema. The starting dose is typically 16 mg/day in divided doses but should be tapered down to the lowest dose that controls the patient's symptoms. Asymptomatic patients should not be started on steroids, as no clinical benefit has been demonstrated in this group of patients [16].

In 2012, the American Society for Radiation Oncology (ASTRO) released a set of guidelines for the management of single and multiple brain metastases. Patients with an expected survival of 3 or more months are recommended for stereotactic radiosurgery (SRS), whole brain radiation therapy (WBRT), or both (all with a level 1 recommendation). Patients with significant mass effect from their metastases are still recommended to undergo surgery followed by WBRT, and patients with a poor prognosis are recommended for WBRT or supportive care only. The National Cancer Comprehensive Network (NCCN) updated its management algorithm in 2018 with treatment recommendations based on "limited" versus "extensive" brain metastases: in patients with newly diagnosed or stable systemic disease and limited brain metastases SRS or WBRT are both appropriate, with SRS as the preferred approach. In patients with limited metastases but disseminated systemic disease with poor systemic treatment options, supportive care or WBRT can be used. In patients with extensive brain metastases, WBRT and SRS are both appropriate, with SRS especially considered for patients with good performance status, low tumor burden, or radio-resistant histologies.

## Surgery

Surgical resection is often considered for patients with a symptomatic or large (>3 cm in diameter) brain metastasis. A controversial retrospective case control study showed improved survival for patients with brain metastases that were treated with resection relative to SRS, and an increased rate of local CNS failures was identified in the cohort treated with SRS as a contributing cause to those patients' poorer survival [17]. Although these larger brain metastases can be treated with SRS, the larger the tumor, the lower the maximal safe marginal radiation dose, the less rapid symptom amelioration, and the lower the probability of tumor control. This will be discussed further in a later section. Many patients with brain metastases are not good candidates for resection because of comorbidities, extracranial cancer progression, or multiple CNS metastases. The resection of multiple metastases is performed less routinely, but with judicious use, survival results comparable to patients who have had a single metastasis resected can be achieved [18]. Several trials have shown that resection alone cannot provide adequate local control of brain metastases, even if en bloc resections are conducted [19, 20]. Radiation, either as WBRT or SRS, will reduce the risk of local tumor recurrence and will be discussed in further detail in the next chapter.

## Radiation

Whole brain radiation therapy (WBRT) has been used for decades for the management of unresectable or multiple brain metastases. In addition to treating macroscopic metastases, WBRT also treats any microscopic disease present at the time of irradiation, preventing symptomatic growth from occurring. WBRT has never been demonstrated to improve survival but appears to reduce metastasis-related symptoms and the risk of death from neurologic causes.

WBRT is delivered with opposed lateral fields with a generous margin around the skull base to include the cribriform plate and meningeal surfaces (Fig. 32.3). For a clinical setup, the isocenter may be placed at the lateral canthus to minimize divergence into the eyes. With CT simulation, the isocenter can be placed in the center of the field, and the lenses, which are sensitive to low-dose radiation, can be blocked to reduce the risk of cataract formation. As cataract formation

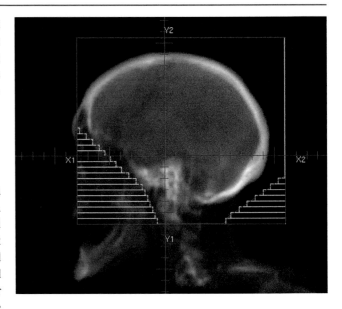

**Fig. 32.3** Beams eye view of a lateral whole brain radiation field on a digitally reconstructed radiograph (DRR)

is a late toxicity of radiation, any potential benefit of lens-blocking is lost in patients with a dismal prognosis.

Six MV X-rays are a default choice for WBRT, but using 10 MV provides similar coverage and better dose homogeneity with a lower integral dose (Fig. 32.4). Higher-energy beams should probably be avoided in patients with leptomeningeal disease, though, as the prescription dose may not optimally cover the most superficial lateral leptomeningeal surfaces. Be that as it may, the leptomeningeal surfaces of the spinal axis will not be treated with WBRT portals, and imaging of the spinal axis with MRI will help disclose whether treatment is needed to prevent neurological compromise from leptomeningeal carcinomatosis outside the cranium.

There are multiple accepted dosing and fractionation schemes for WBRT. Commonly used fractionation schemes in the United States include 30 Gy in 10 fractions, 37.5 Gy in 15 fractions, and 20 Gy in 5 fractions [21]. A comparison of lower doses (10 Gy in 1 fraction, 12 Gy in 2 fractions, and 20 Gy in 5 fractions) to 30 Gy demonstrated no difference in mortality at 6 months [22]. Higher doses have also been evaluated (50 Gy in 20 fractions and 54.4 Gy in 34 fractions) and, again, have not shown any difference in mortality compared to the standard 30 Gy scheme [22]. These protracted courses and higher doses have also not been shown to favorably affect symptom control or toxicity.

As there does not appear to be a difference in outcomes between these fractionation schedules, shorter courses should be preferred for patients with worse survival prognoses. However, delayed neurocognitive sequelae are felt to be worse with fraction sizes >2.5 Gy, so that 3 week courses of therapy may be better for patients with anticipated pro-

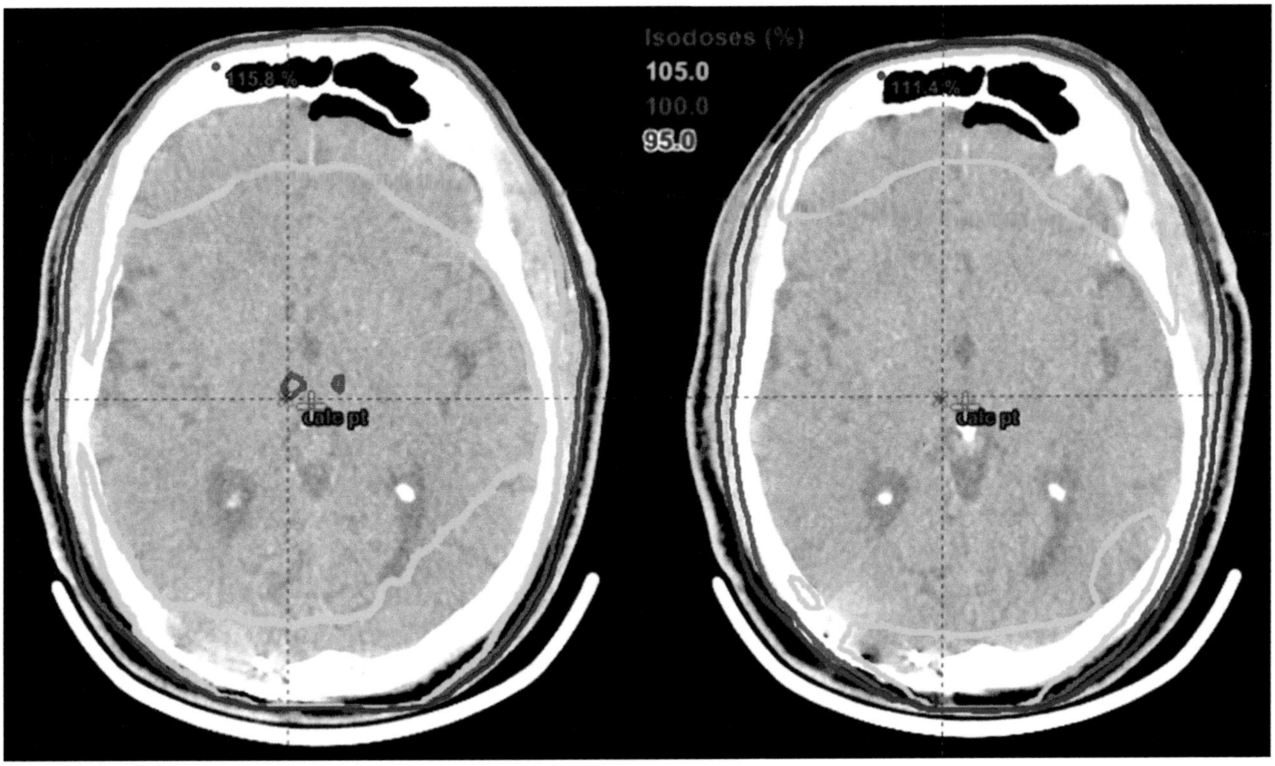

**Fig. 32.4** Dose distribution in a whole brain treatment field using 6 MV (left) versus 10 MV (right) photons. The 10 MV plan has improved dose homogeneity without sacrificing coverage of the peripheral brain parenchyma

tracted survival. Clinical trials have tested approaches to decrease WBRT-associated neurocognitive sequelae with selective dosimetric sparing of the hippocampi and with drugs that decrease hippocampal excitotoxicity [23, 24]. In time, these approaches may be shown to provide incontrovertible benefit for favorable prognosis patients requiring WBRT and become routinely used to lessen WBRT-associated toxicity.

Prior to 2016, there was only one published randomized trial of WBRT versus supportive care alone for symptomatic brain metastases, where patients who received radiation had a median survival of 14 weeks versus 10 weeks for patients who received steroids alone [25]. This study was conducted prior to the availability of CT and MR imaging and included only 48 patients. The recently published international QUARTZ trial was the first randomized controlled trial of WBRT versus optimal supportive care (OSC) in patients with brain metastases from non-small-cell lung cancer [8]. While patients were enrolled if they were deemed ineligible for surgery and radiosurgery, a majority of patients had a KPS of ≥70, and approximately one-third had only a single brain metastasis. Eleven percent of the patients randomized to receive WBRT received no treatment, and the preponderant reason for this was a decline in performance status that precluded WBRT. The primary endpoint was quality-adjusted life years (QALYs), and the authors found no ben-

efit in QALYs between the two arms (41.7 days with WBRT versus 46.4 days with OSC). This study also found that WBRT did not improve survival and overall quality of life or reduce the need for steroid medication compared to the OSC arm, though an apparent survival benefit was seen with WBRT in patients younger than 60 years old.

## WBRT with or without SRS

Tumor response rates after WBRT range from 24 to 55%, and recrudescent symptoms from brain metastases within a few months following WBRT is a frequently encountered problem. Repeated courses of WBRT have been used with additional palliative benefit [26]. Stereotactic radiosurgery (SRS) was hypothesized, through increasing tumor radiation dose, to be able to improve tumor control and survival. SRS is a method of delivering high-dose focal radiation to patients with small tumors in locations where surgery is risky, or in patients with multiple metastases without substantially adding to the radiation dose delivered to normal brain. Treatments can be delivered in a single day; but larger metastases or a large number of metastases may have treatments delivered over up to five sessions. Treatment can be delivered on a variety of platforms and will be discussed further in a separate section.

The addition of SRS to standard WBRT for patients with multiple brain metastases was evaluated in several prospective randomized trials. Andrews et al. published the results of RTOG 9508, where patients with 1–3 brain metastases were treated with WBRT with or without the addition of an SRS boost [27]. Survival was found to be equal in both arms, except for patients who had a single brain metastasis, where survival was improved with an SRS boost. Patients with a single or multiple metastases experienced an improvement in local tumor control with an SRS boost (1-year control of 82% vs 71%); however, this did not translate into a decrease in death from neurologic causes. Patients with an SRS boost were also less dependent on steroids at 6 months. Another study evaluating WBRT with or without an SRS boost for patients with 2–4 brain metastases showed that 100% of patients who had received WBRT alone experienced a local failure at 1 year, versus 8% who received the SRS boost [28]. Despite the equivalent median survival, this study was terminated after the interim analysis because of the improvement in local tumor control in the SRS boost arm.

## SRS with or without WBRT

To reduce the neurocognitive toxicities of radiation, SRS without additional WBRT has been increasingly used for multiple brain metastases. However, omitting WBRT has caused speculative concern about an increased risk of distant brain recurrences leading to symptomatic deterioration, increased rates of neurologic deaths, and decreased survivals. Multiple retrospective analyses were performed to evaluate these outcomes, including a large multi-institutional analysis of nearly 1000 patients that demonstrated no differ-

ence in survival in patients who received SRS alone versus combination therapy [29]. Since then, several randomized controlled trials have been performed to evaluate the safety and efficacy of SRS alone versus SRS with WBRT in the setting of a limited number of brain metastases and have all shown equal survival between the two groups (Table 32.1). The first of these was JROSG 99-1, where patients with 1–4 brain metastases were randomized to WBRT + SRS versus SRS alone [30]. The 1-year tumor recurrence rate was significantly higher with SRS alone (76.4% versus 46.8%), and these patients more frequently required salvage treatment. Toxicity, neurologic preservation, and neurocognitive function (assessed with the Mini-Mental Status Exam) were equal between the two arms. An unplanned secondary analysis of this study evaluating those patients with NSCLC brain metastases demonstrated that patients with a favorable prognosis (DS-GPA scores of 2.5–4.0) had a significantly improved survival with WBRT + SRS versus SRS alone, whereas no benefit was seen in patients with a worse prognostic score [31]. However, similar secondary analyses using phase III trial data from NCCTG N-0574 and EORTC 22952-26001 that also stratified patients with the DS-GPA tool and analyzed survival probabilities based on whether or not patients had received WBRT in addition to SRS showed no survival advantage for receiving WBRT in addition to SRS among any cohorts [32, 33].

The role of WBRT after focal therapy was prospectively evaluated by the EORTC, where patients with 1–3 brain metastases underwent surgery or SRS and were then randomized to observation versus WBRT [34]. Patients who received WBRT experienced improved intracranial control and fewer neurologic deaths; however, this did not translate into a benefit in overall survival or functional independence.

**Table 32.1** Stereotactic radiosurgery with or without whole brain radiation therapy (all values are for 1 year unless otherwise specified)

| Study | Treatment | Local control | Distant brain control | 1-year overall survival | Median survival (months) | Neurologic death | Salvage treatment |
|---|---|---|---|---|---|---|---|
| JROSG 99-1 [30] | SRS | 72.5% | 36.3% | 28.4% | 8.0 | 19.3% | 43% |
| | SRS + WBRT | 88.7% ($p = 0.002$) | 58.5% ($p = 0.003$) | 38.5% | 7.5 | 22.8% | 15% |
| EORTC 22952-26001 [34] | SRS or surgery | 69% (SRS) 41% (surgery) (2 years) | 52% (SRS) 58% (surgery) (2 years) | NR | 10.9 | 44% | 51% |
| | SRS or surgery + WBRT | 81% (SRS) 73% (surgery) (2 years) | 67% (SRS) 77% (surgery) (2 years) | NR | 10.7 | 28% ($p < 0.002$) | 16% |
| MD Anderson [36] | SRS | 67% | 45% | 63% | 15.2 | 40% | 87% |
| | SRS + WBRT | 100% ($p = 0.012$) | 73% ($p = 0.02$) | 21% ($p = 0.003$) | 5.7 | 28% | 7% |
| NCCTG [38] | SRS | 72.8% | 69.9% | NR | 10.4 | NR | 32.4% |
| | SRS + WBRT | 90.1% ($p = 0.003$) | 92.3% ($p < 0.001$) | NR | 7.4 | NR | 7.8% ($p < 0.001$) |

Only significant $p$ values are listed
*NR* not reported

A later analysis of the health-related quality of life (QOL) outcomes in these patients was also reported: patients who underwent observation after focal therapy had improved global health, physical functioning, cognitive functioning, and fatigue (all at different time points) [35].

A separate single-institution study of patients with 1–3 brain metastases who all underwent SRS and were similarly randomized to observation versus additional WBRT, this time with a primary endpoint of neurocognitive preservation, was conducted at the MD Anderson Cancer Center. The study was stopped early because the neurocognitive endpoints were met with significantly improved neurocognitive preservation with SRS alone versus SRS with WBRT. A secondary analysis demonstrated that the patients treated with SRS alone had a significantly higher median survival (15.2 vs 5.7 months with WBRT) [36]. This difference was unexpected, and the data collected for the trial did not permit any answers to be generated about possible unequal rates of extracranial metastatic disease or differing rates of continuing systemic therapy after brain metastasis treatment.

A meta-analysis of these three trials was performed, with a total of 364 evaluable patients (51% treated with SRS alone and 49% treated with SRS with WBRT). In this group, the authors found that the effect of treatment on survival was dependent on age: patients ≤50 years old had significantly better survival when treated with SRS alone (13.6 vs 8.2 months), while patients >50 had no difference in survival with SRS alone or the addition of WBRT. The effect of treatment on distant brain metastases was also correlated with patient age: the risk of distant brain failure did not differ based on treatment in patients ≤50, while it was increased in patients receiving SRS alone in those over 50 [37].

The most recently published randomized controlled trial on the use of SRS with or without the addition of WBRT also evaluated cognitive decline as its primary endpoint. This multicenter trial enrolled 213 patients and found that patients who underwent SRS alone had less cognitive deterioration (63.5% versus 91.7%) and improved quality of life at 3 months. As the previous studies have also shown, patients who underwent whole brain radiation therapy had improved local control and a longer time to intracranial failure; however, median survival was not different between the two groups. For the small group of long-term survivors, lower rates of cognitive deterioration in the SRS only group remained significant at 12 months ($p = 0.04$) [38].

Because of the equivalent survival after SRS with or without the addition of WBRT for a limited number of brain metastases, the omission of WBRT has become more broadly accepted. The current National Comprehensive Cancer Network (NCCN) guidelines for brain metastases recommend SRS with or without WBRT for patients with 1–3 resectable brain metastases and WBRT or SRS for patients with four or more lesions [39]. The ASTRO Choosing

Wisely® recommendations published in 2014 also recommend against the routine addition of WBRT to SRS for patients with limited metastases, with the caveat that careful surveillance is needed to evaluate for the development of distant intracranial metastases [40]. Absent class I data to guide treatment recommendations, it is important to provide patients with brain metastases who are potentially eligible for treatment with SRS alone with adequate information about the potential benefits and morbidities associated with the use of WBRT as an additional therapy [41].

A numerical definition of "limited" or "oligometastatic" and the management for patients with ≥4 brain metastases remains controversial and appears to be dependent upon a number of variables including local expertise and equipment. An expert opinion survey conducted at two radiosurgery meetings asked treating physicians what the maximum number of brain metastases that would be reasonable to treat with SRS alone was, as well as the factors that influence the recommendation of SRS without WBRT [42]. The maximum number of brain metastases that was considered appropriate for SRS alone was 50, while over half of the physicians felt that treating ≥5 lesions with SRS alone was reasonable. There was also a difference in practice patterns based on location, where a less than a quarter of physicians at the meeting in the United States were comfortable treating more than ten metastases with SRS alone, while over half of those in Japan believed this was reasonable. Radiation oncologists were also less likely than neurosurgeons to recommend SRS alone for ≥4 brain metastases. More evidence has since emerged in support of SRS alone for five or more metastases—the Japanese prospective study of 1194 patients treated with SRS alone (JLGK0901) found 10.8-month median survival times in patients with 2–4 and 5–10 brain metastases challenging the convention that SRS alone should be reserved for four or fewer lesions [13].

## Radiation Planning for Single-Fraction SRS

Contouring and planning treatment for multiple metastases does not differ significantly from the techniques used for single metastasis treatment, using thin-slice MR imaging and a T1 sequence with contrast. The notable exception with treating multiple metastases with SRS is the need to take greater care in the planning of SRS to tumors that are spatially close to each other. Avoiding overlap of low-dose regions that sum to total doses >12 Gy may help avoid radiation injury, specifically radiation necrosis, to the normal brain [43]. Many physicians have based single-fraction SRS doses on the results of RTOG 9005, a dose escalation study of recurrent brain metastases or primary brain tumors up to 4 cm in diameter [44]. The maximum tolerated doses were found to be dependent on tumor size, with a recommended dose of 24 Gy to tumors $\leq 2$ cm, 18 Gy to tumors 2.1–3 cm, and 15 Gy for tumors 3.1–4 cm. Using these doses, the rates of total Grade 3 and higher acute and chronic toxicity reached 10, 20, and 14%, respectively. All patients in this study had prior fractionated radiation with a median dose of 60 Gy for primary brain tumors and 30 Gy for metastases, and it can be hypothesized that these or even higher doses may be safe in patients without prior WBRT. In JLGK0901, the prospective study of SRS alone for 1–10 brain metastases, a marginal dose of 22 Gy was used for tumors <4 mL in volume and 20 Gy for tumors between 4 and 10 mL in volume, and the 24-month local control rate was 84.5–90.2% [13]. Brainstem lesions received lower doses, with peripheral doses of 20 Gy for tumors <1 mL, 18 Gy for tumors between 1 and 4 mL, and 16 Gy for tumors between 4 and 10 mL in volume. The 4-year cumulative rate of Grade 3 or higher complications associated with SRS alone in this study was 4%, irrespective of the number of metastases [45].

The risk of increased radionecrosis and other toxicities from escalated doses needs to be balanced with the increased rate of disease control with higher doses. In RTOG 90-05, local tumor control was seen in only 52% of patients. However, this was a combination of patients with primary and metastatic brain tumors, and histopathological evaluation of progressively enlarging lesions after SRS was not routinely performed. In a series of metastases treated with SRS, 1-year local control rates appear to range between 64 and 91% [46]. Higher doses appear to improve the rates of local control, with local failure rates of 27–38% seen when doses <16 Gy are given [47, 48]. Higher doses have also been postulated to be beneficial for certain histologies, including metastases from colorectal cancer and classically radioresistant histologies of melanoma and renal cell carcinoma [49].

## Fractionated SRS

Fractionated SRS (fSRS) had several factors contributing to its development and adoption. A short but incomplete list includes the desire to provide fractionation to help protect normal tissues that could not be adequately excluded from high-dose treatment in the planning of SRS, the desire to avoid stereotactic frame placement, the development of stereotactic kV imaging applications for confirming treatment delivery accuracy, and the need to dosimetrically confirm intensity-modulated treatment planning prior to patient treatment. Also quite important was a definition of SRS in 2006 by the US neurosurgical and radiation oncology professional societies that communicated that SRS could be delivered in up to five fractions. This change was required to clarify professional and technical charges for the procedure as it was being used for patient care in the first decade of the millennium [50].

The delivery of fSRS has been shown to be feasible and to provide good local control of brain metastases [51–53]. While this approach was initiated by physicians using linear accelerators or a robotic radiosurgery system (CyberKnife) which could be used for single or multiple fractions, there has been a recent convergence of capabilities exemplified by the most recent Gamma Knife model (ICON) that can readily provide fractionated treatments for brain metastases, because of the incorporation of mask-based immobilization and kV image guidance on the treatment couch, like a linear accelerator.

Although no prospective randomized trial evaluating single- versus multi-fraction SRS treatment has been published, several phase II and retrospective analyses have been performed. A phase II study evaluated 51 patients treated to either 30 Gy in 5 fractions (if prior WBRT was given) or 35 Gy in 5 fractions, with the dose prescribed to the 90% isodose line. 84.8% of patients had either a partial or complete remission, with larger tumors and larger number of metastases associated with both disease-specific and overall survival [54]. Another study of patients with metastases greater than 2 cm in size received either 27 Gy in 3 fractions or 15–18 Gy in a single fraction—where the majority of patients receiving fSRS had tumors larger than 3 cm—patients receiving fSRS had an improved local control (90% versus 77% at 1 year) [53]. The risk of radionecrosis—a potentially severe complication of radiation therapy that will be discussed later in this section—was also decreased in these larger tumors with the use of fSRS (8% versus 20%). Other fractionation schemes (36 Gy in 6 fractions, 35 Gy in 5 fractions, 40 Gy in 10 fractions) have been used with similar efficacy as single-fraction treatment, with potentially less toxicity [52, 55]. Optimal dose fractionation schemes for 2, 3, 4, and 5 fraction fSRS are not yet well-established from any prospective clinical trials.

Fractionation introduces another variable that must be considered in the treatment of metastases with radiosurgery. Single-fraction treatment is relatively straightforward—both the dose delivered to the margin and the isodose surface that this dose is delivered to are chosen. When fractionation is employed, these two things still must be determined, but the interfraction interval must also be determined. The radiobiological impact of this choice on the tumor and on peritumoral normal brain also must be considered. The impact of treatment on successive days (all treatments completed in a week or less) is likely to be very different than the impact of two or three treatments separated by weeks to a month or more to permit treatment-induced target volume regression to occur. Replanning will be necessary for situations where metastasis regression will occur between fractions. The optimal radiation regimen that accounts for these relatively straightforward variables remains to be defined.

It may be the case that the choice of fractionation regimens will come to depend, in part, on whether systemic checkpoint inhibitors will be used to try to elicit an abscopal response through an autovaccination strategy [56]. Grimaldi et al. have reported that SRS to the brain can result in extracranial abscopal responses in melanoma patients who had progressed through checkpoint inhibitor therapy [57]. Extracranially, there is evidence that a fractionated SRS approach is more immunostimulatory than a single fraction, and here too, the optimal radiation regimen to induce clinical antitumor immunity remains to be defined [58, 59].

## Systemic Therapy

There are an infinite number of variables associated with systemic therapy and how agents may be used to manage systemic disease or to try to affect CNS disease activity. Certain agents do not penetrate the blood-brain barrier well, while others have relatively good CNS penetration. No randomized, controlled trial of WBRT with or without chemotherapy has led to a survival advantage for concomitant therapy, and indeed, though improvements in CNS response rates have been reported, it is generally with increased treatment-related toxicity [60]. Reliable data does not exist about the tolerability of SRS with nearly all systemically administered cancer therapies, and no blanket statements can be made about concomitant use.

In the treatment of systemic disease with agents designed to block the inhibition of the immune system's response to antigens on cancer cells, abscopal responses have been reported to occur in patients treated with radiation to the body. This augmented immune response can help control distant metastatic disease and can also help control the irradiated metastases. The median survival and 2-year survival rate for patients with melanoma brain metastases treated with SRS were 4.9 months and 19.7%, but if ipilimumab (a CTLA-4 inhibitor) was also used, the median survival was 21.9 months and the 2-year survival rate was 47.2% [61]. Increased rates of delayed radiation-induced vasculitic leukoencephalopathy (DRIVL) after SRS can be seen in patients treated with checkpoint inhibitors, but the overall incidence and exactly what patient- and treatment-related factors may predispose a patient to develop this complication are unknown; this complication is also seen in some patients treated with tyrosine kinase inhibitors [62–65]. Studies such as NCT02097732, which investigates SRS to brain metastases before or during ipilimumab induction, will augment our understanding of the optimal timing for combining radiation and immunomodulating therapies. The use of multiple checkpoint inhibitors without any irradiation in patients with melanoma brain metastases has shown results that are impressive (for systemic therapy)--a 46% intracranial response rate and a 17% complete response rate, and has prompted the proposal that nivolumab and ipilimumab be considered as first line therapy for patients with asymptomatic untreated melanoma brain metastases [66].

Although this strategy may avoid any increased risk of radiation necrosis with the use of SRS or diffuse brain injury from the use of WBRT, the potential benefit that may arise from the use of radiation to augment systemic abscopal responses is foregone with this approach.

## Specific Scenarios

### EGFR-Mutated and ALK-Rearranged Lung Cancer

Interestingly, patients who are identified as having brain metastases arising from epidermal growth factor receptor (EGFR)-mutated lung carcinomas will have good systemic and CNS responses to tyrosine kinase inhibitor (TKI) drugs, and this has led to a deferral in some cases of radiation therapy use for multiple brain metastases, as small and asymptomatic metastases may not be deemed readily amenable to radiosurgical treatment because of concerns about the time required to deliver focal treatment to numerous metastases and because of a desire to defer WBRT. A multi-institutional retrospective study has identified that deferral of radiation of brain metastases in patients with EGFR-mutated lung cancer is associated with a worsened survival prognosis [67]. Patients treated with up-front SRS for brain metastases had a better median survival than those treated with up-front WBRT, and both had a median survival superior to patients for whom radiation treatment was deferred in favor of initial systemic TKI therapy (40.8 vs 25.3 vs 20.5 months). Statistical significance was achieved for the comparison between SRS and up-front TKI therapy ($p = 0.0001$) and for SRS or WBRT vs up-front TKI therapy ($p = 0.0015$). This finding, if corroborated with prospective studies, would be among a very few studies that have shown that treatment of a metastatic site with radiation can improve the survival prognosis. ALK-rearranged lung cancers, like those associated with EGFR mutant lung carcinoma also have a good survival prognosis, perhaps because both can be treated with relatively nontoxic targeted therapy in addition to cytotoxic chemotherapy. Studies to investigate the efficacy of CNS-penetrating medications for EGFR-mutated and ALK-rearranged brain metastases (with and without irradiation) are needed; it is likely focal irradiation will be beneficial for patients who do not have disappearance of CNS disease with systemic treatment.

### Small-Cell Lung Cancer

Small-cell lung cancer (SCLC) has a high propensity for intracranial metastases, and patients without brain metastases at diagnosis and a response to systemic therapy benefit from prophylactic cranial irradiation (PCI). Unfortunately, a significant percentage of patients either present with brain metastases or develop metastases after PCI, requiring radiation therapy. Traditionally, WBRT is used in both settings, to treat both the visible disease and the microscopic foci of metastases that are likely present; however, SRS can be considered to delay the neurocognitive toxicities associated with WBRT [29]. A retrospective evaluation of 70 patients in a Japanese institution who had undergone Gamma Knife SRS in the up-front or salvage setting demonstrated comparable survival rates as those who underwent WBRT and prompts consideration of further evaluation of SRS in the up-front setting [68] for patients identified with brain metastases. Because SRS has not yet become a standard of care treatment, the benefits of delaying the neurocognitive toxicity of WBRT must be weighed against a perceived risk of the short-term development of distant brain metastases causing similar neurological consequences.

## Germ Cell Tumors

Germ cell tumors are a rare tumor, with brain metastases found in less than 2% of these patients at the time of presentation; however, an MRI of the brain is not routinely used in the staging workup [69]. The likelihood of brain metastases presenting at the time of diagnosis increases with elevated serum β-hCG, the presence of lung metastases, and widely disseminated disease [70]. These factors should be considered when deciding which patients should undergo an MRI of the brain at the time of diagnosis. In the setting of de novo and relapsed disseminated disease, chemotherapy is recommended as first-line treatment, followed by resection of residual disease if possible. In the case of unresectable disease, stereotactic radiosurgery can be used, and WBRT can be considered for multiple brain metastases [71]. In the rare setting of a solitary brain metastasis at relapse, chemotherapy and resection are recommended, with SRS considered as postoperative therapy. In the setting of brain metastases at relapse, high-dose chemotherapy and multimodality treatment were associated with improved survival [72]. One additional consideration for choriocarcinomas is the increased risk of hemorrhage after chemotherapy is started, and anticoagulation should be held unless the other medical concerns necessitate its use [73].

## Leptomeningeal Carcinomatosis

Leptomeningeal carcinomatosis is an uncommon presentation of intracranial disease—found in 1–5% of patients with solid tumors—where tumor cells travel along the CSF and proliferate along the meninges of the brain and spinal cord (Fig. 32.2). The median survival of patients with leptomeningeal disease is worse than for parenchymal metastatic disease, and treatment usually consists of a combination of WBRT, systemic chemotherapy, and intrathecal chemotherapy. Current MR imaging is able to demonstrate subtler changes and lesser burdens of disease, where patients may be candidates for palliative SRS, as long as the risks of distant dissemination are discussed with the patient. Stereotactic radiosurgery may also be employed as an adjuvant treatment to intrathecal therapy for patients with bulky leptomeningeal disease because of (1) increased risk of toxicity with concurrent WBRT and intrathecal chemotherapy and (2) the low penetration of intrathecal therapy into bulky tumors [74, 75].

## Outcomes

As described above, WBRT offers tumor response rates in up to half of patients, and one study demonstrated that all patients who undergo WBRT alone experienced a local failure at 1 year [28]. The use of stereotactic radiosurgery alone appears to offer local control rates upward of 70% at 1 year (Table 32.1). Multiple studies have demonstrated that a combination of WBRT and SRS, regardless of sequencing, appear to improve the local control rate to over 80–90% at 1 year's time, likely due to the increased dose to the tumor. Additionally, WBRT reduces the risk of distant brain metastases by eliminating microscopic tumor cells and reduces the need for later salvage treatment, but it does not improve survival outcomes.

With SRS alone, single-fraction doses of 18 Gy or higher have been associated with higher rates of local control [76]. These ablative doses appear to offer similar rates of local control for both classically radiosensitive and radioresistant metastases, with local control rates of over 80% at 1 year for both renal cell carcinoma and melanoma [77, 78]. Increased tumor size (likely due to the lower doses that can be safely administered), cerebellar location, and a lower conformity index have been associated with a lower rate of local control [79]. Fractionated SRS may provide greater safety margins through the introduction of the well-recognized radiobiological principles of repair of DNA damage in contiguous normal brain, reassortment of tumor cells into more radiosensitive portions of the cell cycle, reoxygenation of transiently hypoxic tumor cells, and, by keeping overall treatment times at 1 week or less, avoiding any significant repopulation of tumor cells. There are no randomized studies of fSRS and single-fraction SRS for brain metastases that can provide information about important outcomes for normal tissue toxicity or tumor control.

## Radiation Toxicity

### Toxicities of WBRT

Acute toxicity from radiation can occur within weeks of treatment and include symptoms of fatigue, headache, nausea, vomiting, or mental status changes. These are thought to be secondary to increased edema, cytokine release, and disruption of the blood-brain barrier. Erythema and scaling of the scalp and alopecia can also be seen during or within weeks after treatment. Most of these symptoms are usually transient and resolve spontaneously or with glucocorticoids. Subacute toxicities—those occurring 1–6 months after radiation completion, such as headache, fatigue, or somnolence—are attributed to diffuse demyelination. Neurocognitive deterioration after WBRT is also commonly observed and attributed to chronic radiation injury to vital CNS components such as the microvasculature and stem cell compartments [80].

## Radiation Necrosis

Radiation necrosis (or radionecrosis) is a delayed side effect of radiation, which usually occurs 6 months to 2 years after treatment. Although rarely seen with the doses used for WBRT, radionecrosis may occur in up to 50% of lesions treated with stereotactic radiosurgery [43, 81]. This can be asymptomatic and only detected on posttreatment imaging, or it can cause symptoms similar to that of the primary tumors, including seizures and focal deficits. Radionecrosis can present with classic findings on MRI, including an enhancing lesion with central necrosis on T1-weighted images, with low peripheral signal intensity and hyperintensity in the area of central necrosis on T2-weighted images

[82]. This has been described as a "soap bubble" or "green pepper" appearance, with an area of contrast enhancement around a heterogeneous necrotic center (Fig. 32.5). The gold standard for diagnosing radiation necrosis is a biopsy to rule out tumor progression.

Multiple risk factors have been elucidated in the development of radionecrosis. In a study by Korytko et al. on patients receiving Gamma Knife SRS for CNS tumors, the treatment volume >15 cc receiving 12 Gy was found to correlate with a doubling of the risk of symptomatic radiation necrosis to 54% from 20 to 23% [43]. With fractionated radiosurgery delivered over five fractions, delivering more than 4 Gy to volumes $\geq$23 cc was associated with increased radiographic findings of toxicity [54]. Patients who have received WBRT are at greater risk after SRS of developing radionecrosis, and metastases in certain (eloquent) locations are perhaps more likely to develop symptomatic radionecrosis. Systemic use of checkpoint inhibitors and tyrosine kinase inhibitors has been described as elevating the risk of radionecrosis [62–65]. Dose conformity is undoubtedly important, especially for larger lesions, where there will be a larger 12 Gy volume associated with SRS treatment [79].

Symptomatic radionecrosis is often initially managed with steroids. Although some patients respond to short-term steroids, others may require long-term steroids or additional treatment with hyperbaric oxygen, pentoxifylline, antiplatelet agents, or an inhibitor of vascular endothelial growth factor (VEGF). Bevacizumab, a monoclonal antibody against

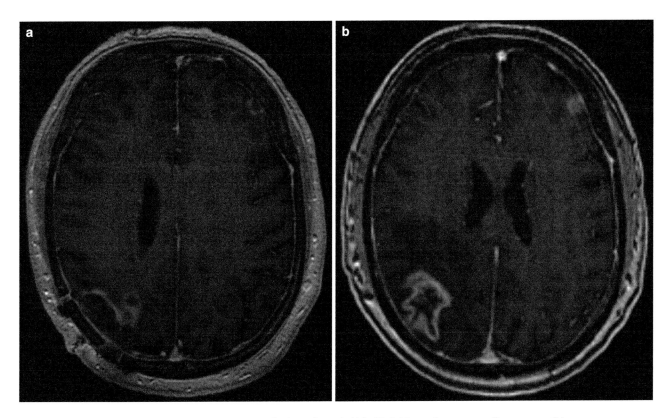

**Fig. 32.5** Radiation necrosis after SRS, classically described as a "soap bubble-like" (**a**) or a "green pepper" appearance (**b**)

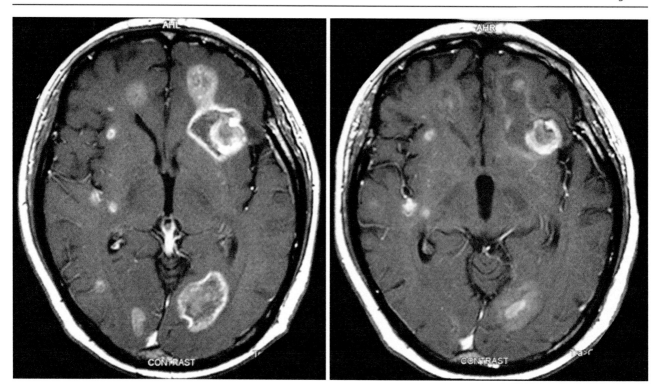

**Fig. 32.6** Radiation necrosis 7 months after SRS (left) and after treatment with two cycles of bevacizumab (right)

VEGF, has been recently demonstrated in a small trial to improve neurologic symptoms and imaging findings and has also been used as a noninvasive approach to manage symptoms [63, 81] (Fig. 32.6). Surgical resection of symptomatic necrosis may be used for emergent symptoms or for progressive disease despite noninvasive therapies. Laser interstitial thermal therapy (LITT) has shown great promise in addressing progressively enlarging and symptomatic lesions that are not amenable (because of location, etc.) to surgical resection [84–85].

## Damage to Other Normal Tissues

While the doses and fractionation schedules used for whole brain radiation are lower than what is expected to cause damage to the optic nerve, cochlea, and brainstem, the doses used in radiosurgery can cause significant toxicity to these organs. Damage to the optic nerve can cause radiation-induced optic neuropathy (RION), which manifests as sudden permanent visual loss occurring as early as 3 months and peaking at 1–1.5 years after treatment [86]. With single-fraction treatments, the doses associated with RION are less clear. A single-institutional study of patients receiving SRS to skull base tumors with no prior radiation demonstrated that no patients receiving ≤12 Gy to the anterior visual pathway developed symptomatic RION and an overall risk of 1% in patients receiving 8 Gy or more to the

pathway [87]. The risk of neuropathy appears to increase to over 10% in patients receiving 12 Gy or more to the optic nerve [88]. The cochlea is sensitive to even lower doses of radiation, where doses of 4.2 Gy and higher to the cochlea were found to predict for worsening hearing after single-fraction treatment [89].

The brainstem also appears more sensitive than the cerebral cortex or cerebellum, and doses should also be limited to this critical structure. Using single-fraction treatment, a maximum point dose of 15 Gy is recommended, while less than 0.5 cc may be allowed to receive 10 Gy [90]. These dose recommendations are more conservative than those used for Gamma Knife SRS of brainstem metastases in JLGK0901, where a marginal dose of 16, 18, or 20 Gy was permitted, based on metastasis volume, with rates of ≥Grade 3 morbidity of only 4% at 4 years' time. In addition to recommendations of maximum doses for single-fraction treatment, the Task Group 101 report also contains critical organ constraints for the brainstem and optic nerves for three- and five-fraction fSRS treatments.

## Neurocognition

Ionizing radiation does not differentiate between normal tissues and tumor tissues, and normal tissue injury from irradiation can lead to neurologic toxicity. In the study published by Chang et al., patients with 1–3 brain metastases were ran-

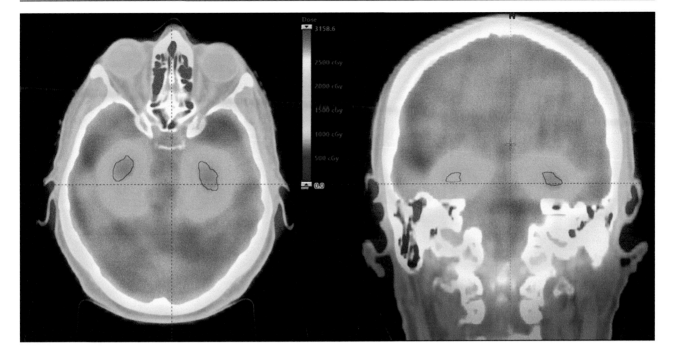

**Fig. 32.7** "Heat Map" dose distribution of whole brain radiation therapy prescribed to deliver 25.0 Gy using intensity-modulated radiation therapy (IMRT) to avoid dose to the hippocampi with prophylactic cranial irradiation

domized to SRS versus SRS with WBRT with a primary endpoint of neurocognitive decline [36]. This study demonstrated a markedly higher probability of decline in learning and memory of patients who received both treatments (52% versus 24% at 4 months), and worse cognitive outcomes occurred despite improved intracranial control. A larger, NCI-supported intergroup study found that patients who received SRS alone experienced less cognitive decline and had an improved quality of life, despite the improved intracranial tumor control rate observed in patients who received additional WBRT [38]. There was no difference in functional independence or median survival between the two arms, which argues for avoidance of WBRT when treating oligometastatic brain metastases with SRS, as recommended by ASTRO.

Based on a hypothesis that ionizing radiation's damage to the microvasculature might be ameliorated with pharmacologic therapies used for microvascular dementia, memantine, an NMDA receptor antagonist with demonstrated efficacy in preventing neurocognitive decline in preclinical models and treating vascular dementia, was prospectively tested in the setting of WBRT for brain metastases. Patients were randomized to receive memantine or placebo starting with radiation and for a total of 24 weeks thereafter [24]. The study did not meet its primary endpoint of finding a difference in delayed recall evaluated with the Hopkins Verbal Learning Test (HVLT) ($p = 0.059$), which was thought to be due to high rates of patient loss at 24 weeks; however, the memantine group drug experienced a longer time to cognitive

decline and improved executive function, processing speed, and delayed recognition.

The neurocognitive decline observed after WBRT has been attributed to damage to hippocampal neural stem cells [91]. This, in addition to a low observed rate of metastasis development in the hippocampal region, led to RTOG 0933, a phase II trial evaluating hippocampal avoidance with WBRT, which found patients who underwent hippocampal avoidance WBRT had improved memory preservation 4 months after radiation relative to historic controls [23]. This study also found that memory preservation was associated with an associated preservation of quality of life. Based on the results of this study and the aforementioned memantine studies, a phase III trial—NRG CC001—has been opened and will evaluate the neurocognitive outcomes after WBRT with memantine and hippocampal avoidance (Fig. 32.7). The hippocampi are likely not the only structures responsible for postradiation neurocognitive decline, and more research into other potentially important subsites, such as the anterior thalami, fornices, and mammillary bodies, is needed.

## Follow-Up

The NCCN guidelines recommend posttreatment imaging with an MRI of the brain every 2–3 months for the first year and then as clinically indicated afterward. Specifically for patients treated with SRS alone, follow-up imaging every

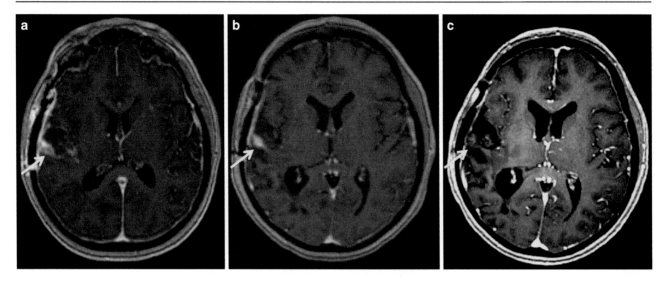

**Fig. 32.8** Evolution of posttreatment changes in a patient who received SRS to a postoperative cavity. A contrast-enhancing area of nodularity is seen on the postsurgical planning MRI (**a**) (denoted with arrow) and remains relatively stable on imaging 2 months after SRS (**b**) with a reduction in enhancement of the surgical cavity. Imaging at 5 months after SRS demonstrates resolution of contrast enhancement in both the cavity and nodular lesion (**c**)

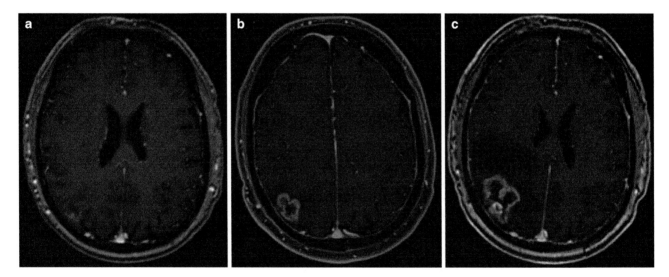

**Fig. 32.9** Posttreatment changes in a patient with metastatic lung cancer who received fractionated SRS. A subtly contrast-enhancing right parietal tumor was seen on initial presentation and treated with fractionated SRS to a dose of 27 Gy in 3 fractions (**a**). A follow-up MRI 2.5 months later demonstrated an increase in the size and enhancement of the right parietal lesion (**b**), and an MR spectroscopy study was performed with results indicating radiation necrosis. An MRI performed 3 months later demonstrated further increase of the right parietal lesion with associated edema, as well as two new areas of intracranial disease (**c**). Surgery was recommended for this lesion, and pathology demonstrated necrosis with no evidence of residual viable tumor

2 months is recommended. A response to treatment can be seen with a reduction in size of a previously seen lesion or loss of contrast enhancement (Fig. 32.8). One challenging task for neuroradiologists is in differentiating postradiation changes and tumor progression. Up to half of patients with brain metastases treated with radiosurgery will experience a transient growth of the mass on imaging within the first 2 years after treatment (Fig. 32.9). In a large series of 500 patients treated with SRS, one third of the patients had a transient increase in lesion size after treatment [92]. Of a subset who underwent a biopsy of their lesions, 22 of 23 patients had findings only of treatment effect without residual viable tumor.

One method to differentiate treatment effect from tumor progression is evaluation of the concordance between the T1 and T2 images, known as "T1/T2 matching." When the border of the lesion on the T2-weighted image does not correspond to the contrast-enhancing lesion, the findings are more likely to be associated with tumor necrosis than tumor progression. In one study, a T1/T2 mismatch had an 83.3% sensitivity and 91.2% specificity for identifying tumor necrosis, while a T1/T2 match had a sensitivity of 93.9% and specificity of 76.9% for identifying tumor recurrence [93].

Other imaging techniques to detect progression versus treatment changes include using perfusion imaging to measure the relative cerebral blood volume (CBV) in the region of interest—tumors are characterized by increased angiogenesis and blood flow, while necrotic tissue has decreased vascularity. Diffusion-weighted imaging (DWI) assesses the movement of water molecules within an environment, with less water movement seen in regions with high cellularity. Areas of tumor recurrence tend to have increased cellularity, translating into restricted water movement. The restriction is measured by the apparent diffusion coefficient (ADC), with lower values seen in tumor recurrence. MR spectroscopy has also been used to quantify the metabolites within a region, including choline, creatinine, and N-acetyl acetate (NAA). Elevated ratios of choline to NAA and to creatinine, as well as decreased ratios of NAA to creatinine, have been found to be indicative of tumor progression [94]. Methionine PET has also been increasingly used to differentiate tumor recurrence versus necrosis after radiosurgery and may be helpful in planning patients for retreatment [95] (Fig. 32.10).

## Management of Recurrent or New Brain Metastases

In patients treated with both focal therapy and WBRT, over half of the patients will develop local and/or distant brain metastases within a year of treatment (Table 32.1).

Retreatment after progression of previously treated metastases or of new brain metastases can include resection, laser interstitial thermal therapy, chemotherapy, or further SRS or WBRT and depends on the prior treatment, extent of systemic disease, and intracranial disease burden and symptoms. For patients with limited disease, focal treatment with surgery or stereotactic radiosurgery has been used after prior focal or whole brain treatment, and the SRS doses used in RTOG 9005 can be used as a guideline after WBRT. Patients who present with limited intracranial disease can undergo salvage with SRS with similar rates of local control, survival, and rates of salvage treatment with SRS or WBRT as the initial treatment course with acceptable rates of toxicity [96, 97]. For patients with more extensive disease, WBRT may be used, and if it is employed after prior WBRT, dose de-escalation to 20 or 25 Gy in ten fractions is common. Several single-institution series have demonstrated that repeat WBRT can reduce neurologic symptoms, with greater benefits seen in patients with better performance statuses, but no prospective trials have evaluated the benefits and harms of repeat WBRT versus a focal treatment or observation [98]. There is a significant concern about the neurocognitive consequences of repeat treatment; however, formal neurocognitive testing has not been performed routinely, and the extent of cognitive decline after re-irradiation has not been well-quantified. Patients with poorer prognostic factors at the time of recurrence—including poor performance status, uncontrolled systemic disease, and extensive brain metastases—should also be offered the option of supportive care, as their survival may be similar with or without radiation [99].

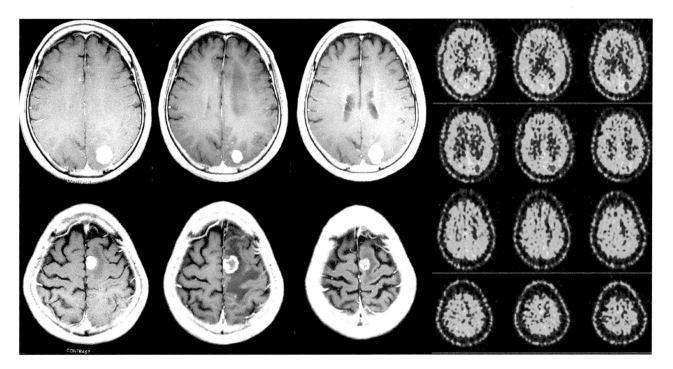

**Fig. 32.10** Progression of two lesions from prior to SRS treatment to 16 months after treatment in left-sided MRI scan images. The top 2 rows of the methionine _PET scan (the color images) show tumor recurrence, while the bottom row shows scar tissue

## Specific Case Scenario

A 62-year-old man with a history of renal cell carcinoma status postprimary tumor resection presented with vertigo. An MRI demonstrated a 1.4 × 1.8 cm mass in the left cerebellum, a 1.0 x 0.7 cm lesion in the left frontal lobe, and a 2.5 × 2.0 cm lesion in the right occipital convexity attached to the dura, all with associated edema. He underwent a suboccipital craniectomy with resection of the cerebellar metastasis and a right occipital craniectomy with pathology from both lesions demonstrating metastatic renal cell carcinoma. He was seen in consultation and agreed to treatment with SRS. An MRI was performed for treatment planning, which redemonstrated the left frontal lesion, two resection cavities, and four new metastases (Fig. 32.11). All metastases and resection beds were contoured on a T1-weighted contrast MRI, and a 1 mm margin was added to create a PTV. The MRI was fused to the CT scan from the patient's simulation. Given the proximity of the tumor volumes to the hippocampi and the patient's otherwise good performance status, a single-isocenter plan was created with standard institutional planning (Fig. 32.12) and with a specific focus on hippocampal avoidance (Fig. 32.13). The minimum target coverage was set at D95% > 100%, and all targets were prescribed to 20 Gy. The maximum point dose (Dmax) to the hippocampi was 9.6 Gy (left) and 12.1 (right) with standard planning (dose-volume histogram in Fig. 32.14a); however, with hippocampal avoidance, these doses were reduced to 4.8 Gy (left) and 5.9 Gy (right) (dose-volume histogram in Fig. 32.14b).

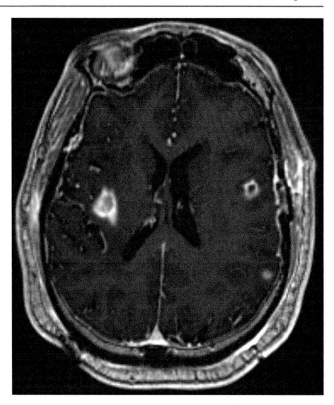

**Fig. 32.11** Post-resection MRI demonstrating multiple new ring-enhancing lesions

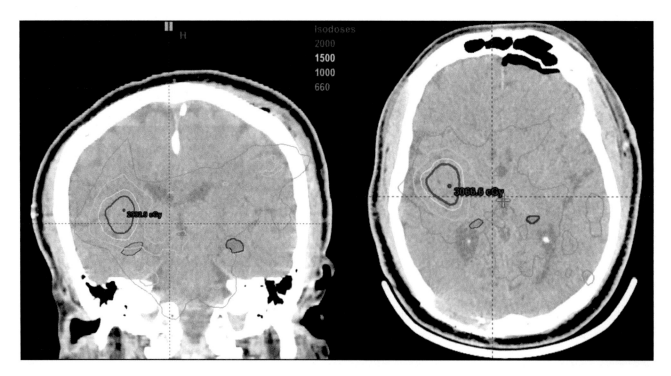

**Fig. 32.12** Single-isocenter LINAC-based SRS plan using standard institutional planning. The hippocampi (purple) were not specifically avoided

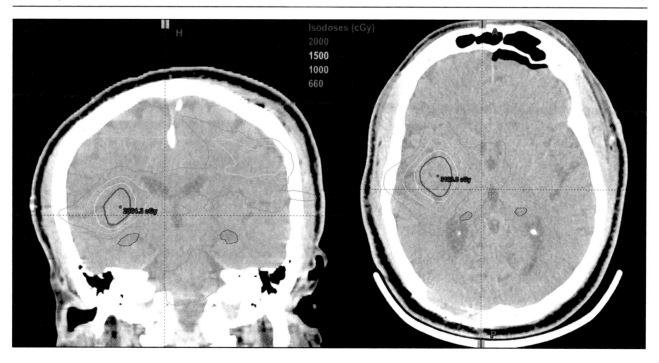

**Fig. 32.13** Single-isocenter LINAC-based SRS plan with hippocampal sparing (hippocampi in purple). Target coverage was not reduced; however, dose to the hippocampi were lowered

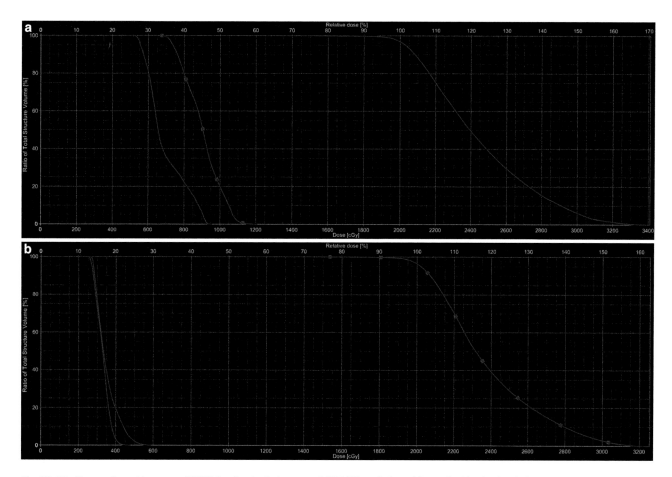

**Fig. 32.14** Dose-volume histogram (DVH) for the single-isocenter LINAC-based plan with standard institutional planning (**a**) versus hippocampal sparing (**b**). The PTV is shown in blue and the hippocampi are shown in purple

## Summary

- Brain metastases outnumber primary brain tumors by tenfold and will affect 20–40% of patients with cancer during their lifetimes.
- The addition of an SRS boost to WBRT for limited disease improves tumor local control without a benefit in survival.
- The addition of WBRT to surgery or SRS can improve intracranial control, but this does not translate into prolonged survival. The addition of WBRT also appears to negatively affect quality of life and neurocognition.
- Hippocampal avoidance and the use of the NMDA antagonist memantine appear to help preserve cognition in patients undergoing radiation for brain metastases, but confirmation of these observations in appropriately rigorous clinical trials is pending.
- Posttreatment effects can be difficult to distinguish from tumor progression, and the use of additional testing, such as cerebral blood volume, MR spectroscopy, and C-11 methionine PET, may be helpful in noninvasive diagnosis.

## Self-Assessment Questions

1. In patients with brain metastases from lung cancer who are not candidates for surgery or stereotactic radiosurgery, whole brain radiation will most likely offer a survival benefit in patients [8]:
   A. With a single brain metastasis
   B. With a KPS >70
   C. Who do not require steroids at presentation
   D. With squamous cell histology
   E. Who are younger than 60 years old

2. In patients with EGFR-mutated lung cancer presenting with multiple asymptomatic brain metastases, patients should undergo [64]:
   A. A targeted tyrosine kinase inhibitor (TKI) followed by SRS
   B. A targeted TKI followed by WBRT
   C. A targeted TKI alone
   D. SRS followed by a targeted TKI
   E. WBRT followed by a targeted TKI

3. All of the following have been demonstrated to reduce neurocognitive toxicities of radiation except [23, 24, 36]:
   A. Hippocampal avoidance during WBRT
   B. Dose reduction of WBRT from 30 Gy in ten fractions to 20 Gy in five fractions
   C. Administration of memantine concurrently with WBRT
   D. Avoidance of WBRT together with SRS

4. In patients undergoing SRS for brain metastases, the addition of WBRT [30, 34, 36, 38]:
   A. Improves overall survival at 1 year
   B. Improves distant brain control at 1 year
   C. Improves quality of life
   D. Improves neurocognition as tested by the HVLT
   E. Is recommended for patients with a limited number of brain metastases by the ASTRO Choosing Wisely® campaign

5. Which of the following imaging characteristics is indicative of postradiation changes versus tumor recurrence [92]?
   A. T1/T2 mismatch on MRI
   B. Increased angiogenesis and cerebral blood volume on perfusion imaging
   C. Elevated ratios of choline to NAA on MR spectroscopy
   D. Decreased levels of NAA to creatinine on MR spectroscopy
   E. Decreased restriction on diffusion-weighted imaging

## Answers

1. E
2. D
3. B
4. B
5. E

## References

1. Wen PY, Loeffler J. Management of brain metastases. Oncology (Williston Park, NY). 1999;13(7):941–54, 57–61; discussion 61–2, 9.
2. Barnholtz-Sloan JS, Sloan AE, Davis FG, et al. Incidence proportions of brain metastases in patients diagnosed (1973 to 2001) in the Metropolitan Detroit Cancer Surveillance System. J Clin Oncol. 2004;22(14):2865–72.
3. Delattre JY, Krol G, Thaler HT, et al. Distribution of brain metastases. Arch Neurol. 1988;45(7):741–4.
4. Arbit E, Wronski M, Burt M, et al. The treatment of patients with recurrent brain metastases. A retrospective analysis of 109 patients with nonsmall cell lung cancer. Cancer. 1995;76(5):765–73.
5. Chamberlain MC. Leptomeningeal metastasis. Semin Neurol. 2010;30(3):236–44.
6. Priedigkeit N, Hartmaier RJ, Chen Y, et al. Intrinsic subtype switching and acquired ERBB2/HER2 amplifications and mutations in breast cancer brain metastases. JAMA Oncol. 2017;3(5):666 71.
7. Zimm S, Wampler GL, Stablein D, et al. Intracerebral metastases in solid-tumor patients: natural history and results of treatment. Cancer. 1981;48(2):384–94.
8. Mulvenna P, Nankivell M, Barton R, et al. Dexamethasone and supportive care with or without whole brain radiotherapy in treating patients with non-small cell lung cancer with brain metastases unsuitable for resection or stereotactic radiotherapy (QUARTZ):

results from a phase 3, non-inferiority, randomised trial. Lancet. 2016;388(10055):2004–14.

9. Gaspar L, Scott C, Rotman M, et al. Recursive partitioning analysis (RPA) of prognostic factors in three Radiation Therapy Oncology Group (RTOG) brain metastases trials. Int J Radiat Oncol Biol Phys. 1997;37(4):745–51.

10. Sperduto PW, Berkey B, Gaspar LE, et al. A new prognostic index and comparison to three other indices for patients with brain metastases: an analysis of 1,960 patients in the RTOG database. Int J Radiat Oncol Biol Phys. 2008;70(2):510–4.

11. Sperduto PW, Chao ST, Sneed PK, et al. Diagnosis-specific prognostic factors, indexes, and treatment outcomes for patients with newly diagnosed brain metastases: a multi-institutional analysis of 4,259 patients. Int J Radiat Oncol Biol Phys. 2010;77(3):655–61.

12. Sperduto PW, Yang TJ, Beal K, et al. Estimating survival in patients with lung cancer and brain metastases: an update of the graded prognostic assessment for lung cancer using molecular markers (lung-molGPA). JAMA Oncol. 2017;3(6):827–31.

13. Yamamoto M, Serizawa T, Shuto T, et al. Stereotactic radiosurgery for patients with multiple brain metastases (JLGK0901): a multi-institutional prospective observational study. Lancet Oncol. 2014;15(4):387–95.

14. Skeie BS, Skeie GO, Enger PO, et al. Gamma Knife surgery in brain melanomas: absence of extracranial metastases and tumor volume strongest indicators of prolonged survival. World Neurosurg. 2011;75(5–6):684–91. discussion 598–603

15. Baschnagel AM, Meyer KD, Chen PY, et al. Tumor volume as a predictor of survival and local control in patients with brain metastases treated with Gamma Knife surgery. J Neurosurg. 2013;119(5):1139–44.

16. Twycross RG. Palliative care formulary. Oxford: Radcliffe Publishing; 2002.

17. Bindal AK, Bindal RK, Hess KR, et al. Surgery versus radiosurgery in the treatment of brain metastasis. J Neurosurg. 1996;84(5):748–54.

18. Bindal RK, Sawaya R, Leavens ME, et al. Surgical treatment of multiple brain metastases. J Neurosurg. 1993;79(2):210–6.

19. Soltys SG, Adler JR, Lipani JD, et al. Stereotactic radiosurgery of the postoperative resection cavity for brain metastases. Int J Radiat Oncol Biol Phys. 2008;70(1):187–93.

20. McPherson CM, Suki D, Feiz-Erfan I, et al. Adjuvant whole-brain radiation therapy after surgical resection of single brain metastases. Neuro Oncol. 2010;12(7):711–9.

21. McTyre E, Scott J, Chinnaiyan P. Whole brain radiotherapy for brain metastasis. Surg Neurol Int. 2013;4(Suppl 4):S236–44.

22. Tsao MN, Lloyd N, Wong RK, et al. Whole brain radiotherapy for the treatment of newly diagnosed multiple brain metastases. Cochrane Database Syst Rev 2012;(4):CD003869.

23. Gondi V, Pugh SL, Tome WA, et al. Preservation of memory with conformal avoidance of the hippocampal neural stem-cell compartment during whole-brain radiotherapy for brain metastases (RTOG 0933): a phase II multi-institutional trial. J Clin Oncol. 2014;32(34):3810–6.

24. Brown PD, Pugh S, Laack NN, et al. Memantine for the prevention of cognitive dysfunction in patients receiving whole-brain radiotherapy: a randomized, double-blind, placebo-controlled trial. Neuro Oncol. 2013;15(10):1429–37.

25. Horton J, Baxter DH, Olson KB. The management of metastases to the brain by irradiation and corticosteroids. Am J Roentgenol Radium Therapy Nucl Med. 1971;111(2):334–6.

26. Wong WW, Schild SE, Sawyer TE, et al. Analysis of outcome in patients reirradiated for brain metastases. Int J Radiat Oncol Biol Phys. 1996;34(3):585–90.

27. Andrews DW, Scott CB, Sperduto PW, et al. Whole brain radiation therapy with or without stereotactic radiosurgery boost for patients with one to three brain metastases: phase III results of the RTOG 9508 randomised trial. Lancet. 2004;363(9422):1665–72.

28. Kondziolka D, Patel A, Lunsford LD, et al. Stereotactic radiosurgery plus whole brain radiotherapy versus radiotherapy alone for patients with multiple brain metastases. Int J Radiat Oncol Biol Phys. 1999;45(2):427–34.

29. Sneed PK, Suh JH, Goetsch SJ, et al. A multi-institutional review of radiosurgery alone vs. radiosurgery with whole brain radiotherapy as the initial management of brain metastases. Int J Radiat Oncol Biol Phys. 2002;53(3):519–26.

30. Aoyama H, Shirato H, Tago M, et al. Stereotactic radiosurgery plus whole-brain radiation therapy vs stereotactic radiosurgery alone for treatment of brain metastases: a randomized controlled trial. JAMA. 2006;295(21):2483–91.

31. Kocher M, Soffietti R, Abacioglu U, et al. Adjuvant whole-brain radiotherapy versus observation after radiosurgery or surgical resection of one to three cerebral metastases: results of the EORTC 22952-26001 study. J Clin Oncol. 2011;29(2):134–41.

32. Chang EL, Wefel JS, Hess KR, et al. Neurocognition in patients with brain metastases treated with radiosurgery or radiosurgery plus whole-brain irradiation: a randomised controlled trial. Lancet Oncol. 2009;10(11):1037–44.

33. Brown PD, Jaeckle K, Ballman KV, et al. Effect of radiosurgery alone vs radiosurgery with whole brain radiation therapy on cognitive function in patients with 1 to 3 brain metastases: a randomized clinical trial. JAMA. 2016;316(4):401–9.

34. Aoyama H, Tago M, Shirato H. Stereotactic radiosurgery with or without whole-brain radiotherapy for brain metastases: secondary analysis of the JROSG 99-1 randomized clinical trial. JAMA Oncol. 2015;1(4):457–64.

35. Churilla TM, Ballman KV, Brown PD, et al. Stereotactic radiosurgery with or without whole-brain radiation therapy for limited brain metastases: a secondary analysis of the North Central Cancer Treatment Group N0574 (Alliance) randomized controlled trial. Int J Radiat Oncol Biol Phys. 2017;99:1173.

36. Churilla TM, Handorf E, Collette S, et al. Whole brain radiotherapy after stereotactic radiosurgery or surgical resection among patients with one to three brain metastases and favorable prognoses: a secondary analysis of EORTC 22952-26001. Ann Oncol. 2017;28(10):2588–94.

37. Soffietti R, Kocher M, Abacioglu UM, et al. A European Organisation for Research and Treatment of Cancer phase III trial of adjuvant whole-brain radiotherapy versus observation in patients with one to three brain metastases from solid tumors after surgical resection or radiosurgery: quality-of-life results. J Clin Oncol. 2013;31(1):65–72.

38. Sahgal A, Aoyama H, Kocher M, et al. Phase 3 trials of stereotactic radiosurgery with or without whole-brain radiation therapy for 1 to 4 brain metastases: individual patient data meta-analysis. Int J Radiat Oncol Biol Phys. 2015;91(4):710–7.

39. NCC Network. Central nervous system cancers (Version 1.2016). [February 7, 2017]; Available from: https://www.nccn.org/professionals/physician_gls/pdf/cns.pdf.

40. Choosing Wisely. American Society for Radiation Oncology. [updated June 21, 2016; June 9, 2017]; Available from: http://www.choosingwisely.org/societies/american-society-for-radiation-oncology/.

41. Mehta MP, Aoyama H, Gondi V. The changing role of whole-brain radiotherapy: demise or time for selective usage? JAMA Oncol. 2017;3:1021.

42. Knisely JP, Yamamoto M, Gross CP, et al. Radiosurgery alone for 5 or more brain metastases: expert opinion survey. J Neurosurg. 2010;113(Suppl):84–9.

43. Korytko T, Radivoyevitch T, Colussi V, et al. 12 Gy Gamma Knife radiosurgical volume is a predictor for radiation necrosis in non-AVM intracranial tumors. Int J Radiat Oncol Biol Phys. 2006;64(2):419–24.

44. Shaw E, Scott C, Souhami L, et al. Single dose radiosurgical treatment of recurrent previously irradiated primary brain tumors and

brain metastases: final report of RTOG protocol 90-05. Int J Radiat Oncol Biol Phys. 2000;47(2):291–8.

45. Yamamoto M, Serizawa T, Higuchi Y, et al. A multi-institutional prospective observational study of stereotactic radiosurgery for patients with multiple brain metastases (JLGK0901 study update): irradiation-related complications and long-term maintenance of mini-mental state examination scores. Int J Radiat Oncol Biol Phys. 2017;99(1):31–40.

46. Swinson BM, Friedman WA. Linear accelerator stereotactic radiosurgery for metastatic brain tumors: 17 years of experience at the University of Florida. Neurosurgery. 2008;62(5):1018–31; discussion 31-2.

47. Varlotto JM, Flickinger JC, Niranjan A, et al. The impact of whole-brain radiation therapy on the long-term control and morbidity of patients surviving more than one year after Gamma Knife radiosurgery for brain metastases. Int J Radiat Oncol Biol Phys. 2005;62(4):1125–32.

48. Jawahar A, Matthew RE, Minagar A, et al. Gamma Knife surgery in the management of brain metastases from lung carcinoma: a retrospective analysis of survival, local tumor control, and freedom from new brain metastasis. J Neurosurg. 2004;100(5):842–7.

49. Skeie BS, Enger PO, Ganz JC, et al. Gamma Knife surgery of colorectal brain metastases: a high prescription dose of 25 Gy may improve growth control. World Neurosurg. 2013;79(3–4):525–36.

50. Surgeons AAoNSaCoN. Statement on coding and reimbursement for stereotactic radiosurgery. 2008 [January 1, 2017.]; Available from: http://www.aans.org/~/media/Files/Legislative%20Activities/Reimbursement/AANS-CNS%20Statement%20on%20SRS%20Coding.ashx?la=en.

51. Higuchi Y, Serizawa T, Nagano O, et al. Three-staged stereotactic radiotherapy without whole brain irradiation for large metastatic brain tumors. Int J Radiat Oncol Biol Phys. 2009;74(5):1543–8.

52. Kim YJ, Cho KH, Kim JY, et al. Single-dose versus fractionated stereotactic radiotherapy for brain metastases. Int J Radiat Oncol Biol Phys. 2011;81(2):483–9.

53. Minniti G, Scaringi C, Paolini S, et al. Single-fraction versus multifraction (3 x 9 Gy) stereotactic radiosurgery for large (>2 cm) brain metastases: a comparative analysis of local control and risk of radiation-induced brain necrosis. Int J Radiat Oncol Biol Phys. 2016;95(4):1142–8.

54. Ernst-Stecken A, Ganslandt O, Lambrecht U, et al. Phase II trial of hypofractionated stereotactic radiotherapy for brain metastases: results and toxicity. Radiother Oncol. 2006;81(1):18–24.

55. Fokas E, Henzel M, Surber G, et al. Stereotactic radiosurgery and fractionated stereotactic radiotherapy: comparison of efficacy and toxicity in 260 patients with brain metastases. J Neurooncol. 2012;109(1):91–8.

56. Demaria S, Coleman CN, Formenti SC. Radiotherapy: changing the game in immunotherapy. Trends Cancer. 2016;2(6):286–94.

57. Grimaldi AM, Simeone E, Giannarelli D, et al. Abscopal effects of radiotherapy on advanced melanoma patients who progressed after ipilimumab immunotherapy. Oncoimmunology. 2014;3:e28780.

58. Schaue D, Ratikan JA, Iwamoto KS, et al. Maximizing tumor immunity with fractionated radiation. Int J Radiat Oncol Biol Phys. 2012;83(4):1306–10.

59. Dewan MZ, Galloway AE, Kawashima N, et al. Fractionated but not single-dose radiotherapy induces an immune-mediated abscopal effect when combined with anti-CTLA-4 antibody. Clin Cancer Res. 2009;15(17):5379–88.

60. Tsao MN, Rades D, Wirth A, et al. Radiotherapeutic and surgical management for newly diagnosed brain metastasis(es): an American Society for Radiation Oncology evidence-based guideline. Pract Radiat Oncol. 2012;2(3):210–25.

61. Knisely JP, Yu JB, Flanigan J, et al. Radiosurgery for melanoma brain metastases in the ipilimumab era and the possibility of longer survival. J Neurosurg. 2012;117(2):227–33.

62. Rauch PJ, Park HS, Knisely JP, et al. Delayed radiation-induced vasculitic leukoencephalopathy. Int J Radiat Oncol Biol Phys. 2012;83(1):369–75.

63. Cohen JV, Kluger HM. Systemic immunotherapy for the treatment of brain metastases. Front Oncol. 2016;6:49.

64. Colaco RJ, Martin P, Kluger HM, et al. Does immunotherapy increase the rate of radiation necrosis after radiosurgical treatment of brain metastases? J Neurosurg. 2016;125(1):17–23.

65. Kim JM, Miller JA, Kotecha R, et al. The risk of radiation necrosis following stereotactic radiosurgery with concurrent systemic therapies. J Neurooncol. 2017;133(2):357–68. https://doi.org/10.1007/s11060-017-2442-8.

66. Long GV, Atkinson V, Lo S, et al. Combination nivolumab and ipilimumab or nivolumab alone in melanoma brain metastases: a multicentre randomised phase 2 study. Lancet Oncol. 2018;19(5):672–81.

67. Magnuson WJ, Yeung JT, Guillod PD, et al. Impact of deferring radiation therapy in patients with epidermal growth factor receptor-mutant non-small cell lung cancer who develop brain metastases. Int J Radiat Oncol Biol Phys. 2016;95(2):673–9.

68. Yomo S, Hayashi M. Is stereotactic radiosurgery a rational treatment option for brain metastases from small cell lung cancer? A retrospective analysis of 70 consecutive patients. BMC Cancer. 2015;15:95.

69. Doyle DM, Einhorn LH. Delayed effects of whole brain radiotherapy in germ cell tumor patients with central nervous system metastases. Int J Radiat Oncol Biol Phys. 2008;70(5):1361–4.

70. Oechsle K, Bokemeyer C. Treatment of brain metastases from germ cell tumors. Hematol Oncol Clin North Am. 2011;25(3):605–13, ix.

71. Gilligan T. Decision making in a data-poor environment: management of brain metastases from testicular and extragonadal germ cell tumors. J Clin Oncol. 2016;34(4):303–6.

72. Feldman DR, Lorch A, Kramar A, et al. Brain metastases in patients with germ cell tumors: prognostic factors and treatment options-DOUBLEHYPHENan analysis from the global germ cell cancer group. J Clin Oncol. 2016;34(4):345–51.

73. Motzer RJ, Bosl GJ. Hemorrhage: a complication of metastatic testicular choriocarcinoma. Urology. 1987;30(2):119–22.

74. Huang TY, Arita N, Hayakawa T, et al. ACNU, MTX and 5-FU penetration of rat brain tissue and tumors. J Neurooncol. 1999;45(1):9–17.

75. Bertke MH, Burton EC, Shaughnessy JN. Stereotactic radiosurgery as part of multimodal treatment in a bulky leptomeningeal recurrence of breast cancer. Cureus. 2016;8(3):e523.

76. Shiau CY, Sneed PK, Shu HK, et al. Radiosurgery for brain metastases: relationship of dose and pattern of enhancement to local control. Int J Radiat Oncol Biol Phys. 1997;37(2):375–83.

77. Kano H, Iyer A, Kondziolka D, et al. Outcome predictors of Gamma Knife radiosurgery for renal cell carcinoma metastases. Neurosurgery. 2011;69(6):1232–9.

78. Mathieu D, Kondziolka D, Cooper PB, et al. Gamma knife radiosurgery in the management of malignant melanoma brain metastases. Neurosurgery. 2007;60(3):471–81. discussion 81–2

79. Garsa AA, Badiyan SN, DeWees T, et al. Predictors of individual tumor local control after stereotactic radiosurgery for non-small cell lung cancer brain metastases. Int J Radiat Oncol Biol Phys. 2014;90(2):407–13.

80. Sheline GE, Wara WM, Smith V. Therapeutic irradiation and brain injury. Int J Radiat Oncol Biol Phys. 1980;6(9):1215–28.

81. Minniti G, Clarke E, Lanzetta G, et al. Stereotactic radiosurgery for brain metastases: analysis of outcome and risk of brain radionecrosis. Radiat Oncol. 2011;6:48.

82. Walker AJ, Ruzevick J, Malayeri AA, et al. Postradiation imaging changes in the CNS: how can we differentiate between treatment effect and disease progression? Future Oncol. 2014;10(7):1277–97.

83. Gonzalez J, Kumar AJ, Conrad CA, et al. Effect of bevacizumab on radiation necrosis of the brain. Int J Radiat Oncol Biol Phys. 2007;67(2):323–6.

84. Chaunzwa TL, Deng D, Leuthardt EC, et al. Laser thermal ablation for metastases failing radiosurgery: a multicentered retrospective study. Neurosurgery. 2018;82(1):56–63.

85. Sharma M, Balasubramanian S, Silva D, et al. Laser interstitial thermal therapy in the management of brain metastasis and radiation necrosis after radiosurgery: an overview. Expert Rev Neurother. 2016;16(2):223–32.

86. Danesh-Meyer HV. Radiation-induced optic neuropathy. J Clin Neurosci. 2008;15(2):95–100.

87. Leavitt JA, Stafford SL, Link MJ, et al. Long-term evaluation of radiation-induced optic neuropathy after single-fraction stereotactic radiosurgery. Int J Radiat Oncol Biol Phys. 2013;87(3):524–7.

88. Mayo C, Martel MK, Marks LB, et al. Radiation dose-volume effects of optic nerves and chiasm. Int J Radiat Oncol Biol Phys. 2010;76(3 Suppl):S28–35.

89. Kano H, Kondziolka D, Khan A, et al. Predictors of hearing preservation after stereotactic radiosurgery for acoustic neuroma. J Neurosurg. 2009;111(4):863–73.

90. Benedict SH, Yenice KM, Followill D, et al. Stereotactic body radiation therapy: the report of AAPM Task Group 101. Med Phys. 2010;37(8):4078–101.

91. Gondi V, Tome WA, Mehta MP. Why avoid the hippocampus? A comprehensive review. Radiother Oncol. 2010;97(3):370–6.

92. Patel TR, McHugh BJ, Bi WL, et al. A comprehensive review of MR imaging changes following radiosurgery to 500 brain metastases. AJNR Am J Neuroradiol. 2011;32(10):1885–92.

93. Kano H, Kondziolka D, Lobato-Polo J, et al. T1/T2 matching to differentiate tumor growth from radiation effects after stereotactic radiosurgery. Neurosurgery. 2010;66(3):486–91; discussion 91–2.

94. Weybright P, Sundgren PC, Maly P, et al. Differentiation between brain tumor recurrence and radiation injury using MR spectroscopy. AJR Am J Roentgenol. 2005;185(6):1471–6.

95. Momose T, Nariai T, Kawabe T, et al. Clinical benefit of 11C methionine PET imaging as a planning modality for radiosurgery of previously irradiated recurrent brain metastases. Clin Nucl Med. 2014;39(11):939–43.

96. Kwon KY, Kong DS, Lee JI, et al. Outcome of repeated radiosurgery for recurrent metastatic brain tumors. Clin Neurol Neurosurg. 2007;109(2):132–7.

97. Koiso T, Yamamoto M, Kawabe T, et al. Follow-up results of brain metastasis patients undergoing repeat Gamma Knife radiosurgery. J Neurosurg. 2016;125(Suppl 1):2–10.

98. Guo S, Balagamwala EH, Reddy C, et al. Clinical and radiographic outcomes from repeat whole-brain radiation therapy for brain metastases in the age of stereotactic radiosurgery. Am J Clin Oncol. 2016;39(3):288–93.

99. Nieder C, Norum J, Dalhaug A, et al. Radiotherapy versus best supportive care in patients with brain metastases and adverse prognostic factors. Clin Exp Metastasis. 2013;30(6):723–9.

# Postoperative Treatment for Brain Metastasis

# 33

G. Laura Masucci and David Roberge

## Summary

With the advancement of systemic therapies leading to an increase in survival, and the improvement in imaging's ability to detect smaller lesions, the incidence of brain metastases is expected to rise. Surgery and radiation remain the main tools in the treatment of brain metastases. In the postoperative setting, the latter can be administered to the whole brain (i.e. WBRT) or in one or few high-dose fractions to the surgical cavity (i.e. radiosurgery). This addition of radiation to the surgical cavity, whether by WBRT or radiosurgery, has been shown to improve local control. However, both adjuvant treatments have been associated with very different side effect profiles. WBRT has been associated with global neurotoxicity, while radiosurgery (SRS) is associated with a risk of local radionecrosis. Decisions regarding adjuvant treatment thus have important consequences.

## Learning Objectives

After reading this chapter, the reader will be able to:

- Describe the role of radiosurgery to the surgical cavity after resection of a brain metastasis.
- Describe the role of adjuvant whole brain radiotherapy after resection of a brain metastasis.
- Recognize the different toxicity profiles of radiosurgery and whole brain radiotherapy.
- Recognize the potential benefit of preoperative radiosurgery compared to postoperative radiosurgery.
- Recognize the potential benefit of fractionated radiosurgery compared to single-fraction radiosurgery.

G. L. Masucci · D. Roberge (✉)
Department of Radiation Oncology, Centre Hospitalier de l'Universite de Montreal (CHUM), Montreal, QC, Canada
e-mail: david.roberge.chum@ssss.gouv.qc.ca

Approximately 15–30% of cancer patients will be diagnosed with brain metastases during the course of their illness [1, 2]. In autopsy series, it has been reported that as much as 60% of patients with lung cancer are affected by asymptomatic brain metastases at the time of their death [3].

Nearly all brain metastases are secondary to haematogenous spread [4] and are located at the junction of the grey and white cerebral matter or at 'watershed areas'. Most are thus located in the cerebral hemispheres. Most metastases arise from breast, lung, kidney, colorectal and skin (melanoma) primary cancers [5]. However, certain primary tumours, namely, gastrointestinal and pelvic tumours, have a tendency of metastasizing to the cerebellum [6, 7].

The improvements in magnetic resonance imaging allowing for earlier detection, combined with recent advances in systemic therapy, will likely result in an increase in the number of treatments for secondary brain lesions. Moreover, with these advances in the control of systemic disease and by consequence in longevity, the effect of radiation on a patient's quality of life has become a preponderant factor in the choice of treatment for patients with brain metastases.

Surgery, when considered as a treatment option, serves multiple purposes. It can provide pathological diagnosis and decrease mass effect and has been associated with an increase in overall survival for selected patients. Often, patients that are deemed fit for surgery have an increased expected survival time; therefore the possible long-term detrimental effects of whole brain radiation on these patients are that much more important.

Despite apparent complete surgical removal of the metastases, local recurrences in the surgical bed are common—occurring in approximately half of patients in the first year of observation. Postoperative WBRT was until recently the only proven means to reduce the incidence of these local recurrences. It has been proven that this type of radiation reduces recurrences in the surgical cavity and elsewhere in the brain [8]. The long-term neurocognitive effects [9] of whole brain radiation therapy, as well as secondary fatigue and alopecia, have encouraged many patients and physicians to opt for radiosurgery, a highly focused radiation treatment administered to the surgical cavity in one or a few high-dose fractions. Such a treatment is associated with less long-term difficulty with memory and concentration, less fatigue and rare focal alopecia. Radiosurgery has the additional advantage of avoiding delay in the initiation of systemic therapy. Radiosurgery does however introduce the possibility of focal radionecrosis.

On one hand, a few retrospective studies have shown, when comparing patients treated with the two modalities, that SRS confers local control approaching that seen with WBRT [10–12]. On the other, a few reports have suggested higher rates of local failure compared to WBRT [13, 14]. In the literature, reported crude LC can range from 35% [13] to 100% [10].

Recently, a multi-institutional phase III trial has been completed to inform what the best treatment option for patients after surgery for brain metastasis would be [15]. Over a 4-year period, 194 patients were randomized between receiving postoperative WBRT (30 Gy in 10 fractions or 37.5 Gy in 15 fractions) and radiosurgery to the surgical cavity with doses ranging from 12 to 20 Gy (based on cavity volume). Patients were allowed to have up to three unresected metastases that were to be treated with SRS in either study arm. Most patients enrolled had a single metastasis (77%). Overall survival, a co-primary endpoint, was similar (11.6 months WBRT vs 12.2 months SRS) in both arms. A main endpoint of this study was cognitive deterioration free survival. As expected, this period was shorter after WBRT vs SRS (median 3.0 vs. 3.7 months) (Fig. 33.1). Cognitive deterioration at 6 months was less frequent (52% vs. 85%) in patients receiving radiosurgery. Overall intracranial control was greater in patients treated with WBRT (72% vs 37% at 12 months) than with SRS. Local control to the surgical bed was higher in the long term with WBRT (Fig. 33.2). Quality of life, functional independence and physical wellbeing measured by patients were better in those treated with SRS. In the absence of survival benefit with either treatment

modality, one needs to consider whether higher intracranial local control with WBRT is worth the price to pay in terms of cognitive toxicity and decline in quality of life.

## Factors Influencing Local Recurrence

In selecting adjuvant treatment for patients with resected brain metastasis, a number of factors can be taken into account. As the different options tend to trade off efficacy with toxicity, an important factor may be the risk of recurrence. A number of studies have tried to clarify which factors could potentially predict local recurrence (LR), distant brain failure (DF) as well as overall survival (OS). The following tables summarize factors predicting local and distant failure throughout the brain (Table 33.1) and overall survival (Table 33.2) for selected studies of cavity radiosurgery.

A few histologies have been associated with an increase in local recurrence after surgery and radiation treatment. Tumours originating from breast cancer [25], gastrointestinal tract, sarcoma and melanoma possibly recur more often [17, 29]. On the other hand, lesions stemming from NSCLC cancers have possibly better outcomes [17].

Preoperative tumour size may also be predictive of local failure [12, 17, 20, 25]. In surgical series, without radiation

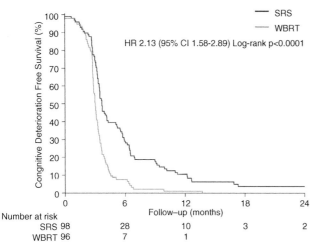

**Fig. 33.1** CDFS with SRS and WBRT. [Courtesy of Dr. Paul Brown]

**Table 33.1** Factors associated with local and distant failure with cavity SRS treatment

|  | Factors associated with local failure | Factors associated with distant failure |
|---|---|---|
| Bilger et al. [16] | Age: older patient NS: KPS, PTV, extracerebral metastases, residual tumour |  |
| Brennan et al. [17] | Histology: NSCLC (better LC) | Location: infratentorial tumour |
|  | Preoperative diameter > 3 cm Deeply located tumours |  |
|  | Dural-pial involvement on pathology NS: radiation dose, time interval between surgery and SRS, surgical cavity diameter and tumour location (infra- vs supratentorial tumour) |  |
| Choi et al. [18] | 2 mm PTV margin (better LC) NS: preoperative lesions diameter, histology, radiation dose, extent of surgical resection | Histology: melanoma Multiple brain metastases NS: extracranial metastases, controlled primary, breast of lung histology, preoperative tumour diameter |
| Doré et al. [19] | NS: extension of resection, histology | NS: GPA score, RPA score, KPS |

**Table 33.1** (continued)

|  | Factors associated with local failure | Factors associated with distant failure |
|---|---|---|
| Hartford et al. [20] | Preoperative diameter > 2 cm NS: tumour diameter, PTV size, radiation dose, extent of resection, number of intracranial metastases | Preoperative diameter > 2 cm |
| Iorio-Morin et al . [21] | Longer surgery to SRS delay (>3 weeks) Lower dose to the PTV NS: type of resection, histology |  |
| Iwai et al . [22] | Dose < 18 gy |  |
| Jagannathan et al. [23] | Greater treated volume |  |
| Jensen et al. [12] | Preoperative diameter > 3 cm | >35 Gy Maximum to cavity large preoperative diameter |
| Karlovits et al. [11] | NS: radiation dose, treated volume, histology, extent of resection |  |
| Mathieu et al. [24] | NS: histology, previous WBRT, time from resection to radiation, extent of resection, radiosurgery volume, margin and maximum dose |  |
| Ojerholm et al. [25] | Histology: breast Infratentorial location Preoperative diameter > 3 cm Residual or recurrent tumour in cavity | Treated volume over 10 cm³ Residual or recurrent tumour in surgical cavity NS: histology, extracranial disease, presence of synchronous metastases |
| Prabhu et al. [26] | Greater treated volume Marginal dose < 18 gy NS: histology, RPA class I, systemic disease, GTR |  |
| Rwigema et al. [27] | Greater treated volume |  |

*NS* not significant, *KPS* Karnofsky performance score, *PTV* planning target volume, *NSCLC* non-small cell lung cancer, *LC* local control, *SRS* radiosurgery treatment, *WBRT* whole brain radiation therapy, *GTR* gross tumour resection, *GPA* graded prognostic assessment, *RPA* recursive partitioning analysis

treatment, larger tumours have been associated with a higher rate of local failure, with lesions measuring more than 3 cm recurring more frequently [5]. A study led by Mahajan et al. [30]from the MD Anderson randomized patients with one to three brain metastasis after GTR (gross total resection) to either surgery followed by observation or postoperative SRS. Lesions with a diameter ≤2.5 cm were associated with better local control (12 months LC: 91%) when compared to larger lesions (2.6–3.5 cm lesions had a 40% 12 month LC; 46% for lesions >3.5 cm). This associa-

**Table 33.2** Factors associated with increased overall survival

|  | Factors associated with overall survival |
|---|---|
| Bilger et al. [16] | KPS > 70%, smaller PTV size |
| Choi et al. [18] | RPA class I KPS ≥ 80 Preoperative tumour diameter |
| Hartford et al. [20] | GPA 1 |
| Jagannathan et al. [23] | No systemic progression |
| Karlovits et al. [11] | Solitary tumour RPA class I No systemic disease on presentation |
| Ogiwara et al. [28] | Systemic disease |
| Ojerholm et al. [25] | Untreated primary |
| Rwigema et al. [27] | Age |

*KPS* Karnofsky performance score, *GPA* graded prognostic assessment, *RPA* recursive partitioning analysis, *PTV* planning target volume.

tion has also been seen with whole brain radiotherapy. It has been reported that, when postoperative radiation is used, local control can be as high as 89% for lesions measuring ≤3 cm preoperatively but can drop as low as 40% for patients with metastasis larger than 3 cm [20]. For patients that do recur, time to the recurrence may also be shorter in patients with lesions >2 cm. Other studies have agreed that local failure seems to be increased in patients with preoperative tumours measuring >3 cm (local failure rate of 39.1% vs 7.5% if lesions ≤3 cm) [12, 17, 25]. In contrast some studies have not found any relationship between preoperative tumour size and the risk of local recurrence after radiation treatment [11, 18, 24, 28].

Metastasis location may, in and of itself, have a role in predicting local failure. Tumours of less than 3 cm but that are superficially located in the brain parenchyma still have a LR failure of more than 10% [17]. For lesions that have both factors (tumours measuring >3 cm and superficially located), the 1-year risk of recurrence can be as high as 53.3% [17]. Local failure seems to be more important with tumours that are located superficially in the parenchyma (1-year LR of 31.3% for superficially vs 5.6% for deeply located tumours) and that have meningeal involvement [17]. In fact, it has been reported that lesions located deep in the parenchyma measuring less than 3 cm with no meningeal involvement have a small chance of recurring 12 months after surgery [17].

The position of metastasis in relationship to the posterior fossa, whether infratentorial or supratentorial, is also related to local recurrence with lesions located in the cerebellum at a higher risk of recurring when compared to supratentorial tumours [17, 25].

As with preoperative tumour, postoperative cavity size and the type of surgery performed can influence local control. In surgical series [5], lesions resected with a *piecemeal* surgery fared worse than tumours that had en bloc resection. This is particularly true for lesions smaller than 9.71 cm³, where patients treated with a *piecemeal* resection were three times more likely to recur than patients treated with a en bloc resection. Without adjuvant radiation treatment, subtotally resected lesions are also more prone to local recurrence with rates of failure of more than 35% vs less than 10% for lesions resected totally [25, 31].

A larger postoperative cavity has been associated with an increase in local recurrence [23, 26]. Cavity volumes of 15.5–21 cm³ are being associated with a higher risk of recurrence when compared to those of less than 10 cm³. However, this association is not seen in all series [11, 28].

One possible advantage of WBRT over cavity SRS is the treatment, if present, of early leptomeningeal disease. The risk of spread to meninges and cerebrospinal fluid seems more important in patients treated with cavity SRS than with postoperative WBRT; however the multi-institutional phase III trial comparing cavity SRS to postoperative WBRT did not see a difference in rates of LMD [15] (Fig. 33.2). The rate of this phenomenon happening after WBRT is 5–12% [29, 32, 33]. Breast cancer as a primary tumour has been reported to be linked to an increase in leptomeningeal disease with as many as 14–28% of patients developing it after surgery [25, 33, 34]. The mere act of surgery has been associated with an increase of LMD in patients. In fact the 1-year risk of LMD was reported to increase from 5.2% without surgical resection to 16.9% with surgery in a review of more than 300 patients treated

for brain metastasis [33]. The type of resection (en bloc vs *piecemeal* resection) may not be predictive of subsequent LMD [34] (Table 33.3).

The association of multiple prognostic factors (age, performance status, primary tumour control and extracranial disease) has been used to develop a recursive partitioning analysis (RPA) for unresected brain metastases treated in RTOG trials. From these factors, three classes have been formed with different prognosis [35]. This RPA classification has been applied to 271 patients with a single brain metastases treated with surgery and postoperative radiation [36]. Of these patients, 84% received WBRT, 21% adjuvant or salvage SRS and 7% had surgery alone. Analysis of these factors in the postoperative setting concluded that age, extracranial metastases, status of primary tumour and the usage of SRS were predictive of overall survival. Median survival of patients with RPA class I was estimated to be 21.4 months, while patients with RPA class 2 and 3 had a median survival of 9 months and 8.9 months. The extent of resection seem to have a slight influence on survival, with GTR resulting in a median survival of 10.6 months vs 8.7 months for patients with a STR. Patients treated with SRS, whether after surgery or as a salvage treatment, fared better than patients treated with WBRT or surgery alone (median survival of 17.1 months). Patients with a RPA class I with a gross total resection had the best median survival (22.3 months) (Table 33.4).

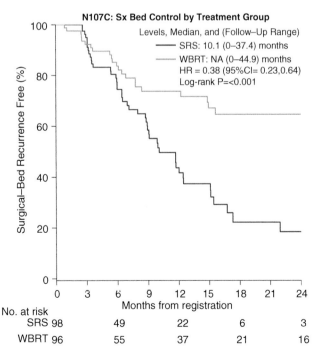

**Fig. 33.2** Local control to surgical bed with SRS vs WBRT. [Courtesy of Dr. Paul Brown]

**Table 33.3** Factors association with leptomeningeal disease

| | Factors associated with leptomeningeal disease |
|---|---|
| Iwai et al. [22] | Location: infratentorial tumour |
| Ojerholm et al. [25] | Histology: breast<br>Location: infratentorial tumour |
| Prabhu et al. [26] | Location: infratentorial tumour |

**Table 33.4** : RPA class and median survival for patients treated with surgery and postoperative radiation

| | Factors | Median survival (GTR) | Median survival (STR) |
|---|---|---|---|
| RPA 1 | Age < 65<br>KPS ≥ 70<br>Controlled primary tumour<br>No extracranial metastases | 22.3 months | 17.7 months |
| RPA 2 | All other patients not included in RPA class 1 or 3 | 9.5 months | 8.5 months |
| RPA 3 | KPS < 70 | 9.1 months | 8.5 months |

*RPA* recursive partitioning analysis, *KPS* Karnofsky performance score, *GTR* gross tumour resection, *STR* subtotal resection

## Whole Brain Radiation Therapy

Whole brain radiation therapy has long been the mainstay of treatment after surgery to minimize recurrence to the surgical cavity or elsewhere in the brain. However this type of treatment has been associated with significant cognitive decline. It has been demonstrated that up to more than 90% of patients [37] develop symptoms interfering with memory and concentration to accomplish everyday tasks.

The use of WBRT has long been justified by the risk of the resected tumour extending beyond the cavity and the possibility of distant metastasis appearing in other areas of the brain.

After resection of a brain metastasis, postoperative WBRT, when compared to surgery alone, allows for a decrease in local failure (LF) (46–59% to 10–28%) and in the incidence of new brain secondary lesions in the brain (37–42% to 14–23%) [38–41]. A randomized trial comparing, in 95 patients with single metastasis, surgery and postoperative WBRT (50.4 Gy in 28 fx) to surgery alone reported a significant decrease in local failure in patients treated with postoperative radiation not only at the surgical cavity (local failure: 46% vs 10%) but also in the rest of the brain (distant failure: 70% vs 18%) [38]. The addition of WBRT also postponed the median time to progression to more than 50 weeks (vs 27 weeks for surgery alone) in the surgical field and to 220 weeks elsewhere in the brain (vs 26 weeks for surgery alone). In this study, WBRT did not improve median overall survival. However, the cause of death of patient that did receive WBRT was less likely to be neurological (14% vs 44% in patients not receiving WBRT). Data from a more recent EORTC trial reported similar outcomes. Eighty-one patients treated with surgery received adjuvant WBRT. When compared to surgery alone, WBRT did not improve overall survival *(10.9 vs 10.7 months; p = 0.71)*. It did however reduce the 2-year local (59% vs 27%) and distant (42% vs 23%) recurrence rates [40].

The combination of WBRT and surgery has also been compared to SRS alone for newly diagnosed brain metastasis. Muacevic et al. [42] accrued 64 patients with lesions ≤3 cm with a good performance status to WBRT + resection vs SRS alone. Median survival was reported to be the same: 9.5 months in the combined arm vs 10.3 months for SRS. However, SRS did provide better local control (96.8% vs 82%). As expected, distance failure was more frequent in patients treated with SRS (25.8% vs 3%).

## Radiosurgery to the Cavity Bed

As discussed previously, WBRT improves local control after surgery. However, because of the possibility of neurotoxicity, radiosurgery to the surgical bed has increasingly been used to prevent failures in the surgical field while minimizing side effects. Radiosurgery allows for the administration of a high dose of radiation in a highly conformal fashion, thus minimizing dose to surrounding brain parenchyma.

Table 33.5 presents the results of selected series of patients treated with radiosurgery to the surgical cavity. The type of device used to administer treatment, the doses and the number of fractions used as well as whether PTV margins are used vary considerably between institutions.

Most commonly, doses used are similar to those used for intact metastases in trials such as RTOG-9005 [47]. They thus usually range from 15 to 24 Gy in one fraction. One-year local control of brain metastasis treated with postoperative radiation to the surgical cavity varies from 54% to almost 95%. There are limited prospective trials assessing the efficacy of radiosurgery to the surgical cavity. A phase III trial led by Mahajan et al. from MD Anderson Cancer Center [30] randomized 132 patients after GTR (gross total resection) of a brain metastasis to either surgery followed by observation or postoperative SRS [30]. One year after surgery, the local tumour recurrence-free rate in the observation arm was 43% vs 72% (in the SRS arm). The median time to local recurrence was 7.6 months in patients observed; it was not reached in patients treated with SRS.

## Distant Failure After Radiosurgery to Cavity

As mentioned previously, WBRT decreases failure elsewhere in the brain. Without any postoperative treatment, 1-year distant failure rates can be as high as 55–65% [18, 25]. This is in keeping with series where patients were treated with radiosurgery to the operative cavity, in which rates of distant failure in the brain are typically 44–55% at 12 months (Table 33.5).

A number of factors have been looked at to explain this recurrence rate. Histologies such as melanoma primary and the presence of multiple brain metastases have been associated with an increase in distant failure [18].

As with local recurrence, brain metastasis with a preoperative size of >2 cm was more predisposed to develop distant failure (32% vs 82% 1-year survival free of distant intracranial recurrence) [20].

## Postoperative Treatment of Large Cavities

One of the main reasons why brain metastases are considered for resection is their size and associated mass effect on surrounding brain tissue. It is therefore not unusual for resection cavities to measure more than 3–4 cm in diameter.

Contrary to smaller targets which are usually treated in one fraction, larger cavities are often treated with doses ranging

**Table 33.5** : Results of selected series of patients treated with radiosurgery to the surgical cavity

| | Number of patients/cavities | Year | Type of SRS | Median dose (Gy) (range) | OS | 1 year LC | DF | Salvage WBRT |
|---|---|---|---|---|---|---|---|---|
| Bilger et al. [16] | 60 pts | 2016 | LA | 30 GTR: 30 Gy/5 fx STR: 35 Gy/7 fx | Median 15 months 1-year OS: 64.5% | 82% | 56% | 50% |
| Brennan et al. [17] | 49 pts | 2014 | LA | 18 (15–22) | Median 14.7 months | 78% | 44% | 65% |
| Broemme et al. [43] | 42/44 | 2013 | LA | 17 (16–18) | Median 15.9 months | 77% | 61% | 38% |
| Choi et al. [18] | 112/120 | 2012 | CK | 20 (12–30) in 1 (51%)—5 fractions | Median 17 months 1 year OS: 62% | 91% | 54% | 28% |
| Do et al. [44] | 30/33 | 2008 | LA | 15 (15–18) in 1 fx or 22–27.5 Gy in 4–6 fx (SRT) (23%) | Median 12 months 51% at 12 months | 82% | 63% | 47% |
| Hartford et al. [20] | 47/49 | 2013 | LA | 10 (8–20) | 53% at 12 months | 86% | 56% | 45% |
| Jagannathan et al. [23] | 47 pts | 2009 | GK | Mean 19 (6–22) | Median 13 months | 94% | 72% | 28% |
| Jensen et al. [12] | 106/112 | 2011 | GK | 17 (11–23) | Median 10.9 months 46.8% at 12 months | 80% | 65% | 37% |
| Iwai et al. [22] | 21 pts | 2008 | GK | 17 (13–20) | Median 20 months | 82% | 48% | 10% |
| Iorio-morin et al. [21] | 110 pts | 2014 | GK | 18 (10–20) | Median 11 months 63% at 12 months | 73% | 54% | 28% |
| Kalani et al. [45] | 68 pts | 2010 | GK | 15 (14–30) | Median 13.2 months | 80% | 60% | 28% |
| Karlovits et al. [11] | 52 pts | 2009 | | 15 (8–18) | Median 15 months | 92% | 55% | 31% |
| Luther et al. [46] | 120 pts | 2013 | GK | 16 | 87% at 12 months | 86% | 40% | 31% |
| Mathieu et al. [28] | 40 pts | 2008 | GK | 16 (11–20) | Median 13 months | 73% | 54% | 16% |
| Ojerholm et al. [25] | 91/96 | 2014 | GK | 16 (12–21) | Median 22.3 months 58% at 12 months | 81% | 64% | 33% |
| Ogiwara et al. [28] | 56 pts | 2012 | GK | Mean 17 (14–20) | Median 20.5 months | 91% | 38% | 14% |
| Prabhu et al. [23] | 62/64 | 2012 | GK | 18 (15–24) | Median 13 months | 84% | 51% | 26% |
| Rwigema et al. [27] | 77 pts | 2011 | CK | 18 median (12–27) | Median 14.5 months 62.5% at 1 year | 76% | 54% | 26% |
| Soltys et al. [15] | 72/76 | 2008 | CK | 18.6 (15–30 Gy in 1 (78%)—5 fx | Median 15.1 months 62.5% at 1 year | 79% | 53% | 19% |
| *Total* | *1262 pts* | | | | | 82% | 55% | *31%* |

*Pts* patients, *CK* CyberKnife, *GK* GammaKnife, *LA* linear accelerator, *LC* local control, *DF* distant failure, *OS* overall survival, *STR* stereotactic radiation therapy

from 24 Gy in three fractions to 36 Gy in six fractions [48–51], with most teams using a planning tumour volume (PTV) of 2–3 mm [48–52]. This margin is supported by the finding that fewer than 5% of recurrences occur beyond 3 mm [52].

A few studies have looked at the outcomes of larger tumours treated with radiosurgery to the surgical cavity with 1-year LC ranging from 77% to 93% [48–51, 53]. In series where the population studied was treated with lesions measuring preoperatively >2 cm, histology of the primary seems to have less of an impact on the rate of recurrence. Brain metastasis stemming from primaries that are usually deemed radiosensitive (i.e. breast and lung) has similar local control (up to 94%) than radioresistant tumours (up to 90% for melanoma, renal cell carcinoma primaries) [49, 50]. For larger cavities, local control does not seem to be associated with the number of fractions or dose used [54].

However, as with smaller cavities, the risk of distant failure seems more important for melanoma vs breast primary (34% vs 65%) and when extracranial disease is present [49]. The rate of distant failure, elsewhere in the brain, is similar to the ones of smaller metastasis, with 40–63% of patients recurring elsewhere in the brain [49–51, 53]. The median survival after treatment of larger brain metastasis is reported to be 5.5–17 months [48–50, 52, 55, 56]. Patients with good KPS and no extracranial disease are expected to have a better survival [49, 50].

## Radiation to Resection Cavity with Whole Brain Radiation Therapy

Combining whole brain radiation therapy and a surgical cavity radiosurgery boost allows for an incremental improvement in intracranial control, possibly reducing the need for strict imaging follow-up. The whole brain component addresses the meninges and eliminates marginal miss, while the radiosurgery provided dose intensity to the area at highest risk of recurrence. However, concern remains that the addition of whole brain radiation increases the risk of neurocognitive toxicity that can be debilitating for some patients.

The combination of WBRT and radiosurgery to the surgical cavity was examined by Roberge et al. [46] in 71 patients. A majority of these patients were treated with WBRT at a dose of 30 Gy in ten fractions with a boost of 10 Gy to the surgical cavity. They reported a 1-year actuarial (censured at the time of the last brain imaging) local control of 91% and few distant metastases with a crude rate of distant failure of 13%.

Others [57] have reported results from a subset of patients treated in their retrospective data. In a series of 39 patients receiving WBRT immediately before a surgical cavity boost, there was not a difference in local control for patients receiving the combined treatment vs radiosurgery alone.

## Preoperative SRS to Metastases

Neoadjuvant SRS is a novel strategy of radiosurgery to brain metastasis. It is advantageous especially for larger lesions that are at a higher risk of relapse after surgery (e.g. lesions >3 cm, in the posterior fossa, of subtotally resected) [58]. It is also thought to possibly reduce tumour seeding during surgical resection [58].

In this type of treatment, radiosurgery is administered, according to guidelines for doses stemming from the RTOG 90-05[47]. Larger tumour, of more than 30 mm, may be treated in 3–5 sessions a few days prior to resection.

Recently, Patel et al. looked at the outcomes of patients treated preoperatively and postoperatively. The rate of local failure was similar in both arms (17.5% at 12 months) [59]. However, larger cavities (with a post op volume > 10 cc) were associated with an increase rate of relapse. The rate of salvage with WBRT was similar in both arms (12% vs 10.9% NS). The rate of LMD however was higher in patients treated postoperatively. The 1-year LMD risk was reported to be 3.2% at 2 years after treatment in the preoperative setting vs 16.6% in patients treated postoperatively. The median survival was found to be a few weeks longer in patients treated with neoadjuvant SRS (17 vs 13.5 months—$p = 0.04$) although the only predictor of OS was the absence of active systemic disease. The results from this study were similar to the ones published by Asher et al. [58] where 1–3 metastasis where treated with SRS preoperatively. In this series, the local control was 85.6% at 1 year. Once more, lesions of a larger volume preoperatively (more than 10 cc), located superficially were associated with a decrease in local control.

## Cavity Dynamics

Removal of lesions measuring more 2 cm may result in a cavity smaller than the original metastasis, this is more evident for lesions that are preoperatively >3 cm [60]. In brain metastasis of this category, a cavity 47% smaller than the original metastasis can be seen [31]. For lesions measuring 2.1–3 cm, a 25.8% decrease in dimension can be noted [31]. While removal of most larger metastasis will lead to a smaller surgical cavity, preoperative lesions (2 cm or less) often are often associated with a cavity larger than the original tumour—as much as 46–56.4% larger [31, 60]. Thus, the resection of larger tumours often produce a cavity volume smaller than the original metastasis, contrary to lesions smaller than 2 cm where tumour resections produce cavities that are larger than the initial tumour. Therefore, it has been suggested that perhaps lesions of less than 2 cm should be considered for SRS without surgery, especially knowing that these lesions respond well to SRS [60].

The ideal interval between treatment with cavity SRS and surgery is yet to be identified. Between initial surgery and SRS, most cavities are stable in size (with less than a 2 cc change in volume); however approximately a quarter of cavities collapse by more than 2 cc and 30% of cavities enlarged by more than 2 cc [31]. Atalar et al. looked at cavity dynamics after resection [60]. They looked at the size of cavities 1 day after surgical intervention and then again at time of radiation planning (median of 20 days after surgery). During this time interval, there was no significant change in volume.

The authors conclude that cavities change the most immediately after surgery and little modification is seen after. Another factor to take into account is the possibility of haemorrhage after surgery, especially with larger cavities [31]. After blood accumulation, a period of a few days to weeks is necessary for its resorption as it can influence cavity size. It is also more cautious to postpone radiation to allow for healing of surgical scar before proceeding with treatment.

It is worth mentioning that a recurrence rate of up to 23% has been reported between time of surgery and treatment with SRS (mean duration between treatments of 30 days) [31]. The potential benefits of waiting for a cavity to reduce in volume are tempered by the suggestion that local recurrences are more common when radiation is not delivered within 6 weeks of surgery [24, 61]. The best time to proceed with cavity SRS may even be within 3 weeks of surgery to minimize local recurrence [21, 62].

Although delays to adjuvant therapy have been associated with an increase in local failure, we find it reasonable to wait at least 10 days from surgery to radiosurgery. Independently of the interval chosen, most radiosurgeons would recommend delivering SRS within a short interval of the planning imaging being acquired to avoid any significant change in cavity size from treatment planning to treatment delivery.

## Adverse Effects of Radiosurgery to the Cavity Bed

The most dreaded side effect from radiosurgery to the cavity is, as with most radiosurgery treatment, radionecrosis. The reported rates of radionecrosis vary from 2% to 10% [15, 18, 21, 25, 26, 49, 52, 55]. For larger metastasis (>3 cm), the rate of radionecrosis can reach up to 9% [48, 49, 54]. The likelihood of patients undergoing surgery to alleviate symptoms of radionecrosis is 1–5% [18, 25, 59]. Prolonged steroid use, however, has been recorded in 3–10% [18, 48, 52, 59]. Bevacizumab to treat radionecrosis is increasingly common as a substitute for surgery, hyperbaric oxygen or protracted steroid use.

The rate of radionecrosis may be lower in patients treated with preoperative radiosurgery. It is estimated to occur in 0–1.5% of patients [58, 59]. This may be explained by the resection of irradiated tissue at the time of surgery.

The number of fractions appears to be related to radiation toxicity. The use of steroids seems to be greater for patients treated with a single fraction [18, 50, 54]. Moreover, the rate of symptomatic radionecrosis has also been reported to be higher in patients treated with one fraction when compared to hypofractionation [55]. The dose administered does not seem to be associated with radiation toxicity (this is not surprising, as dose is typically inversely related to the volume irradiated), neither does the addition of a 2–3 mm PTV margin [14, 18].

Dosimetric factors that have been reported to influence radiation injury are a worse conformality index [59] and the volume irradiated. For fractionated treatments, a volume receiving 24 Gy (V24) > 16.8 cm$^3$ is associated with a radionecrosis risk of 16% vs 2% if <16.8 cm [3, 49]. In single-fraction treatments, a V12 > 20.0 cm$^3$ has been reported to be predictive of an increased risk of radionecrosis (14% vs 4% if V12 < 20.9 cm$^3$) [49].

## Planning for Radiosurgery to Cavity

For linac radiosurgery, patients usually undergo a planning CT and an MRI with gadolinium. For planning purposes, a high-field 3D distortion corrected T1 contrast MRI with isotropic voxels ≤1 mm is ideal. If postoperative radiosurgery is being performed, co-registration of the preoperative MRI is helpful. Planning volumes (GTV, CTV, PTV) are contoured with information from imaging as well as information from the pathologist (i.e. extension to meninges, histology, etc.) and surgeon (Fig. 33.3).

For cavity radiosurgery, most define the clinical tumour volume (CTV) as any contrast-enhancing postoperative changes on the planning MRI. For targets situated deeper in the brain, the full surgical tract is usually not included in the CTV. The surrounding oedema and other abnormalities on any T2 or Flair sequences are not usually taken into account.

When generating the planning tumour volume (PTV) volume, one must consider the patterns of recurrence. Prabhu et al. [26] related that most local failures (73%) after surgery and SRS are located within the treated volume. Less than 10% were considered to be marginal misses, while 18% of lesions relapsed marginally and within treated volume. Therefore, some groups have added a 1–2 mm margin to account for difficulties in delineating some cavities and the possibility of tumour spread in the surrounding brain [63]; others treat only the enhancing margin of the cavity [14, 44, 46]. The value of adding a 2–3 mm PTV has been most prominently promoted by the Stanford group [14, 18]. They concluded that, although this results in less conformal plans, the addition of a margin reduces 1-year local failure (16% vs 3%) while maintaining a similar low risk of toxicity (3% with margin vs 8% without).

The dose providing the best local control in the postoperative setting is still undefined. Some prefer to fractionate all cavities, while others are in favour of a higher per fraction dose. It is important to note that dose limits set by RTOG 90-05 and then used in subsequent trials were determined in patients that had previously received radiation. Therefore, the maximum tolerated dose might be actually higher. Residual tumour in the surgical bed may be hypoxic and require a higher dose of radiation to be sterilized.

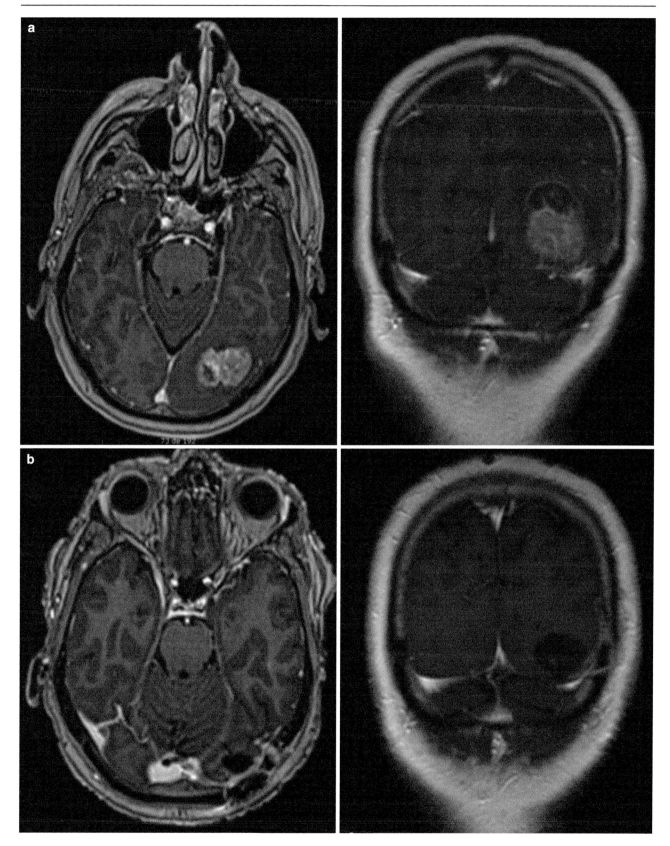

**Fig. 33.3** (a) Axial and coronal preoperative imaging of a 68-year-old patient with renal cell carcinoma and brain metastases, (b) axial and coronal postoperative imaging and (c) planning CT; patient received 24 Gy in 3 fx with a 1 mm PTV, prescribed at the 61% isodose, using the CyberKnife

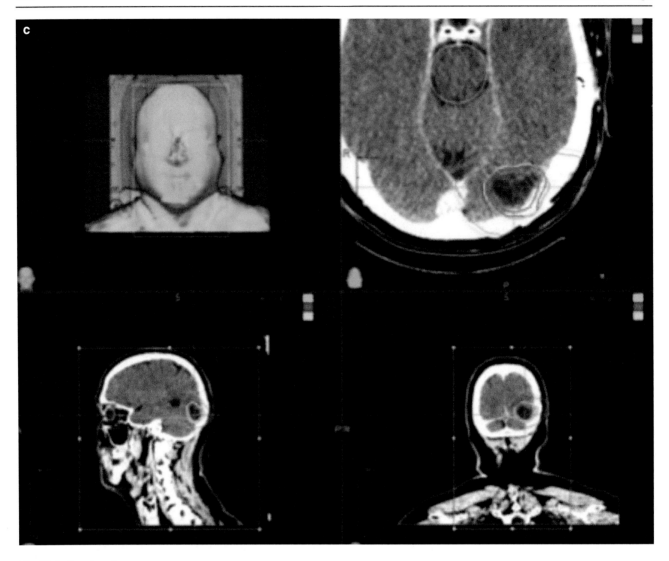

**Fig. 33.3** (continued)

The optimal fractionation scheme to be used to treat operative cavities remains to be settled. Prabhu et al. [26] looked at 64 cavities in 62 patients. Once again, most patients were treated according to doses from RTOG. However, because of the diameter of the residual cavity, 14% of patients were treated in 3–4 fractions, with doses ranging from 24 to 30 Gy. Local failure was seen in 11 out of 64 patients (22% at 12 months). Lesions treated with a marginal dose of less than 18 Gy were more susceptible to recurrence. The fact that lesions were treated in one or more fractions did not seem to influence LC.

## Other Treatment Options

The addition of carmustine wafers to the surgical cavity with WBRT has been studied in a multi-institution study where 25 patients [64] with single metastasis were treated with car-

mustine polymer wafers in the resection cavity followed by WBRT (30 Gy in ten fractions) for most patients. No local failure was reported, and the distant failure rate was similar to historical controls. Two patients were reported to have severe neurological side effects (seizures) related most probably to wafer placement. The addition of iodine-125 seeds to the surgical cavity after GTR has also been attempted and has been reported to provide good local control (96% at 12 months) [65]. *GliaSite* brachytherapy balloon catheter to the surgical cavity has also been tested in a multi-institutional study [66]. Sixty-two patients received, via the *GliaSite* catheter, a dose of 60 Gy to the cavity. Local control rate was estimated to be over 80%, but 13 patients underwent re-resection for possible radionecrosis (69%) or tumour recurrence (31%). An industry-supported trial is evaluating the efficacy of Optune[tm] *tumour-treating fields* for microscopic disease control in patients with limited brain metastases from lung cancer. Although this trial excludes patients having undergone surgery, one would imagine that this would be a logical patient population in which to use this treatment should it be shown effective in preventing brain metastasis recurrence.

## Clinical Case Discussion

A 68-year-old man, with a history of a stage III melanoma diagnosed a year prior, presented to the emergency department with a 2-week history of headaches, accompanied by scotomas.

A CT scan showed (Fig. 33.4) a 20X14mm mass in the occipital lobe, suggestive of a brain metastasis.

An MRI (Fig. 33.5) confirmed the presence of a mass in the occipital lobe of 14 × 23 mm. Patient had a staging CT scan of the chest and the abdomen that did not show any sign of metastatic disease. Patient underwent removal of the brain tumour by craniotomy. Pathology confirmed the presence of a metastases originating from the known melanoma. Postoperative MRI showed complete resection of the lesion (Fig. 33.6). The patient was referred for consideration of radiation therapy. After consideration of possible options, including WBRT and radiation to the surgical cavity, the patient opted for the latter.

A planning MRI was performed and confirmed the complete resection of the tumour. The surgical cavity was contoured on a T1-weighted MRI sequence with contrast

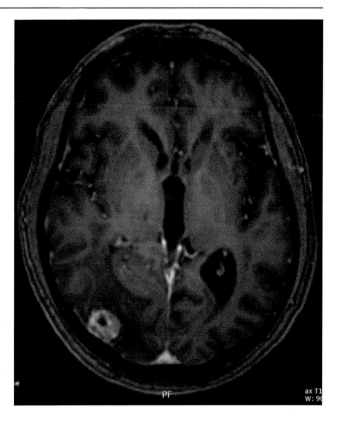

**Fig. 33.5** MRI showing brain lesion

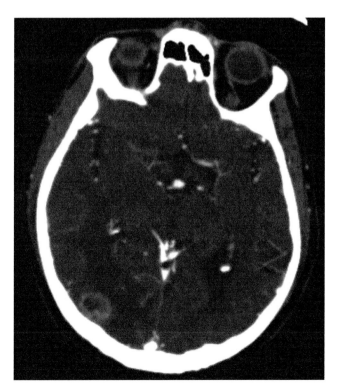

**Fig. 33.4** CT scan showing brain lesion

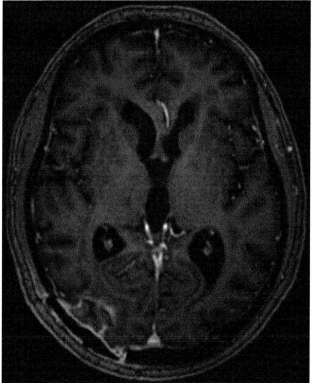

**Fig. 33.6** Postoperative planning MRI showing surgical cavity

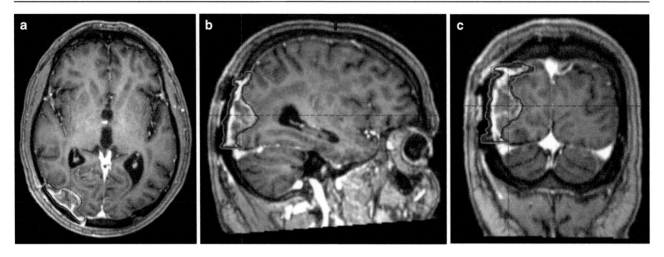

**Fig. 33.7** Planning MRI with treatment volumes (GTV + PTV), in the axial (**a**), sagittal (**b**) and coronal (**c**) views

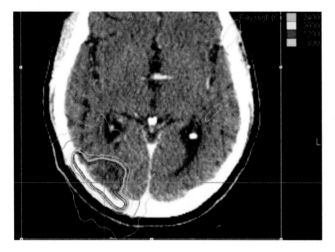

**Fig. 33.8** CT scan with planning volumes and dose administered of 24 Gy in 3 fx

(Fig. 33.7) after fusion with the planning CT scan. A PTV of 1 mm was added. A dose of 24 Gy in 3 fx was prescribed to the 65% isodose (Fig. 33.8). Maximum dose within the PTV was 3692 cGy. Follow-up MRI, 18 months after treatment, showed no recurrence at the treated site.

## Summary

- After surgery for brain metastasis, radiation can be administered using whole brain radiation therapy (i.e. WBRT) or to the surgical cavity alone, typically in one to five fractions.
- The addition of radiation to the surgical cavity, whether by WBRT or radiosurgery, has been shown to improve local control. WBRT is known to decrease distant failure (elsewhere in the brain).

- WBRT and radiation to the surgical cavity have different side effect profiles; WBRT has been associated with global neurotoxicity, while radiation to the cavity, administered in fewer fractions, but at a higher dose per fraction, is associated with an increasing risk of local radionecrosis.

## Self-Assessment Questions

1. True or false. Addition of WBRT to surgical cavity results in improvement of overall survival.

2. WBRT can reduce:
   A. Distant failure
   B. Local failure
   C. The risk of leptomeningeal disease
   D. A and B
   E. All of the above

3. Retrospective comparisons of preoperative SRS to brain metastases to postoperative SRS to the surgical cavity have shown:
   A. A reduction in LMD
   B. Better local control
   C. An increase in OS

4. Radionecrosis:
   A. Is less frequently seen in preoperative radiation compared to postoperative radiation
   B. Can be treated with bevacizumab
   C. Can reach 10% after SRS
   D. All of the above

5. True or false: the addition of a PTV to the surgical cavity possibly reduces local failure

## Answers

1. False
2. E
3. A
4. D
5. True

---

## References

1. Barnholtz-Sloan JS, Sloan AE, Davis FG, et al. Incidence proportions of brain metastases in patients diagnosed (1973 to 2001) in the Metropolitan Detroit Cancer Surveillance System. J Clin Oncol. 2004;22:2865–72.
2. Schouten LJ, Rutten J, Huveneers HA, et al. Incidence of brain metastases in a cohort of patients with carcinoma of the breast, colon, kidney, and lung and melanoma. Cancer. 2002;94:2698–705.
3. Lassman AB, DeAngelis LM. Brain metastases. Neurol Clin. 2003;21:1–23. vii
4. Gavrilovic IT, Posner JB. Brain metastases: epidemiology and pathophysiology. J Neurooncol. 2005;75:5–14.
5. Patel AJ, Suki D, Hatiboglu MA, et al. Factors influencing the risk of local recurrence after resection of a single brain metastasis. J Neurosurg. 2010;113:181–9.
6. Quattrocchi CC, Errante Y, Gaudino C, et al. Spatial brain distribution of intra-axial metastatic lesions in breast and lung cancer patients. J Neurooncol. 2012;110:79–87.
7. Delattre JY, Krol G, Thaler HT, et al. Distribution of brain metastases. Arch Neurol. 1988;45:741–4.
8. Patchell RA, Regine W, Dempsey R, et al. Postoperative radiotherapy in the treatment of single metastases to the brain. JAMA. 1998;290:1485–9.
9. Chang EL, Wefel JS, Hess KR, et al. Neurocognition in patients with brain metastases treated with radiosurgery or radiosurgery plus whole-brain irradiation: a randomised controlled trial. Lancet Oncol. 2009;10:1037–44.
10. Hwang SW, Abozed MM, Hale A, et al. Adjuvant Gamma Knife radiosurgery following surgical resection of brain metastases: a 9-year retrospective cohort study. J Neurooncol. 2010;98:77–82.
11. Brian J, Karlovits Do B, Quigley M, et al. Stereotactic radiosurgery boost to the resection bed for oligometastatic brain disease: challenging the tradition of adjuvant whole-brain radiotherapy. Neurosurg Focus. 2009;27:1–6.
12. Jensen CA, Chan MD, McCoy TP, et al. Cavity-directed radiosurgery as adjuvant therapy after resection of a brain metastasis. J Neurosurg. 2011;114:1585–91.
13. Narayana A, Chang J, Yenice K, et al. Hypofractionated stereotactic radiotherapy using intensity-modulated radiotherapy in patients with one or two brain metastases. Stereotact Funct Neurosurg. 2007;85:82–7.
14. Soltys SG, Adler JR, Lipani JD, et al. Stereotactic radiosurgery of the postoperative resection cavity for brain metastases. Int J Radiat Oncol Biol Phys. 2008;70:187–93.
15. Brown P, Cerhan JH, Anderson SK, et al. N107C/CEC·3 (alliance for clinical trials in oncology/Canadian Cancer Trials Group): phase III trial of post-operative stereotactic radiosurgery (SRS) compared with whole brain radiotherapy (WBRT) for resected metastatic brain disease. Lancet Oncol. 2017;18(8):1049–60
16. Bilgera A, Milanovica D ,Lorenza H, et al. Stereotactic fractionated radiotherapy of the resection cavity in patients with one to three brain metastases. Clin Neurol Neurosurg 2016;142:81–86.
17. Brennan C, Yang TJ, Hilden P, et al. A phase 2 trial of stereotactic radiosurgery boost after surgical resection for brain metastases. Int J Radiat Oncol Biol Phys. 2014;88:130–6.
18. Choi CY, Chang SD, Gibbs IC, et al. Stereotactic radiosurgery of the postoperative resection cavity for brain metastases: prospective evaluation of target margin on tumor control. Int J Radiat Oncol Biol Phys. 2012;84:336–42.
19. Dore M, Martin S, Delpon G, et al. Stereotactic radiotherapy following surgery for brain metastasis: predictive factors for local control and radionecrosis. Cancer Radiother. 2017;21(1):4–9.
20. Hartford AC, Paravati AJ, Spire WJ, et al. Postoperative stereotactic radiosurgery without whole-brain radiation therapy for brain metastases: potential role of preoperative tumor size. Int J Radiat Oncol Biol Phys. 2013;85:650–5.
21. Iorio-Morin C, Masson-Cote L, Ezahr Y, et al. Early gamma knife stereotactic radiosurgery to the tumor bed of resected brain metastasis for improved local control. J Neurosurg. 2014;121(Suppl):69–74.
22. Iwai Y, Yamanaka K, Yasui T, et al. Boost radiosurgery for treatment of brain metastases after surgical resections. Surg Neurol. 2008;69:181–6.
23. Jagannathan J, Yen C-P, Ray DK, et al. Gamma knife radiosurgery to the surgical cavity following resection of brain metastases. J Neurosurg. 2009;111:431–8.
24. Mathieu D, Kondziolka D, Flickinger JC, et al. Tumor bed radiosurgery after resection of cerebral metastases. Neurosurgery. 2008;62:817–23. discussion 23–4
25. OjErholm E, Lee JY, Thawani JP, et al. Stereotactic radiosurgery to the resection bed for intracranial metastases and risk of leptomeningeal carcinomatosis. J Neurosurg. 2014;121:75–83.
26. Roshan Prabhu R, Shu H-K, Hadjipanayis C, et al. Current dosing paradigm for stereotactic radiosurgery alone after surgical resection of brain metastases needs to be optimized for improved local control. Int J Radiat Oncol Biol Phys. 2011;83:e61–6.
27. Rwigema JC, Wegner RE, Mintz AH, et al. Stereotactic radiosurgery to the resection cavity of brain metastases: a retrospective analysis and literature review. Stereotact Funct Neurosurg. 2011;89:329–37.
28. Ogiwara H, Kalakota K, Rakhra SS, et al. Intracranial relapse rates and patterns, and survival trends following post-resection cavity radiosurgery for patients with single intracranial metastases. J Neurooncol. 2012;108:141–6.
29. Suki D, Abouassi H, Patel AJ, et al. Comparative risk of leptomeningeal disease after resection or stereotactic radiosurgery for solid tumor metastasis to the posterior fossa. J Neurosurg. 2008;108:248–57.
30. Mahajan A, Ahmed S, McAleer MF, et al. Postoperative stereotactic radiosurgery versus observation for completely resected brain metastases: results of a prospective randomized study. Lancet Oncol. 2017;18(8):1049–60
31. Jarvis LA, Simmons NE, Bellerive M, et al. Tumor bed dynamics after surgical resection of brain metastases: implications for postoperative radiosurgery. Int J Radiat Oncol Biol Phys. 2012;84:943–8.
32. Suki D, Hatiboglu MA, Patel AJ, et al. Comparative risk of leptomeningeal dissemination of cancer after surgery or stereotactic radiosurgery for a single supratentorial solid tumor metastasis. Neurosurgery. 2009;64:664–74. discussion 74–6
33. Johnson MD, Avkshtol V, Baschnagel AM, et al. Surgical resection of brain metastases and the risk of leptomeningeal recurrence in patients treated with stereotactic radiosurgery. Int J Radiat Oncol Biol Phys. 2016;94:537–43.
34. Atalar B, Modlin LA, Choi CY, et al. Risk of leptomeningeal disease in patients treated with stereotactic radiosurgery targeting the postoperative resection cavity for brain metastases. Int J Radiat Oncol Biol Phys. 2013;87:713–8.
35. Gaspar L, Scott C, Rotman M, et al. Recursive partitioning analysis (RPA) of prognostic factors in three Radiation Therapy Oncology Group (RTOG) brain metastases trials. Int J Radiat Oncol Biol Phys. 1997;37:745–51.

36. Tendulkar R, Liu SW, Barnett G, et al. RPA Classification has prognostic significance for surgically resected single brain metastasis. Int J Radiat Oncol Biol Phys. 2006;66:810–7.

37. Meyers CA, Smith JA, Bezjak A, et al. Neurocognitive function and progression in patients with brain metastases treated with whole-brain radiation and motexafin gadolinium: results of a randomized phase III trial. J Clin Oncol. 2004;22:157–65.

38. Patchell RA, Tibbs PA, Regine WF, et al. Postoperative radiotherapy in the treatment of single metastases to the brain: a randomized trial. JAMA. 1998;280:1485–9.

39. McPherson CM, Suki D, Feiz-Erfan I, et al. Adjuvant whole-brain radiation therapy after surgical resection of single brain metastases. Neuro Oncol. 2010;12:711–9.

40. Kocher M, Soffietti R, Abacioglu U, et al. Adjuvant whole-brain radiotherapy versus observation after radiosurgery or surgical resection of one to three cerebral metastases: results of the EORTC 22952-26001 study. J Clin Oncol. 2011;29:134–41.

41. Nieder C, Schwerdtfeger K, Steudel WI, et al. Patterns of relapse and late toxicity after resection and whole-brain radiotherapy for solitary brain metastases. Strahlenther Onkol. 1998;174:275–8.

42. Muacevic A, Wowra B, Siefert A, et al. Microsurgery plus whole brain irradiation versus Gamma Knife surgery alone for treatment of single metastases to the brain: a randomized controlled multicentre phase III trial. J Neurooncol. 2008;87:299–307.

43. Broemme J, Abu-Isa J, Kottke R, et al. Adjuvant therapy after resection of brain metastases. Frameless image-guided LINAC-based radiosurgery and stereotactic hypofractionated radiotherapy. Strahlenther Onkol. 2013;189:765–70.

44. Do L, Pezner R, Radany E, et al. Resection followed by stereotactic radiosurgery to resection cavity for intracranial metastases. Int J Radiat Oncol Biol Phys. 2009;73:486–91.

45. Kalani MY, Filippidis AS, Kalani MA, et al. Gamma Knife surgery combined with resection for treatment of a single brain metastasis: preliminary results. J Neurosurg. 2010;113(Suppl):90–6.

46. Roberge D, Parney I, Brown PD. Radiosurgery to the postoperative surgical cavity: who needs evidence? Int J Radiat Oncol Biol Phys. 2012;83:486–93.

47. Shaw E, Scott C, Souhami L, et al. Single dose radiosurgical treatment of recurrent previously irradiated primary brain tumors and brain metastases: final report of RTOG protocol 90-05. Int J Radiat Oncol Biol Phys. 2000;47:291–8.

48. Wang C-C, Floyd S, Chang C-C, et al. Cyberknife hypofractionated stereotactic radiosurgery (HSRS) of resection cavity after excision of large cerebral metastasis: efficacy and safety of an 800 cGy 3 3 daily fractions regimen. J Neurooncol. 2012;106:601–10.

49. Minniti G, Esposito V, Clarke E, et al. Multidose stereotactic radiosurgery (9 Gy × 3) of the postoperative resection cavity for treatment of large brain metastases. Int J Radiat Oncol Biol Phys. 2013;86:623–9.

50. Choi CY, Chang SD, Gibbs IC, et al. What is the optimal treatment of large brain metastases? An argument for a multidisciplinary approach. Int J Radiat Oncol Biol Phys. 2012;84:688–93.

51. Al-Omair A, Soliman H, Xu W, et al. Hypofractionated stereotactic radiotherapy in five daily fractions for post-operative surgical cavities in brain metastases patients with and without prior whole brain radiation. Technol Cancer Res Treat. 2013;12:493–9.

52. Vogel J, Ojerholm E, Hollander A, et al. Intracranial control after Cyberknife radiosurgery to the resection bed for large brain metastases. Radiat Oncol. 2015;10:221.

53. Connolly EP, Mathew M, Tam M, et al. Involved field radiation therapy after surgical resection of solitary brain metastases—mature results. Neuro-Oncology. 2013;15:589–94.

54. Kim PK, Ellis T, Stieber VW, et al. Gamma Knife surgery targeting the resection cavity of brain metastasis that has progressed after whole-brain radiotherapy. J Neurosurg. 2006;105(Suppl):75–8.

55. Eaton BR, LaRiviere MJ, Kim S, et al. Hypofractionated radiosurgery has a better safety profile than single fraction radiosurgery for large resected brain metastases. J Neurooncol. 2015;123:103–11.

56. Jeong WJ, Park JH, Lee EJ, et al. Efficacy and safety of fractionated stereotactic radiosurgery for large brain metastases. J Korean Neurosurg Soc. 2015;58:217–24.

57. Luther N, Kondziolka D, Kano H, et al. Predicting tumor control after resection bed radiosurgery of brain metastases. Neurosurgery. 2013;73:1001–6. discussion 6

58. Asher AL, Burri SH, Wiggins WF, et al. A new treatment paradigm: neoadjuvant radiosurgery before surgical resection of brain metastases with analysis of local tumor recurrence. Int J Radiat Oncol Biol Phys. 2014;88:899–906.

59. Patel KR, Burri SH, Asher AL, et al. Comparing preoperative with postoperative stereotactic radiosurgery for resectable brain metastases: a multi-institutional analysis. Neurosurgery. 2016;79:279–85.

60. Atalar B, Choi CY, Harsh GR, et al. Cavity volume dynamics after resection of brain metastases and timing of postresection cavity stereotactic radiosurgery. Neurosurgery. 2013;72:180–5. discussion 5

61. Kondziolka D, Lunsford LD, Flickinger JC. The application of stereotactic radiosurgery to disorders of the brain. Neurosurgery. 2008;62(Suppl 2):707–19. discussion 19–20

62. Strauss I, Corn BW, Krishna V, et al. Patterns of failure after stereotactic radiosurgery of the resection cavity following surgical removal of brain metastases. World Neurosurg. 2015;84:1825–31.

63. Berghoff AS, Preusser M. The future of targeted therapies for brain metastases. Future Oncol. 2015;11:2315–27.

64. Ewend MG, Brem S, Gilbert M, et al. Treatment of single brain metastasis with resection, intracavity carmustine polymer wafers, and radiation therapy is safe and provides excellent local control. Clin Cancer Res. 2007;13:3637–41.

65. Dagnew E, Kanski J, McDermott MW, et al. Management of newly diagnosed single brain metastasis using resection and permanent iodine-125 seeds without initial whole-brain radiotherapy: a two institution experience. Neurosurg Focus. 2007;22:E3.

66. Rogers LR, Rock JP, Sills AK, et al. Results of a phase II trial of the GliaSite radiation therapy system for the treatment of newly diagnosed, resected single brain metastases. J Neurosurg. 2006;105:375–84.

# Vascular Malformation

# 34

John C. Flickinger, Hideyuki Kano, and L. Dade Lunsford

## Learning Objectives

- To understand the risks of morbidity and mortality posed by intracranial AVM and cavernous malformations.
- To understand the risks and benefits of radiosurgery for AVM and cavernous malformations.
- To understand how to optimize radiosurgery of AVM and cavernous malformations.
- To understand when observation may be the best management of intracranial AVM and cavernous malformations.

## Background

Vascular malformations come in several forms and pose different risks to patients. Arteriovenous malformations (AVMs) are congenitally malformed blood vessels that shunt high-pressure oxygenated arterial blood into the venous system without passing through a network of capillaries to oxygenate and nourish tissue which at the same time reduces the high pressure of the blood passing back into the lower-pressure venous system. The high blood pressure in the shunting vessels which lack the strong muscular coating of normal arteries to withstand that pressure leads to the possibility of spontaneous hemorrhage developing over time. The high-pressure bleeding that may develop from intracranial AVM can lead to severe neurological sequelae or death. Dural arteriovenous fistulas/shunts (DAVF) have many similarities to AVM. They may be congenital arteriovenous mal-

formations, but they could also develop from trauma. Cavernous malformations are malformed shunting vessels that occur further down the arterial tree, closer to the capillaries where intravascular pressures are lower. Cavernous malformation bleeds are therefore usually smaller and less likely to result in neurological deficits compared to AVM bleeds. Bleeding from brainstem cavernous malformations, however, can cause significant neurological problems especially after multiple bleeds. Cavernous malformations are usually congenital, but, in some families, affected individuals may develop in increasing numbers of cavernous malformations as they age.

## Epidemiology

The incidence of asymptomatic vascular malformations has been ascertained in several studies. Hospital-based autopsy studies report the prevalence of all brain AVMs which are approximately 600 per 100,000 (0.6%) [1]. Cavernous malformations have been found at a rate of 0.14–0.2% in asymptomatic volunteers undergoing screening brain MR scans [1–3]. The Scottish Intracranial Vascular Malformation Study identified 418 vascular malformations diagnosed in the entire country of Scotland between 1999 and 2000 [1]. The diagnosis rates per 100,000 adults per year (with 95% confidence intervals in parentheses) were 2.27 (1.96–2.62) for all IVMs, 1.12 (0.90–1.37) for brain AVMs, 0.56 (0.41–0.75) for cavernous malformations, 0.43 (0.31–0.61) for venous malformations, and 0.16 (0.08–0.27) for dural AVMs.

## Presentation and Diagnosis

Patients with vascular malformations often present with symptoms from hemorrhage, but other presentations are possible. High-flow arteriovenous malformations with superficial venous drainage can cause pulsatile tinnitus. Transient neurological deficits can occur from seizures, and persistent but potentially

J. C. Flickinger (✉)
Department of Radiation Oncology, UPMC Presbyterian-Shadyside Hospital, University of Pittsburgh School of Medicine, Pittsburgh, PA, USA
e-mail: flickingerjc@msx.upmc.edu; flickingerjc@upmc.edu

H. Kano · L. D. Lunsford
Department of Neurological Surgery, University of Pittsburgh, Pittsburgh, PA, USA

© Springer International Publishing AG, part of Springer Nature 2018
E. L. Chang et al. (eds.), *Adult CNS Radiation Oncology*, https://doi.org/10.1007/978-3-319-42878-9_34

reversible deficits from a vascular steal reduce blood flow to functional brain tissue. Headaches related or unrelated to the AVM may prompt imaging that lead to the discovery of an AVM. Headaches from intravascular hemorrhage are usually severe when they occur from AVMs, while the smaller bleeds from cavernous malformations (compared to AVM) do not seem as likely to cause severe headaches, and the resulting neurological deficits tend to be more limited than with AVM.

## Pathologic and Radiographic Findings

Arteriovenous malformations can be identified on angiography with an early appearing "blush" volume within the AVM nidus where the arteriovenous shunting is taking place, along with the appearance of an early draining vein that is usually distended from high pressure and high flow. Sometimes the high flow rates in the feeding arteries lead to the development of arterial aneurysms. The AVM nidus can often be distinguished from draining veins on MR scans by reviewing both T1 contrast and T2 images, but other times review of angiographic images identifies areas of AVM nidus that were not appreciated on MR imaging. Figure 34.1 shows the appearance of a typical AVM with angiographic and MR imaging.

The draining veins of cavernous malformations are less distended than those from higher pressure AVM. Cavernous malformations that have bled before have easily identifiable hemosiderin rings surrounding the vascular nidus that do not need to be included in the treatment volume. Figure 34.2 shows a cavernous malformation of the brainstem with a typical hemosiderin ring after two prior limited hemorrhagic events.

## Classification, Prognostic, and Predictive Factors

### Bleeding Risk

Large population studies have calculated the overall annual risk of hemorrhage from a cerebral arteriovenous malformation to be about 3%. A 1996 analysis from the University of Pittsburgh analyzed bleeding risk prior to radiosurgery in 315 patients [4]. Multivariate analysis identified three factors associated with hemorrhage: prior hemorrhage (relative risk [RR], 9.09, $P < 0.001$), single draining vein (RR, 1.66, $P < 0.01$), and diffuse (versus compact) AVM morphology (RR, 1.64; 95% CI, 1.12–2.46; $P < 0.01$). From this, four

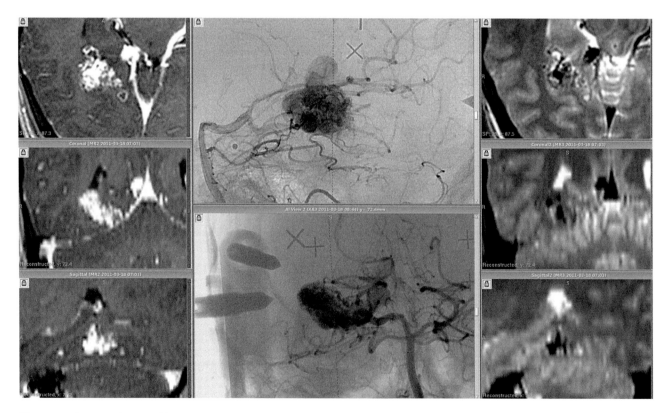

**Fig. 34.1** Diagnostic images with stereotactic biplane angiography (middle two panels) and magnetic resonance (MR) imaging with T1-contrast-enhanced images (left side) and T2 images (right side) for a right medial temporal arteriovenous malformation

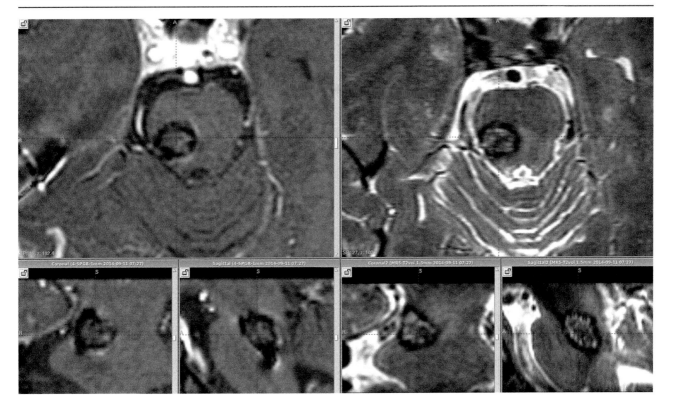

**Fig. 34.2** A typical appearing cavernous malformation of the brainstem in a patient with a history of two prior hemorrhagic events. A dark hemosiderin ring from the prior hemorrhagic events is surrounding the nidus of the cavernous malformation

AVM hemorrhage risk groups were constructed on the basis of the significant factors with annual bleeding rates 0.99%, 2.22%, 3.72%, and 8.94% per year, respectively.

Stapf et al. analyzed bleeding risks in 622 consecutive AVM patients from the prospective Columbia AVM database, just within the time period between time of diagnosis and the start of treatment [5]. Increasing age (hazard ratio [HR] 1.05/year), initial hemorrhage at presentation (HR 5.38), deep brain location (HR 3.25), and exclusive deep venous drainage (HR 3.25) independently predicted subsequent hemorrhage. Annual hemorrhage rates varied from 0.9% for patients with none of the last three factors to 34.4% for patients with all three factors.

## Cavernous Malformations

Studies from the University of Pittsburgh found that cavernous malformations have annual bleeding risks of 0.6%, 4.5%, and 32% per year after 0, 1, and 2 or more bleeds, respectively [6]. Nikoubashman et al. [7] retrospectively categorized 355 cavernous malformations of 70 children and adolescents according to their morphologic appearance on MR imaging and calculated prospective hemorrhage rates on

the basis of survival functions for 255 lesions in 25 patients with a radiologic observation period of >180 days. The presence of acute or subacute blood degradation correlated with increased hemorrhage ($P = 0.036$): the mean annual hemorrhage rates for cavernous malformations with signs of acute or subacute blood degradation products were 23.4% compared to 3.4% without those signs.

## Grading Scales

Several grading scales for AVM have been developed and validated for predicting outcome.

The most widely used scale is the Spetzler-Martin [8] grading scale developed to predict the outcome from surgical resection of AVM. The five-grade Spetzler-Martin scale assigns points according to three different anatomic features of the AVM: diameter (<3 cm [1 point], 3–6 cm [2 points], or >6 cm [3 points]), presence of deep venous drainage (1 point), and "eloquent" location such as the motor, sensory, language, and visual cortex or basal ganglia (1 point). Higher Spetzler-Martin grades correlate with poorer outcomes (lower cure rates and higher complications) from microsurgical resection.

The Pollock-Flickinger score [9] was developed to specifically predict outcome from AVM radiosurgery. It uses the following formula:

$$\text{AVM score} = 0.1^* \text{volume} + 0.02^* \text{age} + 0.5^* \text{location}$$

The Virginia Radiosurgery AVM Scale (VRAS) [10] assigns one of the five grades to AVM based on the sum of points assigned for volume/diameter (<2 cm$^3$ [0 points], 2–4 cm$^3$ [1 point], or >4 cm$^3$ [2 points]), eloquent location (1 point), and history of cerebral hemorrhage (1 point). Grade 1 arteriovenous malformations have 0 points, and grade 5 malformations have 4 points.

## Multimodality Choices for Management Options

The management options for arteriovenous malformations include observation, surgical resection, embolization and radiosurgery. Complete surgical resection solves the problem of having a fragile malformation of blood vessels prone to bleeding by completely removing it, but complete resection comes at the price of possible severe postoperative complications, which vary in probability and magnitude by AVM location, size, and vascular anatomy.

Angiography helps define the AVM nidus, the feeding arteries, and the venous drainage of AVM which allows for planning surgery, radiosurgery, and/or embolization. Angiography also allows for identification and possible coiling of any associated aneurysms to reduce the risk of aneurysmal bleeding while awaiting radiosurgical AVM obliteration. Some AVMs, particularly those supplied through branches of the external carotid, can be obliterated through angiographic embolization. The two main concerns with angiographic AVM embolization are causing vascular infarcts and recanalization of embolized vessels. Preoperative embolization can reduce the risks of hemorrhage during surgical resection. When embolization of superficial arterial AVM feeders is combined with radiosurgery to speed up relief of pulsatile tinnitus and headaches, most institutions prefer post-radiosurgical embolization. Pre-radiosurgical embolization is associated with lower rates of AVM obliteration since it tends to make the nidus less well-defined, and recanalization may develop in embolized portions not targeted by radiosurgery.

The ARUBA trial compared observation of unruptured AVMs with treatment intervention (the choice of embolization, resection, or radiosurgery) [11, 12]. Because the upfront morbidity from surgery, embolization, and radiosurgery was contrasted with the relatively low annual bleeding risk of unruptured AVM with observation, the ARUBA trial found observation was the best management option during their relatively short 33-month mean follow-up period. While this trial could be used to justify observation for older patients with low risk AVMs, the design of the ARUBA trial with a mean follow-up of only 33.3 months was completely inadequate to show the benefit accrued in the long run for definitive management of AVM with surgery or radiosurgery in younger patients.

## Treatment Field Design/Target Delineation

In AVMs the abnormality seen on angiographic, MR, and CT imaging is a combination of AVM nidus, feeding arteries, and enlarged draining veins. The key to planning AVM radiosurgery is to define and target the shunting vessels of the AVM nidus and try to avoid including draining veins as much as possible. This nidus can be seen as the blush or small cloud of contrast appearing in the early phase of the angiogram as seen in Fig. 34.1. As shown in Fig. 34.3, outlines of the nidus on orthogonal 2D angiographic films define a bounding box within co-registered 3D axial MRI images, where the nidus can be accurately defined in 3D space.

For cavernous malformations, the entire hemosiderin ring does not need to be included, only the malformed blood vessels within that ring. Figure 34.4 shows a typical brainstem cavernous malformation with the superimposed radiosurgery treatment plan limited to nidus but not covering the edges of the hemosiderin ring.

## Normal Critical Structure Tolerance Constraints

The standard constraints for normal tissue structures are used for all brain radiosurgery. The maximum tolerated dose for the optic chiasm, optic nerves, and other cranial nerves is normally restricted to a Dmax of 10 Gy in one fraction (or 18 Gy in 3 fractions of 6 Gy each). Brainstem doses are usually limited to 12–13 Gy. Dmax for radiosurgery targets outside the brainstem; however higher doses in the range of 15–18 Gy must be accepted in order to treat AVMs and cavernous malformations that directly involve the brainstem in order to achieve a reasonable chance of obliteration. Mean doses to the cochlea and pituitary gland are usually limited to 4.5 and 7 Gy when possible.

## Complication Avoidance and Radiation Toxicities (Acute and Late)

Prior outcome studies indicate that AVM radiosurgery may be associated with either transient or irreversible adverse radiation effects (ARE) [13–20]. After SRS serial magnetic resonance imaging (MRI), studies indicate that as many as

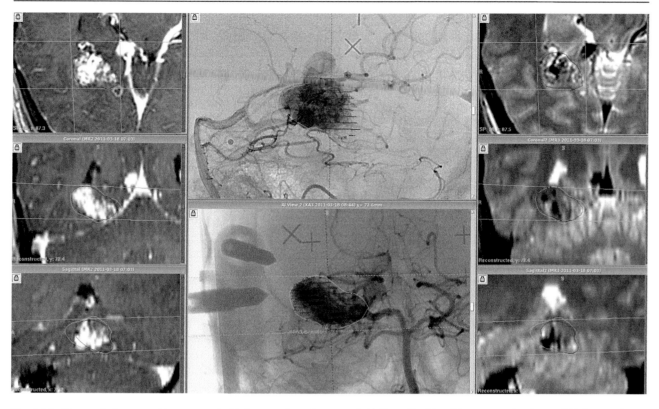

**Fig. 34.3** Diagnostic images with stereotactic biplane angiography (middle two panels) and magnetic resonance (MR) imaging with T1-contrast-enhanced images (left side) and T2 images (right side) for a right medial temporal arteriovenous malformation. The AVM nidus was initially outlined in white on second orthogonal biplane angiography images (middle two panels) and are represented as white lines on the 3D MR images (right and left panels) that help determine border limits for the final 3D MR target outline (in black)

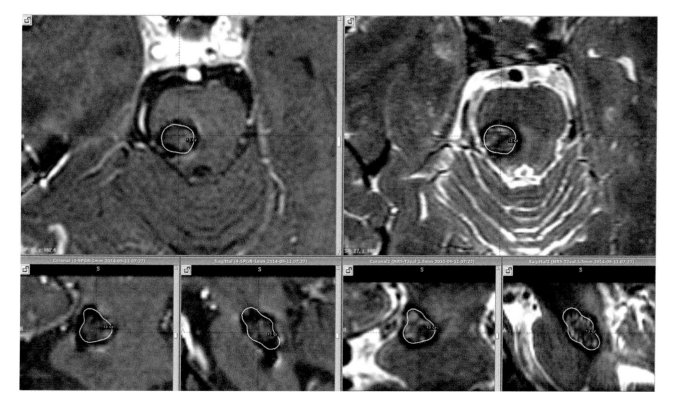

**Fig. 34.4** Radiosurgery treatment plan for a brainstem cavernous malformation with a history of two prior hemorrhagic events. The dark hemosiderin ring surrounding the nidus of the cavernous malformation was not purposely included in the treatment volume

30% of patients develop detectable imaging changes adjacent to the treatment volume [13–20]. Symptomatic ARE develop in 3–11% of patients [13–20]. Prior publications indicate that AVM anatomic location, nidus size, margin dose [5–8, 21], and the brain volume included in 12 Gy are predictive of symptomatic ARE after AVM radiosurgery [13–15]. Flickinger et al. [14, 15] constructed statistical models predicting the risk of irreversible radiation sequelae with a 12 Gy volume, i.e., the volume of tissue (including the AVM target) receiving 12 Gy or more. The relationship between target volume and the occurrence of ARE is considered to be dose dependent. The likelihood of associated symptoms and the type of symptoms that develop depend on the location of the AVM. Flickinger et al. [14, 15] reported that the high-risk group of irreversible symptomatic ARE included the AVM locations in the brainstem and thalamus. Kano et al. [20] later evaluated 755 AVM patients who underwent a single Gamma Knife® SRS procedure with at least a 2-year minimum follow-up. The cumulative rates of symptomatic ARE were 3.2%, 5.8%, 6.7%, and 7.5% at 1, 2, 3, and 5 years, respectively. Factors associated with a higher rate of developing symptomatic ARE included larger AVM volume, higher margin dose, larger 12 Gy volume, higher Spetzler-Martin grade, and higher radiosurgery-based score (RBS). The rates of developing symptomatic ARE were higher in the brainstem (22%) or thalamus (16%), compared to AVMs located in other brain locations (4–8%). The rates of irreversible symptomatic ARE were 0.8%, 1.9%, 2.1%, and 2.8% at 1, 2, 3, and 5 years, respectively. The 5-year cumulative rates of irreversible symptomatic ARE were 9.1% in thalamus, 12.1% in brainstem, and 1.4% in other locations.

Delayed cyst formation or even chronic expanding hematoma after SRS-induced AVM obliteration is an uncommon but well-described phenomenon [19, 22]. Ilyas et al. [10] reported based on pooled data from 22 published studies comprising the incidence analysis that the overall rate of post-SRS delayed cyst formation was 3.0% (78/2619 patients) with a latency period of approximately 7 years. Of the 64 cyst patients with available symptomatology and management data, 21 (32.8%) were symptomatic; 21 cysts (32.8%) were treated with surgical intervention, whereas the remaining 43 (67.2%) were managed conservatively. The risk of radiosurgery causing a malignant tumor to develop in 5–30 years is rare and therefore not well-defined but appears to be in the range of 1/200–1/1000.

## Outcomes

The Spetzler-Martin grading system has been accepted as an accurate method to predict patient outcomes after resection at centers with extensive vascular expertise [23]. Selected reports from such centers indicate that surgery for Spetzler-Martin grade I and II AVMs may be associated with no morbidity or mortality. Not all low-grade AVMs may have the same expectation. For example, a grade II AVM (small with superficial venous drainage) located within the motor cortex may be associated with at least temporary contralateral motor weakness after surgical removal. Kano et al. [15] reported 217 patients with AVMs classified as Spetzler-Martin grade I or II who underwent SRS. The actuarial rates of total obliteration by angiography or MR after one SRS were 58%, 87%, 90%, and 93% at 3, 4, 5, and 10 years, respectively. One of the greatest limitations of SRS for AVMs is the substantial delay in the radiographic obliteration of the lesion, which takes 2–4 years on average [24]. Ding et al. [25] reported on an ARUBA-eligible Spetzler-Martin grades I–II AVM cohort comprised of 232 patients who underwent SRS in multicenter study including seven institutions. The actuarial obliteration rates at 5 and 10 years were 72% and 87%, respectively; annual post-SRS hemorrhage rate was 1.0%; symptomatic and permanent radiation-induced changes occurred in 8% and 1%, respectively; favorable outcome was achieved in 76%; and stroke or death occurred in 10%.

Spetzler-Martin grade III AVMs are a heterogeneous group that includes different subtypes of AVMs according to their size, location in critical brain regions, and venous drainage. Nonetheless relatively few surgical series use a subclassification system to report outcomes of treatment [21, 26, 27]. Kano et al. [28] reported that 474 Spetzler-Martin grade III AVM patients underwent SRS at a median follow-up of 89 months. The total obliteration rates documented by angiography or MR for all Spetzler-Martin grade III AVMs increased from 47% at 3 years to 69% at 4 years, 72% at 5 years, and 77% at 10 years. Small subgroup of Spetzler-Martin grade III was more likely to obliterate than other Spetzler-Martin grade III subgroups. The cumulative rate of hemorrhage was 2.6% at 1 year, 4.4% at 2 years, 5.2% at 3 years, 6.2% at 5 years, and 7.7% at 10 years. Medium/deep subgroup of Spetzler-Martin grade III AVM was significantly higher cumulative rate of hemorrhage. Symptomatic adverse radiation effects were detected in 6%. Ding et al. [2] reported that 891 Spetzler-Martin grade III AVM patients underwent SRS in multicenter study including eight institutions. The actuarial obliteration rates at 5 and 10 years were 63% and 78%, respectively. The annual postradiosurgery hemorrhage rate was 1.2%. Symptomatic and permanent adverse radiation effects were observed in 11% and 4% of the patients, respectively.

In contrast Spetzler-Martin grade IV and V AVMs are associated with higher risks and less success regardless of the option selected [29, 30]. Patibandla et al. [30] reported outcome of 233 Spetzler-Martin grade IV (94.4%) and V (5.6%) patients who underwent single-session SRS in multicenter study including eight institutions at a median follow-up of 84.5 months. The actuarial obliteration rates at 3, 7, 10, and 12 years were 15%, 34%, 37%, and 42%, respectively. The annual post-SRS hemorrhage rate was 3.0%. Symptomatic and permanent adverse radiation effects occurred in 10.7% and 4% of the patients, respectively.

Total obliteration that is confirmed by angiography appears to reduce the cumulative lifetime risk of hemorrhage to approximately 1%, in comparison to an annual hemorrhage risk that varies from 1% to 4% [31]. Whether partial obliteration of AVMs after SRS affects the delayed risk of bleeding remains unclear [22, 31–33]. Approximately 3 years after SRS, patients with residual AVMs are reevaluated to assess whether additional salvage management options (e.g., surgical resection, embolization, and/or repeated SRS) are warranted.

Several studies have shown that approximately 60–70% of patients with incomplete obliteration of AVMs after initial SRS achieve total obliteration after repeat SRS [23, 34, 35]. Kano et al. [36] reported that repeat SRS was performed on 105 patients who had incompletely obliterated AVMs at a median of 40.9 months after initial SRS. The actuarial rate of total obliteration by angiography or MRI after repeat SRS was 35%, 68%, 77%, and 80% at 3, 4, 5, and 10 years, respectively. The cumulative actuarial rates of new AVM hemorrhage after repeat SRS were 1.9%, 8.1%, 10.1%, 10.1%, and 22.4% at 1, 2, 3, 5, and 10 years, respectively, which translate to annual hemorrhage rates of 4.05% and 1.79% of patients developing new post-repeat-SRS bleeds/year. for years 0–2 and 2–10 following repeat SRS. Symptomatic adverse radiation effect developed in five patients (4.7%) after initial SRS and ten patients (9.5%) after repeat SRS.

The management of larger volume (>10 cc) symptomatic AVMs still remains a perplexing clinical challenge. Single-staged SRS of large-volume AVMs was associated with a low rate of obliteration or unacceptable adverse radiation effects. Kano et al. [37] reported that 46 large-volume AVM (>10 cc) patients underwent volume-staged SRS, in which usually 1/3–1/2 of the AVM is treated initially with the remaining portion(s) treated in 1–2 more sessions separated by 3–6 months each (see Fig. 34.5). The rationale for this

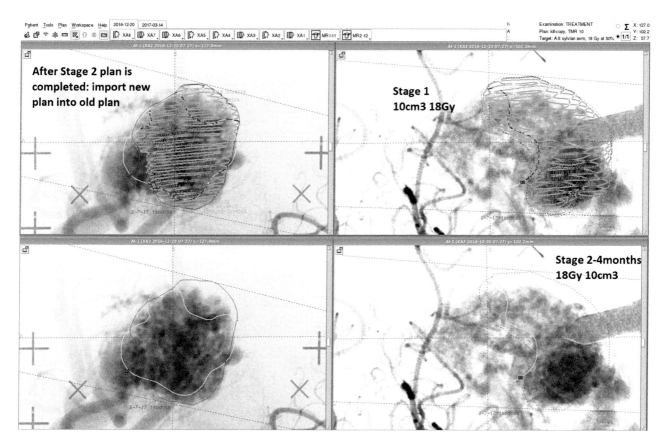

**Fig. 34.5** Staged radiosurgery (SRS) for a 20 cm³ arteriovenous malformation. Frame-based 2D stereotactic angiography was performed along stereotactic magnetic resonance (MR) imaging for the initial stage SRS and were co-registered with the same stereotactic frame. The second stage was performed with stereotactic MR alone. The MR images from the first and second stages can be co-registered with each other, but because of the change in position of the frame between the two sessions, the 2D angiographic images from the first plan cannot be directly displayed with the MR images from the second stage in the second plan. The MR isodose outlines from the second-stage plan can be imported back into the initial stage plan and projected onto the 2D angiographic images as is shown here in the top two panels. An outline of those isodose lines is displayed in the bottom two panels

approach is that the smaller volumes for the individual stages allow higher doses of radiation (usually 16–18 Gy for 8–13 cm³) to be safely given for each portion safely than if the entire portion was irradiated in one session (limited to 13–15 Gy for 16–40 cm³). The actuarial rates of total obliteration after two-staged SRS were 7%, 20%, 28%, and 36% at 3, 4, 5, and 10 years, respectively. The 5-year total obliteration rate after the initial staged volumetric SRS with a margin dose of ≥17 Gy was 62%. Prospective volume-staged SRS for large AVMs has potential benefit but often requires multiple procedures spread over time. In the future, prospective volume-staged SRS followed by innovative embolization strategies (to reduce flow, obliterate fistulas, and occlude associated aneurysms) may further reduce the risk of hemorrhage.

## Follow-Up/Radiographic Assessment

Most centers obtain follow-up MR imaging after AVM or cavernous malformation radiosurgery every 6 months for the first 3 years to look for loss of flow signal indicating probable obliteration and evidence of radiation injury reaction or evidence of limited hemorrhage. If AVM oblitera-

tion looks likely, angiography is recommended to confirm obliteration. It is also reasonable to delay angiography until 4–5 years post-SRS particularly for large AVMs showing a dramatic response, to give more time for obliteration to develop. When AVM remain patent 3–5 years after radiosurgery, they should be considered for either repeat radiosurgery or occasionally surgical resection. If the vascular malformation appears obliterated following radiosurgery, then follow-up MR imaging should be obtained around every 2 years to look for development of post-radiosurgery cyst development or development of a secondary neoplasm.

## Case Summary

A 20-year-old gentleman presented with a history of migraine and symptoms of dizziness. His MRI and angiography disclosed a deep-seated arteriovenous malformation in the right medial temporal lobe with deep venous drainage through the basilar vein of Rosenthal into the internal cerebral vein and straight sinus with no evidence of prior hemorrhage. After discussing the risks and benefits of observation, surgical resection, embolization, and

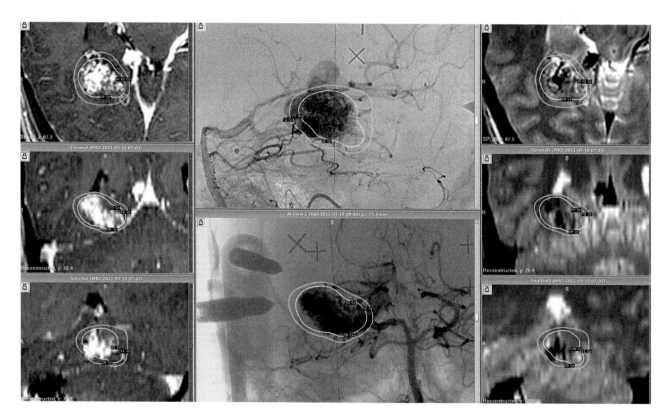

**Fig. 34.6** Radiosurgery treatment plan for the right medial temporal arteriovenous malformation shown in Figs. 34.1 and 34.3. A dose of 20 Gy was prescribed to a 50% isodose treatment volume measuring 4.5 mL with the 12 Gy volume also shown

radiosurgery, he decided to proceed with radiosurgery as shown in Fig. 34.6 (stereotactic magnetic resonance imaging and biplane angiography for a deep right temporal AVM). A dose of 20 Gy was prescribed to a 4.5 mL treatment volume with a maximum dose of 40 Gy. He did not return for follow-up as recommended. Follow up MR imaging 39 months later (Fig. 34.7) was obtained when he

was evaluated by his local neurologist for complaints of a syncopal episode preceded by a visual aura and episodic headaches. His brain MR showed gliosis and T2 signal change around the atrium and occipital horn of the right lateral ventricle where the prior arteriovenous malformation was treated. The signal void of a high-flow arteriovenous malformation present on the pre-radiosurgery images

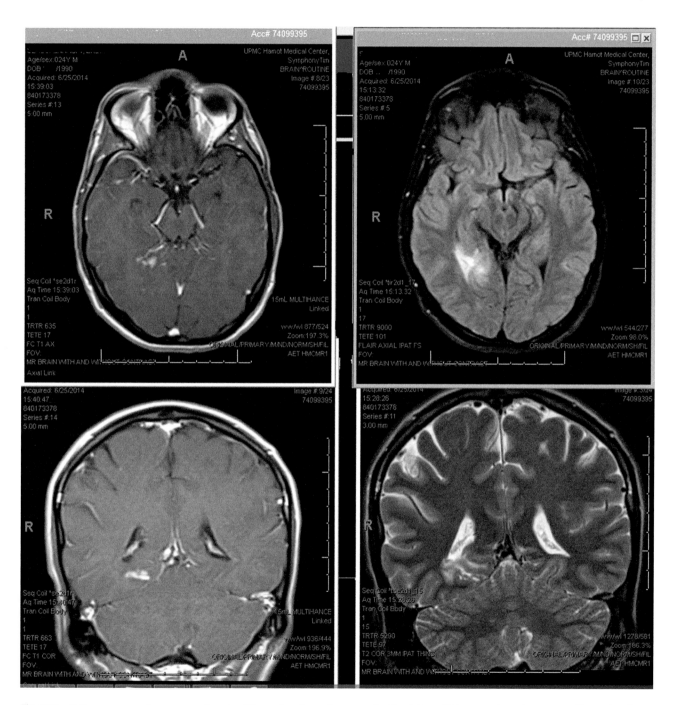

**Fig. 34.7** Follow-up magnetic resonance imaging 39 months after radiosurgery for the right medial temporal arteriovenous malformation shown in Fig. 34.1. The flow void on T2 sequences is no longer present

is no longer evident. The patient was started on anticonvulsants and has not returned for further follow-up imaging such as angiography to confirm obliteration. This example illustrates potential morbidity from arteriovenous malformation radiosurgery and the difficulty keeping follow-up imaging 3–5 years after radiosurgery to confirm obliteration.

## Summary

- Arteriovenous malformations have significant rates of spontaneous hemorrhage, morbidity, and mortality that increase with factors such as age, prior bleeding episodes, deep venous drainage, and brainstem location.
- Embolization of AVM prior to radiosurgery is associated with lower rates of obliteration.
- The risks of post-radiosurgery injury reaction increase with treatment volume and location (brainstem, thalamus, or others).
- Radiosurgical obliteration of AVM larger than 10 cm$^3$ is difficult to achieve with acceptable morbidity. Techniques such as sequential volume-staged radiosurgery appear to improve outcomes.

## Self-Assessment Questions

1. What is the annual risk of bleeding from an arteriovenous malformations?
   A. 1%
   B. 3%
   C. 6%
   D. 10%

2. What is the annual bleeding risk from cavernous malformations with no prior hemorrhage?
   A. 0.6%
   B. 3%
   C. 6%
   D. 10%

3. What does embolization of an arteriovenous malformations prior to radiosurgery achieve?
   A. Improves outcome but reduces treatment volume and thereby lowers complications
   B. Increases the rate of AVM obliteration from subsequent radiosurgcry
   C. Adds additional risk with little benefit in most cases
   D. Helps reduce pulsatile tinnitus and headache from superficial AVM more quickly than radiosurgery alone

4. What did the ARUBA trial of managing AVM with no prior hemorrhage demonstrate at mean follow-up of 33 months?
   A. Observation/medical management of unruptured AVM was associated with best outcome.
   B. Surgical management of unruptured AVM was associated with best outcome.
   C. Embolization of unruptured AVM was associated with best outcome.
   D. Radiosurgery of unruptured AVM was associated with best outcome.

5. The total volume of what dose level is associated with a higher rate of developing symptomatic adverse radiation event when treating AVM with radiosurgery?
   A. 6 Gy
   B. 9 Gy
   C. 12 Gy
   D. 15 Gy

## Answers

1. B
2. A
3. C
4. A
5. C

## References

1. Al-Shahi R, Bhattacharya JJ, Currie DG, et al. Prospective, population-based detection of intracranial vascular malformations in adults: the Scottish Intracranial Vascular Malformation Study (SIVMS). Stroke. 2003;34(5):1163–9. Epub 2003 Apr 17. PubMed PMID: 12702837
2. Katzman GL, Dagher AP, Patronas NJ. Incidental findings on brain magnetic resonance imaging from 1000 asymptomatic volunteers. JAMA. 1999;282:36–9.
3. Yue NC, Longstreth WT Jr, Elster AD, et al. Clinically serious abnormalities found incidentally at MR imaging of the brain: data from the Cardiovascular Health Study. Radiology. 1997;202:41–6.
4. Pollock BE, Flickinger JC, Lunsford LD, et al. Factors that predict the bleeding risk of cerebral arteriovenous malformations. Stroke. 1996;27(1):1–6.
5. Stapf C, Mast H, Sciacca RR, et al. Predictors of hemorrhage in patients with untreated brain arteriovenous malformation. Neurology. 2006;66(9):1350–5.
6. Hasegawa T, McInerney J, Kondziolka D, et al. Long-term results after stereotactic radiosurgery for patients with cavernous malformations. Neurosurgery. 2002;50(6):1190–7. discussion 1197–8
7. Nikoubashman O, Di Rocco F, Davagnanam I, et al. Prospective hemorrhage rates of cerebral cavernous malformations in children and adolescents based on MRI appearance. AJNR Am J Neuroradiol. 2015;36(11):2177–83. https://doi.org/10.3174/ajnr.A4427. Epub 2015 Aug 13

8. Spetzler RF, Martin NA. A proposed grading system for arteriovenous malformations. J Neurosurg. 1986;65(4):476–83.

9. Wegner RE, Oysul K, Pollock BE, et al. A modified radiosurgery-based arteriovenous malformation grading scale and its correlation with outcomes. Int J Radiat Oncol Biol Phys. 2011;79:1147–50.

10. Cohen-Inbar O, Starke RM, Kano H, et al. Stereotactic radiosurgery for cerebellar arteriovenous malformations: an international multicenter study. J Neurosurg. 2017;127(3):512–21. https://doi.org/10.3171/2016.7.JNS161208. Epub 2016 Sep 30

11. Mohr JP, Parides MK, Stapf C, et al. Medical management with or without interventional therapy for unruptured brain arteriovenous malformations (ARUBA): a multicentre, non-blinded, randomised trial. Lancet. 2014;383(9917):614–21. https://doi.org/10.1016/S0140-6736(13)62302-8. Epub 2013 Nov 20

12. Ding D, Starke RM, Kano H, et al. Radiosurgery for cerebral arteriovenous malformations in a randomized trial of unruptured brain arteriovenous malformations (ARUBA)-eligible patients: a multicenter study. Stroke. 2016;47(2):342–9. https://doi.org/10.1161/STROKEAHA.115.011400. Epub 2015 Dec 10

13. Flickinger JC, Kondziolka D, Lunsford LD, et al. A multi-institutional analysis of complication outcomes after arteriovenous malformation radiosurgery. Int J Radiat Oncol Biol Phys. 1999;44:67–74.

14. Flickinger JC, Kondziolka D, Pollock BE, et al. Complications from arteriovenous malformation radiosurgery: multivariate analysis and risk modeling. Int J Radiat Oncol Biol Phys. 1997;38:485–90.

15. Flickinger JC, Lunsford LD, Kondziolka D, et al. Radiosurgery and brain tolerance: an analysis of neurodiagnostic imaging changes after gamma knife radiosurgery for arteriovenous malformations. Int J Radiat Oncol Biol Phys. 1992;23:19–26.

16. Karlsson B, Lax I, Soderman M. Factors influencing the risk for complications following Gamma Knife radiosurgery of cerebral arteriovenous malformations. Radiother Oncol. 1997;43:275–80.

17. Lax I, Karlsson B. Prediction of complications in gamma knife radiosurgery of arteriovenous malformation. Acta Oncol. 1996;35:49–55.

18. Voges J, Treuer H, Sturm V, et al. Risk analysis of linear accelerator radiosurgery. Int J Radiat Oncol Biol Phys. 1996;36:1055–63.

19. Flickinger JC, Kondziolka D, Lunsford LD, et al. Development of a model to predict permanent symptomatic postradiosurgery injury for arteriovenous malformation patients. Arteriovenous Malformation Radiosurgery Study Group. Int J Radiat Oncol Biol Phys. 2000;46:1143–8.

20. Kano H, Flickinger JC, Tonetti D, et al. Estimating the risks of adverse radiation effects after Gamma Knife radiosurgery for arteriovenous malformations. Stroke. 2017;48(1):84–90.

21. de Oliveira E, Tedeschi H, Raso J. Comprehensive management of arteriovenous malformations. Neurol Res. 1998;20:673–83.

22. Karlsson B, Lindquist C, Johansson A, et al. Annual risk for the first hemorrhage from untreated cerebral arteriovenous malformations. Minim Invasive Neurosurg. 1997;40:40–6.

23. Yen CP, Jain S, Haq IU, et al. Repeat Gamma Knife surgery for incompletely obliterated cerebral arteriovenous malformations. Neurosurgery. 2010;67:55–64. discussion 64

24. Solomon RA, Connolly ES Jr. Arteriovenous malformations of the brain. N Engl J Med. 2017;376:1859–66.

25. Ding D, Starke RM, Kano H, et al. Stereotactic radiosurgery for ARUBA (a randomized trial of unruptured brain arteriovenous malformations) eligible Spetzler Martin grade I and II arteriovenous malformations: a multicenter study. World Neurosurg. 2017;102:507–17.

26. Lawton MT. Spetzler-Martin Grade III arteriovenous malformations: surgical results and a modification of the grading scale. Neurosurgery. 2003;52:740–8.; discussion 748–9.

27. Ding D, Starke RM, Kano H, et al. Stereotactic radiosurgery for Spetzler-Martin Grade III arteriovenous malformations: an international multicenter study. J Neurosurg. 2017;126:859–71.

28. Kano H, Flickinger JC, Yang HC, et al. Stereotactic radiosurgery for Spetzler-Martin Grade III arteriovenous malformations. J Neurosurg. 2014;120:973–81.

29. Lawton MT, Kim H, McCulloch CE, et al. A supplementary grading scale for selecting patients with brain arteriovenous malformations for surgery. Neurosurgery. 2010;66:702–13.; discussion 713.

30. Patibandla MR, Ding D, Kano H, et al. Stereotactic radiosurgery for Spetzler-Martin Grade IV and V arteriovenous malformations: an international multicenter study. J Neurosurg. 2017:1–10. https://doi.org/10.3171/2017.3.JNS162635.

31. Maruyama K, Kawahara N, Shin M, et al. The risk of hemorrhage after radiosurgery for cerebral arteriovenous malformations. N Engl J Med. 2005;352:146–53.

32. Maruyama K, Shin M, Tago M, et al. Radiosurgery to reduce the risk of first hemorrhage from brain arteriovenous malformations. Neurosurgery. 2007;60:453–8.; discussion 458–9.

33. Pollock BE, Flickinger JC, Lunsford LD, et al. Hemorrhage risk after stereotactic radiosurgery of cerebral arteriovenous malformations. Neurosurgery. 1996;38:652–9.; discussion 659–61.

34. Karlsson B, Kihlstrom L, Lindquist C, et al. Gamma knife surgery for previously irradiated arteriovenous malformations. Neurosurgery. 1998;42:1–5.; discussion 5–6.

35. Maesawa S, Flickinger JC, Kondziolka D, et al. Repeated radiosurgery for incompletely obliterated arteriovenous malformations. J Neurosurg. 2000;92:961–70.

36. Kano H, Kondziolka D, Flickinger JC, et al. Stereotactic radiosurgery for arteriovenous malformations. Part 3: Outcome predictors and risks after repeat radiosurgery. J Neurosurg. 2012;116:21–32.

37. Kano H, Kondziolka D, Flickinger JC, et al. Stereotactic radiosurgery for arteriovenous malformations. Part 6: Multistaged volumetric management of large arteriovenous malformations. J Neurosurg. 2012;116:54–65.

# Trigeminal Neuralgia

Peter Y. Chen

## Learning Objectives

- Explain the nature of trigeminal neuralgia pain and its unique presentation as compared to other cephalic neuralgias.
- Cite the therapeutic approach to the treatment of trigeminal neuralgia with first-line therapy with pharmacological agents which if refractory or intolerable then to more invasive surgical modes of therapy ranging from operative microvascular decompression to minimally invasive, radiation-based stereotactic radiosurgical approaches including the Gamma Knife.
- Detail the intricate nature of stereotactic radiosurgery with assessment of target localization from MR/CT scanning, the strategic placement of the isocenter for delivery of the single-fraction stereotactic dose, the acceptable dose constraint(s) of surrounding eloquent neurological structures, and expected clinical results of such radiosurgical treatment in contrast to the other modes of available treatment.

## Background Definition/History

Trigeminal neuralgia [TN] or tic douloureux is a facial pain syndrome which involves the fifth cranial nerve also referred to as the trigeminal nerve. The pain is distinct among the cranial neuralgias. The pain of TN can be so violent and unbearable that the term tic douloureux has been used to describe the associated facial contortions and grimaces seen with extreme episodes of the discomfort. Its uniqueness was first denoted

based upon the original description of trigeminal neuralgia in 1783 by an English physician Dr. John Fothergill where he stated "The affection seems to be peculiar to persons advancing in years, and to women more than to men…The pain comes suddenly and is excruciating; it lasts but a short time, perhaps a quarter or half a minute, and then goes off; it returns at irregular intervals, sometimes in half an hour, sometimes there are two or three repetitions in a few minutes…Eating will bring it on some persons. Talking, or the least motion of the muscles of the face affects others; the gentlest touch of a handkerchief will sometimes bring on the pain, whilst a strong pressure on the part has no effect" [1].

The most updated definition of trigeminal neuralgia comes from the Neuropathic Pain Special Interest Group of the International Association for the Study of Pain and the Scientific Panel Pain of the European Academy of Neurology which convened in year 2016 a group of experts in trigeminal neuralgia, diagnostic grading, and evidence-based medicine to review existing descriptors/definitions of trigeminal neuralgia. The goal of the group was to develop a new classification and grading system for trigeminal neuralgia that fits the specific pathophysiology of the disease [2].

The resultant definition and classification of trigeminal neuralgia are as follows and are further delineated in the section on etiology and pathogenesis. The main components of the definition are orofacial pain restricted to one or more divisions of the trigeminal nerve with abrupt onset and typically lasting but a few seconds. The pain paroxysms can always be triggered by innocuous mechanical stimuli or movements. Usually there is no pain between paroxysms, but if pain is continuous, this is considered TN with continuous pain. TN is classified into three categories. Idiopathic TN has no apparent cause.

Classical TN is caused by vascular compression of the trigeminal root. And, secondary TN has causation by a known neurological disease process such as a tumor or multiple sclerosis (Fig. 35.1).

P. Y. Chen
Department of Radiation Oncology, Beaumont Health System, Oakland University-William Beaumont School of Medicine, William Beaumont Hospital, Royal Oak, MI, USA
e-mail: peter.chen@beaumont.edu

© Springer International Publishing AG, part of Springer Nature 2018
E. L. Chang et al. (eds.), *Adult CNS Radiation Oncology*, https://doi.org/10.1007/978-3-319-42878-9_35

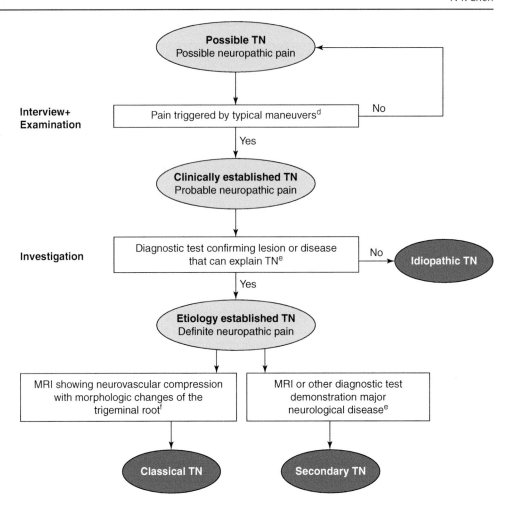

**Fig. 35.1** Schema of the new classification of TN from the Neuropathic Pain Special Interest Group. [Reprinted from Cruccu G, Finnerup NB, Jensen TS, Scholz J, Sindou M, Svensson P, Treede RD, Zakrzewska JM, Nurmikko T. Trigeminal neuralgia: New classification and diagnostic grading for practice and research. Neurology 2016;87:220–228. With permission from Wolters Kluwer Health, Inc.]

Prior to this updated classification of TN, classical TN included all cases of undetermined etiology that is idiopathic along with those cases with vascular compression of the trigeminal nerve. As will be further detailed in the pathophysiology of TN, the unifying mechanism of the TN pain in both the idiopathic or vascular compression presentations is that of demyelination of the nerve fibers of the fifth cranial nerve.

## Epidemiology

With an annual incidence of 4–13 per 100,000, TN is a rare condition which affects females more than males. The male to female prevalence ratio has been reported at 1:1.5–1:1.7 [3, 4]. Despite its low incidence, TN is one of the more commonly seen cranial neuralgias in the elderly with increasing incidence with advancing age; the majority of idiopathic cases are seen after age 50, although they may be seen as early as the 20s or 30s and, rarely, in children [5]. The occurrence of familial cases of TN has rarely been reported; however, the majority of patients have sporadic disease [6].

## Risk Factors

With respect to risk factors for the development of TN, there is variable data that hypertension may be a risk factor [7, 8]. As well, there is some evidence that migraine headaches may be a predisposition to TN [9]. Additionally, approximately 2–5% of patients with multiple sclerosis (MS) develop TN [10], as well as 2–14% of patients with TN have MS [11].

## Pathophysiology

Most cases of TN are either idiopathic or caused by vascular compression of the trigeminal nerve root, usually within a few millimeters of the root entry zone; such vascular impingement has been reported in up to 80% of TN cases. Moreover, investigators have found that the pathophysiological basis of TN is based upon demyelination, nerve microstructural abnormalities, and changes in sodium channels [12, 13].

Indeed, vascular compression in TN can contribute in producing changes in both myelin and neuronal membranes/

sodium channels. Eighty to ninety percent of this compression is by an aberrant loop of an artery or vein especially branches of the superior cerebellar arteries or venous channels [14, 15]. Other entities causing trigeminal nerve compression leading to secondary TN include vestibular schwannoma, meningioma, epidermoid or other cysts, or, rarely, a saccular aneurysm or arteriovenous malformation [16–20]. Thus, the most common cause of classical TN is compression or other morphological changes of the trigeminal nerve by a blood vessel, usually an artery, in the cerebellopontine cistern. This is termed a neurovascular conflict with compression. There are numerous neurophysiological, neuroimaging, and histological studies showing that such compression leads to focal demyelination of primary trigeminal afferents near the entry of the trigeminal root into the pons as the underlying pathophysiological mechanism in TN [21–23]. Demyelinated lesions may set up ectopic impulse generation, possibly causing ephaptic transmission. Ephaptic cross talk between fibers mediating light touch and those involved in pain generation could account for the precipitation of painful attacks by light tactile stimulation of facial trigger zones.

Demyelination of one or more of the trigeminal nerve nuclei may also be caused by multiple sclerosis or other structural lesions of the brainstem. In multiple sclerosis, a plaque of demyelination typically occurs in the root entry zone of the trigeminal nerve [24], although vascular compression also has been noted in these patients [25, 26].

## Clinical Presentation

The pain of TN is stabbing, electric shock-like, and episodic lasting but a few seconds to 1–2 min. Between episodes of pain, there are pain-free periods. Pain may occur several times a day. The pain is usually unilateral, involving one or more branches of the trigeminal nerve, usually the maxillary and mandibular (V2 and V3) divisions. However, bilateral involvement is seen in 5% of cases. When TN is seen with multiple sclerosis, bilaterality may be seen in upward to 20%. Characteristically, the pain is triggered by a variety of external stimuli which precipitate an attack. These include light touch of the face, cold air or wind, chewing, shaving, toothbrushing, face washing, talking, or smiling. With the passage of time, remissions become less, and the intensity of the pain increases. The presentations of TN may be of acute-onset versus a more protracted insidious course of occurrence typified by chronicity.

## Diagnosis/Diagnostic Work-Up

There is no single diagnostic test which is unique in making a diagnosis of TN. From the clinical presentation of a patient who presents with a classic pain pattern of TN, establishment of a diagnosis is not difficult as the symptoms are clear and distinct. Clinically therefore a thorough and detailed historical documentation of presenting symptoms and a complete physical examination should be performed. Specific diagnostic criteria for making a diagnosis of TN as set forth by the International Classification of Headache Disorders, 3rd edition (ICHD-3) [27] for classic TN are as follows:

(a) At least three attacks of unilateral facial pain fulfilling criteria B and C
(b) Occurring in one or more divisions of the trigeminal nerve, with no radiation beyond the trigeminal distribution
(c) Pain has at least three of the following four characteristics:
    Recurring in paroxysmal attacks lasting from a fraction of a second to 2 min
    Severe intensity
    Electric shock-like, shooting, stabbing, or sharp in quality
    At least three attacks precipitated by innocuous stimuli to the affected side of the face (some attacks may be, or appear to be, spontaneous)
(d) No clinically evident neurologic deficit
(e) Not better accounted for by another ICHD-3 diagnosis

Further a practical classification of TN with clinical relevance in the decision-making process of which therapeutic alternative to use on any particular patient delineates a type 1 and type 2 pain pattern along with associated factors describing in part the etiology of the pain [28].

Trigeminal neuralgia type 1 (TN1): This is the classic form of trigeminal neuralgia in which episodic lancinating pain predominates (also known as typical TN).

Trigeminal neuralgia type 2 (TN2): This is the atypical form of trigeminal neuralgia in which more constant pains (aching, throbbing, and/or burning) predominate.

Trigeminal neuropathic pain (TNP): This is pain that results from incidental or accidental injury to the trigeminal nerve or the brain pathways of the trigeminal system.

Trigeminal deafferentation pain (TDP): This is pain that results from intentional injury to the system in an attempt to treat trigeminal neuralgia. Numbness of the face is a constant part of this syndrome, which has also been referred to as anesthesia dolorosa or one of its variants.

Symptomatic trigeminal neuralgia (STN): This is trigeminal neuralgia associated with multiple sclerosis (MS).

Postherpetic neuralgia (PHN): This is chronic facial pain that results from an outbreak of herpes zoster (shingles), usually in the ophthalmic division (V1) of the trigeminal nerve on the face and usually in elderly patients.

Geniculate neuralgia (GeN): This is typified by episodic lancinating pain felt deep in the ear.

Glossopharyngeal neuralgia (GPN): This is typified by pain in the tonsillar area or throat, usually triggered by talking or swallowing.

The diagnosis of TN is purely one made on clinical assessment of the character of the pain, and a key is the description of trigger points of stimuli which bring on the pain. Most commonly the involvement is that of the second and third branches of the trigeminal nerve and rare is the presentation in the ophthalmic branch alone. If the diagnosis of TN is unclear, then to ascertain other possible causes of pain, MRI scanning with and without contrast is of utility in the determination of a compressive component from any adjacent surrounding vascular structures. As well, such MR imaging will aid in identifying such entities as sinusitis, tumors along the trigeminal nerve, pathological enhancement of the trigeminal nerve documenting perineural extension of neoplasm, masses of the cavernous sinus, plaques indicative of multiple sclerosis, and/or thalamic or trigeminal brainstem lesions from lacunar infarcts [29, 30].

Other causes of TN are collagen vascular disorders. Although rare in its occurrence with rheumatic diseases, such as scleroderma (TN reported in up to 5% of patients with this collagen vascular disease) and systemic lupus erythematosus, diagnostic consideration should be in the differential diagnoses in patients with atypical features of facial pain and a systemic presentation of collagen vascular disorder. Appropriate blood work would include a sedimentation rate, antinuclear antibody titer, double-stranded DNA, anti-Sm antibody, lupus erythematosus cell preparation, and complete blood count to look for hematological abnormalities (e.g., hemolytic anemia, leukopenia, thrombocytopenia). Of particular note in assessment of the possibility of scleroderma, creatinine kinase and aldolase levels may be elevated with muscle involvement; additionally, SCL-86 and SCL-70 antibody titers may be present.

Aside from a diagnosis of collagen vascular disorder, baseline blood work with a CBC with differential white count and selected biochemical parameters to include liver function tests and electrolytes are recommended prior to the initiation of any pharmacological agents commonly offered as first-line treatment for TN for drug toxicity monitoring.

## Multimodality Management Approach

Several therapeutic alternatives are available for the treatment of TN. These options include medicinal agents predominantly antiepileptics, surgical alternatives including microvascular decompression (MVD) and percutaneous rhizotomies, and the irradiation approach consisting of stereotactic radiosurgery. The treatment approach taken for any individual TN patient will be dependent on her/his age, comorbid conditions, as well as a personal history of prior therapies received which have been either successful or failed in the control of the TN pain.

## Medicinal Therapy

First-line treatment for classical TN (idiopathic or caused by vascular compression) begins with drug therapy, most frequently with anticonvulsant medication; the gold standard antiepileptic drug is carbamazepine for TN as documented in a Cochrane systemic review based upon two placebo-controlled studies of this anticonvulsant agent in TN [31]. Indeed, treatment of TN as recommended by the American Academy of Neurology (AAN) and the European Federation of Neurological Societies (EFNS) is to start with drugs in patients with classic TN. Of the medicinal alternatives, first line is carbamazepine (CBZ) or oxcarbazepine (OXC) [32]. With first-line carbamazepine (CBZ), the response rate is expected to be in the range of 80–85%.

Dosing of carbamazepine is in the range of 200–1200 mg/day. With the passage of time, higher doses may be required as the effectiveness weans with time [33]. Toxicities of CBZ include drowsiness, nausea, dizziness, diplopia, ataxia, elevation of liver enzymes, hyponatremia along with more serious but uncommon morbidities of allergic rash, myelosuppression, hepatotoxicity, lymphadenopathy, systemic lupus erythematosus, Stevens-Johnson syndrome, and aplastic anemia. In the face of possible toxicities to CBZ, an alternative with a safer profile is oxcarbazepine (OXC) at a dose range of 600–1800 mg/day.

This is a keto-analogue of CBZ with a toxicity profile which is improved over that of CBZ, making OXC a practical alternative to CBZ [34].

Other classes of medications considered for first-line medicinal therapy include other antiepileptic drugs including gabapentin, and pregabalin. Muscle relaxants such as baclofen and clonazepam are alternatives to consider. Tricyclic antidepressants have also been shown in selected studies to be effective, these including amitriptyline and nortriptyline.

If ineffective control of TN is experienced with both CBZ and OXC or adverse effects become intolerable, alternative medicinal therapies which would be considered second line are lamotrigine and pimozide which are possibly effective in the control of TN [30]. Several other medical therapies have more limited data with less certain effectiveness including, phenytoin, tocainide, tizanidine, valproate, and botulinum toxin injections.

If a trial of medicinal therapy is attempted with failure of at least three drug trials [32] and persistent TN is documented or the toxicity profile of the agent under use is not tolerated by the subject, the patient should be considered for a number of surgical approaches to treatment according to the candidate's medical status, age, and/or preference. A surgical procedure may also be considered for those who have had a prior intervention which failed or those with recrudescence of pain after a prior successful surgery.

## Surgical Alternatives

Indeed, in assessing the long-term control of TN with medicinal therapy, eventually as many as 50% of TN patients will become refractory to drug therapy and require alterative therapeutic management to achieve pain relief [35]. Surgical interventions for TN are used to either relieve compression which results in aberrant nerve activity with resultant pain (nerve preserving) or destroy/ablate selective nerve fibers which mediate the pain (nerve damaging).

Whether one chooses a nerve preservation procedure or a surgery which leads to ablation of pain nerve fibers, each of the surgical interventions is clinically assessed for the degree of TN pain relief by an objective scale as formulated by the Barrow Neurological Institute (BNI) [36]. TN pain severity based on this scale is scored both before and serially after any procedure/treatment between levels I and V per the BNI pain intensity scoring criteria: I, no pain; II, occasional pain, not requiring medication; IIIa, no pain, continued medication; IIIb, some pain, controlled with medication; IV, some pain, not controlled with medication; and V, severe pain/no pain relief.

In the assessment of the effectiveness of any of the surgical interventions, the attainment of a BNI score of I, II, or IIIa–b is considered a treatment success, while a BNI score of IV or V after any of the procedural treatments is denoted a treatment failure.

## Microvascular Decompression

Microvascular decompression (MVD) is the only operative procedure which is nerve preserving but is the most invasive of the surgical procedures and highest risk requiring general anesthesia in order to perform a retrosigmoid craniotomy and microsurgical exploration of the posterior fossa for removal or separation of vascular structures, oftentimes an ectatic superior cerebellar artery, away from the trigeminal nerve [37]. Advances in endoscopic neurosurgical techniques have led to minimizing the MVD procedure with a smaller scalp incision, less muscle dissection, and smaller bony exposure, leading to less postoperative headaches at 1 month, with no loss of the effectiveness of the surgical MVD on pain relief of TN [38].

Although no randomized trials have ever been formally conducted to prospectively compare the various surgical interventions for TN, many series which have reported on the clinical results of MVD consistently reveal excellent pain relief in the range of 80% with complete resolution, while another 10% achieve partial relief. The time course is frequently complete response immediately after MVD with durable long-lasting resolution not only at 1-year (approximately 85% with good to excellent pain relief on low dose or no medication, respectively) but 10-year results of nearly 70% with good to excellent relief [39]. A recent systematic review of MVD has confirmed, in 26 publications with nearly 7000 TN patients so treated, a mean postoperative complete symptomatic pain relief with a success rate of 83.5% [40]. These clinical results from several published series documenting the effectiveness of MVD for TN are summarized and highlighted in Table 35.1 [41–49]. The complication rate of MVD has been low with incisional infection in 1.3%, facial palsy rate of 2.9%, facial numbness in 9.1%, hearing change noted in 1.9%, and a rare CSF leak in 1.6%.

**Table 35.1** Microvascular decompression (MVD) for TN

| Study | Time period | N (m:f) | Duration, mo | Age, y | Vessel(s) causing compression | Success rate pain-free (%) | Redo MVD | Follow-up mo |
|---|---|---|---|---|---|---|---|---|
| Broggi (2000) [41] | 1990–1998 | 146 (75:71) | 24 | 56 | A 51.4%, V 13.1%, A + V 35.6% | 85% | 4.7% | 38 |
| Lee (2000) [42] | 1988–1998 | 393 (64:329) | 84 | 15–80 | V | 81.3% | 26.2% | 12 |
| Kalkanis (2003) [43] | 1996–2000 | 1326 (NR) | NR | 57 | NR | NR | NR | NR |
| Revuelta-Gutierrez (2006) [44] | 1984–2004 | 668 (NR) | 7.6 | 33–77 | NR | NR | NR | NR |
| Sindou (2009) [45] | 1983–1999 | 330 (165:165) | 8.2 | 28–84 | SCA 77%, AICA 6%, SCA + AICA 17% | 80% | 3.1% | 98.4 |
| Bond (2010) [46] | 1994–2009 | 119 (61:58) | NR | 60 | SCA 61%, AICA 6%, SCA + AICA 17% | 90% | NR | 39.6 |
| Zhong (2012) [47] | 2002–2011 | 1274 (NR) | NR | 8–90 | SCA 41%, AICA 29%, V 35% PICA 9%, VA 6% | 88.3% | 3.6% | 36 |
| Sandel (2013) [48] | 1999–2009 | 243 (98:145) | 7.3 | 63.1 | SCA 41%, AICA 29%, V 35%, PICA 9%, VA 6% | 88.3% | 3.6% | 36 |
| Zhang (2013) [49] | 2001–2005 | 154 (NR) | NR | NR | A + V | 84% | NR | 67.2 |

*AICA* anterior inferior cerebral artery, *PICA* posterior inferior cerebellar artery, *VA* vertebral artery, *SCA* superior cerebellar artery, *BA* basilar artery, *V* this study only focused on vein, *N (M:F)* number (male: female), duration, history of symptoms (months), *A* artery, *V* vein, *redo MVD* reoperation, *M* average or range month, *y* average or range year, *NR* not reported

## Percutaneous Rhizotomies

For those patients with contraindications to surgery or prefer not to undergo a craniotomy for MVD, other surgical procedures directed at ablating selectively the nerve pain fibers are available.

These various ablative techniques include cutting or destroying the trigeminal nerve via rhizotomy which entails a number of percutaneous surgical procedures done by passing a cannula through the foramen ovale to access and allow lesioning of the trigeminal nerve ganglion or root using one of several alternatives. These include radio-frequency thermocoagulation rhizotomy (RFTR) which ablates the nerve fibers by heat, balloon compression (BC) which uses a Fogarty catheter to mechanically compress the Gasserian ganglion, and chemical rhizotomy with either alcohol or glycerol (GR) injected into the trigeminal cistern to cause ablation of the pain fibers [50]. The 2008 AAN/EFNS practice parameter identified and reported on the clinical results of these ablative procedures for TN. The analysis revealed that initial pain relief was seen in 90% of patients so treated with rapid resolution of the pain similar to the time course of relief attained with MVD, but the pain-free rates diminished by year 1 to 68–85%, by 3 years to 54–64%, and by year 5 to approximately 50% [30]. The major complication after any of the rhizotomy procedures is perioperative meningitis rarely in 0.2%. Dysesthesia variably described as a burning, heavy, or aching feeling is seen postoperatively in 12%. Longer-term morbidity includes localized sensory loss of the trigeminal distribution in nearly 50%, corneal numbness in 4%, and anesthesia dolorosa approximating 4% [30].

If a patient is determined to be refractory to medical therapy or has intolerable morbidity from the prescribed drugs, surgical procedures/options available are to be considered. If more invasive surgery such as MVD or rhizotomy does not provide pain relief, stereotactic radiosurgery (SRS) provides an alternative approach. Indeed, SRS is minimally invasive, being an ablative treatment using single-fraction high-dose radiation which has been proven to be effective and safe in the treatment of TN.

## Irradiation Approach

The irradiation approach to treating TN known as Stereotactic Radiosurgery (SRS) is performed with delivery of single-fraction radiation doses using various technologies such as the Gamma Knife, CyberKnife, and linear accelerators (linacs) converted with specialized hardware to deliver such stereotactic treatment.

Of the forms of SRS available for TN, the one that has had the most scientific investigations for documentation of accuracy, effectiveness, and safety is the Gamma Knife (GK).

In detailing the evolution of Gamma Knife in the treatment of TN, numerous observational studies have been published. Although to date no randomized phase III clinical trials have been undertaken to compare Gamma Knife Stereotactic Radiosurgery (GK SRS) with the other treatment modalities for TN, the many predominantly single-institutional experiences in the use of GK SRS provide important clinical data and insights of the utility of this modality for TN. This GK SRS data will be reviewed sequentially with the following clinical highlights in mind: (a) delineation of the effectiveness of GK SRS in TN in the short and long term; (b) assessment of the safety of surrounding eloquent neurological tissues to the doses required for pain relief of TN; (c) denotation of the important technical details of GK dose delivery, specifically, review of dose-response data for pain control, volume of trigeminal nerve treated, and importantly the appropriate target location site along the trigeminal nerve treated; (d) differentiation of any treatment modifications needed for treating a multiple sclerosis (MS) patient with TN compared to a patient without MS; (e) description of the utility of repeat treatment (done once or even twice) after the initial radiosurgical fraction if a patient fails to respond long-term to an initial GK treatment; (f) assessment retrospectively of existing clinical data which have undertaken comparative analyses of GK SRS with other modalities for TN as a surrogate for nonexistent phase III clinical trials comparing the various surgical modalities; (g) follow-up of patients after the GK SRS delivery of the prescription dose; and (h) description of the standard protocol used for the treatment of a TN patient with documented refractoriness to medicinal and/or other surgical forms of therapy.

## Effectiveness of SRS for TN

Patients worldwide have been treated for TN with GK SRS since the first two were treated by Dr. Lars Leksell in 1953 but not published until 1971 [51]. Selected single-institutional studies published since 1996 with long-term results of GK SRS in treatment of TN have demonstrated at 1 year between 47% and 90% pain relief as defined by BNI scores of I–IIIB (Table 35.2) [52–63]. For GK SRS, a minimum dose of 70 Gy has been found necessary for efficacy of pain control, this having been established in 1996 by a multicenter trial [64].

Maximal median doses delivered to the trigeminal nerve ranged from 80 to 90 Gy in a single fraction.

Each of these series has over 100 patients, and each demonstrates both the short- and long-term effectiveness, although the durability of pain relief at 5 years does fall off into the range of 44–65%.

Predictors of durable pain relief include the type of presenting pain with typical presentations responding better than atypical, the post-GK SRS BNI score, and whether or not there is post-GK SRS facial numbness [54]. One series performed a detailed analysis of a cohort of 149 patients treated for medicinally refractory TN finding that the strongest predictors of long-lasting pain relief were age ≥ 70 years and a post-GK treatment BNI pain intensity score of I or II compared to a BNI score of III (93% vs 38% at 3 years,

**Table 35.2**  Gamma Knife stereotactic radiosurgery (GK SRS) for TN

| Study | N | Median maximum dose (Gy) | Median follow-up (mo) | Pain-free (%) | Recurrence (%) | Median time to recurrence | Sensory dysfunction (%) |
|---|---|---|---|---|---|---|---|
| Regis et al. (2015) [52] | 497 | 85 | 43.8 | BNI1: 6 mo: 91.8 5y 64.9 | 34.4 | 24 | 14.5 |
| Lucas et al. (2014) [54] | 446 | 90 | 21.2 | BNI1–3B: 1y: 84.5 5y: 46.9 BNI1: 1y: 62.9 5y: 22.0 | 45.1 | 55.2 | 42.0 |
| Marshall et al. (2012) [55] | 448 | 88 (mean) | 20.9 | BN1–3B: 1y: ~75 5y: ~50 | 40.0 | 58.4 | 42.0 |
| Kondziolka et al. (2010) [53] | 503 | 80 | 24.0 | BNI1–3B: 1y: 80.0 5y: 46.0 | 42.9 | 48 | 10.5 |
| Baschnagel, et al. (2013) [56] | 149 | 80 | 27 | Initial relief: 92 1y: 76 2y: 69 3y: 60 | 32 | | 25 |
| Dhople et al. (2009) [57] | 112 | 70–80 | 5.6 | Initial relief: 81 1y: 60 3y: 41 5y: 34 | 28 | | 6 |
| Balamucki et al. (2006) [58] | 239 | >80 | 17 | Initial relief: 50 | 23 | | – |
| Sheehan et al. (2005) [59] | 151 | 70–80 | 19 | Initial relief: 44 1y: 47 3y: 34 | 24 | | 19 |
| Urgosik et al. (2005) [60] | 107 | 70–80 | 60 | Initial relief: 80 | 25 | | 20 |
| Pollock et al. (2002) [61] | 117 | 70–80 | 26 | Initial relief: 59 1y: 57 3y: 55 | 16 | | 25 |
| Maesawa et al. (2001) [62] | 220 | 70–80 | 24 | 1y: 63 3y: 57 | 14 | | 10 |
| Brisman et al. (2000) [63] | 172 | 70–80 | 6 and 12 | Initial relief: 90 | – | | – |

$p < 0.01$ [56]. Another factor predictive of durability of radiosurgical pain response includes GK SRS being the first procedure/treatment the TN patient has ever received (other than for the failed pharmaceutical therapeutics) with receipt of such treatment within 3 years of pain onset [65]. Of note, as opposed to the immediate pain relief obtained through a rhizotomy procedure or MVD, with GK SRS, there is a latency period before the pain relief is noted by the patient. On average, the median reported time which the majority of patients (89%) responded to the GK SRS was 1 month, with total pain relief achieved at a median of 5 months [53].

## SRS Treatment Morbidity and the Avoidance of Toxicity

The major morbidity of GK SRS for TN is that of resultant facial numbness related to the dose delivered to a portion of the adjacent brainstem. In assessing normal tissue dose tolerances to nearby surrounding neurological structures such as the brainstem, much of the dose-volume effects to eloquent tissues are well elaborated for standard dose-fractionation schemes. For example, legacy RTOG has introduced the dose tolerance limit for brainstem to be 60 Gy at maximum point (defined as a volume greater than 0.03 cc) for conventional fractionated radiation therapy. The Quantitative Analyses of Normal Tissue Effects in the Clinic (QUANTEC) report has concluded that the risk of brainstem complications increases markedly at doses greater than 64 Gy [66].

For stereotactic radiosurgery, few studies have been published on brainstem toxicity with clearly defined data. The limited published experience has been with single-fraction SRS treatment of vestibular schwannoma where a peripheral brainstem dose of <12.5 Gy has been associated with low (<5%) risk [66]. Higher-dose single-fraction data (15–20 Gy) can be found in SRS for brainstem metastases, but long-term results of neurological morbidity have been limited by the poor prognosis for long-term survival of such patients. Thus, based upon the low rate of brainstem neuropathy or necrosis for SRS treatment of vestibular schwannoma, QUANTEC has established <12.5 max dose to the brainstem for SRS treatment but states that future investigation(s) of detailed long-term experience/data of brainstem dose-volume and outcome data for such patients are needed.

There are currently no definitive criteria regarding more subtle dose-volume effects or effects after SRS for the high doses delivered in the treatment of TN except for one in-depth analysis emphasizing the dose-volume effect rather than single-point doses being delivered to the brainstem [67]. Gamma Knife radiosurgery of trigeminal neuralgia (TGN) treatment typically prescribes 75–90 Gy to 100%. A single isocenter with the 4-mm-diameter collimators without blocking is placed at the trigeminal nerve with typically the 12–20 Gy isodose line/volume just touching the brainstem. The brainstem may receive in extremely small volumes a dose anywhere between 20% and 50% of the prescribed maximal dose delivered to the trigeminal nerve. Indeed, the dose falloff is so steep that a dose of 44.5 Gy just at the periphery of the brainstem to a volume of 0.01 mm$^3$ (to the brainstem) would deliver a dose to a 10 mm$^3$ volume of brainstem of 11 Gy (acceptable to most treating GK SRS clinicians), this extremely rapid decrement in dose gradient occurring in a linear distance of between 2 and 3 mm [67].

Resultant mild to moderate facial numbness is seen after TN radiosurgery, but radionecrosis is rarely seen [67]. Scoring of this morbidity is likewise done with a BNI scale as follows: grade I, no facial numbness; grade II, mild facial numbness that is not bothersome; grade III, somewhat bothersome facial numbness; and grade IV, very bothersome facial [36]. The dose falloff is so steep and the delivery so accurate that brainstem volumes of 0.1–0.5 cm$^3$ receive lower planned and delivered doses compared with other radiation-related treatment delivery [67]. Such reported facial numbness reaches a maximal at 3 months in as many as 49% of patients, with the majority with BNI numbness scores of II–III [68]. The trend is that of decreasing incidence with time with the vast majority of patients often not finding the post-GK SRS numbness bothersome or disabling [52].

In essence, brainstem morbidity in the setting of TN treatment should be considered as a dose-volume effect, and not based upon a maximal single-point dose. Additionally, brainstem dose tolerance may be heterogeneous in that one region compared to another may have differing acute and late effects from a given dose and volume of in vivo tissue irradiated [67]. Thus, the delineation of one dose constraint for the entire brainstem may not reflect what differing partial volumes and regions the brainstem may tolerate in terms of radiation dose. Importantly, the continued acquisition of dose-volume-outcome data remains of paramount importance in settings such as GK SRS treatment of TN in order to further elucidate brainstem response to single-fraction SRS treatment regimens.

For practical purposes, when a maximal dose of 80 Gy is prescribed to the target trigeminal nerve, treatment planning is done such that the resultant brainstem dose-volume histogram reveals 1 mm$^3$ or less of the brainstem receives a dose of less than 15 Gy [Brainstem $_D$1 mm$^3$] and that 10 mm$^3$ or less receive a dose of less than 12 Gy [69]

## SRS Dose Prescription

In a recent retrospective analysis of dose response in the treatment of TN with GK SRS done at two institutions, 870 were treated typically using a single 4 mm isocenter localized at the dorsal root entry zone of the trigeminal nerve. The patients so treated were analyzed in three groups based upon the treatment doses: ≤82 Gy (352 patients), 83–86 Gy (85 patients), and ≥90 Gy (433 patients). The majority had typical TN (95%). Overall, the 4-year rate of good to excellent pain relief was 87%; stratified by treatment doses delivered, the 4-year rate of pain response was 79%, 82%, and 92% in patients treated to ≤82 Gy, 83–86 Gy, and ≥ 90 Gy, respectively. Consistent with these findings, those patients receiving ≤82 Gy had an increased risk of pain failure compared with ones treated to ≥90 Gy (hazard ratio 2.0, $P = 0.0007$) [70]. In terms of reported morbidity across the treatment-dose groups, facial numbness rates were similar among patients treated to doses ≥83 Gy [70]. The authors conclude that dose escalation in the GK SRS treatment of TN to >82 Gy is associated with an improvement in response as well as duration of pain relief.

Similarly, in a report of 130 patients who underwent radiosurgery for classical TN, all were treated with GK SRS to a median maximal dose of 85 Gy (range 70–90 Gy) with the 4-mm-diameter collimator helmet used. The isocenter was localized to a position in the anterior cisternal portion of the trigeminal nerve at a median distance of 8 mm (range = 4.9–14) anterior to the emergence of the trigeminal nerve. With all patients having follow-up of at least 7 years (median = 9.9, range = 7–14.5), a total of 122 patients (93.8%) attained pain-free status (median delay = 15 days) after the GK SRS (BNI score I–IIIa). The probability of remaining pain-free without requiring medication at 3, 5, 7, and 10 years was 77.9%, 73.8%, 68%, and 51.5%, respectively [71]. Indeed at 10 years, of the initial 130 patients, 67.7% were free of any recurrent pain requiring further new surgery (BNI class I–IIIa). The new-onset hypesthesia rate was 20.8% (median delay of onset = 12 months), and only one patient (0.8%) reported very bothersome hypesthesia.

## SRS Optimization of the Therapeutic Ratio

In an attempt to optimize the therapeutic ratio of achieving the optimal pain relief while minimizing treatment-induced neuropathy predominantly manifested by facial numbness, a proposed plan for personalized dose planning for TN has been investigated. Based upon the premise that the radiobiological effect of radiation is determined by the amount of energy delivered to the tissue (integral dose [ID] = mean dose × target volume) and is directly associated with the nerve volume, the authors studied retrospectively the trigeminal nerve volume treated as a function of the ID delivered.

In order to evaluate the effect of delivered ID on the outcome of TN radiosurgery, the investigators measured the postganglionic ID within the SRS target and retrospectively stratified patients into three groups: low (<1.4 mJ), medium (1.4–2.7 mJ), and high (>2.7 mJ) ID [with integral dose measured in mJ].

Clinical outcomes, which included pain status (scored using the BNI pain scale) and sensory dysfunction (scored using the BNI numbness scale), were evaluated at a median follow-up of 71 months.

Patients who were treated with a medium ID had superior pain relief either with or without medications ($p = 0.006$). In the medium ID group, the rates of complete pain relief without medications at 1, 3, and 6 years after SRS were 67%, 54%, and 33%, respectively, while the rates in the rest of the cohort were 55%, 36%, and 19%, respectively [72]. Patients given a high ID had a higher rate of post-SRS trigeminal sensory deterioration ($p < 0.0001$). At 1, 3, and 6 years after SRS, the high ID group had an estimated rate for developing sensory dysfunction of 35%, 45%, and 50%, respectively, while the rates in patients receiving low and medium IDs were 3%, 4%, and 9%, respectively. The optimal clinical outcome (maximum pain relief and minimal trigeminal sensory dysfunction) was obtained in patients who had received a medium ID. The authors conclude that with current dose selection methods, nerve volume affects long-term clinical outcomes in patients with TN who have undergone SRS. This study suggests that the prescribed SRS dose should be customized for each TN patient based on the nerve volume [72].

## Target Localization and Isocenter Placement

Placement of the GK SRS isocenter along the length of the trigeminal nerve for treatment of TN has varied across centers. The dorsal root entry zone (DREZ), a transition area on the trigeminal nerve from peripheral myelin to central myelin, has on a theoretical basis been considered to be more susceptible to radiation damage or vascular compression [14, 64]. But, clinical reports of isocenter placement vary from more anterior cisternal locations toward Meckel's cave to more posterior locales toward the DREZ. Variable results have been reported on the effectiveness of pain relief along with facial numbness based upon the isocenter target location [73]. In studies where dose has been kept relatively constant, generally in the range of 80 Gy (maximal dose), the target isocenter location is usually determined by the clinical

experience of the radiosurgical team members. With the general dictum that dose to brainstem will determine the risk of late treatment sequelae of facial numbness, the placement of the isocenter in the anterior cisternal portion of the nerve has led to a reported diminished rate of numbness as low as 10% at 1 year after the GK SRS treatment [74]. Figure 35.2 demonstrates two different isocenter placements along the trigeminal nerve, one more anterior toward Meckel's cave with the second posterior adjacent to the DREZ. Given the desire for the most optimal therapeutic ratio of pain relief while minimizing the risk of treatment-related sensory dysfunction, the variability of isocenter placement may become more standardized once the integral dose based upon nerve volume effect is more thoroughly investigated and understood, thus giving more objective parameters upon which to determine the optimal isocenter target location [72].

## SRS Target Delineation/Field Design

Another technical variable related to the isocenter which has been analyzed is the use of a single isocenter or that of two. The premise investigated was whether or not a longer length of nerve treated would lead to more effective pain control. In a prospective randomized fashion, GK SRS with one versus two isocenters was studied with the results showing no significant difference in the effectiveness of pain relief with use of two isocenters but a higher complication rate of sensory neuropathy [75].

## SRS for MS Patients

Patients with multiple sclerosis (MS)-related TN have been effectively treated with GK SRS. Reported response rates have ranged from 57% to 97% with long-term pain relief similar to that achieved with idiopathic or classic TN. In one of the largest reported series of MS-related TN with GK SRS delivered maximal doses between 70 and 90 Gy, response [with BNI scores I–IIIb] was seen at some point in 97.3% of patients. Over time, reported pain control was maintained in 82.6%, 73.9%, and 54.0% of patients after 1, 3, and 5 years, respectively [76]. In terms of complications from GK treatment, morbidity was low at a rate of 5.4% of non-disabling facial paresthesias.

## Repeat SRS Treatment for Recurrent TN After Initial GK SRS

A systemic review of repeat GK SRS for recurrent TN has been undertaken with the assessment that despite variable treatment techniques, doses, time intervals between the first and second single-fraction treatments, and differences in

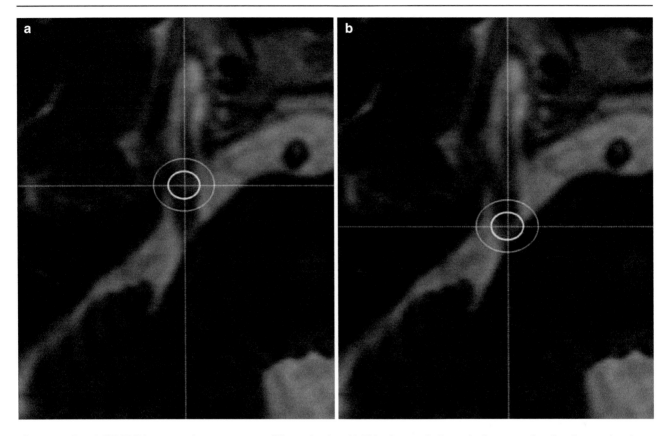

**Fig. 35.2** Virtual GK SRS isocenter placements at two different locales. (**a**) This pictograph shows the isocenter placed at the anterior cistern toward Meckel's cave (**b**) Pictograph denoting the posterior locale of the GK SRS isocenter toward the DREZ

selection criteria for the second SRS treatment, repeat irradiation is safe and effective however with the caveat of a substantial increase in the hypesthesia rate [77].

Specifically, with repeat radiosurgery, for achieving greater than 50% relief of initial pain, the median was 88% (range 60–100%); the median rate for new hypesthesia after repeat GKS was 33% (range 11–80%), considerably higher than that reported after first GK SRS (6–54%) [77]. The suggested alternative therapeutic approach due to this higher toxicity is for the consideration of other surgical approaches such as MVD as the first intention therapy for recurrent TN after first GK SRS.

If in the event that no other surgical alternative is available, then a second GK SRS would be evaluated and cautiously recommended.

If after a second GK SRS treatment the patient recurs with further TN and other treatment alternatives have been thoroughly assessed but deemed unsuitable as an option for the patient, a third GK SRS has been reported in a limited number of patients to be safe and effective with acceptable morbidity. The initial reported pain relief was seen in 94% of the cases with the latency of 2.9 months. At a mean follow-up of 22.9 months, 77% of patients have durable pain control with no reported further sensory loss in any of the cases undergoing the third GK SRS [78]. These findings suggest that third time GK SRS is a satisfactory option entailing low risk for patients

with medically and surgically refractory TN, especially those on chronic anticoagulation and/or antiplatelet therapy.

## Comparative Analysis of SRS vs Other Surgical Alternatives for TN

As no randomized controlled phase III trials have ever been done comparing the various surgical approaches for TN including that of any of the invasive procedures such as MVD or rhizotomy to that of the minimally invasive radiation-based GK SRS, retrospective comparative analyses have been done to demonstrate comparable effectiveness of the modalities. In analyzing the efficacy along with patient satisfaction of MVD and GK SRS for TN, in one clinical review, there were no significant differences in pain relief and patient satisfaction when the two modalities were compared [79]. However, two other reports affirm that MVD offers quicker, higher, and longer pain-free results compared with GK SRS, but the former has more morbidity associated with an open, invasive craniotomy including cerebrospinal fluid leak, cranial neuropathies, wound infection, deep vein thrombosis, and pulmonary embolism [80, 81].

Further, comparative studies have shown both rhizotomy and GK SRS to be effective treatments to achieve pain control (defined as BNI pain scale scores of I–IIIb) in TN, with rhizotomy resulting in faster onset of pain relief, while GK SRS achieved pain relief with a latency period of upward to a median of 6 months [82]. As well, there has been a trend toward a higher proportion of pain relief among patients who underwent GK SRS, but a higher rate of complications is reported with rhizotomy than GK SRS [83]. Compared with GK SRS data, limited long-term published data are available for both Cyberknife and linac-based SRS for TN. One representative cohort of patients treated with Cyberknife demonstrated initial pain relief in 67% with a median time to pain control of 14 days [84, 85]. Posttreatment numbness was seen in 47%. The use of higher doses of radiation and the treatment of a longer length of nerve led to both better pain relief but a higher hypesthesia rate. The presence of posttreatment numbness was predictive of better pain control. At a mean follow-up of 2 years, 50% of patients had durable pain relief without need for any pain medications. Two linac-based SRS for TN with published long-term results reveal a pattern of pain control and secondary hypesthesia similar to that of GK SRS for TN. One of the linac-based series using a BrainLAB Novalis device equipped with a commercially available 4 mm collimator treated 22 patients who underwent first-time treatment and 10 who were undergoing retreatment for recurrence of pain following various other surgically based treatments. The target for dose delivery was the most proximal segment of the cisternal portion of the trigeminal nerve which received 85–90 Gy administered in a 5- or 7-noncoplanar arc single-isocenter plan with the 4 mm circular collimator. In patients undergoing a second, repeat radiosurgery, the prescribed target dose was 60 Gy. Good to excellent results scored as BNI grade I, II, or III from a baseline of BNI of IV/V were achieved in 78% of patients. The median time to pain relief was 6 weeks.

Long-term results of pain relief were not reported at the 1- and 2-year mark. New-onset trigeminal dysfunction following treatment was seen in two patients [86]. In a second reported linac-based series, 179 patients were treated on a dedicated Novalis linac unit; of the treated patients, 169 had serial recorded pain scores. With doses ranging from 70 to 90 Gy maximal, the initial pain control was noted in 79.3%. Average time to relief was 1.92 months. Of those with essential TN, sustained pain control was seen in 93.9% at 12 months and 82.6% at 3 years. For all patients treated, pain recurrence was noted in 19.0% [87].

## Follow-Up of GK SRS for TN

Specific imaging follow-up will not typically be required unless the patient develops new apparently unrelated neurological symptoms. Patients should be followed at 2 weeks initially and then every 3–6 months for clinical assessments for 2 years and then every 1–3 years. At the time of follow-up, subjective and objective pain assessment need be obtained with a standardized measurement tool such as the

Barrow Neurological Institute (BNI) pain score scale, and any medication use or discontinuation, along with any toxicities, should be documented whenever possible. Trigeminal pain medications (in the absence of patient intolerance) should generally not be discontinued or tapered until the trigeminal pain is gone. The patient's clinical status should be documented and recorded at each outpatient visit.

## Stereotactic Radiosurgical Technique and Procedure for Treatment of TN

### Patient Selection/Indications for GK SRS Treatment

Patient selection for GK SRS treatment is based on a clinical diagnosis of TN with prior MRI imaging to assess for any vascular or other secondary compression of the trigeminal nerve. First-line therapy is that of medicinal treatments with the antiepileptics progressing onto second- and third-line drugs as needed. If the patient is refractory to medical management, the various surgical alternatives are presented to the patient. Indications for proceeding with GK SRS are when patients become refractory to maximal medical therapeutics and/or surgical management, medically not suitable for surgical intervention (such as on anticoagulation therapy) or personally choose GK SRS over other surgical modalities such as microvascular decompression (MVD) or rhizotomy when medical refractoriness is documented. MVD should be strongly considered in young patients. Young patients should be appropriately counseled regarding the durability of MVD vs Gamma Knife prior to proceeding with GK even in the setting of patient choice. Prior to treatment, the Barrow Neurological Institute (BNI) pain score as well as medications for trigeminal pain should be documented.

### Imaging Protocol for GK SRS Treatment

All patient GK SRS treatments begin with placement/fixation of a Leksell titanium stereotactic frame with local anesthesia at four pin insertion sites. A fiducial box specific to each imaging modality is placed on the frame and fitted to both the MRI and CT scan tables. A non-contrast CT scan and a contrast-enhanced MRI are obtained, the former to assure that there is no anatomical distortion with the MR imaging. An axial MP-RAGE (or equivalent) post-contrast sequence with 1-mm-thick slices and a T2-weighted high-resolution 3D gradient echo constructive interference in steady state (CISS) sequence are both acquired. For patients who are unable to undergo MRI scanning due to such contraindications as a pacemaker, metal within a critical body site, and the like, a CT cisternogram to define the trigeminal nerve is appropriate.

## GK SRS Treatment Planning

The Leksell GammaPlan, a 3D-based treatment planning system with multiview, is utilized by the treating radiation oncologist, neurosurgeon, and medical physicist to formulate an optimal treatment plan. The most common technique utilized is a single 4 mm isocenter along the long axis of the nerve. The utilization of a single or multiple isocenters as well as the location of the isocenter placement is based upon the preference of the treating clinicians. Typically, the isocenter is placed along the middle to anterior 1/3 of the nerve to deliver the prescribed dose to the target volume located between the root entry zone posteriorly and Meckel's cave anteriorly; dependent upon the experience and expertise of the treating clinician, more posterior placement of the isocenter toward the DREZ may be preferred.

The recommended dose in cases without a prior history of stereotactic radiosurgery to the trigeminal nerve is 40 Gy to the 50% isodose volume (80 Gy maximum dose). A maximum dose of 70 Gy appears to be the minimum effective dose for radiosurgery-naïve patients, but doses as high as 90 Gy maximum dose have been used. In assessing the dose-volume histograms on treatment plans for TN, the maximal dose to the DREZ is limited to between 20% and 50% of the prescription dose.

For repeat procedures/treatments (instances where there is an initial response to radiosurgery, but symptoms later recur), a dose of 30–35 Gy to the 50% isodose line (60–70 Gy maximum dose) should be considered. For retreatment cases the isocenter is ideally placed at a different location usually more anteriorly toward Meckel's cave in contradistinction to the original isocenter placement of the initial treatment.

## Illustrative TN Case Treated by GK SRS

A 67-year-old female presented in January of 2010 after a fall while getting up and hit her nose along the edge of a table. Since that time she has noted severe left-sided facial pain. She described the hemifacial pain as "stabbing and hot," lasting 15 min to an hour or so, occurring every 2–3 h. There were no specific triggers, but she did report that when she turned her head, sometimes this would trigger the pain. Her pain score was 8 of 10 to 10 of 10 occurring in the V2 distribution along the cheek and occasionally with pain of the left eye. CT of the head and the maxillofacial region indicated no evidence of fracture. With various medications, including Tegretol 100 mg BID, Neurontin, Lyrica, Trileptal, and Topamax, there was only partial alleviation of the pain, but she reported significant side effects, including anxiety and weight gain, especially with Lyrica. An MRI and MRA of the brain done in March 2010 indicated no enhancing

mass or vascular lesions at the CP angle cistern or of the left trigeminal nerve. The patient reported seeing an ENT surgeon, neurologist, and dentist, but none were able to control the pain. After nearly 1½ years, she was seen by the Anesthesia Pain Service in June 2011. Keppra was prescribed at 500 mg BID. Similar to the other medications, she reported significant anxiety and weight gain.

The *neurologic exam* revealed no focal lateralizing signs and no elicitable triggers of the left-sided facial pain. As she failed outpatient therapy with medications over an extended period of time, she was seen by a neurosurgeon in collaboration with a radiation oncologist along with a second neurologist and underwent GK SRS in late September of 2011. Upon arrival to the Gamma Knife Center, the patient was met by the GK SRS team and had placement of an IV line and received light sedation, as well as Decadron along with GI prophylaxis. The patient had placement of a Leksell stereotactic localization frame via local anesthesia under the guidance of the neurosurgical team. The patient then underwent MR as well as CT scan imaging for 3D target localization and GK 3D treatment planning. The images from both the MR and the CT scans were transferred to the GK treatment planning system. A single isocenter with the 4-mm-diameter collimators was placed along the middle third of the left trigeminal nerve; this delivered a prescribed dose of 40 Gy to the 50% isodose volume (max dose of 80 Gy) (Fig. 35.3). The conformality index was 2.37 with treatment volume of 0.096 cc. The mean dose to the brainstem was 1.3 Gy with a maximal brainstem dose of 20.1 Gy. The volume of brainstem receiving 8 Gy (V8) was 1%, while V5 was 2% and V3 of 8%.

Over the course of 1 month, the TN had decreased from a pre-GK SRS BNI score of IV down to IIIa with eventual slow taper of Keppra to a BNI score of II. However, recrudescence of the TN occurred in mid-June of 2012 with a BNI score of IV in the same left hemifacial distribution. GK retreatment was deemed appropriate. On retreatment with GK SRS in late July of 2012, the same imaging and treatment protocol was followed, but most remarkably the MR scan for the GK retreatment revealed *enhancement* of the middle third portion of the left trigeminal nerve identical to the location of the first GK SRS treatment target volume where a single-fraction dose of 40 Gy to the 50% isodose volume (80 Gy max dose) was delivered (Fig. 35.4). As this was retreatment, a dose reduction to 35 Gy prescribed to the 50% isodose volume (70 Gy max dose) was delivered to a locale anterior to the enhancement region seen on MRI with a single isocenter using the 4-mm-diameter collimators positioned anteriorly toward Meckel's cave (Fig. 35.5). The mean and maximal brainstem doses were 0.8 and 4.4 Gy, respectively. With the second treatment, she had substantial pain relief within 6 weeks of the repeat GK SRS, down to a BNI score of IIIa with eventual tapering of her prior chronic doses of Keppra. Figure 35.6 shows the

**Fig. 35.3** The 40 Gy isodose volume depicted from the first GK SRS treatment of the illustrative patient case with the isocenter of the 4-mm-diameter collimators placed at the midportion of the trigeminal nerve

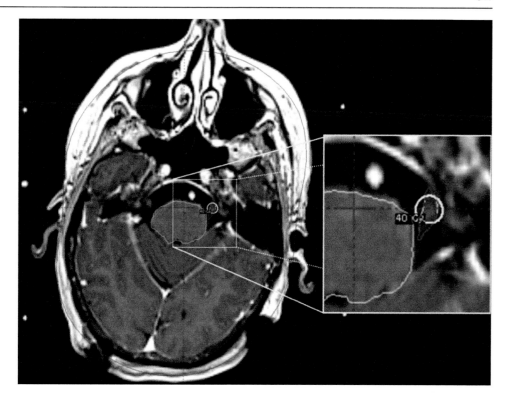

**Fig. 35.4** The planning MR scan of the illustrative case for the retreatment with GK SRS of the left trigeminal nerve. Note the enhancement in the midportion of the nerve corresponding to the exact location of the first GK SRS treatment target site

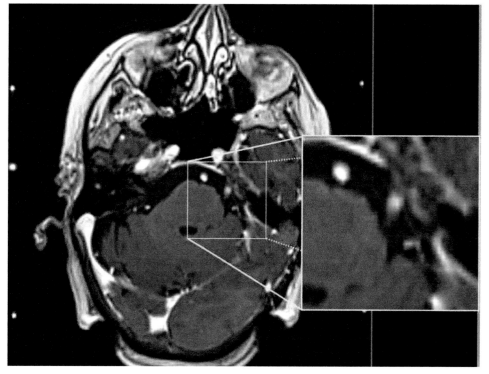

two GK SRS treatment isocenters overlayed on one treatment planning MR scan to demonstrate the geometric placement of the two different isocenters along the long axis of the left trigeminal nerve.

## Summary

- Trigeminal neuralgia (TN) is a syndrome featured by unilateral, paroxysmal, stabbing facial pain involving the fifth

**Fig. 35.5** Dose distribution of the 35 Gy isodose volume anterior to the enhancing target site of the first GK SRS dose delivery region along the left trigeminal nerve. This second isocenter with the 4-mm-diameter collimators was accurately placed and planned anteriorly toward Meckel's cave in order not to overlap geometrically as well as dosimetrically with the first GK treatment site

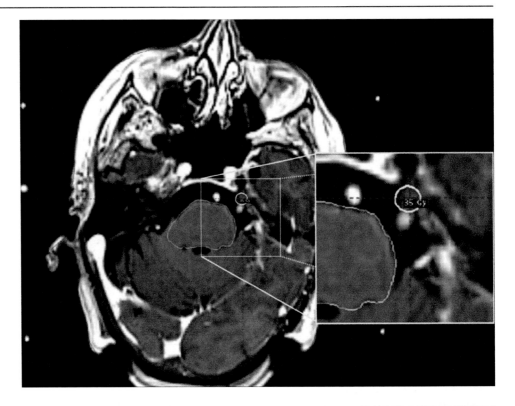

**Fig. 35.6** Composite GK SRS treatment plan of the first and second isodose distributions from the initial and retreatment isocenter placements with resultant first treatment 40 Gy isodose volume (blue) along with the second treatment 35 Gy isodose volume (yellow)

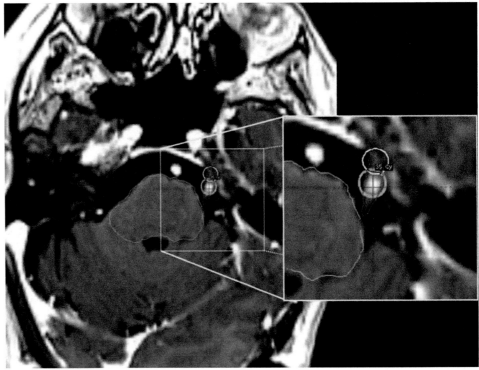

cranial or trigeminal nerve. Known also as tic douloureux which describes the contortions of the face due to the intensity of the pain, aggravating factors which may trigger the pain include a myriad of external stimuli including light touch of the face, cold air or wind, chewing, shaving, tooth brushing, face washing, talking, or smiling.

Therefore, in making the diagnosis, a detailed, meticulous history of symptoms associated with TN is paramount.

- TN is usually present with no apparent cause, that is, idiopathic or can be caused when the trigeminal nerve is being compressed by a vascular structure [either an artery or vein]. Neuroimaging is performed to exclude secondary causes such as tumors or plaques from multiple sclerosis.

- Therapeutically the standard paradigm of treatment begins with medicinal therapy. First-line pharmacological treatment is with carbamazepine which is considered the gold standard drug for TN. Alternatives include oxcarbazepine with other antiepileptics and muscle relaxants to be considered if response to carbamazepine is less than ideal. Most patients respond well to such medicinal therapeutics.

- If medications are no longer controlling the pain or are poorly tolerated, surgical alternatives are available. These include microvascular decompression (MVD) the most invasive of the surgical options due to the need for an operative craniotomy; less invasive percutaneous rhizotomies incorporating the use of alcohol, glycerol, or heat.

- For TN cases refractory to both medicinal therapy as well as surgical alternatives, radiation-based single-fraction Stereotactic Radiosurgery (SRS) is a treatment option to be considered. Such SRS is delivered most commonly with the Gamma Knife but also with linac-based systems or with the CyberKnife.

## Self-Assessment Questions

1. In a patient presenting with classic symptoms of an idiopathic case of trigeminal neuralgia (TN), aside from a careful history and physical exam, what diagnostic testing would be deemed as advisable in the diagnostic work-up of this patient [30]?
   A. An EEG to assess for seizure activity as the basis of the TN
   B. An urgent head CT scan to assess for any hemorrhagic lesion leading to the TN
   C. MRI scan of the brain to determine any vascular or neoplastic anomaly resulting in TN
   D. Widescreen blood work to include ANA, LE prep, and SCL antibody titers to assess for a rheumatic cause of TN
   E. Skull X-ray along with a C-spine film to ascertain any bony changes resulting in TN

2. In the pathophysiology of TN, the basic causation of TN is felt to be caused by which combination of factors [13]?
   A. Calcium channels, muscle depolarization, elevated aldolase levels
   B. Sodium potassium pump, elevated creatine kinase levels, musculature fibrillations
   C. Migraine variant, EEG spikes, elevated magnesium levels
   D. ANA positive, sed rate elevation, antismooth muscle antibodies
   E. Sodium channels, demyelination, nerve microstructural changes

3. First-line treatment of idiopathic TN consists of which of the following therapeutic interventions [32]?
   A. Immediate surgery with transection of the involved trigeminal nerve
   B. Glycerol rhizotomy followed by thermocoagulation
   C. Medicinal therapy with carbamazepine
   D. Endoscopically directed microvascular decompression
   E. Single-fraction Gamma Knife SRS to a dose maximal of 80 Gy

4. For Gamma Knife SRS, the acceptable dose constraint to the adjacent brainstem while an appropriate maximal dose of 80 Gy is prescribed to trigeminal nerve for TN is which of the following [69]?
   A. The same as the prescribed dose of 80 Gy maximal
   B. 30 Gy or less to 10 mm³ of the brainstem
   C. A point dose of 40 Gy to the surface of the brainstem
   D. 12 Gy or less to 10 mm³ of the brainstem
   E. 15 Gy median dose to the entire contoured brainstem

5. In GK treatment planning for a TN case refractory to medicinal therapy, what combination of isocenter collimator diameter and isocenter placement is most ideal for optimal control of the TN pain while minimizing the risk of causing secondary facial numbness [72]?
   A. Isocenter with the 8-mm-diameter collimators placed at the root entry zone
   B. Isocenter with the 4-mm-diameter collimators localized at the cavernous sinus
   C. Isocenter with the 8-mm-diameter collimators placed at the foramen ovale
   D. Isocenter with the 4-mm plus the 8-mm-diameter collimators localized at the Gasserian ganglion
   E. Isocenter with the 4-mm-diameter collimators placed at the midportion of the trigeminal nerve midway between the root entry zone and Meckel's cave

## Answers

1. C
2. E
3. C
4. D
5. E

**Acknowledgments** The author extends sincere appreciation to the GK physicist Ann Maitz, MS, for the acquisition of GK treatment plan/dose-volume histogram data for the illustrative case presentation; 3D imaging expert Kenneth A. Richey, BSRT, R, CT, MR, for his design/formulation of the MR images for the figures; resident Leonid Zamdborg, MD, for his unending technical software support; and, last but not least, secretary Ann Karmo for her clerical skills in the details of manuscript style/publication guidelines.

# References

1. Fothergill J. Of a painful affection of the face. In: Anonymous medical observations and inquiries by a Society of Physicians in London, London, 1776. p. 129–142.
2. Cruccu G, Finnerup NB, Jensen TS, et al. Trigeminal neuralgia: new classification and diagnostic grading for practice and research. Neurology. 2016;87:220–8.
3. Katusic S, Williams DB, Beard CM, et al. Epidemiology and clinical features of idiopathic trigeminal neuralgia and glossopharyngeal neuralgia: similarities and differences, Rochester, Minnesota, 1945–1984. Neuroepidemiology. 1991;10:276–81.
4. Maarbjerg S, Gozalov A, Olesen J, et al. Trigeminal neuralgia—a prospective systematic study of clinical characteristics in 158 patients. Headache. 2014;54:1574–82.
5. Childs AM, Meaney JF, Ferrie CD, et al. Neurovascular compression of the trigeminal and glossopharyngeal nerve: three case reports. Arch Dis Child. 2000;82:311–5.
6. Fleetwood IG, Innes AM, Hansen SR, et al. Familial trigeminal neuralgia. Case report and review of the literature. J Neurosurg. 2001;95:513–7.
7. Pan SL, Yen MF, Chiu YH, et al. Increased risk of trigeminal neuralgia after hypertension: a population-based study. Neurology. 2011;77:1605–10.
8. Teruel A, Ram S, Kumar SK, et al. Prevalence of hypertension in patients with trigeminal neuralgia. J Headache Pain. 2009;10:199–201.
9. Lin KH, Chen YT, Fuh JL, et al. Increased risk of trigeminal neuralgia in patients with migraine: a nationwide population-based study. Cephalalgia. 2016;36(13):1218–27.
10. O'Connor AB, Schwid SR, Herrmann DN, et al. Pain associated with multiple sclerosis: systematic review and proposed classification. Pain. 2008;137:96–111.
11. Truini A, Barbanti P, Pozzilli C, et al. A mechanism-based classification of pain in multiple sclerosis. J Neurol. 2013;260:351–67.
12. Seeburg DP, Northcutt B, Aygun N, et al. The role of imaging for trigeminal neuralgia: a segmental approach to high-resolution MRI. Neurosurg Clin N Am. 2016;27:315–26.
13. Siqueira SR, Alves B, Malpartida HM, et al. Abnormal expression of voltage-gated sodium channels Nav1.7, Nav1.3 and Nav1.8 in trigeminal neuralgia. Neuroscience. 2009;164:573–7.
14. Love S, Coakham HB. Trigeminal neuralgia: pathology and pathogenesis. Brain. 2001;124:2347–60.
15. Hamlyn PJ. Neurovascular relationships in the posterior cranial fossa, with special reference to trigeminal neuralgia. 2. Neurovascular compression of the trigeminal nerve in cadaveric controls and patients with trigeminal neuralgia: quantification and influence of method. Clin Anat. 1997;10:380–8.
16. Cheng TM, Cascino TL, Onofrio BM. Comprehensive study of diagnosis and treatment of trigeminal neuralgia secondary to tumors. Neurology. 1993;43:2298–302.
17. Linskey ME, Jho HD, Jannetta PJ. Microvascular decompression for trigeminal neuralgia caused by vertebrobasilar compression. J Neurosurg. 1994;81:1–9.
18. Ildan F, Gocer AI, Bagdatoglu H, et al. Isolated trigeminal neuralgia secondary to distal anterior inferior cerebellar artery aneurysm. Neurosurg Rev. 1996;19:43–6.
19. Figueiredo PC, Brock M, De Oliveira AMJ, et al. Arteriovenous malformation in the cerebellopontine angle presenting as trigeminal neuralgia. Arq Neuropsiquiatr. 1989;47:61–71.
20. Mohanty A, Venkatrama SK, Rao BR, et al. Experience with cerebellopontine angle epidermoids. Neurosurgery. 1997;40:24–9. discussion 29–30
21. Rappaport ZH, Govrin-Lippmann R, Devor M. An electron-microscopic analysis of biopsy samples of the trigeminal root taken during microvascular decompressive surgery. Stereotact Funct Neurosurg. 1997;68:182–6.
22. Lutz J, Thon N, Stahl R, et al. Microstructural alterations in trigeminal neuralgia determined by diffusion tensor imaging are independent of symptom duration, severity, and type of neurovascular conflict. J Neurosurg. 2016;124:823–30.
23. Obermann M, Yoon MS, Ese D, et al. Impaired trigeminal nociceptive processing in patients with trigeminal neuralgia. Neurology. 2007;69:835–41.
24. Gass A, Kitchen N, MacManus DG, et al. Trigeminal neuralgia in patients with multiple sclerosis: lesion localization with magnetic resonance imaging. Neurology. 1997;49:1142–4.
25. Truini A, Prosperini L, Calistri V, et al. A dual concurrent mechanism explains trigeminal neuralgia in patients with multiple sclerosis. Neurology. 2016;86:2094–9.
26. Meaney JF, Watt JW, Eldridge PR, et al. Association between trigeminal neuralgia and multiple sclerosis: role of magnetic resonance imaging. J Neurol Neurosurg Psychiatry. 1995;59:253–9.
27. Headache Classification Committee of the International Headache Society (IHS). The international classification of headache disorders, 3rd edition (beta version). Cephalalgia. 2013;33:629–808.
28. Eller JL, Raslan AM, Burchiel KJ. Trigeminal neuralgia: definition and classification. Neurosurg Focus. 2005;18:E3.
29. Cruccu G, Gronseth G, Alksne J, et al. AAN-EFNS guidelines on trigeminal neuralgia management. Eur J Neurol. 2008;15:1013–28.
30. Gronseth G, Cruccu G, Alksne J, et al. Practice parameter: the diagnostic evaluation and treatment of trigeminal neuralgia (an evidence-based review): report of the Quality Standards Subcommittee of the American Academy of Neurology and the European Federation of Neurological Societies. Neurology. 2008;71:1183–90.
31. Wiffen PJ, Derry S, Moore RA, et al. Carbamazepine for acute and chronic pain in adults. Cochrane Database Syst Rev. 2011;(1):CD005451. https://doi.org/10.1002/14651858.CD005451.pub2.
32. Al-Quliti KW. Update on neuropathic pain treatment for trigeminal neuralgia. The pharmacological and surgical options. Neurosciences (Riyadh). 2015;20:107–14.
33. Campbell FG, Graham JG, Zilkha KJ. Clinical trial of carbazepine (tegretol) in trigeminal neuralgia. J Neurol Neurosurg Psychiatry. 1966;29:265–7.
34. Martinez W, Ingenito A, Blakeslee M, et al. Efficacy, safety, and tolerability of oxcarbazepine monotherapy. Epilepsy Behav. 2006;9:448–56.
35. Katusic S, Beard CM, Bergstralh E, et al. Incidence and clinical features of trigeminal neuralgia, Rochester, Minnesota, 1945–1984. Ann Neurol. 1990;27:89–95.
36. Rogers CL, Shetter AG, Fiedler JA, et al. Gamma knife radiosurgery for trigeminal neuralgia: the initial experience of The Barrow Neurological Institute. Int J Radiat Oncol Biol Phys. 2000;47:1013–9.
37. Jannetta PJ. Microsurgical management of trigeminal neuralgia. Arch Neurol. 1985;42:800.
38. Lee JY, Pierce JT, Sandhu SK, et al. Endoscopic versus microscopic microvascular decompression for trigeminal neuralgia: equivalent pain outcomes with possibly decreased postoperative headache after endoscopic surgery. J Neurosurg. 2016;126(5):1676–84.

39. Barker FG 2nd, Jannetta PJ, Bissonette DJ, et al. The long-term outcome of microvascular decompression for trigeminal neuralgia. N Engl J Med. 1996;334:1077–83.

40. Xia L, Zhong J, Zhu J, et al. Effectiveness and safety of microvascular decompression surgery for treatment of trigeminal neuralgia: a systematic review. J Craniofac Surg. 2014;25:1413–7.

41. Broggi G, Ferroli P, Franzini A, et al. Microvascular decompression for trigeminal neuralgia: comments on a series of 250 cases, including 10 patients with multiple sclerosis. J Neurol Neurosurg Psychiatry. 2000;68:59–64.

42. Lee SH, Levy EI, Scarrow AM, et al. Recurrent trigeminal neuralgia attributable to veins after microvascular decompression. Neurosurgery. 2000;46:356–61. discussion 361–2

43. Kalkanis SN, Eskandar EN, Carter BS, et al. Microvascular decompression surgery in the United States, 1996 to 2000: mortality rates, morbidity rates, and the effects of hospital and surgeon volumes. Neurosurgery. 2003;52:1251–61. discussion 1261–2

44. Revuelta-Gutierrez R, Lopez-Gonzalez MA, Soto-Hernandez JL. Surgical treatment of trigeminal neuralgia without vascular compression: 20 years of experience. Surg Neurol. 2006;66:32–6. discussion 36

45. Sindou M, Leston JM, Le Guerinel C, et al. Treatment of trigeminal neuralgia with microvascular decompression. Neurochirurgie. 2009;55:185–96.

46. Bond AE, Zada G, Gonzalez AA, et al. Operative strategies for minimizing hearing loss and other major complications associated with microvascular decompression for trigeminal neuralgia. World Neurosurg. 2010;74:172–7.

47. Zhong J, Li ST, Zhu J, et al. A clinical analysis on microvascular decompression surgery in a series of 3000 cases. Clin Neurol Neurosurg. 2012;114:846–51.

48. Sandel T, Eide PK. Long-term results of microvascular decompression for trigeminal neuralgia and hemifacial spasms according to preoperative symptomatology. Acta Neurochir. 2013;155:1681–92. discussion 1692

49. Zhang H, Lei D, You C, et al. The long-term outcome predictors of pure microvascular decompression for primary trigeminal neuralgia. World Neurosurg. 2013;79:756–62.

50. Lopez BC, Hamlyn PJ, Zakrzewska JM. Systematic review of ablative neurosurgical techniques for the treatment of trigeminal neuralgia. Neurosurgery. 2004;54:973–82. discussion 982–3

51. Leksell L. Sterotaxic radiosurgery in trigeminal neuralgia. Acta Chir Scand. 1971;137:311–4.

52. Regis J, Tuleasca C, Resseguier N, et al. Long-term safety and efficacy of Gamma Knife surgery in classical trigeminal neuralgia: a 497-patient historical cohort study. J Neurosurg. 2016;124:1079–87.

53. Kondziolka D, Zorro O, Lobato-Polo J, et al. Gamma Knife stereotactic radiosurgery for idiopathic trigeminal neuralgia. J Neurosurg. 2010;112:758–65.

54. Lucas JT Jr, Nida AM, Isom S, et al. Predictive nomogram for the durability of pain relief from gamma knife radiation surgery in the treatment of trigeminal neuralgia. Int J Radiat Oncol Biol Phys. 2014;89:120–6.

55. Marshall K, Chan MD, McCoy TP, et al. Predictive variables for the successful treatment of trigeminal neuralgia with gamma knife radiosurgery. Neurosurgery. 2012;70:566–72. discussion 572–3

56. Baschnagel AM, Cartier JL, Dreyer J, et al. Trigeminal neuralgia pain relief after gamma knife stereotactic radiosurgery. Clin Neurol Neurosurg. 2014;117:107–11.

57. Dhople AA, Adams JR, Maggio WW, et al. Long-term outcomes of Gamma Knife radiosurgery for classic trigeminal neuralgia: implications of treatment and critical review of the literature. Clinical article. J Neurosurg. 2009;111:351–8.

58. Balamucki CJ, Stieber VW, Ellis TL, et al. Does dose rate affect efficacy? The outcomes of 256 gamma knife surgery procedures for trigeminal neuralgia and other types of facial pain as they relate to the half-life of cobalt. J Neurosurg. 2006;105:730–5.

59. Sheehan J, Pan HC, Stroila M, et al. Gamma knife surgery for trigeminal neuralgia: outcomes and prognostic factors. J Neurosurg. 2005;102:434–41.

60. Urgosik D, Liscak R, Novotny J Jr, et al. Treatment of essential trigeminal neuralgia with gamma knife surgery. J Neurosurg. 2005;102(Suppl):29–33.

61. Pollock BE, Phuong LK, Gorman DA, et al. Stereotactic radiosurgery for idiopathic trigeminal neuralgia. J Neurosurg. 2002;97:347–53.

62. Maesawa S, Salame C, Flickinger JC, et al. Clinical outcomes after stereotactic radiosurgery for idiopathic trigeminal neuralgia. J Neurosurg. 2001;94:14–20.

63. Brisman R. Gamma knife radiosurgery for primary management for trigeminal neuralgia. J Neurosurg. 2000;93(Suppl 3):159–61.

64. Kondziolka D, Lunsford LD, Flickinger JC, et al. Stereotactic radiosurgery for trigeminal neuralgia: a multiinstitutional study using the gamma unit. J Neurosurg. 1996;84:940–5.

65. Mousavi SH, Niranjan A, Huang MJ, et al. Early radiosurgery provides superior pain relief for trigeminal neuralgia patients. Neurology. 2015;85:2159–65.

66. Mayo C, Yorke E, Merchant TE. Radiation associated brainstem injury. Int J Radiat Oncol Biol Phys. 2010;76:S36–41.

67. Xue J, Goldman HW, Grimm J, et al. Dose-volume effects on brainstem dose tolerance in radiosurgery. J Neurosurg. 2012;117(Suppl):189–96.

68. Matsuda S, Nagano O, Serizawa T, et al. Trigeminal nerve dysfunction after Gamma Knife surgery for trigeminal neuralgia: a detailed analysis. J Neurosurg. 2010;113(Suppl):184–90.

69. Massager N, Lorenzoni J, Devriendt D, et al. Gamma knife surgery for idiopathic trigeminal neuralgia performed using a far-anterior cisternal target and a high dose of radiation. J Neurosurg. 2004;100:597–605.

70. Kotecha R, Kotecha R, Modugula S, et al. Trigeminal neuralgia treated with stereotactic radiosurgery: the effect of dose escalation on pain control and treatment outcomes. Int J Radiat Oncol Biol Phys. 2016;96:142–8.

71. Regis J, Tuleasca C, Resseguier N, et al. The very long-term outcome of radiosurgery for classical trigeminal neuralgia. Stereotact Funct Neurosurg. 2016;94:24–32.

72. Mousavi SH, Niranjan A, Akpinar B, et al. A proposed plan for personalized radiosurgery in patients with trigeminal neuralgia. J Neurosurg. 2017;128(2):452–9.

73. Xu Z, Schlesinger D, Moldovan K, et al. Impact of target location on the response of trigeminal neuralgia to stereotactic radiosurgery. J Neurosurg. 2014;120:716–24.

74. Regis J, Metellus P, Hayashi M, et al. Prospective controlled trial of gamma knife surgery for essential trigeminal neuralgia. J Neurosurg. 2006;104:913–24.

75. Flickinger JC, Pollock BE, Kondziolka D, et al. Does increased nerve length within the treatment volume improve trigeminal neuralgia radiosurgery? A prospective double-blind, randomized study. Int J Radiat Oncol Biol Phys. 2001;51:449–54.

76. Zorro O, Lobato-Polo J, Kano H, et al. Gamma knife radiosurgery for multiple sclerosis-related trigeminal neuralgia. Neurology. 2009;73:1149–54.

77. Tuleasca C, Carron R, Resseguier N, et al. Repeat Gamma Knife surgery for recurrent trigeminal neuralgia: long-term outcomes and systematic review. J Neurosurg. 2014;121(Suppl):210–21.

78. Tempel ZJ, Chivukula S, Monaco EA 3rd, et al. The results of a third Gamma Knife procedure for recurrent trigeminal neuralgia. J Neurosurg. 2015;122:169–79.

79. Nanda A, Javalkar V, Zhang S, et al. Long term efficacy and patient satisfaction of microvascular decompression and gamma

knife radiosurgery for trigeminal neuralgia. J Clin Neurosci. 2015;22:818–22.

80. Brisman R. Microvascular decompression vs. gamma knife radiosurgery for typical trigeminal neuralgia: preliminary findings. Stereotact Funct Neurosurg. 2007;85:94–8.

81. Pollock BE, Schoeberl KA. Prospective comparison of posterior fossa exploration and stereotactic radiosurgery dorsal root entry zone target as primary surgery for patients with idiopathic trigeminal neuralgia. Neurosurgery. 2010;67:633–8. discussion 638–9

82. Mathieu D, Effendi K, Blanchard J, et al. Comparative study of Gamma Knife surgery and percutaneous retrogasserian glycerol rhizotomy for trigeminal neuralgia in patients with multiple sclerosis. J Neurosurg. 2012;117(Suppl):175–80.

83. Henson CF, Goldman HW, Rosenwasser RH, et al. Glycerol rhizotomy versus gamma knife radiosurgery for the treatment of tri-geminal neuralgia: an analysis of patients treated at one institution. Int J Radiat Oncol Biol Phys. 2005;63:82–90.

84. Fariselli L, Marras C, De Santis M, et al. Cyberknife radiosurgery as a first treatment for idiopathic trigeminal neuralgia. Neurosurgery. 2009;64:A96–A101.

85. Villavicencio AT, Lim M, Burneikiene S, et al. Cyberknife radiosurgery for trigeminal neuralgia treatment: a preliminary multicenter experience. Neurosurgery. 2008;62:647–55. discussion 647–55

86. Chen JC, Girvigian M, Greathouse H, et al. Treatment of trigeminal neuralgia with linear accelerator radiosurgery: initial results. J Neurosurg. 2004;101(Suppl 3):346–50.

87. Smith ZA, Gorgulho AA, Bezrukiy N, et al. Dedicated linear accelerator radiosurgery for trigeminal neuralgia: a single-center experience in 179 patients with varied dose prescriptions and treatment plans. Int J Radiat Oncol Biol Phys. 2011;81:225–31.

**Part XIV**

**Radiation Associated Complications**

# Brain Radionecrosis

Caroline Chung and Timothy J. Kaufmann

## Abbreviations

| | |
|---|---|
| AUC | Area under the curve |
| AVM | Arteriovenous malformation |
| CBV | Cerebral blood volume |
| CFT | Category fluency test |
| Cho | Choline |
| CMMSE | Cantonese version of the Mini-Mental Status Examination |
| Cr | Creatine |
| DCE | Dynamic contrast-enhanced |
| DSC | Dynamic susceptibility-weighted contrast-enhanced |
| DWI | Diffusion-weighted imaging |
| EANO | European Association of Neuro-Oncology |
| FDG | Fluorodeoxyglucose |
| FLAIR | Fluid-attenuated inversion recovery |
| HBOT | Hyperbaric oxygen therapy |
| HIF-1α | Hypoxia-inducible factor-1 alpha |
| HKLLT | Hong Kong List Learning Test |
| HR-QOL | Health-related quality of life |
| IMRT | Intensity-modulated radiotherapy |
| KPS | Karnofsky Performance Status |
| Lac | Lactate |
| LENT-SOMA | Late Effects Normal Tissue Task Force-Subjective, Objective, Management, Analytic |
| Lip | Lipid |
| LITT | Laser interstitial thermal therapy |
| MDASI-BT | MD Anderson Symptom Inventory for brain tumor |
| MRS | MR spectroscopy |
| NAA | N-Acetylasparate |
| PSR | Percent signal recovery |
| PTX | Pentoxifylline |
| RANO | Response Assessment in Neuro-Oncology Criteria |
| rCBV | Relative cerebral blood volume |
| ROC | Receiver operating characteristic |
| ROIs | Regions of interest |
| SRS | Stereotactic radiosurgery |
| VEGF | Vascular endothelial growth factor |
| WMS-III VR | Visual Reproduction subtest of the Wechsler Memory Scale-III |

## Learning Objectives

- To learn the typical clinical presentation of brain radionecrosis.
- To understand the diagnostic tests that can be done to help with diagnosis of brain radionecrosis while recognizing their limitations.
- To understand the proposed pathophysiological mechanism associated with the development of brain radionecrosis.
- To review the management options for symptomatic brain radionecrosis and supporting data, including the typical first-line treatment and potentially promising treatment that are under investigation.

## Incidence

Brain radionecrosis (tissue death caused by radiation) is a complication that may follow radiotherapy to all or part of the brain [1, 2]. It is most commonly observed following radiosurgery treatments to the brain or high-dose fractionated radiotherapy treatments for primary or secondary brain tumors. Brain radionecrosis can also develop following high-

C. Chung (✉)
Department of Radiation Oncology, University of Texas MD Anderson Cancer Center, Houston, TX, USA
e-mail: cchung3@mdanderson.org

T. J. Kaufmann
Department of Radiology, Mayo Clinic, Rochester, MN, USA

© Springer International Publishing AG, part of Springer Nature 2018
E. L. Chang et al. (eds.), *Adult CNS Radiation Oncology*, https://doi.org/10.1007/978-3-319-42878-9_36

dose radiation targeted to non-CNS tumors that are in close approximation to brain tissue, such as nasopharyngeal carcinoma.

The incidence of brain radionecrosis is rising as a result of the growing use of stereotactic radiosurgery, administration of higher doses of radiation during initial therapy, and increasing use of salvage radiation therapy for brain and head and neck cancers, which results in higher cumulative radiation doses over the course of a patient's care. The overall risk of radionecrosis following fractionated radiotherapy to the brain or head and neck area is not well estimated in the current era of intensity-modulated radiotherapy (IMRT). With more conformal radiation delivery techniques, the patterns and distribution of brain radionecrosis appear to be more focal than previously observed [3]. Stereotactic radiosurgery is a highly precise radiation treatment that is delivered over only one to five fractions (treatment sessions). Following single-fraction brain radiosurgery, the risk of radionecrosis has been estimated at about 10% at 1 year, but the incidence appears to rise with longer follow-up or with additional radiation treatments in the same region [1, 4, 5].

Studies report the incidence of radionecrosis to range from 2% to 40% depending on the dose utilized, volume of the target lesion, and duration of follow-up after radiosurgery [1, 4–11]. Typically, radionecrosis presents between 6 and 24 months following single-fraction radiosurgery [1, 4–11].

## Presentation and Symptoms

### Diagnosis

To date, the diagnosis of brain radionecrosis has largely been clinical, based on clinical and radiological presentation. The clinical presentation is dependent on the region of the brain that is affected by radionecrosis. For example, radionecrosis affecting the motor strip can present with unilateral weakness of an upper and/or lower extremity, whereas radionecrosis within the occipital lobe may present with visual symptoms. Head and neck cancer patients tend to develop radionecrosis in the temporal lobes and present with deterioration in short-term memory and emotional lability. A subset of patients can develop significant rapid neurological deterioration and rarely can even cause death in some cases. When patients are suspected to have brain radionecrosis clinically, various radiological investigations are used to help confirm this diagnosis, and these are reviewed in the subsequent section ("Radiographic Findings").

Although pathological diagnosis is considered the "gold standard" for diagnosis of tumor in most oncologic situations, biopsy of these lesions has failed to have 100% sensitivity or specificity due to sampling error and histological ambiguity related to the common presence of both tumor cells (which may or may not be viable) and necrosis. Further

description of the pathological findings is provided in the section, "Pathological Findings." As biopsy is an invasive procedure with imperfect diagnostic capabilities, efforts have been made to improve the noninvasive diagnostic approaches using various imaging techniques. This includes the use of qualitative and quantitative measures from conventional magnetic resonance imaging (MRI) and use of perfusion and diffusion MRI, MR spectroscopy, positron emission tomography (PET), and diffusion-weighted imaging. However, each of these imaging modalities has its particular limitations and yields imperfect accuracy in the diagnosis of radiation necrosis vs. viable tumor. The majority of studies which have evaluated these imaging techniques in this setting have also suffered from substantial methodological limitations, such as retrospective design, relatively small subject numbers, and a tarnished reference standard for lesion pathology (e.g., imaging studies themselves, the clinical course, stereotactic biopsy with its inherent sampling limitations, admixture of viable tumor and radiation necrosis, and ambiguous histopathology). Therefore, many have suggested that the best sensitivity and specificity can be achieved by using a combination of these imaging measures in the diagnosis of brain radionecrosis [12–15].

## Radiographic Findings

### Conventional MRI

Conventional or structural MRI, including T1-weighted, T2-weighted, and post-gadolinium T1-weighted imaging, is necessary in following brain tumors and assessing for changes in lesion size and mass effect. However, following relatively high-dose radiation, both radiation-related injury including necrosis and viable, recurrent tumor may present as an enhancing necrotic mass with surrounding edema at conventional MRI.

As radiation therapy induces injury to other cell types than neoplastic, such as endothelial cells and oligodendrocytes, it is expected that effects on those cells may be seen at imaging, such as increased interstitial or vasogenic edema and extravascular, extracellular leakage of IV gadolinium (enhancement). The time course after radiation does affect imaging findings and histopathology, as tissue injury evolves [16]. In high-grade gliomas, the differentiation of pseudoprogression and radiation necrosis is an important and difficult topic which has been much discussed elsewhere and is beyond the scope of this chapter, though both entities could be considered radiation-induced changes, perhaps on a spectrum [16]. Suffice it to say, pseudoprogression in gliomas is most common in the first 3 months after the end of radiotherapy [17], and radiation necrosis is more common thereafter, though there is overlap. In stereotactic radiosurgery (SRS)-treated metastases, it has been shown that 54% of patients have one or more of their lesions increase in size following SRS [18], and many of these lesions will ultimately represent radiation necrosis.

The post-contrast MR appearances of "cut green pepper" and "soap bubble" have previously been used to suggest radiation necrosis rather than viable tumor, but enhancement patterns or morphologic features like these have since been found to not reliably distinguish between the two for metastases [15] and have also had sensitivity and specificity limitations for gliomas [19]. Periventricular enhancing foci within a radiation port are typical of radiation-induced injury, given the vulnerability of that watershed zone to ischemia following vascular injury [19]; however, high-grade gliomas do not infrequently spread in the subependymal region as well.

Some have made the observation that some recurrent metastases following SRS have a component of T2-hypointensity within a larger enhancing lesion and that the closer to 1.0 is the ratio of T2-hypointense nodule diameter to overall contrast-enhancing lesion diameter, the more likely the lesion is to represent recurrent metastasis rather than radiation necrosis [15, 20]. This ratio has been termed the "lesion quotient," and it has been suggested that a lesion quotient of 0.3 is likely to be radiation necrosis, and over 0.3 is likely to represent an admixture of tumor and necrosis or pure recurrent tumor [15]. However, this metric was not replicated by another group using similar methods [21]. The variability in what constitutes a lesion component which is hypointense on T2-weighted imaging likely relates to inconsistent results of this measure.

Another study of SRS-treated metastases has suggested that a larger volume ratio of edema to enhancing lesion is predictive of radionecrosis [22]. Another recent study also suggested reliable differentiation between radiation necrosis and

recurrent metastasis through evaluating the change of border and interior contrast enhancement over 55 minutes following IV gadolinium contrast injection [23]. Additional data to validate the findings of both these studies' are still required.

## Perfusion MRI

Neoangiogenesis and increased microvascular density are characteristic of malignancies, in contradistinction to necrotic tissue. Although both tumor and necrosis may have leaky capillaries which allow IV gadolinium to leak into the interstitium (and thereby contrast enhance at MRI), the volume of venules and capillaries (cerebral blood volume, CBV) is expected to be greater in viable tumor than in radiation necrosis for both treated glioma and metastases.

Following radiosurgery and high-dose radiotherapy to the brain, relative cerebral blood volume (rCBV) as measured from dynamic susceptibility-weighted contrast-enhanced (DSC) MRI has shown promise as a single imaging measure in distinguishing radionecrosis from progressive tumor in both gliomas and metastases [13, 14, 24, 25]. However, appropriate cutoff values of rCBV would be very technique-dependent, with variability introduced by many factors, including how one draws regions of interest (ROIs), if gadolinium preload is given, which pulse sequence parameters are chosen (e.g., flip angle in gradient echo-based DSC), and what software is used and with which options (e.g., leakage correction) [26]. Importantly, it is also noted that conflicting data exists on the ability of rCBV to distinguish progressive glioma from pseudoprogression (i.e., rather than frank radiation necrosis) [16] (see Fig. 36.1).

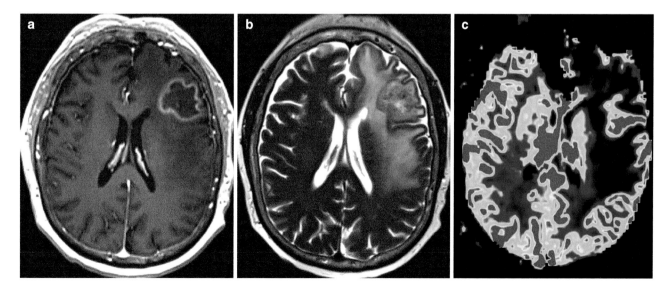

**Fig. 36.1** Representative axial MR images of radionecrosis in the left frontal lobe: (**a**) ring-enhancing centrally necrotic lesion on T1-weighted MR, (**b**) vasogenic edema around the lesion appearing as hyperintense region on T2-weighted imaging, (**c**) relative cerebral blood volume map showing a deficit in the region of the ring-enhancing lesion, consistent with radionecrosis rather than active tumor. [Courtesy of Dr. Derek Johnson]

## MR Spectroscopy

MR spectroscopy (MRS) is able to estimate the amounts of particular biochemicals within the brain and brain lesions. For example, as an oversimplification, N-acetylasparate (NAA) is a marker of intact neurons, choline (Cho) is a marker of membrane turnover, creatine (Cr) is a general reference marker of metabolism, and lactate (Lac) is a marker of anaerobic metabolism. MRS can be performed as single voxel or as multivoxel, but multivoxel is generally preferred for mass lesions, particularly those which might have spatially variable biochemistry [27, 28]. Normal brain normally has relatively high NAA and Cr and Cho peaks. Malignancies show diminished NAA but may have preserved or elevated Cho and may have elevated lipid (Lip)/Lac peaks. Elevated Cho may be seen in early radiation-induced injury (and resemble that of viable tumor) [29], but as radiation necrosis evolves, Cho would be expected to drop, leaving a predominance of only Lip/Lac [28].

In the hands of experienced users, MRS has shown good accuracy in differentiating both recurrent metastasis and glioma from radiation necrosis, though with limited numbers of patients [27, 29–32]. It is also noted that proposed metabolite ratio thresholds in the literature for this differentiation have been myriad [28].

Limitations of MR spectroscopy include its extra time of acquisition, as it is usually asked to be performed on top of a full structural MRI exam, its sampling limitations (even if multivoxel MRS is performed, it is usually limited to one or two slices in the brain), its vulnerability to nondiagnostic quality near areas of magnetic field inhomogeneity such as near the skull base, and its variability in interpretation and the use of ratio cutoffs. Standardization of imaging acquisition and metabolite ratio threshold selection is needed, as well as prospective validation of these techniques. As for all imaging techniques in this sphere, there is the ever-present issue of admixture of tumor and necrosis.

## PET Imaging

PET imaging holds the promise of differentiating between viable tumor and treatment-induced changes in the brain based on their differential metabolism [33]. $^{18}$F-FDG-PET has most commonly been used for brain imaging, and tumors with substantial biological activity would be expected to take up FDG (fluorodeoxyglucose) as they would glucose. However, the normal background brain uptake of FDG is also unfortunately high, especially in the cortex, which complicates image analysis and can mask lesion uptake. For this

reason, some centers perform delayed PET imaging of the brain in hopes of detecting differential washout of tumor relative to normal brain. $^{18}$F-FDG PET has had moderate but limited success in differentiating between radionecrosis and both recurrent malignant glioma and metastasis [34–38] (see Figs. 36.2, 36.3, and 36.4).

Conversely, amino acid PET (e.g., $^{11}$C-methionine/$^{11}$C-MET, $^{18}$F-fluorodopa/$^{18}$F-FDOPA, and $^{18}$F-fluoroethyltyrosine/$^{18}$F-FET) have lower native brain uptake relative to metabolically active tumor, and therefore viable tumor conspicuity may be greater with these PET exams [39–42]. Tumors may have differentially increased amino acid tracer uptake related to increased active transport of amino acids across their cell membranes, increased protein synthesis, disruption of the blood brain barrier, and/or related to their microvascular density and perfusion.

A recent study in 18 metastases showed that $^{11}$C-methionine PET outperformed $^{18}$F-FDG PET, dynamic contrast-enhanced (DCE) permeability, and diffusion-weighted imaging (DWI) in differentiating recurrent metastases from radiation necrosis, with an area under the curve (AUC) in receiver operating characteristic (ROC) analysis of 0.90 [38]. $^{18}$F-FET, including with time-activity curve analysis, has produced accuracies of 88–93% in differentiating recurrent metastasis from radiation necrosis 88–93% [43, 44]. $^{18}$F-DOPA PET has produced an accuracy of 83% in this determination [45]. The joint Response Assessment in Neuro-Oncology Criteria (RANO) and European Association of Neuro-Oncology (EANO) guidelines paper for PET imaging in treated gliomas references studies which have shown the superiority of these three amino acid PET radiotracers over MRI in differentiating tumor recurrence from treatment-induced changes, as well as the general superiority of amino acid tracers over 18F-FDG in gliomas [33].

Amino acid PET radiotracers are not yet FDA-approved for the diagnosis of recurrent brain metastases vs. radiation necrosis, however. Relatedly, clinical availability and lack of reimbursement have been particular limitations in the use of amino acid PET radiotracers to date. The short half-life of $^{11}$C also presents difficulties for many centers because its use requires an on-site cyclotron to produce it. Although the $^{18}$F-labeled amino acid tracers could be shipped, without an on-site cyclotron needed, the lack of reimbursement in clinical use has limited their widespread implementation. However, academic centers' success with these agents prompts one to hope that these barriers to implementation can be overcome. As with any imaging technique for response assessment in posttreatment glioma or metastasis, it must be kept in mind that accuracy will always be limited at least by the frequent admixture of tumor and necrosis.

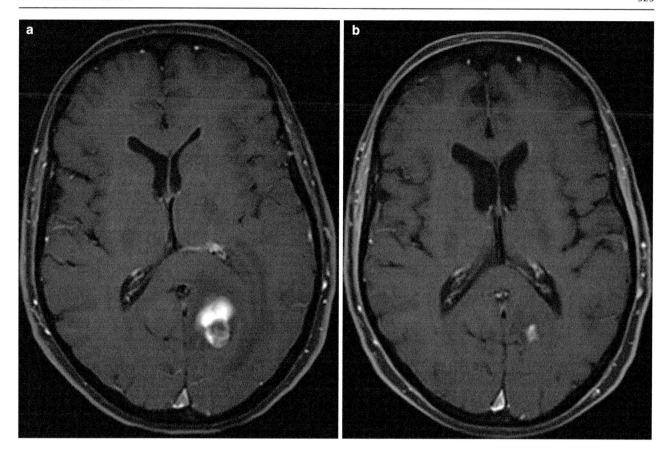

**Fig. 36.2** Axial post-contrast T1-weighted MR images of a 65-year-old female with metastatic lung adenocarcinoma with solitary enhancing left parieto-occipital metastasis (**a**). WBRT was given, followed by SRS. By 3 months after SRS, the mass had substantially decreased in size (**b**). [Courtesy of Dr. Derek Johnson]

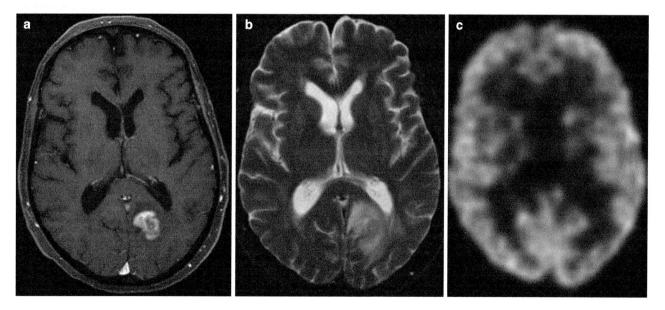

**Fig. 36.3** At 8 months after SRS, however, the enhancing lesion had progressed in size (**a**), and the diameter of nodular hypointensity on T2-weighted imaging was over half that of the enhancing lesion (**b**). However, 18F-FDG PET at this time did not show obvious hypermetabolism in the mass (**c**)

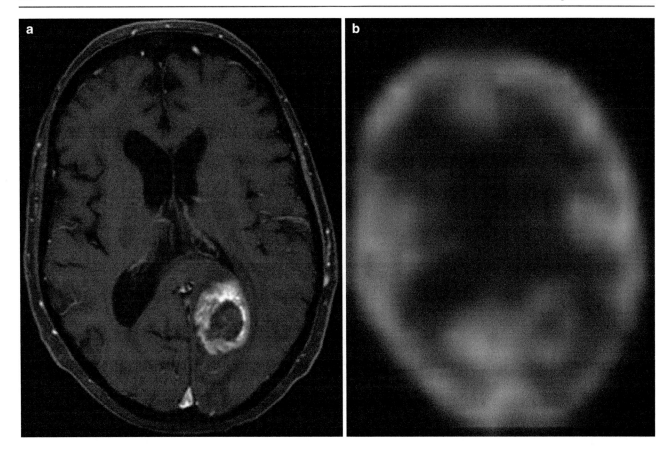

**Fig. 36.4** The lesion was followed for 4 more months, now 1 year after SRS. The lesion continued to increase in size and became more necrotic (**a**). At this point, the contrast-enhancing portion of the mass was hypermetabolic on FDG-PET (**b**), though only the white matter portion of the lesion is clearly abnormally increased above background brain. The mass was resected and was recurrent, viable metastasis. Assuming that tumor progression had begun by 8 months after SRS, this case demonstrates the variable accuracy of FDG-PET

## Imaging Summary

The presence of an enhancing, necrotic lesion with surrounding edema in the brain poses a diagnostic dilemma after high-dose radiation, for both treated gliomas and metastases. Conventional MR imaging is limited or ineffective in distinguishing between the two possibilities. Other functional or mechanistic MRI techniques, and PET imaging, show promise in distinguishing between viable, recurrent tumor and radiation necrosis. Others have also investigated the use of DWI and $^{201}$Tl-SPECT and DCE permeability imaging in irradiated tumor response assessment. However, each of these imaging techniques is imperfect, because of limitations intrinsic to them as well as due to the fact that postradiation lesions frequently represent an admixture of viable tumor and necrosis and would therefore be expected to give conflicting or ambiguous findings at imaging. Therefore, a multimodality imaging approach is advocated in the posttreatment setting to maximize accuracy. If imaging results are congruent in their being suggestive of one diagnosis or the other, this naturally increases our confidence in them. Further imaging improvements and validation of existing imaging techniques are needed, however.

## Pathological Findings

Although the pathophysiology of brain radionecrosis is not well understood, the general proposed mechanism suggests that the process starts with local vascular disruption in the region of high-dose radiation. This results in vasogenic edema and vascular compromise that can lead to tissue hypoxia, which in turn upregulates hypoxia-inducible factor-1 alpha (HIF-1α), a known transactivator of vasoactive proteins including vascular endothelial growth factor (VEGF) [46–48]. As VEGF can induce fenestrations in capillary endothelial cells and interfere with tight junction assembly of the blood-brain barrier, the downstream effects of upregulated VEGF can include cumulative edema, hypoxia, and tissues necrosis [49]. Bevacizumab is a humanized murine monoclonal antibody that can selectively inhibit VEGF and has been clinically used to treat various solid tumors through the proposed mechanism of inhibiting tumor angiogenesis [50].

Some studies have specifically described the histopathological findings of coagulation necrosis as a result of induced vascular damage. The histological description within these studies includes the presence of telangiectasia, atypical appearance of endothelial cells, vascular thickening and proliferation, as well as focal hemorrhage. Studies have also reported immunoreactive cells including reactive astrocytes that are attracted to necrotic tissue and cause granuloma formation within areas of radionecrosis [51, 52].

Initial therapy for symptomatic brain radionecrosis is typically high-dose corticosteroids [53]. If symptoms continue to progress despite the initiation of high-dose corticosteroids, surgical resection may be considered [54].

## Management of Condition

### Medical Therapy

#### Corticosteroids
Generally patients are only treated for brain radionecrosis that is symptomatic. Corticosteroids are the typical first-line treatment, as they effectively reduce the brain edema and thereby improve the edema-related symptoms. Corticosteroids can also inhibit the pro-inflammatory processes involved in radionecrosis [2]. Patients are often started on a moderate to high of corticosteroids and are given a gradual tapering schedule. However, as the corticosteroids are withdrawn, some patients may experience a rebound of brain edema and related symptoms. Some patients may be unable to completely taper of corticosteroids, and prolonged use of corticosteroids can be associated with significant toxicities that include but are not limited to glucose intolerance, steroid myopathy, iatrogenic Cushing's syndrome, and increase risk of infections [2].

### Antiangiogenic Agent: Bevacizumab

Several recent reviews have highlighted the promising responses of brain radionecrosis to bevacizumab, based on both retrospective and small prospective studies [55, 56]. In a review by Lubelski et al., 30 of 30 patients had radiographic improvement with bevacizumab treatment for brain radionecrosis following radiotherapy for high-grade glioma across seven studies. In this review, 16 of 23 patients had clinical symptom data and reported symptomatic improvement [56]. A subsequent review of 71 patients across 16 studies treated with bevacizumab for brain radionecrosis after radiation for any brain tumor reported radiographic response in 97% of patients and improvement in performance status in 79% of patients [55].

Two small prospective single-arm studies of bevacizumab for brain radionecrosis have evaluated 9 patients [57] and 17

patients [58]. Yonezawa et al. reported a 65% mean reduction in edema, measured as the volume of T2-weighted fluid-attenuated inversion recovery (FLAIR) hyperintensity on MR images, and 80% mean reduction in the volume of contrast enhancement on the post-gadolinium T1-weighted MR images. Clinically, seven of these nine patients had an improvement in Karnofsky Performance Status (KPS) [57]. Wang et al. reported 48.8% mean reduction in hyperintense volume on T2-FLAIR and 54.9% mean reduction in the volume of enhancements on the post-gadolinium T1-weighted MR images and KPS improvement in 16 of 17 patients [58].

There has been one small randomized, double-blind, placebo-controlled trial of bevacizumab 7.5 mg/kg every 3 weeks × 2 cycles versus placebo q 3 weeks × 2 cycles for adult patients who developed a radiological diagnosis of brain radionecrosis following radiotherapy for brain or head and neck cancer at least months prior to study entry. If patients were taking corticosteroids prior to study participation, they were required to be on a stable dose for at least 1 week prior to starting study treatment. The primary endpoint of the trial was radiological response, defined 25% or greater reduction in brain edema, measured as the volume of T2-FLAIR hyperintensity on MRI, at 6 weeks following study treatment compared with pretreatment [59]. Using this response criteria, 100% of patients randomized to bevacizumab had a radiological response and also have reduction in post-gadolinium enhancement. In contrast, of the patients receiving placebo, five patients experienced clinical and radiological progression, and two patients had radiological progression without worsening symptoms. Despite the radiological response, no differences were noted between treatment arms in terms of neurocognitive function or symptom severity measured using MD Anderson Symptom Inventory for brain tumor (MDASI-BT).

An ongoing double-blind, randomized, placebo-controlled phase II trial is comparing the symptomatic improvement achieved by bevacizumab + corticosteroids vs. corticosteroids + placebo (BeSt) for symptomatic brain radionecrosis after radiosurgery for brain metastases (A221208). Eligible patients require a radiological diagnosis of brain radionecrosis 3–24 months following radiosurgery for brain metastases and symptoms requiring at least dexamethasone 4 mg a day (or equivalent dose of alternative corticosteroid). The radiological features required for a radiological diagnosis of radionecrosis for this trial include a lesion quotient <0.3 and relative cerebral blood volume (rCBV) <1.5 and percent signal recovery (PSR) ≥ 76%. Patients are randomized to bevacizumab 10 mg/kg IV days 1 and 15 × 4 cycles and corticosteroids (dose adjusted by the treating physician to manage symptoms) or placebo and corticosteroids (dose adjusted by the treating physician to manage symptoms). The primary objective is to determine whether patients treated with bevacizumab will have greater improvement in symptoms, measured using MDASI-BT, compared with standard corticosteroid therapy. This trial will also evaluate the adverse effects associated with corticosteroids and bevacizumab, health-related quality of life (HR-QOL), duration of corticosteroids required, and time to maximum radiographic response as well as correlative serum/urine biomarkers and imaging biomarkers that predict for treatment response.

## Antioxidants Agents

### Edaravone

Edaravone (3-methyl-1-phenyl-2-pyrazolin-5-one) is an effective free radical scavenger that has been used to treat a wide range of oxidative stress-related neurological diseases such as cerebral ischemia [60]. As oxidative damage is a known mechanism of radiation injury, Tang et al. completed an open-label, randomized trial to evaluate the protective effects of edaravone versus corticosteroids for patients who developed brain radionecrosis following radiation for nasopharyngeal cancer. Patients were randomized to edaravone 30 mg po twice daily for 14 days versus methylprednisolone 500 mg IV × 3 days followed by tapering oral prednisone [60]. The primary response, defined as at least 25% reduction in edema measured as the volume of T2-hyperintensity at 3 months, was observed in 40 patients (55.6%) in the edaravone group versus 23 patients (35.4%) in the corticosteroid group ($p = 0.025$). Unlike bevacizumab, the enhancing volume did not decrease more significantly with edaravone compared with corticosteroids ($p = 0.468$) [60]. Patients receiving edaravone reported greater improvement in their symptoms, measured using the Late Effects Normal Tissue Task Force-Subjective, Objective, Management, Analytic (LENT-SOMA) scale, but the open-label design of the study may have influenced this finding.

### Vitamin E and Pentoxifylline

Vitamin E (or tocopherol) is another free radical scavenger that has been investigated in the treatment of radiation injury. Pentoxifylline (PTX) is a methylxanthine derivative that decreases blood viscosity thereby increasing blood circulation and tissue oxygenation, which has been investigated in combination with vitamin E for the treatment of late toxicities of radiotherapy. In a small retrospective study, 11 patients with brain radionecrosis following brain radiation for brain metastases, meningioma, or arteriovenous malformation (AVM) were treated with the combination of PTX and vitamin E. All but one patient had radiological improvement, and this patient was eventually confirmed to have progressive tumor rather than radionecrosis [61].

A prospective non-randomized study allowed adult patients who had developed radiological evidence of temporal lobe necrosis following radiotherapy for nasopharyngeal cancer to choose between vitamin E 1000 IU twice daily for up to 1 year versus no active treatment. Patients were assessed at baseline and at 1 year using the Cantonese version of the Mini-Mental Status Examination (CMMSE), Hong Kong List Learning Test (HKLLT), Visual Reproduction subtest of the Wechsler Memory Scale-III (WMS-III VR), Category fluency test (CFT), and computerized Cognitive Flexibility Test [62]. A small improvement in global cognitive function on CMMSE of 5.33% was seen in patients who received vitamin E compared with no improvement in the control group ($p = 0.007$). Assessment of verbal learning using HKLLT demonstrated that the treatment group had a 27.24% improvement at 1 year versus no improvement in the control group. There was no difference in attention, language, or executive function between the two groups at baseline or at 1 year [62].

## Hyperbaric Oxygen Therapy (HBOT)

Although hyperbaric oxygen therapy is attempted for some patients with brain radionecrosis, there is limited data to support its use with only small retrospective case reports and case studies [63]. One prospective single-arm study is evaluating hyperbaric oxygen therapy for brain radionecrosis (NCT02714465) in patients aged 10–75 years old with clinical and radiological signs of radionecrosis following radiosurgery. On this trial, patients will receive up to 40 sessions of HBOT if they show radiological response after the first 24 sessions.

## Local Therapies

### Surgery

Although surgical resection is frequently used to clinically address progressive radionecrosis, there are no prospective trials that report the efficacy of surgery for brain radionecrosis. In a small retrospective series of 24 patients previously treated with high-dose radiotherapy for nasopharyngeal cancer who developed contrast-enhancing lesions in the temporal lobes (16 unilateral, 8 bilateral), surgical resection of contrast-enhancing lesions was associated with radiological improvement in brain edema on CT or MRI in 15 patients who completed serial imaging. Of the 24 patients, one patient required a second surgical resection for locally recurrent necrosis [64]. In another retrospective series of 15 patients who developed radionecrosis after radiosurgery, surgical resection resulted in improvement of symptoms, reduction in brain edema, and associated ability to reduce or discontinue corticosteroids [65].

## Laser Interstitial Thermal Therapy (LITT)

Laser interstitial thermal therapy (LITT) uses light energy to create tissue heating around a laser fiber which is surgically inserted into the brain. Some have used LITT for a progressing and symptomatic enhancing lesion in the setting of prior SRS for brain metastasis, as it was felt that LITT would be an effective treatment of whatever the lesion may be (i.e., radiation necrosis or recurrent tumor) [66]. Following this concept, a prospective single-arm study has evaluated the effect of LITT in patients with growing enhancing lesions that were previously treated with SRS [67]. This study has reported promising local control of 75.8% (13 of 15 lesions) and dramatic reductions in enhancing lesion volume to less than 10% of the pretreated volume in seven of the treated lesions [67]. Although the results from a small, single-arm study will not support a change in practice, these promising findings encourage further prospective investigation of LITT for brain radionecrosis.

## Case Illustration

Figures 36.5, 36.6, 36.7, and 36.8.

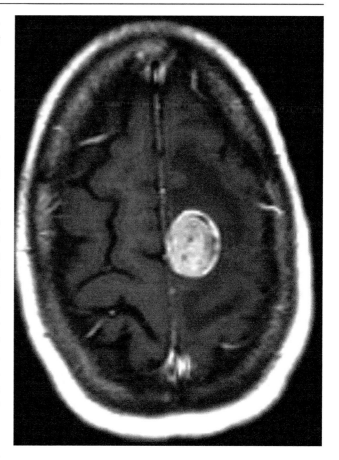

**Fig. 36.5** A 56-year-old female presented with melanoma metastatic to the left frontal lobe (axial post-gadolinium T1-weighted MRI). This was resected, followed by LINAC-based stereotactic radiosurgery to the resection cavity 1 month later (20 Gy in one fraction)

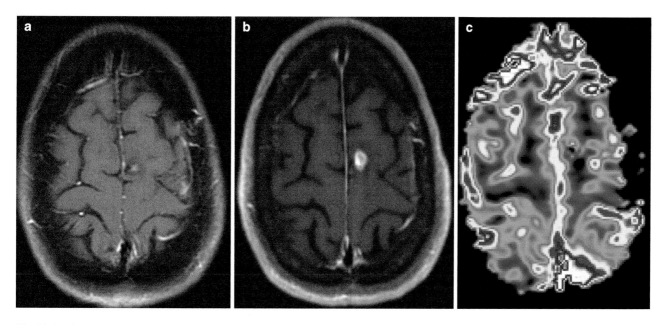

**Fig. 36.6** 14 months following SRS, a new contrast enhancing nodule developed at the site of resection (**a**). This slowly enlarged over the following 8 months (**b**), though there was not abnormally increased blood volume within it on DSC perfusion imaging (**c**)

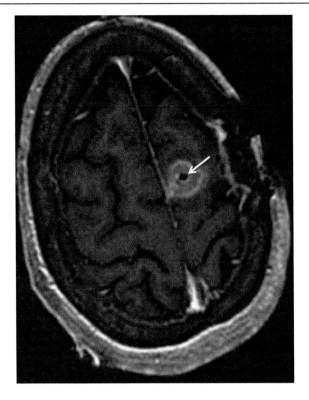

**Fig. 36.7** Stereotactic needle biopsy of the enhancing lesion was performed at 22 months after SRS, immediately followed by MR-guided LITT of the enhancing lesion. Histopathology revealed necrosis, vascular hyaline changes, and gliosis, consistent with radiation effect and no viable metastatic melanoma. Post-gadolinium MPRAGE immediately following laser ablation depicts the thinly peripherally enhancing treatment zone with the still present laser cannula (arrow, to focal dark spot) seen in cross section in the center of the treatment zone

## Summary

- The risk of radionecrosis has been estimated at about 10% at 1 year following radiosurgery, but the cumulative incidence appears to rise with longer follow-up.
- On conventional brain MRI, brain radionecrosis typically appears as an enhancing, necrotic lesion with surrounding edema, which is often indistinguishable from active tumor.
- Beyond conventional brain MR images, perfusion MRI, spectroscopy, and PET imaging may help differentiate tumor progression from brain radionecrosis.
- The proposed mechanism that triggers the radionecrosis process is local vascular disruption followed by ongoing upregulation of vasoactive proteins including hypoxia-inducible factor-1 alpha (HIF-1α) and vascular endothelial growth factor (VEGF).
- On histopathology, there is often an admixture of tumor cells and necrosis, which makes it challenging to definitively diagnose brain radionecrosis pathologically.
- First-line treatment is typically corticosteroids, as they effectively reduce the brain edema, and they have anti-inflammatory effect.
- Other treatments that are currently under investigation include anti-vascular agents such as bevacizumab and antioxidant agents including edaravone, vitamin E, and pentoxifylline. Additional treatments under investigation include hyperbaric oxygen therapy and local surgical therapies such as laser interstitial thermal therapy.

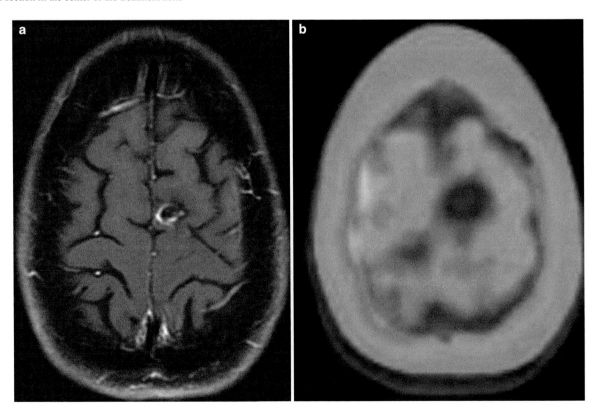

**Fig. 36.8** Follow-up MRI (**a**) and FDG PET-CT (**b**) 13 months after LITT, showing a stable, thinly peripherally enhancing treatment zone which corresponds to a photopenic defect on PET

## Self-Assessment Questions

1. What is the estimate risk of developing brain radionecrosis at 1 year following radiosurgery treatment?
   A. 1%
   B. 3%
   C. 10%
   D. 50%

2. Which of the following molecular factors are considered a major contributor to the development and progression of brain radionecrosis?
   A. EGFR
   B. VEGF
   C. PD-1
   D. ALK

3. A patient presents with headache and recurrent left arm numbness 9 months after prior radiosurgery for a brain metastasis in the right parietal lobe. An MRI shows a recurrent enhancing lesion with surrounding edema. What characteristics on conventional MRI favor a diagnosis of recurrent tumor rather than radionecrosis?
   A. "Soap bubble" appearance on the post-contrast T1-weighted MRI
   B. Lesion quotient = 0.2
   C. Lesion quotient = 0.9
   D. Larger volume ratio of edema to enhancing lesion

4. A patient presents with headache and recurrent left arm numbness 9 months after prior radiosurgery for a brain metastasis in the right parietal lobe. An MRI shows a recurrent enhancing lesion with surrounding edema. What is an additional imaging study that may help determine whether this lesion is radionecrosis or recurrent tumor?
   A. Dynamic susceptibility-weighted contrast-enhanced (DSC) MRI
   B. MR spectroscopy
   C. PET scan using an amino acid tracer
   D. All of the above

5. A patient presents with headache and recurrent left arm numbness 9 months after prior radiosurgery for a brain metastasis in the right parietal lobe. An MRI shows a recurrent enhancing lesion with surrounding edema. Given that the patient is symptomatic, you would offer which of the following as initial therapy:
   A. Surgical resection
   B. Corticosteroids
   C. Bevacizumab
   D. Laser interstitial thermal therapy (LITT)

## Answers

1. C
2. B
3. C
4. D
5. B

## References

1. Blonigen BJ, Steinmetz RD, Levin L, et al. Irradiated volume as a predictor of brain radionecrosis after linear accelerator stereotactic radiosurgery. Int J Radiat Oncol Biol Phys. 2010;77(4):996–1001.
2. Giglio P, Gilbert MR. Cerebral radiation necrosis. Neurologist. 2003;9(4):180–8.
3. Suh JH. Stereotactic radiosurgery for the management of brain metastases. N Engl J Med. 2010;362(12):1119–27.
4. Kohutek ZA, Yamada Y, Chan TA, et al. Long-term risk of radionecrosis and imaging changes after stereotactic radiosurgery for brain metastases. J Neurooncol. 2015;125(1):149–56.
5. Shaw E, Scott C, Souhami L, et al. Single dose radiosurgical treatment of recurrent previously irradiated primary brain tumors and brain metastases: final report of RTOG protocol 90-05. Int J Radiat Oncol Biol Phys. 2000;47(2):291–8.
6. Kocher M, Soffietti R, Abacioglu U, et al. Adjuvant whole-brain radiotherapy versus observation after radiosurgery or surgical resection of one to three cerebral metastases: results of the EORTC 22952-26001 study. J Clin Oncol. 2011;29(2):134–41.
7. Aoyama H, Shirato H, Tago M, et al. Stereotactic radiosurgery plus whole-brain radiation therapy vs stereotactic radiosurgery alone for treatment of brain metastases: a randomized controlled trial. JAMA. 2006;295(21):2483–91.
8. Korytko T, Radivoyevitch T, Colussi V, et al. 12 Gy gamma knife radiosurgical volume is a predictor for radiation necrosis in non-AVM intracranial tumors. Int J Radiat Oncol Biol Phys. 2006;64(2):419–24.
9. Minniti G, Clarke E, Lanzetta G, et al. Stereotactic radiosurgery for brain metastases: analysis of outcome and risk of brain radionecrosis. Radiat Oncol. 2011;6:48.
10. Ohtakara K, Hayashi S, Nakayama N, et al. Significance of target location relative to the depth from the brain surface and high-dose irradiated volume in the development of brain radionecrosis after micromultileaf collimator-based stereotactic radiosurgery for brain metastases. J Neurooncol. 2012;108(1):201–9.
11. Schüttrumpf LH, Niyazi M, Nachbichler SB, et al. Prognostic factors for survival and radiation necrosis after stereotactic radiosurgery alone or in combination with whole brain radiation therapy for 1-3 cerebral metastases. Radiat Oncol. 2014;9:105.
12. Barajas RF Jr, Chang JS, Segal MR, et al. Differentiation of recurrent glioblastoma multiforme from radiation necrosis after external beam radiation therapy with dynamic susceptibility-weighted contrast-enhanced perfusion MR imaging. Radiology. 2009;253(2):486–96.
13. Barajas RF, Chang JS, Sneed PK, et al. Distinguishing recurrent intra-axial metastatic tumor from radiation necrosis following gamma knife radiosurgery using dynamic susceptibility-weighted contrast-enhanced perfusion MR imaging. AJNR Am J Neuroradiol. 2009;30(2):367–72.
14. Hoefnagels FWA, Lagerwaard FJ, Sanchez E, et al. Radiological progression of cerebral metastases after radiosurgery: assessment of

perfusion MRI for differentiating between necrosis and recurrence. J Neurol. 2009;256(6):878–87.

15. Dequesada IM, Quisling RG, Yachnis A, et al. Can standard magnetic resonance imaging reliably distinguish recurrent tumor from radiation necrosis after radiosurgery for brain metastases? A radiographic-pathological study. Neurosurgery. 2008;63(5):898–903, discussion 904

16. Ellingson BM, Chung C, Pope WB, et al. Pseudoprogression, radionecrosis, inflammation or true tumor progression? Challenges associated with glioblastoma response assessment in an evolving therapeutic landscape. J Neurooncol. 2017;134(3):495–504.

17. Wen PY, Macdonald DR, Reardon DA, et al. Updated response assessment criteria for high-grade gliomas: response assessment in neuro-oncology working group. J Clin Oncol. 2010;28(11):1963–72.

18. Patel TR, McHugh BJ, Bi WL, et al. A comprehensive review of MR imaging changes following radiosurgery to 500 brain metastases. AJNR Am J Neuroradiol. 2011;32(10):1885–92.

19. Kumar AJ, Leeds NE, Fuller GN, et al. Malignant gliomas: MR imaging spectrum of radiation therapy- and chemotherapy-induced necrosis of the brain after treatment. Radiology. 2000;217(2):377–84.

20. Kano H, Kondziolka D, Lobato-Polo J, et al. T1/T2 matching to differentiate tumor growth from radiation effects after stereotactic radiosurgery. Neurosurgery. 2010;66(3):486–91. discussion 491–2

21. Stockham AL, Tievsky AL, Koyfman SA, et al. Conventional MRI does not reliably distinguish radiation necrosis from tumor recurrence after stereotactic radiosurgery. J Neurooncol. 2012;109(1):149–58.

22. Leeman JE, Clump DA, Flickinger JC, et al. Extent of perilesional edema differentiates radionecrosis from tumor recurrence following stereotactic radiosurgery for brain metastases. Neuro Oncol. 2013;15(12):1732–8.

23. Wagner S, Lanfermann H, Eichner G, et al. Radiation injury versus malignancy after stereotactic radiosurgery for brain metastases: impact of time-dependent changes in lesion morphology on MRI. Neuro Oncol. 2017;19(4):586–94.

24. Hu LS, Baxter LC, Smith KA, et al. Relative cerebral blood volume values to differentiate high-grade glioma recurrence from posttreatment radiation effect: direct correlation between image-guided tissue histopathology and localized dynamic susceptibility-weighted contrast-enhanced perfusion MR imaging measurements. AJNR Am J Neuroradiol. 2009;30(3):552–8.

25. Mitsuya K, Nakasu Y, Horiguchi S, et al. Perfusion weighted magnetic resonance imaging to distinguish the recurrence of metastatic brain tumors from radiation necrosis after stereotactic radiosurgery. J Neurooncol. 2010;99(1):81–8.

26. Willats L, Calamante F. The 39 steps: evading error and deciphering the secrets for accurate dynamic susceptibility contrast MRI. NMR Biomed. 2013;26(8):913–31.

27. Chernov M, Hayashi M, Izawa M, et al. Differentiation of the radiation-induced necrosis and tumor recurrence after gamma knife radiosurgery for brain metastases: importance of multi-voxel proton MRS. Minim Invasive Neurosurg. 2005;48(4):228–34.

28. Chernov MF, Ono Y, Abe K, et al. Differentiation of tumor progression and radiation-induced effects after intracranial radiosurgery. Acta Neurochir Suppl. 2013;116:193–210.

29. Nakajima T, Kumabe T, Kanamori M, et al. Differential diagnosis between radiation necrosis and glioma progression using sequential proton magnetic resonance spectroscopy and methionine positron emission tomography. Neurol Med Chir (Tokyo). 2009;49(9):394–401.

30. Kimura T, Sako K, Tanaka K, et al. Evaluation of the response of metastatic brain tumors to stereotactic radiosurgery by proton magnetic resonance spectroscopy, 201TlCl single-photon emission computerized tomography, and gadolinium-enhanced magnetic resonance imaging. J Neurosurg. 2004;100(5):835–41.

31. Truong MT, St Clair EG, Donahue BR, et al. Results of surgical resection for progression of brain metastases previously treated by gamma knife radiosurgery. Neurosurgery. 2006;59(1):86–97. discussion 86–97

32. Kamada K, Saguer M, Möller M, et al. Combined study of ischemic brain conditions using magnetencephalography and proton magnetic resonance spectroscopy imaging. Biomed Tech (Berl). 1997;42(Suppl):188–90.

33. Albert NL, Weller M, Suchorska B, et al. Response assessment in neuro-oncology working group and European Association for Neuro-Oncology recommendations for the clinical use of PET imaging in gliomas. Neuro Oncol. 2016;18(9):1199–208.

34. Nihashi T, Dahabreh IJ, Terasawa T. Diagnostic accuracy of PET for recurrent glioma diagnosis: a meta-analysis. AJNR Am J Neuroradiol. 2013;34(5):944–50. S1–11

35. Van Laere K, Ceyssens S, Van Calenbergh F, et al. Direct comparison of 18F-FDG and 11C-methionine PET in suspected recurrence of glioma: sensitivity, inter-observer variability and prognostic value. Eur J Nucl Med Mol Imaging. 2005;32(1):39–51.

36. Chao ST, Suh JH, Raja S, et al. The sensitivity and specificity of FDG PET in distinguishing recurrent brain tumor from radionecrosis in patients treated with stereotactic radiosurgery. Int J Cancer. 2001;96(3):191–7.

37. Lai G, Mahadevan A, Hackney D, et al. Diagnostic accuracy of PET, SPECT, and arterial spin-labeling in differentiating tumor recurrence from necrosis in cerebral metastasis after stereotactic radiosurgery. AJNR Am J Neuroradiol. 2015;36(12):2250–5.

38. Tomura N, Kokubun M, Saginoya T, et al. Differentiation between treatment-induced necrosis and recurrent tumors in patients with metastatic brain tumors: comparison among 11C-methionine-PET, FDG-PET, MR permeability imaging, and MRI-ADC-preliminary results. AJNR Am J Neuroradiol. 2017;38(8):1520–7.

39. Chen W, Silverman DH, Delaloye S, et al. 18F-FDOPA PET imaging of brain tumors: comparison study with 18F-FDG PET and evaluation of diagnostic accuracy. J Nucl Med. 2006;47(6):904–11.

40. Herrmann K, Czernin J, Cloughesy T, et al. Comparison of visual and semiquantitative analysis of 18F-FDOPA-PET/CT for recurrence detection in glioblastoma patients. Neuro Oncol. 2014;16(4):603–9.

41. Takenaka S, Asano Y, Shinoda J, et al. Comparison of (11)C-methionine, (11)C-choline, and (18)F-fluorodeoxyglucose-PET for distinguishing glioma recurrence from radiation necrosis. Neurol Med Chir (Tokyo). 2014;54(4):280–9.

42. Terakawa Y, Tsuyuguchi N, Iwai Y, et al. Diagnostic accuracy of 11C-methionine PET for differentiation of recurrent brain tumors from radiation necrosis after radiotherapy. J Nucl Med. 2008;49(5):694–9.

43. Ceccon G, Lohmann P, Stoffels G, et al. Dynamic O-(2-18F-fluoroethyl)-L-tyrosine positron emission tomography differentiates brain metastasis recurrence from radiation injury after radiotherapy. Neuro Oncol. 2017;19(2):281–8.

44. Galldiks N, Stoffels G, Filss CP, et al. Role of O-(2-(18) F-fluoroethyl)-L-tyrosine PET for differentiation of local recurrent brain metastasis from radiation necrosis. J Nucl Med. 2012;53(9):1367–74.

45. Lizarraga KJ, Allen-Auerbach M, Czernin J, et al. (18)F-FDOPA PET for differentiating recurrent or progressive brain metastatic tumors from late or delayed radiation injury after radiation treatment. J Nucl Med. 2014;55(1):30–6.

46. Nonoguchi N, Miyatake S, Fukumoto M, et al. The distribution of vascular endothelial growth factor-producing cells in clinical radiation necrosis of the brain: pathological consideration of their potential roles. J Neurooncol. 2011;105(2):423–31.

47. Nordal RA, Nagy A, Pintilie M, et al. Hypoxia and hypoxia-inducible factor-1 target genes in central nervous system radiation injury:

a role for vascular endothelial growth factor. Clin Cancer Res. 2004;10(10):3342–53.

48. Plateel M, Dehouck MP, Torpier G, et al. Hypoxia increases the susceptibility to oxidant stress and the permeability of the blood-brain barrier endothelial cell monolayer. J Neurochem. 1995;65(5):2138–45.

49. Roberts WG, Palade GE. Increased microvascular permeability and endothelial fenestration induced by vascular endothelial growth factor. J Cell Sci. 1995;108(Pt 6):2369–79.

50. Presta LG, Chen H, O'Connor SJ, et al. Humanization of an anti-vascular endothelial growth factor monoclonal antibody for the therapy of solid tumors and other disorders. Cancer Res. 1997;57(20):4593–9.

51. Moravan MJ, Olschowka JA, Williams JP, et al. Cranial irradiation leads to acute and persistent neuroinflammation with delayed increases in T-cell infiltration and CD11c expression in C57BL/6 mouse brain. Radiat Res. 2011;176(4):459–73.

52. Zhao W, Robbins ME. Inflammation and chronic oxidative stress in radiation-induced late normal tissue injury: therapeutic implications. Curr Med Chem. 2009;16(2):130–43.

53. Gonzalez J, Kumar AJ, Conrad CA, et al. Effect of bevacizumab on radiation necrosis of the brain. Int J Radiat Oncol Biol Phys. 2007;67(2):323–6.

54. McPherson CM, Warnick RE. Results of contemporary surgical management of radiation necrosis using frameless stereotaxis and intraoperative magnetic resonance imaging. J Neurooncol. 2004;68(1):41–7.

55. Tye K, Engelhard HH, Slavin KV, et al. An analysis of radiation necrosis of the central nervous system treated with bevacizumab. J Neurooncol. 2014;117(2):321–7.

56. Lubelski D, Abdullah KG, Weil RJ, et al. Bevacizumab for radiation necrosis following treatment of high grade glioma: a systematic review of the literature. J Neurooncol. 2013;115(3):317–22.

57. Yonezawa S, Miwa K, Shinoda J, et al. Bevacizumab treatment leads to observable morphological and metabolic changes in brain radiation necrosis. J Neurooncol. 2014;119(1):101–9.

58. Wang Y, Pan L, Sheng X, et al. Reversal of cerebral radiation necrosis with bevacizumab treatment in 17 Chinese patients. Eur J Med Res. 2012;17:25.

59. Levin VA, Bidaut L, Hou P, et al. Randomized double-blind placebo-controlled trial of bevacizumab therapy for radiation necrosis of the central nervous system. Int J Radiat Oncol Biol Phys. 2011;79(5):1487–95.

60. Tang Y, Rong X, Hu W, et al. Effect of edaravone on radiation-induced brain necrosis in patients with nasopharyngeal carcinoma after radiotherapy: a randomized controlled trial. J Neurooncol. 2014;120(2):441–7.

61. Williamson R, Kondziolka D, Kanaan H, et al. Adverse radiation effects after radiosurgery may benefit from oral vitamin E and pentoxifylline therapy: a pilot study. Stereotact Funct Neurosurg. 2008;86(6):359–66.

62. Chan AS, Cheung M-C, Law SC, et al. Phase II study of alpha-tocopherol in improving the cognitive function of patients with temporal lobe radionecrosis. Cancer. 2004;100(2):398–404.

63. Pasquier D, Hoelscher T, Schmutz J, et al. Hyperbaric oxygen therapy in the treatment of radio-induced lesions in normal tissues: a literature review. Radiother Oncol. 2004;72(1):1–13.

64. Wong ST, Loo KT, Yam KY, et al. Results of excision of cerebral radionecrosis: experience in patients treated with radiation therapy for nasopharyngeal carcinoma. J Neurosurg. 2010;113(2):293–300.

65. Telera S, Fabi A, Pace A, et al. Radionecrosis induced by stereotactic radiosurgery of brain metastases: results of surgery and outcome of disease. J Neurooncol. 2013;113(2):313–25.

66. Patel NV, Mian M, Stafford RJ, et al. Laser interstitial thermal therapy technology, physics of magnetic resonance imaging thermometry, and technical considerations for proper catheter placement during magnetic resonance imaging-guided laser interstitial thermal therapy. Neurosurgery. 2016;79(Suppl 1):S8–S16.

67. Rao MS, Hargreaves EL, Khan AJ, et al. Magnetic resonance-guided laser ablation improves local control for postradiosurgery recurrence and/or radiation necrosis. Neurosurgery. 2014;74(6):658–67. discussion 667

# Spinal Cord Tolerance and Risk of Radiation Myelopathy

# 37

Majed Alghamdi, Shun Wong, Paul Medin, Lijun Ma,
Young Lee, Sten Myrehaug, Chia-Lin Tseng,
Hany Soliman, David A. Larson, and Arjun Sahgal

## Learning Objectives

- To review the clinical features, pathophysiology, and histopathology of radiation myelopathy.
- To review the radiobiology of spinal cord and radiobiological issues specific to stereotactic body radiotherapy.
- To review the clinical and dosimetric factors affecting the risk of radiation myelopathy based on animal models and available clinical data.
- To appreciate current research strategies to mitigate the risk of radiation myelopathy.
- To know the current safe practice and dose constraints for spinal cord with conventional and stereotactic body radiotherapy.

M. Alghamdi
Department of Radiation Oncology, Sunnybrook Odette Cancer
Centre, University of Toronto, Toronto, ON, Canada

Faculty of Medicine, Al Baha University, Al Baha, Saudi Arabia

S. Wong · Y. Lee · S. Myrehaug · C.-L. Tseng
H. Soliman · A. Sahgal (✉)
Department of Radiation Oncology, Sunnybrook Odette Cancer
Centre, University of Toronto, Toronto, ON, Canada
e-mail: Arjun.Sahgal@sunnybrook.ca

P. Medin
Department of Radiation Oncology, University of Texas
Southwestern, Dallas, TX, USA

L. Ma · D. A. Larson
Department of Radiation Oncology, University of California San
Francisco, San Francisco, CA, USA

## Introduction

Radiation myelopathy (RM) is a rare and devastating sequela from overdosing the spinal cord with radiation. Traditionally, the dose permitted to the spinal cord has been set to a conservative constraint based predominantly on animal data and expert opinion, given the few cases of human RM reported in the literature. One of the earliest investigations specific to human data was reported by Wong et al. who summarized all known cases of RM at the Princess Margaret Hospital (Toronto, Canada) and provided a threshold for safe practice specific to conventional radiation [1]. Based on homogeneous wide-field radiation exposure to the spinal cord, it was concluded that an equivalent dose in 2 Gy fractions (EQD2) of 50 Gy would yield a negligible risk of RM. Since that paper and work done by Emami and colleagues [2], RM has been considered a rare event when the spinal cord is constrained to an EQD2 ≤ 50 Gy. Insofar that with modern radiation technology, in the event of the complication when accepted constraints are respected, the explanation is likely not associated with dose exposure but an inherent patient-specific genetic radiosensitivity or an error in dose delivery.

With the advent of stereotactic body radiation therapy (SBRT) for spinal metastases, this complication reemerged, and an alarm was raised specific to this form of treatment. SBRT is defined as "*The precise delivery of highly conformal and image-guided hypofractionated external beam radiotherapy, delivered in a single or few fraction(s), to an extracranial body target with doses at least biologically equivalent to a radical course when given over a protracted conventionally (1.8–3.0 Gy/fraction) fractionated schedule*" [3]. In essence, a very high total dose in few fractions is prescribed to a small volume target with defined boundaries resulting in a much greater heterogeneity of the dose distribution than traditionally accustomed. With respect to the organs at risk (OAR), SBRT is also fundamentally distinct from conventional external beam radiation. The critical OAR, namely, the spinal cord in the setting of spine SBRT, is exposed to lower doses than that prescribed to the target. In order to maximize coverage at the tumor-spinal cord interface, steep dose gradients of approximately 15–20% decrease per millimeter are required (Fig. 37.1).

The tight interface gradient results in the ability to set a dose constraint to a small volume of the OAR that could exceed traditional limits, while the majority of the OAR volume is exposed to a subclinical dose with respect to tolerance. Some indeed exploited this technical paradigm as a means to dose escalate the maximum point dose within the spinal cord, proposing that the spinal cord is organized more as a mixed (series and parallel component) OAR as opposed to the traditionally accepted notion that the spinal cord is strictly an organ in series. As a result, much higher doses to small volumes of spinal cord that would be considered safe were delivered in order to maximize target coverage, and RM was indeed observed [4–6]. Importantly, this was despite the majority of the spinal cord volume exposed to a sub-threshold dose.

The increasing clinical experience with spine SBRT has resulted in further knowledge of both the radiobiology and dose tolerance of the spinal cord which will be summarized in this chapter. We will also summarize those guidelines for safe spine SBRT practice which were developed based on careful dosimetric analysis of cases of RM and controls specific to SBRT [4–6]. Ultimately, when dose limits are respected for conventional or SBRT practice, this complication is regarded again as a rare event.

## Structure and Function of the Spinal Cord

The origin of the spinal cord is from the level of the foramen magnum and is a continuation of the medulla oblongata. It extends caudally, typically, to the bottom of first lumbar vertebra where the cauda equina begins. The spinal cord runs within the vertebral canal and is surrounded by three meninges, the dura mater, the arachnoid mater and the pia mater. Cerebrospinal fluid runs in the subarachnoid space. The vertebral canal is formed by the vertebral column which consists of 33 vertebrae (7 cervical, 12 thoracic, 5 lumbar, 5 sacral, and 4 fused coccygeal bones) separated by intervertebral discs. Laterally, intervertebral foramina between two adjacent vertebrae allow for exiting of the spinal nerves.

Spinal nerves are formed by two roots (motor and sensory); each of them consists of many rootlets that attach the nerve root to the spinal cord. There are 31 pairs of spinal nerves (8 cervical, 12 thoracic, 5 lumbar, 5 sacral, and 1 coccygeal) along the entire length of the cord.

On cross section, spinal cord has both gray and white matter. Gray matter forms an inner H-shape with anterior and posterior horns. The rest of the cord is part of the white matter. Ascending tracts through the spinal cord include lateral spinothalamic tract (pain and temperature pathways), anterior spinothalamic tract (crude touch and pressure pathways), and posterior white column (discriminative touch, vibratory sense, and conscious muscle joint sense pathways). The major descending tracts through the cord include anterior and lateral corticospinal tracts (motor).

## Radiation Myelopathy (RM)

### Clinical Features

After irradiation exposure to the spinal cord, there may be a transient early-delayed (subacute) toxicity known as *Lhermitte's syndrome*. It is usually observed 2–4 months after radiation and is clinically characterized by transient electrical shock-like paresthesias radiating from the neck to the extremities, often precipitated by neck flexion (*Lhermitte's sign*) and resolves spontaneously over a few months [7]. Although, this syndrome is diagnosed clinically, magnetic resonance imaging (MRI) may be required to exclude other potential causes of neurological symptoms including disease progression. The development of Lhermitte's does not translate to an increased risk of developing RM.

RM generally refers to an irreversible toxicity that usually occurs 6–12 months after completing radiation treatment, and longer latent periods (>2 years) have also been reported [8]. Clinical presentation depends on the affected area of the spinal cord. Cervical RM can be fatal in 70% of cases [9]. Symptoms and signs are usually progressive and consistent with those associated with upper motor neuron lesions including paraplegia, paraparesis, spasticity, Brown-Sequard syndrome, hyperreflexia, hypertonia, Babinski sign, and sphincteric dysfunction. Sensory changes can include diminished sensations of spinothalamic tract (pain, temperature, and crude touch) and posterior column tract (proprioception, vibration, and fine touch).

As RM is a diagnosis of exclusion, correlation of the patient's clinical manifestation with anatomical treated region of the spinal cord and radiation dose is essential, along with excluding disease recurrence or progression. This is usually achieved by imaging tests, typically MRI. Signal changes associated with RM include hyperintense signals on T2-weighted MR images and iso- or hypointense signals on T1-weighted MR images, with or without variable patterns of enhancement due to necrosis (Fig. 37.2) [10, 11]. At present, other imaging modalities including FDG-PET scans remain investigational [12].

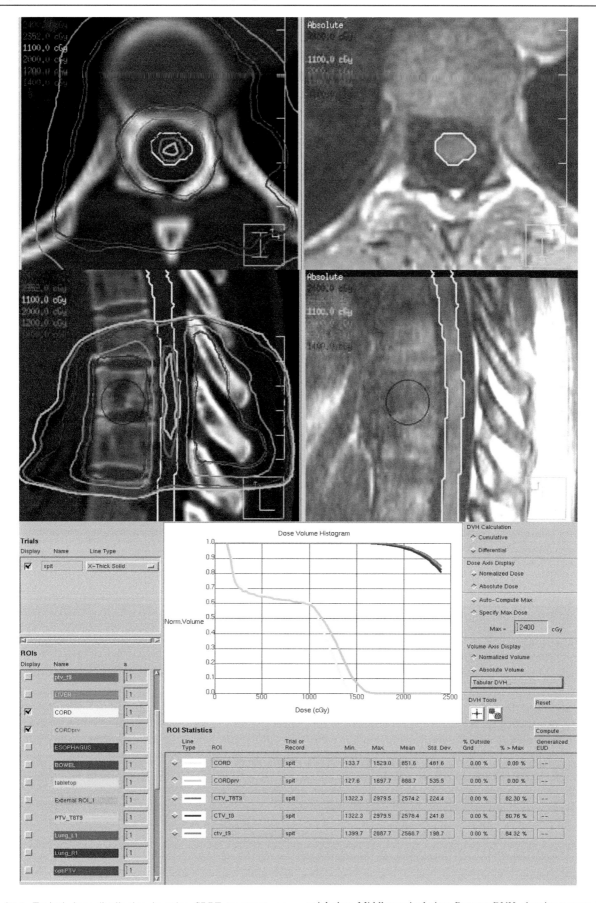

**Fig. 37.1** Typical dose distribution in spine SBRT treatment prescribed 24 Gy in 2 fractions with a point maximum dose constraint set to the spinal cord planning organ-at-risk volume (PRV) of 17 Gy. Top:
axial view. Middle: sagittal view. Bottom: DVH, showing a steep dose falloff with a maximum dose to the cord of 1529 cGy and to cord PRV of 1697.7 cGy, while the maximum dose within the PTV is 2979.5 cGy

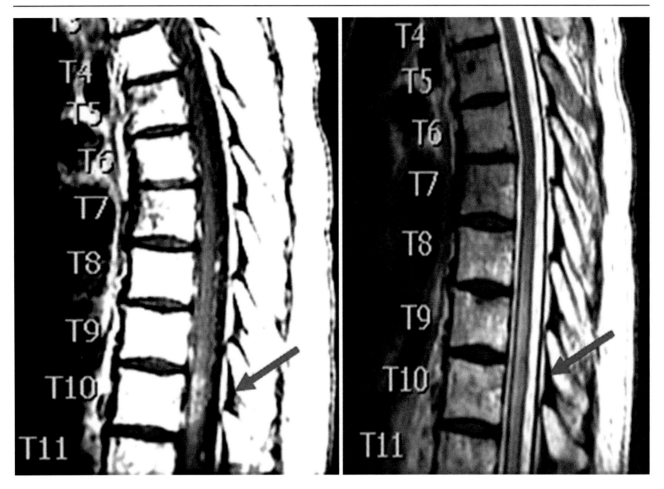

**Fig. 37.2** MRI findings of RM. This patient had been treated with conventional radiation and a dose of 30 Gy in ten fractions with a point maximum dose (Pmax) of 33 Gy within the spinal canal at the level of T10. Three months later, the patient was conventionally re-irradiated with 25 Gy in ten fractions to the same region with a Pmax of 26 Gy within the spinal canal. Seven months later the patient developed a sensory level from T10 caudally. MRI revealed on the left moderate enhancement within the spinal cord at T10 (arrow) on the sagittal T1-weighted image with gadolinium and on the right hyperintense signal (arrow) seen on the sagittal T2

## Pathophysiology and Histopathology

The molecular and cellular events underlying RM are considered as a damage continuum that remains incompletely understood. Although these events, such as changes in the gene expression profile, start almost immediately after irradiation, histopathological features are late findings. It is widely accepted that the targets of radiation injury include oligodendrocytes and vascular endothelial cells, resulting primarily in demyelination and disruption of blood-spinal cord barrier (BSCB), respectively [7]. Endothelial cell apoptosis is an early molecular event following irradiation that could result in early disruption of BSCB. It is a p53-independent process and involves ceramide generation as a result of acid sphingomyelinase activation secondary to radiation-induced endothelial membrane damage. The involvement of this process in late radiation damage is an area of controversy and remains to be explored. There is evidence that vascular endothelial growth factor (VEGF) upregulation and hypoxia play a role in late disruption of BSCB. In *Lhermitte's syndrome*, demyelination is transient due to reversible inhibition of oligodendrocytes proliferation and is not associated with developing a permanent RM [13].

Animal studies showed that the histopathological findings of irradiation injury to the spinal cord following inhomogeneous partial volume, and homogenous irradiation, are essentially the same [7]. While demyelination is typically confined to white matter, along with reactive gliosis and necrosis, vascular endothelial cell injury can be observed in either white or gray matter.

## Radiobiology

The clinical response of normal tissue to radiation is dependent on many factors including intrinsic radiosensitivity, total dose, dose per fraction, overall treatment time, dose rate, type of tissue, volume of irradiated tissue, baseline tissue function, and the use of radiosensitizers or radioprotectors.

A pervasive radiobiologic concept is the organization of normal tissues into functional subunits (FSU), defined as the largest tissue volume or unit of cells that can be regenerated from a single surviving congenic cell [14]. Based on this model, organ dysfunction is dependent on the arrangement of FSU into serial or parallel arrangements within the organ; in addition, the model affords for mixed proportions of serial and parallel arrangements. The spinal cord has been considered a serial organ (FSU are arranged in a linear fashion); hence, the risk of RM has been considered dependent on the dose to even a single FSU, as opposed to dose received by a partial volume. This notion of FSU is much debated and will be discussed in subsequent sections.

## Mathematical Radiobiologic Modeling of Spinal Cord Data

The linear-quadratic (LQ) model is the most widely used model in experimental and clinical radiobiology, largely due to its simplicity. It is the basis for the *biologic effective dose* (BED) calculation that equates dose-fractionation schemes into a single number. The BED facilitates comparisons of different dose-fractionations schemes in terms of expected efficacy (tumor BED) and both acute and late toxicity (normal tissue BED). It is calculated as:

$$BED = nd \left(1 + \frac{d}{\alpha/\beta}\right).$$

where $n$ is the number of fractions and $d$ is the dose per fraction. For the spinal cord, extensive experimental data have shown that the fractionation sensitivity for RM could be described by an $\alpha/\beta$ value of approximately 2 or 3 Gy, and most use 2 as a conservative estimate [1, 4, 15]. For tumor, most use an $\alpha/\beta$ of 10. For example, 30 Gy in ten fractions, assuming an $\alpha/\beta$ of 2 Gy for the fractionation sensitivity of

the spinal cord gives a BED of $10 * 3(1 + \frac{3}{2}) = 75$ Gy$_2$. For

tumor, with an $\alpha/\beta$ of 10 Gy, the BED = 39 Gy$_{10}$. In the case of 24 Gy in two fractions, which is typical of SBRT practice, and limiting the spinal cord planning organ-at-risk volume (PRV) to 17 Gy in two fractions, the BED is 89.3 Gy$_2$ for the spinal cord tolerance and 52.8 Gy$_{10}$ with respect to tumor efficacy. Therefore, one can appreciate that SBRT dose escalates the tumor with respect to BED and represents greater dose exposure to the spinal cord.

More recently it is increasingly recognized that standardization of reporting is needed, and the BED should be equated in a 2 Gy equivalent known as the EQD2. It is considered more practical as it converts dose/fractionation

into a dose fractionation size that is more familiar to radiation oncologists. EQD2 equation is given as:

$$EQD2 = nd \left(\frac{d + \alpha/\beta}{2 + \alpha/\beta}\right)$$

For example, 30 Gy in ten fractions yields an EQD2 of 37.5 Gy$_2$ for RM ($\alpha/\beta = 2$ Gy) and an EQD2 of 32.5 Gy$_{10}$ for tumor ($\alpha/\beta = 10$ Gy). Using 24 Gy in two fractions and a 17 Gy dose limit to the cord PRV, the EQD2 is 44.6 Gy$_2$ for RM ($\alpha/\beta = 2$ Gy) and 44 Gy$_{10}$ for the tumor ($\alpha/\beta = 10$Gy).

The LQ is reasonably accurate for conventional fractionation (1.8–3 Gy); however, its predictive capacity for tolerance specific to very high dose per fraction (>15 Gy per fraction) regimens, inherent to SBRT, has been questioned. When considering re-treatment, one should also always keep in mind that the LQ does not take into account the time interval between courses, and a longer time interval between courses may be associated with increasing recovery and increased tolerance.

Lyman et al. developed a model describing a power-law relationship between the irradiated volume and dose tolerance assuming uniform irradiation [16]. This model was extended to inhomogeneous irradiation resulting in the Lyman-Kutcher-Burman (LKB) model [17]. While this model has its value in conventional radiation, Daly et al. reported an overestimation of the risk of RM with the LKB method in predicting spinal cord tolerance specific to spine SBRT [18]. In that study, patients with hemangioblastoma were treated with 20 Gy in single fraction or 20–25 Gy in two to three fractions, resulting in point maximum doses within the spinal cord of 22.7 and 22 Gy, respectively. Using Emami parameters and an $\alpha/\beta$ of 3 Gy, the model resulted in a 54% risk of RM, while the observed rate was 4%. Although the sample size of the patient population was limited, the data indicate caution in extrapolating existing models to extreme hypofractionation regimens.

Modifications have been incorporated into the LQ model to allow for better estimate of BED for extreme hypofractionation as in the case of SBRT. For example, Wang et al. introduced a generalized LQ model in which the original LQ model was modified to account for reduced sublethal damage at high doses per fraction compared to conventional fractionation [19, 20]. It is important to appreciate that all models have their own caveats and limitations and should be used with caution in clinic. Despite the issues with the original LQ model, it remains one with the least number of assumptions and provides a number to guide safe practice. Further research is needed to develop more accurate models for safe clinical practice that are clinically validated.

## Radiobiological Issues Related to Spinal Cord Tolerance and SBRT

SBRT allows for maximal dose delivery to a target close to the spinal cord while limiting its dose. Inherent to SBRT dose distributions, small volumes (e.g., a point maximum volume or 0.1 cc) of spinal cord can be exposed to the higher doses with a rapid dose drop-off such that larger volumes (e.g., 0.5, 1, 2 cc) receive very low doses (Fig. 37.1).

The BED method assumes that a surface dose enclosing a volume of interest is sufficient in surrogating the biological response of the entire contoured organ regardless of the distribution of hot spots within the target or OAR, which is again an inherent characteristic of SBRT. Thus, the concern regarding using this method to estimate cord tolerance when a small part of the cord receives high dose while most of the cord receives near-zero dose was raised. Sahgal and Ma developed a generalized BED (gBED) method to account for the gradient of dose deposition within small inhomogeneously irradiated structure volume [21]. When this method was applied to a data set of patients with and without RM, it was found that the gBED resulted in a statistically significant difference in mean gBED, at both the point maximum volume and 0.1 cm$^3$ volume as compared to the point maximum volume only when using the straight BED approach.

The use of the BED has also been applied to the re-treatment scenario. One approach is to simply sum the BED of both courses to provide an estimate of what is safe for the re-treatment course and the cumulative exposure. However, the simple approach of adding the individual BEDs from different courses may not yield an accurate cumulative BED as the locations of hot spots can vary. In an attempt to overcome this issue, Ma et al. also developed a gBED method specific for repeat SBRT [22]. One of the key findings of the gBED model was that when dealing with doses to sufficiently small volumes of interest such as point maximum and 0.1 cc doses etc., both serial and parallel structures converge to similar behavior that may be modeled with the same mathematical formulas. As a result, the point maximum cumulative EQD2 can be used as a conservative value to guide safe spine SBRT re-treatments. A major shortcoming regardless of the model, and all known models in this regard, is the inability to model the influence of the time interval between the two courses. Clinical and preclinical data are consistent with evidence for significant time-dependent recovery of occult damage. At present, there is no robust and simple method to incorporate the influence of long-term time-dependent recovery into the BED model.

## Preclinical Studies of Spinal Cord Tolerance

Preclinical studies in rodents and small animals involving direct spinal cord radiation to determine tolerance have provided important insights with respect to human cord tolerance. However, direct extrapolation of animal data to the human spinal cord should be considered with caution.

Animal studies are costly and involve extensive ethical considerations including reduction in the number of animals to the absolute minimum required to yield statistical power a priori. Irradiation parameters of interest have been the subject of rodent studies and include variation in radiation dose, dose per fraction, dose rate, energy, region and length of irradiated cord, radiation technique, homogeneity of the dose distribution, and irradiation under general anesthesia. One unknown that remains a cause for concern is the difference in biology/radiobiology of the spinal cord between that of rodents/small animals and humans. A common conception is that the pig spinal cord likely approximates best that of the human. The complexity of modern radiation techniques and the ability to mimic new irradiation conditions in small animals add to the cost and complexity of animal studies, and only recently has it been possible to perform such experiments. In addition, the traditional endpoint in animal studies for tolerance is the dose resulting in a 50% rate of RM (ED50) based on clinical observation of motor dysfunction, while 5% rate of RM (ED5) is more relevant for human clinical practice. However, unlike clinical studies, histopathological examination of irradiated cord segments is usually available for correlation to the clinical observation and represents strength of animal-based experiments. Lastly, most animal data stems from rat irradiation; however, recent studies in pigs have provided evidence of spinal cord tolerance in the setting of modern radiation distributions inherent to SBRT.

## De Novo Radiation

### Uniform Versus Nonuniform Irradiation (Lateral Dose-Volume Effect)

"Uniform" irradiation refers to the delivery of a homogeneous dose distribution throughout the irradiated cord, while the "lateral dose-volume effect" refers to nonuniform radiation across an axial cross section of the spinal cord resulting in partial-volume irradiation. Historically, uniform irradiation to the spinal cords of rats, guinea pigs, and mice to lengths >16 mm has consistently yielded similar single dose ED50 of approximately 20 Gy [23–30].

Recently, rodents were exposed in a series of experiments with uniform and nonuniform spinal cord irradiation using a proton beam. The hypothesis being that partial-volume irradiation would yield a greater ED50 versus uniform irradiation. One potential mechanism of the increased tolerance stems from experimental data that suggests the potential for oligodendrocytes and their precursors to migrate a distance of 2–3 mm and effectively remyelinate the radiation-induced damage [31, 32]. In these rat-based experiments, a greater ED50 of 30 Gy was observed as compared to 20 Gy for the nonuniform and uniform irradiation, respectively [33, 34]. Interestingly, the ED50 for uniform irradiation was consistent with previous photon-based data.

Medin et al. exposed 4.5–7 cm of Yucatan minipig spinal cord with uniform irradiation to point maximum doses of 17.5, 19.5, 22, and 24.1 Gy in a single fraction [30]. ED50 in that study was 20.2 Gy. In another study, the same group performed spinal cord partial-volume (nonuniform) irradiation using 6 MV SBRT technique [35]. In that study, minipigs were irradiated with doses of 47, 36, 24, 22, 20, 18, 16, and 12 Gy in a single fraction prescribed to the 90% isodose line covering a target positioned lateral to spinal cord. In the resulting dose distribution, the 90%, 50%, and 10% isodose line were traversing ipsilateral, central, and contralateral spinal cord. Fourteen out of twenty-six pigs developed clinical and histological RM with a follow-up of at least 1 year. The ED50 for the maximal dose to the spinal cord was 20 Gy. Although, there was less debilitating neurologic and histopathologic morbidity with nonuniform irradiation, the ED50 was similar between uniform and nonuniform irradiation in these two experiments.

These results indicate that there may not be a dramatic effect associated with nonuniform radiation when applied to a species closer to the human spinal cord.

## Longitudinal Dose-Volume Effects (Length Effect)

### Homogeneous Dose Distribution

Animal data has shown that ED50 values decrease by approximately fourfold when the irradiated spinal cord length is increased from 2 to 20 mm [28], while no such effect is observed when the irradiated length is increased from 25 to 100 mm [36]. Hopewell et al. investigated irradiated rat spinal cord lengths from 4 to 16 mm and observed a similar length effect as Bijl et al. [25] Considering the observations from all studies of the length effect, it is likely that the length effect is only observed for lengths <1.6 cm. This may be significant for clinical SBRT to very small targets near the spinal cord, but most clinicians are reluctant to escalate the dose to the spinal cord beyond currently perceived tolerance thresholds for larger volumes [18, 37].

### Inhomogeneous Dose Distribution (Bath and Shower Effect)

Bath and shower effect refers to a phenomenon observed when irradiating a smaller and central segment of the cord to a higher dose (shower), concurrently with a lower dose to a longer segment (bath) that includes the shower volume. Bijl et al. irradiated rat spinal cords with protons using a 20 mm field length for bath doses, which contained a smaller central shower field of 2, 4, or 8 mm. The bath doses were 4 or 18 Gy, and the shower doses were variable in single fractions. For the 2 mm shower length, the ED50 was 61.2 Gy in shower-bath experiments, compared to 87.8 Gy in single

field (only shower) for a 4 Gy bath dose, and was significantly lower when the bath dose was increased to 18 Gy [28, 38]. This effect was only observed for the 2 and 4 mm, but not for 8 mm, field size that received shower doses. When the experiment was conducted using a bath area (10 mm) cephalad to the shower area (2 mm), hence both arranged longitudinally, the resultant ED50 was 68.6 Gy. The authors suggested that this effect is less likely explained by migration of stem progenitor cells, which can only travel 2–3 mm. This interesting effect likely has no implication in the clinic.

### Regional Variation in Cord Tolerance

Using an irradiated cord length of 20 mm, Bijl et al. irradiated with protons the lateral and central cervical spinal cord in rats [34]. The ED50 values were 28.9 Gy and 33.4 Gy for the lateral wide and lateral tight irradiations, respectively. The ED50 was as high as 71.9 Gy when only the central spinal cord was irradiated, compared with 20.4 Gy for the homogeneously irradiated 20-mm length of cervical spinal cord. The authors concluded that lateral white matter is more radiosensitive than central gray matter. This observation is consistent with that fact that most radiation-induced lesions are almost exclusively seen in white matter in animal studies.

There are no conclusive animal-based data to suggest a difference in radiation tolerance between the cervical and thoracic spinal cord. However, in a modeling study by Schultheiss et al., based on human clinical published data, a best fit dose-response curve suggested the thoracic spine to be "theoretically" less radiosensitive than the cervical cord which was found to have a lower $\alpha/\beta$ of 0.87 Gy [39].

## Re-irradiation

### Re-irradiation with Conventional Doses

The seminal animal study reporting re-irradiation tolerance of the spinal cord in animals was published in 1993 by Ang et al. [40]. Twelve asymptomatic rhesus monkeys were re-irradiated to cumulative doses of 83.6, 92.4, or 101.2 Gy, 2 years following 70.4 Gy. Another group of 15 animals were re-irradiated to cumulative doses of 83.6, 92.4, 101.2, or 110 Gy, 2 years after a prior 44 Gy treatment. In all cases, radiation was given in 2.2 Gy daily fractions. Only two animals in each group developed RM at 2-year follow-up after re-irradiation. It was concluded that there was significant recovery of occult damage after initial treatment with the most conservative model estimating a 61% recovery of tolerance by a year posttreatment [41].

Data from re-irradiation studies of rat spinal cord also showed significant occult damage recovery [24, 42]. Similar findings were demonstrated in a guinea pig myelopathy model [43]. There is evidence that recovery is dependent on the size and total dose of the first treatment in addition to the interval between the two courses [24]. Wong et al. found an increase in latent time to paralysis when re-irradiation occurs >8 weeks after initial treatment [42].

## Re-irradiation with Single Dose Following Conventional Treatment

In rats, Wong et al. observed an ED50 of a single dose of 19 Gy with no prior radiation. Following re-irradiation after 20 weeks, an ED50 of 17 Gy was found following initial radiation with 2.15 Gy × 10 fractions, 15.7 Gy following a course of 2.15 Gy × 20 fractions, and 14 Gy after 2.15 Gy × 30 fractions and 11.8 Gy after 2.15 Gy × 36 fractions. This observation is important as it indicates that re-irradiation tolerance of spinal cord in rats decreases as initial radiation dose increases [24].

## Re-irradiation with SBRT Following Conventional Treatment

Medin et al., using SBRT technique similar to that used in clinic, re-irradiated the cervical spine of pigs with 14.9, 17.1, 19, 21.2, 23.4, or 25.4 Gy, 1 year after initial radiation treatment at the same level with 30 Gy in ten fractions [44]. The re-treatment mimicked SBRT as a partial volume was re-irradiated. A steep dose-response curve was observed with an ED50 for maximum dose of 19.7 Gy. Comparing this finding to the ED50 of de novo irradiated pigs in their historic companion study (ED50 = 20), the authors concluded that tolerance of the spinal cord of pigs to re-irradiation SBRT doses was not significantly lower than cord tolerance in de novo radiosurgery.

## Re-irradiation with Single Dose Following Hypofractionated Treatment and Effect of Timing Interval

Wong et al. irradiated adult rats using two or three fractions of 9 Gy or three fractions of 10.25 Gy [42]. At day 4, weeks 6, 8, 12, 20, 28, or 40, animals were re-irradiated with graded doses in single fractions. ED50 gradually increased with increasing time intervals (ranging from 14.1 to 16.2 Gy) in animals initially receiving 9 Gy × 2 fractions. Similarly, ED50 increased from 10 to 14.7 Gy as the time interval increased between the two courses of radiation. In the group received initially irradiated with 10.25 Gy × 3 fractions, the ED50 ranged from 5.8 to 13.3 Gy, again as time intervals increased so did the ED50.

## Clinical Data of Spinal Cord Tolerance

Generally, the available clinical data on radiation tolerance of spinal cord is sparse and largely based on retrospective analyses.

## De Novo Spinal Cord Tolerance with Conventionally Fractionated Radiation

In 1991, Emami et al. published a landmark literature review of normal tissue tolerance with conventionally fractionated doses at 1.8–2.0 Gy per day [2]. With respect to spinal cord tolerance, 50 and 70 Gy were recommended as associated with a 5% and 50% risk of transverse myelitis at 5 years, respectively. 60 and 75 Gy to the whole cauda equina were determined to carry a 5-year risk of clinically apparent nerve damage of 5% and 50%, respectively. It is important to note that the data was largely absent to make these recommendations, and these threshold values are based on expert opinion.

Given the significant advances in radiation therapy including 3D CRT and modern dosimetry, the Quantitative Analysis of Normal Tissue Effects in the Clinic (QUANTEC) report was published in 2010 [45]. Based on the updated literature review, a RM risk of 0.2%, 6%, and 50% was associated with 50, 60, and 69 Gy when delivered with conventional fractionation. The endpoints of QUANTEC were clearly defined as grade 2 myelitis or higher as per Common Terminology Criteria for Adverse Events v3.0.

There may be potential to dose escalate safely beyond these accepted dose limits; however, this is not recommended outside of specialized quaternary centers. For example, Delaney et al. showed no cases of RM following high doses of conventional photon or proton irradiation for chordoma and chondrosarcoma cases at a median follow-up of 7.3 years [46]. Radiation doses in this study were ≤72 GyRBE in 25 patients and 67.6–77.4 GyRBE in another 25 patients (GyRBE for protons = Gy × 1.1). The actual doses received by spinal cord were not reported, however; the study dose limits were reported separately with 54 GyRBE to the center of the spinal cord, 63 GyRBE to the surface of the spinal cord, and 70.2 GyRBE to the cauda equina except at tumor contact where the dose was limited to 77.4 GyRBE [47].

## Spinal Cord Tolerance to De Novo Stereotactic Body Radiation Therapy (SBRT)

According to a logistic regression model for nine cases of RM compared to controls, Sahgal et al. estimated a 5% or less risk of RM when the maximum point dose (Pmax) to the thecal sac (surrogate for the true spinal cord) was limited to 12.4 Gy in single fraction, 17 Gy in two fractions, 20.3 Gy in three fractions, 23 Gy in four fractions, and 25.3 Gy in five fractions [6]. Although QUANTEC recommended a cord dose of 13 Gy in single fraction and 20 Gy in three fractions to be associated with a clinically acceptable rate of myelopathy (<1%), this was based on the consensus expert opinion, and no actual data were presented to derive the risk estimate [45].

Daly et al. reported on a cohort of 19 patients with 27 spinal hemangioblastoma tumors treated with single SRS or SBRT in 2–3 fractions [37]. Median doses of SRS and SBRT were 20 Gy and 18–25 Gy, respectively. Pmax to the cord were 22.7 Gy in SRS patients and 14.1 Gy in SBRT patients. Only one patient with a history of von Hippel-Lindau developed grade 2 unilateral foot drop 5 months later after 20 Gy in single faction to T10 with the spinal cord maximum dose of 17.8 Gy. Two other patients developed grade 1 sensory deficit 3 years after a prescribed dose of 18 Gy in single fraction to T7 and 18 months after 20 Gy in two fractions to T11 in another patient. No details specific to the cord dose in these two cases were reported. These data highlight the inherent heterogeneity in spinal cord dose tolerance. At present, there is a spectrum of radiosensitivity but no ability to determine a priori who we can dose escalate and who in others we need to be conservative.

## Spinal Cord Tolerance to Re-irradiation with Conventional Fractionation

Based on early reported cases of RM by Wong et al., a cumulative BED of <120 $Gy_2$ is considered a safe dose limit resulting in an ~5% risk of RM [1]. In a subsequent analysis based on the same data but expanded controls, a cumulative BED of 135.5 $Gy_2$ (EQD2 67.7 $Gy_2$) was considered safe when neither radiation course exceeds a BED of 98 $Gy_2$ (EQD2 49 $Gy_2$) and a longer than 6-month interval between courses respected [15].

## Spinal Cord Tolerance to Re-irradiation with SBRT

### Following Previous Conventional External Beam Radiation

Based on a DVH analysis of the thecal sac doses in patients who did and did not develop RM, Sahgal et al. recommended a re-irradiation spinal cord (contoured based on the thecal sac) Pmax BED normalized to a 2 Gy equivalent BED (termed nBED in the paper which is the same as EQD2 when an $\alpha/\beta = 2$ Gy) of 20–25 $Gy_2$ with the caveat that the total Pmax EQD2 of 70 $Gy_2$ is respected which is again assuming

a spinal cord $\alpha/\beta$ of 2 Gy and a time interval of at least 5 months between courses [5].

One of the largest re-irradiation SBRT series to date was published by Hashmi et al. [48]. At 8-month follow-up, there were no observed RM cases in 215 patients. The median SBRT re-irradiation total dose was 18 Gy delivered in a single fraction 13.5 months following a median conventional palliative radiation regimen of 30 Gy in ten fractions. In that series, the cumulative median Pmax EQD2 to the spinal cord PRV (1.5–2 mm)/thecal sac was 60.8 $Gy_2$ and 24.6 $Gy_2$ specific to the SBRT re-treatment regimen. These clinical data support the Sahgal et al. recommendations.

### Following Previous SBRT

Data for re-irradiation with SBRT following a previous SBRT treatment is limited. However, a single-institution experience of 32 spinal segments, treated with 30 Gy in four fractions at a median time interval of 12.9 months after a prior treatment of 24 Gy in two fractions observed no RM or cauda equina toxicity [49]. The re-irradiation Pmax EQD2 to the cord PRV was 21.9 $Gy_2$, and the cumulative was 51.3 $Gy_2$. Pmax EQD2 to the thecal sac (at the level of cauda equina) for tumors in the lumbar-sacral region was 23.5 $Gy_2$ for re-treatment and 54.6 $Gy_2$ for the cumulative EQD2.

## Extreme Re-treatment (>Two Courses of Radiation)

Again, human data for cord tolerance to multiple courses of radiation therapy with at least one SBRT treatment are severely lacking. In the abovementioned case series, 24 spinal segments had been irradiated with conventional radiation therapy with doses in the range of 22.5–37.5 Gy prior to the subsequent two SBRT treatments [49]. Median cumulative Pmax EQD2 (considering $\alpha/\beta$ of 2 Gy) to spinal cord PRV was 73.9 $Gy_2$ and to thecal sac (for cauda equina) was 80.4 $Gy_2$. Again, there were no observed cases of RM or cauda equina toxicity.

## Strategies to Mitigate RM

Over the last decade, with the improved understanding of the mechanisms of radiation-induced spinal cord injury, research has focused on strategies to mitigate and treat the injury. Research strategies are largely based on either reducing the secondary damage or repairing the primary damage through restoration of neural cells. The former can be achieved by targeting hypoxia with vascular endothelial growth factor (VEGF) inhibitors (i.e., bevacizumab) [50] or reducing disruption of blood-spinal cord barrier (BSCB) by using steroids or antibodies against intracellular adhesion molecules [51]. Valproic acid and fluoxetine have been proven to act as neuroprotectors. Erythropoietin has anti-inflammatory and neuroprotective properties [52, 53]; however, the increased risk of thromboembolic disease has limited its use in cancer patients [53]. Hyperbaric oxygen therapy was used for some neurological diseases and RM based on anecdotal reports [54, 55]. Currently, research on stem cell therapy to repair radiation-induced neural cell injury is ongoing with early encouraging results in animal models. The reader is referred to the recent review reported by Wong et al. for more details [7].

## Suggested Considerations and Guidelines for Safe Practice

1. Contouring: for conventional treatment, we recommend contouring the spinal canal. In case of treating spinal tumors with SBRT, we recommend contouring spinal cord and adding a 1.5 mm PRV to account for setup uncertainties or contour the thecal sac with no applied PRV margin. Contours should be extended at least one vertebral body above and below the treated level. At the level of the cauda equina, we recommend contouring the entire thecal sac. Cord and thecal sac contouring should be performed using fused thin slice volumetric axial T1- and T2-weighted MRI and correlated with thin slice (1.0–2.0 mm slice thickness) CT simulation scan. Caution should be taken when treating the cervical spine, as fusion of the MRI can be difficult due to the curvature of the c-spine. For post-op SBRT treatments, a treatment planning myelogram can help if visualization of the cord is obscured by metal instrumentation. The interested reader should refer to the Sahgal et al. Canadian Association of Radiation Oncology recommendations for spine SBRT [3] and a recent overview of spine SBRT response determination by Thibault et al. as led by Sahgal on behalf of the SPIne Neuro-Oncology (SPINO) response assessment group [56].

2. Treatment delivery: IMRT/VMAT can shape the high dose around the spinal cord. Image guidance with associated six degree-of-freedom patient alignment correction capability is recommended for spine SBRT treatments. We recommend daily cone beam CT (CBCT) scans with a threshold of 1 mm and 1° and matching to the spinal canal. The spine SBRT technique at the University of Toronto has been extensively scrutinized and reported by Hyde et al. [57].

3. Dose limits: Table 37.1 summaries suggested dose limits for spinal conventional and SBRT de novo and re-treatment. Practical case scenarios are provided in Table 37.2. Figures 37.3, 37.4, 37.5, and 37.6 show reported RM doses in relation to suggested dose limits.

**Table 37.1** Suggested dose limits for the spinal cord

| Treatment | Organ at risk | Suggested dose limits (maximum point dose) |
|---|---|---|
| De novo conventional radiation | Spinal canal | 50–60 Gy in 1.8–2.0 Gy per fractions [45] |
| De novo SBRT (1–5 fractions with >5 Gy/fraction) | Cord PRV or thecal sac | (EQD2 = 44.7 $Gy_2$) [6, 45]<br>12.4 Gy in single fraction<br>17 Gy in two fractions<br>20.3 Gy in three fractions<br>25.3 in five fractions |
| Re-treatment conventional radiation (<5 Gy/fraction) | Spinal canal | 1. Cumulative EQD2 should be limited to 67.5 $Gy_2$<br>2. Neither course to exceed 49 $Gy_2$<br>3. ≥6-month interval between courses respected [15] |
| Re-treatment SBRT | Cord PRV or thecal sac | 1. Cumulative EQD2 < 70 $Gy_2$<br>2. Second course not to exceed an EQD2 of 25 $Gy_2$<br>3. Point maximum EQD2/cumulative EQD2 < 50%<br>4. ≥5-month interval between courses [5] |

**Table 37.2** Clinical scenarios of using suggested dose limits for re-treatment

| Clinical scenario | EQD2 cord limit |
|---|---|
| Prior treatment to thoracic spinal metastasis with 30 Gy/10 fx using a parallel opposed AP/PA beam arrangement. Spinal cord received 33 Gy (110%) in ten fractions (EQD2 43.7 $Gy_2$). Re-treatment with *conventional radiation* was indicated for local progression after 7 months | – Using the suggested cumulative EQD2 dose constraint for spinal canal of 67.5 $Gy_2$, the maximum EQD2 remaining for the re-treatment:<br>67.5–43.7 = 23.8 $Gy_2$<br>– Options for re-irradiation include:<br>20 Gy/5 fx giving an EQD2 of 30 $Gy_2$ or 20Gy/8 fx giving an EQD2 of 22.5 $Gy_2$<br>– 20 Gy/8 fx is considered a safer approach for re-treating this patient attempt should be made to avoid or minimize hot spots to the spinal cord in the re-treatment setting |

**Table 37.2** (continued)

| Clinical scenario | EQD2 cord limit |
|---|---|
| Prior radiation with 20 Gy/5 fx using a parallel opposed AP/PA beam arrangement for thoracic spinal bony metastasis from prostate cancer. The spinal cord had received a point maximum dose of 22 Gy (110% of prescribed dose) in 5 fx (EQD2 = 35.2 $Gy_2$). Two years later, he developed symptomatic in-field local recurrence. The patient was a candidate for SBRT re-treatment | – Using the above dose limit criteria, suggested safe dose constraints for SBRT re-treatment are:<br>*Cord PRV limit for single fx:* 8.9 Gy<br>– Re-treatment EQD2 = 24.25 $Gy_2$ (<25 $Gy_2$)<br>– Cumulative EQD2 = 35.2 + 24.25 = 59.45 $Gy_2$ (<70 $Gy_2$)<br>– Point maximum EQD2 for re-treatment/cumulative EQD2 = 40.8% (<50%)<br>*Cord PRV limit for 2 frx:* 12.2 Gy<br>– Re-treatment EQD2 = 24.71 $Gy_2$ (<25 $Gy_2$)<br>– Cumulative EQD2 = 59.91 $Gy_2$ (<70 $Gy_2$)<br>– Point maximum EQD2 for re-treatment/cumulative EQD2 = 41.2% (<50%)<br>*Cord PRV limit for 3 frx:* 14.5 Gy<br>– Re-treatment EQD2 = 24.65 $Gy_2$ (<25 $Gy_2$)<br>– Cumulative EQD2 = 59.85 $Gy_2$ (<70 $Gy_2$)<br>– Point maximum EQD2 for re-treatment/cumulative EQD2 = 41.2% (<50%)<br>*Cord PRV limit for 4 frx:* 16.2 Gy<br>– Re-treatment EQD2 = 24.5 $Gy_2$ (<25 $Gy_2$)<br>– Cumulative EQD2 = 59.7 $Gy_2$ (<70 $Gy_2$)<br>– Point maximum EQD2 for re-treatment/cumulative EQD2 = 41% (<50%)<br>*Cord PRV limit for 5 frx:* 17.9 Gy<br>– Re-treatment EQD2 = 24.97 $Gy_2$ (<25 $Gy_2$)<br>– Cumulative EQD2 = 60.2 $Gy_2$ (<70 $Gy_2$)<br>– Point maximum EQD2 for re-treatment/cumulative EQD2 = 41.5% (<50%)<br>– The preferred treatment at the University of Toronto is 24 Gy in 2 fx with a cord prv limit of 12.2 Gy |
| Prior SBRT with 24 Gy/2 fx to thoracic spine with the spinal cord PRV maximum dose 17 Gy (EQD2 = 44.63 $Gy_2$). Re-treatment with a second course of SBRT was indicated for isolated local recurrence 6 months later | – Re-treatment with 30 Gy/4 fx with a limit to the cord PRV of 16.2 Gy (EQD2 = 24.5 $Gy_2$) gives a cumulative EQD2 of 69.13 $Gy_2$ (<70 $Gy_2$)<br>– The second course EQD2 is <25 $Gy_2$ and the point maximum EQD2/cumulative EQD2 = 35.4% (<50%)<br>– This is the preferred regimen at the University of Toronto in accordance with the data from Thibault et al. [49] |

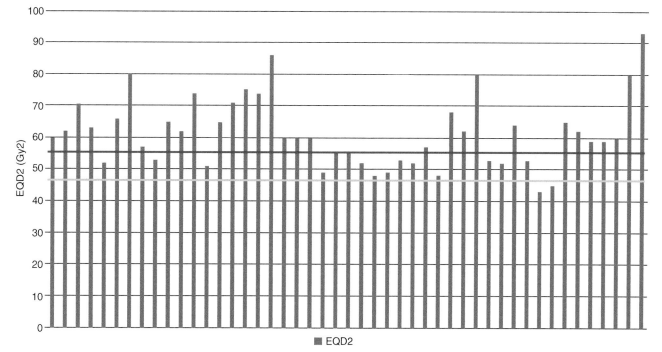

**Fig. 37.3** Spinal cord EQD2 following conventional fractionation radiation doses (de novo treatment) that have resulted in RM as derived from the literature. QUANTEC dose limits associated with 0.2% risk of myelopathy and 6% are shown in green and red, respectively

## Summary

- Radiation myelopathy is a diagnosis of exclusion. A correlation of clinical and MRI findings can confirm the diagnosis.
- The spinal cord is considered a serial organ with respect to radiation sensitivity. The LQ model is an accepted model to predict sensitivity; however, there are limita-

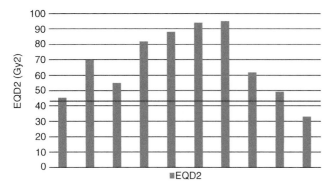

**Fig. 37.4** Spinal cord EQD2 that has resulted in RM specific to hypofractionated regimens and de novo SBRT. The recommended EQD2 of 44.7 $Gy_2$ is represented by the red line, and at this EQD2 the risk of RM is 5% or less

tions when extreme SBRT is applied. Although newer models may be more applicable, they require clinical validation.
- Radiobiological factors that determine the spinal cord sensitivity include dose, dose per fraction, uniform vs. nonuniform, homogenous vs. inhomogeneous radiation, previous radiation exposure, and the timing interval between radiation courses.
- Research is undergoing to find clinically acceptable strategies to mitigate the risk of radiation injury to the spinal cord.
- Following suggested SBRT practice guidelines and respecting the dose limits provided in Table 37.1, the risk of radiation myelopathy is considered to be below 5% and clinically acceptable.

## Self-Assessment Questions

1. Radiation myelopathy:
   A. Doesn't occur when safe dose constraint are used
   B. Occurs only after re-treatment of spinal cord
   C. Is a diagnosis of exclusion
   D. Is effectively treated with bevacizumab

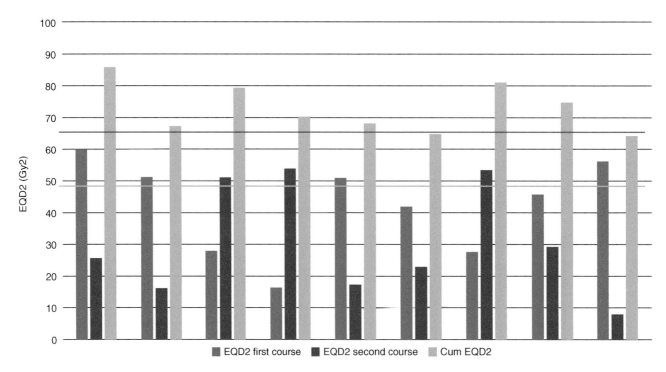

**Fig. 37.5** Spinal cord EQD2 that has resulted in RM with re-irradiation using conventional fractionation (<5 Gy/fraction). The recommended cumulative EQD2 should be <67.5 $Gy_2$ (BED 135 $Gy_2$) as indicated by red line and neither course to exceed 49 $Gy_2$ (BED 98 $Gy_2$) as indicated by green line

**Fig. 37.6** Spinal cord EQD2 that have resulted in RM after re-irradiation with at least one course of hypofractionation (>5 Gy/fraction). The recommended cumulative EQD2 < 70 Gy$_2$ is shown as the red line, and the second course not to exceed EQD2 of 25 Gy$_2$ is shown as the green line

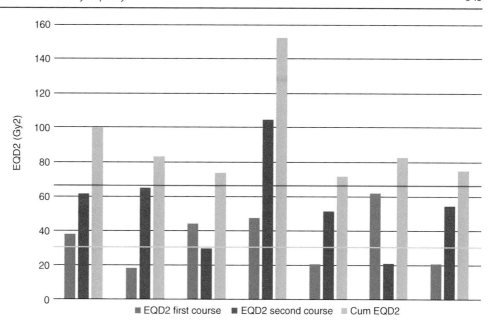

2. Data have shown that α/β ratio for late toxicity of spinal cord is:
   A. 2
   B. 10
   C. 4
   D. 3

3. Regarding ED50 in animal data:
   A. It is the most important single measured outcome
   B. Similar in all species
   C. Higher for partial spinal irradiation in rats
   D. Similar in both uniform and partial irradiation in pigs

4. Spinal cord dose of 60 Gy in 30 daily fractions (conventional radiation fraction sizes) is associated with RM risk of:
   A. 50%
   B. 0.2%
   C. 6%
   D. 5%

5. Safe re-treatment with SBRT involves:
   A. Cumulative EQD2 <67 Gy$_2$, second course not to exceed an EQD2 of 25 Gy$_2$, Pmax EQD2/cumulative EQD2 <50%, and ≥5-month interval between courses
   B. Cumulative EQD2 <70 Gy$_2$, second course not to exceed an EQD2 of 25 Gy$_2$, Pmax EQD2/cumulative EQD2 <50%, and ≥5-month interval between courses

C. Cumulative EQD2 <70 Gy$_2$, second course not to exceed an EQD2 of 20 Gy$_2$, Pmax EQD2/cumulative EQD2 <50%, and ≥5-month interval between courses
D. Cumulative EQD2 <70 Gy$_2$, second course not to exceed an EQD2 of 25 Gy$_2$, Pmax EQD2/cumulative EQD2 <50%, and ≥6-month interval between courses

## Answers

1. C
2. A
3. D
4. C
5. B

**Conflicts of Interest** Arjun Sahgal: Grants from Elekta AB and educational honoraria from previous educational seminars from Elekta AB, Varian Medical Systems, Accuray and Medtronic kyphoplasty division.

## References

1. Wong CS, Van Dyk J, Milosevic M, et al. Radiation myelopathy following single courses of radiotherapy and retreatment. Int J Radiat Oncol Biol Phys. 1994;30(3):575–81.
2. Emami B, Lyman J, Brown A, et al. Tolerance of normal tissue to therapeutic irradiation. Int J Radiat Oncol Biol Phys. 1991;21(1):109–22.

3. Sahgal A, Roberge D, Schellenberg D, et al. The Canadian association of radiation oncology scope of practice guidelines for lung, liver and spine stereotactic body radiotherapy. Clin Oncol (R Coll Radiol). 2012;24(9):629–39.

4. Sahgal A, Ma L, Gibbs I, et al. Spinal cord tolerance for stereotactic body radiotherapy. Int J Radiat Oncol Biol Phys. 2010;77(2):548–53.

5. Sahgal A, Ma L, Weinberg V, et al. Reirradiation human spinal cord tolerance for stereotactic body radiotherapy. Int J Radiat Oncol Biol Phys. 2012;82(1):107–16.

6. Sahgal A, Weinberg V, Ma L, et al. Probabilities of radiation myelopathy specific to stereotactic body radiation therapy to guide safe practice. Int J Radiat Oncol Biol Phys. 2013;85(2):341–7.

7. Wong CS, Fehlings MG, Sahgal A. Pathobiology of radiation myelopathy and strategies to mitigate injury. Spinal Cord. 2015;53(8):574–80.

8. Schultheiss TE, Higgins EM, El-Mahdi AM. The latent period in clinical radiation myelopathy. Int J Radiat Oncol Biol Phys. 1984;10(7):1109–15.

9. Schultheiss TE, Stephens LC, Peters LJ. Survival in radiation myelopathy. Int J Radiat Oncol Biol Phys. 1986;12(10):1765–9.

10. Wang PY, Shen WC, Jan JS. Serial MRI changes in radiation myelopathy. Neuroradiology. 1995;37(5):374–7.

11. Philippens ME, Gambarota G, van der Kogel AJ, et al. Radiation effects in the rat spinal cord: evaluation with apparent diffusion coefficient versus T2 at serial MR imaging. Radiology. 2009;250(2):387–97.

12. Uchida K, Nakajima H, Takamura T, et al. Neurological improvement associated with resolution of irradiation-induced myelopathy: serial magnetic resonance imaging and positron emission tomography findings. J Neuroimaging. 2009;19(3):274–6.

13. Esik O, Csere T, Stefanits K, et al. A review on radiogenic Lhermitte's sign. Pathol Oncol Res. 2003;9(2):115–20.

14. Withers HR, Taylor JM, Maciejewski B. Treatment volume and tissue tolerance. Int J Radiat Oncol Biol Phys. 1988;14(4):751–9.

15. Nieder C, Grosu AL, Andratschke NH, et al. Proposal of human spinal cord reirradiation dose based on collection of data from 40 patients. Int J Radiat Oncol Biol Phys. 2005;61(3):851–5.

16. Lyman JT. Complication probability as assessed from dose-volume histograms. Radiat Res Suppl. 1985;8:S13–9.

17. Kutcher GJ, Burman C. Calculation of complication probability factors for non-uniform normal tissue irradiation: the effective volume method. Int J Radiat Oncol Biol Phys. 1989;16(6):1623–30.

18. Daly ME, Luxton G, Choi CY, et al. Normal tissue complication probability estimation by the Lyman-Kutcher-Burman method does not accurately predict spinal cord tolerance to stereotactic radiosurgery. Int J Radiat Oncol Biol Phys. 2012;82(5):2025–32.

19. Wang JZ, Huang Z, Lo SS, et al. A generalized linear-quadratic model for radiosurgery, stereotactic body radiation therapy, and high-dose rate brachytherapy. Sci Transl Med. 2010;2(39):39ra48.

20. Huang Z, Mayr NA, Yuh WT, et al. Reirradiation with stereotactic body radiotherapy: analysis of human spinal cord tolerance using the generalized linear-quadratic model. Future Oncol. 2013;9(6):879–87.

21. Sahgal A, Ma L, Fowler J, et al. Impact of dose hot spots on spinal cord tolerance following stereotactic body radiotherapy: a generalized biological effective dose analysis. Technol Cancer Res Treat. 2012;11(1):35–40.

22. Ma L, Kirby N, Korol R, et al. Assessing small-volume spinal cord dose for repeat spinal stereotactic body radiotherapy treatments. Phys Med Biol. 2012;57(23):7843–51.

23. Lo YC, McBride WH, Withers HR. The effect of single doses of radiation on mouse spinal cord. Int J Radiat Oncol Biol Phys. 1992;22(1):57–63.

24. Wong CS, Poon JK, Hill RP. Re-irradiation tolerance in the rat spinal cord: influence of level of initial damage. Radiother Oncol. 1993;26(2):132–8.

25. Hopewell JW, Morris AD, Dixon-Brown A. The influence of field size on the late tolerance of the rat spinal cord to single doses of X rays. Br J Radiol. 1987;60(719):1099–108.

26. Knowles JF. The effects of single dose X-irradiation on the Guinea-pig spinal cord. Int J Radiat Biol Relat Stud Phys Chem Med. 1981;40(3):265–75.

27. Knowles JF. The radiosensitivity of the Guinea-pig spinal cord to X-rays: the effect of retreatment at one year and the effect of age at the time of irradiation. Int J Radiat Biol Relat Stud Phys Chem Med. 1983;44(5):433–42.

28. Bijl HP, van Luijk P, Coppes RP, et al. Dose-volume effects in the rat cervical spinal cord after proton irradiation. Int J Radiat Oncol Biol Phys. 2002;52(1):205–11.

29. Scalliet P, Landuyt W, van der Schueren E. Repair kinetics as a determining factor for late tolerance of central nervous system to low dose rate irradiation. Radiother Oncol. 1989;14(4):345–53.

30. Medin PM, Foster RD, van der Kogel AJ, et al. Spinal cord tolerance to single-session uniform irradiation in pigs: implications for a dose-volume effect. Radiother Oncol. 2013;106(1):101–5.

31. Franklin RJ, Gilson JM, Blakemore WF. Local recruitment of remyelinating cells in the repair of demyelination in the central nervous system. J Neurosci Res. 1997;50(2):337–44.

32. Withers R. Migration and myelination. Int J Radiat Oncol Biol Phys. 2003;57(1):9–10.

33. van Luijk P, Bijl HP, Coppes RP, et al. Techniques for precision irradiation of the lateral half of the rat cervical spinal cord using 150 MeV protons [corrected]. Phys Med Biol. 2001;46(11):2857–71.

34. Bijl HP, van Luijk P, Coppes RP, et al. Regional differences in radiosensitivity across the rat cervical spinal cord. Int J Radiat Oncol Biol Phys. 2005;61(2):543–51.

35. Medin PM, Foster RD, van der Kogel AJ, et al. Spinal cord tolerance to single-fraction partial-volume irradiation: a swine model. Int J Radiat Oncol Biol Phys. 2011;79(1):226–32.

36. van den Aardweg GJ, Hopewell JW, Whitehouse EM. The radiation response of the cervical spinal cord of the pig: effects of changing the irradiated volume. Int J Radiat Oncol Biol Phys. 1995;31(1):51–5.

37. Daly ME, Choi CY, Gibbs IC, et al. Tolerance of the spinal cord to stereotactic radiosurgery: insights from hemangioblastomas. Int J Radiat Oncol Biol Phys. 2011;80(1):213–20.

38. Bijl HP, van Luijk P, Coppes RP, et al. Influence of adjacent low-dose fields on tolerance to high doses of protons in rat cervical spinal cord. Int J Radiat Oncol Biol Phys. 2006;64(4):1204–10.

39. Schultheiss TE. The radiation dose-response of the human spinal cord. Int J Radiat Oncol Biol Phys. 2008;71(5):1455–9.

40. Ang KK, Price RE, Stephens LC, et al. The tolerance of primate spinal cord to re-irradiation. Int J Radiat Oncol Biol Phys. 1993;25(3):459–64.

41. Ang KK, Jiang GL, Feng Y, et al. Extent and kinetics of recovery of occult spinal cord injury. Int J Radiat Oncol Biol Phys. 2001;50(4):1013–20.

42. Wong CS, Hao Y. Long-term recovery kinetics of radiation damage in rat spinal cord. Int J Radiat Oncol Biol Phys. 1997;37(1):171–9.

43. Mason KA, Withers HR, Chiang CS. Late effects of radiation on the lumbar spinal cord of Guinea pigs: re-treatment tolerance. Int J Radiat Oncol Biol Phys. 1993;26(4):643–8.

44. Medin PM, Foster RD, van der Kogel AJ, et al. Spinal cord tolerance to reirradiation with single-fraction radiosurgery: a swine model. Int J Radiat Oncol Biol Phys. 2012;83(3):1031–7.

45. Kirkpatrick JP, van der Kogel AJ, Schultheiss TE. Radiation dose-volume effects in the spinal cord. Int J Radiat Oncol Biol Phys. 2010;76(3 Suppl):S42–9.

46. DeLaney TF, Liebsch NJ, Pedlow FX, et al. Long-term results of phase II study of high dose photon/proton radiotherapy in the management of spine chordomas, chondrosarcomas, and other sarcomas. J Surg Oncol. 2014;110(2):115–22.

47. DeLaney TF, Liebsch NJ, Pedlow FX, et al. Phase II study of high-dose photon/proton radiotherapy in the management of spine sarcomas. Int J Radiat Oncol Biol Phys. 2009;74(3):732–9.

48. Hashmi A, Guckenberger M, Kersh R, et al. Re-irradiation stereotactic body radiotherapy for spinal metastases: a multi-institutional outcome analysis. J Neurosurg Spine. 2016;25:1–8.

49. Thibault I, Campbell M, Tseng CL, et al. Salvage stereotactic body radiotherapy (SBRT) following in-field failure of initial SBRT for spinal metastases. Int J Radiat Oncol Biol Phys. 2015;93(2):353–60.

50. Nordal RA, Wong CS. Molecular targets in radiation-induced blood-brain barrier disruption. Int J Radiat Oncol Biol Phys. 2005;62(1):279–87.

51. Nordal RA, Wong CS. Intercellular adhesion molecule-1 and blood-spinal cord barrier disruption in central nervous system radiation injury. J Neuropathol Exp Neurol. 2004;63(5):474–83.

52. Brines ML, Ghezzi P, Keenan S, et al. Erythropoietin crosses the blood-brain barrier to protect against experimental brain injury. Proc Natl Acad Sci U S A. 2000;97(19):10526–31.

53. Tonia T, Mettler A, Robert N, et al. Erythropoietin or darbepoetin for patients with cancer. Cochrane Database Syst Rev. 2012;12:CD003407.

54. Helms A, Evans AW, Chu J, et al. Hyperbaric oxygen for neurologic indications action plan for multicenter trials in; stroke, traumatic brain injury, radiation encephalopathy & status migrainosus. Undersea Hyperb Med. 2011;38(5):309–19.

55. Calabro F, Jinkins JR. MRI of radiation myelitis: a report of a case treated with hyperbaric oxygen. Eur Radiol. 2000;10(7):1079–84.

56. Thibault I, Chang EL, Sheehan J, et al. Response assessment after stereotactic body radiotherapy for spinal metastasis: a report from the SPIne response assessment in neuro-oncology (SPINO) group. Lancet Oncol. 2015;16(16):e595–603.

57. Hyde D, Lochray F, Korol R, et al. Spine stereotactic body radiotherapy utilizing cone-beam CT image-guidance with a robotic couch: Intrafraction motion analysis accounting for all six degrees of freedom. Int J Radiat Oncol Biol Phys. 2012;82(3):e555–62.

# Radiation Optic Neuropathy

**38**

Andrea L. H. Arnett and Kenneth Wing Merrell

## Learning Objectives

- Understand common symptoms and physical findings of RION and retinopathy.
- Review basic pathophysiology, workup, and risk factors.
- Review radiation tolerance of retina and optic structures.
- Management of symptoms and therapeutic outcomes.

## Background and Epidemiology

Radiation-induced retinopathy and radiation-induced optic neuropathy (RION) are rare and disabling late-onset complications of ocular irradiation. Both can lead to profound and irreversible vision loss and substantial disability and are thus critically important to consider in the treatment of any intracranial or base of skull disease. RION and retinopathy are infrequently reported within the prospective literature, and true incidence is uncertain.

Most information regarding radiation tolerance of the retina and optic pathway is limited to retrospective reviews and case reports, often of extracranial disease sites with conventional fractionation. Adding further complexity to the topic is frequent utilization of hypofractionated radiotherapy, single or fractionated stereotactic radiosurgery (SRS), and charged-particle radiation with higher linear energy transfer (LET). Further research is needed to define dose constraints for emerging advanced radiation modalities. Ultimately, precise radiation planning and prevention are paramount, as existing treatment options for RION and retinopathy have limited efficacy.

## Diagnosis

Radiation-induced retinopathy and RION should be considered in the clinical setting of a patient with visual field deficits who

A. L. H. Arnett · K. W. Merrell (✉)
Department of Radiation Oncology, Mayo Clinic,
Rochester, MN, USA
e-mail: Merrell.kenneth@mayo.edu

has received cranial radiation treatment, with appropriate latency often beyond 6 months. Characteristic retinal changes associated with radiation-induced retinopathy can be observed via direct fundoscopic exam in conjunction with visual field testing [1, 2]. In contrast, diagnosis of RION is often more challenging than retinopathy and is typically approached as a diagnosis of exclusion. The key differential diagnosis in RION is that of potential tumor recurrence. For example, if the treated tumor was in the vicinity of the optic chiasm, both RION and compressive symptoms related to tumor progression may present as bilateral hemianopia, which may be difficult to distinguish on initial evaluation (see Case Illustration 1) [3]. In general, tumor recurrence is often associated with slowly progressive vision loss, in contrast to a more rapid course of vision loss in RION. In addition to temporal time frame of onset, the corresponding lack of residual or recurrent disease or optic nerve or chiasm enhancement on MRI supports a diagnosis of RION.

Other causes of vision loss should also be considered, including arachnoid adhesions, retinal detachment, vitreous hemorrhage, macular degeneration, and giant cell arteritis, many of which are independent of radiation treatment [4]. In addition, comorbid conditions such as vascular disorders, diabetic retinopathy, and hypertension can both increase the risk of radiation-induced optic complications and independently lead to visual dysfunction, adding further complexity to the diagnostic process [1, 5].

## Diagnostic Tests

All patients who receive significant radiation dose to optic structures should undergo baseline ophthalmologic evaluation and regular follow-up examination. Testing should include direct fundoscopy (Fig. 38.1, a–e), as well as regular visual field assessment to detect visual deficits that may be clinically undetectable (see Case Illustration [1]. Electrophysiologic evaluation may be warranted in suspected cases. Visual evoked potential (VEP) or visual evoked response (VER) is determined via measurement

© Springer International Publishing AG, part of Springer Nature 2018
E. L. Chang et al. (eds.), *Adult CNS Radiation Oncology*, https://doi.org/10.1007/978-3-319-42878-9_38

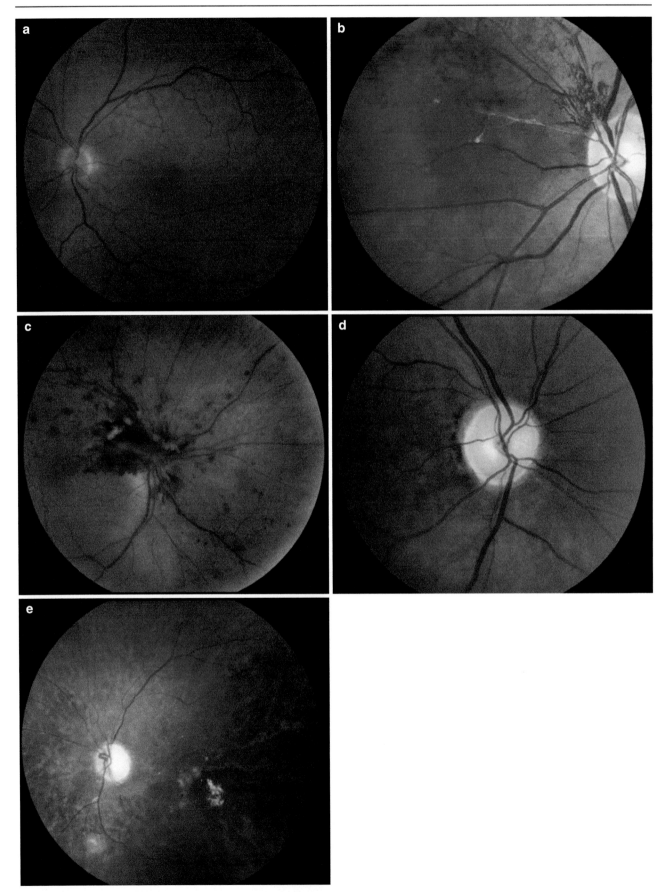

**Fig. 38.1** Fundoscopic images of radiation-induced retinopathy (**b–d**) and optic neuropathy (**e**); (**a**) normal retina with normal retinal vascular anatomy; (**b**) retinal hemorrhage; (**c**) cotton-wool spots and hard exudates; (**d**) neovascularization; (**e**) optic disc pallor due to optic nerve atrophy

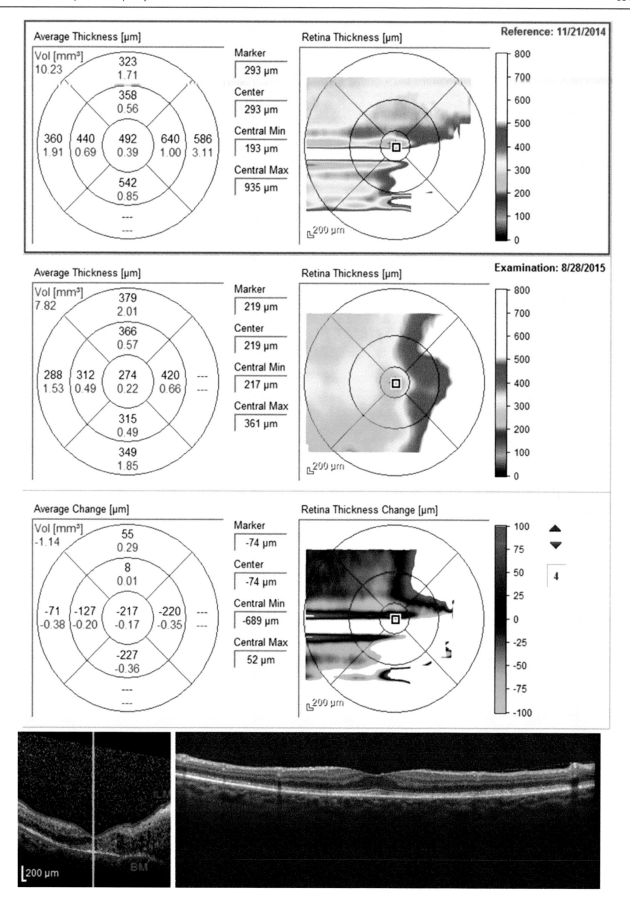

**Fig. 38.2** Ocular coherence tomography (OCT) evaluation of the retina and fovea

of the electrical signal recorded at the scalp, over the occipital cortex, in response to light stimulus. It can be used to evaluate the integrity of the afferent visual pathway and allow comparison between both eyes and bilateral cerebral hemispheres [6]. Unilateral abnormalities may reflect optic neuropathy and may assist in localization of lesions in the absence of obvious retinal lesions. While the application of this diagnostic method is limited in the standard clinical setting, reports have suggested VEP may be abnormal months before the patient with RION reports loss of vision [7, 8].

Routine imaging performed for surveillance of tumor response may also be useful in monitoring for structural changes in the optic pathway. CT scan is of limited diagnostic utility for assessment of subtle abnormalities and small optic pathway lesions, whereas MRI has a higher degree of sensitiv-

ity for detection of changes within the optic pathway (see Case Illustration). Orbital imaging protocols can be employed to obtain detailed and specialized views of the chiasm and post-chiasmal structures of the orbit. In addition, optical coherence tomography (OCT) (Fig. 38.2), fluorescein angiography (Fig. 38.3), and ocular ultrasound (Fig. 38.4) can be used to assess the integrity of the retina and posterior segment [2, 9].

## Presentation and Symptoms

Knowledge of the anatomical structure and networking of neural pathways can assist with localization of specific lesions based on clinical presentation. A basic summary of the structures of the eye and the optic pathway is presented in Figs. 38.5 and 38.6, respectively. The lamina cribrosa demarcates the

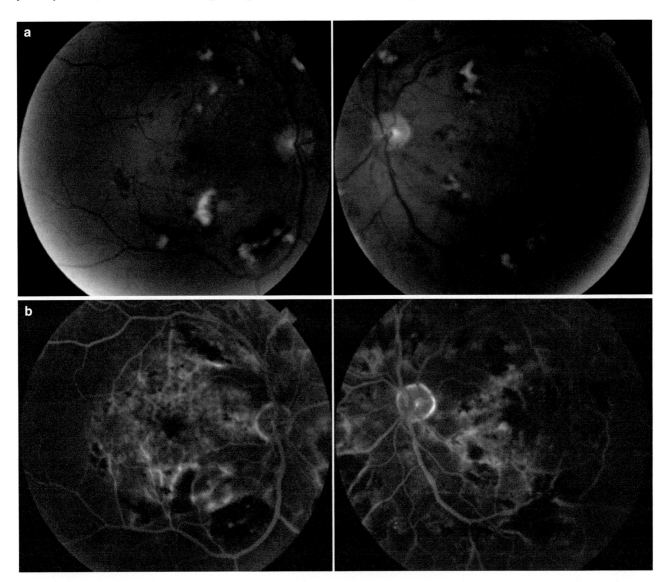

**Fig. 38.3** Neovascularization following radiation-induced retinal injury; (**a**) fundoscopic imaging of the retina and associated vasculature, demonstrating pigmentary changes, hemorrhage, and cotton-wool spots; (**b**) fluorescein angiography of the same retinae, exhibiting areas of reduced perfusion and capillary dropout [Reprinted from Gupta A, Dhawahir-Scala F, Smith A, Young L, Charles S. Radiation retinopathy: case report and review. BMC Ophthalmol. 2007;7:6. With permission from Creative Commons: https://creativecommons.org/licenses/by/2.0/]

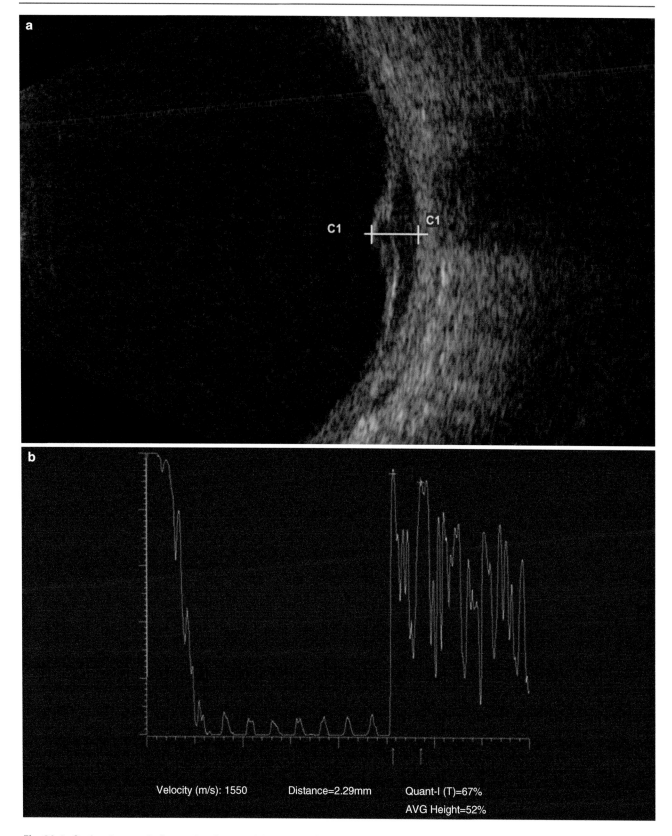

Velocity (m/s): 1550          Distance=2.29mm          Quant-I (T)=67%
                                                       AVG Height=52%

**Fig. 38.4** Ocular ultrasound of a uveal melanoma; (**a**) representative planar imaging of the uveal lesion; (**b**) quantification of retinal depth and depth of melanoma

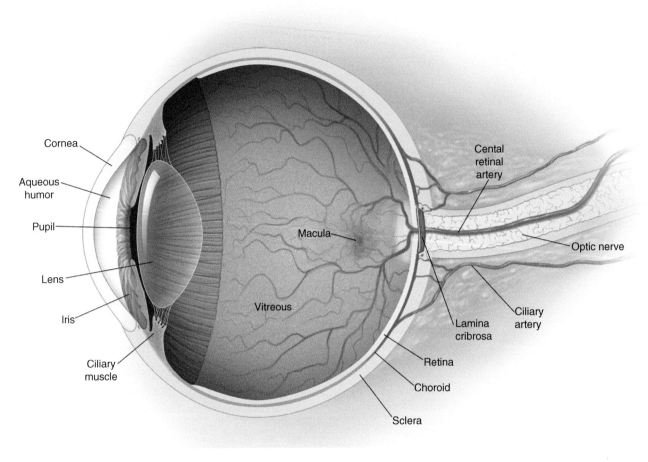

**Fig. 38.5** Basic anatomy of the eye and optic nerve head. The lamina cribrosa supports the optic nerve head as it exits the optic disc . Courtesy of Mayo Clinic ©

posterior boundary of the optic disc and facilitates the exit of the optic nerve from the retina. Lesions anterior to the lamina cribrosa typically are associated with retinitis and radiation-induced retinopathy, whereas lesions posterior to this junction result in RION. As illustrated in Fig. 38.6, a light stimulus enters the eye and is refracted and inverted as it passes through the cornea and lens. Thus, lesions involving the medial retina will present as temporal visual field deficits and vice versa. Signals from the retina are transmitted via the optic nerve as it exits through the optic disc. The right and left nerves converge at the optic chiasm where retinal ganglion cell axons from the contralateral nasal field cross to opposite hemispheres and travel to the left and right visual cortices, respectively. Thus lesions within the optic chiasm may cause bitemporal hemianopsia or complete blindness (Fig. 38.6b, c). Posterior to the chiasm, neurons branch along the left and right optic tracts and ultimately terminate within the lateral geniculate nucleus of the visual cortex. Lesions within the optic tracts may lead to varying degree of partial vision loss in both eyes (Fig. 38.6e, f).

The degree of change in visual acuity and timing of presentation is variable. Radiation-induced retinopathy typically presents with gradual vision loss in comparison with a

more rapid onset in RION, but both may present with severe, acute loss [2, 10]. Onset of visual loss has been reported from 2 months to more than 9 years after radiation exposure [1, 4], with peak incidence between 6 months and 3 years' posttreatment (Fig. 38.7) [4]. Severe loss, graded as no light perception, is reported to occur in up to 45% of RION cases at initial presentation [10–12]. Radiation dose can influence both the absolute risk and time delay to presentation, as shown in a number of series demonstrating shorter latency with higher radiation dose [11–13]. Patients may describe transient episodes of vision loss or indistinct visual disturbances for several weeks prior to the acute event.

Clinical and radiographic findings differ between radiation-induced retinopathy and RION. For patients with retinopathy, fundoscopic exam may demonstrate microaneurysms, retinal edema, exudates, cotton-wool spots, and macular edema (Fig. 38.1, a–d). Other common findings include telangiectasia with vascular sheathing, and more extreme cases can present with hemorrhage and vetreous detachment [1, 2, 14]. In contrast, RION is more often a retrobulbar complication and less likely to be detectable via normal ophthalmoscopy. Lesions anterior to the lamina cribrosa will present

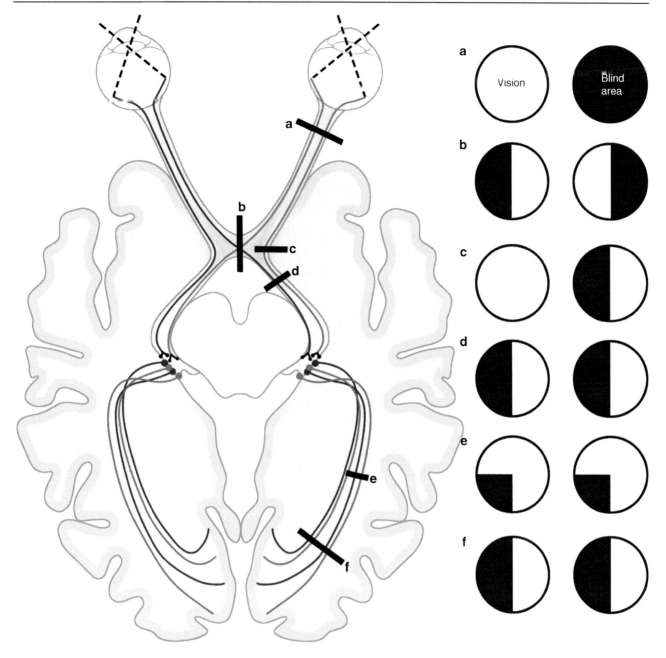

**Fig. 38.6** Schematic of the visual pathway and corresponding visual field deficits based on location of optic lesion. Courtesy of Mayo Clinic ©

with swelling of the optic nerve head and are more commonly seen with retinopathy, rather than RION. After the acute presentation, atrophy of the optic nerve leads to pallor and cupping of the optic disc, which can be observed via fundoscopic exam within 8–10 weeks of symptom manifestation (Fig. 38.1e).

## Radiographic Findings

CT imaging in the setting of both retinopathy and RION is often normal, but other imaging modalities may provide additional information to aid in diagnosis. Magnetic reso-

nance imaging (MRI) may demonstrate changes in optic nerve and chiasm enhancement on post-gadolinium T1-weighted images (see case Illustration 1). Further image refinement can be obtained with fat-suppressed RARE (rapid acquisition with relaxation enhancement) sequence imaging [15]. However, MRI findings may be non-specific and may be difficult to distinguish from other causes of optic neuritis and optic neuropathy, including multiple sclerosis, sarcoidosis, or other neoplastic processes involving the optic structures. OCT can provide good visualization of the vitreoretinal interface and posterior segment inflammation (Fig. 38.2). It is also used to study retinal detachment in conjunction with ocular ultrasound and has high utility in differentiating

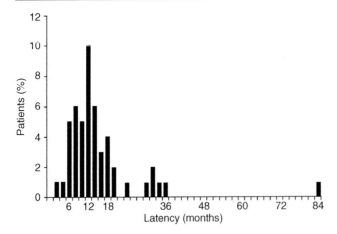

**Fig. 38.7** Frequency and latency of patients who developed optic neuropathy following irradiation of the optic nerve. [Reprinted from Borruat FX, Schatz NJ, Glaser JS, Feun LG, Matos L. Visual recovery from radiation-induced optic neuropathy. The role of hyperbaric oxygen therapy. J Clin Neuroophthalmol. 1993;13 (2):98–101. Wolters Kluwer Health, Inc.]

between potential causes of rapid-onset vision loss [9]. OCT in the setting of radiation-induced retinopathy and retinitis may demonstrate diffuse macular edema, cystoid changes, and choroidal neovascularization [2, 14].

Fundus fluorescein angiography is useful for visualization of choroidal and retinal neovascularization, retinal vasculitis, and areas of capillary non-perfusion (Fig. 38.3b). Inflamed capillaries allow leakage of the dye into adjacent tissues, making this approach particularly appropriate for the evaluation of retinitis [9]. Typical findings consistent with radiation-induced retinopathy include perifoveal capillary loss, masking of signal due to retinal hemorrhage, regions of capillary dropout with areas of non-perfusion, and changes in perfusion of the optic nerve head [1, 14, 16].

## Pathogenesis

The pathogenesis of radiation-induced retinopathy is more clearly characterized than RION. In radiation-induced retinopathy, radiation leads to damage of retinal capillary endothelial cells and ultimately results in significantvasculopathy. Unlike the pattern of loss seen with diabetic retinopathy, capillary pericytes remain preserved in the initial response to radiation injury. Adjacent capillary endothelial cells migrate to the regions of damaged epithelium in an attempt to repair injured tissues (Fig. 38.8). However, the proliferative response is inadequate for endothelial recovery and leads to chronic injury and activation of the clotting cascade. This, in turn, leads to vascular occlusion, microaneurysms, telangiectasia, and regions of retinal ischemia with exudates, edema, and hemorrhage [17–20].

RION is thought to be primarily related to radionecrosis within white matter tracts. This process likely involves damage to the microvasculature supplying the optic pathways, disruption of the blood brain barrier, and subsequent damage to glial cell progenitors following irradiation. These hypotheses have been explored in both animal models and human tissues. Nagayama et al. [21] characterized histopathologic changes in the optic chiasm in adult rats treated with a single dose of 20 Gy to the chiasm and optic nerves. Shortly after irradiation of the optic chiasm, an increase in apoptotic oligodendrocytes was observed. The authors speculated that the acute loss of oligodendrocytes may contribute to chronic white matter changes. However, it remains to be determined whether this observation is linked to the progressive demyelination that occurs as optic neuropathy progresses.

Vascular injury and depletion of endothelial cells have been documented in irradiated optic nerves taken from patients who underwent enucleation after receiving radiation doses of 55–70 Gy (Fig. 38.8) [22]. Based on histopathologic analysis and cross-sectional quantification, the authors reported an inverse correlation between radiation dose and number of endothelial cells in irradiated optic nerves. The vascular hypothesis of nerve injury is also supported by animal studies which demonstrate a moderate neuroprotective benefit after administration of the angiotensin-converting enzyme (ACE) inhibitor, ramipril [23]. This drug is primarily used in the treatment of hypertension and causes blood vessel relaxation via inhibition of the renin-angiotensin-aldosterone system. However, efficacy of ACE inhibitor therapy in the setting of RION remains to be validated in human subjects.

## Associated Risk Factors

A number of risk factors are known to increase susceptibility to radiation-induced retinopathy and RION. Several reports in the literature describe the synergistic effect of diabetic neuropathy, hypertension, and radiation-induced retinal injury [1, 24, 25]. The combined injury to capillary endothelial cells from radiation treatment and pre-existing vascular comorbidities may lead to the development of RION and retinopathy at doses of radiation considered low risk for injury [14]. Chemotherapy agents can also lead to radiation-independent optic nerve toxicity and have been documented after administration of vincristine and cisplatin therapy [26–28]. Furthermore, studies suggest pre-existing injuries to the optic nerve and chiasm, related to either surgical manipulation or presurgical compression by tumor, can predispose the optic apparatus to radiation-induced injury. In an animal model of compressive injury, a balloon was surgically placed to compress the optic chiasm and proximal optic nerve in

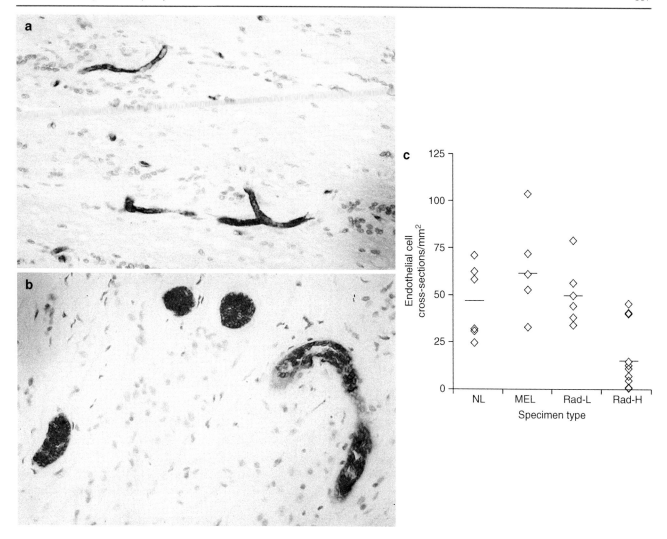

**Fig. 38.8** Endothelial cell loss in irradiated optic nerves. Paraffin-embedded sections of optic nerves taken from enucleated human eyes treated with 3.5 Gy (**a**) and 70 Gy (**b**), stained for an endothelial cell marker. Optic nerves treated with high-dose radiation (**b**) show engorged and dysmorphic vessels; (**c**), quantification of endothelial cells per mm². Higher dose was significantly associated with reduction in optic nerve endothelial cells. Normal eyes (NL), unirradiated eyes with melanoma (MEL), <10 Gy (Rad-L), and >55 Gy (Rad-H). [Reprinted from Levin LA, Gragoudas ES, Lessell S. Endothelial cell loss in irradiated optic nerves. Ophthalmology. 2000;107 (2):370–4. With permission from Elsevier].

adult cats followed by radiation to the optic nerves and chiasm. Animals that underwent compressive surgery showed abnormalities in VEP at lower doses of radiation than those that did not [29, 30].

## Normal Critical Structure Tolerance and Constraints

Radiation-associated damage to the optic nerve, optic chiasm, and retina is infrequently reported within the literature for patients with a variety of brain tumors. This may be a function of exclusion of patients with tumors adjacent to or involving organs at risk, indetermination with respect to radiation-induced toxicity and tumor progression, and often shortened life span related to the natural history of glioma progression. Further, many prospective studies classify all forms of radionecrosis without unique specification to the location within the brain. Therefore, RION and retinopathy may be underreported in prospective, clinical trials. In addition, radiosensitivity of the retina, optic nerves, and chiasm differs, adding to the difficulty in interpretation of reports of toxicity without information regarding tumor location and individual dose to each organ at risk. As this information is not readily available or reported from prospective clinical trials, most information regarding radiation tolerance of the retina and optic pathway is limited to retrospective reviews and case reports, often of extracranial disease sites. Adding further complexity to the topic is frequent utilization of hypofractionated radiotherapy, single or fractionated stereotactic radiosurgery (SRS), and charged-particle radiation with higher linear energy transfer (LET).

## Retina

At the onset of 3D conformal radiation planning, Emami et al. set out to provide guidance for specific organ tolerance estimates through a systematic literature review and expert opinion consensus [31]. Specific organ at risk tolerance was reported as "TD 5/5" or "TD 50/5," which refers to the probability of 5 or 50% complication rates within 5 years of radiotherapy, respectively. These estimates were limited to adult patients with conventionally fractionated radiotherapy (1.8–2.0 Gy/day). Retina and optic pathway injury were estimated based on any volume of irradiation, and partial volume analysis was not performed. From these estimates, a patient with a retinal dose of 45 Gy would have a 5 year rate of complete ipsilateral blindness of 5%. Likewise, a patient with any volume of the retina receiving 65 Gy or more would have a 50% risk of complete ipsilateral blindness at 5 years after completion of radiation treatment.

Estimates of retinal toxicity by Emami et al. were based upon small, retrospective series of radiation retinopathy in patients with high-dose radiation to at least half of the posterior pole of the eye [32–34]. From this collection of studies, patients who receive retinal doses between 60 Gy and more than 70 Gy almost universally developed monocular blindness. In contrast, while patients who receive 45–50 Gy to the retina may have clinically detectable retinal damage, vision loss was infrequently observed. As such, it was estimated the normal tissue complication curve would be relatively flat below 45 Gy with a steep incline between 50 and 60 Gy. While many institutions and clinical studies utilize these estimates for dose constraints in modern radiation therapy, it must be acknowledged that these estimates are based on small cohorts of patients without prospective validation.

Despite these limitations, several studies corroborate these estimated dose constraints. Parsons et al. evaluated 64 patients with head and neck cancers who received radiation to the retina with ophthalmologic follow-up of 3 years or more [35]. A total of 26 patients developed radiation retinopathy with visual acuity of 20/200 or worse. No patients with retinal doses less than 45 Gy developed retinopathy, but similar to the Emami estimates, there was a steady increase in incidence for retinal doses above 45 Gy (Fig. 38.9). Aside from retinal dose, other predictors of radiation retinopathy include concurrent use of chemotherapy, diabetes mellitus, and daily fraction greater than 1.9 Gy per day. In a similar analysis by Takeda et al., no patients who received less than 50 Gy to the retina experienced radiation retinopathy [13]. Of patients with retinal doses greater than 50 Gy, the complication rate was greatest when more than 60% of the retina was radiated, suggesting both the maximum dose and volume of retina irradiated are important. Additionally, these studies showed that the onset of retinopathy after irradiation

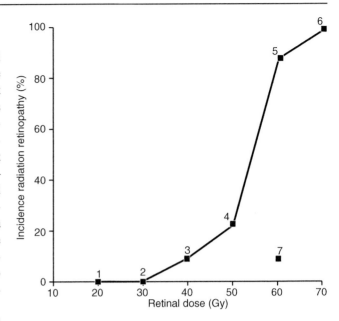

**Fig. 38.9** Incidence of radiation retinopathy as a function of retinal dose. [Reprinted from Parsons JT, Bova FJ, Fitzgerald CR, Mendenhall WM, Million RR. Radiation retinopathy after external-beam irradiation: analysis of time-dose factors. Int J Radiat Oncol Biol Phys. 1994;30 (4):765–73. With permission from Elsevier]

occurred most frequently between 1 and 3 years, but higher doses of radiation may be associated with a more rapid and progressive course [13, 35, 36].

With the rapid dose falloff associated with SRS, treatment of common parenchymal lesions within the brain is unlikely to result in significant retinal dose. However, SRS has been utilized as management for both choroidal melanoma and age-related macular degeneration (AMD), providing response data for single-fraction and fractionated SRS (fSRS). The INTREPID trial was designed as a comparison of SRS (16 Gy vs. 24 Gy) and sham treatment to evaluate response in patients with AMD [37, 38]. Following completion of treatment or placebo, fundoscopic examination was performed to identify microvascular abnormalities. With 2 years of follow-up, microvascular abnormalities were observed in 6 control eyes compared to 29 eyes treated with SRS, of which 18 (9 with each dose regimen) were attributed to SRS. However, only 2 of the 18 events in the treated cohort were observed to impact the patient's vision. Thus, the authors concluded that the risk of foveal microvascular abnormality and visual changes at 2 years was 1% at a dose of 16–24 Gy in a single fraction.

In the management of uveal melanoma, prescription dose to the periphery of the tumor is much greater than that which has been utilized for AMD, ranging from 50 to 70 Gy with internal maximal doses as high as 120 Gy [38, 39]. Incidence of radiation-induced retinopathy with high-dose SRS ranges from 22% to 65% [40–42]. Dinca et al. compared dose-response for uveal melanoma with SRS and reported higher rates of retinopathy for patients receiving 50–70 Gy (42% incidence) compared to 45 Gy (35% incidence) and 35 Gy (26% incidence) [42]. Experience with fSRS for uveal melanoma is also associated with high rates of radiation retinopathy. For example, 5-fraction fSRS (10–14 Gy/fraction) is associated with rates of retinopathy ranging from 58% to 81% [43–45]. The use of similar total dose delivered over 10 fractions does not appear to decrease the risk of retinopathy [46].

Radiation-induced retinopathy is a frequent side effect seen in the management of choroidal melanoma with low-dose rate brachytherapy. Similar to retinopathy caused by external beam radiation therapy, plaque brachytherapy has similar clinical presentation and temporal onset. In an analysis of 1300 patients, Gündüz et al. reported the incidence of radiation retinopathy of 43% with evidence of dose-response [47]. Retinopathy rates were low for patients with fovea doses less than 35 Gy, but increasing incidences were observed between 35 and 70 Gy (HR = 1.7) and above 70 Gy (HR = 2.4) [48].

Current clinical protocols often mandate inclusion of both retinae as contoured organs at risk. Similar to dose constraints established by Emami et al. in 1991, most studies limit maximal doses to the retina to less than 45 Gy. For example, in RTOG 0539, which includes target doses of both 54 and 60 Gy, the dose constraints to the retina are 45 Gy and 50 Gy (max point dose of 0.03 cc), respectively. For conventionally fractionated daily radiotherapy, a maximum dose of 45–50 Gy would result in a low and acceptable risk of radiation retinopathy. For patients receiving a single fraction of SRS, doses up to 24 Gy to small volumes appear safe and are associated with low risk of retinopathy. As retinal dose increases beyond 35 Gy in single-fraction SRS, the risk of retinopathy also increases substantially. As most intracranial SRS treatments are less than 24 Gy to the periphery, significant rates of retinopathy are unlikely to be observed. It is unclear whether fractionation of SRS decreases the risk of retinopathy.

## Optic Nerve and Chiasm

Emami et al., in a systematic review of available literature and expert opinion, estimated the 5-year risk of RION, including both the optic nerve and chiasm, to be 5% at doses of 50 Gy or less [31]. As dose increases above 65 Gy, the estimated risk was 50%. Similar to retinal toxicity estimates, risk assessment was based on any volume of dose to the optic nerve or chiasm. While 50 Gy was selected as the threshold dose for the optic nerve and chiasm TD 5/5, it is important to note that RION was observed with dosing between 42 and 70 Gy, emphasizing the variable range

throughout which RION can occur. This reflects the limitations of these data, which were based on small, retrospective reviews with heterogeneous tumor types as well as dose and fractionation (165–280 cGy/fraction).

Further research has improved our knowledge regarding dose constraints of optic structures with conventionally fractionated radiation indicating that optic nerve threshold tolerance is likely greater than initially estimated by Emami et al. (Table 38.1). Parsons et al., in an analysis of extracranial head and neck cancer, analyzed ocular toxicity for 131 patients receiving fractionated external beam radiotherapy [49]. Only patients whose optic nerve received doses in excess of 60 Gy or more experience RION. Fraction size was found to be a significant predictor, as patients who received ≥1.9 Gy per day had a higher rate of optic neuropathy than those receiving lower doses per day (47% vs. 11%, respectively) (Fig. 38.10). Similarly, Martel et al. compared average maximum dose for patients with and without RION [50]. Patients with RION had a mean maximal dose of 63 Gy compared to 56 Gy for those without. A single patient developed an optic chiasm injury with maximum dose of 59.5 Gy, compared to a maximum average dose of 53.7 Gy for patients without. Further, Jiang et al. observed no cases of RION for patients with optic nerve and chiasm doses less than 50 Gy

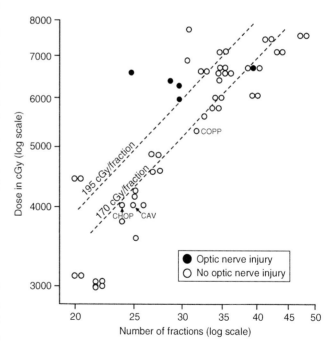

**Fig. 38.10** Impact of total dose and dose per fraction on incidence of radiation-induced optic neuropathy. Concurrent chemotherapy use is indicated with CHOP, CAV, and COPP [Reprinted from Parsons JT, Bova FJ, Fitzgerald CR, Mendenhall WM, Million RR. Radiation optic neuropathy after megavoltage external-beam irradiation: analysis of time-dose factors. Int J Radiat Oncol Biol Phys. 1994;30 (4):755–63. With permission from Elsevier]

**Table 38.1** Reported incidence of radiation-induced optic neuropathy

| Study | Patients (N) | Disease site | Prescription dose (range) and dose/fraction (range) | RION incidence | Dose detail (range) |
|---|---|---|---|---|---|
| Parsons et al. [49] | 131 | Head-and-neck cancer (NOS) | 55 to >75 Gy 1.2–2.6 Gy/fx | 0/21 5/7 1/16 1/15 6/73 | 55 to <65 Gy, <1.9 Gy/fx 55 to <65 Gy, >1.9 Gy/fx 55 to <60 Gy, <70 y 60 to <65 Gy, <70 y 65 to >75 Gy, <70 y |
| Martel et al. [50] | 20 | Paranasal sinus cancer | 50.4–70.2 Gy 1.8 Gy/fx | 1/20 (OC) 6/20 (ON) | 59.5 Gy 63.1 Gy (47.5–75.5) |
| Jiang et al. [51] | 219 | Paranasal sinus cancer | NR | 1/39 (ON) 20/59 (ON) 4/110 (OC) 9/66 (OC) | 50–60 Gy, 2.1 Gy/fx 61–78 Gy, 2.2 Gy/fx 50–60 Gy, 2.1 Gy/fx 61–76 Gy, 2.2 Gy/fx |
| Bhandare et al. [52] | 273 | Nasopharynx, paranasal sinus, and nasal cavity cancer | <50 Gy to >70 Gy 1.8 Gy/fx QD or 1.1–1.2 Gy/fx BID | 3/27 16/90 1/14 4/69 | 50 to <60Gy, 1.8 Gy/fx 60 to >70 Gy, 1.8 Gy/fx 50 to <60 Gy, 1.1 to 1.2 Gy/fx BID 60 to <70 Gy, 1.1 to 1.2 Gy/fx BID |

Selected studies of fractionated external beam radiotherapy highlighting documented cases of RION and dose and fractionation range when this occurred. Some data was estimated from tables, figures, and text. Abbreviations: *N* number, *RION* radiation-induced optic neuropathy, *fx* fractions, *OC* optic chiasm, *ON* optic nerve
[Reprinted from Mayo C, Martel MK, Marks LB, Flickinger J, Nam J, Kirkpatrick J. Radiation dose-volume effects of optic nerves and chiasm. International journal of radiation oncology, biology, physics. 2010;76(3 Suppl):S28–35. With permission from Elsevier].

[51]. In contrast, the risk of RION increased as optic nerve or chiasm dose increased to 50–60 Gy (5% risk) or 61–78 Gy (30% risk). Bhandare et al. suggested twice-daily fractionation was associated with decreased risk of RION in patients with optic nerve or chiasm dose >63 Gy compared to conventional daily fractionation, though this is an uncommon clinical practice for CNS tumors [52].

The impact of charged-particle therapy, with doses reported as cobalt gray equivalent (CGE), on risk of RION has largely been consistent with dose-response studies from photon radiotherapy. While radiation planning with physical and biologic dosimetry with higher LET of proton or carbon ions is not fully understood, one must take into account the end-of-range biologic enhancement of the beam, especially when treating tumors adjacent to the optic structures. Despite biologic uncertainties and limited experience, most studies with proton or carbon ion therapy directed at tumors adjacent to optic nerves report similar rates of RION, with optic nerve and chiasm doses ranging from 50 to 60 CGE [53–59].

Similar to fractionated radiotherapy, optic nerve and chiasm dose tolerance for single-fraction SRS is based on retrospective studies. In one of the first reports on the topic, Tishler et al. observed no cases of RION for patients receiving single-fraction SRS to or near the cavernous sinus when the optic apparatus was limited to less than 8 Gy [60]. In comparison, RION was observed at a rate of 24% when dose to the optic apparatus exceeded 8 Gy. While many institutions have adopted 8 Gy as a maximal point dose constraint, this can present a significant challenge when attempting to achieve a dose sufficient for tumor control in lesions immediately adjacent to optic structures. Subsequent studies have questioned the tolerance of the optic apparatus, including Leber et al., who reported no cases of RION with optic apparatus dose of 10 Gy or less but did report increasing incidence with doses of 10–15 Gy (26.7% incidence) and 15 Gy or more (77.8% incidence) [8]. In a large series from the Mayo Clinic, Stafford et al. reviewed 218 single-fraction SRS treatments to the sellar and parasellar regions [61]. A total of four patients (1.9%) developed RION, correlating with a 1.1% risk for RION with doses to the optic apparatus less than or equal to 12 Gy. The risk of RION was 6.9% when dose exceeded 12 Gy (2 of 29 patients). Of the patients with RION, three had prior fractionated radiotherapy (median dose 50.4 Gy). Pollock et al. reviewed 133 patients with single-fraction SRS for pituitary adenomas, with exclusion of patients with previous radiotherapy, and observed no cases of RION with 46% of optic apparatus receiving point doses greater than 10 Gy and 11% with doses greater than 12 Gy [62].

Few studies, with limited follow-up, are available with recommended dose constraints for fSRS. Hiniker et al. reviewed 326 patients with perioptic tumors who received SRS with a single (total dose, 12–25 Gy), three (total dose, 18–33 Gy), or five (total dose, 18–40 Gy) fractions of SRS [63]. To achieve RION risk of less than 1%, patients treated with three or five fractions would be limited to a maximum dose of 20.9 Gy or 26.1 Gy to the optic apparatus, respectively. These constraints are similar to previous reports from Timmerman et al. and the AAPM Task Group 101 (Table 38.2) [64].

In a Quantitative Analyses of Normal Tissue Effects in the Clinic (QUANTEC) report regarding RION, Mayo et al. performed a systematic review of dose-volume data with recommended guidelines of optic pathway constraints for conventionally fractionated and single-fraction SRS [65]. In contrast to the Emami TD5/5 estimates, for patients who received conventionally fractionated external beam radiotherapy, the risk of RION was estimated to be close to "near zero" for patients receiving 50 Gy to the optic structures. As the dose increased to beyond 50 Gy to 55 Gy, the risk of optic neuropathy was estimated to be "unusual." The estimated risk for patients receiving maximum doses of 55–60 Gy and >60 Gy was 3–7% and 8–20%, respectively (Fig. 38.11). For patients receiving single-fraction SRS, the risk of RION is low for a maximum dose less than 10–12 Gy. The Emami and QUANTEC recommendations, as well as other retrospective data, represent guidelines that can be utilized for radiation planning. However, these recommendations are based on best available data, which remains limited to mostly retrospective reviews and case reports. As such, each patient must be considered individually, taking into account patient risk factors and comorbidities, total target dose and dose per fraction, location of tumor, and the patient's willingness to accept risk of complications.

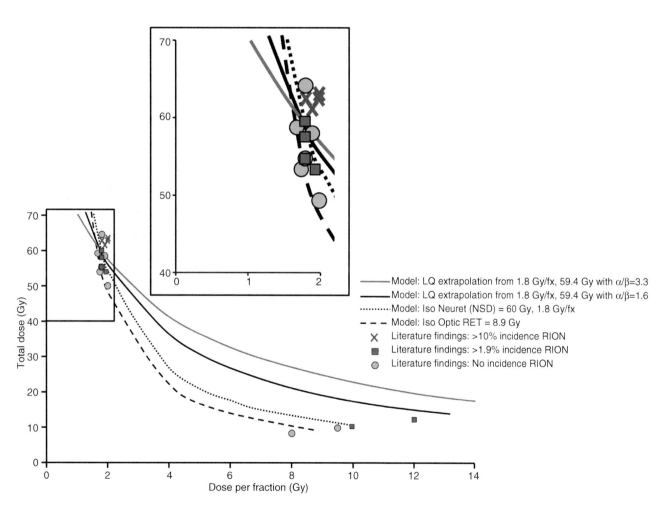

**Fig. 38.11** Extrapolation of radiation-induced optic neuropathy (RION) incidence with isoeffect linear-quadratic and biologically effective threshold models for prediction of RION. The symbols represent the presence or absence of documented RION. With limited data, extrapolation from multiple to single fractionation is unreliable. **Inset:** magnified view of graph in range of typical fractionation (1.8–2 Gy/fx). [Reprinted from Mayo C, Martel MK, Marks LB, Flickinger J, Nam J, Kirkpatrick J. Radiation dose-volume effects of optic nerves and chiasm. International journal of radiation oncology, biology, physics. 2010;76(3 Suppl):S28–35. With permission from Elsevier]

**Table 38.2** Expert recommendations of stereotactic radiosurgery dose constraints for the optic pathway

| | Hiniker et al. [63] | | Timmerman et al. [79] | | AAPM TG 101(64) | | Stafford et al. [61] |
|---|---|---|---|---|---|---|---|
| Number of fractions | Dmax for 1% RION risk (Gy) | Dmax for 5% RION risk (Gy) | Volume max (<0.2 cc) (Gy) | Max point dose (Gy) | Threshold dose (Gy) | Max point dose (Gy) | Dmax for 1% RION risk (Gy) |
| 1 | 12.7 | 17.5 | 8 | 10 | 8 | 10 | 12 |
| 3 | 20.9 | 29.1 | 15 | 19.5 | 15.3 | 17.4 | – |
| 5 | 26.1 | 36.6 | 20 | 25 | 23 | 25 | – |

Selected studies with expert recommendations for optic pathway dose constraints with the use of either single- or multiple-fraction stereotactic radiosurgery.

## Treatment Options

Unfortunately, few treatment options with limited success exist for patient with radiation retinopathy and RION. For management of radiation-induced retinopathy, the goal is to reduce macular edema and vascular overgrowth. Treatment options with some available evidence include focal laser photocoagulation, photodynamic therapy, and intravitreal triamcinolone or bevacizumab injection. Focal laser therapy uses high-intensity wavelength source resulting in thermal denaturing of ocular tissue. Mixed results are reported for photocoagulation, with most reporting modest gains in the first 6 months of treatment with subsequent visual deterioration to baseline within 2 years [66, 67]. Photodynamic therapy, which utilizes intravenous infusion of verteporfin followed by irradiance with a laser, has also been evaluated in a small number of clinical studies and has demonstrated potential efficacy of treatment [68]. Intravitreal injection of triamcinolone acetonide was utilized in a prospective, non-randomized study of 31 patients with radiation retinitis after plaque brachytherapy [69]. Within 1 month after injection, visual acuity was improved in 91% of patients, though most had gradual decline in visual acuity within 6 months after injection. Further, corticosteroid injection into the vitreous space is associated with cataract progression and glaucoma. Intravitreal injection of bevacizumab, a VEGF-A inhibitor, has been used off label for neovascularization in patients with diabetic retinopathy and retinal vein occlusions. Similar to intravitreal triamcinolone acetonide injection, bevacizumab is associated with short-term improvement in visual acuity with deterioration within several months [70, 71]. Despite physical findings of improvement in macular edema within 6 weeks, many patients will not experience improvement in vision, likely related to persistent capillary perfusion deficits. Very limited data is available regarding hyperbaric oxygen therapy and pentoxifylline for the management of radiation-induced retinopathy.

For the management of RION, most patients receive high-dose intravenous corticosteroid treatment. The rationale of corticosteroid use is to reduce vasogenic edema, which is often observed on MR imaging in association with other optic changes within the optic structures. However, it is uncertain whether the observed edematous changes are a direct cause of visual injury. Some investigators have evaluated the role of anticoagulation to improve blood flow to areas of radiation necrosis [72]. While a small number of successes with anticoagulation are reported in the literature, a case of RION occurring while a patient was actively receiving anticoagulation also exists [73]. Several case reports indicate that hyperbaric oxygen therapy (HBO), with increase in partial pressure of oxygen, may potentially improve revascularization of damaged capillaries and lead to improved vision loss in RION. Side effects related to HBO are infrequent but include barotrauma, lenticular myopia, seizures, and pulmonary toxicity. In a systematic review of the literature, Levy et al. reviewed several case reports of HBO for RION [74]. Successful treatments with HBO are associated with rapid initiation of treatment within 72 hours after onset and partial pressures greater than 2.4 ATM. Despite these measures, success rates remain low, with vision loss typically progressing despite aggressive treatment. Systemic bevacizumab use, with and without pentoxifylline, has also been reported to achieve durable reversal of visual deficits and improvement in optic nerve contrast enhancement on MR imaging [75–78]. Other treatment options, such as administration of ACE inhibitors, have shown promise in animal models, but validation in human subjects is needed.

Radiation-induced retinopathy and RION are rare and devastating complications of intracranial radiotherapy. Few treatment options, with modest results, are available. Patients should be informed of the likelihood of poor outcomes despite intervention, to enable educated decision-making regarding costly treatment options. Ultimately, preventative strategies with advanced radiation planning and delivery will likely prove to be of greatest benefit.

## Case Illustration

### Radiation-Induced Optic Neuropathy

A 71-year-old female with a history of hypertension, glaucoma, and benign paroxysmal positional vertigo presented to the emergency department with an acute episode of dizziness, nausea, and mild headache. She described episodes of positional vertigo that occurred sporadically for approximately 15 years prior to presentation to the emergency department. No other neurologic symptoms were reported by the patient, and findings on physical exam were normal. A non-contrast CT scan of the head was obtained (Fig. 38.12a) which showed a left parasellar mass, with no evidence of intracranial hemorrhage. Subsequent MRI (Fig. 38.12b) confirmed the presence of a left suprasellar, extra-axial mass invading the cavernous sinus, with extension into the midbrain cistern along the tentorium. It was noted to encase the left ICA, but did not occlude the vessel. Imaging was consistent with meningioma.

The patient opted to proceed with radiation treatment at an outside institution. The lesion was treated via static-field IMRT to a dose of 54 Gy in 30 fractions (Fig. 38.13). Maximum dose to the right and left optic nerves and optic chiasm was 54.49 Gy, 56.03 Gy, and 56.45 Gy, respectively. The patient developed mild fatigue and partial, transient alopecia, but treatment was generally well-tolerated. No further worsening of her neurologic symptoms occurred, and the transient vertigo resolved during treatment.

Eleven months after treatment, the patient noted discomfort and reduced vision in her left eye. Her vision continued to worsen over the next several weeks, despite symptomatic management. Steroid therapy was initiated, and she was referred to our clinic for further evaluation. On physical exam, she was noted to have reduced visual acuity bilaterally, the left worse than the right, and right homonymous hemianopia. Fundoscopic exam showed bilateral optic disc pallor and a left afferent pupillary defect. Visual acuity was 20/40 in the right eye and 20/80 in the left. No retinal lesions were noted on OCT, and intraocular pressure was unchanged compared to prior evaluations. Visual field testing was performed, which showed severely reduced light perception in the left eye, in both temporal and nasal fields, and a substantial deficit in the temporal field of the right eye (Fig. 38.14). A gadolinium-enhanced MRI was obtained, which showed bilateral T2 hyperintensity in the pre-chiasmal optic nerves, as well as mild, bilateral T1 enhancement in the same region of the optic nerves (Fig. 38.15). The original intracranial lesion showed no evidence of progression, and the left optic nerve showed no signs of compression.

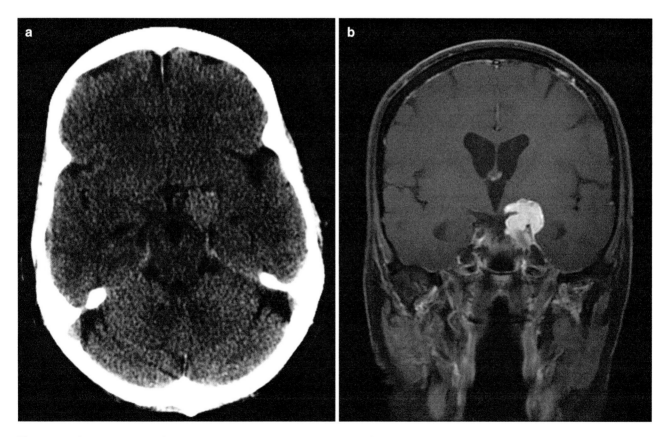

**Fig. 38.12** Non-contrast axial CT (**a**) and coronal T1 post gadolinium MRI (**b**) demonstrating a well-circumscribed extra-axial lesion in the suprasellar region, invading the cavernous sinus and encasing the supraclinoid left internal carotid artery

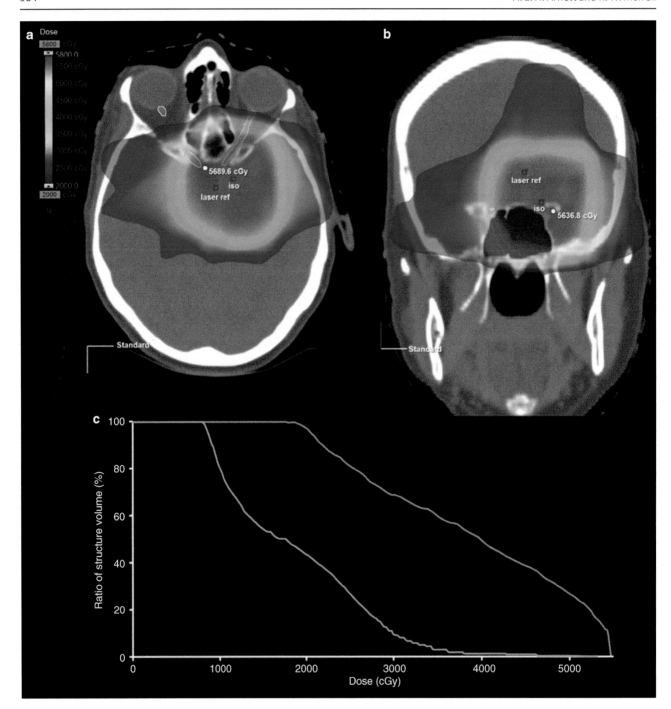

**Fig. 38.13** Axial (**a**) and coronal (**b**) slice of radiation planning CT scan with dose-wash representation of radiation dose distribution. The right and left optic nerve contour is indicated in green and orange, respectively. Dose-volume histogram (**c**) for the right (green) and left (orange) optic nerve

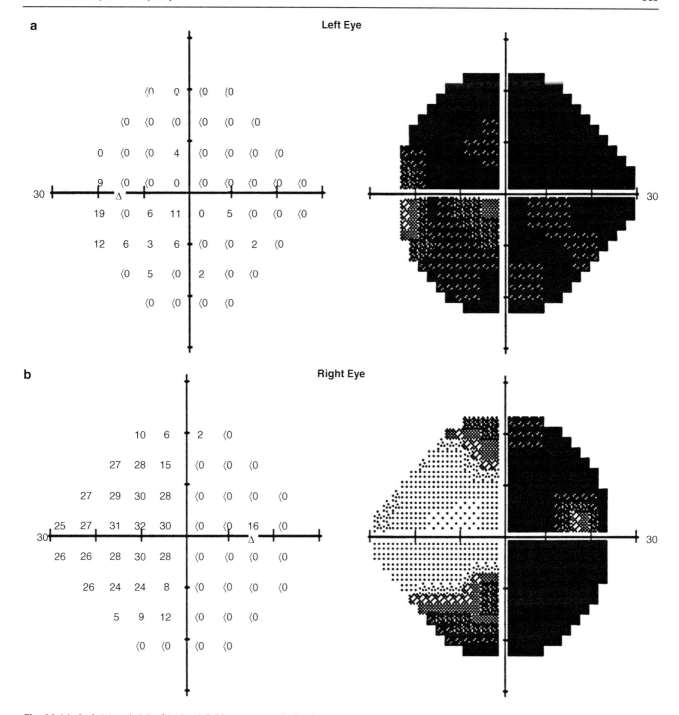

**Fig. 38.14** Left (**a**) and right (**b**) visual field assessment, indicating severe deficits throughout the left eye, as well as a left-sided homonymous hemianopsia

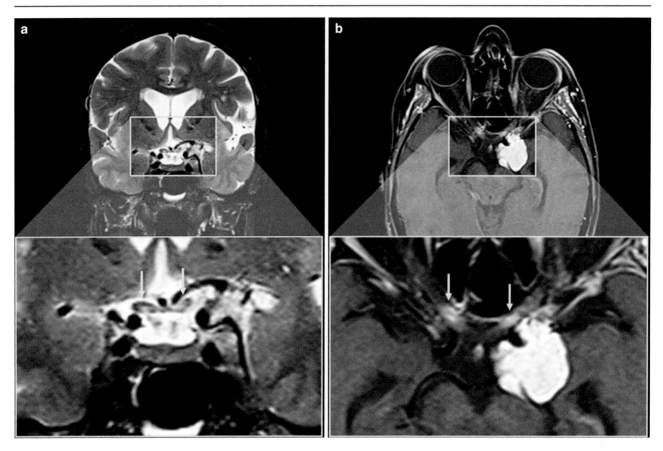

**Fig. 38.15** Coronal T2 MRI (**a**) demonstrating bilateral hyperintensity of the optic nerves at the junction with the optic chiasm; axial T1 post-gadolinium-enhanced MRI (**b**) exhibiting an enhancing left suprasellar mass corresponding to the previously treated melanoma. Bilateral enhancement of the proximal optic nerve is shown. **Insets:** magnified views of the optic lesions

Given the findings on MRI and chronology of symptoms, as well as the absence of tumor progression or retinal pathology, the patient was diagnosed with radiation-induced optic neuropathy. She was started on pentoxifylline for further management. At follow-up, her vision remained stable and did not worsen after initiation of treatment. However, she unfortunately did not demonstrate improvement of visual field deficits.

## Retinopathy

A 78-year-old male presented with a 4-week history of left orbital swelling. A contrast CT scan and MRI of the orbit demonstrated an infiltrative lesion involving the medial aspect of the left orbit, with encasement of the superior rectus, superior oblique, and medial rectus musculature. Tumor was noted to extend along the medial surface of the globe, with extension through the cribriform plate and along the inferomedial aspect of the left frontal lobe. Biopsy of the lesion was consistent with diffuse large B cell lymphoma. MRI of the spine showed no additional lesions, and CSF samples were negative. He underwent

treatment with six cycles of CHOP chemotherapy and showed a good response to treatment. The size of the orbital mass was substantially reduced after treatment, and the post-chemotherapy MRI showed no evidence of mass effect within the orbit.

The patient subsequently received involved-field radiation at a dose of 30.6 Gy in 17 fractions. He developed mild dry eye and grade 1 erythema in the treatment field. His vision remained stable until 6 years after completion of radiation treatment, at which point he began to notice intermittent double vision and underwent a full ophthalmologic evaluation. Visual acuity was 20/30 on the right and 20/60 on the left. OCT exam and assessment of the macula (Fig. 38.16) showed evidence of cystoid retinal edema, pigmentary changes, and retinal hemorrhage in the vicinity of the macula. He was treated with triamcinolone and bevacizumab injections and reported subsequent improvement of vision, with no further episodes of double vision. Follow-up OCT obtained 3 months later showed decreased but persistent edema in the vicinity of the left macula. This remained stable on subsequent follow-up exams. He showed no recurrence of his lymphoma and stable vision at 15 years posttreatment.

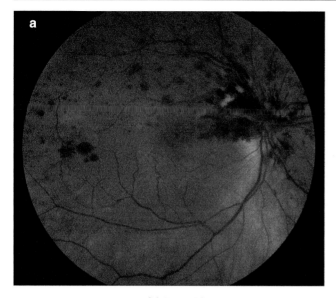

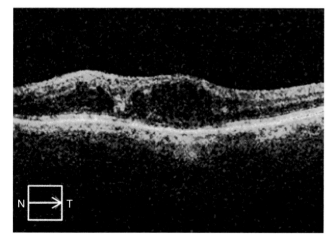

**Fig. 38.16** Fundoscopic exam (**a**) revealed extensive retinal hemorrhages involving the optic disc, as well as pigmentary changes; ocular coherence tomography (OCT) (**b**) findings consistent with macular edema, cystoid changes, and increased cross-sectional depth

## Callout Text Boxes

### Section: Diagnosis

#### Fundoscopic Findings of Radiation Retinopathy

- Exudates.
- Retinal edema.
- Macular edema.
- Microaneurysms.
- Cotton-wool spots.
- Telangiectasia with vascular sheathing.
- Hemorrhage and vitreous detachment.

### Section: Pathogenesis

#### Risk Factors Associated with Radiation-Induced Optic Neuropathy

- Diabetes mellitus.
- Hypertension.
- Chemotherapy.
- Optic nerve compression or injury.
- Dose per fraction.

## Summary

- Radiation-induced retinopathy and optic neuropathy are rare, but devastating, consequences of intracranial and skull base radiotherapy.
- Radiation retinopathy is often a slow, progressive process characterized by physical exam findings of microaneurysms, retinal edema, exudates, cotton-wool spots, and macular edema.
- Typical presentation for radiation-induced optic neuropathy includes rapid-onset changes in visual acuity with optic nerve and/or chiasm enhancement on post-gadolinium T1-weighted images.
- Radiation retinopathy is rare with retinal doses below 45–50 Gy for conventionally fractionated radiotherapy.
- Radiation-induced optic neuropathy is unusual for doses below 55 Gy for conventionally fractionated radiotherapy.
- Limited treatment options exist for radiation-induced retinopathy and optic neuropathy, and treatments are often ineffective.

## Self-Assessment Questions

1. What are typical findings of radiation retinopathy?
   A. Rapid onset immediately after completion of radiotherapy.
   B. Normal-appearing retina on fundoscopic examination.
   C. Microaneurysms, cotton-wool spots, and macular edema on fundoscopic examination.
   D. Usually self-limited.

2. What visual lesion would be anticipated for a radiation-induced optic neuropathy occurring within the optic chiasm?
   A. Complete right eye blindness.
   B. Bitemporal hemianopsia or complete blindness.
   C. Complete left eye blindness.
   D. Superior quadrant quadrantanopsia.

3. Which is not a known risk factor for development of radiation-induced optic neuropathy?
   A. Congestive heart failure.
   B. Diabetes.
   C. Mass effect on the optic nerve.
   D. High total dose or dose per fraction.

4. When attempting to treat a temporal lobe glioma to a dose of 60 Gy, which of the following dose constraints would most likely result in adequate tumor coverage and low risk of radiation-induced optic neuropathy?
   A. Optic nerve max dose 45 Gy with 75% coverage of PTV.
   B. Optic nerve max of 50 Gy with 85% coverage of PTV.
   C. Optic nerve max dose of 53 Gy with 100% coverage of PTV.
   D. Optic nerve max dose of 60 Gy with 100% coverage of PTV.

5. Which of the following are true regarding treatment options for radiation-induced optic neuropathy?
   A. Available treatments are very effective and most patients recover complete vision.
   B. No treatment is needed as this is a self-limited process.
   C. There are no known adverse effects from the available treatment options.
   D. Despite attempted treatments with interventions such as systemic corticosteroids, bevacizumab, and hyperbaric oxygen, most patients will have little to no improvement in visual acuity.

## Answers

1. C
   On fundoscopic examination, findings may include microaneurysms, retinal edema, exudates, cotton-wool spots, macular edema, telangiectasia with vascular sheathing, and more extreme cases potentially hemorrhage and vitreous detachment.

2. B
   Damage to the optic chiasm may impact the retinal ganglion cell axons from the contralateral nasal field or if severe enough may impact axons from the temporal fields resulting in complete blindness.

3. A
   Congestive heart failure is not known to increase risk of radiation-induced option neuropathy.

4. C
   Answer C provides the best coverage of tumor with prescription dose while maintaining optic nerve dose in an optimal level. Per the QUANTEC report, radiation-induced optic neuropathy was felt to be "unusual" with doses between 50 and 55 Gy [65].

5. D
   Despite best efforts and aggressive management, most patients will not have improvements in visual acuity. Management of radiation-induced optic neuropathy is associated with risk of adverse events. Patients should be educated on the likelihood of success of the treatment as well as the potential risks of treatment.

## References

1. Viebahn M, Barricks ME, Osterloh MD. Synergism between diabetic and radiation retinopathy: case report and review. Br J Ophthalmol. 1991;75(10):629–32.
2. Reichstein D. Current treatments and preventive strategies for radiation retinopathy. Curr Opin Ophthalmol. 2015;26(3):157–66.
3. Zimmerman CF, Schatz NJ, Glaser JS. Magnetic resonance imaging of radiation optic neuropathy. Am J Ophthalmol. 1990;110(4):389–94.
4. Kline LB, Kim JY, Ceballos R. Radiation optic neuropathy. Ophthalmology. 1985;92(8):1118–26.
5. Kaushik M, Pulido JS, Schild SE, et al. Risk of radiation retinopathy in patients with orbital and ocular lymphoma. Int J Radiat Oncol Biol Phys. 2012;84(5):1145–50.
6. Alexander KR, Rajagopalan AS, Seiple W, et al. Contrast response properties of magnocellular and parvocellular pathways in retinitis pigmentosa assessed by the visual evoked potential. Invest Ophthalmol Vis Sci. 2005;46(8):2967–73.
7. Leber KA, Bergloff J, Langmann G, et al. Radiation sensitivity of visual and oculomotor pathways. Stereotact Funct Neurosurg. 1995;64(Suppl 1):233–8.
8. Leber KA, Bergloff J, Pendl G. Dose-response tolerance of the visual pathways and cranial nerves of the cavernous sinus to stereotactic radiosurgery. J Neurosurg. 1998;88(1):43–50.

9. Gupta V, Al-Dhibi HA, Arevalo JF. Retinal imaging in uveitis. Saudi J Ophthalmol. 2014;28(2):95–103.

10. Danesh-Meyer HV. Radiation-induced optic neuropathy. J Clin Neurosci. 2008;15(2):95–100.

11. Borruat FX, Schatz NJ, Glaser JS, et al. Visual recovery from radiation-induced optic neuropathy. The role of hyperbaric oxygen therapy. J Clin Neuroophthalmol. 1993;13(2):98–101.

12. Roden D, Bosley TM, Fowble B, et al. Delayed radiation injury to the retrobulbar optic nerves and chiasm. Clinical syndrome and treatment with hyperbaric oxygen and corticosteroids. Ophthalmology. 1990;97(3):346–51.

13. Takeda A, Shigematsu N, Suzuki S, et al. Late retinal complications of radiation therapy for nasal and paranasal malignancies: relationship between irradiated-dose area and severity. Int J Radiat Oncol Biol Phys. 1999;44(3):599–605.

14. Gupta A, Dhawahir-Scala F, Smith A, et al. Radiation retinopathy: case report and review. BMC Ophthalmol. 2007;7:6.

15. Gass A, Moseley IF. The contribution of magnetic resonance imaging in the differential diagnosis of optic nerve damage. J Neurol Sci. 2000;172(Suppl 1):S17–22.

16. Hayreh SS. Evaluation of optic nerve head circulation: review of the methods used. J Glaucoma. 1997;6(5):319–30.

17. Avery RB, Diener-West M, Reynolds SM, et al. Histopathologic characteristics of choroidal melanoma in eyes enucleated after iodine 125 brachytherapy in the collaborative ocular melanoma study. Arch Ophthalmol. 2008;126(2):207–12.

18. Krebs IP, Krebs W, Merriam JC, et al. Radiation retinopathy: electron microscopy of retina and optic nerve. Histol Histopathol. 1992;7(1):101–10.

19. Archer DB, Gardiner TA. Ionizing radiation and the retina. Curr Opin Ophthalmol. 1994;5(3):59–65.

20. Krema H, Xu W, Payne D, et al. Factors predictive of radiation retinopathy post (125)iodine brachytherapy for uveal melanoma. Can J Ophthalmol. 2011;46(2):158–63.

21. Nagayama K, Kurita H, Nakamura M, et al. Radiation-induced apoptosis of oligodendrocytes in the adult rat optic chiasm. Neurol Res. 2005;27(4):346–50.

22. Levin LA, Gragoudas ES, Lessell S. Endothelial cell loss in irradiated optic nerves. Ophthalmology. 2000;107(2):370–4.

23. Ryu S, Kolozsvary A, Jenrow KA, et al. Mitigation of radiation-induced optic neuropathy in rats by ACE inhibitor ramipril: importance of ramipril dose and treatment time. J Neurooncol. 2007;82(2):119–24.

24. Stitt AW, Anderson HR, Gardiner TA, et al. The combined effects of diabetes and ionising radiation on the rat retina: an ultrastructural study. Curr Eye Res. 1994;13(1):79–86.

25. Krema H, Somani S, Sahgal A, et al. Stereotactic radiotherapy for treatment of juxtapapillary choroidal melanoma: 3-year follow-up. Br J Ophthalmol. 2009;93(9):1172–6.

26. Wang MY, Arnold AC, Vinters HV, et al. Bilateral blindness and lumbosacral myelopathy associated with high-dose carmustine and cisplatin therapy. Am J Ophthalmol. 2000;130(3):367–8.

27. Sanderson PA, Kuwabara T, Cogan DG. Optic neuropathy presumably caused by vincristine therapy. Am J Ophthalmol. 1976;81(2):146–50.

28. Griffin JD, Garnick MB. Eye toxicity of cancer chemotherapy: a review of the literature. Cancer. 1981;48(7):1539–49.

29. Girkin CA, Comey CH, Lunsford LD, et al. Radiation optic neuropathy after stereotactic radiosurgery. Ophthalmology. 1997;104(10):1634–43.

30. Deng X, Yang Z, Liu R, et al. The maximum tolerated dose of gamma radiation to the optic nerve during gamma knife radiosurgery in an animal study. Stereotact Funct Neurosurg. 2013;91(2):79–91.

31. Emami B, Lyman J, Brown A, et al. Tolerance of normal tissue to therapeutic irradiation. Int J Radiat Oncol Biol Phys. 1991;21(1):109–22.

32. Shukovsky LJ, Fletcher GH. Retinal and optic nerve complications in a high dose irradiation technique of ethmoid sinus and nasal cavity. Radiology. 1972;104(3):629–34.

33. Byers RM. Management of head and neck cancer: a multidisciplinary approach. By Rodney R. Million and Nicholas J. Cassisi, 649 pp, illus, J. B. Lippincott co., Philadelphia, PA, 1984. Head Neck Surg. 1985;7(3):260.

34. Nakissa N, Rubin P, Strohl R, et al. Ocular and orbital complications following radiation therapy of paranasal sinus malignancies and review of literature. Cancer. 1983;51(6):980–6.

35. Parsons JT, Bova FJ, Fitzgerald CR, et al. Radiation retinopathy after external-beam irradiation: analysis of time-dose factors. Int J Radiat Oncol Biol Phys. 1994;30(4):765–73.

36. Wara WM, Irvine AR, Neger RE, et al. Radiation retinopathy. Int J Radiat Oncol Biol Phys. 1979;5(1):81–3.

37. Jackson TL, Chakravarthy U, Kaiser PK, et al. Stereotactic radiotherapy for neovascular age-related macular degeneration: 52-week safety and efficacy results of the INTREPID study. Ophthalmology. 2013;120(9):1893–900.

38. Jackson TL, Chakravarthy U, Slakter JS, et al. Stereotactic radiotherapy for neovascular age-related macular degeneration: year 2 results of the INTREPID study. Ophthalmology. 2015;122(1):138–45.

39. Langmann G, Pendl G, Klaus M, et al. Gamma knife radiosurgery for uveal melanomas: an 8-year experience. J Neurosurg. 2000;93(Suppl 3):184–8.

40. Wackernagel W, Holl E, Tarmann L, et al. Visual acuity after gamma-knife radiosurgery of choroidal melanomas. Br J Ophthalmol. 2013;97(2):153–8.

41. Kang DW, Lee SC, Park YG, et al. Long-term results of gamma knife surgery for uveal melanomas. J Neurosurg. 2012;117(Suppl):108–14.

42. Dinca EB, Yianni J, Rowe J, et al. Survival and complications following gamma knife radiosurgery or enucleation for ocular melanoma: a 20-year experience. Acta Neurochir. 2012;154(4):605–10.

43. Dunavoelgyi R, Zehetmayer M, Gleiss A, et al. Hypofractionated stereotactic photon radiotherapy of posteriorly located choroidal melanoma with five fractions at ten Gy--clinical results after six years of experience. Radiother Oncol. 2013;108(2):342–7.

44. Dunavoelgyi R, Georg D, Zehetmayer M, et al. Dose-response of critical structures in the posterior eye segment to hypofractioned stereotactic photon radiotherapy of choroidal melanoma. Radiother Oncol. 2013;108(2):348–53.

45. Somani S, Sahgal A, Krema H, et al. Stereotactic radiotherapy in the treatment of juxtapapillary choroidal melanoma: 2-year follow-up. Can J Ophthalmol. 2009;44(1):61–5.

46. Al-Wassia R, Dal Pra A, Shun K, et al. Stereotactic fractionated radiotherapy in the treatment of juxtapapillary choroidal melanoma: the McGill University experience. Int J Radiat Oncol Biol Phys. 2011;81(4):e455–62.

47. Gunduz K, Shields CL, Shields JA, et al. Radiation retinopathy following plaque radiotherapy for posterior uveal melanoma. Arch Ophthalmol. 1999;117(5):609–14.

48. Finger PT, Chin KJ, Yu GP, et al. Risk factors for radiation maculopathy after ophthalmic plaque radiation for choroidal melanoma. Am J Ophthalmol. 2010;149(4):608–15.

49. Parsons JT, Bova FJ, Fitzgerald CR, et al. Radiation optic neuropathy after megavoltage external-beam irradiation: analysis of time-dose factors. Int J Radiat Oncol Biol Phys. 1994;30(4):755–63.

50. Martel MK, Sandler HM, Cornblath WT, et al. Dose-volume complication analysis for visual pathway structures of patients with

advanced paranasal sinus tumors. Int J Radiat Oncol Biol Phys. 1997;38(2):273–84.

51. Jiang GL, Tucker SL, Guttenberger R, et al. Radiation-induced injury to the visual pathway. Radiother Oncol. 1994,30(1):17–25.

52. Bhandare N, Monroe AT, Morris CG, et al. Does altered fractionation influence the risk of radiation-induced optic neuropathy? Int J Radiat Oncol Biol Phys. 2005;62(4):1070–7.

53. Weber DC, Lomax AJ, Rutz HP, et al. Spot-scanning proton radiation therapy for recurrent, residual or untreated intracranial meningiomas. Radiother Oncol. 2004;71(3):251–8.

54. Ares C, Hug EB, Lomax AJ, et al. Effectiveness and safety of spot scanning proton radiation therapy for chordomas and chondrosarcomas of the skull base: first long-term report. Int J Radiat Oncol Biol Phys. 2009;75(4):1111–8.

55. Weber DC, Rutz HP, Pedroni ES, et al. Results of spot-scanning proton radiation therapy for chordoma and chondrosarcoma of the skull base: the Paul Scherrer Institut experience. Int J Radiat Oncol Biol Phys. 2005;63(2):401–9.

56. Pommier P, Liebsch NJ, Deschler DG, et al. Proton beam radiation therapy for skull base adenoid cystic carcinoma. Arch Otolaryngol Head Neck Surg. 2006;132(11):1242–9.

57. Noel G, Habrand JL, Mammar H, et al. Combination of photon and proton radiation therapy for chordomas and chondrosarcomas of the skull base: the Centre de Protontherapie D'Orsay experience. Int J Radiat Oncol Biol Phys. 2001;51(2):392–8.

58. Demizu Y, Murakami M, Miyawaki D, et al. Analysis of vision loss caused by radiation-induced optic neuropathy after particle therapy for head-and-neck and skull-base tumors adjacent to optic nerves. Int J Radiat Oncol Biol Phys. 2009;75(5):1487–92.

59. Hasegawa A, Mizoe JE, Mizota A, et al. Outcomes of visual acuity in carbon ion radiotherapy: analysis of dose-volume histograms and prognostic factors. Int J Radiat Oncol Biol Phys. 2006;64(2):396–401.

60. Tishler RB, Loeffler JS, Lunsford LD, et al. Tolerance of cranial nerves of the cavernous sinus to radiosurgery. Int J Radiat Oncol Biol Phys. 1993;27(2):215–21.

61. Stafford SL, Pollock BE, Leavitt JA, et al. A study on the radiation tolerance of the optic nerves and chiasm after stereotactic radiosurgery. Int J Radiat Oncol Biol Phys. 2003;55(5):1177–81.

62. Pollock BE, Link MJ, Leavitt JA, et al. Dose-volume analysis of radiation-induced optic neuropathy after single-fraction stereotactic radiosurgery. Neurosurgery. 2014;75(4):456–60. discussion 60

63. Hiniker SM, Modlin LA, Choi CY, et al. Dose-response modeling of the visual pathway tolerance to single-fraction and hypofractionated stereotactic radiosurgery. Semin Radiat Oncol. 2016;26(2):97–104.

64. Benedict SH, Yenice KM, Followill D, et al. Stereotactic body radiation therapy: the report of AAPM task group 101. Med Phys. 2010;37(8):4078–101.

65. Mayo C, Martel MK, Marks LB, et al. Radiation dose-volume effects of optic nerves and chiasm. Int J Radiat Oncol Biol Phys. 2010;76(3 Suppl):S28–35.

66. Kinyoun JL, Zamber RW, Lawrence BS, et al. Photocoagulation treatment for clinically significant radiation macular oedema. Br J Ophthalmol. 1995;79(2):144–9.

67. Hykin PG, Shields CL, Shields JA, et al. The efficacy of focal laser therapy in radiation-induced macular edema. Ophthalmology. 1998;105(8):1425–9.

68. Bakri SJ, Beer PM. Photodynamic therapy for maculopathy due to radiation retinopathy. Eye (Lond). 2005;19(7):795–9.

69. Shields CL, Demirci H, Dai V, et al. Intravitreal triamcinolone acetonide for radiation maculopathy after plaque radiotherapy for choroidal melanoma. Retina. 2005;25(7):868–74.

70. Mason JO 3rd, Albert MA Jr, Persaud TO, et al. Intravitreal bevacizumab treatment for radiation macular edema after plaque radiotherapy for choroidal melanoma. Retina. 2007;27(7):903–7.

71. Finger PT. Radiation retinopathy is treatable with anti-vascular endothelial growth factor bevacizumab (Avastin). Int J Radiat Oncol Biol Phys. 2008;70(4):974–7.

72. Glantz MJ, Burger PC, Friedman AH, et al. Treatment of radiation-induced nervous system injury with heparin and warfarin. Neurology. 1994;44(11):2020–7.

73. Landau K, Killer HE. Radiation damage. Neurology. 1996;46(3):889.

74. Levy RL, Miller NR. Hyperbaric oxygen therapy for radiation-induced optic neuropathy. Ann Acad Med Singap. 2006;35(3):151–7.

75. Finger PT, Chin KJ. Antivascular endothelial growth factor bevacizumab for radiation optic neuropathy: secondary to plaque radiotherapy. Int J Radiat Oncol Biol Phys. 2012;82(2):789–98.

76. Finger PT. Anti-VEGF bevacizumab (Avastin) for radiation optic neuropathy. Am J Ophthalmol. 2007;143(2):335–8.

77. Chahal HS, Lam A, Khaderi SK. Is pentoxifylline plus vitamin E an effective treatment for radiation-induced optic neuropathy? J Neuroophthalmol. 2013;33(1):91–3.

78. Farooq O, Lincoff NS, Saikali N, et al. Novel treatment for radiation optic neuropathy with intravenous bevacizumab. J Neuroophthalmol. 2012;32(4):321–4.

79. Timmerman RD. An overview of hypofractionation and introduction to this issue of seminars in radiation oncology. Semin Radiat Oncol. 2008;18(4):215–22.

# Cerebral Atrophy and Leukoencephalopathy Following Cranial Irradiation

# 39

Morgan Prust and Jorg Dietrich

## Learning Objectives

- To learn about delayed adverse effects of cranial irradiation on the central nervous system.
- To recognize common clinical syndromes induced by cranial irradiation, such as leukoencephalopathy, brain atrophy, and cognitive impairment.
- To review common risk factors associated with delayed adverse effects of cranial irradiation.
- To review the current understanding of potential mechanisms underlying delayed neurotoxic effects of cranial irradiation.
- To learn about potential management strategies to prevent and treat neurotoxic syndromes following cranial irradiation.

## Introduction

As survival of primary and secondary malignancies of the central nervous system improves with the efficacy of anticancer therapies, the delayed adverse effects of radiotherapy have been increasingly recognized as an important clinical problem facing patients and clinicians seeking to maximize both survival and quality of life in the posttreatment period.

Complications of cranial irradiation are conventionally categorized into early manifestations, including acute and early delayed radiation injury, and chronic manifestations, or late radiation injury [1]. Early manifestations include fatigue, alopecia, dermatitis, cerebral edema, and the somnolence syndrome and typically manifest within weeks (acute) to

6 months (early delayed). While debilitating, these changes are typically transient and reversible. Manifestations of late radiation injury, including leukoencephalopathy, hydrocephalus, and cerebral atrophy, typically manifest after 6 months and in some cases years after treatment and can be associated with severe, debilitating, and usually irreversible clinical sequelae. These include progressive cognitive impairment, urinary incontinence, and gait dysfunction [2–6]. The current chapter will focus on the pathophysiology, diagnosis, and management of delayed leukoencephalopathy and cerebral atrophy.

## Pathophysiology

A variety of pathophysiologic mechanisms have been implicated in late radiation injury, including neurovascular toxicity, neuroinflammation, and damage to diverse neural cell types.

It is known from preclinical studies that radiation induces vascular endothelial damage and endothelial cell apoptosis [7]. This may lead to fibrinoid necrosis of small vessels, in turn giving rise to capillary leakage, cerebral edema, spongiosis, and rarefaction of the white matter [2, 8]. Cerebrovascular mortality from stroke and intracerebral hemorrhage is increased in patients who have received cranial irradiation [9–11]. The adverse vascular effects of delayed radiation injury may be mediated by local tissue ischemia and the release of vascular endothelial growth factor (VEGF) [12].

Indeed, inhibition of VEGF with the monoclonal antibody bevacizumab has been shown to attenuate the radiographic abnormalities associated with delayed radiation necrosis and has been used in patients suffering from this complication [13].

A growing literature from preclinical and clinical studies also implicates damage to neuronal and glial progenitor cells within the dentate gyrus of the hippocampus, subventricular zone, and subcortical white matter as an important cause of delayed radiation injury and cognitive decline [14–20].

M. Prust · J. Dietrich (✉)
Department of Neurology, Division of Neuro-Oncology,
Massachusetts General Hospital, Harvard Medical School,
Boston, MA, USA
e-mail: Dietrich.Jorg@mgh.harvard.edu

© Springer International Publishing AG, part of Springer Nature 2018
E. L. Chang et al. (eds.), *Adult CNS Radiation Oncology*, https://doi.org/10.1007/978-3-319-42878-9_39

Specifically, the hippocampal dentate gyrus is an important region for adult neurogenesis and critical for the maintaining of the cellular hippocampal architecture that underlies learning and memory, spatial processing, and pattern separation [21–28]. Not surprisingly, disruption of adult hippocampal neurogenesis has been identified as a potential cause of radiation-induced cognitive impairment [19]. In addition, the subventricular zone (SVZ) and parenchymal white matter, known to harbor self-renewing glial progenitor cells essential to neuroplasticity, myelination, and endogenous neural repair, have been shown to be sensitive to the effects of radiation, and their depletion may contribute to the delayed cognitive decline, demyelination, and cerebral atrophy that commonly afflict long-term survivors [16, 29–31].

In an effort to minimize radiation-induced damage to hippocampal structures relevant to learning and memory, hippocampal-sparing radiotherapy techniques have been developed and appear to improve long-term cognitive outcomes in patients with brain metastases, though this may or may not be an option depending on the extent and distribution of a patient's disease [32]. A phase III study is ongoing to corroborate the results of this phase II trial.

Lastly, the role of inflammatory changes has been increasingly recognized as a key factor in radiation-induced neurotoxicity. Radiation is known to induce microglial activation and release of neurotoxic cytokines including tumor necrosis factor alpha (TNF-$\alpha$) and interleukin-1 beta (IL-1$\beta$) [14, 33–37]. These inflammatory changes likely contribute to neurovascular damage and direct cytotoxicity, though the precise role of the inflammatory process in delayed radiation injury remains an area of current investigation.

## Risk Factors

A variety of risk factors predicting delayed radiation injury have been established. Chief among them are radiation dose, fractionation schedule, the use of concurrent medications, and underlying patient-specific factors. Radiation doses of more than 20 Gy are considered sufficient to cause white matter changes on magnetic resonance imaging (MRI)  in patients surviving longer than 1 year (Fig. 39.1). Doses of 72 Gy or higher are associated with increased risk for focal radiation necrosis in at least 5% of patients, though radiation necrosis can also be encountered

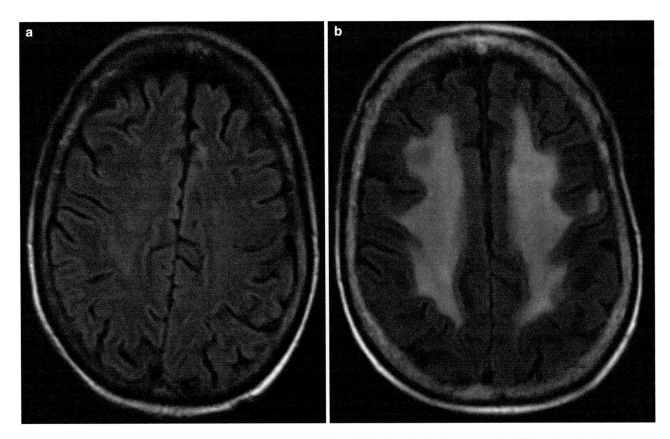

**Fig. 39.1** MRI scan of a 66-year-old female with metastatic non-small cell lung cancer, treated with whole brain radiation (35 Gy). (**a**) Axial T2/FLAIR MRI scan prior to radiation therapy without evidence of leukoencephalopathy. (**b**) Axial T2/FLAIR MRI scan 3–4 years after whole brain radiation therapy showing diffuse subcortical leukoencephalopathy. The patient was symptomatic with cognitive decline and gait difficulties

with lower radiation doses and with some heterogeneity among brain regions in their inherent propensity for tissue damage (Fig. 39.2). There is also evidence that fraction sizes exceeding 2 Gy are more commonly associated with delayed neurotoxicity [38–41].

Aside from the absolute radiation dose and fraction size, it is well established that whole brain radiation therapy (WBRT) confers significantly greater risk for delayed toxicities than partial radiation therapy. Regimens that combine WBRT and stereotactic radiosurgery (SRS) appear to induce the greatest declines in performance across an array of neurocognitive domains in surviving patients [42–44]. Recognition of these risk factors has led to a shift in practice toward smaller fraction sizes and, when possible, focal rather than whole brain regimens that attempt to spare vulnerable structures [32, 45].

While radiation therapy alone can cause delayed injury, the concurrent use of chemotherapy appears to significantly increase the risk of complications in survivors, perhaps as a result of synergistic injury to the blood-brain barrier, white matter tracts, or brain regions with neurogenic potential [31, 46].

Patient-specific factors also appear to be important predictors of long-term outcomes following radiation therapy. Young patients are particularly vulnerable to late injury, presumably due to disruption of normal neurodevelopmental processes and neural networks that rely on rapid cell division and progenitor cell function [16]. In a recent study in medulloblastoma patients treated with craniospinal irradiation, the cumulative incidence of neurovascular injury was highest in patients treated at age younger than 20 and followed a progressive pattern in the absence of additional treatment [47].

Elderly patients are also particularly vulnerable to late injury, likely as a result of premorbid age-related brain changes including microvascular disease and cerebral atrophy, which may serve to lessen patient's neurologic and cognitive reserve [2]. Indeed, patients with pre-existing white matter changes at the time of treatment are more likely to develop progressive white matter changes on MRI at a given radiation dose than patients without white matter changes at the time of treatment [48]. Patients with pre-existing demyelinating diseases such as multiple sclerosis may also be more vulnerable to radiation-induced neurotoxicity [49].

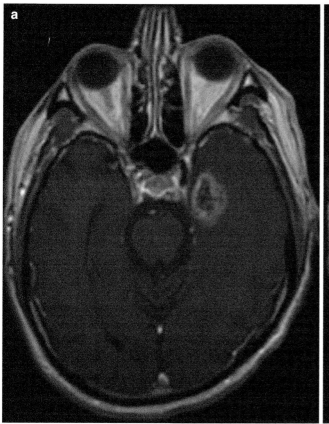
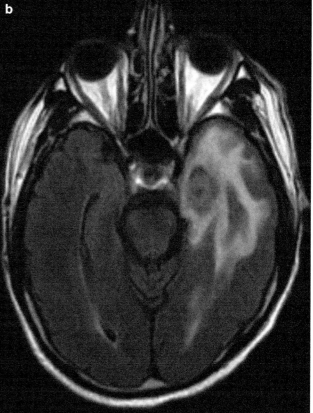

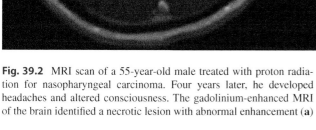

**Fig. 39.2** MRI scan of a 55-year-old male treated with proton radiation for nasopharyngeal carcinoma. Four years later, he developed headaches and altered consciousness. The gadolinium-enhanced MRI of the brain identified a necrotic lesion with abnormal enhancement (**a**) with associated cerebral edema and focal leukoencephalopathy characterized by T2/FLAIR signal hyperintensity surrounding the enhancing lesion (**b**), consistent with delayed radiation necrosis

## Leukoencephalopathy

Leukoencephalopathy, or diffuse white matter injury, is one of the most commonly encountered delayed complications of radiation therapy. Its incidence is not clearly known and varies widely among published case series, though conservative estimates indicate a range from 5 to 30% in patients undergoing radiation therapy alone, with higher rates in patients receiving concurrent chemotherapy or a combination of WBRT and SRS [2, 50, 51].

Leukoencephalopathy was initially recognized in patients undergoing high-dose radiation therapy for cerebral metastatic disease. For instance, in a series of 12 patients who were radiographically considered cured of CNS malignancy following WBRT, DeAngelis and colleagues found that all patients developed a delayed, insidious, and progressive syndrome of neurologic and cognitive decline [52]. Onset ranged from 5 to 36 months of treatment and was typically characterized by non-specific symptoms including dizziness, fatigue, and headache. Development of an overt neurocognitive syndrome was common, beginning with mild memory impairment and progressing to disorientation, confusion, and ultimately severe dementia. Gait abnormalities were universal, initially manifesting as mild gait instability and progressing to disabling ataxia resulting in frequent falls and traumatic injuries. Urinary urgency, progressing to urinary incontinence, was found in half of the patients. Other symptoms that have been recognized

in association with radiation-induced leukoencephalopathy include personality changes, neuropsychiatric abnormalities, Parkinsonism, tremor, and seizures [50, 51, 53–55].

An increasing variety of imaging modalities has been used to detect and follow the progression of radiation-induced leukoencephalopathy, though MRI and computed tomography (CT) remain the most commonly employed [5, 56, 57]. MRI is generally preferred for patient evaluation, as it is more sensitive than CT to detect structural changes. Leukoencephalopathy typically appears as increased signal with the periventricular and deep white matter on T2-weighted MRI sequences. Increased diffusivity is seen on diffusion-weighted imaging (DWI), reflecting an increase in the free movement of water as hydrophobic structures degenerate in response to radiation damage. In early stages of this syndrome, T2 hyperintensity may only be seen as capping the frontal and occipital horns of the lateral ventricles. As the disease process ensues, however, those changes typically evolve into confluent and patchy white matter hyperintensity extending from the ventricles to the corticomedullary junction. Foci of contrast enhancement may develop, reflecting disruption of the blood-brain barrier. CT may be used in patients who are unable to undergo MRI due to an implanted device or some other contraindication. The CT signature of leukoencephalopathy is diffuse white matter hypodensity (Fig. 39.3) that typically does not enhance with iodinated contrast.

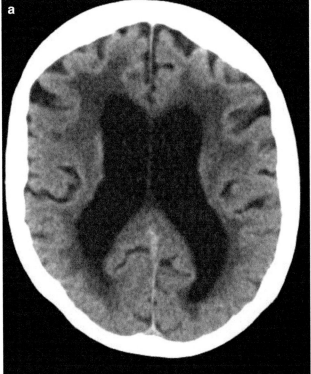
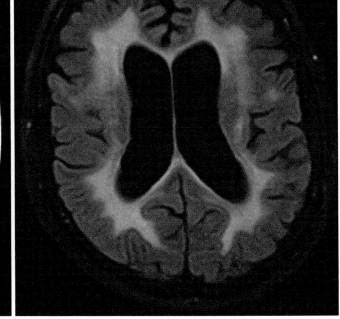

**Fig. 39.3** CT and MRI scan of a 70-year-old female treated with whole-brain radiation therapy for lung cancer. Two to three years after radiation therapy, an axial computed tomography (CT) scan shows ventricular enlargement and periventricular hypodensities (**a**), consistent with diffuse subcortical leukoencephalopathy, which can be better visualized on a corresponding axial T2/FLAIR MRI scan (**b**)

The histopathologic hallmarks of leukoencephalopathy include loss of blood-brain barrier integrity and demyelination. Injury to the blood-brain barrier, as discussed above, leads to increase in capillary permeability and chronic vasogenic edema. Injury to the white matter and oligodendroglia that serve to maintain myelin integrity leads to demyelination and replacement of hydrophobic myelin tracts with spongiform vacuoles and gliosis [2, 4, 52]. The combined effect of these changes is an increase in free tissue water, which underlies the T2 hyperintense signal on MRI and the hypodense signal on CT.

In its most severe form, a necrotizing leukoencephalopathy may develop, typically in patients who have received combined radiation and chemotherapy [53]. The latency between treatment and onset of leukoencephalopathy tends to be shorter than for patients treated with radiation therapy alone. Vascular injury is prominent in necrotizing leukoencephalopathy, leading to a higher degree of coagulative necrosis relative to milder forms, and in addition to the MRI features described above, patients may display tumorlike enhancement or disseminated hemorrhagic changes (Fig. 39.4). These findings portend a poor prognosis and are typically irreversible and progressive [4].

Leukoencephalopathy is frequently associated with worsening communicating hydrocephalus, which can be seen on MRI or CT as an enlargement of the ventricles out of proportion to cerebral atrophy, with evidence of increased periventricular edema, also known as transependymal flow, which results from a pressure gradient driving fluid from the ventricular space into the periventricular tissue [54]. Hydrocephalus is thought to result from leptomeningeal fibrosis and disruption of CSF resorption by the arachnoid villi, leading to communicating hydrocephalus. It is there-fore perhaps not surprising that there is such overlap between the clinical manifestations of radiation leukoencephalopathy and those of normal pressure hydrocephalus, in which the hallmark features include dementia, ataxia, and urinary incontinence. Relief of intracranial pressure by means of ventriculoperitoneal shunting (VPS) is a possible intervention for hydrocephalus associated with radiation leukoencephalopathy and has been shown to improve symptoms and quality of life in a subset of patients [50, 58]. In one early series, Thiessen and DeAngelis demonstrated a 6-month duration in symptomatic benefit (primarily in ataxia and urinary incontinence, with minimal effect on cognitive outcomes), though without a demonstrable prolongation of survival [52, 54].

## Cerebral Atrophy and Neurocognitive Decline

Cerebral atrophy is a concerning and frequent manifestation of delayed radiation injury [59–63] (Fig. 39.5). In a landmark early study, Constine and colleagues found evidence on MRI and CT of ventricular expansion and enlarged sulci in approximately half of patients [2]. Cerebral atrophy has long been considered a late change, typically observed in advanced stages of radiation-induced neurotoxic injury [1]. More recent studies, however, suggest that atrophy may already begin within weeks of treatment onset, continuing to progress for months after completion of treatment. The ventricles may expand to as much as double their pretreatment volume in some cases [30].

Loss of both white and gray matter contributes to the decrease in total brain volume [62]. Within the white matter,

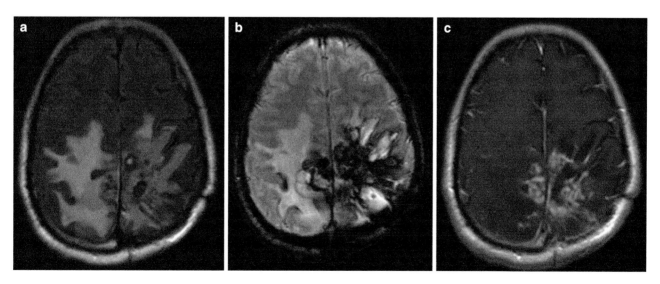

**Fig. 39.4** Axial MRI scan of a 42-year-old male with a left parieto-occipital IDH-mutant glioblastoma, treated with involved-field radiation therapy and concurrent chemotherapy with temozolomide. Approximately 3–5 years later, he developed progressive T2/FLAIR signal abnormalities within both parieto-occipital lobes (**a**), associated with interval hemorrhages best seen on gradient echo (GRE) sequences (**b**) and abnormal enhancement on T1 post-contrast MRI (**c**). Under the initial assumption of recurrent disease, he underwent repeat surgery. Pathology revealed hemorrhagic tissue necrosis in the absence of solid tumor, consistent with delayed treatment effects

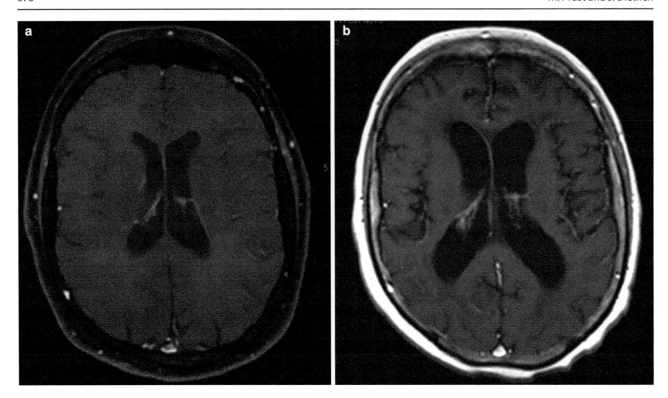

**Fig. 39.5** MRI scan of a 72-year-old female with neuroendocrine carcinoid lung cancer treated with prophylactic whole brain radiation. She developed cognitive decline and gait difficulties 3–4 years after cranial irradiation. (**a**) Contrast-enhanced axial T1-weighted MRI scan at time of whole brain radiation therapy. (**b**) Contrast-enhanced axial T1-weighted MRI scan 4 years after radiation therapy, showing significant global brain atrophy and enlargement of ventricular spaces

radiation-induced demyelination and spongiform vacuolization, coupled with injury to neural progenitor cell-mediated endogenous neural repair, lead to diffuse gliosis and contraction of the white matter space. While the mechanism of cortical atrophy is less well understood, it is thought that vascular injury to distal perforating arteries plays a central role to its pathophysiology [4].

The precise relationship between cerebral atrophy and neurocognitive performance remains under current investigation, though more recent studies suggest preferential vulnerability of hippocampal structures [64] and of cortical areas relevant for higher cognitive function to radiation treatment [65].

It has been established that higher degrees of cortical atrophy are associated with poorer cognitive outcomes and overall performance status [66, 67]. Outcomes are worse after WBRT compared to partial radiation therapy and appear to be particularly unfavorable for patients undergoing regimens that combine WBRT and SRS [42, 55]. In one recent series, Brown and colleagues found that 92% of patients undergoing WBRT and SRS experienced cognitive decline compared to 64% of patients receiving SRS alone. Early recall, delayed recall, and verbal fluency were particularly affected [43].

Treatment of late cognitive decline is generally supportive and relies on a combination of pharmacotherapy and neuro-cognitive rehabilitation. There are mixed data to support the use of neurostimulants. For instance, low-dose methylphenidate appears to improve attention and social cognition in patients with known neurocognitive impairment following WBRT [68–70]. Acetylcholinesterase inhibitors, including donepezil, have also been shown to yield significant improvements in attention, concentration, memory, and mood, with the greatest benefit conferred to those with low baseline cognitive scores [71]. While the data for such treatment strategies is equivocal, these medications are generally well tolerated and may be reasonable to consider in selected patients for whom non-pharmacologic treatments have failed.

The use of memantine, an inhibitor of the glutamatergic NMDA receptor, to prevent radiation-induced cognitive impairment following whole-brain radiation therapy has recently been studied in a randomized and prospective clinical trial and was associated with improved cognitive function over time and a reduced rate of decline in executive function, memory, and processing speed [72]. A phase III study is ongoing to corroborate these results.

Future strategies to prevent or minimize the neurotoxic effects of radiation on the brain are likely to include radiation dose alterations, modifications of the radiation field, delay of radiation therapy, and combined use of pharmacological and non-pharmacological interventions aiming at neuroprotection and enhanced brain repair.

## Conclusions and Key Points

Radiation therapy remains an essential treatment modality and means of prolonging survival in patients with CNS malignancy. It is, however, associated with an array of early and delayed complications. As more patients achieve longer survival periods with the increasing efficacy of anticancer therapies, the delayed neurotoxicities of cranial irradiation represent an important challenge in an effort to not only maximizing survival but also quality of life.

- Early complications of CNS radiation occur within weeks to 6 months of treatment onset, including side effects such as cerebral edema, and are typically transient and reversible. Late complications typically occur after 6 months and include leukoencephalopathy, cerebral atrophy, and progressive neurocognitive decline.
- Radiation causes injury to the CNS through a variety of pathophysiologic mechanisms, including (a) damage to large and small cerebral blood vessels; (b) depletion of neural progenitor cell populations leading to impaired neurogenesis, gliogenesis, and endogenous cellular repair; and (c) inflammatory changes including cytokine release and microglial activation.
- An individual patient's risk for developing delayed central nervous system toxicity depends on the total radiation dose administered, the fraction size, the extent of radiation (whole brain versus partial), the concurrent use of chemotherapy, and independent patient specific factors including age and premorbid functional status.
- Leukoencephalopathy is characterized clinically by progressive neurocognitive decline and may also result in urinary incontinence and gait instability. On a cellular level, chronic vasogenic edema and loss of white matter are seen, resulting in gliosis and vacuolization that appear on MRI as confluent patches of T2 white matter hyperintensity. It is often complicated by hydrocephalus, for which ventriculoperitoneal shunting may be considered in selected patients.
- Cerebral atrophy results from white matter destruction, as above, and loss of gray matter, possibly due to neural progenitor cell damage and chronic ischemia secondary to radiation-associated vasculopathy. While patients may respond to neurostimulants, acetylcholinesterase inhibitors, and cognitive rehabilitation, the neurocognitive impairment that accompanies these delayed complications can be profound and is commonly irreversible.

## Self-Assessment Questions

1. Which of the following is NOT a common feature of delayed radiation injury?
   A. Hydrocephalus.
   B. Cerebral atrophy.
   C. Cerebral edema.
   D. Leukoencephalopathy.

2. Radiation-induced leukoencephalopathy is characterized on neuroimaging by all of the following features EXCEPT:
   A. Diffuse white matter hypodensity on CT.
   B. Increased T2 white matter intensity on MRI.
   C. Multifocal subcortical infarcts.
   D. Patchy foci of contrast enhancement.

3. Ventriculoperitoneal shunting in radiation-induced leukoencephalopathy has been shown to:
   A. Prolong patient survival by an average of 6 months.
   B. Improve cognitive outcomes.
   C. Improve quality of life without prolonging survival.
   D. Increase the rate of fatal CNS infection.

4. The following medications have a role in supportive treatment for neurocognitive decline after radiation therapy EXCEPT:
   A. Acetylcholinesterase inhibitors.
   B. NMDA receptor antagonists.
   C. Atypical antipsychotics.
   D. Psychostimulants.

5. Which of the following is NOT an established risk factor for delayed radiation injury?
   A. Patient age.
   B. Radiation dose and fractionation schedule.
   C. Patient gender.
   D. Concurrent chemotherapy.

## Answers

1. C
2. C
3. C
4. C
5. C

## References

1. Belka C, Budach W, Kortmann RD, et al. Radiation induced CNS toxicity–molecular and cellular mechanisms. Br J Cancer. 2001;85(9):1233–9.

2. Constine LS, Konski A, Ekholm S, et al. Adverse effects of brain irradiation correlated with MR and CT imaging. Int J Radiat Oncol Biol Phys. 1988;15(2):319–30.

3. Crossen JR, Garwood D, Glatstein E, et al. Neurobehavioral sequelae of cranial irradiation in adults: a review of radiation-induced encephalopathy. J Clin Oncol. 1994;12(3):627–42.

4. Valk PE, Dillon WP. Radiation injury of the brain. AJNR Am J Neuroradiol. 1991;12(1):45–62.

5. Douw L, Klein M, Fagel SS, et al. Cognitive and radiological effects of radiotherapy in patients with low-grade glioma: long-term follow-up. Lancet Neurol. 2009;8(9):810–8.

6. Arrillaga-Romany IC and Dietrich J. Imaging finings in cancer therapy-associated neurotoxicity. Seminars in Neurology. 2012; 32(3):476–86.

7. Wong CS, Van der Kogel AJ. Mechanisms of radiation injury to the central nervous system: implications for neuroprotection. Mol Interv. 2004;4(5):273–84.

8. Murphy ES, Xie H, Merchant TE, et al. Review of cranial radiotherapy-induced vasculopathy. J Neurooncol. 2015;122(3):421–9.

9. Campen CJ, Kranick SM, Kasner SE, et al. Cranial irradiation increases risk of stroke in pediatric brain tumor survivors. Stroke. 2012;43(11):3035–40.

10. Mueller S, Fullerton HJ, Stratton K, et al. Radiation, atherosclerotic risk factors, and stroke risk in survivors of pediatric cancer: a report from the childhood cancer survivor study. Int J Radiat Oncol. 2013;86(4):649–55.

11. Mueller S, Sear K, Hills NK, et al. Risk of first and recurrent stroke in childhood cancer survivors treated with cranial and cervical radiation therapy. Int J Radiat Oncol. 2013;86(4):643–8.

12. Nordal RA, Nagy A, Pintilie M, et al. Hypoxia and hypoxia-inducible factor-1 target genes in central nervous system radiation injury: a role for vascular endothelial growth factor. Clin Cancer Res. 2004;10(10):3342–53.

13. Torcuator R, Zuniga R, Mohan YS, et al. Initial experience with bevacizumab treatment for biopsy confirmed cerebral radiation necrosis. J Neurooncol. 2009;94(1):63–8.

14. Monje ML, Mizumatsu S, Fike JR, et al. Irradiation induces neural precursor-cell dysfunction. Nat Med. 2002;8(9):955–62.

15. Rola R, Raber J, Rizk A, et al. Radiation-induced impairment of hippocampal neurogenesis is associated with cognitive deficits in young mice. Exp Neurol. 2004;188(2):316–30.

16. Dietrich J, Monje M, Wefel J, et al. Clinical patterns and biological correlates of cognitive dysfunction associated with cancer therapy. Oncologist. 2008;13(12):1285–95.

17. Hernández-Rabaza V, Llorens-Martín M, Velázquez-Sánchez C, et al. Inhibition of adult hippocampal neurogenesis disrupts contextual learning but spares spatial working memory, long-term conditional rule retention and spatial reversal. Neuroscience. 2009;159(1):59–68.

18. Hellström NAK, Björk-Eriksson T, Blomgren K, et al. Differential recovery of neural stem cells in the subventricular zone and dentate gyrus after ionizing radiation. Stem Cells. 2009;27(3):634–41.

19. Monje M, Dietrich J. Cognitive side effects of cancer therapy demonstrate a functional role for adult neurogenesis. Behav Brain Res. 2012;227(2):376–9.

20. Boström M, Kalm M, Karlsson N, et al. Irradiation to the young mouse brain caused long-term, progressive depletion of neurogenesis but did not disrupt the neurovascular niche. J Cereb Blood Flow Metab. 2013;33(6):935–43.

21. Squire LR, Ojemann JG, Miezin FM, et al. Activation of the hippocampus in normal humans: a functional anatomical study of memory. Proc Natl Acad Sci U S A. 1992;89(5):1837–41.

22. Burgess N, Maguire EA, O'Keefe J. The human hippocampus and spatial and episodic memory. Neuron. 2002;35(4):625–41.

23. Ekstrom AD, Kahana MJ, Caplan JB, et al. Cellular networks underlying human spatial navigation. Nature. 2003;425(6954):184–8.

24. Kempermann G. The neurogenic reserve hypothesis: what is adult hippocampal neurogenesis good for? Trends Neurosci. 2008;31(4):163–9.

25. Clelland CD, Choi M, Romberg C, et al. A functional role for adult hippocampal neurogenesis in spatial pattern separation. Science. 2009;325(5937):210–3.

26. Deng W, Aimone JB, Gage FH. New neurons and new memories: how does adult hippocampal neurogenesis affect learning and memory? Nat Rev Neurosci. 2010;11(5):339–50.

27. Knoth R, Singec I, Ditter M, et al. Murine features of neurogenesis in the human hippocampus across the lifespan from 0 to 100 years. Callaerts P, editor. PLoS One. 2010;5(1):e8809.

28. Richard GR, Titiz A, Tyler A, et al. Speed modulation of hippocampal theta frequency correlates with spatial memory performance. Hippocampus. 2013;23(12):1269–79.

29. Peissner W, Kocher M, Treuer H, et al. Ionizing radiation-induced apoptosis of proliferating stem cells in the dentate gyrus of the adult rat hippocampus. Brain Res Mol Brain Res. 1999;71(1):61–8.

30. Prust MJ, Jafari-Khouzani K, Kalpathy-Cramer J, et al. Standard chemoradiation for glioblastoma results in progressive brain volume loss. Neurology. 2015;85(8):683–91.

31. Correa DD, Shi W, Abrey LE, et al. Cognitive functions in primary CNS lymphoma after single or combined modality regimens. Neuro Oncol. 2012;14(1):101–8.

32. Gondi V, Pugh SL, Tome WA, et al. Preservation of memory with conformal avoidance of the hippocampal neural stem-cell compartment during whole-brain radiotherapy for brain metastases (RTOG 0933): a phase II multi-institutional trial. J Clin Oncol. 2014;32(34):3810–6.

33. Mizumatsu S, Monje ML, Morhardt DR, et al. Extreme sensitivity of adult neurogenesis to low doses of X-irradiation. Cancer Res. 2003;63(14):4021–7.

34. Monje ML, Toda H, Palmer TD. Inflammatory blockade restores adult hippocampal neurogenesis. Science. 2003;302(5651):1760–5.

35. Han W, Umekawa T, Zhou K, et al. Cranial irradiation induces transient microglia accumulation, followed by long-lasting inflammation and loss of microglia. Oncotarget. 2015;7(50):82305–23.

36. Morganti JM, Jopson TD, Liu S, et al. CCR2 antagonism alters brain macrophage polarization and ameliorates cognitive dysfunction induced by traumatic brain injury. J Neurosci. 2015;35(2):748–60.

37. Moravan MJ, Olschowka JA, Williams JP, et al. Cranial irradiation leads to acute and persistent neuroinflammation with delayed increases in T-cell infiltration and CD11c expression in C57BL/6 mouse brain. Radiat Res. 2011;176(4):459–73.

38. Tomio L, Romano M, Zanchin G, et al. Ultrarapid high-dose course of prophylactic cranial irradiation in small-cell lung cancer: evaluation of late neurologic morbidity in 16 long-term survivors. Am J Clin Oncol. 1998;21(1):84–90.

39. Laack NN, Brown PD. Cognitive sequelae of brain radiation in adults. Semin Oncol. 2004;31(5):702–13.

40. Lawrence YR, Li XA, el Naqa I, et al. Radiation dose-volume effects in the brain. Int J Radiat Oncol Biol Phys. 2010;76(3 Suppl):S20–7.

41. Dietrich J, Gondi V, Mehta M. Delayed complications of cranial irradiation. In: UpToDate, Waltham, MA, 05(2), 2018.

42. Chang EL, Wefel JS, Hess KR, et al. Neurocognition in patients with brain metastases treated with radiosurgery or radiosurgery plus whole-brain irradiation: a randomised controlled trial. Lancet Oncol. 2009;10(11):1037–44.

43. Brown PD, Jaeckle K, Ballman KV, et al. Effect of radiosurgery alone vs radiosurgery with whole brain radiation therapy on cognitive function in patients with 1 to 3 brain metastases. JAMA. 2016;316(4):401.

44. Brown PD, Buckner JC, O'Fallon JR, et al. Effects of radiotherapy on cognitive function in patients with low-grade glioma mea-

sured by the folstein mini-mental state examination. J Clin Oncol. 2003;21(13):2519–24.

45. Sun A, Bae K, Gore EM, et al. Phase III trial of prophylactic cranial irradiation compared with observation in patients with locally advanced non–small-cell lung cancer: neurocognitive and quality-of-life analysis. J Clin Oncol. 2011;29(3):279–86.

46. Prabhu RS, Won M, Shaw EG, et al. Effect of the addition of chemotherapy to radiotherapy on cognitive function in patients with low-grade glioma: secondary analysis of RTOG 98-02. J Clin Oncol. 2014;32(6):535–41.

47. Roongpiboonsopit D, Kuijf HJ, Charidimou A, et al. Evolution of cerebral microbleeds after cranial irradiation in medulloblastoma patients. Neurology. 2017;88(8):789–96.

48. Sabsevitz DS, Bovi JA, Leo PD, et al. The role of pre-treatment white matter abnormalities in developing white matter changes following whole brain radiation: a volumetric study. J Neurooncol. 2013;114(3):291–7.

49. Miller RC, Lachance DH, Lucchinetti CF, et al. Multiple sclerosis, brain radiotherapy, and risk of neurotoxicity: the Mayo clinic experience. Int J Radiat Oncol. 2006;66(4):1178–86.

50. Perrini P, Scollato A, Cioffi F, et al. Radiation leukoencephalopathy associated with moderate hydrocephalus: intracranial pressure monitoring and results of ventriculoperitoneal shunting. Neurol Sci. 2002;23(5):237–41.

51. Lai R, Abrey LE, Rosenblum MK, et al. Treatment-induced leukoencephalopathy in primary CNS lymphoma: a clinical and autopsy study. Neurology. 2004;62(3):451–6.

52. DeAngelis LM, Delattre JY, Posner JB. Radiation-induced dementia in patients cured of brain metastases. Neurology. 1989;39(6):789–96.

53. Cummings M, Dougherty DW, Mohile NA, et al. Severe radiation-induced leukoencephalopathy: case report and literature review. Adv Radiat Oncol. 2016;1(1):17–20.

54. Thiessen B, DeAngelis LM. Hydrocephalus in radiation leukoencephalopathy: results of ventriculoperitoneal shunting. Arch Neurol. 1998;55(5):705–10.

55. Monaco EA, Faraji AH, Berkowitz O, et al. Leukoencephalopathy after whole-brain radiation therapy plus radiosurgery versus radiosurgery alone for metastatic lung cancer. Cancer. 2013;119(1):226–32.

56. Dietrich J, Klein JP. Imaging of cancer therapy–induced central nervous system toxicity. Neurol Clin. 2014;32(1):147–57.

57. Mamlouk MD, Handwerker J, Ospina J, et al. Neuroimaging findings of the post-treatment effects of radiation and chemotherapy of malignant primary glial neoplasms. Neuroradiol J. 2013;26(4):396–412.

58. Fischer CM, Neidert MC, Péus D, et al. Hydrocephalus after resection and adjuvant radiochemotherapy in patients with glioblastoma. Clin Neurol Neurosurg. 2014;120:27–31.

59. Swennen MHJ, Bromberg JEC, Witkamp TD, et al. Delayed radiation toxicity after focal or whole brain radiotherapy for low-grade glioma. J Neurooncol. 2004;66(3):333–9.

60. Omuro AMP, Ben-Porat LS, Panageas KS, et al. Delayed neurotoxicity in primary central nervous system lymphoma. Arch Neurol. 2005;62(10):1595–600.

61. Shibamoto Y, Baba F, Oda K, et al. Incidence of brain atrophy and decline in mini-mental state examination score after whole-brain radiotherapy in patients with brain metastases: a prospective study. Int J Radiat Oncol Biol Phys. 2008;72(4):1168–73.

62. Karunamuni R, Bartsch H, White NS, et al. Dose-dependent cortical thinning after partial brain irradiation in high-grade glioma. Int J Radiat Oncol. 2016;94(2):297–304.

63. Ailion AS, King TZ, Wang L, et al. Cerebellar atrophy in adult survivors of childhood cerebellar tumor. J Int Neuropsychol Soc. 2016;22(5):501–11.

64. Seibert TM, Karunamuni R, Bartsch H, et al. Radiation dose–dependent hippocampal atrophy detected with longitudinal volumetric magnetic resonance imaging. Int J Radiat Oncol. 2017;97(2):263–9.

65. Seibert TM, Karunamuni R, Kaifi S, et al. Cerebral cortex regions selectively vulnerable to radiation dose-dependent atrophy. Int J Radiat Oncol. 2017;97(5):910–8.

66. Gondi V, Paulus R, Bruner DW, et al. Decline in tested and self-reported cognitive functioning after prophylactic cranial irradiation for lung cancer: pooled secondary analysis of radiation therapy oncology group randomized trials 0212 and 0214. Int J Radiat Oncol. 2013;86(4):656–64.

67. Kiehna EN, Mulhern RK, Li C, et al. Changes in attentional performance of children and young adults with localized primary brain tumors after conformal radiation therapy. J Clin Oncol. 2006;24(33):5283–90.

68. Mulhern RK, Khan RB, Kaplan S, et al. Short-term efficacy of methylphenidate: a randomized, double-blind, placebo-controlled trial among survivors of childhood cancer. J Clin Oncol. 2004;22(23):4795–803.

69. Meyers CA, Weitzner MA, Valentine AD, et al. Methylphenidate therapy improves cognition, mood, and function of brain tumor patients. J Clin Oncol. 1998;16(7):2522–7.

70. Page BR, Shaw EG, Lu L, et al. Phase II double-blind placebo-controlled randomized study of armodafinil for brain radiation-induced fatigue. Neuro Oncol. 2015;17(10):1393–401.

71. Rapp SR, Case LD, Peiffer A, et al. Donepezil for irradiated brain tumor survivors: a phase III randomized placebo-controlled clinical trial. J Clin Oncol. 2015;33(15):1653–9.

72. Brown PD, Pugh S, Laack NN, et al. Memantine for the prevention of cognitive dysfunction in patients receiving whole-brain radiotherapy: a randomized, double-blind, placebo-controlled trial. Neuro Oncol. 2013;15(10):1429–37.

# Hypopituitarism

# 40

Sara J. Hardy, Ismat Shafiq, Michael T. Milano,
G. Edward Vates, and Louis S. Constine

## Learning Objectives

- To describe late effects from radiation to the hypothalamic-pituitary axis.

## Background

## Introduction

Endocrinopathy related to cancer or cancer treatment is one of the most treatable late effects occurring in cancer survivors; however, lack of recognition of hypopituitarism can lead to significant impact on quality of life and survival for patients. It is important to be aware of consequences to the hypothalamic-pituitary axis following radiation treatment and make early referrals to the appropriate specialists.

S. J. Hardy · M. T. Milano
Department of Radiation Oncology, University of Rochester
Medical Center, Rochester, NY, USA

I. Shafiq
Division of Endocrinology and Metabolism, University of
Rochester, Rochester, NY, USA

G. E. Vates
Department of Neurosurgery, University of Rochester Medical
Center, Rochester, NY, USA

L. S. Constine (✉)
Department of Radiation Oncology, University of Rochester
Medical Center, Rochester, NY, USA

Department of Pediatrics, University of Rochester Medical Center,
Rochester, NY, USA
e-mail: Louis_constine@urmc.rochester.edu

## Normal Hypothalamic-Pituitary Axis (HPA)

The hypothalamus and pituitary constitute a unique portion of the central nervous system. They communicate not only through synaptic connections with the rest of the brain but through the release of humoral substances. In that way, they link the neural and endocrine systems. This allows the hypothalamus to be a key regulator of body homeostasis, including temperature, appetite, thirst, sexual behavior, and fear [1].

The hypothalamus is located below the thalamus, forming the walls and floor of the interior portion of the third ventricle (Fig. 40.1). It is located immediately posterior to the optic chiasm. The mammillary bodies form the posterior portion of the hypothalamus. The infundibulum arises from between the optic chiasm and mammillary bodies and continues as the pituitary stalk. The pituitary gland lies within the pituitary fossa. It is bound by the anterior clinoid process and posterior clinoid process, which, along with the intervening portions of the sphenoid bone, form the sella turcica. Just beneath the floor of the sella turcica is the sphenoid sinus. The pituitary fossa is bounded on both sides by the cavernous sinus. The pituitary lies just behind and inferior to the optic chiasm [1].

The hypothalamus contains two types of neurosecretory cells: neurohypophysial neurons, which release vasopressin and oxytocin, and hypophysiotropic neurons, which secrete releasing and inhibitory hormones in the portal hypophyseal vessels. The releasing and inhibitory hormones regulate secretion of hormones from the anterior pituitary glandular cells. The anterior pituitary gland produces six important hormones: adrenocorticotropic hormone (ACTH), growth hormone (GH), prolactin, thyroid-stimulating hormone (TSH), luteinizing hormone (LH), and follicle-stimulating hormone (FSH). The posterior pituitary does not contain glandular cells; rather, it contains the axons and terminals of the neurohypophysial neurons mentioned previously that are located in the hypothalamus. The axon terminals in the posterior pituitary release the hormones oxytocin and antidiuretic hormone (vasopressin or ADH) into the circulation [1].

**Fig. 40.1** Anatomic image of the normal hypothalamic-pituitary axis

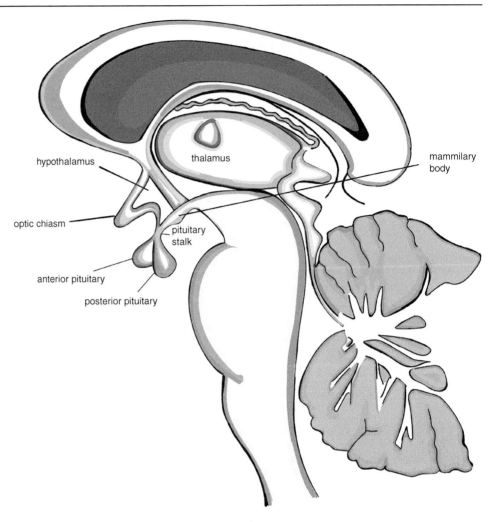

**Table 40.1** Hypothalamic-releasing factors

| Factor | Effect | Function |
| --- | --- | --- |
| Thyrotropin-releasing hormone | Stimulates release of TSH | Stimulates thyroid to make thyroxine (T4) and triiodothyronine (T3) |
| Growth hormone-releasing hormone | Stimulates release of GH | Induces the liver, kidneys, and other organs to produce somatomedins or insulin-like growth factors |
| Gonadotropin-releasing hormone | Stimulates release of LH and FSH | Modulates puberty, menses, sexual drive |
| Corticotropin-releasing hormone | Stimulates release of ACTH | Stimulates the adrenal gland to make cortisol |
| Dopamine | Inhibits release of prolactin | Modulates lactation |
| Somatostatin | Inhibits release of GH and TSH | Regulates thyroid and growth hormones |

The hormones originating in the anterior and posterior pituitary serve a variety of important functions (Table 40.1). Deficiency or excess of these hormones leads to specific clinical syndromes, which can vary according to the age of the individual and the degree of change in hormone release.

GH induces the liver, kidneys, and other organs to produce somatomedins or insulin-like growth factors, which promote increased growth of long bones and bone mineralization and affect body composition (muscle mass and fat deposition). GH release is controlled by GH-releasing hormone (GHRH) and somatostatin. In healthy children and adults, GH secretion is pulsatile and occurs 2–6 times per day [2]. In adolescents, there are additional pulses and these pulses have higher peaks.

ACTH (corticotropin) stimulates the adrenal cortex to produce corticosteroid hormones, particularly cortisol, a glucocorticoid, and to a lesser extent the mineralocorticoid hormone, aldosterone. Both hormones help to maintain blood pressure, control electrolyte balance, and promote glucose mobilization into the bloodstream [1]. Secretion of ACTH normally peaks in the morning before a person awakens, and it increases with stress.

Prolactin causes the mammary glands to produce milk. The primary hypothalamic factor controlling prolactin release is dopamine, which is an inhibitory factor.

TSH stimulates the thyroid gland to make thyroxine (T4) and triiodothyronine (T3), which promote cell metabolism. The secretion of TSH from the anterior pituitary is stimulated by thyrotropin-releasing hormone and inhibited by somatostatin and dopamine from the hypothalamus.

LH and FSH are responsible for the menstrual cycle and oogenesis in females and regulate the testicular hormones and spermatogenesis in males. As noted above, it is produced in the anterior pituitary and regulated by the hypothalamus. The hypothalamic stimulus is inhibited between 6 months of age and onset of puberty.

Oxytocin causes contractions of the smooth muscle in the breast to allow for release of milk and contractions of the uterus during labor. ADH (vasopressin) promotes water retention by the kidneys and allows concentration of urine.

## Neuroendocrine Dysfunction in Brain Tumor Patients

One of the complexities of hypothalamic-pituitary dysfunction in brain tumor patients is that there can be multiple contributing factors including mass effect from the tumor and treatment effects from chemotherapy, surgery, and radiation. Studies have shown that there is a high incidence of neuroendocrinopathies in pediatric patients with brain tumors [3]. In some cases, pathology due to mass effect from the tumor, such as hydrocephalus, correlates strongly to abnormalities in neuroendocrine testing [4]. Additionally, there is some evidence that patients who are treated with chemotherapy alone have a high risk of neuroendocrine dysfunction. A study which reviewed patients with childhood cancers ($n = 362$) found that in patients treated with chemotherapy alone for non-CNS tumors ($n = 31$), 48% developed GH deficiency, 52% developed TSH deficiency, and 32% developed pubertal abnormalities [5]. More recently, ipilimumab, an immune system modulator, has been found to potentially cause autoimmune hypophysitis causing panhypopituitarism [6].

## Radiation and Hypothalamic-Pituitary Axis Injury

Cranial irradiation has also been shown to be a significant contributor to abnormalities of the hypothalamic-pituitary axis (HPA). Historically, hypopituitarism has been noted in children treated with prophylactic cranial radiation for acute lymphoblastic leukemia, total body irradiation in preparation for bone marrow transplant, and after radiation therapy for brain tumors that directly or incidentally exposed the hypothalamic-pituitary axis [7, 8]. Radiation-induced hypopituitarism is also often seen after radiation for pituitary adenomas [9, 10]. Additionally, radiation-induced hypopituitarism can be seen with inclusion of the HPA in the radiation field in a variety of cancers including nasopharyngeal cancer, retinoblastoma, base of skull tumors, and craniopharyngioma. Constine et al. reported radiation dose and frequency of HPA injury after review of 32 patients who received cranial radiation for brain tumors, after receiving a dose of 39.6–70.2 Gy to the hypothalamic-pituitary region [11]. A recent meta-analysis of 18 studies showed a 66% prevalence of any form of hypopituitarism in adult patients after cranial radiation therapy for nasopharyngeal and intracerebral tumors [7]. Much of the data comes from cranial irradiation for childhood cancers. Hudson et al. were able to show that disorders of the hypothalamic-pituitary-adrenal axis occurred in 13.8% of childhood cancer survivors who received cranial irradiation [12]. A report from the St Jude Lifetime Cohort Study published in 2015 showed an estimated point prevalence of 46.5% for growth hormone deficiency, 10.8% for LH/FSH deficiency, 7.5% for TSH deficiency, and 4% for ACTH deficiency [13].

The main cause of hypopituitarism after radiation therapy is thought to be direct neuronal damage from ionizing radiation with resultant cell death [8]. This is supported by the differences in radiosensitivity of different components of the HPA. However, there may also be a chronic inflammatory response and vascular damage, which can cause ischemic damage to neurons and reactive gliosis [8, 14–16]. Clinical studies demonstrate that the GH axis is the most vulnerable to damage followed by the gonadotrophin, adrenal, and thyroid hormone axes [17–19]. Cranial irradiation in the range of 18–50 Gy will often result in isolated GH deficiency, while higher doses of radiation such as those used for skull base tumors or nasopharyngeal carcinoma will often result in multiple anterior pituitary deficiencies [8, 20].

Radiation damage is thought to occur both to the hypothalamus and anterior pituitary with higher doses in excess of 40 Gy. There is some controversy regarding where the predominant site of damage occurs at lower doses. Early studies suggested the site of injury is mainly the hypothalamus, since GHRH can still stimulate release of GH in patients and gonadotropin-releasing hormone can still stimulate release of LH and FSH [11, 21–25]. However, recent studies by Darzy et al. also suggested direct pituitary damage with compensatory increase in hypothalamic GHRH release. In irradiated patients, pituitary responsiveness to GHRH decreases with time. It was postulated that somatotroph dysfunction in the pituitary was due to atrophy after the loss of GHRH. However, Darzy et al. showed that patients who have undergone cranial irradiation continue to have spontaneous GH release in both baseline and stressed states. This implies that GHRH stimulation is still present despite hypothalamic dysfunction due to compensatory increase in hypothalamic GHRH release. Thus, pituitary dysfunction cannot be completely attributed to the loss of GHRH, and there may be combined damage to both the hypothalamus and pituitary [26–29].

Fractionation is also thought to modulate radiation damage to the HPA. Growth hormone deficiency (GHD) is frequently seen in in children who receive total body irradiation with single doses of 8–11 Gy, which supports the importance of fraction size even in the setting of low total doses [30]. However, the evidence for fraction size-dependent HPA damage is mixed. Two early studies [31, 32] showed that children treated with larger fraction sizes had a higher prevalence of GHD. However, Thomas et al. [33] and another study by Brauner et al. [34] did not show that larger fraction size increased risk. Another series [19] demonstrated that biological equivalent dose was correlated with risk of GHD.

Multiple studies have found that younger age at time of radiation therapy is a risk factor for neuroendocrine abnormalities after radiation therapy. GH deficiency was seen frequently in children treated with TBI but not in adults treated with similar schedules [19, 35–39].

Additionally, studies have found that increased time from treatment was a risk factor. A meta-regression analysis from Mulder (2009) showed that impaired GH responses could occur within the first 12 months after treatment was completed but were still detected after longer follow-up periods of 8–32 years [30].

## Clinical Syndromes

### Growth Hormone Deficiency
Growth hormone deficiency is the most common and often the only hormonal deficiency noted after cranial irradiation. The deficiency is most notable in children, where there is a reduction in growth velocity, leading to short stature. There may also be fasting hypoglycemia. Adults with GH deficiency may experience decrease in muscle mass and increased adipose tissue [40, 41].

### Gonadotropin Deficiency
Deficiency of the gonadotropins can cause oligomenorrhea or amenorrhea in women and low testosterone concentrations in men [42]. In children, it can cause delayed or arrested pubertal development [43]. In adults, lack of normal gonadotropin function can cause infertility, sexual dysfunction, and decreased libido [41].

### Early Sexual Maturation
Central precocious puberty is defined as early activation of the hypothalamic-pituitary-gonadal axis leading to onset of puberty prior to age 8 or 9 in girls and boys, respectively. This can lead to premature closure of growth plates leading to decreased adult height. Further, precocious puberty can cause psychosocial dysfunction [43].

### TSH Deficiency
Central hypothyroidism refers to deficiency of thyroid hormone due to dysfunction of the pituitary, hypothalamus, or hypothalamic-pituitary portal circulation. Thyroid hormone deficiency can be subclinical and cause no significant dysfunction. However, it can cause symptoms such as fatigue, constipation, cold intolerance, and weight gain. In children, poor linear growth and delayed puberty can occur with TSH deficiency [41].

### ACTH Deficiency
ACTH deficiency, also known as central adrenal insufficiency, can cause fatigue, weakness, nausea, vomiting, anorexia, and abdominal cramping. Additionally, patients with ACTH deficiency may develop life-threatening complications in the setting of severe illness including hypoglycemia and hypotensive shock [43].

### Hyperprolactinemia
Hyperprolactinemia (caused by loss of hypothalamic inhibition of prolactin release) can cause amenorrhea, infertility, and/or decreased libido [42].

There is mixed evidence about whether certain types of deficiencies appear before others. Some studies suggest that GH deficiency is the first to emerge after injury to HPA, followed by deficiencies of gonadotropin, ACTH, and TSH [44, 45]. However, other studies suggest that these deficiencies can occur in any order [2, 3, 11, 45, 46].

## Tolerances

### Growth Hormone Deficiency

Growth hormone deficiency is the most common and often the only anterior pituitary deficit seen after cranial irradiation. GH deficiency is thought to be largely due to loss of the growth hormone-releasing hormone neurons in the arcuate nucleus of the hypothalamus. It has been seen after conventional fractionated radiation therapy with doses ≥18 Gy and following doses as low as 9–10 Gy given in a single dose [47, 48]. Merchant et al. in [49] were able to demonstrate that growth hormone deficiency was likely to develop within 36 months of exposure to the hypothalamus/pituitary in patients receiving ≥20 Gy [49]. Data suggests that nearly all children treated with doses >35 Gy will develop GH deficiency [37]. Cranial radiation 18–50 Gy will most commonly result in isolated GH deficiency [8].

Merchant et al. [50] examined the correlation between the dosimetry of the hypothalamus and the peak GH value after cranial irradiation in children. They recorded the volume of the hypothalamus receiving 0–20 Gy, 20–40 Gy, or 40–60 Gy as well as the change in GH. They found that using the volumes receiving a particular dose range, it was possible to predict the change in GH level [50]. A pooled study with a hypothalamic-pituitary dose ranging from 13 to 65 Gy showed that radiation-induced growth hormone deficiency had a prevalence of 35% [30].

Interestingly, the radiation threshold dose for GHD is higher in adults, and for any given dose, the incidence of GHD is lower than in children [51].

## LH/FSH Deficiency

There is no detailed information regarding the threshold dose, which causes LH/FSH deficiency. However, it is rare at HPA doses <40 Gy, and there is a progressive increase in incidence as the dose to the HPA exceeds 50 Gy [11, 52].

## Precocious Puberty

This phenomenon was initially described in patients treated with cranial irradiation to 24–45 Gy but is most commonly seen in patients given CNS prophylaxis for leukemia (Table 40.2). At doses >50 Gy, the prevalence of early puberty decreases as the incidence of gonadotropin deficiency increases [43]. Interestingly, radiation-induced precocious puberty is only seen in girls with radiation doses 18–24 Gy but affects both sexes equally at higher doses of 25–50 Gy [58, 59, 62, 65]. Triggers can also include tumors near the HPA [43]. The mechanism is thought to be related to disinhibition of cortical influences on the hypothalamus and a reduction in GABAergic tone [8].

## TSH Deficiency

The TSH axis is the most resistant to radiation damage [8]. At doses below 40 Gy, TSH deficiency is very unusual. The incidence increases substantially when the HPA dose exceeds 50 Gy [11].

## ACTH Deficiency

Clinically relevant ACTH deficiency is uncommon in patients receiving HPA irradiation <50 Gy [41]. Following doses >50 Gy, the incidence of ACTH deficiency varies from 18 to 35% during follow-up periods ranging from 5 to >15 years [11, 46, 51]. The incidence of ACTH deficiency may be higher in older patients compared to children and adolescents [41].

**Table 40.2** Neuroendocrine dysfunction with different fractionated radiation therapy doses

| Type of radiation therapy/typical dose | Tumor type | Type of neuroendocrine dysfunction |
| --- | --- | --- |
| Total body radiation 7–12 Gy | Leukemia and lymphoma | Isolated growth hormone deficiency, mainly seen in children [8, 38, 53, 54] |
| Prophylactic cranial radiation 18–25 Gy | Leukemia | Isolated growth hormone deficiency in a significant proportion of children Compensated growth hormone deficiency in adults Precocious puberty (girls only) [8, 35, 36, 55–58] |
| Intracranial radiation therapy 30–50 Gy | Brain tumors, not including pituitary or parasellar tumors | Growth hormone deficiency in at least 27–67% Precocious puberty (both sexes) ACTH in 3–4% Gonadotropin deficiency in 20–27% TSH deficiency in 3–9% Hyperprolactinemia [8, 9, 11, 59–62] |
| Extracranial radiation therapy 50–70 Gy | Nasopharyngeal carcinoma and skull base tumors | Growth hormone deficiency in almost all patients at 5 years Gonadotropin deficiency in 29% at 5 years, 36% at 10 years Hypothyroidism in 30% at 5 years, 63% at 10 years ACTH deficiency in 19% at 5 years, 28% at 10 years Hyperprolactinemia in 72% at 5 years, 84% at 10 years [8, 46, 63] |
| Intracranial radiation therapy, pituitary and parasellar only 30–50 Gy | Pituitary adenomas and parasellar tumors | Growth hormone deficiency in almost all patients at 5 years Gonadotropin deficiency in up to 19–60% TSH deficiency in up to 40% ACTH deficiency in 33–60% Hyperprolactinemia in 20–50% [8–10, 64] |

## Hyperprolactinemia

Elevation of prolactin levels is less frequent in patients treated with HPA irradiation under 40–45 Gy (Table 40.2). Mild increases are commonly observed with radiation doses greater than 50 Gy, particularly in women [11, 20]. The overall incidence of hyperprolactinemia varies from 20 to 50% [11, 46, 51].

## Stereotactic Radiation Therapy

Stereotactic radiation therapy was developed to reduce the volume of normal tissue exposed to therapeutic radiation dose while delivering high-dose conformal radiation to tumor sites. There is evidence supporting its use for multiple tumor types including functional and nonfunctional pituitary adenomas [66–70]. With stereotactic radiation therapy to the pituitary gland, the risk of hypopituitarism is thought to be mainly related to anterior pituitary pathology rather than the hypothalamus as radiation dose to the hypothalamus appears to be low [67]. Deterioration in pituitary function is usually reported after a mean radiation dose >15 Gy for the gonadotropic and thyrotropic axes and 18 Gy for the adrenocorticotropic axes [68, 70].

Data are accumulating regarding the risk of hypopituitarism after both single-fraction and multiple-fraction stereotactic radiation therapy. Factors influencing risk of hypopituitarism potentially include single versus multiple fraction, volume treated, and dose. One study compared hypopituitarism after fractionated stereotactic radiation therapy and after single-fraction stereotactic radiosurgery. Mitsumori et al. did not find that there was a significantly different rate of hypopituitarism in either group; however, there was a short-term follow-up. The rates of freedom from new pituitary hormone replacement were 21.1% in the fractionated SRT group and 22.1% for the SRS group [71]. The other studies, which do not make a direct comparison, have not thus far shown a clear benefit to fractionated stereotactic radiotherapy for pituitary adenomas [8]. It has been shown that hypopituitarism after Gamma Knife radiosurgery increases with larger tumor volumes. Pollock et al. showed that the 5-year risk of hypopituitarism was 18% at 5 years for patients who are treated with a tumor volume of 4 cm or less and 58% at 5 years for patients with a tumor volume of >4 cm. The risk of hypopituitarism also increases with higher doses, such as the higher doses required for secretory pituitary adenomas [70, 72–74]. There is also some evidence that higher radiation doses to the pituitary stalk can increase risk of hypopituitarism [75].

## Screening

Hypopituitarism is a highly treatable complication of cranial radiation therapy seen in both adults and children. Cancer survivors should be monitored for symptoms of neuroendocrinopathy. Many symptoms can be subtle, so routine yearly surveillance is indicated in patients who are at high risk of pituitary dysfunction [76].

**Table 40.3** Screening and management of hypopituitarism in children and adults

| Syndrome | Common symptoms (adults) | Common symptoms (children) | Screening | Typical replacement | Typical dose |
|---|---|---|---|---|---|
| Central adrenal insufficiency | Fatigue, weakness, nausea, vomiting, anorexia, abdominal cramping, complications in setting of severe illness such as hypotension or hypoglycemia | Same | Serum cortisol levels at 8–9 AM, corticotropin stimulation test | Hydrocortisone | 15–20 mg total daily dose |
| Central hypothyroidism | Fatigue, constipation, cold intolerance, weight gain | Poor linear growth, delayed puberty | Serum free T4 and TSH | Levothyroxine | Titrate to serum free T4 levels in the mid to upper half of the reference range |
| GH deficiency | Decrease in muscle mass and increased adipose tissue, fasting hypoglycemia | Children: Reduction in growth velocity, short stature | GH stimulation testing (single GH measurements are not helpful) | GH | Starting dose 0.2–0.4 mg/d for patients younger than 60 years, 0.1–0.2 for patients older than 60 years, then titrate using IGF-1 levels |
| Central hypogonadism in males | Infertility, sexual dysfunction, decreased libido, decreased bone density, decreased energy, decreased muscle mass | Delayed or arrested pubertal development | Serum testosterone, FSH, and LH (perform in the absence of illness and before 10 AM after overnight fast) | Testosterone | Varies by means of administration |
| Central hypogonadism in females | Oligomenorrhea or amenorrhea, infertility, sexual dysfunction, decreased libido | Delayed or arrested pubertal development | Serum estradiol, FSH, and LH | Estrogen | Same |

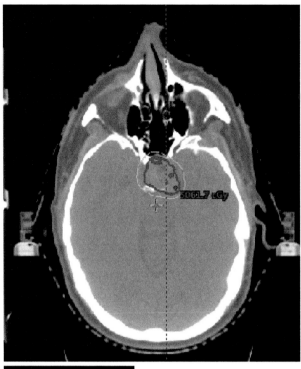
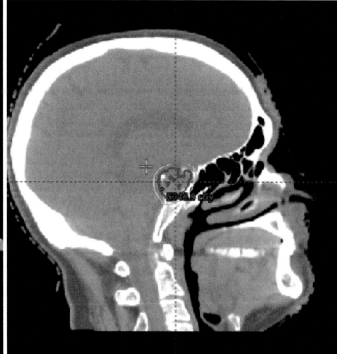

Isodoses (cGy)
5000
4500

**Fig. 40.2** Treatment plan for a 44-year-old man with recurrent pituitary adenoma. After repeat resection, adjuvant radiation was recommended due to the prior recurrence and residual tumor seen in the left cavernous sinus. He was treated with 4500 cGy in 180 cGy fractions to surgical bed with a simultaneous integrated boost to 5000 cGy in 200 Gy fractions to gross residual disease. The 5000 cGy (red) and 4500 cGy (green) isodose lines are shown in axial and sagittal planes above

Survivors of childhood cancer should be monitored for changes in growth rate, failure to thrive, or altered onset of puberty. This includes assessment of Tanner stage, weight, BMI, nutritional status, and height. Free T4 and TSH should also be measured.

## Management

Management of hypopituitarism is typically carried out through endocrine replacement therapy [76]. Table 40.3 summarizes common replacement strategies for specific syndromes.

## Case Study

A 44-year-old male presented with hypopituitarism. He was found to have pituitary mass and underwent transsphenoidal resection. Pathology was consistent with pituitary adenoma. However, there was residual tumor in the left cavernous sinus, and 4 years later, the mass had grown significantly. He underwent repeat transsphenoidal resection, which again left significant residual gross disease. Given his history, he was referred for adjuvant radiation therapy. He was treated with 4500 cGy in 180 cGy fractions to surgical bed with a simultaneous integrated boost to 5000 cGy in 200 cGy fractions to gross residual disease (Fig. 40.2). He developed growth hormone deficiency and hypogonadism within a year after radiation. Over the next 2–3 years, he gradually developed joint pain and muscle weakness. Labs showed adrenal insufficiency and hypothyroidism. He was managed by endocrinology with serial bloodwork and hormone replacement.

## Summary

- Radiation-induced hypopituitarism is a side effect commonly seen in cranial radiation affecting the hypothalamic-pituitary axis.
- The growth hormone axis is particularly sensitive and is frequently the only site affected with lower-dose fractionated radiation therapy.

- At higher doses, multiple axes can be affected, including gonadotropins, TSH, ACTH, and prolactin.
- For fractionated radiation therapy, both hypothalamic and pituitary cells are currently thought to be sites of damage. For radiosurgery and fractionated stereotactic radiation therapy, the pituitary is felt to be the main site of damage.
- The mechanism of damage to the HPA is thought to be direct neuronal damage from ionizing radiation therapy.
- Factors that affect risk in fractionated radiation therapy include total dose, fraction size, age at time of radiation, and length of time after radiation therapy.
- Factors that affect risk of stereotactic radiation therapy include total dose, volume radiated, and radiation dose to the pituitary stalk.
- Clinical syndromes from radiation-induced hypopituitarism include growth hormone deficiency, gonadotropin deficiency, precocious puberty, central adrenal insufficiency, TSH deficiency, and hyperprolactinemia.
- Screening for hypopituitarism and referral to appropriate specialists can avoid unnecessary morbidity in this patient population.

## Self-Assessment Questions

1. What axis is the most sensitive to radiation therapy?
   A. Gonadotropins.
   B. TSH.
   C. ACTH.
   D. Growth hormone.

2. How does radiation treatment cause hyperprolactinemia?
   A. Loss of hypothalamic inhibition.
   B. Damage to the pituitary.
   C. Mechanism is unknown.

3. What are factors that affect the risk of hypopituitarism from fractionated radiation therapy?
   A. Total dose, fraction size, age at time of radiation, duration of time after radiation.
   B. Fraction size only.
   C. Total dose and fraction size only.

4. Which factors affect the risk of hypopituitarism from stereotactic radiation?
   A. Total dose.
   B. Volume irradiated.
   C. Radiation dose to the pituitary stalk.
   D. All of the above.
   E. a and c.

5. Which clinical syndromes can occur with radiation-induced changes to the hypothalamic-pituitary axis?
   A. Precocious puberty.
   B. Central adrenal insufficiency.
   C. TSH deficiency.
   D. Hyperprolactinemia.
   E. Any of the above.

## Answers

1. D. Growth hormone deficiency is the most common and often the only anterior pituitary deficit seen after cranial irradiation because it is the most sensitive to radiation. Interestingly, the radiation threshold dose for GHD is higher in adults, and for any given dose, the incidence of GHD is lower than in children [8, 51].
2. A. Hyperprolactinemia is thought to be caused by loss of hypothalamic inhibition of prolactin release [42].
3. A. Total dose, fraction size, age at time of radiation, and duration of time after radiation all modulate radiation damage to the HPA [19, 30–32, 35].
4. D. Factors that alter risk of hypopituitarism after stereotactic radiation therapy include total dose, volume radiated, and radiation dose to the pituitary stalk [8, 70–75].
5. E. Radiation therapy can cause neuroendocrine dysfunction, and there are reports of hyperprolactinemia, precocious puberty in children, central adrenal insufficiency, central hypothyroidism, GH deficiency, and hypogonadism in the literature [8, 11, 41].

## References

1. Blumenfeld H. Neuroanatomy through clinical cases. Sunderland, MA: Sinauer Associates, Inc.; 2002.
2. Rose SR, Municchi G. Six-hour and four-hour nocturnal sampling for growth hormone. J Pediatr Endocrinol Metab. 1999;12:167–73.
3. Merchant TE, Williams T, Smith JM, et al. Preirradiation endocrinopathies in pediatric brain tumor patients determined by dynamic tests of endocrine function. Int J Radiat Oncol Biol Phys. 2002b;54:45–50.
4. Merchant TE, Lee H, Zhu J, et al. The effects of hydrocephalus on intelligence quotient in children with localized infratentorial ependymoma before and after focal radiation therapy. J Neurosurg. 2004;101:159–68.
5. Rose SR, Schreiber RE, Kearney NS, et al. Hypothalamic dysfunction after chemotherapy. J Pediatr Endocrinol Metab. 2004;17:55–66.
6. Corsello SM, Barnabei A, Marchetti P, et al. Endocrine side effects induced by immune checkpoint inhibitors. J Clin Endocrinol Metab. 2013;98:1361–75.
7. Appelman-Dijkstra NM, Kokshoorn NE, Dekkers OM, et al. Pituitary dysfunction in adult patients after cranial radiotherapy: systematic review and meta-analysis. J Clin Endocrinol Metab. 2011;96:2330–40.

8. Darzy KH. Radiation-induced hypopituitarism. Curr Opin Endocrinol Diabetes Obes. 2013;20:342–53.
9. Littley MD, Shalet SM, Beardwell CG, et al. Hypopituitarism following external radiotherapy for pituitary tumours in adults. Q J Med. 1989;70:145–60.
10. Rim CH, Yang DS, Park YJ, et al. Radiotherapy for pituitary adenomas. Long term outcome and complications. Radiat Oncol J 2011a;29:156–63.
11. Constine LS, Woolf PD, Cann D, et al. Hypothalamic-pituitary dysfunction after radiation for brain tumors. N Engl J Med. 1993;328:87–94.
12. Hudson MM, Ness KK, Gurney JG, et al. Clinical ascertainment of health outcomes among adults treated for childhood cancer. JAMA. 2013;309:2371–81.
13. Chemaitilly W, Li Z, Huang S, et al. Anterior hypopituitarism in adult survivors of childhood cancers treated with cranial radiotherapy: a report from the St Jude lifetime cohort study. J Clin Oncol. 2015;33:492–500.
14. Chiang CS, Hong JH, Stalder A, et al. Delayed molecular responses to brain irradiation. Int J Radiat Biol. 1997;72:45–53.
15. Nishioka H, Hirano A, Haraoka J, et al. Histological changes in the pituitary gland and adenomas following radiotherapy. Neuropathology. 2002;22:19–25.
16. Nishioka H, Ito H, Haraoka J, et al. Histological changes in the hypofunctional pituitary gland following conventional radiotherapy for adenoma. Histopathology. 2001;38:561–6.
17. Agha A, Sherlock M, Brennan S, et al. Hypothalamic-pituitary dysfunction after irradiation of nonpituitary brain tumors in adults. J Clin Endocrinol Metab. 2005;90:6355–60.
18. Darzy KH, Aimaretti G, Wieringa G, et al. The usefulness of the combined growth hormone (GH)-releasing hormone and arginine stimulation test in the diagnosis of radiation-induced GH deficiency is dependent on the post-irradiation time interval. J Clin Endocrinol Metab. 2003;88:95–102.
19. Schmiegelow M, Lassen S, Poulsen HS, et al. Cranial radiotherapy of childhood brain tumours: growth hormone deficiency and its relation to the biological effective dose of irradiation in a large population based study. Clin Endocrinol. 2000;53:191–7.
20. Constine LS, Rubin P, Woolf PD, et al. Hyperprolactinemia and hypothyroidism following cytotoxic therapy for central nervous system malignancies. J Clin Oncol. 1987;5:1841–51.
21. Achermann JC, Brook CG, Hindmarsh PC. The GH response to low-dose bolus growth hormone-releasing hormone (GHRH(1-29) NH2) is attenuated in patients with longstanding post-irradiation GH insufficiency. Eur J Endocrinol. 2000;142:359–64.
22. Crosnier H, Brauner R, Rappaport R. Growth hormone response to growth hormone-releasing hormone (hp GHRH1-44) as an index of growth hormone secretory dysfunction after prophylactic cranial irradiation for acute lymphoblastic leukemia (24 grays). Acta Paediatr Scand. 1988;77:681–7.
23. Grossman A, Savage MO, Blacklay A, et al. The use of growth hormone-releasing hormone in the diagnosis and treatment of short stature. Horm Res. 1985;22:52–7.
24. Lustig RH, Schriock EA, Kaplan SL, et al. Effect of growth hormone-releasing factor on growth hormone release in children with radiation-induced growth hormone deficiency. Pediatrics. 1985;76:274–9.
25. Oberfield SE, Kirkland JL, Frantz A, et al. Growth hormone response to GRF 1-44 in children following cranial irradiation for central nervous system tumors. Am J Pediatr Hematol Oncol. 1987;9:233–8.
26. Darzy KH, Thorner MO, Shalet SM. Cranially irradiated adult cancer survivors may have normal spontaneous GH secretion in the presence of discordant peak GH responses to stimulation tests (compensated GH deficiency). Clin Endocrinol. 2009;70:287–93.
27. Darzy KH, Pezzoli SS, Thorner MO, et al. Cranial irradiation and growth hormone neurosecretory dysfunction: a critical appraisal. J Clin Endocrinol Metab. 2007;92:1666–72.
28. Darzy KH, Murray RD, Gleeson HK, et al. The impact of short-term fasting on the dynamics of 24-hour growth hormone (GH) secretion in patients with severe radiation-induced GH deficiency. J Clin Endocrinol Metab. 2006;91:987–94.
29. Darzy KH, Pezzoli SS, Thorner MO, et al. The dynamics of growth hormone (GH) secretion in adult cancer survivors with severe GH deficiency acquired after brain irradiation in childhood for nonpituitary brain tumors: evidence for preserved pulsatility and diurnal variation with increased secretory disorderliness. J Clin Endocrinol Metab. 2005;90:2794–803.
30. Mulder RL, Kremer LC, van Santen HM, et al. Prevalence and risk factors of radiation-induced growth hormone deficiency in childhood cancer survivors: a systematic review. Cancer Treat Rev. 2009;35:616–32.
31. Brauner R, Fontoura M, Zucker JM, et al. Growth and growth hormone secretion after bone marrow transplantation. Arch Dis Child. 1993;68:458–63.
32. Shalet SM, Price DA, Beardwell CG, et al. Normal growth despite abnormalities of growth hormone secretion in children treated for acute leukemia. J Pediatr. 1979;94:719–22.
33. Thomas BC, Stanhope R, Plowman PN, et al. Endocrine function following single fraction and fractionated total body irradiation for bone marrow transplantation in childhood. Acta Endocrinol. 1993;128:508–12.
34. Brauner R, Adan L, Souberbielle JC, et al. Contribution of growth hormone deficiency to the growth failure that follows bone marrow transplantation. J Pediatr. 1997;130:785–92.
35. Brauner R, Czernichow P, Rappaport R. Greater susceptibility to hypothalamopituitary irradiation in younger children with acute lymphoblastic leukemia. J Pediatr. 1986;108:332.
36. Brennan BM, Rahim A, Mackie EM, et al. Growth hormone status in adults treated for acute lymphoblastic leukaemia in childhood. Clin Endocrinol. 1998;48:777–83.
37. Clayton PE, Shalet SM. Dose dependency of time of onset of radiation-induced growth hormone deficiency. J Pediatr. 1991;118:226–8.
38. Littley MD, Shalet SM, Morgenstern GR, et al. Endocrine and reproductive dysfunction following fractionated total body irradiation in adults. Q J Med. 1991;78:265–74.
39. Melin AE, Adan L, Leverger G, et al. Growth hormone secretion, puberty and adult height after cranial irradiation with 18 Gy for leukaemia. Eur J Pediatr. 1998;157:703–7.
40. Salomon F, Cuneo RC, Hesp R, et al. The effects of treatment with recombinant human growth hormone on body composition and metabolism in adults with growth hormone deficiency. N Engl J Med. 1989;321:1797–803.
41. Sklar CA, Constine LS. Chronic neuroendocrinological sequelae of radiation therapy. Int J Radiat Oncol Biol Phys. 1995;31:1113–21.
42. Tonorezos ES, Hudson MM, Edgar AB, et al. Screening and management of adverse endocrine outcomes in adult survivors of childhood and adolescent cancer. Lancet Diabetes Endocrinol. 2015;3:545–55.
43. Barnes N, Chemaitilly W. Endocrinopathies in survivors of childhood neoplasia. Front Pediatr. 2014;2:101.
44. Shalet SM. Radiation and pituitary dysfunction. N Engl J Med. 1993;328:131–3.
45. Spoudeas HA. Growth and endocrine function after chemotherapy and radiotherapy in childhood. Eur J Cancer. 2002;38:1748–59. discussion 1760-1
46. Lam KS, Tse VK, Wang C, et al. Effects of cranial irradiation on hypothalamic-pituitary function--a 5-year longitudinal study in patients with nasopharyngeal carcinoma. Q J Med. 1991;78:165–76.

47. Rappaport R, Brauner R. Growth and endocrine disorders secondary to cranial irradiation. Pediatr Res. 1989;25:561–7.

48. Sklar CA. Growth and pubertal development in survivors of childhood cancer. Pediatrician. 1991;18:53–60.

49. Merchant TE, Rose SR, Bosley C, et al. Growth hormone secretion after conformal radiation therapy in pediatric patients with localized brain tumors. J Clin Oncol. 2011;29:4776–80.

50. Merchant TE, Goloubeva O, Pritchard DL, et al. Radiation dose-volume effects on growth hormone secretion. Int J Radiat Oncol Biol Phys. 2002a;52:1264–70.

51. Samaan NA, Schultz PN, Yang KP, et al. Endocrine complications after radiotherapy for tumors of the head and neck. J Lab Clin Med. 1987;109:364–72.

52. Bajorunas DR, Ghavimi F, Jereb B, et al. Endocrine sequelae of antineoplastic therapy in childhood head and neck malignancies. J Clin Endocrinol Metab. 1980;50:329–35.

53. Ogilvy-Stuart AL, Clark DJ, Wallace WH, et al. Endocrine deficit after fractionated total body irradiation. Arch Dis Child. 1992;67:1107–10.

54. Spoudeas HA, Hindmarsh PC, Matthews DR, et al. Evolution of growth hormone neurosecretory disturbance after cranial irradiation for childhood brain tumours: a prospective study. J Endocrinol. 1996;150:329–42.

55. Brauner R, Rappaport R. Precocious puberty secondary to cranial irradiation for tumors distant from the hypothalamo-pituitary area. Horm Res. 1985;22:78–82.

56. Costin G. Effects of low-dose cranial radiation on growth hormone secretory dynamics and hypothalamic-pituitary function. Am J Dis Child. 1988;142:847–52.

57. Kirk JA, Raghupathy P, Stevens MM, et al. Growth failure and growth-hormone deficiency after treatment for acute lymphoblastic leukaemia. Lancet. 1987;1:190–3.

58. Leiper AD, Stanhope R, Kitching P, et al. Precocious and premature puberty associated with treatment of acute lymphoblastic leukaemia. Arch Dis Child. 1987a;62:1107–12.

59. Lannering B, Jansson C, Rosberg S, et al. Increased LH and FSH secretion after cranial irradiation in boys. Med Pediatr Oncol. 1997a;29:280–7.

60. Livesey EA, Hindmarsh PC, Brook CG, et al. Endocrine disorders following treatment of childhood brain tumours. Br J Cancer. 1990;61:622–5.

61. Madaschi S, Fiorino C, Losa M, et al. Time course of hypothalamic-pituitary deficiency in adults receiving cranial radiotherapy for primary extrasellar brain tumors. Radiother Oncol. 2011;99:23–8.

62. Ogilvy-Stuart AL, Clayton PE, Shalet SM. Cranial irradiation and early puberty. J Clin Endocrinol Metab. 1994;78:1282–6.

63. Pai HH, Thornton A, Katznelson L, et al. Hypothalamic/pituitary function following high-dose conformal radiotherapy to the base of skull: demonstration of a dose-effect relationship using dose-volume histogram analysis. Int J Radiat Oncol Biol Phys. 2001;49:1079–92.

64. Rush S, Cooper PR. Symptom resolution, tumor control, and side effects following postoperative radiotherapy for pituitary macroadenomas. Int J Radiat Oncol Biol Phys. 1997;37:1031–4.

65. Quigley C, Cowell C, Jimenez M, et al. Normal or early development of puberty despite gonadal damage in children treated for acute lymphoblastic leukemia. N Engl J Med. 1989;321:143–51.

66. Castinetti F, Nagai M, Morange I, et al. Long-term results of stereotactic radiosurgery in secretory pituitary adenomas. J Clin Endocrinol Metab. 2009;94:3400–7.

67. Feigl GC, Pistracher K, Berghold A, et al. Pituitary insufficiency as a side effect after radiosurgery for pituitary adenomas: the role of the hypothalamus. J Neurosurg. 2010;113(Suppl):153–9.

68. Jezkova J, Marek J, Hana V, et al. Gamma knife radiosurgery for acromegaly--long-term experience. Clin Endocrinol. 2006;64:588–95.

69. Leenstra JL, Tanaka S, Kline RW, et al. Factors associated with endocrine deficits after stereotactic radiosurgery of pituitary adenomas. Neurosurgery. 2010;67:27–32. discussion 32-3

70. Vladyka V, Liscak R, Novotny J Jr, et al. Radiation tolerance of functioning pituitary tissue in gamma knife surgery for pituitary adenomas. Neurosurgery. 2003;52:309–16. discussion 316-7

71. Mitsumori M, Shrieve DC, Alexander E 3rd, et al. Initial clinical results of LINAC-based stereotactic radiosurgery and stereotactic radiotherapy for pituitary adenomas. Int J Radiat Oncol Biol Phys. 1998;42:573–80.

72. Jane JA Jr, Vance ML, Woodburn CJ, et al. Stereotactic radiosurgery for hypersecreting pituitary tumors: part of a multimodality approach. Neurosurg Focus. 2003;14:e12.

73. Sheehan JP, Xu Z, Lobo MJ. External beam radiation therapy and stereotactic radiosurgery for pituitary adenomas. Neurosurg Clin N Am. 2012;23:571–86.

74. Vladyka V, Liscak R, Simonova G, et al. Radiosurgical treatment of hypophyseal adenomas with the gamma knife: results in a group of 163 patients during a 5-year period. Cas Lek Cesk. 2000;139:757–66.

75. Feigl GC, Bonelli CM, Berghold A, et al. Effects of gamma knife radiosurgery of pituitary adenomas on pituitary function. J Neurosurg. 2002;97:415–21.

76. Fleseriu M, Hashim IA, Karavitaki N, et al. Hormonal replacement in hypopituitarism in adults: an endocrine society clinical practice guideline. J Clin Endocrinol Metab. 2016;101:3888–921.

# Neurocognitive Changes

Jane H. Cerhan, Alissa M. Butts, Michael W. Parsons, and Paul D. Brown

## Learning Objectives

- Describe the causes of cognitive decline in patients with cancer.
- Recognize that many cancer patients have cognitive impairment before treatment.
- Describe the cognitive impact of systemic therapy.
- Describe the cognitive impact of both whole brain radiotherapy and focal radiotherapy.
- Describe treatments or treatment techniques to alleviate or decrease the risk of cognitive decline after radiotherapy.
- Describe the role of neuropsychological assessment in the clinic and in research.

Cognitive functioning is a critical component of overall quality of life and key to performance of most activities of daily living [1]. Indeed, cognitive impairment is often more stressful for patients and caregivers than impairment in physical functioning [2]. In patients with brain tumors, cognitive changes can precede changes on neuroimaging, and thus cognitive assessment may present an important surveillance tool [3]. In this chapter, we will review the impact of cancer and cancer treatment, including radiotherapy, on cognitive functioning. Then, we will turn to discussion of the purposes and elements of formal neuropsychological evaluation and interpretation of neuropsychological results in the clinic and in research.

J. H. Cerhan (✉) · A. M. Butts
Department of Psychiatry and Psychology, Mayo Clinic, Rochester, MN, USA
e-mail: Cerhan.jane@mayo.edu

M. W. Parsons
Burkhardt Brain Tumor Center, Cleveland Clinic, Cleveland, OH, USA

P. D. Brown
Department of Radiation Oncology, Mayo Clinic, Rochester, MN, USA

## Cancer-Related Cognitive Impairment

Persons with cancer are at risk for cognitive impairment prior to any potentially neurotoxic treatment or direct neurologic involvement. Some reviews have estimated that up to 30% of cancer patients may experience cognitive symptoms prior to any treatment [4]. This finding was noted in early studies of chemotherapy-related cognitive symptoms [5, 6]. For example, in a pilot study of 18 women with breast carcinoma, Wefel et al. [7] found that a third of patients performed below normal levels on at least one measure in a neuropsychological test battery after surgery but prior to any adjunctive treatment. A similar study conducted with a slightly larger sample but a shorter test battery found that 21% of the sample had at least one impaired cognitive test score prior to treatment.

Further demonstration of the neurocognitive impact of cancer has come from the arena of cognitive neuroscience. Cimprich et al. [8] used functional MRI (FMRI) to compare brain activity of women with breast cancer (who had not yet undergone systemic treatment) with a healthy control group. They found that cancer patients activated a broader network of brain areas and performed more poorly on a working memory task than control subjects. This pattern suggested that the patients may be recruiting additional brain networks to perform the task and was taken as indicative of inefficient neurocognitive processing, a pattern that has been demonstrated in other conditions that compromise cognitive function, such as aging of the brain [9]. The etiology of these cognitive symptoms is not well understood, but hypotheses have included aberrant DNA repair mechanisms, [10] imbalance of cytokines interfering with brain function, or possibly fatigue-related issues [8].

## Cognitive Symptoms Related to Brain Tumor

When cancer involves the brain, either as the primary site of disease or through metastases, cognitive deficits are even more prevalent [11–15]. Rates vary across studies, based primarily on tumor type and the sensitivity of cognitive testing employed, but the literature suggests that measurable cognitive deficits occur in up to 90% of patients [14, 16, 17]. The nature and degree of cognitive impact are related to tumor location, overall tumor burden, rate of growth, and the extent of surrounding edema.

Supratentorial tumors are more likely to be associated with cognitive deficits than infratentorial lesions, with left frontal and temporal masses often producing the most disruptive cognitive problems [18]. In general, left lateralized lesions are more likely to be associated with verbal deficits and right hemisphere tumors with visuospatial deficits [18, 19]. However, brain tumors can disrupt the functioning of both local and larger-scale neural networks, which can produce deficits that differ from those predicted by tumor location alone [20]. Even leptomeningeal metastases can be associated with significant neurologic morbidity, including the presence of functional and cognitive deficits [21].

Tumor "momentum," or rate of growth, is another important predictor of cognitive impact. Although early studies of the relationship between tumor histology and cognitive function failed to demonstrate an effect of tumor grade [22], more recent studies have clarified the relationship. In a comparison of patients with left temporal gliomas, grade IV tumors were more likely to produce impairment on tests of memory and language than grade II or III tumors [23]. A recent study further demonstrated that the likelihood of cognitive impairment is greater in those patients whose gliomas harbor the more aggressive IDH-1 wild-type genotype [24]. It appears that, although cognitive deficits are fairly common in patients with low-grade gliomas prior to resection or other treatment [19]. The slow-growing or more infiltrative nature of these lesions is less disruptive to the surrounding neural networks or perhaps encourages neural reorganization [25].

## Cognitive Effects of Systemic Treatment

Cognitive impact of chemotherapy for cancers that have *not* metastasized to the brain has been the subject of intense research scrutiny over the past 15–20 years. A comprehensive review of this literature is beyond the scope of this chapter, but the vast majority of meta-analyses demonstrate small to moderate effects of chemotherapy on cognitive function [26–32]. However, there has been a controversy about the consistency with which these effects have been found [33], perhaps because the size of the cognitive effects tends to be modest. In some cases, it appears that methodologic issues may lead to an absence of findings. For instance, studies that compare the performance of cancer patients to population-based norms are less likely to demonstrate cognitive differences than those that examine subjects both before and after

chemotherapy treatment and demonstrate within-subject changes [34]. Studies that restrict the definition of cognitive impairment to the severe range [35] have been insensitive to the deficits typically identified in the majority of studies.

Extensive preclinical research has demonstrated neurotoxic effects of many systemic chemotherapy agents. Although the mechanisms by which chemotherapies affect the brain are not clearly delineated, possibilities include myelin toxicity, disruption of the neurovascular niche, oxidative stress, pro-inflammatory effects, and destruction of neural progenitor cells in the hippocampal and subventricular zone (see [36] for a review). Noninvasive neuroimaging studies in human subjects have demonstrated that chemotherapy treatment affects brain gray matter volume [37], white matter integrity [38, 39], brain activity at rest [40, 41], and functional brain activation during the performance of cognitive tasks [42]. The consistency of the findings from bench to clinical research paradigms supports the notion that there is a measurable cognitive impact of chemotherapy on cognitive function. What is less clear, however, is what individual variables may predispose some patients to develop these cognitive problems, while others are completely unaffected.

Antiangiogenic agents may have less cognitive impact than other chemotherapy agents because they target vasculature on the abluminal side of the blood-brain barrier. The literature on antiangiogenic agents to date does not generally include assessment of cognitive or functional outcome beyond adverse events and performance status [43], and some trials include only screening measures of cognitive function, such as the Montreal Cognitive Assessment (MoCA; [44, 45]). A small study of sunitinib, an agent with antiangiogenic properties, as an alternative to whole brain radiotherapy in patients with 1–3 brain metastases included cognitive outcomes [46]. Sixty-four percent of the patients in the study had cognitive impairment in at least one domain at baseline, but there was no decline in cognitive performance at 2-month follow-up. A small subset of subjects followed longer (>6 months) continued to show stable or improved cognitive functioning. Further integration of cognitive outcome measurement in future studies of antiangiogenic agents in the treatment of brain metastases is needed.

The explosion of targeted agents in the treatment of systemic cancer has raised hope for the promise of more efficacious and specific targeting of brain metastases as well. Interestingly, genomic analysis of brain metastases has shown that many tumors harbor clinically actionable mutations that are distinct from those detected in the primary cancer [47]. However, at this early stage of development, the large-scale studies evaluating efficacy of targeted treatments for brain metastases have generally not included the assessment of cognitive or other functional outcomes [48].

In the future, combination therapy that includes surgery or biopsy to identify actionable mutations, possible treatment with laser interstitial thermal therapy, and followed by treatment with targeted agents may provide improved survival and tumor recurrence for patients with brain metastases. As such advances take place, the assessment of cognitive outcomes and quality of life for these patients will become even more important.

## Radiation Treatment and Cognition

Characterization of the cognitive risks of radiotherapy is a moving target with evolution of therapeutic dosages and approaches. Often, by the time long-term follow-up has occurred, new techniques have usurped the strategies used in the target subjects [49]. The actual rate of cognitive injury is highly dependent on the specific characteristics of the sample studied (e.g., high-grade or low-grade glioma, metastases, acute, subacute, long-term, etc.), the sensitivity of the instruments used [50, 51], and the type, location, and spatial extent of therapy [52].

Furthermore, the relative risk of cognitive impact on a given patient depends on a range of factors. For example, the impact of radiation on an infant's developing brain is different from the impact radiation has on a young adult brain or older adult brain. As described in the previous section, the overlay of radiation effects on cognitive deficits associated with the tumor (or extracranial disease) itself and any prior or concurrent treatments are also important factors to consider. The effects radiation can have on cognition may vary in acute and later stages of survival. Finally, in a recent review, Wefel et al. [53] discuss the heterogeneity of cognitive deficits associated with genetic variation. Greene-Schloesser et al. [54] found remarkable variability in radiation effect across disease states and concluded "It is distinctly possible that the molecular, cellular, and microanatomic events that lead to radiation-induced cognitive impairment are different for SCLC, nasopharyngeal cancer, low-grade glioma, benign non-parenchymal brain tumor, primary brain tumor and metastatic brain tumor patients".

Overall, the impact of radiation on cognition is complex, requiring appreciation of neurocognitive systems, the individual difference factors that contribute to cognitive symptoms, and the role of neuroplasticity in symptom expression over time. In the remainder of this section, we will review cognitive effects of whole brain radiation followed by discussion of more focal approaches to dosing radiation and prevention and mitigation of cognitive effects.

Whole brain radiotherapy (WBRT) can be associated with cognitive decline. Traditionally, a distinction has been made between early-delayed and late-delayed neurocognitive effects of WBRT. The former emerges between 1 and 6 months posttreatment and is thought to be a reversible process of de- and re-myelination. Late-delayed effects, which

are often permanent or even progressive, may become apparent after 6 months [55, 56]. Makale et al. [52] propose that the precursors to long-term injury are set in motion early. Similarly, Onodera et al. [57] found that impairment at 4 months after WBRT, while often transient, predicts development of late-delayed effects. The cognitive domains most often impacted include attention and processing speed, likely due to effects on frontal-subcortical white matter pathways, and memory given selective effects on the hippocampi [58]. Predicting the impact on individuals, though, is particularly challenging. By definition, patients receiving WBRT have serious disease and multiple cognitive risk factors. The risk of developing a severe progressive dementia has previously been estimated to be between 1.9% and 5.1%, [59] but methodologies have changed considerably, and the current risk is likely lower. In particular, the use of high daily fractions is thought to be detrimental.

Given the risks of WBRT, there is momentum toward more focal radiation approaches whenever possible [11]. In a recent large multicenter phase III clinical trial [60], 213 individuals with 1–3 brain metastases were randomized to either WBRT plus stereotactic radiosurgery (SRS) or SRS alone. Patients who received only SRS had better and more stable cognitive functioning as well as greater self-reported quality of life at 3 and 12 months, despite the fact that the WBRT group had better tumor control [60]. There was no difference between groups in median overall survival (7.4 months for SRS + WBRT vs 10.4 months for SRS alone). Cognitive deterioration at 3 months was 19% after SRS alone compared to 46% with SRS plus WBRT ($p < 0.01$), with a decline defined as a drop of 1.5 SD on at least two cognitive tests. Other studies have similarly shown that individuals with brain metastases treated with SRS alone have better neurocognitive outcomes compared to those treated with SRS + WBRT [61].

With less malignant disease, cognitive deficits can often be minimized or avoided completely using focal treatment. In a prospective trial, Laack et al. [62] followed low-grade glioma patients treated with standard doses of conformal radiotherapy and found cognitive functioning was stable after up to 3 years of follow-up. The study employed a comprehensive neuropsychological battery and included a pretreatment exam to control for baseline deficits [62]. In another prospective trial, 95 patients with arteriovenous malformation (AVM) who underwent extensive neuropsychological testing before and up to 3 years after SRS showed no cognitive declines, and many subjects showed improvement in intelligence, attention, and memory over the trial period [63].

Because of the physical properties of proton beam therapy, involving low entry dose with maximal dose of energy at the depth of the tumor and nearly zero exit dose, less healthy tissue is exposed and thus holds potential for limiting neurocognitive impact than in traditional photon beam therapy [64]. In a controlled study by Sherman et al. using a comprehensive test battery, 20 patients treated with proton beam therapy for low-grade glioma showed cognitive stability for up to 5 years of follow-up [65].

## Mitigating and Protective Interventions

As discussed, more focal methods of radiotherapy (i.e., intensity-modulated radiation therapy, SRS, proton beam, etc.) can minimize the risk of cognitive impact. Additional approaches to prevent or mitigate cognitive decline will be discussed in this section. For example, WBRT has been modified to selectively avoid the hippocampal region (hippocampal avoidance HA-WBRT) given its known role in memory and its neuronal stem cell compartment [66, 67]. An association between radiation therapy to the bilateral hippocampi and poor memory performance on neuropsychological testing has been shown [68]. A phase II trial evaluating HA-WBRT found better preservation of memory functioning in patients with brain metastases compared to historical controls [67, 69], although an ongoing phase III trial is needed to confirm these results. Similar findings were reported by Tsai et al. [70] who found preserved immediate recall of verbal information in those who received HA-WBRT compared to those who received traditional WBRT, but there were no group differences in delayed recall scores.

The use and development of pharmacologic agents to protect against radiation-induced cerebral injury is a growing area of interest, including memantine, which acts on the glutamatergic system by blocking NMDA receptor [71]. Brown et al. [72] found those who received memantine during WBRT showed longer time to cognitive decline than those who did not receive memantine. The memantine group also had stronger performance on measures of executive functioning 16 weeks later and better processing speed and delayed recognition at 24 weeks.

Treating cognitive symptoms that arise *after* treatment requires evaluation of multiple potential contributing factors including but not limited to radiation effect. For example, fatigue is extremely common in patients with brain tumor; small studies suggest positive symptomatic effect of psychostimulants such as methylphenidate [73] and modafinil [74]. Donepezil, an acetylcholinesterase inhibitor, has been examined as a potential treatment for postradiation cognitive symptoms. A phase III trial found patients receiving donepezil had better performances on tests of memory and motor speed. An interaction analysis suggested donepezil was particularly beneficial for those who had lower baseline cognitive performances [75].

Another potential treatment model involves using neural stem cells and oligodendrocyte progenitor cells as agents to provide either neuroprotective or restorative effects for radiation-induced cognitive decline. The proposed mechanism includes a combination of cell replacement and trophic factors that hypothetically contribute to improved white matter integrity and ultimately preserved or improved cognitive functioning as shown in animal models [76].

Cognitive rehabilitation interventions for patients with brain tumor are typically extensions of methods developed for other neurologic injuries, such as stroke and traumatic brain injury [77]. Very few studies have looked specifically at rehabilitation in patients with brain tumor [78] or specifically postradiotherapy [71]. In one randomized controlled trial, Gehring et al. [79] evaluated a cognitive rehabilitation intervention in patients with glioma and cognitive concerns whose disease was in remission. The intervention consisted of a computerized attention training program and one-on-one sessions reviewing cognitive compensatory strategies. Patients who received the intervention did better than controls on select neuropsychological tests (attention and verbal memory) and reported less subjective mental fatigue at 6 months. About 60% of Gehring et al.'s subjects had previous radiation treatment. Recently, Riggs et al. [80] reported promising preliminary data demonstrating increased white matter integrity and hippocampal volumes as well as improved reaction times following a physical exercise intervention in young adults who had been treated with radiation during childhood. Overall, rehabilitation interventions, both individually and in multimodality programs, show promise and have demonstrated some efficacy, particularly in patients treated for non-brain cancers, but more randomized controlled trials are greatly needed [81].

## Neuropsychological Assessment

Neuropsychological assessment and imaging are complementary in understanding the clinical status of patients with brain injury or disease. In spite of advances in imaging technology, cognitive deficits can often be present with no abnormality on imaging, and conversely patients with tumors and other cerebral lesions can sometimes have normal cognitive functioning [82]. A thorough neuropsychological evaluation can inform care in many ways, starting with detecting dysfunction and then monitoring the impact of treatment and potential side effects. Surveillance is another important role, as changes in cognitive functioning have been found to often precede brain tumor changes seen on imaging [3]. Neuropsychological assessment can also be useful in discriminating between neurocognitive symptoms due to neurologic versus psychological factors such as depression. This is important given different treatment implications and the fact that depression is a risk factor for treatment non-compliance [83] and shortened length of survival [84]. Finally, the results of a neuropsychological evaluation can inform rehabilitation interventions and issues like return to work, making independent decisions, managing ADLs, and driving.

Asking patients about cognitive symptoms is extremely important clinically, especially given the close relationship to quality of life. However, subjective report is not a good proxy for neuropsychological assessment. Subjective report usually does not correlate, or correlates only weakly, with actual cognitive performance measured with neuropsychological tests. This has been found time and again in numerous patient populations including patients with brain tumor [85]. Reasons for this are not entirely known, but subjective cognitive complaints often relate more strongly than neuropsychological test scores to factors such as mood, personality, and fatigue [86]. Another factor could include declining insight with disease progression. As such, patients might actually overestimate cognitive difficulties early in the course when the symptoms are new and underestimate them later [87]. As a result, neuropsychological testing is important to measure and monitor cognitive functioning objectively.

Neuropsychological testing usually consists of mostly paper-and-pencil tasks administered one-on-one by a psychologist or technician. Proper examiner training is key to a valid and reliable result. Standardized test administration is the cornerstone of the neuropsychological evaluation because normative data is only applicable when the test is given to patients exactly as it was given to the norm group. An easy example to consider is a basic word-list learning task where the examiner reads a list to the subject and asks them to try to memorize as many words as they can. If the list is standardized at a presentation rate of one word per 2 seconds, but the list is read more quickly, the test becomes too hard, the norms no longer apply, and it becomes essentially a different test.

Appropriate tests have well-established psychometric properties, including reliability and validity for the particular use. Reliability refers to the consistency of scores on the test and thus freedom from error. Reliability is a basic requirement and a prerequisite to validity [88]. Validity is a multidimensional concept that is often misunderstood. When a test has been successfully administered to a population, it shows *feasibility*. In contrast, *validity* is established through an accumulation of evidence that a test truly measures what it purports to measure or predict [89]. The validity of a test can vary by purpose as well as population. In other words, validity is a function of the interpretation or specific *use* of a test, not just the test itself [90]. Convergent validity is demonstrated by showing a sufficiently robust correlation between the test and other measures of the same construct (i.e., "gold standard"). Discriminant validity is equally important, wherein the test shows a lack of (or less) correlation with measures of different constructs [91, 92]. The American Psychological Association stipulates that establishing validity for an intended purpose is the joint responsibility of pub-

lishers and test users, and the existence of published norms is not enough [93]. Board certified neuropsychologists are familiar with validity models and how to apply them to appropriate test selection for research and clinical purposes with specific patient groups.

Thorough neuropsychological evaluations aim to sample from all major cognitive domains in order to monitor and harness the patient's strengths as well as to identify deficits (Fig. 41.1). As discussed earlier, domain of dysfunction in the context of brain tumors and/or radiation is not always predictable. Distant, diffuse, as well as localized effects can occur. Thorough testing also allows the examiner to monitor change in areas that might not initially be impacted. In fact, it is most desirable to obtain pretreatment baseline testing whenever possible because cognitive profiles in the general population vary widely (i.e., everyone has a unique pattern of strengths and weaknesses). Timing of this pretreatment exam is often challenging because the window between diagnosis and treatments like surgery is often small and filled with high

- Orientation
- Validity (effort)
- Baseline indicators (premorbid attainment)
- Basic Attention
- Complex Attention/Working Memory
- Memory
  - Verbal
    - Learning, Delayed Recall, Recognition
  - Visual
    - Learning, Delayed Recall, Recognition
- Language
  - World Fluency
  - Naming
  - Comprehension
  - Writing
- Visual Spatial
  - Perceptual
  - Constructional
- Processing and Psychomotor Speed
- Executive Functions
  - Reasoning
  - Problem solving
  - Cognitive Flexibility
- Mood and Adjustment
- Quality of Life

**Fig. 41.1** Domains assessed in a comprehensive clinical neuropsychological evaluation

emotion and medical appointments. But, in the absence of baseline testing, it can be more difficult to determine the etiology of deficits, disentangling the effects of surgery, radiation, tumor, medications, fatigue, mood factors, and developmental cognitive pattern.

## Testing for Research

Neurocognitive status is increasingly being recognized as a key outcome measure in research involving brain tumor and radiation [94, 95]. For most research purposes, a full neuropsychological battery is neither practical nor necessary. Early clinical trials often used the Mini-Mental State Exam (MMSE) [96, 97]. However, this measure has proven insensitive to the types of cognitive changes most common in brain tumor populations, [50, 51] and single tests used alone have high misclassification rates [98]. More recently, a three-test battery has been used often in brain tumor trials [99].

This battery employs three well-validated tests tapping the key domains of processing speed [100], memory [101], language [102], and executive function [100]. By expanding the assessment from 10 min (MMSE) to 25 min, six interpretable subscores are generated, allowing more granularity of interpretation and options for statistical analyses. This compares with one unitary score with the MMSE which is essentially a blunt instrument for these purposes. This three-test battery has generated very robust outcomes in controlled clinical trials while also facilitating comparison and data pooling across trials using the same tests [103]. A great many other tests have also been used effectively in studies, and batteries should always be tailored to the research question in a given trial.

In selecting cognitive tests for research studies, there is a natural tension between longer exams which provide greater sensitivity and shorter exams which might be more cost efficient or less burdensome for patients. Using computerized or device-based tasks can be attractive because of the perceived ease of use and electronic data generated. Caution is advised, however, as many such tests are developed and marketed without establishing requisite psychometric properties, representative normative data, and population-specific validity, thus limiting the interpretability of the results [91]. Computerized tasks often rely on processing speed which is one, but not the only, important aspect of cognition impacted by systemic therapy or radiation. Neuropsychologists are cautious about introducing new tests because evidence supporting psychometric properties and validity for various uses is a cumulative process that can take years.

## Test Interpretation

Neuropsychological test scores are converted to standard scores derived from the normal curve, using normative data from a relevant reference group. Often scores are adjusted for age, gender, and/or education, depending on how much those factors impact the ability being assessed. One familiar standard score is the Wechsler intelligence quotient (IQ), which has a mean of 100 and a standard deviation of 15. Thus, an IQ of 100 is at the 50th percentile relative to the normative population, and 68% of persons in the population have IQ scores between 85 and 115 [104]. The most common standard score used in research is the standard deviation (SD) unit or "z-score" (X = 0 SD = 1) [105]. All neuropsychological test scores can be converted to z-score units to facilitate comparison across tests, but care is required because of potential differences in normative groups used. Broadly speaking, a score 2 SD below the mean of the normal population is considered in the impaired range, with 1.5–2 SD considered a trend [106]. As such, an IQ score 1.5 SD below the mean (~77) is in the "borderline" range.

When considering results of a battery of tests, as in a neuropsychological evaluation, the likelihood of an isolated score being in the impaired range in normal persons increases with the number of tests administered (as in type I error), while sensitivity to detect impairment also increases. The significance of any low score depends on many other factors as well, including the patient's background and baseline level of functioning, purpose of the exam, emotional state and effort on the test, pattern of other scores within the same domain, and diagnostic patterns related to symptom profiles. If a patient has a low-normal intellectual baseline (e.g., IQ of 85), then test scores in most cognitive domains would be *predicted* to cluster around 1 SD below average (or a z-score of −1) and then would need to be more than a standard deviation below *that* to be considered impaired. For someone with superior intelligence, an average score could represent a significant decline from baseline. In a clinical exam, the neuropsychologist establishes an estimated baseline for the patient, considering background information and certain test scores, and compares results to that standard. A complex range of other factors go into interpreting neuropsychological profiles that can have 40 or 50 subscores or more, and neuropsychologists gain expertise in pattern analysis [106].

## Measuring Change

Often it is necessary to follow patients or research subjects over time to monitor cognitive change. There are two key issues in determining whether a test score change is significant. The first is to determine whether the change represents *true* change in the patient, versus indicating change based on practice effects, test unreliability or other measurement error, or patient-related variables like education, fatigue, medications, or poor motivation [107, 108]. Because of the myriad factors to consider, there is not agreement on the best way to define real change [109]. Clinicians will generally look for changes of at least 1 SD or more. But, again where multiple tests are given, a smaller change seen across more tests in a domain might be more indicative of true change than a dramatic change on one test. Statistical methods have been developed to help identify true change, including standardized regression-based methods [110, 111] and the Reliable Change Index using the standard error of differences between test and retest scores [112]. However, both can be especially complex to implement in lengthy test batteries, and they are not yet in wide clinical use [107, 113].

After considering whether there is true change, the second issue is whether a change is *clinically* significant. When is a change noticeable to patients? When does it impact their lives? The answer is of course complex. This can really vary depending on the person and the ability being assessed. For example, a professional actuary might notice a very small decline in arithmetic ability that is not noticeable to most people. People depend on other abilities such as memory, processing speed, and language fluency to varying degrees in daily life as well. In broad terms, though, most clinicians would agree that a 1 SD change is likely to be noticeable, and 1.5–2 SD is likely to have marked real-life impact.

In many research trials, mean cognitive scores are already below normal at baseline because subjects enter the study with disease. Thus, for example, say a patient whose premorbid baseline was average enrolls in a brain tumor clinical trial. If this subject's memory score is already a standard deviation below their own personal baseline due to disease, they are probably already noticing the change and needing to use compensatory memory strategies such as writing things down. If that subject then loses *another* standard deviation during the trial, they now have memory functioning in the significantly impaired range and could expect to have very disabling memory difficulty in daily life.

## Case Example

### Background

This 67-year-old Caucasian woman was a retired teacher, living alone when she was diagnosed with non-small cell lung cancer with brain metastases. She initially underwent whole brain radiation therapy (30 Gy in 10 fx) and was treated with systemic chemotherapy but had progressive disease in the CNS and subsequently (19 months after initial diagnosis) underwent multistage gamma knife radiosurgery (GKRS) as well as (repeat) radiation therapy to the posterior fossa (30 Gy in 12 fx). Six months later, brain imaging revealed progression of a lesion in the corpus callosum, for which she underwent repeat GKRS. Neuropsychological evaluation was requested 6 weeks later to characterize cognitive concerns raised by the family and to inform management strategies.

## Neuropsychological Evaluation

Upon the interview, the patient acknowledged minimal cognitive symptoms that she felt were most likely due to normal aging. The patient's family expressed a great deal more concern and provided numerous examples including forgetting conversations, repeating herself often, and losing track in conversation wherein she would disengage and start playing on her phone. They noted poor judgment, including purposely leaving the stove on while she napped and insisting on carrying laundry down the stairs despite significant balance problems. Her affect was flat; she seemed to lack interest or initiative to engage in her usual activities and would not initiate basic self-care activities, such as bathing or brushing her teeth.

These behavioral changes first became noticeable around 1 year after her initial radiation treatment (WBRT) and had been progressive, with a substantial decline in the past few months. The family expressed concern about possible depression. However, the patient denied depressed mood. She felt her children were nagging her and was bothered by her loss of independence. Imaging (Fig. 41.2) showed progressive widespread white matter damage and cerebral atrophy over a 2-year period during which she had multiple radiation treatments.

## Results

The graph in Fig. 41.3 represents the patient's performance in various domains of cognitive function on an abbreviated (1 h) test battery. The patient showed severe impairments in memory and mild impairment in speed of processing and executive function. The patient's substantial behavior change, including lack of insight, impulsivity, and apathy, reflects an additional element of frontal-executive dysfunction not well captured by traditional cognitive tests.

## Impression

The pattern of cognitive impairment and behavior change strongly implicated frontal/subcortical dysfunction, consistent with the widespread imaging changes. This was a typical example of radiation-induced dementia following WBRT noting she also received multiple courses of radiosurgery and repeat cranial radiation. It is possible that some improvement and recovery of function could occur as she recovered from her most recent radiation treatment, but there are concerns she may have a continued decline in cognition and behavior, consistent with a neurodegenerative process.

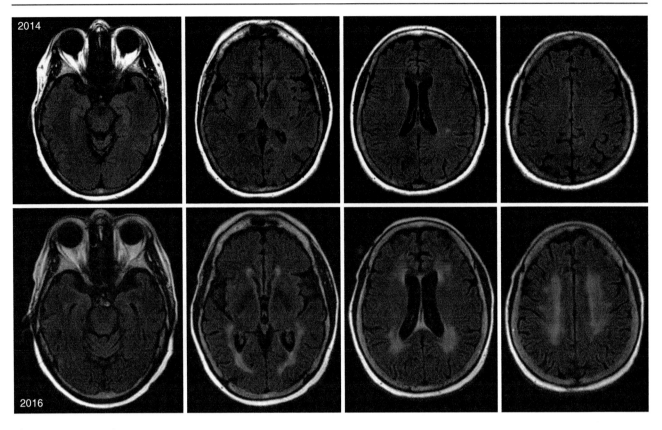

**Fig. 41.2** Brain imaging

**Fig. 41.3** Cognitive function

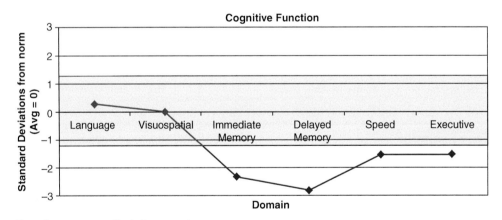

Key : the grey area reflects the normal range

## Recommendations

1. Supervision in daily life. Her impulsivity and impaired insight made it unlikely that she would consistently implement appropriate cognitive compensatory strategies or set limits on herself for safety alone and her memory impairment would limit new learning.

2. Social work consultation to provide guidance to the family regarding respite care resources, community services, and support for their caregiving burden.
3. Patient and family education regarding brain tumor and dementia.
4. Reevaluation after several months to determine whether there is a progressive process.

## Summary

- Many patients with cancer experience cognitive changes that impact their quality of life.
- A significant subset of patients with non-brain cancers experience cognitive symptoms even prior to any systemic treatment. Others experience changes during or after treatment, and preclinical research has demonstrated neurotoxic effects of many chemotherapy agents. Cognitive effects (or "chemobrain") are usually modest, and it is not clear why some patients are more susceptible.
- Most patients with brain tumors have cognitive decline. Specific cognitive functions impacted can be referable to tumor location but also can be produced by disruption of complex networks, making the nature of dysfunction less predictable.
- Higher-grade brain tumors have greater cognitive impact, as slow-growing tumors may be less disruptive to surrounding neurons and networks.
- The impact of radiation treatment on cognition depends on a variety of factors including radiation dosage and type, tumor type and location, and patient factors such as genetics and age.
- Whole brain radiotherapy carries significant cognitive risk, whereas when more focal treatments such as SRS, IMRT, and proton beam therapy are used, cognitive impact can be minimized and often avoided altogether.
- Interventions to minimize radiation impact on cognitive, such as hippocampal sparing (with WBRT) and memantine, show promise. Post-therapy treatments include cognitive rehabilitation and addressing other factors that can impact cognition such as depression and fatigue.
- Neuropsychological assessment delineates cognitive deficits more accurately than imaging or patient self-report alone. Testing is even more useful when a pretreatment baseline is obtained.
- Clinical neuropsychological assessment will sample a wide variety of cognitive domains in order to best delineate focal, distant, and diffuse effects, as well as implications for occupational activities and daily living. Testing for research typically utilizes more abbreviated batteries that must still have sufficient breadth and sensitivity to change.

## Self-Assessment Questions

1. Cognitive symptoms have *not* been related to which of the following features of brain tumors?
   A. Tumor location
   B. MGMT methylation status
   C. IDH-1 mutation status
   D. Tumor size

2. Which of the following statements most accurately captures the state of the literature regarding chemotherapy-induced cognitive symptoms?
   A. Cognitive symptoms are severe and pervasive.
   B. The evidence in support of cognitive symptoms is inconsistent.
   C. The majority of studies demonstrate small to moderate cognitive side effects in group studies.
   D. The mechanisms of chemotherapy-induced cognitive deficits are well understood.

3. The validity of a neuropsychological test:
   A. Is independent from reliability
   B. Varies based on the purpose of testing
   C. Requires accumulation of evidence
   D. B and C
   E. None of the above

4. The correlation between patient report of cognitive symptoms and the results of objective cognitive testing is generally:
   A. Negative
   B. Strong
   C. Weak

5. Which form of radiation therapy presents the greatest risk of cognitive impairment?
   A. Whole brain radiotherapy
   B. Radiosurgery
   C. Intensity-modulated radiotherapy (IMRT)

## Answers

1. B
2. C
3. D
4. C
5. A

## References

1. Li J, Bentzen SM, Li J, et al. Relationship between neurocognitive function and quality of life after whole-brain radiotherapy in patients with brain metastasis. Int J Radiat Oncol Biol Phys. 2008;71:64–70. https://doi.org/10.1016/j.ijrobp.2007.09.059.

2. Farace E, Shaffrey ME. Relationship of neurocognitive impairment to QOL in malignant brain tumor patients (abstract). J Neuropsychiatry Clin Neurosci. 2000;13:1.

3. Meyers CA, Hess KR. Multifaceted end points in brain tumor clinical trials: cognitive deterioration precedes MRI progression. Neuro Oncol. 2003;5:89–95. https://doi.org/10.1215/S1522-8517-02-00026-1.

4. Janelsins MC, Kesler SR, Ahles TA, et al. Prevalence, mechanisms, and management of cancer-related cognitive impairment. Int Rev Psychiatry. 2014;26:102–13. https://doi.org/10.3109/09540261.2013.864260.

5. Wefel JS, Lenzi R, Theriault RL, et al. The cognitive sequelae of standard-dose adjuvant chemotherapy in women with breast carcinoma: results of a prospective, randomized, longitudinal trial. Cancer. 2004;100:2292–9. https://doi.org/10.1002/cncr.20272.

6. Cimprich B. Attentional fatigue following breast cancer surgery. Res Nurs Health. 1992;15:199–207.

7. Wefel JS, Saleeba AK, Buzdar AU, et al. Acute and late onset cognitive dysfunction associated with chemotherapy in women with breast cancer. Cancer. 2010;116:3348–56. https://doi.org/10.1002/cncr.25098.

8. Cimprich B, Reuter-Lorenz P, Nelson J, et al. Prechemotherapy alterations in brain function in women with breast cancer. J Clin Exp Neuropsychol. 2010;32:324–31. https://doi.org/10.1080/13803390903032537.

9. Reuter-Lorenz P. New visions of the aging mind and brain. Trends Cogn Sci. 2002;6:394.

10. Ahles TA, Root JC, Ryan EL. Cancer- and cancer treatment-associated cognitive change: an update on the state of the science. J Clin Oncol. 2012;30:3675–86. https://doi.org/10.1200/jco.2012.43.0116.

11. Chang EL, Wefel JS, Hess KR, et al. Neurocognition in patients with brain metastases treated with radiosurgery or radiosurgery plus whole-brain irradiation: a randomised controlled trial. Lancet Oncol. 2009;10:1037–44. https://doi.org/10.1016/S1470-2045(09)70263-3.

12. Herman MA, Tremont-Lukats I, Meyers CA, et al. Neurocognitive and functional assessment of patients with brain metastases: a pilot study. Am J Clin Oncol. 2003;26:273–9. https://doi.org/10.1097/01.coc.0000020585.85901.7c.

13. Mehta MP, Rodrigus P, Terhaard CH, et al. Survival and neurologic outcomes in a randomized trial of motexafin gadolinium and whole-brain radiation therapy in brain metastases. J Clin Oncol. 2003;21:2529–36. https://doi.org/10.1200/jco.2003.12.122.

14. Meyers CA, Smith JA, Bezjak A, et al. Neurocognitive function and progression in patients with brain metastases treated with whole-brain radiation and motexafin gadolinium: results of a randomized phase III trial. J Clin Oncol. 2004;22:157–65. https://doi.org/10.1200/jco.2004.05.128.

15. Sherman AM, Jaeckle K, Meyers CA. Pretreatment cognitive performance predicts survival in patients with leptomeningeal disease. Cancer. 2002;95:1311–6. https://doi.org/10.1002/cncr.10816.

16. Taphoorn MJ, Klein M. Cognitive deficits in adult patients with brain tumours. Lancet Neurol. 2004;3:159–68. https://doi.org/10.1016/s1474-4422(04)00680-5.

17. Gerstenecker A, Nabors LB, Meneses K, et al. Cognition in patients with newly diagnosed brain metastasis: profiles and implications. J Neurooncol. 2014;120:179 85. https://doi.org/10.1007/s11060-014-1543-x.

18. Tucha O, Smely C, Preier M, et al. Cognitive deficits before treatment among patients with brain tumors. Neurosurgery. 2000;47:324–33. discussion 333-324

19. Racine CA, Li J, Molinaro AM, et al. Neurocognitive function in newly diagnosed low-grade glioma patients undergoing surgical resection with awake mapping techniques. Neurosurgery.

20. 2015;77:371–9.; discussion 379. https://doi.org/10.1227/NEU.0000000000000779.

20. Derks J, Reijneveld JC, Douw L. Neural network alterations underlie cognitive deficits in brain tumor patients. Curr Opin Oncol. 2014;26:627–33. https://doi.org/10.1097/cco.0000000000000126.

21. Lee EQ. Nervous system metastases from systemic cancer. Continuum (Minneap Minn). 2015;21:415–28. https://doi.org/10.1212/01.con.0000464178.81957.18.

22. Kayl AE, Meyers CA. Does brain tumor histology influence cognitive function? Neuro Oncol. 2003;5:255–60. https://doi.org/10.1215/S1152851703000012.

23. Noll KR, Sullaway C, Ziu M, et al. Relationships between tumor grade and neurocognitive functioning in patients with glioma of the left temporal lobe prior to surgical resection. Neuro Oncol. 2015;17:580–7. https://doi.org/10.1093/neuonc/nou233.

24. Wefel JS, Noll KR, Rao G, et al. Neurocognitive function varies by IDH1 genetic mutation status in patients with malignant glioma prior to surgical resection. Neuro Oncol. 2016;18:1656–63. https://doi.org/10.1093/neuonc/now165.

25. Duffau H, Herbet G, Moritz-Gasser S. Toward a pluri-component, multimodal, and dynamic organization of the ventral semantic stream in humans: lessons from stimulation mapping in awake patients. Front Syst Neurosci. 2013;7:44. https://doi.org/10.3389/fnsys.2013.00044.

26. Anderson-Hanley C, Sherman ML, Riggs R, et al. Neuropsychological effects of treatments for adults with cancer: a meta-analysis and review of the literature. J Int Neuropsychol Soc. 2003;9:967–82. https://doi.org/10.1017/s1355617703970019.

27. Falleti MG, Sanfilippo A, Maruff P, et al. The nature and severity of cognitive impairment associated with adjuvant chemotherapy in women with breast cancer: a meta-analysis of the current literature. Brain Cogn. 2005;59:60–70. https://doi.org/10.1016/j.bandc.2005.05.001.

28. Hodgson KD, Hutchinson AD, Wilson CJ, et al. A meta-analysis of the effects of chemotherapy on cognition in patients with cancer. Cancer Treat Rev. 2013;39:297–304. https://doi.org/10.1016/j.ctrv.2012.11.001.

29. Jansen CE, Miaskowski C, Dodd M, et al. A metaanalysis of studies of the effects of cancer chemotherapy on various domains of cognitive function. Cancer. 2005;104:2222–33. https://doi.org/10.1002/cncr.21469.

30. Jim HS, Phillips KM, Chait S, et al. Meta-analysis of cognitive functioning in breast cancer survivors previously treated with standard-dose chemotherapy. J Clin Oncol. 2012;30:3578–87. https://doi.org/10.1200/jco.2011.39.5640.

31. Ono M, Ogilvie JM, Wilson JS, et al. A meta-analysis of cognitive impairment and decline associated with adjuvant chemotherapy in women with breast cancer. Front Oncol. 2015;5:59. https://doi.org/10.3389/fonc.2015.00059.

32. Stewart A, Bielajew C, Collins B, et al. A meta-analysis of the neuropsychological effects of adjuvant chemotherapy treatment in women treated for breast cancer. Clin Neuropsychol. 2006;20:76–89. https://doi.org/10.1080/138540491005875.

33. Lindner OC, Phillips B, McCabe MG, et al. A meta-analysis of cognitive impairment following adult cancer chemotherapy. Neuropsychology. 2014;28:726–40. https://doi.org/10.1037/neu0000064.

34. Donovan KA, Small BJ, Andrykowski MA, et al. Cognitive functioning after adjuvant chemotherapy and/or radiotherapy for early-stage breast carcinoma. Cancer. 2005;104:2499–507. https://doi.org/10.1002/cncr.21482.

35. Schagen SB, Muller MJ, Boogerd W, et al. Change in cognitive function after chemotherapy: a prospective longitudinal study in breast cancer patients. J Natl Cancer Inst. 2006;98:1742–5. https://doi.org/10.1093/jnci/djj470.

36. Dietrich J, Prust M, Kaiser J. Chemotherapy, cognitive impairment and hippocampal toxicity. Neuroscience. 2015;309:224–32. https://doi.org/10.1016/j.neuroscience.2015.06.016.

37. McDonald BC, Conroy SK, Smith DJ, et al. Frontal gray matter reduction after breast cancer chemotherapy and association with executive symptoms; a replication and extension study. Brain Behav Immun. 2013;30(Suppl):S117–25. https://doi.org/10.1016/j.bbi.2012.05.007.

38. Abraham J, Haut MW, Moran MT, et al. Adjuvant chemotherapy for breast cancer: effects on cerebral white matter seen in diffusion tensor imaging. Clin Breast Cancer. 2008;8:88–91. https://doi.org/10.3816/CBC.2008.n.007.

39. Deprez S, Amant F, Yigit R, et al. Chemotherapy-induced structural changes in cerebral white matter and its correlation with impaired cognitive functioning in breast cancer patients. Hum Brain Mapp. 2011;32:480–93. https://doi.org/10.1002/hbm.21033.

40. Bruno J, Hosseini SM, Kesler S. Altered resting state functional brain network topology in chemotherapy-treated breast cancer survivors. Neurobiol Dis. 2012;48:329–38. https://doi.org/10.1016/j.nbd.2012.07.009.

41. Horky LL, Gerbaudo VH, Zaitsev A, et al. Systemic chemotherapy decreases brain glucose metabolism. Ann Clin Transl Neurol. 2014;1:788–98. https://doi.org/10.1002/acn3.121.

42. McDonald BC, Conroy SK, Ahles TA, et al. Alterations in brain activation during working memory processing associated with breast cancer and treatment: a prospective functional magnetic resonance imaging study. J Clin Oncol. 2012;30:2500–8. https://doi.org/10.1200/jco.2011.38.5674.

43. Besse B, Le Moulec S, Mazieres J, et al. Bevacizumab in patients with nonsquamous non-small cell lung cancer and asymptomatic, untreated BRAIN metastases (BRAIN): a nonrandomized, phase II study. Clin Cancer Res. 2015;21:1896–903. https://doi.org/10.1158/1078-0432.ccr-14-2082.

44. Nasreddine ZS, Phillips NA, Bedirian V, et al. The Montreal cognitive assessment, MoCA: a brief screening tool for mild cognitive impairment. J Am Geriatr Soc. 2005;53:695–9. https://doi.org/10.1111/j.1532-5415.2005.53221.x.

45. Centre Hospitalier Intercommunal Creteil (sponsor). Therapeutic strategies in patients with non-squamous non-small cell lung cancer with brain metastases (METAL2) (ClinicalTrials.gov identifier NCT02162537). ClinicalTrials.gov. 2017. Accessed 2017. Available at: https://clinicaltrials.gov/ct2/show/NCT02162537.

46. Ahluwalia MS, Chao ST, Parsons MW, et al. Phase II trial of sunitinib as adjuvant therapy after stereotactic radiosurgery in patients with 1-3 newly diagnosed brain metastases. J Neurooncol. 2015;124:485–91. https://doi.org/10.1007/s11060-015-1862-6.

47. Brastianos PK, Carter SL, Santagata S, et al. Genomic characterization of brain metastases reveals branched evolution and potential therapeutic targets. Cancer Discov. 2015;5:1164–77. https://doi.org/10.1158/2159-8290.cd-15-0369.

48. Robert C, Karaszewska B, Schachter J, et al. Improved overall survival in melanoma with combined dabrafenib and trametinib. N Engl J Med. 2015;372:30–9. https://doi.org/10.1056/NEJMoa1412690.

49. Brown PD, Cerhan JH. Same, better, or worse? Neurocognitive effects of radiotherapy for low-grade gliomas remain unknown. Lancet Neurol. 2009;8:779–81. https://doi.org/10.1016/S1474-4422(09)70205-4.

50. Sun A, Bae K, Gore EM, et al. Phase III trial of prophylactic cranial irradiation compared with observation in patients with locally advanced non-small-cell lung cancer: neurocognitive and quality-of-life analysis. J Clin Oncol. 2011;29:279–86. https://doi.org/10.1200/JCO.2010.29.6053.

51. Meyers CA, Wefel JS. The use of the mini-mental state examination to assess cognitive functioning in cancer trials: no ifs, ands,

buts, or sensitivity. J Clin Oncol. 2003;21:3557–8. https://doi.org/10.1200/JCO.2003.07.080.

52. Makale MT, McDonald CR, Hattangadi-Gluth JA, et al. Mechanisms of radiotherapy-associated cognitive disability in patients with brain tumours. Nat Rev Neurol. 2017;13:52–64. https://doi.org/10.1038/nrneurol.2016.185.

53. Wefel JS, Noll KR, Scheurer ME. Neurocognitive functioning and genetic variation in patients with primary brain tumours. Lancet Oncol. 2016;17:e97–e108. https://doi.org/10.1016/S1470-2045%2815%2900380-0.

54. Greene-Schloesser D, Robbins ME. Radiation-induced cognitive impairment--from bench to bedside. Neuro Oncol. 2012;14(Suppl 4):iv37–44. https://doi.org/10.1093/neuonc/nos196

55. Schultheiss TE, Stephens LC. Invited review: permanent radiation myelopathy. Br J Radiol. 1992;65:737–53. https://doi.org/10.1259/0007-1285-65-777-737.

56. Taphoorn MJB, Niël CG. Low-grade gliomas. In: Meyers CA, Perry JR, editors. Cognition and cancer. New York, NY: Cambridge University Press; 2008. p. 142.

57. Onodera S, Aoyama H, Tha KK, et al. The value of 4-month neurocognitive function as an endpoint in brain metastases trials. J Neurooncol. 2014;120:311–9. https://doi.org/10.1007/s11060-014-1550-y

58. McDuff SG, Taich ZJ, Lawson JD, et al. Neurocognitive assessment following whole brain radiation therapy and radiosurgery for patients with cerebral metastases. J Neurol Neurosurg Psychiatry. 2013;84:1384–91. https://doi.org/10.1136/jnnp-2013-305166.

59. DeAngelis LM, Delattre JY, Posner JB. Radiation-induced dementia in patients cured of brain metastases. Neurology. 1989;39:789–96.

60. Brown PD, Jaeckle K, Ballman KV, et al. Effect of radiosurgery alone vs radiosurgery with whole brain radiation therapy on cognitive function in patients with 1 to 3 brain metastases: a randomized clinical trial. JAMA. 2016;316:401–9. https://doi.org/10.1001/jama.2016.9839.

61. Chang JE, Robins HI, Mehta MP. Therapeutic advances in the treatment of brain metastases. Clin Adv Hematol Oncol. 2007;5:54–64.

62. Laack NN, Brown PD, Ivnik RJ, et al. Cognitive function after radiotherapy for supratentorial low-grade glioma: a north central cancer treatment group prospective study. Int J Radiat Oncol Biol Phys. 2005;63:1175–83. https://doi.org/10.1016/j.ijrobp.2005.04.016.

63. Steinvorth S, Wenz F, Wildermuth S, et al. Cognitive function in patients with cerebral arteriovenous malformations after radiosurgery: prospective long-term follow-up. Int J Radiat Oncol Biol Phys. 2002;54:1430–7.

64. Dennis ER, Bussiere MR, Niemierko A, et al. A comparison of critical structure dose and toxicity risks in patients with low grade gliomas treated with IMRT versus proton radiation therapy. Technol Cancer Res Treat. 2013;12:1–9. https://doi.org/10.7785/tcrt.2012.500276.

65. Sherman JC, Colvin MK, Mancuso SM, et al. Neurocognitive effects of proton radiation therapy in adults with low-grade glioma. J Neurooncol. 2016;126:157–64.

66. Marsh JC, Ziel GE, Diaz AZ, et al. Integral dose delivered to normal brain with conventional intensity-modulated radiotherapy (IMRT) and helical tomotherapy IMRT during partial brain radiotherapy for high-grade gliomas with and without selective sparing of the hippocampus, limbic circuit and neural stem cell compartment. J Med Imaging Radiat Oncol. 2013;57:378–83. https://doi.org/10.1111/1754-9485.12048.

67. Gondi V, Tome WA, Mehta MP. Why avoid the hippocampus? A comprehensive review. Radiother Oncol. 2010;97:370–6. https://doi.org/10.1016/j.radonc.2010.09.013.

68. Gondi V, Hermann BP, Mehta MP, et al. Hippocampal dosimetry predicts neurocognitive function impairment after fractionated stereotactic radiotherapy for benign or low-grade adult brain tumors. Int J Radiat Oncol Biol Phys. 2012;83:e487–93. https://doi.org/10.1016/j.ijrobp.2011.10.021.

69. Gondi V, Pugh SL, Tome WA, et al. Preservation of memory with conformal avoidance of the hippocampal neural stem-cell compartment during whole-brain radiotherapy for brain metastases (RTOG 0933): a phase II multi-institutional trial. J Clin Oncol. 2014;32:3810–6. https://doi.org/10.1200/JCO.2014.57.2909.

70. Tsai PF, Yang CC, Chuang CC, et al. Hippocampal dosimetry correlates with the change in neurocognitive function after hippocampal sparing during whole brain radiotherapy: a prospective study. Radiat Oncol. 2015;10:253. https://doi.org/10.1186/s13014-015-0562-x.

71. Day J, Zienius K, Gehring K, et al. Interventions for preventing and ameliorating cognitive deficits in adults treated with cranial irradiation. Cochrane Database Syst Rev. 2014;12:CD011335. https://doi.org/10.1002/14651858.CD011335.pub2.

72. Brown PD, Pugh S, Laack NN, et al. Memantine for the prevention of cognitive dysfunction in patients receiving whole-brain radiotherapy: a randomized, double-blind, placebo-controlled trial. Neuro-oncol. 2013;15:1429–37. https://doi.org/10.1093/neuonc/not114.

73. Meyers CA, Weitzner MA, Valentine AD, et al. Methylphenidate therapy improves cognition, mood, and function of brain tumor patients. J Clin Oncol. 1998;16:2522–7. https://doi.org/10.1200/JCO.1998.16.7.2522.

74. Gehring K, Patwardhan SY, Collins R, et al. A randomized trial on the efficacy of methylphenidate and modafinil for improving cognitive functioning and symptoms in patients with a primary brain tumor. J Neurooncol. 2012;107:165–74. https://doi.org/10.1007/s11060-011-0723-1.

75. Rapp SR, Case LD, Peiffer A, et al. Donepezil for irradiated brain tumor survivors: a phase III randomized placebo-controlled clinical trial. J Clin Oncol. 2015;33:1653–9. https://doi.org/10.1200/JCO.2014.58.4508.

76. Burns TC, Awad AJ, Li MD, et al. Radiation-induced brain injury: low-hanging fruit for neuroregeneration. Neurosurg Focus. 2016;40:E3. https://doi.org/10.3171/2016.2.FOCUS161.

77. Locke DEC, Cerhan JH, Malec JF. Behavioral strategies and rehabilitation. In: Meyers CA, Perry JR, editors. Cognition and cancer. New York, NY: Cambridge University Press; 2008.

78. Locke DE, Cerhan JH, Wu W, et al. Cognitive rehabilitation and problem-solving to improve quality of life of patients with primary brain tumors: a pilot study. J Support Oncol. 2008;6:383–91.

79. Gehring K, Sitskoorn MM, Gundy CM, et al. Cognitive rehabilitation in patients with gliomas: a randomized, controlled trial. J Clin Oncol. 2009;27:3712–22. https://doi.org/10.1200/JCO.2008.20.5765.

80. Riggs L, Piscione J, Laughlin S, et al. Exercise training for neural recovery in a restricted sample of pediatric brain tumor survivors: a controlled clinical trial with crossover of training versus no training. Neuro Oncol. 2017;19:440–50. https://doi.org/10.1093/neuonc/now177.

81. Treanor CJ, McMenamin UC, O'Neill RF, et al. Non-pharmacological interventions for cognitive impairment due to systemic cancer treatment. Cochrane Database Syst Rev. 2016;8:CD011325. https://doi.org/10.1002/14651858.CD011325.pub2.

82. Harvey PD. Clinical applications of neuropsychological assessment. Dialogues Clin Neurosci. 2012;14:91–9.

83. DiMatteo MR, Lepper HS, Croghan TW. Depression is a risk factor for noncompliance with medical treatment: meta-analysis of the effects of anxiety and depression on patient adherence. Arch Intern Med. 2000;160:2101–7.

84. Litofsky NS, Farace E, Anderson F Jr, et al. Glioma outcomes project I. Depression in patients with high-grade glioma: results of the Glioma outcomes project. Neurosurgery. 2004;54:358–66. discussion 366-357

85. Gehring K, Taphoorn MJ, Sitskoorn MM, et al. Predictors of subjective versus objective cognitive functioning in patients with stable grades II and III glioma. Neurooncol Pract. 2015;2:20–31. https://doi.org/10.1093/nop/npu035.

86. Comijs HC, Deeg DJ, Dik MG, et al. Memory complaints; the association with psycho-affective and health problems and the role of personality characteristics. A 6-year follow-up study. J Affect Disord. 2002;72:157–65.

87. Kinsinger SW, Lattie E, Mohr DC. Relationship between depression, fatigue, subjective cognitive impairment, and objective neuropsychological functioning in patients with multiple sclerosis. Neuropsychology. 2010;24:573–80. https://doi.org/10.1037/a0019222.

88. Brennan RL, editor. Educational measurement. 4th ed. Lanham, MD: Rowman & Littlefield Publishers; 2006.

89. Messick S. Validity of psychological assessment: validation of inferences from persons' responses and performances as scientific inquiry into score meaning. Am Psychol. 1995;50:741–9.

90. Cronbach LJ. Test validation. In: Thorndike RL, editor. Educational measurement. 2nd ed. Washington, DC: American Council on Education; 1971. p. 443–507.

91. Bauer RM, Iverson GL, Cernich AN, et al. Computerized neuropsychological assessment devices: joint position paper of the American academy of clinical neuropsychology and the national academy of neuropsychology. Arch Clin Neuropsychol. 2012;27:362–73. https://doi.org/10.1093/arclin/acs027.

92. Downing SM, Haladyna TM, editors. Handbook of test development. Mahway, NJ: Lawrence Erlbaum Associates, Publishers; 2006.

93. American Educational Research Association, American Psychological Association, National Council on Measurement in Education. Standards for educational and psychological testing. Washington, DC: American Educational Research Association; 2014.

94. Lin NU, Lee EQ, Aoyama H, et al. Challenges relating to solid tumour brain metastases in clinical trials, part 1: patient population, response, and progression. A report from the RANO group. Lancet Oncol. 2013;14:e396–406. https://doi.org/10.1016/s1470-2045(13)70311-5.

95. Lin NU, Wefel JS, Lee EQ, et al. Challenges relating to solid tumour brain metastases in clinical trials, part 2: neurocognitive, neurological, and quality-of-life outcomes. A report from the RANO group. Lancet Oncol. 2013;14:e407–16. https://doi.org/10.1016/s1470-2045(13)70308-5.

96. Brown PD, Buckner JC, Uhm JH, et al. The neurocognitive effects of radiation in adult low-grade glioma patients. Neuro Oncol. 2003;5:161–7. https://doi.org/10.1215/S1152-8517-02-00043-1.

97. Folstein MF, Folstein SE, McHugh PR. "Mini-mental state". A practical method for grading the cognitive state of patients for the clinician. J Psychiatr Res. 1975;12:189–98.

98. Spreen O, Benton AL. Comparative studies of some psychological tests for cerebral damage. J Nerv Ment Dis. 1965;140:323–33.

99. Gilbert MR, Dignam JJ, Armstrong TS, et al. A randomized trial of bevacizumab for newly diagnosed glioblastoma. N Engl J Med. 2014;370:699–708. https://doi.org/10.1056/NEJMoa1308573.

100. Reitan RM. Trail making test: manual for administration and scoring. Reitan Neuropsychological Laboratory: South Tucson, AZ; 1992.

101. Brandt J. The Hopkins verbal learning test: development of a new memory test with six equivalent forms. Clin Neuropsychol. 1991;5:125–42.

102. Benton AL, Hamsher K. Multilingual aphasia examination. Manual of instructions. 2nd ed. Iowa City, IA: AJA Associates; 1989.

103. Joly F, Giffard B, Rigal O, et al. Impact of cancer and its treatments on cognitive function: advances in research from the Paris international cognition and cancer task force symposium and update since 2012. J Pain Symptom Manag. 2015;50:830–41. https://doi.org/10.1016/j.jpainsymman.2015.06.019.

104. Wechsler D. The wechsler adult intelligence scale, 4th ed. (WAIS-IV). Pearson Assessment: San Antonio, TX; 2009.

105. Anastasi A, Urbina S. Psychologial testing. 7th ed. Pearson: New York, NY; 1997.

106. Lezak MD, Howieson DB, Bigler ED, et al. Neuropsychological assessment. 5th ed. Oxford, England, UK: Oxford University Press; 2012.

107. Attix DK, Story TJ, Chelune GJ, et al. The prediction of change: normative neuropsychological trajectories. Clin Neuropsychol. 2009;23:21–38. https://doi.org/10.1080/13854040801945078.

108. Heilbronner RL, Sweet JJ, Attix DK, et al. Official position of the American Academy of clinical neuropsychology on serial neuropsychological assessments: the utility and challenges of repeat test administrations in clinical and forensic contexts. Clin Neuropsychol. 2010;24:1267–78. https://doi.org/10.1080/138540 46.2010.526785.

109. Strauss E, Sherman EMS, Spreen O. A compendium of neuropsychological tests. 3rd ed. Oxford, England, UK: Oxford University Press; 2006.

110. Crawford JR, Garthwaite PH, Denham AK, et al. Using regression equations built from summary data in the psychological assessment of the individual case: extension to multiple regression. Psychol Assess. 2012;24:801–14. https://doi.org/10.1037/a0027699.

111. Hinton-Bayre AD. Deriving reliable change statistics from test-retest normative data: comparison of models and mathematical expressions. Arch Clin Neuropsychol. 2010;25:244–56. https://doi.org/10.1093/arclin/acq008.

112. Chelune GJ. Assessing reliable neuropsychological change. In: Franklin R, editor. Prediction in forensic and neuropsychology: new approaches to psychometrically sound assessment. Mahway, NJ: Lawrence Erlbaum Associates, Inc.; 2003.

113. Duff K. Evidence-based indicators of neuropsychological change in the individual patient: relevant concepts and methods. Arch Clin Neuropsychol. 2012;27:248–61. https://doi.org/10.1093/arclin/acr120.

# Cranial Nerve Palsies, Vascular Damage, and Brainstem Injury

# 42

Aryavarta M. S. Kumar and Simon S. Lo

## Learning Objectives

- To learn the basic principles of detection and diagnosis of radiation-induced cranial nerve palsies, vascular damage, and brainstem injury.
- To learn the incidence of radiation-induced cranial nerve palsies, vascular damage, and brainstem injury.
- To learn the management of radiation-induced cranial nerve palsies, vascular damage, and brainstem injury.

Radiation therapy to brain and spine tumors can provide effective local control. However, balancing the potential short- and long-term complications from treatment is important. The main strategy toward radiation-associated complications is prevention; however, the following may be used to help the practitioner in assessing and treating a patient who has developed complications. This chapter will specifically cover cranial nerve (CN) injury (except radiation-induced optic neuropathy which is to be covered in Chap. 38), vascular injury, and brainstem injury.

## Detection and Diagnosis

The detection of radiation injury is primarily based on patient-reported side effects and clinical examination. Establishing a baseline physical examination, and baseline visual field testing if indicated, is important to make comparisons. Close clinical observation is recommended after radiation therapy. Typically, a follow-up visit approximately 1 month after completing radiation therapy is recommended to assess for any short-term side effects. Two to three

monthly follow-up visits after the initial visit are typical for the first 2 years, but shorter follow-up times are recommended if patients have complications requiring closer monitoring.

During the office visit, a complete history and physical examination, along with specific attention to the neurological examination, should take place. Symptoms from cranial nerve deficits will likely be reported by the patient, and the presenting sign will depend on the cranial nerve involved. Similarly, brainstem injury will likely be associated with sensory or motor deficits or gait imbalance. If a patient has a vascular injury, stroke-like symptoms will likely be the presenting signs. In almost all situations, the history and physical examination including a detailed neurologic examination will likely detect the findings. It is possible for radiation-induced cranial nerve or the brainstem injury to occur without a significant presenting symptom, and a careful neurologic examination may elicit those signs.

Typically, brain MRI is ordered at follow-up visits to evaluate response to treatment. T1, T2, and FLAIR sequences are important for diagnosis with the frequency determined by tumor type. Typically, contrast enhancement of a cranial nerve on T1 sequence may indicate latent inflammation. Any abnormal enhancement, demyelination, and edema should be investigated. Sometimes, the diagnosis of radiation-induced complication can be made before a presenting sign, and in this scenario, imaging is vital to early diagnosis. MRI can also help determine whether the neurologic deficits are caused by tumor progression or radiation effects.

## Tests to Evaluate

- Detailed history.
- Clinical examination.
- Neurological examination.
- Ophthalmologic examination/visual field testing.
- Review of prior radiation therapy plan(s).

A. M. S. Kumar
Department of Radiation Oncology, Louis Stokes Cleveland VA Medical Center, Cleveland, OH, USA

S. S. Lo (✉)
Department of Radiation Oncology, University of Washington Medical Center, Seattle, WA, USA
e-mail: simonslo@uw.edu

© Springer International Publishing AG, part of Springer Nature 2018
E. L. Chang et al. (eds.), *Adult CNS Radiation Oncology*, https://doi.org/10.1007/978-3-319-42878-9_42

- CT with and without contrast.
- Angiography.
- Brain MRI (with and without contrast).
- PET/MRI perfusion.

## Presentation, Symptoms, and Data from the Literature

### Optic Neuropathy

This will be covered in Chap. 38.

### CN III, IV, V, and VI

Patients with III, IV, and VI nerve palsies typically present with double vision, and the direction of gaze where it occurs depends on the nerves involved. When III nerve palsy is present, it can be accompanied by complete ptosis and pupillary dilatation of the affected side. Patients with V nerve injury present with paresthesia or anesthesia of the affected dermatome of the ipsilateral face. Careful neurologic examination should be performed to confirm the diagnosis. Radiological evaluation with MRI of the brain and skull base is also paramount to rule out tumor progression or recurrence. Data from studies on cavernous sinus tumors and pituitary adenomas provide us with the information on toxicity with cranial nerves III, IV, V, and VI [1]. In general for standard total doses for CNS indications using standard fractionation (1.8–2 Gy per fraction), there has been little reported cranial nerve deficits [2].

When compared to the doses received by the optic nerve, cranial nerves III, IV, V, and VI are generally able to tolerate higher single doses of radiation without developing toxicity. In a series by Witt et al., data on 1255 patients who underwent SRS for pituitary adenoma with the marginal dose delivered ranging from 14 to 34 Gy in 1 fraction were analyzed [1]. With the cavernous sinus adjacent and receiving a high radiation dose, the cranial nerves in the cavernous sinus received relatively high radiation doses, and the overall incidence of permanent III, IV, or VI neuropathy was 0.4% [1]. The incidence of cranial nerve V toxicity was 0.2% in this study. In a study by Spiegelmann et al., 102 patients with cavernous sinus meningiomas were treated with 12–17.5 Gy in a single fraction using linear accelerator (LINAC)-based SRS, and the reported incidence of cranial nerve V and VI deficits was <2% [3].

Cranial nerve V can also be exposed to a substantial level of radiation when SRS is used for the treatment of vestibular schwannoma and trigeminal neuralgia. Based on an earlier SRS series on vestibular schwannomas that used a dose of 14–20 Gy, the reported incidence of cranial nerve V deficit was 16% [4] which was much higher than studies using doses of 12–13 Gy which reported cranial nerve V deficit rates ranging between 2% and 8% [5–7]. Based largely on retrospective series, the risks of radiation-induced dysfunction of cranial nerves III, IV, V, and VI are typically low with SRS using commonly used doses and dose constraints.

Data on tolerance of cranial nerves III, IV, V, and VI are more limited for HSRT. In a phase II study where 14 patients with cavernous sinus hemangiomas were treated with HSRT to a dose of 21 Gy in 3 fractions, among the 6 patients with cranial nerve deficits, they either showed complete recovery or improvement of function, and none had radiation-induced cranial nerve toxicities [8]. Colleagues from Johns Hopkins University treated patients with vestibular schwannomas with HSRT to 25 Gy in 5 fractions, and the observed rate of cranial nerve V deficit was 7% [9]. In a Japanese study where HSRT was used for vestibular schwannoma delivering 18–21 Gy in 3 fractions or 25 Gy in 5 fractions, there was no observed cranial nerve V deficit at a median follow-up of 80 months [10]. In Georgetown University study of HSRT for vestibular schwannoma, a dose of 25 Gy in 5 fractions was given, and the rate of V nerve complication was 5.5% [11]. A series that treated pituitary metastases to 31 Gy in 5 fractions did not report any cranial nerve complications [12].

### CN VII and CN VIII

When VII nerve palsy occurs, patients typically present with ipsilateral facial weakness with no sparing of the frontalis muscle, drooling of saliva, and inability to completely close the ipsilateral eye. Facial nerve dysfunction can be scored using House-Brackmann facial nerve grading system with six grades (grades I–VI) [13]. Radiation-induced VIII nerve injury manifests as ipsilateral hearing loss. As this nearly exclusively occurs in patients who receive radiation therapy for vestibular schwannoma, tumor progression must be ruled out using MRI prior to establishing the diagnosis of radiation-induced VIII nerve injury. An audiometry test is used to document the hearing loss.

Vestibular schwannoma outcomes also provide us with some toxicity data for cranial nerves VII and VIII. In an early series from the University of Pittsburgh, the hearing retention rate was only 47% when a dose of 14–20 Gy in 1 fraction was used for Gamma Knife SRS and the risk of VII nerve injury was 15% [4]. As a result of these findings, the dose has been decreased to 12–13 Gy in one fraction, and this has improved the hearing preservation rate to 44%–88% with Gamma Knife- or LINAC-based SRS, while maintaining excellent local control [5–7]. The risk of VII nerve deficit was also reduced to <5% [5–7]. With proton-based SRS delivering 12 CGE, cranial nerve V and VII preservation rates were excellent. However, the hearing preservation rates were only 30% [6, 14]. This effect of proton radiation needs further investigation. Putz et al. reviewed 107 patients treated with single dose or fractionated SRS and reported long-term hearing preservation in 72%, while worsening of facial nerve function in 1.7% (1 patient) treated with primary radiation alone [15].

Data on VII and VIII nerve deficits from HSRT are more limited. Song et al. published their HSRT experience for vestibular schwannoma at Johns Hopkins University using a regimen of 25 Gy in 5 fractions and with follow-up times of 6–44 months; the rates of hearing preservation and VII nerve deficits were 75% and 0, respectively [9]. Morimoto et al. reported a study where 26 vestibular schwannomas were treated with the regimens of 18–21 Gy in 3 fractions or 25 Gy in 5 fractions using CyberKnife-based HSRT. The overall VII and VIII nerve preservation rates were 92% and 50%, respectively [10]. Another study from Taiwan using a regimen of 18 Gy in 3 fractions reported a serviceable hearing retention rate of 81.5% with a mean follow-up of 61.1 months [16]. At Georgetown University, a regimen of 25 Gy in 5 fractions was generally used, and the hearing preservation rate was 73% at 5 years, and the rate of VII deficits was 0 [11]. Using a regimen of 18 Gy in 3 fractions for vestibular schwannomas, the University of Pittsburgh group reported a 53.5% hearing retention rate [17]. A Dutch study of 129 patients comparing SRS and HSRT for vestibular schwannomas used 10–12.5 Gy in 1 fraction (SRS) or 20–25 Gy in 5 fractions (HSRT). The rates of preservation of cranial nerves VII and VIII were 93% and 75% for the SRS group and 97% and 61% for the HSRT group, respectively [18]. From this small study, the authors concluded that there was no significant difference in control rates or toxicity.

## CN IX, X, XI, and XII

Radiation injury to IX, X, XI, and XII nerves is rare and occurs mainly in patients who receive radiation therapy to their glomus jugulare tumors. A diagnosis can be made through careful history taking and neurologic examination. As in other radiation-induced cranial injuries, it is important to rule out tumor progression by obtaining a thin-slice MRI of the brain including a T1 fat-suppressed sequence with gadolinium.

Studies on glomus tumors outcomes help us understand toxicity related to cranial nerves IX, X, XI, and XII. There are two meta-analyses reviewing SRS outcomes for glomus tumors [19, 20]. In the University of California, San Francisco (UCSF), study, there were 339 patients treated with SRS alone, and the rates of IX, X, XI, and XII nerve deficits were 9.7%, 9.7%, 12%, and 8.7%, respectively [20]. However, there is no dosimetric data for analysis. In the meta-analysis from Johns Hopkins University, no toxicity data were reported [19]. Ibrahim et al. reported on 75 patients who received a median marginal dose of 18 Gy in 1 fraction for glomus jugulare tumors with 12 patients (16% of patients) reporting new symptoms or progression of previous symptoms [21]. Only two of these patients had long-term changes in CN X and CN VII with tumor that was controlled radiographically. All the other patients who developed new symptoms had transient CN nerve deficits that improved with steroids. Previous deficits, larger tumor volume, and previous surgery were associated with a significantly higher risk of CN deficits after radiosurgery.

For standard fractionation, doses of up to 45–50.4 Gy in 25–28 fractions are used with minimal attributable toxicity to the cranial nerves. Data are even more limited on IX, X, XI, and XII nerve toxicities caused by HSRT. In a study from University of Texas Southwestern Medical Center where 31 patients with skull base glomus tumors were treated with HSRT to a dose of 25 Gy in 5 fractions, no grade 3 IX, X, XI, and XII nerve toxicities were observed with a median follow-up of 24 months [22]. Schuster et al. published outcomes for 18 patients with no reported toxicity for doses up to 21 Gy in 3 fractions [23].

## Vascular Injury

Radiation vasculopathy is a well-known complication of radiotherapy and can cause significant morbidity in patients. When radiation injury causes narrowing of the large vessels in the circle of Willis, moyamoya syndrome, an uncommon complication characterized by the formation of abnormal collateral channels, can occur although the risk is much higher when radiotherapy is given at the age younger than 5 years [24]. Vascular injury may not manifest itself for many years after radiotherapy is delivered, and in many cases, patients may be asymptomatic. When stenosis of a large artery such as the internal carotid artery occurs, patients may present with stroke-like symptoms.

Internal carotid arteries can be exposed to high doses when radiation is prescribed for cavernous sinus meningiomas and pituitary adenomas. Witt et al., reporting on SRS for pituitary adenomas, found that among the 1255 patients evaluated in the studies, there were only three cases of internal carotid artery occlusion or stenosis [1]. In one case, the internal carotid artery SRS dose was estimated to be less than 20 Gy. They recommended keeping <50% of the circumference receiving prescribed dose while the internal carotid artery itself not receive a maximum point dose higher than 30 Gy in 1 fraction [1].

For HSRT, among the studies on pituitary adenoma or cavernous sinus tumors, no vascular injury was observed when regimens of 21 Gy in 3 fractions or 25 Gy in 5 fractions were used [8, 25, 26]. Using HSRT to treat giant cavernous sinus hemangiomas, there were no reported vascular complications in a group of 31 patients that received 21 Gy in 3 fractions or 22 Gy in 4 fractions [27].

## Brainstem Injury

The clinical manifestation of radiation-induced brainstem injury depends on the location of the necrosis. For instance, a necrotic focus in the cerebral peduncle will lead to contralateral hemiparesis caused by damage to the ipsilateral corticospinal tract, whereas a necrotic focus in the abducens nucleus will lead to ipsilateral abducens palsy. To establish a diagnosis, the correlation of the radiation plan with the MRI findings and neurologic examination findings is necessary.

The brainstem has historically been viewed as a more delicate structure, but more recent data suggest that going to higher doses with small volumes is possible [28]. In general, using conventional fractionation, doses of 54 Gy to large brainstem volumes is considered safe, and small volumes to doses approaching 60 Gy are also considered acceptable. The risk profile increases substantially however with doses above 64 Gy. While the brainstem tolerance to conventional radiotherapy is better studied, data on the brainstem tolerance to SRS and HSRT are more limited. Mayo et al. published a comprehensive review on radiation-induced brainstem injury as part of the Quantitative Analyses of Normal Tissue Effects in the Clinic (QUANTEC) project in 2010 [28] and concluded that a maximum single dose of 12.5 Gy to the brainstem carries a <5% risk of brainstem injury [28]. Other studies of SRS delivering doses of 15–20 Gy to brainstem metastases report very low incidence of complications [28]. It is possible that some of these patients did not live long enough to develop any reportable toxicity. Therefore, when using radiation in patients who may have a long life expectancy, caution is advised. Dose volume effects have also been studied for patients being treated for trigeminal neuralgia, and small volumes of brainstem going to doses of around 45 Gy in a single fraction are tolerated well [29]. In general, keeping the brainstem dose as low as possible and when needed a very small volume going to higher doses is generally viewed as acceptable.

Data on brainstem injury from HSRT are drawn from studies of skull base tumors. An early HSRT study for benign and malignant tumors at different intracranial locations using 42 Gy in 6 fractions observed late and serious brainstem complications in 4 of 77 (5%) patients treated [30]. The treatment plans in general were not conformal relative to modern planning, and it was expected that a large volume of the brainstem received prescription dose [30]. Technology has evolved, and more conformal treatment planning is readily performed now, rendering data from earlier HSRT studies not applicable to modern HSRT.

Modern series report low toxicity for brainstem injury. In the phase II study of HSRT for cavernous sinus hemangiomas, Wang and colleagues observed no brainstem injury with a brainstem dose of 19.8 Gy (range 12.4–22.8 Gy) in 3 fractions [8]. In a follow-up study using HSRT for cavernous sinus hemangiomas [27] delivering doses of 21 Gy in 3 fractions and 22 Gy in 4 fractions, no brainstem injury was observed. A Japanese study reviewed their HSRT experience for vestibular schwannoma, and no brainstem injury was observed when the maximum brainstem dose was limited to 35 Gy in 5 fractions or 27 Gy in 3 fractions [10]. The study from Georgetown University reported zero incidence of brainstem injury with HSRT regimens of 25 Gy in 5 fractions or 21 Gy in 3 fractions for vestibular schwannoma [11]. Using 25 Gy in 5 fractions, colleagues from Johns Hopkins observed no brainstem injury [9]. From TG101, maximum brainstem dose is recommended to be <23.1Gy in 3 fractions and 31Gy in 5 fractions [31].

## Radiographic Findings

When a patient presents with a new neurologic deficit, it is important to rule out recurrent tumor or secondary malignancy as a cause. The standard diagnostic test is MRI of the brain with and without gadolinium. Since the fat signal in the skull base can obscure the visualization of the cranial nerves, a fat-suppressed T1 sequence with gadolinium is frequently included.

For cranial nerve injury, MRI may show abnormal enhancement in the involved cranial nerve, particularly after SRS (Fig. 42.1b, c) [32]. In one study, over 1/3 of the cases showed abnormal V nerve enhancement after SRS to a dose of 70–90 Gy in one fraction prescribed to 100%. In patients with vestibular schwannomas who are treated with SRS and later develop V and VII nerve deficits and progressive VIII nerve deficit (hearing loss), MRI may show stable, centrally necrotic, or enlarged tumor. Tumor response to treatment does not always predict CN function.

Patients with radiation-induced large vessel vasculopathy may present with stroke-like symptoms, and CT or MR angiogram may show stenosis or occlusion of a large artery [33] (Fig. 42.2). MRI may show features of an acute infarct. Radiation-induced aneurysm has occurred in rare circumstances [34].

For brainstem injury or necrosis, MRI typically shows abnormal enhancement and T2 signal intensity corresponding to the high-dose zone [35]. Figure 42.1a, c show enhancement after SRS for trigeminal neuralgia. Figure 42.3 shows an example of radiation necrosis of the brainstem after radiotherapy for nasopharyngeal carcinoma. Interested readers are encouraged to refer to Chap. 33 which covers brain radionecrosis.

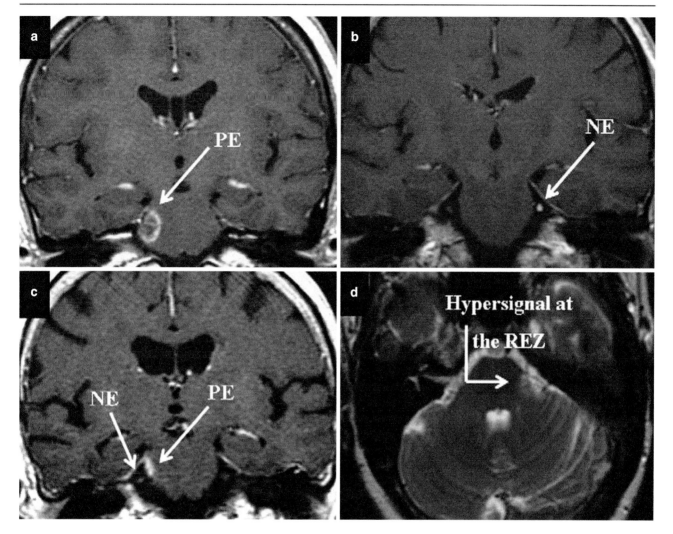

**Fig. 42.1** Three patterns of abnormal gadolinium enhancement observed at the follow-up MRI scans after linear accelerator-based SRS for trigeminal neuralgia: pons enhancement at the root entry zone (**a**), trigeminal nerve enhancement (**b**), pons and nerve enhancement (**c**). The hypersignal on the T2-weighted image corresponds strictly to the area of gadolinium enhancement (**d**). [Reprinted from Gorgulho A, De Salles AA, McArthur D, Agazaryan N, Medin P, Solberg T, et al. Brainstem and trigeminal nerve changes after radiosurgery for trigeminal pain. Surg Neurol. 2006;66(2):127–35; discussion 35. With permission from Elsevier]

## Pathologic Findings

There are typically no biopsies or resected tissue for analysis of the diagnosis in patients with CN injury, brainstem injury, and vascular injury. In an animal study, trigeminal nerves of baboons were irradiated to 80–100 Gy, and progressive focal damage of the nerve was found [36]. The histologic changes at 6 months consisted of demyelination, axonal degeneration, and necrosis and depended on the maximum radiation dose delivered. One nerve that was irradiated to 100 Gy showed near-complete nerve width necrosis [36]. In a case report, Szeifert et al. reported on the autopsy results of a patient treated with SRS twice to the same trigeminal nerve. The first SRS treatment delivered 90 Gy in 1 fraction at 100% at the pars triangularis of the trigeminal nerve, and the second SRS treatment delivered 70 Gy in 1 fraction at 100%

close to the root entry zone [37]. The first and second SRS treatments occurred 11 months and 26 days before the patient's death, respectively. On pathologic examination, the nerve showed a focused fibrotic lesion with hyaline-degenerated collagen bundles and scattered fibrocytes at the site treated during the first SRS session. The inside of the fibrotic lesion did not show S100 immunoreactivity which was present surrounding the lesion. A necrotic center with tissue debris and fibrinoid material was present at the root entry zone with no S100 positivity inside but with it in the tissues surrounding the lesion [37]. The above findings showed that ablative radiation affects all nerve fibers regardless of myelination.

The most significant vascular injury from radiation is the injury to a large vessel such as the internal carotid artery from cranial radiotherapy. When radiation-induced

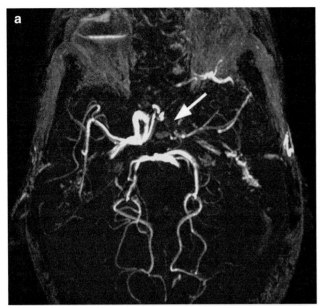

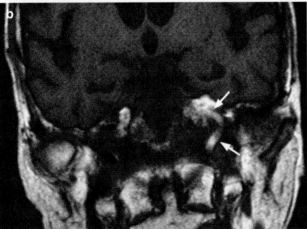

**Fig. 42.2** Radiation-induced thrombosis of the left internal carotid artery. (**a**) Absence of the artery on the 3D time-of-flight magnetic resonance angiography (TOF MRA; arrow) and (**b**) a high-signal thrombus on the coronal T1-weighted image (arrows). [Reprinted from King AD, Ahuja AT, Yeung DK, Wong JK, Lee YY, Lam WW, et al. Delayed complications of radiotherapy treatment for nasopharyngeal carcinoma: imaging findings. Clin Radiol. 2007;62(3):195–203. With permission from Elsevier]

vasculopathy occurs, there are subintimal foam cells and myointimal proliferation, fibrous thickening and hyalinization of the subintima, thickening of the elastica, fibrous thickening of the adventitia, and loose connective tissue thickening leading to luminal occlusion [38]. There are very few autopsy reports documenting radiation-induced injury of the internal carotid artery. Tonomura and colleagues published the case report of an 87-year-old patient who received head and neck radiotherapy 27 years prior to his presentation with a stroke [39]. Ultrasound examination of the carotid showed diffusely increased thickness of the intima-media of the common carotid artery and severe left internal carotid

stenosis. MRI showed an acute ischemic stroke in the left frontal lobe on diffusion-weighted images. The patient succumbed to aspiration pneumonia, and an autopsy was performed. Microscopic examination of the left internal carotid artery showed transmural fibrosis, focal intramural necrosis with diffuse decreased thrombomodulin expression, and fibrin thrombus on the vessel wall [39] (Fig. 42.4). Although the internal carotid artery examined was extracranial, it was the same vessel intracranially. One can extrapolate that the changes from radiation injury of the intracranial portion of the internal carotid artery will be the same.

In another case report, colleagues from Mayo Clinic operated on a patient 10 months after failed SRS, and two adjacent veins and the superior cerebellar artery were noted to have focal changes consistent with atheromatous disease, consistent with radiation injury [40].

For brainstem injury/necrosis, the pathologic findings are typical of those for brain necrosis and readers are encouraged to refer to Chap. 33 which covers brain radionecrosis.

## Management of Complications

The mechanisms of cranial nerve damage typically involve scar tissue formation, edema, fibrosis, and ischemia, and time course can span several months after radiation is completed.

Most cranial nerve injury relates to the optic nerve as it is more sensitive; however, treatment options for other cranial nerve injuries can follow a similar treatment paradigm. Radiation-induced optic neuropathy is covered in Chap. 38.

Corticosteroids are typically initiated to help reduce acute inflammation or edema caused by radiotherapy or SRS. However, it should be noted that steroid efficacy is not consistent for cranial nerve injury. There are no standard dose recommendations, but titrating the dose to a schedule avoiding the steroid-induced side effects is important. Patients may need to stay on corticosteroids for a prolonged course for symptomatic control. If there is minimal improvement after a prolonged course of steroid therapy, it is important to balance the risks and benefits of continuation of the treatment. Hyperbaric oxygen for symptomatic control in the acute phase of radiation-induced cranial nerve injury may be considered, but data are very limited with regard to its efficacy in reversing the deficits.

Apart from the management of cranial nerve injury itself, the functional impairment as a result of this also warrants attention, depending on the cranial nerve(s) involved. Patients who have diplopia from radiation injury to the cranial nerves in the cavernous sinus should be evaluated by an ophthalmologist for the management of the double vision. Patients who have V and VII nerve injury should also be managed by an ophthalmologist to avoid corneal abrasion. In

**Fig. 42.3** Dose distributions and imaging of brainstem necrosis. Contrast-enhanced T1-weighted axial and sagittal MR image showing areas of brainstem necrosis. Axial and sagittal CT image showing dose distribution. Both cases of brainstem necrosis were located in the right pons within the high-dose irradiated field. (**a**) The 41-year-old male (pt #1). (**b**) The 43-year-old female (pt #2). [Reprinted from Li YC, Chen FP, Zhou GQ, Zhu JH, Hu J, Kang DH, et al. Incidence and dosimetric parameters for brainstem necrosis following intensity modulated radiation therapy in nasopharyngeal carcinoma. Oral Oncol. 2017;73:97–104. with permission from Elsevier]

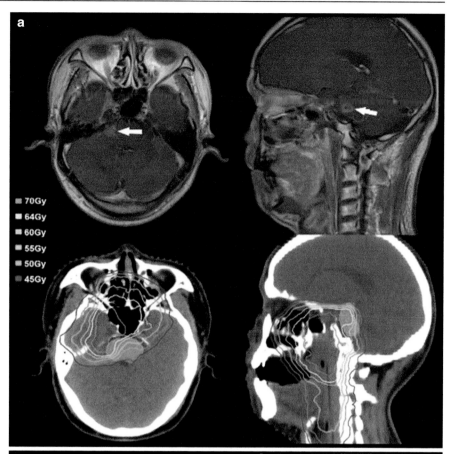

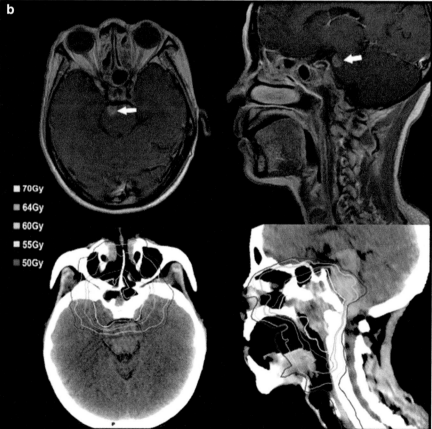

**Fig. 42.4** Microscopic examination of autopsied cross sections of a carotid artery stenosis after radiation therapy showing increased intimal layer thickness (*) with intramural necrosis (†) and thrombus (‡) on hematoxylin-eosin (H&E) staining (**a**); bar = 1 mm. Transmural fibrosis was observed by Elastica van Gieson staining (**b**). The endothelial layer was not stained for thrombomodulin (**c**) compared with atherosclerotic coronary artery (**d**). A thrombus consisting of fibrin was stained red with Masson trichrome stain (**e**); bar = 100 μm. [Reprinted from Tonomura S, Shimada K, Funatsu N, Kakehi Y, Shimizu H, Takahashi N. Pathologic Findings of Symptomatic Carotid Artery Stenosis Several Decades after Radiation Therapy. Journal of Stroke and Cerebrovascular Diseases. 2018:1–3. with permission from Elsevier]

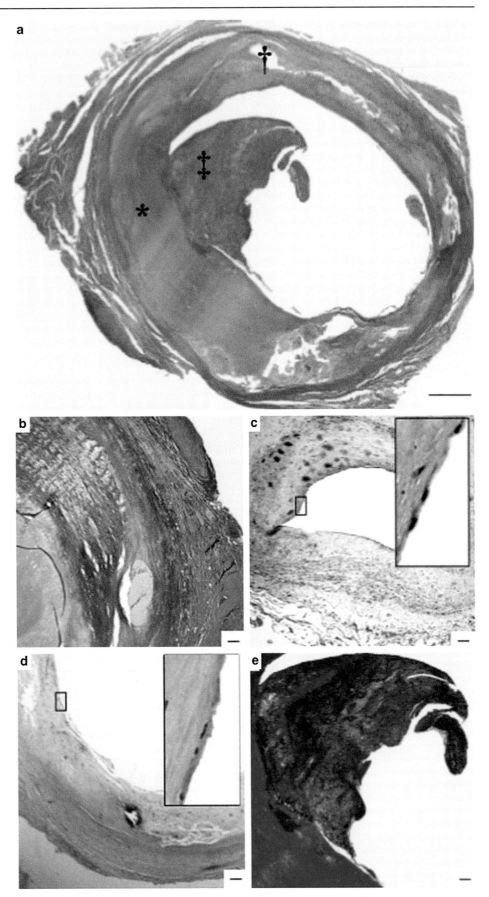

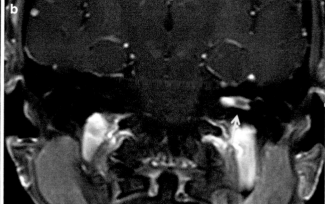

**Fig. 42.5** Left vestibular schwannoma (yellow arrow) before treatment (**a**); MRI of the brain obtained 6 months after SRS showed mild increase in the size of the left vestibular schwannoma (yellow arrow) with some central necrosis, now filling the left internal acoustic meatus completely (**b**)

patients with progressive hearing loss after SRS for vestibular schwannoma, an otolaryngology consultation is warranted for the monitoring of the auditory function. If there is injury to the last four cranial nerves (IX, X, XI, and XII nerves), swallowing function may be affected, and an evaluation by a speech pathologist is indicated.

There is very little data on successful treatments of vascular injury caused by radiation in the CNS. Many of the same medical treatment strategies have been employed and have provided anecdotal success. For brainstem injury, the treatment is similar to that for radiation necrosis occurring elsewhere in the brain. The mainstay of treatment is steroid therapy with success in some cases [41]. Bevacizumab has been used for radiation necrosis with some success, but the data are still limited [42]. A recent systematic review has demonstrated promising results in the 125 patients who received bevacizumab for radiation necrosis of the brain parenchyma [42]. However, the authors concluded that prospective trials would be needed to properly evaluate the role of bevacizumab as an efficacious agent against radiation necrosis and to better define the optimal scheduling, dosage, and duration of bevacizumab. Interested readers are encouraged to refer to Chap. 33 on brain radionecrosis.

## Case Study

This is a patient who presented with gradual onset of left-side tinnitus, gait imbalance, and mild decrease in left-side sensorineural high frequency hearing by 20 dB. MRI showed a small left vestibular schwannoma which was treated with stereotactic radiosurgery delivering 13 Gy in 1 fraction at 50% isodose line. Two weeks after SRS, the patient developed worsening of left-sided hearing and vertigo and was subsequently given dexamethasone 4 mg QID. There was some improvement of vertigo and left-sided hearing in the next 2 months, and dexamethasone was tapered off. Over the next 4 months, the patients noticed hearing machine noise and increased tearing of the left eye. There was some residual left-sided hearing, but the constant machine noise rendered it not serviceable. Repeat MRI of the brain in 6 months showed slight enlargement of the left vestibular schwannoma with central necrosis which was regarded as treatment effect (Fig. 42.5).

## Summary

- The goal of reducing radiation-associated complications begins with high-quality radiation planning.
- Patient history, clinical examination, and updated and comparative imaging can help identify a toxicity associated with radiation by ruling out tumor progression or other changes.
- Cranial nerve III, IV, V, VI, VII, VIII, IX, X, XI, and XII deficits are rare, and generally speaking toxicity can result many years after radiation is completed. There are no specific constraints used for these cranial nerves.
- Brainstem injury can result in devastating changes to a patient. Conventional radiation maximum point doses can be close to 60 Gy but only to a small volume. Maximum SRS doses are typically less than 12.5 Gy. However, even very small volumes can safely receive a higher single-fraction dose as evidenced by the data on trigeminal neuralgia patients receiving SRS.
- Vascular complications can occur, and while practice patterns are evolving, for SRS, a maximum point dose less than 30 Gy is recommended. For pituitary adenomas, also attempting to keep less than 50% of the circumference of

the internal carotid artery receiving prescription dose is recommended.

- Treatment of cranial nerve deficits and other radiation-associated complications in the central nervous system is evolving but with very little data on efficacy. Corticosteroids have been used with occasional success, but the efficacy of hyperbaric oxygen is not well documented for cranial nerve injury.
- Bevacizumab has been used for radiation necrosis with some apparent success, but further research is needed to properly evaluate the role of bevacizumab as an efficacious agent against radiation necrosis and to better define the optimal scheduling, dosage, and duration of the drug.

## Self-Assessment Questions

1. What is the approximate rate of VII nerve injury after SRS for vestibular schwannoma using 13 Gy in 1 fraction?
   A. 5%
   B. 15%
   C. 25%
   D. 35%

2. What cranial nerve(s) are at risk when SRS is used to treat a macroadenoma?
   A. CN II
   B. CN III, IV, and VI
   C. CN VII and VIII
   D. CN IX, X, XI, and XII

3. In treated acoustic neuromas, which of the following statements is false?
   A. SRS doses of 12–13 Gy in 1 fraction are typically prescribed.
   B. Local control at 12–13 Gy is comparable to local control with 14–20 Gy doses.
   C. Rates of CN VII toxicity are no different with SRS doses of 13 and 18 Gy.
   D. While additional investigation is needed, initial published data show that proton radiation has a higher rate of CN VII and VIII injury compared to SRS.

4. The risk of brainstem injury with a maximum dose of 12.5 Gy in 1 fraction is
   A. <5%
   B. <10%
   C. 10–15%
   D. 15–20%

5. When treating a glomus tumor with radiation, what CNs are the closest and potentially at risk for injury?
   A. CN II
   B. CN III, IV, V, and VI
   C. CN VIII and VIII
   D. CN IX, X, XI, and XII

## Answers

1. A [6]
2. B [1]
3. C [6]
4. A [28]
5. D [20]

## References

1. Witt TC. Stereotactic radiosurgery for pituitary tumors. Neurosurg Focus. 2003;14(5):e10.
2. Loeffler JS, Shih HA. Radiation therapy in the management of pituitary adenomas. J Clin Endocrinol Metab. 2011;96(7):1992–2003.
3. Spiegelmann R, Cohen ZR, Nissim O, et al. Cavernous sinus meningiomas: a large LINAC radiosurgery series. J Neurooncol. 2010;98(2):195–202.
4. Kondziolka D, Lunsford LD, McLaughlin MR, et al. Long-term outcomes after radiosurgery for acoustic neuromas. N Engl J Med. 1998;339(20):1426–33.
5. Petit JH, Hudes RS, Chen TT, et al. Reduced-dose radiosurgery for vestibular schwannomas. Neurosurgery. 2001;49(6):1299–306. discussion 306-7
6. Murphy ES, Suh JH. Radiotherapy for vestibular schwannomas: a critical review. Int J Radiat Oncol Biol Phys. 2011;79(4):985–97.
7. Flickinger JC, Kondziolka D, Niranjan A, et al. Acoustic neuroma radiosurgery with marginal tumor doses of 12 to 13 Gy. Int J Radiat Oncol Biol Phys. 2004;60(1):225–30.
8. Wang X, Liu X, Mei G, et al. Phase II study to assess the efficacy of hypofractionated stereotactic radiotherapy in patients with large cavernous sinus hemangiomas. Int J Radiat Oncol Biol Phys. 2012;83(2):e223–30.
9. Song DY, Williams JA. Fractionated stereotactic radiosurgery for treatment of acoustic neuromas. Stereotact Funct Neurosurg. 1999;73(1-4):45–9.
10. Morimoto M, Yoshioka Y, Kotsuma T, et al. Hypofractionated stereotactic radiation therapy in three to five fractions for vestibular schwannoma. Jpn J Clin Oncol. 2013;43(8):805–12.
11. Karam SD, Tai A, Strohl A, et al. Frameless fractionated stereotactic radiosurgery for vestibular schwannomas: a single-institution experience. Front Oncol. 2013;3:121.
12. Chon H, Yoon K, Kwon DH, et al. Hypofractionated stereotactic radiosurgery for pituitary metastases. J Neurooncol. 2017;132(1):127–33.
13. Fattah AY, Gurusinghe AD, Gavilan J, et al. Facial nerve grading instruments: systematic review of the literature and suggestion for uniformity. Plast Reconstr Surg. 2015;135(2):569–79.
14. Weber DC, Chan AW, Bussiere MR, et al. Proton beam radiosurgery for vestibular schwannoma: tumor control and cranial nerve toxicity. Neurosurgery. 2003;53(3):577–86. discussion 86-8
15. Putz F, Muller J, Wimmer C, et al. Stereotactic radiotherapy of vestibular schwannoma: hearing preservation, vestibular function,

and local control following primary and salvage radiotherapy. Strahlenther Onkol. 2017;193(3):200–12.

16. Tsai JT, Lin JW, Lin CM, et al. Clinical evaluation of CyberKnife in the treatment of vestibular schwannomas. Biomed Res Int. 2013;2013:297093.

17. Vivas EX, Wegner R, Conley G, et al. Treatment outcomes in patients treated with CyberKnife radiosurgery for vestibular schwannoma. Otol Neurotol. 2014;35(1):162–70.

18. Meijer OW, Vandertop WP, Baayen JC, et al. Single-fraction vs. fractionated linac-based stereotactic radiosurgery for vestibular schwannoma: a single-institution study. Int J Radiat Oncol Biol Phys. 2003;56(5):1390–6.

19. Guss ZD, Batra S, Limb CJ, et al. Radiosurgery of glomus jugulare tumors: a meta-analysis. Int J Radiat Oncol Biol Phys. 2011;81(4):e497–502.

20. Ivan ME, Sughrue ME, Clark AJ, et al. A meta-analysis of tumor control rates and treatment-related morbidity for patients with glomus jugulare tumors. J Neurosurg. 2011;114(5):1299–305.

21. Ibrahim R, Ammori MB, Yianni J, et al. Gamma knife radiosurgery for glomus jugulare tumors: a single-center series of 75 cases. J Neurosurg. 2017;126(5):1488–97.

22. Chun SG, Nedzi LA, Choe KS, et al. A retrospective analysis of tumor volumetric responses to five-fraction stereotactic radiotherapy for paragangliomas of the head and neck (glomus tumors). Stereotact Funct Neurosurg. 2014;92(3):153–9.

23. Schuster D, Sweeney AD, Stavas MJ, et al. Initial radiographic tumor control is similar following single or multi-fractionated stereotactic radiosurgery for jugular paragangliomas. Am J Otolaryngol. 2016;37(3):255–8.

24. Desai SS, Paulino AC, Mai WY, et al. Radiation-induced moyamoya syndrome. Int J Radiat Oncol Biol Phys. 2006;65(4):1222–7.

25. Killory BD, Kresl JJ, Wait SD, et al. Hypofractionated CyberKnife radiosurgery for perichiasmatic pituitary adenomas: early results. Neurosurgery. 2009;64(2 Suppl):A19–25.

26. Nguyen JH, Chen CJ, Lee CC, et al. Multisession gamma knife radiosurgery: a preliminary experience with a noninvasive, relocatable frame. World Neurosurg. 2014;82(6):1256–63.

27. Wang X, Zhu H, Knisely J, et al. Hypofractionated stereotactic radiosurgery: a new treatment strategy for giant cavernous sinus hemangiomas. J Neurosurg. 2018;128(1):60–7.

28. Mayo C, Yorke E, Merchant TE. Radiation associated brainstem injury. Int J Radiat Oncol Biol Phys. 2010;76(3 Suppl):S36–41.

29. Xue J, Goldman HW, Grimm J, et al. Dose-volume effects on brainstem dose tolerance in radiosurgery. J Neurosurg. 2012;117(Suppl):189–96.

30. Clark BG, Souhami L, Pla C, et al. The integral biologically effective dose to predict brain stem toxicity of hypofractionated stereotactic radiotherapy. Int J Radiat Oncol Biol Phys. 1998;40(3):667–75.

31. Benedict SH, Yenice KM, Followill D, et al. Stereotactic body radiation therapy: the report of AAPM task group 101. Med Phys. 2010;37(8):4078–101.

32. Gorgulho A, De Salles AA, McArthur D, et al. Brainstem and trigeminal nerve changes after radiosurgery for trigeminal pain. Surg Neurol. 2006;66(2):127–35. discussion 35

33. King AD, Ahuja AT, Yeung DK, et al. Delayed complications of radiotherapy treatment for nasopharyngeal carcinoma: imaging findings. Clin Radiol. 2007;62(3):195–203.

34. Matsumoto H, Minami H, Yamaura I, et al. Radiation-induced cerebral aneurysm treated with endovascular coil embolization. A case report. Interv Neuroradiol. 2014;20(4):448–53.

35. Li YC, Chen FP, Zhou GQ, et al. Incidence and dosimetric parameters for brainstem necrosis following intensity modulated radiation therapy in nasopharyngeal carcinoma. Oral Oncol. 2017;73:97–104.

36. Kondziolka D, Lacomis D, Niranjan A, et al. Histological effects of trigeminal nerve radiosurgery in a primate model: implications for trigeminal neuralgia radiosurgery. Neurosurgery. 2000;46(4):971–6. discussion 6-7

37. Szeifert GT, Salmon I, Lorenzoni J, et al. Pathological findings following trigeminal neuralgia radiosurgery. Prog Neurol Surg. 2007;20:244–8.

38. Brant-Zawadzki M, Anderson M, DeArmond SJ, et al. Radiation-induced large intracranial vessel occlusive vasculopathy. AJR Am J Roentgenol. 1980;134(1):51–5.

39. Tonomura S, Shimada K, Funatsu N, et al. Pathologic findings of symptomatic carotid artery stenosis several decades after radiation therapy. J Stroke Cerebrovasc Dis. 2018;27(3):e39–41.

40. Maher CO, Pollock BE. Radiation induced vascular injury after stereotactic radiosurgery for trigeminal neuralgia: case report. Surg Neurol. 2000;54(2):189–93.

41. Sloan AE, Arnold SM, St Clair WH, et al. Brain injury: current management and investigations. Semin Radiat Oncol. 2003;13(3):309–21.

42. Delishaj D, Ursino S, Pasqualetti F, et al. Bevacizumab for the treatment of radiation-induced cerebral necrosis: a systematic review of the literature. J Clin Med Res. 2017;9(4):273–80.

# 3-D Conformal Therapy and Intensity-Modulated Radiation Therapy/Volumetric-Modulated Arc Therapy

# 43

Raymond Chiu, Nicole McAllister, and Fahad Momin

## Learning Objectives

- Identify field parameters that need to be adjusted for 3D conformal radiotherapy plans.
- Choose appropriate field modifiers to generate ideal dose distributions in forward planning.
- Identify field parameters that are required for intensity-modulated radiation therapy plans.
- Determine the effectiveness of using planning structures during inverse planning.
- Select useful objectives in the treatment planning system to optimize a plan.
- Explain the differences between intensity-modulated radiation therapy and volumetric-modulated arc therapy plans.
- Evaluate a treatment plan to determine acceptability.
- Apply planning strategies for gliomas, hippocampal avoidance whole brain radiation therapy, craniospinal irradiation, craniopharyngioma, and pituitary tumors.

## Three-Dimensional Conformal Radiotherapy (3D-CRT)

Advances in technology have allowed central nervous system (CNS) treatment planning to be accurate and patient-specific. One of the early treatment planning methods is called 3D-CRT. By utilizing modern imaging modalities, such as computed tomography (CT) and magnetic resonance imaging (MRI), treatment planners can fuse these image sets so that physicians can delineate tumors and normal tissue structures accurately and quickly. Contouring these structures is necessary for the creation of conformal plans which treat the tumor and minimize damage to healthy normal tis-

sue and organs [1]. Since each tumor is different, treatment planners must adjust field parameters to create the most optimal plan, so it is important to know how each parameter affects the plan quality.

Creating 3D-CRT treatment plans is considered forward planning as the planner must select all the parameters to develop a treatment plan. These parameters include beam energy, gantry, collimator, and couch angles, field size, field modifiers, prescription normalization, isocenter location, and beam weighting. Keep in mind, these parameters are for one treatment field only, so additional fields have their own settings. In addition, many CNS plans require more than three fields. Since there are many variables to consider, this type of planning involves trial and error and can be overwhelming, so following an iterative approach can be helpful.

1. Beam energy
   Most linear accelerators have low- and high-energy photon beams, so it is important to select the correct energy. Using a low-energy beam ($\leq 10$ MV) is usually the default treatment energy and has several advantages. First, low-energy photons are not as penetrating as high-energy photons, so the exit dose is lower [2]. Minimizing the exit dose is important so that normal tissue areas beyond the planning target volume (PTV) do not receive higher doses than necessary. Second, the penumbra is smaller for low-energy beams than high-energy beams. Since the goal is to have the penumbra outside the PTV, the field aperture needs to be enlarged to satisfy this goal [2]. As a result of opening up the field, some extra normal tissue is treated, but this amount is still less than what is required for high-energy beams to cover the PTV. Last, low-energy beams have no neutron production. If physicians are concerned about additional doses from neutron production, it is best to avoid using high-energy photons (Figs. 43.1 and 43.2).

2. Despite low-energy beams being commonly used in many CNS plans, there are benefits to using high-energy beams ($\geq 15$ MV). The penetration power is higher than

R. Chiu (✉) · N. McAllister · F. Momin
Department of Radiation Oncology, Keck School of Medicine of University of Southern California, Los Angeles, CA, USA
e-mail: chiuraym@usc.edu

© Springer International Publishing AG, part of Springer Nature 2018
E. L. Chang et al. (eds.), *Adult CNS Radiation Oncology*, https://doi.org/10.1007/978-3-319-42878-9_43

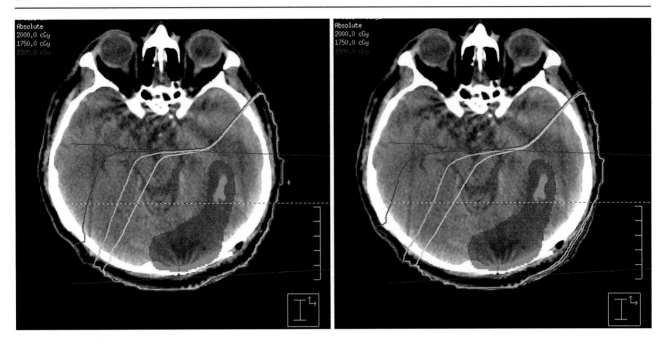

**Fig. 43.1** An axial slice showing the beam energy effect on isodose lines between 6 MV (left) and 15 MV (right). A left lateral field (red) shows the greatest differences between the energies. The red-shaded contour is the PTV, and 20 Gy, 17.5 Gy, and 15 Gy isodose lines are blue, green, and pink lines, respectively

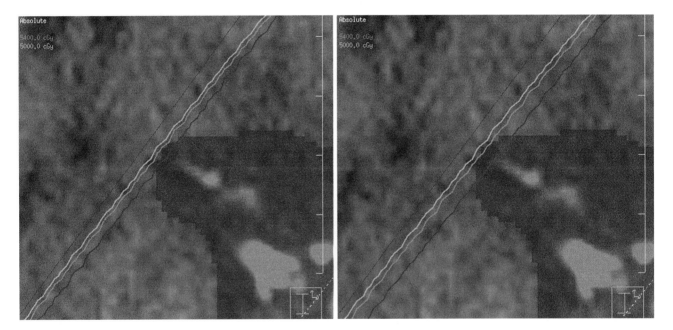

**Fig. 43.2** The penumbra effect between 6 MV (left) and 15 MV (right) photon fields on a transverse slice. The field edge is pink, and the PTV is the red shade. The red, orange, and green lines represent 60 Gy, 54 Gy, and 50 Gy isodose lines, respectively

low-energy photons, so hotspots ($\geq 105\%$ of prescription dose) in and around the PTV can be minimized. Some physicians prefer to minimize hotspots, so this penetration power is beneficial. In addition, surface doses are lower as the dose buildup region is deeper into the tissue [2]. Since some tumors are deep, higher doses in

superficial areas can be avoided by using high-energy photons.

3. Gantry angle

There are many angles to choose from, so it may be helpful to select optimal beam paths. In general, the most optimal beam paths are ones that treat minimal normal tissues to reach the PTV. These fields usually enter the same side as the PTV. For example, if the PTV is located in the right hemisphere of the brain, it is unlikely that left-sided beams provide a better dose distribution than right-sided beams. However, a combination of left- and right-sided fields may be useful if the PTV is centrally located. Since the gantry rotates in one plane, more beam paths are available when the couch angle is changed from the default, which is usually zero degrees.

4. Collimator angle

Choosing an appropriate collimator angle can reduce dose leakage from the multi-leaf collimator (MLC) and improve the dose distribution created by a wedge. Although the MLC can form many conformal shapes, a consequence is dose transmission through and between leaves. So, choosing a collimator angle that minimizes the number of leaves required to form the shape and reduces the travel distance of each leaf is imperative. Usually, a suitable setting has the leaves running parallel to the smallest PTV diameter. A good technique to visualize an appropriate angle is turning on the PTV in 3-D and looking at the beam's eye view (BEV). However, when a wedge is used, it may not be desirable to have the MLCs running in this configuration because a benefit of the wedge is to push dose to another region. In this scenario, priority should be given to the wedge to maximize its usefulness (Fig. 43.3).

5. Couch angle

By changing the couch angle from the default position, treatment fields become noncoplanar, and additional beam paths are available. Since noncoplanar beams are not confined to a single plane, sharper dose gradients can be achieved. Also, additional beam paths that treat the PTV without going through much normal tissues become possible. However, there are drawbacks when the couch is rotated. First, low doses (<40% of prescription dose) are spread out in different planes. As a result, the integral dose may increase when noncoplanar fields are utilized. Second, most couch rotations are controlled inside the treatment room only. Since a radiation therapist must enter the treatment room to rotate the couch, radiation therapists and patients may become frustrated as the treatment time is prolonged. Last, machine collisions with the couch table or patient are possible depending on the selected gantry and couch angles. To prevent any surprises or untoward events, perform a dry run of gantry and couch angle combinations to ensure safe and deliverable treatment plans.

6. Field size

Setting appropriate field sizes ensures that the PTV is covered while reducing the amount of normal tissue treated. Ideally, a treatment field is opened enough to cover the PTV only. However, the beam penumbra makes it difficult to create this type of treatment field. Therefore, an extra margin or block margin structure needs to be created and used to set up the field block. Usually, a uniform margin of 0.5–0.7 cm around the PTV is enough to have the penumbra outside the PTV [1]. When coplanar fields are used, there may be times when the superior and inferior margins are still tight, so opening up these areas by 1 cm from the PTV resolves any issues. Alternatively, noncoplanar fields can be used instead of this expansion.

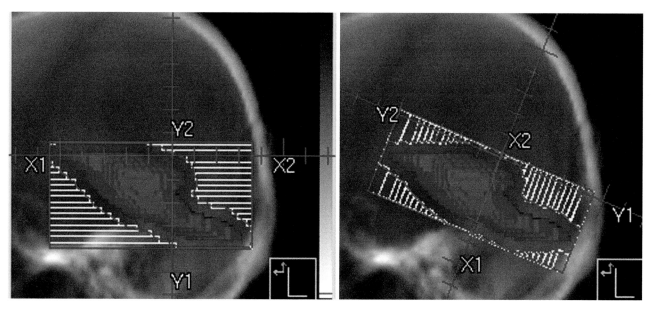

**Fig. 43.3** Beam's eye view of two fields with different collimator angles and PTV in 3-D. The field on the left has several leaves traveling a long distance compared to the field on the right. Since the field on the right has less dose leakage, the collimator angle is optimal

7. Field modifiers

By using modifiers in the path of the beam, dose distributions may be improved. One common modifier is the wedge. There are two types called physical wedge and electronic dynamic wedge, and both of them perform similarly. They are primarily used to push dose from one region to another. To understand how to push dose, turn on a hotspot in 3-D and look at the BEV. Then, visualize a line that connects this hotspot to a low-dose region. Rotate the collimator so that the $x$- or $y$-axis runs parallel to this line, and the wedge's heel is placed on the hotspot side. As a result, the hotspot is shifted away from the heel, and the dose on the toe side increases. A preferred hotspot location is the PTV's center so be careful not to over wedge a field.

Another feature of wedges is that they act as tissue compensators. When the treatment area has different tissue thicknesses, areas with less tissue receive higher doses. For example, the top of the head has more hotspots than the middle of the brain. Areas that lack tissue can be compensated by the wedge's heel. As a result, the dose becomes better distributed as the heel acts as tissue material to attenuate these higher doses.

Sometimes, wedges are not able to produce a desirable plan, so MLCs can be used instead. A method to utilize MLC for blocking hotspots is called field-in-field (FIF) technique [3]. To block hotspots using FIF, copy a field, turn on a reasonable hotspot in 3-D, and look at the BEV. A reasonable hotspot is larger than $2 \times 2$cm but should not cover the entire treatment field. Then, draw a block that covers this isodose cloud. In Philips Pinnacle treatment planning system (TPS), when the user adds a

block, the block action is either expose or block, depending on how the block is drawn. Also, the priority needs to be set to one if there are other blocks in the field. In Varian Eclipse TPS, the shaper tool can be used in conjunction with the select MLC leaves tool to tweak the block. After calculating this new field, which is called the subfield, take some beam weighting from the primary field, and add it to this subfield. By shifting dose away from the primary field, the doses in the open region are preserved, and the hotspot decreases in size as the weight of the subfield increases. Continue adding more weight until the prescription isodose line begins to break up. If there are still hotspots remaining, copy a different field, and repeat the same steps to create the subfield. Sometimes, the hotspot shape cannot be blocked effectively because the MLC runs along the $x$-axis. In this scenario, the collimator needs to be rotated to provide a better path for the MLC. However, the collimator rotates slowly so try to minimize using different angles (Fig. 43.4).

Besides blocking hotspots, FIF technique can be used for patching in additional dose to a certain region. To visualize which region needs more dose, contour areas that need to be increased, and turn it on in 3-D. Copy a field and using the BEV, design the field to surround this patch contour only. The same tools used for blocking in Philips Pinnacle and Varian Eclipse TPS can be applied to this scenario too. When the field is finished calculating, instead of taking weight from the primary field, change the plan normalization to add new weight. In Pinnacle TPS, change the prescribe method from prescribe to set monitor units. In Eclipse TPS, change the

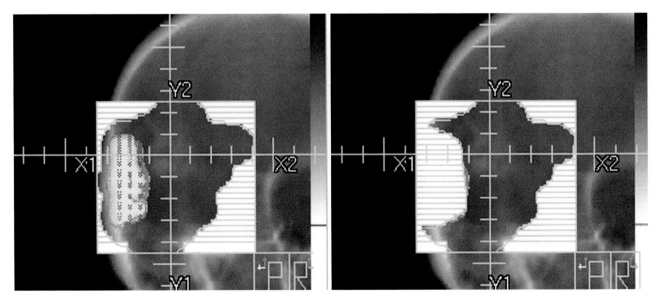

**Fig. 43.4** Beam's eye view of the primary (left) and subfield (right) with the hotspot in yellow. The MLC is shaded white to demonstrate how to design a subfield when using FIF technique

plan normalization mode to plan normalization value. In both treatment planning systems, there is an option to manually enter a monitor unit (MU) in the field, so enter the minimum amount of MU needed for delivery. Evaluate the dose distribution, and increase the MU if this region is not receiving adequate dose. As a consequence, areas within and around the subfield receive more dose, so additional hotspots may appear. If the entrance dose from the subfield becomes hotter than desired, copy a different field, and create another subfield to evenly distribute the patch dose.

Although having multiple subfields may increase treatment delivery time, each TPS has its own method of shortening this time when using FIF. In Pinnacle TPS, switching the beam type from "static" to "step and shoot" MLC allows the use of control points which act as subfields. Although "step and shoot" MLC can be used when FIF are used to block regions, these control points cannot be used to patch dose. However, in Eclipse TPS, by right-clicking on the plan and selecting "merge subfields," all subfields become merged with the primary beam. So, when the radiation therapists load the plan on the treatment machine, they should see the primary field only.

8. Prescription normalization

The overall doses in the plan can be scaled to affect PTV coverage and hotspots. Since each TPS has its own normalization methods, finding an appropriate method helps achieve a desirable plan sooner. Prescribing to a point dose is the most common method used in Pinnacle TPS. If further tweaking is necessary, the point location and the prescription percentage can be adjusted. For example, placing a calculation/reference point in a dose breakup region or reducing the prescription percentage increases the doses in the plan. Although normalizing to a point dose is common in Eclipse TPS too, it has a method that adjusts the isodose line percentage automatically to achieve the desired target coverage. Under the "plan normalization mode," there is an option for 100% covers 100% of the target volume. As long as this volume is set to the correct structure, tweaking these percentages helps scale the doses. However, if this contour is not created appropriately, this normalization may lead to suboptimal results, so careful contouring is recommended when using this mode.

9. Isocenter location

There are not many variations in where the isocenter should be placed. Typically, the isocenter is located in the **center** of the PTV. The treatment field can fully cover the target and is likely to be symmetrical at this location. Alternatively, the isocenter can be moved to another spot to control how the treatment field diverges. One technique is called "half-beam block" and involves

placing the isocenter at the edge of the block margin. As a result, the collimator jaws can be closed down to the center, so there is no divergence into other regions. An advantage to using "half-beam block" is that field matching becomes easier to do. For example, if the patient previously received radiation near the current treatment site, minimizing the divergence is important to reduce overlap doses. However, a drawback is that the maximum field size becomes smaller as only one collimator jaw can be opened. So, this blocking method is suitable for targets ≤20 cm in one dimension.

10. Beam weighting

Isodose lines shift according to how the treatment fields are weighted. Typically, equally weighted fields spread out the dose distribution evenly. However, there may be situations where equally weighted fields might not work. For example, if the lesion is located on one side, the plan might be better by increasing the weighting on the ipsilateral fields. This method has the potential to reduce the normal tissue doses. Regarding other scenarios, any field percentage can be used to change the weights to create a balanced dose distribution.

## Intensity-Modulated Radiation Therapy (IMRT)

The process of setting target goals in the TPS to shape the isodose lines and dose volume histogram (DVH) to the desired outcome is referred to as inverse planning. When this type of planning is combined with static gantry fields, the treatment technique is considered IMRT. Creating IMRT plans requires the planner to select the proper number of beams and field parameters similarly to 3D-CRT planning. However, selecting appropriate field modifiers and beam weights is unnecessary because the TPS has a function called the optimizer which handles this process. The TPS optimizer uses the planning goals entered by the planner and generates a fluence map for each beam. Then, this map is then converted to MLC block patterns. Consequently, these additional block patterns increase the total MU compared to 3D-CRT. In order to use the optimizer efficiently, generating planning structures and entering reasonable objectives are necessary.

1. Beam energy

In contrast to 3D-CRT, IMRT plans should only use low-energy photon beams (≤10 MV). When high-energy beams are used, the increased energy leads to higher neutron production. The additional neutron dose is undesirable, so using high-energy fields can be problematic. Although the penetrating power is reduced using low-energy fields, the TPS optimizer can still create a reasonable plan.

2. Gantry and Couch Angles

For an optimal IMRT plan, the use of five or more beams is used to create a uniform dose distribution around the target. Similar to 3D-CRT, choosing beams which are closer to the target helps reduce the amount of normal tissue irradiation. It is important to remember that increasing the number of beams increases the integral dose to the surrounding tissues and prolongs treatment time. The use of parallel opposed beams should be avoided to maximize the variation in the fluence map generated by the TPS. While using only coplanar beams may produce an adequate plan, one or more noncoplanar beams may be used to keep the intermediate doses conformal. Specifically for CNS planning, vertex fields are commonly introduced to avoid entering through the patient's face while keeping the dose conformal.

3. Planning

When creating an IMRT plan, it is important to create structures that help shape doses around the PTV and limit doses to critical organs. Planning organ at risk volume (PRV) structures are created to put a margin on structures, such as the brainstem or spinal cord, to reduce the uncertainty in the doses delivered to them [3]. When dose-limiting structures overlap the PTV, a planning PTV (pPTV) is often created. To create the pPTV, copy the PTV, and subtract the dose-limiting structure with a margin of 1–3 mm to avoid conflicting priorities in the optimization window that may lead to unreasonable dose gradients [4]. An additional planning structure may be created to ensure the area of the PTV that is overlapping with a critical structure still gets dose within tolerance to the critical structure. When generating a simultaneous integrated boost (SIB) plan, it is important to create a pPTV for the lower dose PTV. Subtracting the higher dose level PTV with a 1 mm margin from the lower dose level PTV minimizes conflicting objectives in the TPS optimizer for regions that share the same voxel.

In addition to using planning structures, the TPS optimizer needs to know how to handle regions outside the PTV. Therefore, to help tighten doses and make plans more conformal, structures called rings are created. In Eclipse TPS, a useful ring can be created by using a normal tissue objective (NTO). Eclipse introduces the NTO parameter in the optimization window. The normal starting priority is 100 and can be adjusted depending on the result. If the target is more uniform in shape, a higher priority can be used to be tighter on constraints. However, if the PTV coverage starts to decrease, lowering the priority may be helpful. Regarding the other NTO parameters, a good starting point for the "distance from target" is 0.3–0.5 cm with start and end doses of 105% and 60%, respectively. Next, the falloff for uniform structures can be 0.5 and greater. Typically, manually adjusting the NTO

works better than the automated values. Since NTO is an Eclipse exclusive feature, Pinnacle users need to manually create rings. Usually, a minimum of two rings is required. The table below lists the structures and how to create them. In the optimizer, add a max dose constraint for the ring, and set it at 98% of prescription dose. For normal tissue, add a max DVH constraint, and set it at 50% of prescription dose at 1% volume. Additional rings can be used to control other dose levels, and these structures can be created similar to the ring. Remember to update the normal tissue contour so that this structure is the outermost ring (Table 43.1 and Figs. 43.5 and 43.6).

A typical Pinnacle TPS optimization involves using different types of objectives. For PTV structures, min dose, uniform dose, and max dose objectives are used and set to prescription dose except for max dose which should be 105% of prescription dose. If there are pPTVs that overlap critical structures, use a min dose that is at least 5% below the dose tolerance of the critical structure. For critical structures and rings, max dose and max DVH objectives are used. To lower mean doses, max EUD

**Table 43.1** Structures necessary to help create rings

| Planning Structures | Description | Purpose |
|---|---|---|
| PTV Exp | PTV + 0.1 cm | Placeholder |
| Ring | PTV Exp + 0.5 cm using create ring ROI | Controls high doses |
| External | Patient's body or external contours | Placeholder |
| Normal tissue | External minus both PTV Exp and ring | Controls low doses |

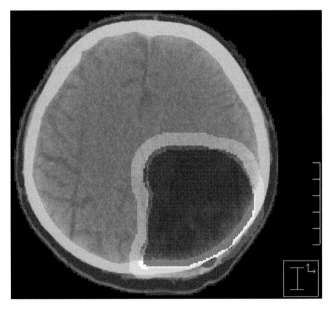

**Fig. 43.5** Planning structures on an axial slice. The PTV, ring, and normal tissue are shaded red, cyan, and orange, respectively

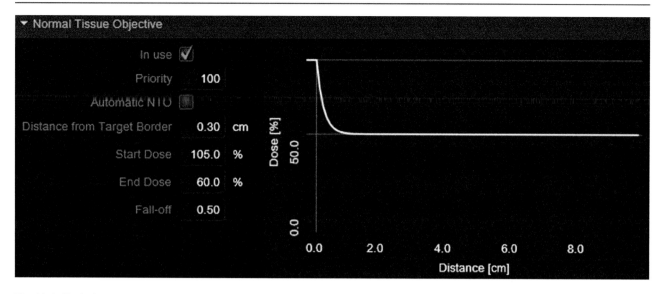

**Fig. 43.6** Typical parameters entered in the normal tissue objective for Eclipse

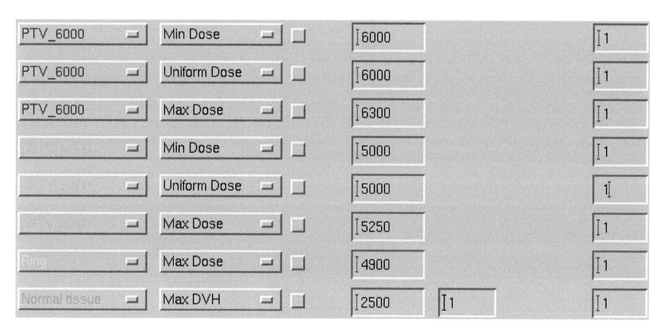

**Fig. 43.7** Starting objectives entered into Pinnacle for a SIB plan. The prescription doses are 50 Gy and 60 Gy

(equivalent uniform dose) performs better than using max DVH. So, the general optimizing workflow starts with entering objectives and weights of 1 for all types of PTV structures and rings. After the first run and dose computation, evaluate the doses to critical structures, and start adding objectives for them. Then, reset the beams and optimize again. When this run has finished, evaluate the plan again and focus on getting adequate coverage. Increasing coverage can be accomplished by increasing the weight or dose on PTV contours or relaxing ring objectives. After several runs and coverage is appropriate, focus on organ sparing by changing the weight or dose. Finally, carefully change the weight or dose for the rings to tighten the isodose lines.

However, if the target coverage is already low, tightening the doses may not be helpful. Once the plan calculation has completed and meets the planning criteria, the physician can be notified to review the plan (Fig. 43.7).

Similar to Pinnacle TPS, IMRT optimization in Eclipse TPS consists of min, max, and gEUD (generalized equivalent uniform dose) dose objectives. Min dose objectives are used for target structures, such as PTVs and pPTVs, whereas max dose objectives are used to reduce hotspots in PTVs and carve dose around normal tissue organs. Setting min dose objectives slightly higher, such as 103% of prescription dose, helps ensure adequate coverage, while setting the max dose objective around 105% of prescription dose minimizes the hotspots inside the PTV. It is important to know that the priorities are relative to one another. For example, the maximum priority value in Eclipse TPS is 1000, but the same planning results can be accomplished by setting the highest priority at 100. For the initial run, using just PTV objectives and the NTO feature allows the planner to evaluate how much to push on the normal tissue structures. After the initial run, evaluate the DVH, and slowly push on the secondary structures with the max dose and gEUD functions until the desired outcome is reached. Continue to evaluate the DVH throughout the optimization process to maintain a balance between target coverage and critical structure sparing. To have the optimization DVH reflect more accurately to the final dose DVH, initiate an intermediate dose calculation, which performs a final dose calculation algorithm during the optimization stage (Fig. 43.8).

After final calculation, sometimes both TPS optimizers generate a suboptimal plan, so slice-by-slice adjustments may be necessary. Dose painting is a technique which involves contouring certain isodose lines and setting an objective to increase or decrease the prevalence of that isodose line. Therefore, this technique can help achieve an improved dose distribution by increasing coverage and decreasing doses to critical structures. For example, regions of the PTV that are missing coverage can be contoured and given a minimum dose objective. Similarly, parts of critical structures receiving a high dose can be drawn and given a maximum dose objective. Since these spot contours are drawn on individual slices, dose painting can be time-consuming. Also, the results are not guaranteed. As a result, this method is effective for small changes only.

## Volumetric-Modulated Arc Therapy (VMAT)

A treatment technique that is becoming more widely utilized is VMAT. Treatment plans using this technique have similar target coverage and dose sparing to IMRT but have shorter delivery times. The treatment planning process follows a similar approach to IMRT as the optimizer creates conformal dose distributions. However, VMAT plans take longer to compute than IMRT because there are more parameters that need to be considered by the TPS, such as the variable motion of the gantry, MLC block patterns, and dose rate [2, 5]. Therefore, carefully setting up the VMAT field parameters in the beginning saves time from having to redo plans caused by mistakes in initial parameter settings.

The number of fields in VMAT plans to produce a desirable plan is fewer than other treatment techniques. Two arcs, one moving clockwise and the other moving counterclockwise, are sufficient to provide optimal PTV coverage and organ sparing. In fact, several studies have compared the differences between single and two arc plans and found similar results [5–9]. Although adding an additional arc may increase the delivery time about 1.5 min according to Vanetti et al. [8], the benefits in dose distribution may outweigh this drawback.

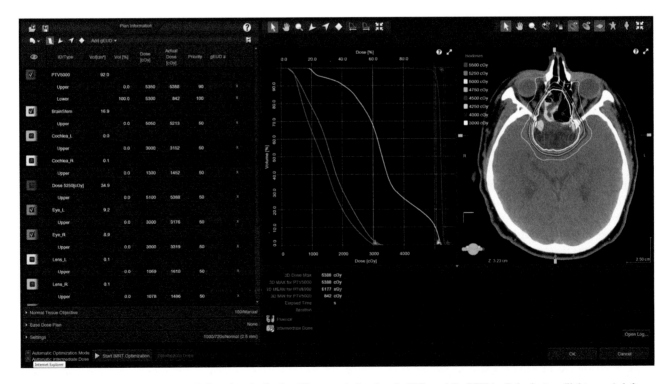

**Fig. 43.8** Final objectives entered into Eclipse for a brain plan. The prescription dose is 50Gy and the PTV (red), brainstem (light green), left eye (green), and right eye (pink) are displayed on the DVH

Sometimes, using noncoplanar arcs are beneficial because rotating or kicking the couch can create optimal dose distributions around the target [5, 9, 13, 16]. However, it is important to keep in mind that adding a noncoplanar arc increases the treatment time as the couch has to be rotated mid-treatment, similar to other treatment techniques. Other arc adjustments involve determining whether to use a partial or full rotation. This decision is not easily determined, so tweaking this arc path has a significant outcome on the plan quality.

The arc path can be chosen similarly to how IMRT field angles are selected. Gantry start and stop angles define the arc path, and optimal paths are usually located on the ipsilateral side of the PTV. However, arcs with some contralateral paths may be beneficial in certain situations, such as a centrally located or irregular-shaped PTV that requires more modulation. Sometimes when these paths become large, the arc needs to be split to avoid entrance doses in certain regions. For example, entering the patient's face may be unnecessary and undesirable, so one can stop the arc before it enters this region. In Pinnacle TPS, a separate arc needs to be created in order to treat on the other side of the avoidance region. In contrast, Eclipse TPS has a handy feature inside the optimizer to define an avoidance sector. By entering the gantry start and stop angles for this sector, the radiation beam turns off as the gantry rotates over this region and turns back on after passing this sector. Defining an appropriate arc range is a delicate balance as large arc paths tend to spread out low dose as the field enters more normal tissue. However, small arc ranges may inhibit the optimizer from finding an ideal solution, so the plan quality may suffer.

An important field parameter in VMAT plans that needs to be carefully adjusted is the collimator angle. When MLCs are utilized, there is radiation leakage between adjacent MLC leaves, and this observation is known as "tongue and groove effect" [10]. This effect is more apparent with VMAT compared to other treatment techniques. To minimize this leakage, treatment fields usually have a collimator angle between 10 and 45° depending on the shape of the PTV in the BEV. When two arcs are used, the collimator angle is adjusted so that one arc has the complementary angle of the other. For example, if the clockwise arc has a collimator angle of 45°, then the counterclockwise arc should have a collimator angle of 315°. However, there are situations when the angles deviate from this range to improve dose sparing of organs at risk (OAR). In one study, 0° or 90° provides better organ sparing for paraspinal treatments [10]. Another study suggests using 95° and 265° for hippocampal avoidance whole brain radiation therapy [11]. Since critical structures are blocked differently depending on the MLC orientation, multiple collimator configurations may need to be explored to create an optimal plan.

Since the collimator is rotated, and many gantry angles are used for treatment, the field size may have to be opened larger than expected to cover the target. The best way to set the collimator jaws is by using the BEV and rotating the gan-try around. However, there are times that the arc needs to be split. Since the maximum MLC travel distance is about 14.5 cm from the most protracted to retracted leaf, field sizes larger than this number can create issues for the optimizer because there are regions that the MLC cannot reach [2]. To minimize these regions, set the maximum field size to 18 cm by adjusting one of the X jaws for each arc. For example, if the X1 and X2 jaws are 10 cm, one arc should have an X1 jaw of 8 cm, and the second arc should have an X2 jaw of 8 cm. As a result, the TPS optimizer struggles less trying to overcome the MLC limitation and may improve the dose distribution and homogeneity compared to leaving the jaws opened greater than 18 cm [5].

## Plan Evaluation

A systematic review of treatment plans allows for consistency and efficiency. Regardless of treatment technique, all plans can be evaluated the same way using the following guidelines:

1. PTV coverage and PTV hotspots ($\geq$105% of prescription dose) on the DVH.
2. Doses to critical structures on the DVH.
3. Maximum dose location on CT slices.
4. Prescription isodose line conformality on CT slices.
5. 30Gy isodose line conformality on CT slices.
6. Hotspot locations on CT slices.
7. Low to intermediate dose streaking on CT slices (Figs. 43.9–43.11).

## Planning Strategies: Glioma

A class solution was developed for glioma treatment planning to help save time and provide some standardization for plan quality. At the University of Texas MD Anderson Cancer Center, Likhacheva et al. implemented an IMRT class solution based on tumor location [12]. To begin the planning process, the brain was divided up into the following regions: right and left frontal, right and left temporal, right and left parietal-occipital, right and left clival, midline clival, midbrain, cerebellum, and brainstem. Depending on which region the tumor was located in, specific gantry and couch angles were used. Next, four planning structures were created and used in the Pinnacle TPS optimizer with standardized objectives. After a few iterations, the treatment plan was finalized. Compared to manually generated plans, Likhacheva et al. found that the class solution plans were equal or better when evaluating the Radiation Therapy Oncology Group (RTOG) conformity index, mean brain dose, and brain volume receiving 30 Gy [12]. In addition, the investigators found that the treatment planning time for dosimetrists of all

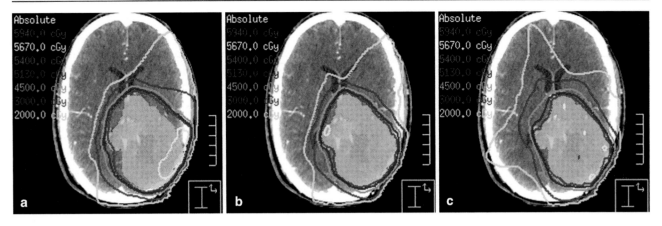

**Fig. 43.9** Transverse slices of 3D-CRT (**a**), IMRT (**b**), and VMAT (**c**) plans. Each plan has a prescription dose of 54 Gy, and the PTV is shaded in green. Both 3D-CRT and IMRT plans use noncoplanar beams, whereas the VMAT plan uses coplanar arcs. The yellow, red, blue, orange, pink, and cyan lines represent 56.7 Gy, 54 Gy, 51.3 Gy, 45 Gy, 30 Gy, and 20 Gy isodose lines

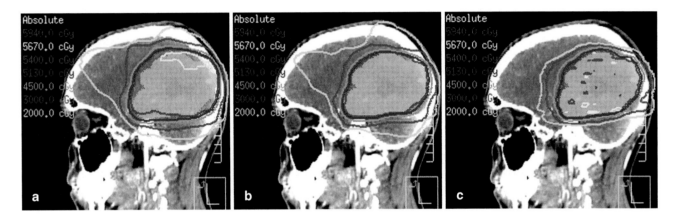

**Fig. 43.10** Sagittal slices of the same 3D-CRT (**a**), IMRT (**b**), and VMAT (**c**) plans. The yellow, red, blue, orange, pink, and cyan lines represent 56.7 Gy, 54 Gy, 51.3 Gy, 45 Gy, 30 Gy, and 20 Gy isodose lines

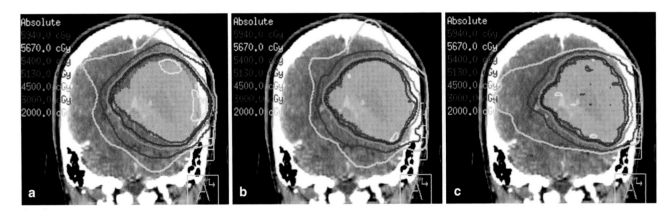

**Fig. 43.11** Coronal slices of the same 3D-CRT (**a**), IMRT (**b**), and VMAT (**c**) plans. The yellow, red, blue, orange, pink, and cyan lines represent 56.7 Gy, 54 Gy, 51.3 Gy, 45 Gy, 30 Gy, and 20 Gy isodose lines

levels of experience reduced significantly [12]. So, utilizing a class solution benefited patients in terms of plan quality and start times (Table 43.2, 43.3, and 43.4).

Although this class solution has been developed for IMRT, applying the same field angle selections to 3D-CRT provides a decent starting point for treatment planners. Instead of creating planning structures, field modifiers, such as wedges or FIF, should be used to generate an acceptable plan. By following the instructions listed for wedges and FIF

**Table 43.2** Beam parameters for each brain region based on glioma class solution developed by Likhacheva et al. Angles are listed as gantry-couch where gantry angle of 0° is the anterior-posterior beam and couch angles of 0°and 90° represent default position and table rotated counterclockwise, respectively

| Region | Field 1 | Field 2 | Field 3 | Field 4 | Field 5 | Field 6 | Field 7 |
|---|---|---|---|---|---|---|---|
| Rt frontal | 230–000 | 300–000 | 045–315 | 060–270 | 315–045 | – | – |
| Lt frontal | 130–000 | 060–000 | 045–315 | 060–270 | 315–045 | – | – |
| Rt temporal | 300–000 | 230–000 | 285–085 | 055–315 | 305–045 | – | – |
| Lt temporal | 060–000 | 130–000 | 075–270 | 305–045 | 055–315 | – | – |
| Rt parietal-occipital | 235–000 | 170–000 | 270–060 | 330–030 | 090–285 | – | – |
| Lt parietal-occipital | 125–000 | 190–000 | 090–310 | 030–330 | 270–055 | – | – |
| Rt clival | 290–015 | 260–345 | 300–045 | 315–090 | 330–300 | – | – |
| Lt clival | 070–345 | 100–015 | 060–315 | 315–090 | 030–060 | – | – |
| Midline clival | 100–000 | 075–345 | 060–300 | 300–060 | 045–270 | – | – |
| Midbrain | 035–270 | 090–315 | 040–350 | 270–350 | 270–045 | 320–010 | 090–010 |
| Cerebellum | 290–000 | 230–000 | 070–000 | 130–000 | 065–310 | 295–050 | – |
| Brainstem | 230–000 | 120–000 | 270–045 | 300–045 | 060–315 | 090–315 | – |

**Table 43.3** Planning structures listed by Likhacheva et al. to be used in the TPS optimizer for glioma treatment planning

| Planning Structures | Description |
|---|---|
| Planning PTV | PTV minus boost PTV |
| PTV Exp 1 cm | PTV + 1 cm |
| Ring | PTV Exp 1 cm minus PTV |
| External | Patient's body or external contours |
| Normal tissue | External minus PTV Exp 1 cm |

**Table 43.4** Class solution planning objectives that were used by Likhacheva et al. and entered in Pinnacle

| Structure | Objective | Dose | Percent | Weight |
|---|---|---|---|---|
| Boost PTV | Min dose | Prescription #1 | – | 100 |
| Boost PTV | Uniform dose | Prescription #1 + 2% | – | 100 |
| Planning PTV | Min dose | Prescription #2 | – | 100 |
| Planning PTV | Uniform dose | Prescription #2 + 2% | – | 3 |
| Ring | Max DVH | Prescription #2 | 1 | 5 |
| Normal tissue | Max dose | 2900 | – | 25 |
| Normal tissue | Max DVH | 2400 | 2 | 25 |

in the 3D-CRT section of this chapter, the PTV coverage and dose homogeneity can be improved.

Regarding frontotemporal gliomas, noncoplanar VMAT was shown to be equivalent to noncoplanar IMRT. Panet-Raymond et al. compared these two techniques by creating two plans [13]. The VMAT plan consisted of a coplanar arc with a collimator angle of 45° and no avoidance regions and a noncoplanar arc with 180° rotation at a couch angle of 90°. The IMRT plan had seven fields where two to four fields were noncoplanar, and the couch angles were limited to one to two angles. The authors found that the doses to critical structures and PTV coverage were similar [13]. However, compared to IMRT, VMAT reduced the number of MU and treatment time but increased the planning time [13]. In the end, both techniques had to be evaluated for each patient to determine the best course of action.

## Case Study: Plan Comparison between Coplanar VMAT and Noncoplanar IMRT for a Right Frontoparietal Glioblastoma Multiforme Lesion

A 67-year-old male with a history of prostate cancer presented with seizures which affected his left hand coordination and caused left face and arm numbness and dysarthria. He received an MRI scan that showed a 2.5 × 2.5 × 2.3 cm contrast enhancing mass in the right precentral gyrus. The pathology came back as glioblastoma, IDH-wildtype. So, he underwent a gross total resection with a plan to treat with chemoradiation involving Temodar and daily radiation to 60 Gy in 30 fractions. A five-field noncoplanar IMRT SIB plan was created using the class solutions from Table 43.2 using Pinnacle TPS.

During plan evaluation, the physician asked to see a plan with a short treatment time. So, the dosimetrist created a coplanar VMAT plan to compare and used two 168 degree arcs sweeping on the patient's right. Also, the planning objectives in the optimization were kept similar. After adjusting the normalization to maintain similar PTV coverages, the doses to critical structures were different. Compared to the IMRT plan, the VMAT plan had lower maximum doses to the left lens, eyes, brainstem, cochleas, and spinal cord because these structures were not in the exit dose region as much as the IMRT plan. Conversely, higher mean doses to the optic nerves, optic chiasm, pituitary, and brain tissue were noticed because the exit dose had a larger contribution to these organs in the VMAT plan. Since both plans had doses to the organs at risk far below dose tolerances, the physician felt comfortable treating with VMAT. In this case, class solutions helped provide a good starting point to explore other planning options (Figs. 43.12–43.16).

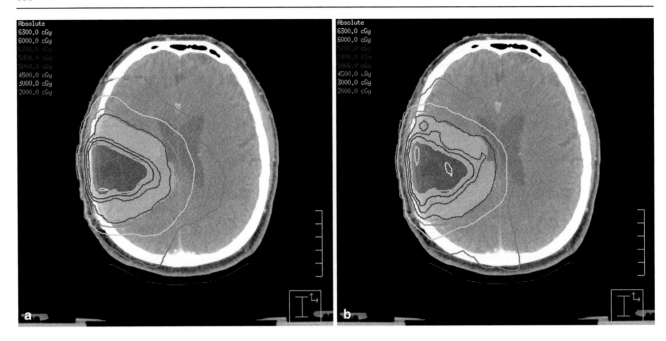

**Fig. 43.12** Axial slices of VMAT (**a**) and IMRT (**b**) plans. The PTV_6000 and PTV_5000 are shaded in red and green, respectively. The yellow, green, blue, pink, red, orange, cyan, and dark green lines represent 63 Gy, 60 Gy, 57 Gy, 54 Gy, 50 Gy, 45 Gy, 30 Gy, and 20 Gy isodose lines

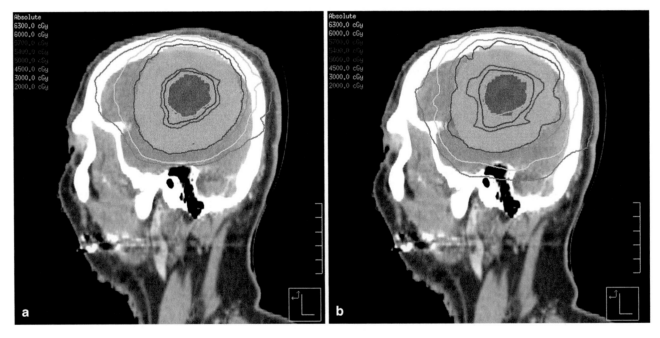

**Fig. 43.13** Sagittal slices of the same VMAT (**a**) and IMRT (**b**) plans. The yellow, green, blue, pink, red, orange, cyan, and dark green lines represent 63 Gy, 60 Gy, 57 Gy, 54 Gy, 50 Gy, 45 Gy, 30 Gy, and 20 Gy isodose lines

## Planning Strategies: Hippocampal Avoidance Whole Brain Radiation Therapy (HA-WBRT)

Shen et al. developed a VMAT class solution for hippocampal sparing that is simple to implement and satisfied the RTOG 0933 protocol guidelines [11]. First, creating six planning structures, which were sPTV1, sPTV2, sPTV3, sPTVu, PTVsup, and PTVinf, were necessary to create three optimization regions. Then, they chose an isocenter placed in the center of sPTV2 and created two arcs with full rotation. For the superior arc, the gantry rotated from 179° to 181° with a collimator angle of 265°, and collimator jaws fitted to 0.5 cm margin around PTVsup.

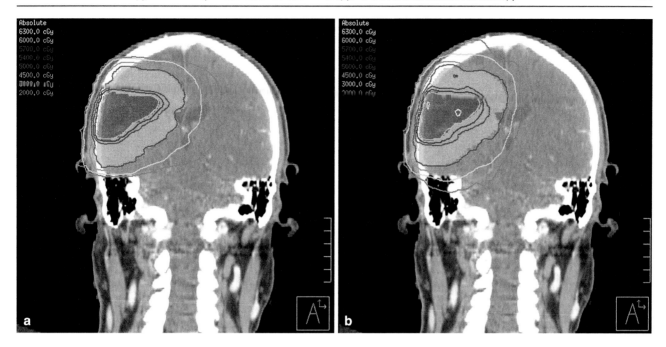

**Fig. 43.14** Coronal slices of the same VMAT (**a**) and IMRT (**b**) plans. The yellow, green, blue, pink, red, orange, cyan, and dark green lines represent 63 Gy, 60 Gy, 57 Gy, 54 Gy, 50 Gy, 45 Gy, 30 Gy, and 20 Gy isodose lines

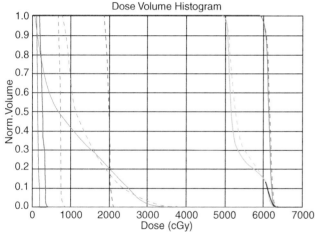

**Fig. 43.15** DVH of the VMAT (solid line) and IMRT (dashed line) plans. The left cochlea (pink), right cochlea (sky blue), brainstem (orange), PTV_5000 (green), and PTV_6000 (red) structures are displayed

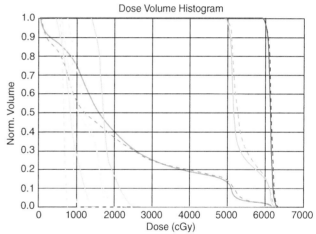

**Fig. 43.16** DVH of the VMAT (solid line) and IMRT (dashed line) plans. The left optic nerve (cyan), right optic nerve (yellow), optic chiasm (yellow green), brain tissue (violet), PTV_5000 (green), and PTV_6000 (red) structures are displayed

For the inferior arc, the gantry rotated from 181° to 179° with a collimator angle of 95°, and collimator jaws fitted to 0.5 cm margin around PTVinf. Shen et al. confirmed that the total field length in the *x*-direction was <15 cm. Once the fields were set, using standard objectives in Eclipse TPS helped expedite the planning time. The authors found that having two arcs overlap on sPTV2 allowed the MLC to shield the hippocampal avoidance region [11]. This blocking was visualized by examining the MLC patterns in the BEV. Also, PTV coverage remained unaffected with this arrangement, so this class

solution met the protocol guidelines in terms of target coverage and normal tissue sparing (Table 43.5).

For institutions without VMAT capabilities, IMRT had the ability to spare the hippocampus as well. After performing a 3-D search space, Gondi et al. determined an optimal field arrangement which involved nine noncoplanar fields [14]. The field setup and observed tissue doses helped Gondi et al. develop RTOG 0933 [14]. However, using noncoplanar fields had drawbacks as mentioned earlier in the 3D-CRT section of this chapter. As an alternative to noncoplanar fields, Siglin et al. found that placing a patient on a 30-degree

**Table 43.5** Class solution planning structures that were used by Shen et al. for hippocampal sparing

| Planning Structures | Description |
|---|---|
| sPTV1 | Part of PTV within 0.5 cm ring around hippocampal avoidance region |
| sPTV2 | Part of PTV in same axial planes as sPTV1 but excludes sPTV1 |
| sPTVu | One superior slice of PTV above sPTV2, one inferior slice of PTV below sPTV2, and part of PTV within 0.3 cm margin around optic nerves and optic chiasm |
| sPTV3 | Whole brain PTV minus sPTV1, sPTV2, and sPTVu |
| PTVsup | Superior portion of sPTV3, superior slice of sPTVu, and sPTV2 |
| PTVinf | Inferior portion of sPTV3, inferior slice of sPTVu, and sPTV2 |

**Table 43.6** Noncoplanar IMRT fields that Gondi et al. utilized and modified for deliverability. Angles based on Varian Standard coordinate system

| Field | Gantry angle (°) | Couch angle (°) |
|---|---|---|
| 1 | 150 | 140 |
| 2 | 230 | 150 |
| 3 | 360 | 225 |
| 4 | 76 | 190 |
| 5 | 131 | 196 |
| 6 | 171 | 96 |
| 7 | 275 | 150 |
| 8 | 223 | 196 |
| 9 | 221 | 90 |

inclined headboard improved the ability of the TPS optimizer to block the hippocampus and optic structures when using coplanar fields [15]. In fact, this beam arrangement produced similar results to the nine-field setup [15]. So, if the patient could tolerate this head position, coplanar IMRT was a simpler and faster delivery technique (Table 43.6).

## Planning Strategies: Craniospinal Irradiation (CSI)

Craniospinal irradiation treatment planning is complex and involves attention to detail. A typical 3D-CRT plan involves lateral brain fields and posterior spine fields with a prone setup. The divergence of the brain and spine fields can be matched to avoid overlap. However, if two spine fields are necessary to cover the entire spine PTV, overlapping fields become an issue. One method to address this issue is to shift the field junctions after a third of the prescription dose has been delivered to minimize underdose and overdose regions. To begin beam setup, proper isocenter locations are important. The brain isocenter is placed midline in the center of the brain, the upper spine isocenter is placed in the midpoint between the top of the shoulders and the middle of the spinal column, and the lower spine isocenter is placed in the midpoint between the middle of the spinal column and the

coccyx. One should adjust the brain, upper spine, and lower spine isocenter coordinates to be in the same sagittal and coronal planes so that when the radiation therapists set up the patient, the only shift to get to the different isocenters is a couch table in or out motion. Then, one can add a lateral brain field and design it similarly to a whole brain field. Lowering the inferior border to be slightly above the shoulders to avoid entering through the oropharynx is ideal. One should try to keep the Y collimator jaws divisible by 0.5 cm so that there are no discrepancies between the treatment plan and portal images. Next, one should add the upper spine field and raise the superior border to match the brain's inferior border. An exact match involves a collimator rotation for the brain field and moving the upper spine isocenter in the superior/inferior dimension only. Once the match is complete, one can adjust the MLC block so that the spine PTV is covered and the anterior normal tissue is shielded. On the upper spine field, tweak the lateral border to cover the spine PTV, and set the inferior border to have a symmetrical jaw setting to the superior border. Next, add the lower spine field, and raise the superior edge so that this edge and the inferior border of the upper spine intersect in the **middle** of the spinal cord. This intersection can be visualized in the sagittal plane. Then, move the lateral and inferior edges of the lower spine field to cover the spine PTV. It is best to keep the Y collimator jaws divisible by 0.5 cm and to be somewhat symmetrical, so one should move the lower spine isocenter in the superior/inferior direction to achieve that result. After these adjustments, make sure the intersection between the upper and lower spine fields is still in the middle of the spinal cord. Once all the fields have been tweaked appropriately, dose calculation may proceed.

There are several steps necessary to create an optimal treatment plan after the fields have been calculated. First, create calculation points for the spine fields, and place it as far anterior as possible within tissue and at least 2 cm away from field edge. Then, adjust the prescription normalization for the brain, upper spine, and lower spine so that the prescription dose covers the PTV. Next, use FIF to minimize hotspots in the brain and to conform the prescription isodose line to the spine PTV. To pull back the isodose lines in the spinal region, start from the superior axial slices, and locate the slices where the prescription isodose line starts moving away from the target and where this line starts moving back toward the target and almost touches the anterior side of the PTV. Sometimes, the isodose line never moves back so use the last axial slice that is within the upper spine field. On the BEV of an upper spine subfield, create a MLC block that covers those transverse slices and slowly increase the beam weight. Continue to add weight from the primary beam to the subfield until this isodose line touches the anterior edge of the PTV, and lock the subfield's weight. Create another subfield and repeat the same steps to make the prescription dose skim the PTV. When these improvements to the upper spine

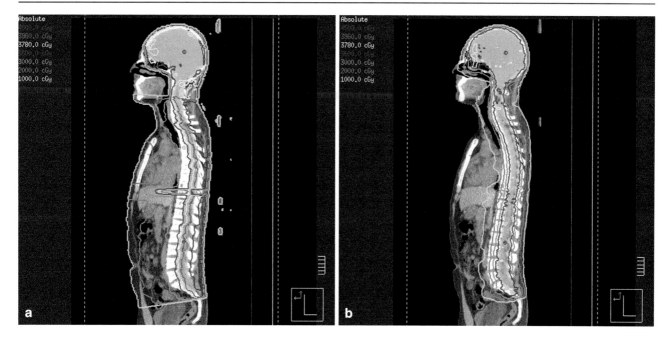

**Fig. 43.17** Sagittal slices of 3D-CRT (**a**) and VMAT (**b**) CSI plans. The PTV is shaded green, and the prescription dose is 36 Gy (red line). For each junction, the 3D-CRT plan consists of two brain fields and two spine fields using FIF technique. There are three junctions in this plan to create a total of 12 fields. The VMAT plan consists of two brain arcs, two upper spine arcs, and two lower spine arcs with no junction shifts

are completed, perform the same steps to the lower spine region. Once all the FIFs have been created, copy this plan, and create another one to shift the field junctions superiorly by 0.5 cm. So, the inferior border of the brain field and the superior border of the upper spine field move superiorly by 0.5 cm. Similarly, the inferior border of the upper spine field and the superior border of the lower spine field move superiorly. Copy this new plan and shift the junctions superiorly one more time. The end result is three plans with three different field junction areas.

To avoid having to create different junction shift plans and improve patient comfort, VMAT can be used to feather the dose in the junction areas using a supine setup. When utilizing this technique, the isocenter placements follow the same principles used in 3D-CRT. Since VMAT fields require collimator angle rotations, the field borders cannot be an exact match, but the TPS optimizer compensates this issue to minimize underdose and overdose regions. Regarding the field borders, the inferior border of the brain arcs should be above the shoulders, and the superior border of the upper spine arcs overlaps the brain arcs by about 3 cm. In the spine region, the upper spine and lower spine arcs overlap by about 3–4 cm, and the collimator jaws for each arc should be as symmetrical as possible, so slight isocenter adjustments may be necessary. In terms of arc rotation, each region has a clockwise and counterclockwise arc. Also, the brain arcs have full rotation but exclude entering portions of the patient's face or 30° on each side of an anterior-posterior beam. The spine arcs have arc paths that sweep 120° posteriorly or 60° on each side of a posterior-anterior field. Once

the field setup is complete, a planning PTV needs to be created for each arc section. By using the BEV as a guide, create a brain PTV, upper spine PTV, and lower spine PTV. Separating the PTVs allows the TPS optimizer to focus on each region so that the doses in the field overlap areas are smoothed out. Then, add the typical starting objectives to these planning PTVs to the TPS optimizer. By allowing the optimization process to find solutions to feather the junctions, multiple plans are avoided (Fig. 43.17).

The issue with 3D-CRT and VMAT techniques is that low doses spread out to the anterior normal tissues. Ideally, there should be very little dose delivered to these tissues. Fortunately with the advances in technology, proton therapy is the best option to accomplish this goal as the Bragg peak allows the dose to be delivered at the end of the range [2]. Specifically, pencil beam scanning optimizes many individual pencil beams so that the treatment field has optimally weighted Bragg peaks to create a homogenous dose distribution [2]. By using a posterior field only, prescription dose can cover the target, and the remaining dose stops before reaching anterior tissues (Figs. 43.18 and 43.19).

## Planning Strategies: Craniopharyngioma

Similar 3D-CRT and IMRT strategies used for gliomas could be applied to craniopharyngiomas, but using VMAT for this disease required a different approach. Uto et al. compared the differences between coplanar and noncoplanar VMAT plans [16]. The coplanar plans had two full arcs rotating

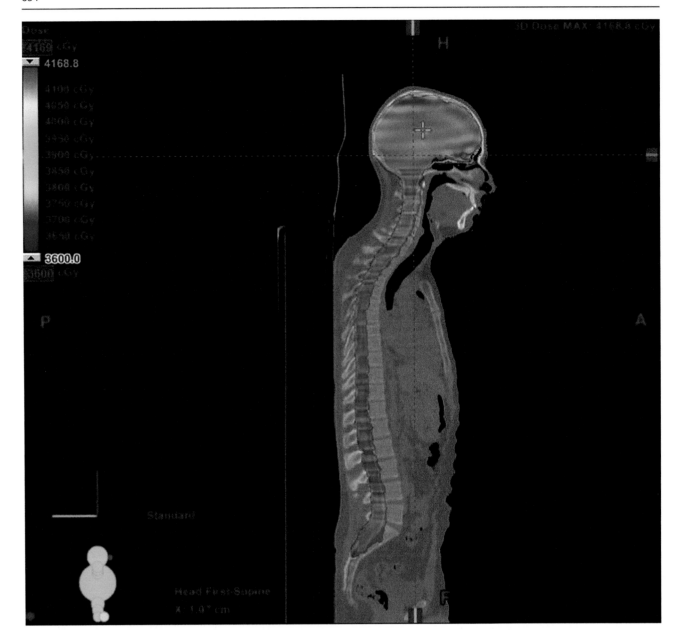

**Fig. 43.18** Sagittal slice of a proton CSI plan treating to 36 Gy. The dose is displayed in color wash and ranges from 36 Gy (blue) to 41.6 Gy (red). The plan consists of one brain, one upper spine, and one lower spine field. The fields are modulated using pencil beam scanning

clockwise and counterclockwise with collimator angles of 45° and 315°. The noncoplanar plans had one coplanar arc at a couch angle of 0° with full rotation and avoided entering the eyes and two noncoplanar arcs at couch angles 45° and 315°. Also, no collimator rotation was necessary. Uto et al. found that rotating the couch provided better sparing of the hippocampus and a slightly better homogeneity index [16]. In addition, the authors suggested that organs at risk in the same level as the PTV received lower doses from noncopla-

nar VMAT plans [16]. So, this dose sparing was achieved without losing PTV coverage.

## Planning Strategies: Pituitary Tumors

Some institutions had been using 3D-CRT to treat pituitary tumors, but the temporal lobes received a high dose. Parhar et al. investigated the possibility of reducing the dose to the

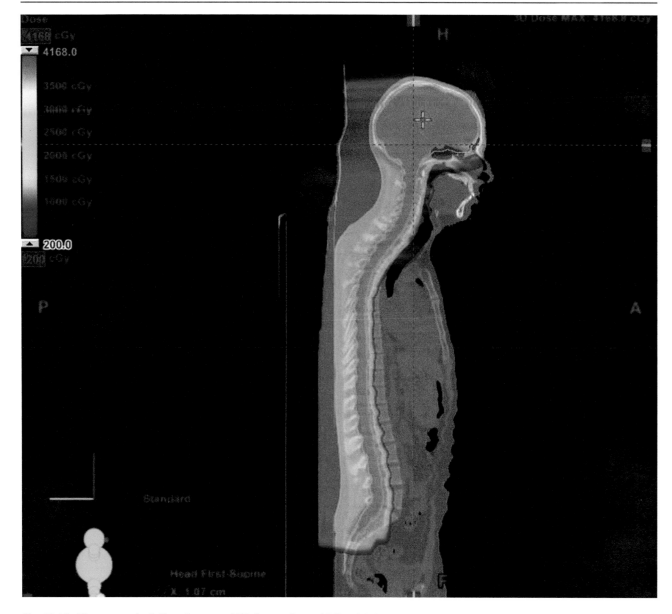

**Fig. 43.19** The same sagittal slice of a proton CSI plan treating to 36 Gy with the dose color wash ranging from 2 Gy (blue) to 41.6 Gy (red)

temporal lobes by using IMRT [17]. The authors noticed that most 3D-CRT plans had two lateral beams and one midline superior anterior oblique (SAO) beam [17]. So, Parhar et al. tried a five-field IMRT approach using the same three fields in 3D-CRT but adding right and left SAO fields. When the authors compared these techniques, the IMRT plans spared the temporal lobes better especially in the intermediate doses of 15–25 Gy [17]. Also, the PTV coverage and brain integral dose were not compromised [17]. Therefore, the five-field IMRT technique was able to improve the plan quality for this disease.

## Normal Tissue Tolerances

Regardless of treatment technique, the dose limits to critical structures are based on the fractionation scheme. In addition, many institutions use different constraints, so there is no definite answer on which limits are the best to use. For further information on tissue constraints, Selek and Chang have listed dose effects on several CNS critical structures [18]. Before planning, consult with the radiation oncologist to determine the planning criteria. For conventional fractionation, the following table lists typical constraints (Table 43.7).

**Table 43.7** Radiation dose limits to CNS structures when conventional fractionation is used

| Structure | Max Dose (Gy) | Max Dose to a Volume | Mean Dose (Gy) | Reference |
|---|---|---|---|---|
| Brainstem | 54 | 60Gy to 1% | – | RTOG 0225 |
| Cochlea | – | 55Gy to 5% | – | RTOG 0615 |
| Ears (inner/middle) | – | – | 50 | RTOG 0225 |
| Eyes | 50 | – | 35 | RTOG 0615 & RTOG 0225 |
| Lacrimal gland | 30 | – | – | Batth et al. |
| Lens | 7 | Avoid direct exposure | – | RTOG 0513 & RTOG 0539 |
| Optic chiasm | 54 | 60Gy to 1% | – | RTOG 0225 |
| Optic nerves | 54 | 60Gy to 1% | – | RTOG 0225 |
| Retina | 50 | – | – | RTOG 0539 |
| Spinal cord | 45 | 48Gy to 0.03 cc | – | RTOG 0623 & RTOG 0619 |
| Temporal lobes | 60 | 65Gy to 1% | – | RTOG 0225 |

## Summary

- 3D-CRT is considered forward planning as it involves many steps for the planner to create a treatment plan. Therefore, the TPS assists the planner but cannot create an optimal dose distribution.
- Inverse planning, such as IMRT and VMAT, relies on the user to set desired points on the DVH to create a plan. Since the TPS runs the optimization process, the planning time can be long as many MLC patterns need to be created for conformal dose delivery and organ sparing.
- VMAT produces the same plan quality as IMRT, and patients have reduced treatment delivery times.
- IMRT class solution for gliomas helps shorten planning times and improves plan quality.
- VMAT class solution for hippocampal sparing provides the same benefits seen in glioma planning.
- Any technique can be used for CSI, but the best option is one where clinicians feel comfortable planning and treating.
- Craniopharyngioma treatment planning can follow the same approach as glioma planning except for VMAT which requires noncoplanar arcs to achieve similar plan quality.
- A five-field IMRT technique has lower doses to the temporal lobes than 3D-CRT for pituitary treatments.

## Self-Assessment Questions

1. Why are low-energy photon beams preferred for IMRT/VMAT plans?
   A. Neutron dose does not exist.
   B. Low-energy beams require less MU.
   C. Faster treatment delivery.
   D. TPS models low-energy beams better than high-energy beams.

2. What is a drawback of using noncoplanar fields?
   A. Sharper dose gradients.
   B. Potentially undeliverable fields without a dry run.
   C. Inability to spare critical structures.
   D. Inability to treat using IMRT/VMAT.

3. What is the main purpose to rotate the collimator 10–45° for VMAT?
   A. VMAT is designed to work only within this range.
   B. Shorten treatment delivery.
   C. Minimize tongue and groove effect.
   D. The TPS optimizer creates optimal plans using these collimator angles only.

4. Why are junction shifts not required for IMRT/VMAT CSI plans?
   A. The patient setup is more reproducible than 3D-CRT.
   B. IMRT/VMAT plans are complicated already, so adding junction shifts will add another layer of complexity.
   C. There are no field matching issues to compensate for.
   D. The TPS optimizer modulates the overlap region, so the junction areas are smoothed out.

5. What is the best course of action for a patient that has vision intact and a portion of PTV 60Gy overlapping the optic chiasm?
   A. Use IMRT/VMAT to cover the entire PTV to prescription dose.
   B. Create planning PTV structures.
   C. Use proton therapy to cover the entire PTV to prescription dose.
   D. Cover the PTV with less than 60Gy.

## Answers

1. A
2. B
3. C
4. D
5. B

## References

1. Prado KL, Starkschall G, Mohan R. Three-dimensional conformal radiation thearpy. In: Khan FM, Gerbi BJ, editors. Treatment planning in radiation oncology. 3rd ed. Philadelphia: Wolters Kluwer/Lippincott Williams & Wilkins Health; 2012. p. 169–200.
2. Khan FM, Gibbons JP Jr. Khan's the physics of radiation therapy. 5th ed. Philadelphia: Lippincott Williams & Wilkins/Wolters Kluwer; 2014.
3. Marinetti T, Dong L. Delivery of precision radiation therapy: IMRT, IGRT, proton beam therapy. In: Chao KSC, Wang TJC, Marinetti T, editors. Practical essentials of intensity modulated radiation

therapy. 3rd ed. Philadelphia: Wolters Kluwer Health/Lippincott Williams & Wilkins; 2014. p. 43–77.

4. Nedzi LA, Choe KS, Pompos A, et al. Cancers of the central nervous system. In: Khan FM, Gerbi BJ, editors. Treatment planning in radiation oncology. 3rd ed. Philadelphia: Wolters Kluwer/Lippincott Williams & Wilkins Health; 2012. p. 628–47.

5. Boyer AL, Ezzell GA, Yu CX. Intensity-modulated radiation therapy. In: Khan FM, Gerbi BJ, editors. Treatment planning in radiation oncology. 3rd ed. Philadelphia: Wolters Kluwer/Lippincott Williams & Wilkins Health; 2012. p. 201–28.

6. Yuan J, Lei M, Yang Z, et al. Dosimetric comparison between intensity-modulated radiotherapy and RapidArc with single arc and dual arc for malignant glioma involving the parietal lobe. Mol Clin Oncol. 2016;5(1):181–8.

7. Davidson MTM, Masucci GL, Follwell M, et al. Single arc volumetric modulated arc therapy for complex brain gliomas: is there an advantage as compared to intensity modulated radiotherapy or by adding a partial arc? Technol Cancer Res Treat. 2012;11(3):211–20.

8. Vanetti E, Clivio A, Nicolini G, et al. Volumetric modulated arc radiotherapy for carcinomas of the oro-pharynx, hypo-pharynx and larynx: a treatment planning comparison with fixed field IMRT. Radiother Oncol. 2009;92(1):111–7.

9. Roa DE, Schiffner DC, Zhang J, et al. The use of RapidArc volumetric-modulated arc therapy to deliver stereotactic radiosurgery and stereotactic body radiotherapy to intracranial and extracranial targets. Med Dosim. 2012;37(3):257–64.

10. Yang J, Tang G, Zhang P, et al. Dose calculation for hypofractionated volumetric-modulated arc therapy: approximating continuous arc delivery and tongue-and-groove modeling. J Appl Clin Med Phys. 2016;17(2):4989–99.

11. Shen J, Bender E, Yaparpalvi R, et al. An efficient volumetric arc therapy treatment planning approach for hippocampal-avoid-ance whole-brain radiation therapy (HA-WBRT). Med Dosim. 2015;40(3):205–9.

12. Likhacheva A, Palmer M, Du W, et al. Intensity modulated radiation therapy class solutions in Philips pinnacle treatment planning for central nervous system malignancies: standardized, efficient, and effective. Pract Rad Oncol. 2012;2(4):e145–53.

13. Panet Raymond V, Ansbacher W, Zavgorodni S, et al. Coplanar versus noncoplanar intensity-modulated radiation therapy (IMRT) and volumetric-modulated arc therapy (VMAT) treatment planning for fronto-temporal high-grade glioma. J Appl Clin Med Phys. 2012;13(4):3826–35.

14. Gondi V, Tolakanahalli R, Mehta MP, et al. Hippocampal-sparing whole-brain radiotherapy: a "how-to" technique using helical tomotherapy and linear accelerator–based intensity-modulated radiotherapy. Int J Radiat Oncol Biol Phys. 2010;78(4):1244–52.

15. Siglin J, Champ CE, Vakhnenko Y, et al. Optimizing patient positioning for intensity modulated radiation therapy in hippocampal-sparing whole brain radiation therapy. Pract Rad Oncol. 2014;4(6):378–83.

16. Uto M, Mizowaki T, Ogura K, et al. Non-coplanar volumetric-modulated arc therapy (VMAT) for craniopharyngiomas reduces radiation doses to the bilateral hippocampus: a planning study comparing dynamic conformal arc therapy, coplanar VMAT, and non-coplanar VMAT. Radiat Oncol. 2016;11(1):86.

17. Parhar PK, Duckworth T, Shah JN, et al. Decreasing temporal lobe dose with five-field intensity-modulated radiotherapy for treatment of pituitary macroadenomas. Int J Radiat Oncol Biol Phys. 2010;78(2):379–84.

18. Selek U, Chang EL. Skull base and CNS glial tumors. In: Chao KSC, Wang TJC, Marinetti T, editors. Practical essentials of intensity modulated radiation therapy. 3rd ed. Philadelphia: Wolters Kluwer Health/Lippincott Williams & Wilkins; 2014. p. 43–77.

# Linac-Based Stereotactic Radiosurgery and Hypofractionated Stereotactic Radiotherapy

# 44

Evan M. Thomas, Richard A. Popple, Markus Bredel, and John B. Fiveash

## Definition of Stereotactic Radiosurgery and Hypofractionated Stereotactic Radiotherapy

Stereotactic radiosurgery (SRS) is a minimally invasive technique by which focal delivery of high-dose radiation is used to selectively ablate tissue within the central nervous system (CNS) without the necessity of direct physical contact with tissue. It was developed in the 1940s by Swedish neurosurgeon Lars Leksell, Gamma Knife inventor and the universally recognized father of radiosurgery. Leksell himself defined the term as "a technique for the non-invasive destruction of intracranial tissues or lesions that may be inaccessible or unsuitable for open surgery" [1]. Historically, the term SRS was principally deployed to describe intracranial treatment of lesions with the brain or skull base; however, the designation has since expanded to encompass treatment of spinal lesions as well. In conventional radiotherapy, delivery of the prescription dose is divided into a high number of small fractions to exploit the differential sensitivity between more rapidly dividing malignant CNS tissue and healthy CNS tissue. SRS fundamentally differs from conventional treatment in that a single high dose is delivered to the desired target, with as sharp of a dose gradient as possible between the target and surrounding tissue.

The designation *stereotactic* originated in 1908 in a publication by British neurosurgeon, Victor Horsley, and mathematician/physiologist, Robert Clarke, which demonstrated the first three-dimensional (3D) neurosurgical targeting technique, used at the time to localize and study monkey cerebellar function. The term was an amalgamation of the Greek στερεός (stereos), meaning "solid," and the New Latin suffix *–taxis*, meaning arrangement [2]. In practice, it is the application of a systematic coordinate system, usually Cartesian, onto human anatomy or a human anatomical structure such as the brain. The label *radiosurgery* may have originated about the same time as stereotaxy, during a lecture by Dr. Francis Hernaman-Johnson to the Royal Society of Medicine wherein he exposited upon combined applications of the recently discovered X-ray with surgical techniques [3, 4]. The application of the term radiosurgery as we know it today, however, was not minted until some years later, when in 1951, Dr. Leksell first published his technique in the seminal publication "The stereotaxic method and radiosurgery of the brain" [5] (Fig. 44.1).

After SRS was demonstrated to be feasible on, and was ported to linear accelerator platforms (discussed in more depth later), the obvious application of fractionated therapy with stereotactic precision was pursued. However, an invasive frame for daily treatments was not feasible. Therefore, in order to achieve this paradigm, the Brown-Roberts-Wells frame (which had been developed for CT-guided stereotactic procedures [6]) was modified into the Gill-Thomas-Cosman device which was the first relocatable stereotactic frame [7]. The convenience of a relocatable frame soon facilitated the coupling of CT-imaged treatments and also made easier the division of radiosurgical treatments into multiple fractions. In that, Leksell's pioneering approach to non-operative neurosurgical intervention represented the awakening of the field of radiosurgery, neurosurgeons and radiation oncologists alike agreed. However, there was deliberation between the two specialties on how to officially designate radiation treatment to the brain divided into multiple fractions. *Fractionated stereotactic radiosurgery (FSRS)* was originally preferred by neurosurgeons, and *hypofractionated stereotactic radiotherapy (fSRT or hfSRT)* was preferred by many radiation oncologists [8]. Hypofractionated stereotactic radiosurgery (hf-SRS) has also been used (Fig. 44.2).

The distinction between terms remains blurred, and there is great inconsistency throughout the literature. In radiation oncology parlance, standard fractionation refers to division

E. M. Thomas (✉) · R. A. Popple · M. Bredel · J. B. Fiveash
Department of Radiation Oncology, University of Alabama at Birmingham, Birmingham, AL, USA
e-mail: emthomas@uabmc.edu

© Springer International Publishing AG, part of Springer Nature 2018
E. L. Chang et al. (eds.), *Adult CNS Radiation Oncology*, https://doi.org/10.1007/978-3-319-42878-9_44

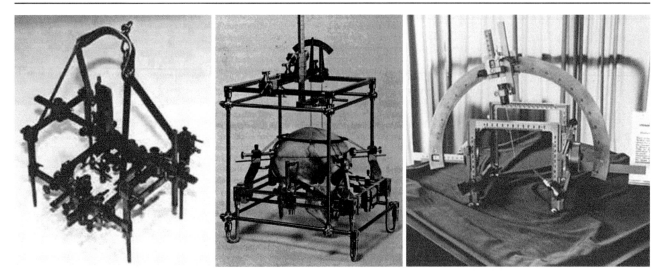

**Fig. 44.1** Evolution of early stereotactic apparatuses (left to right): Horsley-Clark frame, first stereotactic apparatus, conceived to study monkey cerebellar function, circa 1908; Spiegel-Wycis Model I, adaptation of the Horsley-Clarke frame for human use, circa 1945; First version of the Leksell stereotactic frame. Left & Right: [Reprinted from Heller C, Yu C, Apuzzo MLJ. Techniques of Stereotactic Radiosurgery. In: Chin LS, Regine WF (eds). Principles and Practice of Stereotactic Radiosurgery. New York, NY: Springer; 2008: 25–30. With permission from Springer Nature.]. Middle: [Reprinted from Grunert P. From the idea to its realization: the evolution of minimally invasive techniques in neurosurgery. Minimally invasive surgery 2013: Article ID 171369. with permission from Creative Commons License 3.0: https://creativecommons.org/licenses/by/3.0/]

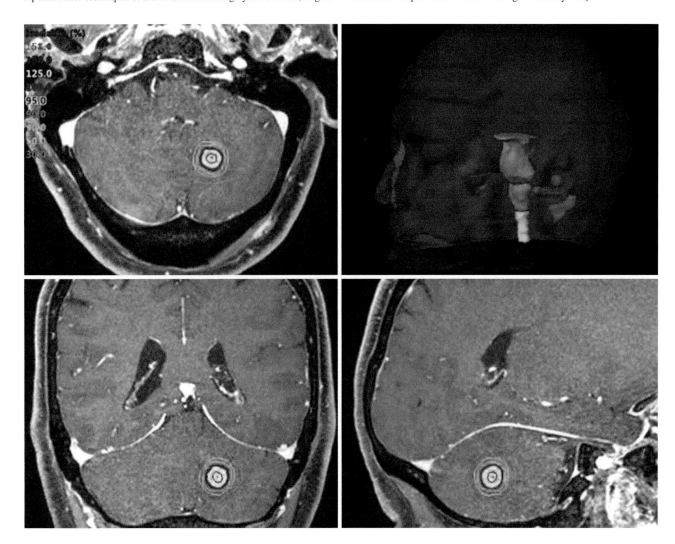

**Fig. 44.2** Radiosurgical isodose distribution for a single brain metastasis treated with a linear accelerator

of radiation treatment into fractions of 1.8–2 Gy per day, 5 days per week, for typically 5–7 weeks. Hypofractionation refers to treatments of >2 Gy per day and ≤5 days per week, for a reduced duration of time. The traditional purpose of hypofractionation is to reduce duration of treatment, with the theoretical benefit of reduced likelihood or severity of acute radiation toxicity, but potential cost of reduced tumor control and increased likelihood or severity of late effects [9]. In practice, the effects of hypofractionation on tumor control, acute toxicity, and late toxicity are heavily dependent on the type of tissue being targeted, the type of tissue(s) adjacent the target, the prescription dose selected, and the degree of hypofractionation. The application of stereotactic targeting and advances in high-resolution imaging localization, precision patient setup, and techniques facilitating rapid dose falloff allow for very high biologically equivalent doses to be delivered to targets and low doses to be delivered to adjacent tissues. This may mitigate the theoretical tumor control disadvantages of hypofractionation for stereotactic treatments as higher absolute doses to tumor become more achievable for a given surrounding normal tissue toxicity limit.

In the practice of radiosurgery for metastases and benign tumors, the decision to hypofractionate is most frequently a decision to *increase* the number of fractions from one to more than one (usually three or five) when the size of a lesion or its proximity to a critical structure like the brainstem or optic chiasm causes concern [10, 11]. For malignant brain tumors such as high-grade gliomas, where the established standard of care is 60 Gy conventionally fractionation [12], the decision to hypofractionate lies more with reducing the impact of a 6-week treatment on quality of life.

The ASTRO Model Policy guideline for SRS is an important reference for practitioners. It defines radiosurgery as "radiation therapy delivered in one to five fractions via stereotactic guidance, with approximately 1 mm targeting accuracy to intracranial targets and selected tumors around the base of skull" [13]. Based on this designation, a large number of entries in the literature on fSRT or hfSRT could be classified as SRS. The debate on hypofractionation of SRS remains ongoing within the literature. For the purposes of consistency within this chapter, the authors will refer to all stereotactic treatments as radiosurgery or SRS, except where hypofractionation is a salient consideration, where it will be referred to as hfSRT.

We have established that there are multiple fractionations that can be classified as SRS, and there are multiple platforms on which they can be delivered. There are however designated required elements for a treatment to be appropriately considered SRS. Table 44.1 enumerates them. The neoplastic indications for SRS supported by ASTRO Model Policy are listed in Table 44.2.

**Table 44.1** Mandatory components of SRS treatment per ASTRO Model Policy

| |
|---|
| 1  Position stabilization (attachment of a frame or frameless) |
| 2  Imaging for localization (CT, MRI, angiography, PET, etc.) |
| 3  Computer-assisted tumor localization (i.e., "image guidance") |
| 4  Treatment planning – Number of isocenters; number, placement, and length of arcs or angles; number of beams, beam size and weight, etc. |
| 5  Isodose distributions, dosage prescription, and calculation |
| 6  Setup and accuracy verification testing |
| 7  Simulation of prescribed arcs or fixed portals |
| 8  Radiation treatment delivery |

**Table 44.2** Indications and limitations of coverage and/or medical necessity

| |
|---|
| Primary and secondary tumors involving the brain parenchyma, meninges/dura, or immediately adjacent bony structures |
| Benign brain tumors such as meningiomas, acoustic neuromas, other schwannomas, pituitary adenomas, pineocytomas, craniopharyngiomas, glomus tumors, or hemangioblastomas |
| As a boost treatment for larger cranial or spinal lesions that have been treated initially with external beam radiation therapy or surgery (e.g., sarcomas, chondrosarcomas, chordomas, and nasopharyngeal or paranasal sinus malignancies) |
| Metastatic brain, independent of the number of lesions if other positive clinical indications exist, with stable systemic disease, Karnofsky performance status 40 or greater (and expected to return to 70 or greater with treatment), and otherwise reasonable survival expectations, *or* ECOG performance status of 3 or less (or expected to return to 2 or less with treatment) |
| Relapse in a previously irradiated cranial where the additional stereotactic precision is required to avoid unacceptable vital tissue radiation |

## Principles and Techniques of Linac-Based Stereotactic Radiosurgery and Hypofractionated Stereotactic Radiotherapy

### History

Since its advent in the early 1950s, neurosurgeons and radiation oncologists have investigated a number of devices and techniques for SRS. Although the Gamma Knife (Elekta AB, Stockholm, Sweden) became, and still is, the most commonly utilized tool for radiosurgery, it was not the first employed for the task. That distinction belongs to the linear accelerator, although in a much different form than we are familiar with today. Lars Leksell first investigated radiosurgery with an old orthovoltage linear accelerator in 1951 [5] and published his first case report in 1955 [14]. His initial treatment attempts were principally directed toward what we now define as functional radiosurgery. He had a particular fascination with treating pathologies afflicting great pain, namely, trigeminal neuralgia and cancer pain [15] (Fig. 44.3).

He reflects on the experience in a 1981 lecture to the Society of British Neurological Surgeons [1]:

> "The first attempt to supplant the electrodes with ionizing radiation was made in the early fifties, with X-rays. It was tempting to try and reduce the hazards of open surgery and by the administration of a single heavy dose of radiation it appeared possible to destroy any deep brain structure, without risk of bleeding or infection."

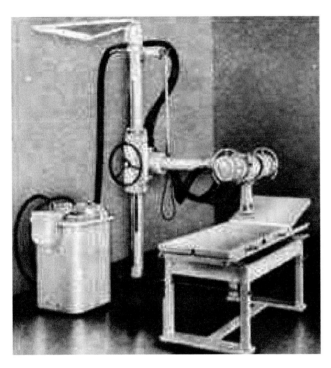

**Fig. 44.3** Photogram of an old orthovoltage teletherapy unit, the Siemens Stabilapan

Even very early on in development, it was obvious that the dosimetry of orthovoltage beams was not ideal for targets that could lie deep within the brain. As Leksell noted in the 1951 concept paper:

> "At present X-rays and gamma rays would seem to be the most promising and the easiest to apply. It is clear, however, that the radiation in the 200 kilovolt range used here should be replaced by radiation of higher energy. This would give a better depth dose, especially with the extremely small fields used here, and also a better definition of the beam" [5].

The isodose distributions of a 200 kVp orthovoltage beam, a cobalt-60 beam, and a 10M V X-ray beam are shown in Fig. 44.4 (isodose distributions of 10 cm × 10 cm fields for (A) 200 kVp, SSD = 50 cm, HVL = 1 mm Cu; (B) cobalt-60, SSD–80 cm; (C) 10 MV X-rays, SSD = 100 cm).

Leksell soon began experimenting with proton beams for stereotactic ablation within the brain but found working with the synco-cyclotron too cumbersome. His eventual solution was the stereotactic gamma unit. The original unit, deployed in 1968, was intended for ablation of fiber tracts and nuclei deep within the brain and produced discoid lesions with excellent dose falloff. Its utility for additional applications such as tumors and AVMs was quickly realized. The demand for the revolutionary technique was immediate, and Leksell founded Elekta in 1972 to commercialize the product. The second prototype gamma unit (Elekta AB, Stockholm, Sweden) installed at Karolinska University Hospital in 1974 was designed to produce more spheroid dose distributions. Commercial units thereafter were marketed as the Gamma Knife. The Gamma Knife (Elekta AB, Stockholm, Sweden) and its specifics are covered in further detail in Chapter 45.

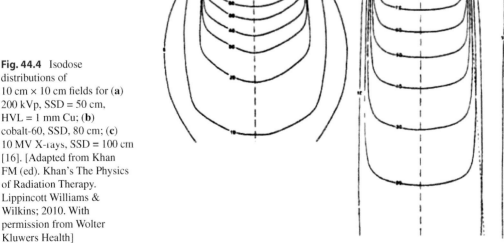

**Fig. 44.4** Isodose distributions of 10 cm × 10 cm fields for (**a**) 200 kVp, SSD = 50 cm, HVL = 1 mm Cu; (**b**) cobalt-60, SSD, 80 cm; (**c**) 10 MV X-rays, SSD = 100 cm [16]. [Adapted from Khan FM (ed). Khan's The Physics of Radiation Therapy. Lippincott Williams & Wilkins; 2010. With permission from Wolter Kluwers Health]

Linacs had for some time been commonly used to treat intracranial neoplasms, but the appeal of completing treatment in a single or highly reduced number of fractions quickly prompted exploration of the platform for SRS. Argentinian neurosurgeon Betti et al. was the first to describe the coupling of a stereotactic headframe with a linear accelerator for radiosurgery, followed shortly thereafter by Colombo et al. in Vicenza, Italy. Drs. Winston and Lutz at the Brigham and Women's Hospital in Boston were the first in the United States to deploy the approach, where it quickly became such mainstay for intracranial radiosurgical applications by Loeffler and colleagues that the first dedicated linac for SRS was established [17–23]. Early Linac-based SRS approaches rotated the patient in a chair under the gantry or about the patient in a single arc, which can produce a spherical dose distribution at the prescription isodose line, but concentrate the dose falloff in the axial plane of delivery. Generation of a spherical dose distribution with a linear accelerator, similar to Gamma Knife, requires the entry of the beam through both a large number of different angles and in different planes. This requires rotation of both the gantry and the patient, usually sequentially. Physicist Podgorsak at McGill University investigated doing both, simultaneously, which he dubbed dynamic radiosurgery [24] (Fig. 44.5).

Led by William Friedman, Frank Bova, and others, the University of Florida was an early pioneer in linac radiosurgery. From the late 1980s onward, they amassed extensive experience treating a variety of pathologies with cone-based SRS. Early treatments used a single isocenter, but increased experience led them to utilize sphere packing of multiple isocenters for improved conformality of non-spherical targets.

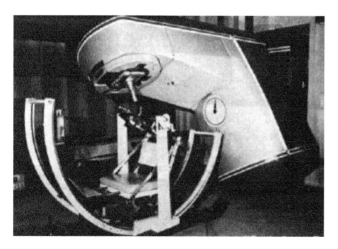

**Fig. 44.5** First application of a linac with stereotactic targeting for radiosurgery at El Instituto Médico Antártida – Rosario in Buenos Aires, Argentina by Betti et al. [Reprinted from Betti O, Derechinsky V. Hyperselective encephalic irradiation with linear accelerator. In: Gybels J, Hitchcock E., Ostertag C, Rossi GF, Siegfried J, Szikla G (eds). Advances in Stereotactic and Functional Neurosurgery 6: Vienna, Austria: Springer; 1984:385–90. With permission form Springer Nature]

The value of their experience and contributions to the field of linac radiosurgery cannot be overstated.

In 1993, Brainlab entered into a partnership with Varian Medical Systems with the intent of creating a linac dedicated to radiosurgery. A Varian 600SR was modified with the addition of a micro MLC to create the Novalis radiosurgery platform, and in 1997 the first shaped-beam dedicated radiosurgery platform was installed at UCLA.

John Adler, former neurosurgery trainee at Brigham and Women's Hospital and radiosurgical fellow under Lars Leksell, was convinced the notion of high-dose single-fraction radiosurgery could be applied to extracranial sites, such as the spine. With a team of engineers, he married a compact linear accelerator powered by an X-band RF source to a Japanese industrial Fanuc robotic arm and created the CyberKnife (Accuray Inc., Sunnyvale, CA, USA), which has become synonymous with the term robotic radiosurgery [25]. The versatile CyberKnife (Accuray Inc., Sunnyvale, CA, USA) robotic arm's six axes of freedom allow it access to almost any treatment path (Figs. 44.6 and 44.7).

The next major advent in linac radiosurgery was the use of the dynamic MLC to improve the plan quality of treatments with non-spherical targets. The difficulty of treating non-spherical targets was not a new one. The initial solution was to treat the target with the smallest sphere that would encompass all of the target volume. Radiosurgeons quickly realized that using multiple spheres or sphere packing could cover the target volume with less full dose coverage of healthy adjacent tissue. Multi-isocenter plans, however, could be complex to plan and very time-consuming to treat, particularly if multiple collimator/cone sizes were necessary to generate an acceptable treatment plan. Static MLC plans had been used for conformal arc plans since very early for large targets. Soon dynamic MLC (or IMRT) approaches were being used to increase target conformity for non-spherical lesions [27–29]. These treatments were functionally step-and-shoot IMRT treatments with radiosurgical doses and fractionation.

In 1995, Cedric Yu of the University of Maryland proposed simultaneously coupling dynamic MLC leaf movement with gantry movement in order to increase the efficiency and improve upon the general workflow of tomotherapy, which he called intensity-modulated arc therapy (IMAT) [30]. Unfortunately, it was an idea ahead of its time and saw minimal adoption. Yu's solution could only optimize a beam intensity for every 5° of an arc, required successive arc deliveries if multiple beam intensities were desired, and necessitated beam cessation if the gantry reached a position and the leaves could not travel to their predesignated position for that control point. Each beam cessation required a manual restart of radiation. This led to treatments, even in ideal scenarios, taking as much time or sometimes longer than conventional conformal arc, or dynamic MLC step and shoot plans. A typical arc could take approximately 15 min. Ten years later, Karl

**Fig. 44.6** Original art from US Patent and Trade Office application for the CyberKnife robotic radiosurgery system [26]. [Reprinted from Adler JR. Apparatus for and method of performing stereotaxic surgery. Google Patents; 1993]

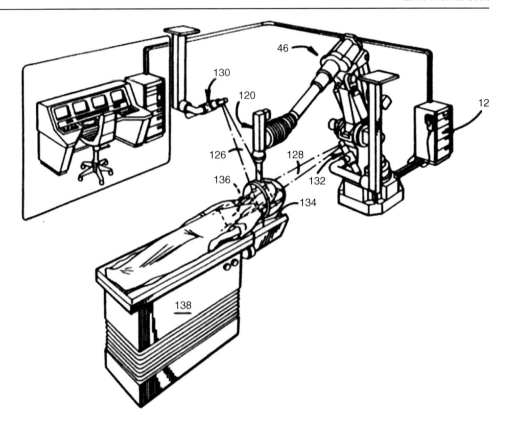

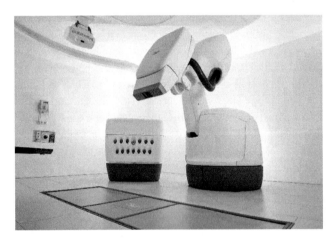

**Fig. 44.7** Modern CyberKnife with M6 MLC at the European CyberKnife Center in Munich, Germany. [Reprinted from https://commons.wikimedia.org/wiki/Category:Cyberknife#/media/File:Cyberknife_M6_und_MLC.jpg With permission from Creative Commons Attribution: https://creativecommons.org/licenses/by-sa/4.0/deed.en]

Otto, armed with a decade of improvements not only in MLC engineering but also the >2$^5$ factor increase in CPU clock speed (and thus brute-force algorithm solving capability) accurately predicted by Moore's law, was able to overcome the barriers faced by Yu. His technique was dubbed volumetric modulated arc therapy (VMAT) and allowed complete treatment in one arc in the minimum gantry rotation period of 1 min [31]. Three factors are optimized and varied throughout the arc treatment: MLC shaping, intensity (dose rate), and gantry speed. Although initially demonstrated for conventionally fractionated prostate and head/neck cancer treatments, the technique was quickly explored for virtually every radiotherapy site in the body, including SRS.

The principle and most obvious benefits of VMAT were in treatment efficiency, particularly when coupled with flattening filter-free (FFF) delivery (discussed later). FFF delivery on a linear accelerator with 10 MV and 6 MV beams facilitated maximum dose rates of approximately 2400 and 1400 Gy/min, respectively. For comparison, the maximum dose rate of a Gamma Knife (Elekta AB, Stockholm, Sweden) with a new source is about 3.3 Gy/min; this decays with the installed cobalt-60 sources whose half-life is 5.3 years. Clinically this translated into radiation oncologists being able to treat a single target with radiosurgery in less than 10 min, inclusive of setup time. The benefit to patients, oncologists, and neurosurgeons was clear. Now, each of the three major remaining linear accelerator vendors (Varian, Elekta, Accuray) offers FFF treatment options of their platforms. Both Varian and Elekta adapted VMAT technology to their existing, capable linear accelerators and have included it in all platforms released since.

After linac-based VMAT SRS demonstrated its utility for single targets, the natural progression was to investigate its feasibility for multiple brain metastasis plans. Whole brain radiation therapy (WBRT) had been the standard of care for many years for multiple metastasis patients; however, a growing body of literature has been steadily supplanting the role of WBRT with SRS, particularly in light of its comparative decreased effect on associated neurocognitive effects [32].

Initial VMAT plans for multiple metastasis plans on linac platforms were generally comparable in terms of conformity but markedly inferior in dose falloff and low-dose spill compared with a Gamma Knife (Elekta AB, Stockholm, Sweden) plans for the same case, particularly when a single isocenter was being used for linac plans [33–35]. Subsequently, advances in VMAT optimization algorithms, linac-accessory

features, treatment geometry selection, and treatment planning strategies, together rendered it feasible to generate plans of equivalent clinical quality on either platform [36–38] (Fig. 44.8).

The high efficiency and quality of linac SRS, coupled with the flexibility of the linac to treat all disease sites, have resulted in large growth in utilization of the platform for radiosurgery, particularly in community centers. From 2003 to 2011, the proportion of patients receiving SRS with a linac rose from 0% to 22% and 11% to 38% in academic and community centers, respectively. Extrapolating from the trend,

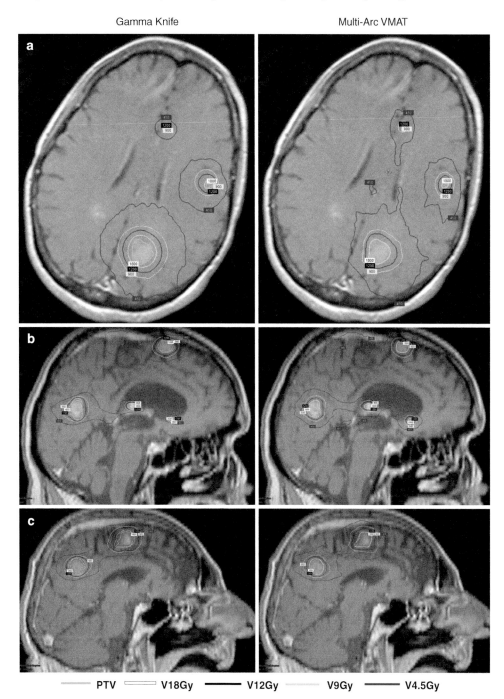

**Fig. 44.8** Isodose curve comparison between Gamma Knife and VMAT for (**a**) nine metastasis, (**b**) six metastasis, and (**c**) two metastasis SRS plans each receiving 18 Gy in single fraction to all targets. [Reprinted from Thomas EM, et al. Comparison of plan quality and delivery time between volumetric arc therapy (RapidArc) and Gamma Knife radiosurgery for multiple cranial metastases. Neurosurgery 2014;75(4): 409–418. With permission from Oxford University Press]

by 2020, the majority of patients in the United States will receive their SRS on a linear accelerator [39].

## Important SRS/hfSRT Concepts

There are several metrics that are commonly used to evaluate the quality of SRS treatment plans. The conformity/conformality index (CI) is used to quantify how tightly the prescription isodose volume (PIV) is delivered to the target or targets. The RTOG (or Shaw) CI is simply the ratio of the prescription isodose to the target volume [40]. This index is simple and easy to calculate but can erroneously imply a high-quality plan if the treatment planning position does not align the dose with target or if the PIV undercovers the target. The Paddick CI addresses these considerations by including in its metric the proportion of prescription dose the target receives. The Paddick gradient index (GI) is a simple ratio of the volume of tissue receiving 50% of the prescription dose to the volume receiving the prescription dose. It is generally useful in assessing how rapidly the prescription dose falls off to a moderate isodose range but suffers in that a plan with a poor conformity can erroneously appear to have better gradient than a more conformal plan with identical 50% isodose volume. A better simple metric is simply the ratio of 50% isodose volume to the target volume or 50% falloff ratio. The volume of tissue receiving 12 Gy in a single fraction is known as the $V_{12Gy}$. This has become an important surrogate for prediction of symptomatic radionecrosis, with the risk of symptomatic radionecrosis approaching 50% for $V_{12Gy}$ region >10 cc. This association was first demonstrated for Gamma Knife treatments [41, 42] but has been validated for linac radiosurgery treatments as well [43, 44]. For fractionated treatments between 2 and 5 fractions, $V_{18Gy}$ has been shown to be a predictor of radionecrosis with risk rising from 4 to 14% when $V_{18Gy} > 21$ cc [45]. The homogeneity index measures the ratio of the maximum dose within target volume to prescribed dose [40]. For a given case, single or multiple targets, a properly planned linac SRS/hfSRT plan is of equivalent quality to a Gamma Knife plan [37] (Table 44.3).

## Linac SRS/hfSRT Treatment Planning Considerations

The hallmark principle of radiosurgery is minimizing the exposure of normal tissue to a clinically relevant dose threshold through focused delivery of dose. The amount of surrounding tissue exposed to a given dose level is minimized when the surface area to volume ratio of that dose distribution is minimized. Mathematically, this is achieved by a spherical dose distribution. Treatment strategy for a tumor within the CNS can be divided into either conformal or organ avoidance. A conformal plan assumes equivalent value and sensitivity of tissue in all directions and attempts to deliver the tightest dose distribution possible around each target. An organ avoidance plan is employed when the target is adjacent to a critical structure. In this type of plan, rapidity of dose falloff is sacrificed in one or more directions for the purpose of increasing falloff between the target and critical structure. All linac SRS/hfSRT plans are improved through the use of noncoplanar treatment approaches, which improve the three-dimensional dose falloff by decreasing the aspect ratio of the dose distribution. Arc-based plans utilize at least two arcs. Complex plans with higher numbers of targets benefit from a greater number of arcs. Modern VMAT plans are inversely optimized and utilize a single isocenter, even in treatments of multiple targets. Four arcs seem to be sufficient, even for very large numbers of targets [46]. Dynamic conformal arc plans are forward optimized and historically used a separate isocenter for each target. Modern treatment planning systems (TPS) now facilitate treatment up to ten targets with a single isocenter [47] (Fig. 44.9).

As with all inversely optimized treatment plans, single-isocenter VMAT SRS plan quality is sensitive to planning approach and geometry. The authors have described a detailed technique for high-quality multiple-target, single-isocenter VMAT radiosurgery which has been widely validated [38]. For VMAT SRS/hfSRT plans, the authors recommend the following to maximize plan quality:

- Use at least one noncoplanar arc in addition to an axial arc.
- Use concentric rind structures to emphasize dose falloff at clinically relevant dose levels.

**Table 44.3** Important radiosurgery metrics

| | |
|---|---|
| $\text{RTOG CI} = \dfrac{\text{PIV}}{\text{TV}}$ | TV: Target volume |
| | CI: Conformity/conformality index |
| $\text{Paddick CI} = \dfrac{\text{TV}^2_{\text{PIV}}}{\text{TV} \times \text{PIV}}$ | PIV: Prescription isodose volume |
| | GI: Gradient index |
| $\text{Paddick GI} = \dfrac{\text{PIV}_{50\%}}{\text{PIV}}$ | $\text{PIV}_{50\%}$: Volume receiving 50% of prescription isodose |
| | $\text{TV}_{\text{PIV}}$: Target volume receiving prescription isodose |
| $50\% \text{ Falloff Ratio} = \dfrac{\text{PIV}_{50\%}}{\text{TV}}$ | HI: Homogeneity index |
| $V_{12Gy}$ (cc) = tissue volume receiving 12Gy | |
| $\text{HI} = \dfrac{D_{\max}}{D_{\text{Rx}}}$ | |

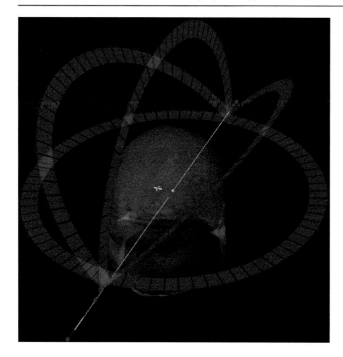

**Fig. 44.9** Depiction of four-arc geometry for single-isocenter VMAT treatment of nine metastases

- Do not penalize hotspots/heterogeneity within tumor volume (increases moderate/low isodose spill).
- Inclusion of optimization criteria that reflect any desired outcomes of plan quality (e.g., if low isodose spill is considered clinically relevant, an optimization criterion should be included).

Vendors have also recognized the increased interest in multiple metastasis SRS and are now producing dedicated treatment planning solutions to maximize quality of treatments and minimize inter-planner variability. Elements™ (Brainlab) and HyperArc (Varian Medical Systems) are two such available software suites.

## Clinical Applications of Stereotactic Radiosurgery and Hypofractionated Stereotactic Radiotherapy

### Hypofractionation

HSRT has become an effective strategy for preserving the excellent local control of SRS but reducing the likelihood of late toxicity in treatment of large targets or targets with nearby sensitive structures. The most common structures for which a nearby target might prompt consideration of hypofractionation are the brainstem, spinal cord, optics, and cochlea.

Recent studies have shown that there may be an improved ratio of tumor control to toxicity risk for hypofractionation of treatment in several treatment applications, including large brain metastases, meningiomas, vestibular schwannomas, and gliomas. An in-depth discussion of the radiobiological considerations of SRS versus hfSRT is beyond the scope of this chapter, but for those interested, Kirkpatrick et al. have done so [48].

## Benign Tumors

### Vestibular Schwannomas (Acoustic Neuromas)

Vestibular schwannomas are tumors derived from Schwann cells (neurilemmas) that occur most commonly intracranially in the vestibular section of vestibulocochlear nerve (CNVIII). They represent 8–10% of all intracranial tumors in adults but comprise a majority of cerebellopontine angle tumors. Bilateral incidence is a hallmark feature of neurofibromatosis type II commonly tested on medical licensing exams. The biology and treatment of vestibular schwannomas are covered in extensive detail in Chapter 4. Among all benign indications for SRS, vestibular schwannoma is among the most common. In general, local control is quite good (>95%) if complete tumor removal can be achieved with microsurgical resection. Local control rates drop significantly (80–85%) in the setting of subtotal resection. Patients who are poor surgical candidates or in whom the neurosurgeon does not feel they can achieve total resection should be considered for SRS (Fig. 44.10).

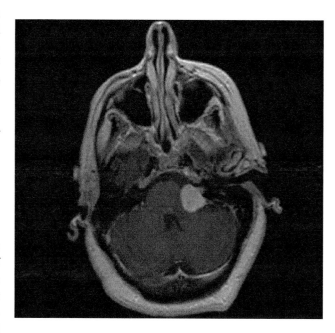

**Fig. 44.10** Moderate-sized schwannoma of left vestibulocochlear nerve, an excellent candidate for hfSRT [49]. [Reprinted from https://commons.wikimedia.org/wiki/File:Vestibular-schwannoma-003.jpg. With permission from Creative Commons Attribution:https://creativecommons.org/licenses/by-sa/3.0/deed.en]

**Table 44.4** Local control for vestibular schwannomas in dedicated linac SRS series

| Series | No. Pts | Median F/U (yrs) | Rx (Gy) | LC (%) |
|---|---|---|---|---|
| Badakhshi | 190 | 3 | 13.5 | 88 |
| Combs | 30 | 6 | 13 | 91 |
| Foote | 149 | 5 | 14 | 87 |
| Friedman | 390 | 5 | 13 | 90 |
| Hsu | 75 | 5 | 15 | 92 |
| Okunaga | 46 | 5 | 14 | 100 |
| Roos | 65 | 4 | 13 | 95 |
| Rutten | 26 | 5 | 12 | 95 |
| Spiegelmann | 48 | 3 | 14 | 98 |
| Suh | 29 | 5 | 16 | 94 |

The local control rates for vestibular schwannomas treated with linac SRS are compiled in Table 44.4 [50–58]. There has been no prospective comparison with Gamma Knife or fractionated radiosurgery, but pooled analyses show similar rates of local control and hearing preservation among those who still possessed it prior to treatment. Combs et al. compared the 30 patients who received linac SRS with 170 who received standard fractionation SRT (57.6 Gy/32fx), and there was no difference in control or maintenance of pretreatment hearing; however, SRS with doses >13 Gy was associated with decreased hearing preservation [51]. There are conflicting data as to whether cochlear dose is associated with maintenance of pretreatment hearing. Two series reported higher rates of pretreatment hearing maintenance with limitation of the cochlea dmax or central cochlear dose <4 Gy [59, 60]; others have not found it borne out in multivariate analysis. In the absence of incontrovertible evidence otherwise, it seems prudent to limit the cochlear dmax if it does not compromise tumor coverage to at least 12 Gy.

For larger vestibular schwannomas, hypofractionation can be used as a means of increasing likelihood of hearing preservation or other at-risk cranial nerves. The outcomes for hfSRT are less mature, with shorter follow-up, but in general show similar local control (83–100%) and good rates of hearing preservation (50–82%) when compared with single fraction. Regimens used are typically 18–21 Gy in 3 fractions or 25 Gy in 5 fractions [61–66].

## Meningiomas

Meningiomas are classified as benign tumors but known be very locally aggressive if high grade or recurrent/refractory to treatment. Grading is according to World Health Organization (WHO) from I to III, based on morphologic and several other pathologic criteria. They are the most common benign tumor of primary brain tissue. Their biology and treatment are covered in great detail in the first chapter. Surgical resection is generally the treatment of choice; however, in non-operative candidates or candidates with unresectable tumors, SRS is

often used. As with schwannomas, recurrence after surgery is associated with the adequacy of the resection, which is scored according to the Simpson grading criteria, I–V [67]. By definition, complete resection of a meningioma includes removal or obliteration of dural attachment. Grade I resection is ideal and represents total resection including the tumor's dural attachment and any abnormal bone. Grade II is defined by complete resection of the tumor and coagulation without removal of the dural attachment. Grades III–V represent varying degrees of incomplete resection. There are no randomized trials comparing surgery with SRS, but each modality appears to yield similar rates of progression-free survival for small- to medium-sized lesions. Table 44.5 displays the local control rates for several of the larger series utilizing linac for SRS. Many of these patients had had previous treatment [68–74] (Fig. 44.11).

For meningiomas thought to be at high risk of SRS complication, either because of size or critical structure proximity, hfSRT has been utilized. Local control rates are similar to those appropriately treated with SRS prescriptions with the caveat of fewer data and less mature follow-up. In a Stanford CyberKnife series of 27 patients with meningiomas of mean size 7.7 cm$^3$ located within <3 mm of optic apparatus, Adler et al. reported 94% local control and vision preservation rate with mean dose 20.3 (range, 15–30) Gy in median 3 fractions (range, 1–5) [76].

## Pituitary Adenomas

Pituitary adenomas are benign neoplasms that typically arise from the anterior portion of the hypophysis. Posterior pituitary adenomas have been known to occur but are very rare. Indication for radiosurgery depends on a large degree on the type of adenoma, if it is functioning (producing excess hormone), what type of hormone it is overproducing, and its proximity to the optic pathway. If the tumor is too close to the optic pathway (<3 mm) and radiation is indicated, fractionated therapy is typically selected to minimize risk of optic pathway damage.

For a nonfunctioning pituitary adenoma, the primary treatment is surgery; if the adenoma recurs after surgery and repeat surgery is contraindicated or not desired, SRS is considered to prevent regrowth. Prescription doses have ranged from 12 to 20 Gy. Indications for SRS in functional adenomas depend on the hormone being secreted. The goal of SRS for all functional adenomas is not only tumor control, but biochemical control as well. This requires a higher dose, and 20–25 Gy is usually selected. For ACTH-secreting tumors (Cushing's disease), surgery is preferred, even to medical therapy. The approach of choice is transsphenoidal resection, but if this is contraindicated or has failed, SRS is the next indication. The decision tree is similar for somatotropin-secreting adenomas. Surgery is preferred to medical therapy;

**Table 44.5** Local control for meningiomas in dedicated linac SRS series

| Series | No. Pts | Median Age (yr) | Median F/U (mo) | Median GTV (cc) | Rx Dose (Gy) | LC (%) | AE (%) |
|---|---|---|---|---|---|---|---|
| Hadelsberg (2014) | 74 | 60 | 49 | 6.9 | 13 | 90.6 | 10.8 |
| Correa [68] | 32 | 55 | 73 | 6 | 14 | 100 | N/A |
| Spiegelmann [69] | 102 | 57 | 67 | 7 | 13.5 | 98 | 4.90 |
| Pollock [69] | 62 | 58 | 64 | 2.4 | 17.7 | 95 | 9.68 |
| Torres [70] | 63 | 57 | 40.6 | 12.7 | 15.7 | 92 | 6.34 |
| Shafron [71] | 70 | 58 | 23 | 10 | 12.7 | 100 | 2.86 |
| Rodolfo [72] | 127 | 61.5 | 31 | 4.1 | 15 | 84.3 | 4.7 |

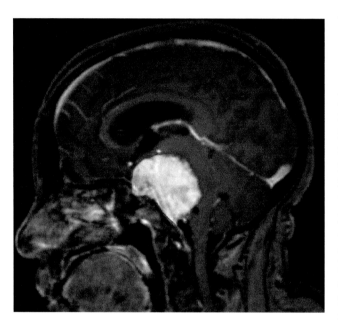

**Fig. 44.11** Sagittal T1 contrasted view of a large parasellar meningioma [75]. [Reprinted from File:Tumor Meningioma3.JPG. https://commons.wikimedia.org/wiki/File:Tumor_Meningioma3.JPG. With permission from Creative Commons Attribution 3.0: https://creativecommons.org/licenses/by-sa/3.0/deed.en]

but alternatively in this case, medical therapy is indicated prior to SRS. Prolactinomas have such an excellent response rate to dopamine agonist therapy that very few patients require surgery for their management. Most of these respond well to surgery. Those that do not respond to or cannot undergo surgery can be considered for SRS. Again, the dose-limiting structure is the optic complex. Radiation should be fractionated if cannot be appropriately spared (fSRT). Control rates for pituitary adenomas treated with SRS are generally very high. The majority of published SRS experience is with Gamma Knife (Elekta AB, Stockholm, Sweden), but there are a few small series of linac-treated patients which are outlined in Table 44.6.

hfSRT local control rates are similar albeit with fewer data and less mature follow-up. Iwata et al. reported 98% local control with only 4.1% new-onset hypopituitarism in 100 patients treated with either 21 Gy/3fx or 25 Gy/5fx [77].

# Malignant Tumors

## Intracranial Metastasis

Brain metastases are the primary indication for intracranial malignancy SRS. Metastases represent the most common intracranial neoplasm in adults. Two large autopsy series involving people who expired secondary to a cancer diagnosis revealed the prevalence of intracranial metastasis to be 25% and 26% [78, 79]. Estimates of brain metastasis vary widely. A commonly cited figure is 80,000–170,000 per year within the United States, but the true figure is unknown as all of the population-based estimates and autopsy series are old and suffer from methodological shortcomings [80]. Nevertheless, cerebral metastases are extremely common and are the most frequent indication for SRS. The most common histologies of brain metastasis are lung, melanoma, renal, breast, and colorectal. Metastases from lung primaries represent 30 to 60% of all cases.

We do know that the incidence is increasing. This is likely due to better and more frequent MR surveillance of people with cancer, increased availability of high-quality MRI, and also increased median survival duration of persons with cancers with high intracranial metastasis potential (e.g. NSCLC, melanoma).

Diagnosis of brain metastasis retains a poor prognosis, however, perhaps not so poor as it once was. The recursive partitioning analysis (RPA) is a prognostic index that was developed based on KPS, primary tumor control, and presence of extracranial metastasis in 1200 patients treated between 1985 and 2005 in 3 clinical trials [81]. Recently an updated GPA derived from 2186 patients diagnosed between 2006 and 2014 was released specifically for NSCLC to account for the availability of new agents to many patients with adenocarcinoma with targetable mutations. The longest median survival estimate has now been extended from 7.1 months to nearly 4 years for patients with excellent performance status, four or fewer metastases, no extracranial disease, and an EGFR or ALK mutation. Nonadenocarcinoma patients do have increased estimated median survival compared with the previous RPA, but the increase is much

**Table 44.6** Local control for pituitary adenomas in dedicated linac SRS series

| Series | No. Pts | Median F/U (mo) | Median GTV (cc) | Rx Dose (Gy) | LC (%) | AE (%) | Incidence of new hypopituitarism (%) |
|---|---|---|---|---|---|---|---|
| Puataweepong (2016) | 21 | 62 | | | 93 | – | 4.7 |
| Runge (2012) | 61 | 83 | 3.5 | 13 | 98 | 1.6 | 9.8 |
| Wilson (2012) | 51 | 37 | 2.4 | 14 | 100 | 2 | – |
| Mitsumori (1998) | 18 | 48 | 1.9 | 15 | 100 | 0 | 5.5 |
| Yoon (1998) | 24 | 49.2 | – | 21.1 | 95.8 | – | – |

**Table 44.7** Comparison of historical and recent survival in patients with NSCLC and brain metastases

| | 1985–2005 | 2006–2014 | |
|---|---|---|---|
| | All NSCLC, DS-GPA | Nonadenocarcinoma NSCLC lung-molGPA[a] | Adenocarcinoma NSCLC lung-molGPA[a] |
| Lung GPA score | MS, mo Patients, no. (%) | MS, mo Patients, no. (%) | MS, mo Patients, no. (%) |
| 0.0–1.0 | 3.0 254 (14) | 5.3 175 (26) | 6.9 337 (22) |
| 1.5–2.5 | 5.5 705 (38) | 9.8 324 (49) | 13.7 664 (44) |
| 2.5–3.5 | 9.4 713 (40) | 12.8 166 (25) | 26.5 455 (30) |
| 3.5–4.0 | 14.8 161 (9) | 0 | 46.8 65 (4) |
| Overall | 7.0 1833 (100) | 9.2 665 (100) | 15.2 1521 (100) |

Abbreviations: *DS* diagnosis specific, *GPA* graded prognostic assessment, *MS* median survival, *NSCLC* non-small cell lung cancer
[a]The lung-molGPA is the updated DS-GPA designed from the data in the present study

**Fig. 44.12** Kaplan-Meier curves showing survival by the lung-molGPA for adenocarcinoma NSCLC. [Reprinted from Sperduto PW, Yang TJ, Beal K, Pan H, Brown PD, Bangdiwala A, et al. Estimating survival in patients with lung cancer and brain metastases: an update of the graded prognostic assessment for lung cancer using molecular markers (Lung-molGPA). JAMA oncology. 2017;3(6):827–31. With permission from American Medical Association]

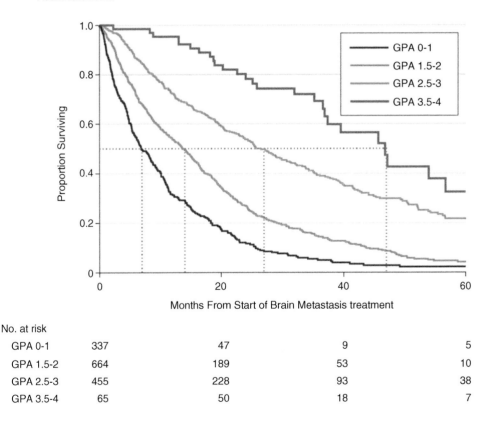

smaller in magnitude than adenocarcinoma patients, even those who do not have a targetable mutation [82] (Table 44.7 and Fig. 44.12).

Utilization of SRS for brain metastases has significantly increased throughout the past several years. Recent level I evidence has shown that for the most common etiology of brain metastasis, NSCLC, addition of WBRT to SRS, may improve local control in patients with one to three mets but with no benefit to overall survival and substantial cost to neurocognitive function and quality of life [83]. Increased MRI availability allows for routine post-SRS surveillance in brain metastasis patients, and salvage SRS can be used for distant intracranial progression. Prospective data also support use of SRS rather than WBRT for patients with four or more brain mets. In the JLGK0901 study, for patients receiving upfront SRS for ten or fewer metastases, there were no differences in local recurrence, appearance of new lesions, risk of neurologic death, or overall survival in patients with two to four mets versus five to ten mets [84].

Local control of brain metastases with SRS is very good. The most important factors predicting local control are likely lesion size and prescription dose. The platform on which brain metastases are treated has not been shown to affect the outcome of treatment. A multitude of historical data show equivalent local control between SRS on Gamma Knife (Elekta AB, Stockholm, Sweden), gantry-based linac, or CyberKnife (Accuray Inc., Sunnyvale, CA, USA). Recent randomized prospective data from Scorsetti et al. further support the equivalence in LC and OS between Gamma Knife (Elekta AB, Stockholm, Sweden) and linac SRS for brain mets [85].

## Malignant/High-Grade Gliomas

The use of SRS in gliomas is mostly limited to the treatment of recurrent disease or providing a boost in combination with conventionally fractionated radiation. RTOG 9305, a Phase III study, generated level I data on the efficacy of SRS in patients with newly diagnosed GBM. This trial randomized 203 patients with supratentorial GBM with <4 cm to external beam radiation therapy (60 Gy) plus BCNU with or without upfront SRS boost [86]. Single-fraction SRS doses depended on tumor size but ranged from 15 to 24 Gy. There was no difference in median, 2-year and 3-year overall survivals, or in failure patterns between the two treatment arms. Quality of life and cognitive outcomes were comparable. RTOG 0023, a Phase II study, enrolled 76 patients with newly diagnosed supratentorial GBM with <6 cm of residual contrast-enhancing tumor to receive accelerated radiation therapy combining EBRT with weekly SRS boost [PMID: 16750317] [87]. Patients were treated with 50 Gy conventional radiation therapy plus BCNU with four fractionated stereotactic radiosurgery boost fractions of either 5 or 7 Gy administered once weekly during the final 4 weeks. While the regimen was feasible and well tolerated, there was no survival benefit compared to the historical RTOG database for the entire cohort but for a subset of patients undergoing complete or near-complete resection. Both trials were conducted in an era that predates the current standard of care management, which includes concurrent and adjuvant Temozolomide. While these studies provide compelling negative results for the use of SRS in newly diagnosed GBM, there is some retrospective and single-institution evidence suggesting a potential local control or overall survival benefit for combining SRS with EBRT in newly diagnosed GBM as well as in the recurrent disease setting [88]. Evidence for the use of SRS in low-grade gliomas is sparse and limited to single-institution experiences [89–92].

## Physical Characteristics and Technical Considerations of Modern Linear Accelerator Platforms

### Radiation Production and Delivery with a Linear Accelerator

Within radiation oncology, radiation can be broadly divided in two categories: *ionizing and nonionizing*. Although there are a number of types of nonionizing radiation with important applications with radiation oncology, for radiation to be therapeutically useful, it must be ionizing. Conventionally, a photon can be regarded as ionizing if possesses energy of between 10 and 33 eV, which is approximately the energy necessary to liberate a loosely bound outer shell electron. The energies used for therapeutic radiation are typically 4 MeV–20 MeV, most commonly 6 MeV and 10 MeV. At these energies, the predominant interaction between the photon and a tissue medium is Compton scattering.

Modern commercial linear accelerators in radiation oncology use X-ray photons for treatment. This is in contrast to the Gamma Knife (Elekta AB, Stockholm, Sweden) platform, which, as its name suggests, uses gamma ray photons for treatment. There is often confusion regarding the difference between gamma rays and X-rays. This is understandable as the distinction actually has no universally agreed upon consensus. Some physicists have conventionally ascribed the difference as differing origins of the two types of photons. In this convention, gamma rays by definition originate from the nucleus as a result of an interaction within the nucleus of an atom; X-rays by definition are emitted by electrons via one of their potential interactions with matter or an electromagnetic field. Another convention defines them based on their typical characteristic spectra of energies, gamma rays being higher energy, or lower wavelength than X-rays. Each convention has its disadvantages. For example, an inconsistency of the photon origin paradigm would be that in an electron-positron annihilation reaction, there is no nucleus involved in the reaction but the photons produced are universally referred to as gamma rays. An inconsistency of the energy spectrum paradigm is that X-rays generated in a modern electron tube can and do have far higher energies than photons universally referred to gamma photons (e.g., the 1.022 MeV gamma photons emitted in the previous annihilation example). The salient point is that the distinction is purely semantic and largely immaterial. Once an ionizing photon has left its source, its only important feature is its energy [93].

A modern C-arm medical linear accelerator is pictured below (Fig. 44.13). An electron gun injects pulses of elec-

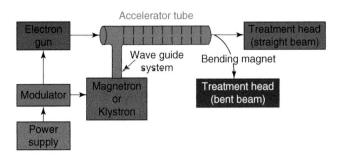

**Fig. 44.13** Schematic of a modern medical linear accelerator. [Adapted from Khan FM (ed). Khan's The Physics of Radiation Therapy. Lippincott Williams & Wilkins; 2010. With permission from Wolter Kluwers Health]

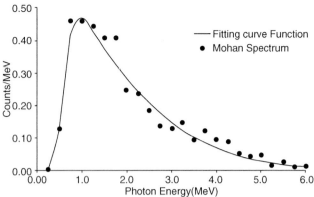

**Fig. 44.14** Relative fluence of photon energy range for a 10 MV linac. Bremsstrahlung X-rays produced by collision of electrons with a target may possess any energy within the range of 0 to the energy of the incident electron. [Reprinted from Tartar A. Monte Carlo simulation approaches to dose distributions for 6 MV photon beams in clinical linear accelerator. Biocybernetics and Biomedical Engineering 2014;34(2): 90–100. With permission from Elsevier]

trons into an accelerating waveguide tube. Microwave pulses generated with a klystron are used to accelerate the electrons through a multi-cavity waveguide. Once the electrons exit the waveguide, in a C-arm linac, a magnet bends their path 270° after which their path ends in impact with a target made of a high-z material such as tungsten. In a non-C-arm linac (i.e., CyberKnife, Accuray Inc., Sunnyvale, CA, USA), the electrons exit the waveguide and proceed directly to the high-z target.

The electrons' sudden deceleration at the target causes the production of bremsstrahlung X-rays. X-rays produced via bremsstrahlung are not monoenergetic and exist on a continuous spectrum of energies ranging from 0 to the energy of the incident electron, typically 4–18 MV. The photon flux intensity distribution (Fig. 44.14) depends on the z-value of the target, and the energy of the incident electron is governed by Kramer's law [94]. In diagnostic X-ray imaging, the energies utilized are in 40–150 keV range, and target material characteristic X-ray transitions in this energy range cause peaks within the spectrum. The peaks are not consequential to therapeutic X-ray considerations [16].

In practice, the most common energies utilized for linac radiosurgery are 6 MV and 10 MV. At energies >10 MV, the probability of photoneutron production from interaction of X-rays and linac head materials significantly increases, greatly complicating shielding and patient dosimetry considerations [16].

From the target, the X-ray beam then passes a flattening filter which both homogenizes the beam profile and hardens the beam (raises the average energy of the beam by filtering out low energy X-rays). After the flattening filter, the beam passes through an ionization chamber which measures various characteristics of the X-ray beam such as dose rate and axis symmetry. Once the X-ray beam exits the ionization chamber, it is collimated by an upper and lower set of "jaws." Each set of jaws can move independently of the other in the x and y direction. Thereafter, the beam passes through a multi-leaf collimator. The multi-leaf collimator is an array of

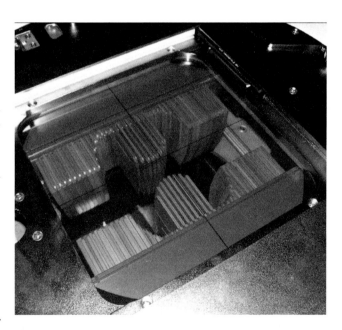

**Fig. 44.15** Photograph of the final multi-leaf collimator on a modern linac. The entire collimator can rotate 360°, and each of the leaves can move independently of not only its paired leaf, but all the other leaves as well [Reprinted from https://commons.wikimedia.org/wiki/File:Multi_leaf_collimator.jpg. With permission from Creative Commons Attribution 2.5: https://creativecommons.org/licenses/by-sa/2.5/deed.en]

paired tungsten "leaves" which can move independently of all the other leaves in order to shape the beam. Motion of the leaves during treatment allows intensity-modulated radiation therapy (IMRT). Motion of the gantry and leaves during treatment is known as volumetric modulated arc therapy (VMAT). These concepts are previously covered in Chapter 43 (Fig. 44.15).

## Flattening Filter-Free Delivery

In recent years, many centers have begun to operate their linac without the flattening filter or in FFF mode. Fu et al. [95] and Vassiliev et al. [96] were the first to investigate the dosimetric effects of operating the beam without a flattening filter on the Varian Clinac 21EX. As it turned out, there were several advantages to doing so. Most importantly, operating the beam without the flattening filter considerably increases the dose rate. Dose output of the 6 MV FFF increases by a factor of 2.3 and 10 MV FFF by a factor of 4.0 with respect to each beam's flattened counterpart. For standard fractions, the difference may not be clinically meaningful; however, for single and hypofractionated radiosurgical treatments, the dose output increase confers a large reduction in treatment time [97–101] (Fig. 44.16).

Hoogeman et al. assessed the time dependence of intrafraction motion in a study of 32 patients receiving intracranial radiation on the CyberKnife (Accuray Inc., Sunnyvale, CA, USA) system and noted a clear positive correlation with patient drift and time of treatment. Drift was very small for short treatments, but as treatment duration approached 15 min, drift vector magnitude began to approach clinical significant values [102]. Kim et al. assessed the likelihood of patient motion as a function of time in 33 treatments of single-fraction spinal radiosurgery and found that over a mean treatment time of 19 min, the potential magnitude of motion was 0.15 mm/min, or up to a total of 3 mm through the entirety of treatment [103].

Another advantage of FFF treatment is there is a large decrease in the amount of head scatter as well as the number of photoneutrons produced when the X-ray beam does not have to traverse a high-z filter. Fry et al. reported a 20% reduction in neutron fluence/monitor unit for an 18 MV beam and a 69% decrease in total neutron dose associated with FFF treatment for a standard prostate IMRT course [103]. Although the reductions are more modest for lower energy beams, this still translates to reduced far field peripheral dose to the patient. Moreover, because of the aforementioned factors, design of a vault specifically for a flattening filter-free linac may require less shielding material [104].

## Importance of Six Degrees of Freedom (6DOF) Immobilization, Setup, Verification, and Intrafraction Motion Monitoring

All modern radiosurgery platforms are capable of highly conformal plans that are delivered at very high-dose rates. It is obvious that proper three-dimensional orientation of the patient and verification of the positioning are critical in radiosurgery. In the early days of linac radiosurgery, a stereotactic frame was employed for fixation of the patient. This had the advantage of excellent rigid immobilization, but the necessity of local anesthesia rendered it impractical

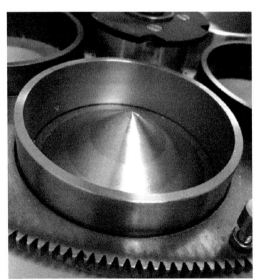
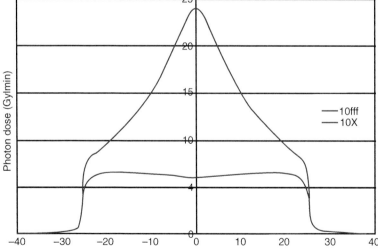

**Fig. 44.16** (left) Flattening filter on a rotating carousel. The carousel is rotated according to the desired treatment mode depending on if photons or electrons are being used for treatment. Some modern linear accelerator carousels included an aperture enabling unflattened photon delivery. (right) Comparison of the dose rate for a 10 MV FFF beam with a 10 MV flattened beam. The 10 MV FFF facilitates a fourfold increase in dose rate. Left: [Image courtesy of Geoff Budgell]. Right: [Adapted from Prendergast BM, Dobelbower MC, Bonner JA, et al. Stereotactic body radiation therapy (SBRT) for lung malignancies: preliminary toxicity results using a flattening filter-free linear accelerator operating at 2400 monitor units per minute. Radiation Oncology 2013;8: 273. With permission from Creative Commons License: https://creativecommons.org/licenses/by/2.0/]

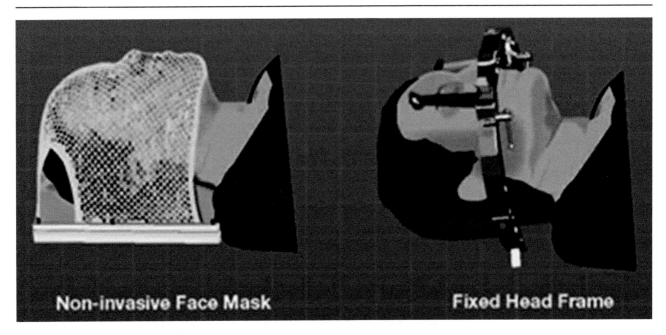

**Fig. 44.17** Comparison of patient immobilization with a thermoplastic mask and fixed head frame

for prolonged treatments and inconvenient for hypofractionated courses. Although stereotactic frames are still used in some centers for radiosurgery, thermoplastic masks have become the immobilization method of choice for many centers. Early thermoplastic masks suffered from insufficient rigidity and allowed up to 2 mm of patient motion in the mask [105]. The most recent masks incorporate more rigid thermoplastics and have been measured to allow less than 1 mm of motion (Fig. 44.17).

Advanced robotic couches now facilitate rotational alignment in addition to alignment in the three translational dimensions. For a single spherical lesion, being treated with a spherical isodose distribution, there is theoretically minimal effect to rotational misalignment as long as the isocenter is in the correct $x$, $y$, and $z$ position. However, for treatment of irregularly shaped lesions, there are important consequences to rotational misalignment. Figure 44.18 shows an example of compromised target coverage that would have occurred without rectification of rotational misalignment. In single-isocenter treatment of multiple targets with radiosurgery, rotational alignment is even more critical. Even with perfect $x$, $y$,

and $z$ alignment to isocenter, rotational error can cause miss of an intended target(s). For this reason, 6DOF correction is recommended for all radiosurgery, particularly for multiple metastases. To this same end, monitoring of motion is recommended during radiosurgery. Each of the current flagship platforms (Accuray, CyberKnife, Elekta Versa HD, Varian Edge) from the principal medical linac vendors catered to radiosurgery offers an intrafraction motion monitoring solution. A third-party vendor (Brainlab) offers the ExacTrac™ ceiling-mounted kV imager system which can be used with either Elekta or Varian linacs. In the CyberKnife and Brainlab systems, kV X-rays are periodically obtained from ceiling-mounted imagers and compared with digitally reconstructed radiographs (DRRs) from the 3D treatment planning CT volume. The Varian Edge solution employs an optical surface monitoring system (OSMS) which uses ceiling-mounted cameras with 3D meshing to assess the constancy of the face's position during treatment. When properly integrated, both ceiling-mounted kV imaging and OSMS solutions offer submillimetre accuracy monitoring of patient displacement.

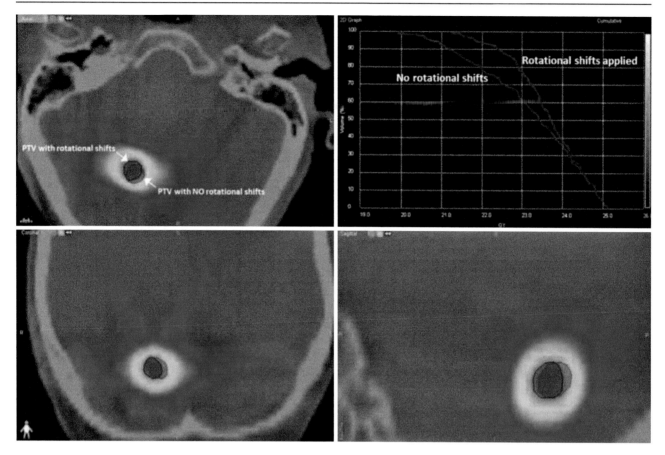

**Fig. 44.18** Dosimetric impact of not applying pitch and roll corrections on PTV coverage. Note that 22 Gy prescription coverage for this lesion would have been 80% instead of 95% which had rotational corrections not been applied [106]. [Reprinted from Dhabaan A, Schreibmann E, Siddiqi A, Elder E, Fox T, Ogunleye T, et al. Six degrees of freedom CBCT-based positioning for intracranial targets treated with frameless stereotactic radiosurgery. Journal of Applied Clinical Medical Physics. 2012;13(6):215–25. With permission from Creative Commons License 3.0: https://creativecommons.org/licenses/by/3.0/]

## Workflow in Linac-Based Radiosurgery

The process for a linac SRS/hfSRT treatment begins with a CT simulation in an SRS quality mask. An MRI is also typically required for treatment planning, particularly for metastases. If renal function permits, we recommend iodine- and gadolinium-based contrasted sequences, respectively. We recommend no larger than 1 mm slice thickness in both CT and MR imaging for stereotactic planning. Many modern MRI's are capable of acquiring 3D sequences. These sequences take longer to acquire, but because the entire volume is excited in single RF and gradient pulses, the resulting data set is less susceptible to interpolation error. The next step is fusion of the MR data set to the CT data set. In departments that rely on diagnostically acquired MRIs for treatment planning, having a 3D MR is particularly useful as it is difficult to coordinate patients being separately imaged with identical degrees of neck extension. After fusion, the target volume(s) and organs at risk are contoured in the TPS. The desired type of plan is then designed within the TPS by a dosimetrist or physicist based on the machine/TPS capabilities and physician preference. Once a plan is designed and approved by the treating physician, a physicist will perform patient-specific quality

**Pre-treatment**

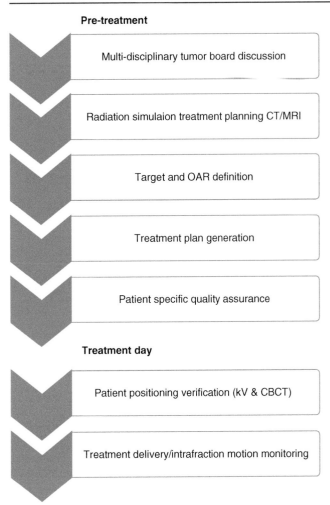

Multi-disciplinary tumor board discussion

Radiation simulaion treatment planning CT/MRI

Target and OAR definition

Treatment plan generation

Patient specific quality assurance

**Treatment day**

Patient positioning verification (kV & CBCT)

Treatment delivery/intrafraction motion monitoring

**Fig. 44.19** Workflow for typical intracranial radiosurgery case

assurance (QA) on the plan to verify that the machine will deliver within an acceptable range what the TPS predicts.

On the day of treatment, the patient is immobilized in the same position and mask in which their CT simulation was performed. An initial set of orthogonal kV images are obtained, from which the patient is aligned to the prescribed isocenter. Some treatment planning systems are capable of generating automatic shift recommendations based on comparison of kV images to digitally reconstructed radiographs (DRRs) of the patient. Serial kV imaging is performed until the treating physician is satisfied with the patient's positioning. If available, a cone beam CT is acquired which can help assess rotational error that may not be obvious from orthogonal kV imaging. Once the treatment commences, motion is monitored according to the available IGRT solution. If there is patient motion beyond the predetermined acceptable amount (usually 0.5–1 mm), the treatment is halted, and the patient's position is reestablished before treatment resumes. Treatment time varies according to number of isocenters, dose rate, and number of arcs (or nodes for CyberKnife) and may range from less than 5 min to more than 45 min (Fig. 44.19).

## Quality Assurance in Linac-Based Radiosurgery

Because of the nature of a solitary fraction treatment with a high dose in or adjacent to the central nervous system, inaccuracy in any number of factors can lead to severe deleterious treatment-related toxicity to the patient or lack of tumor control or both. One of the most important aspects in maintaining a safe and effective linac radiosurgery program is comprehensive and routine quality assurance of all aspects of the program by a medical physicist experienced in SRS. Failure of any aspect of a program to pass QA should be cause for immediate pause of any treatments and determination whether there is any possibility of patient being harmed or having been harmed.

A number of guidelines and recommendations have been developed by multiple task groups to aide physicists in development, deployment, and maintenance of robust QA measures within their own programs. The following are resources available to assist with quality assurance:

- IAEA-TECDOC-989: quality assurance in radiotherapy [107]
- RTOG: radiosurgery quality assurance guidelines [40]
- AAPM TG 40 report: comprehensive QA for radiation oncology [108]
- AAPM TG 42 report: stereotactic radiosurgery [109]
- AAPM TG 55 report: radiochromic film dosimetry [110]
- AAPM TG 68 report: intracranial stereotactic positioning systems [111]
- AAPM TG 142 report: quality assurance of medical accelerators [112]
- AAPM TG 101 report: stereotactic body radiation therapy [113]
- Quality and safety considerations in SRS and SBRT (ASTRO white paper) [114]

QA for stereotactic radiosurgery can be loosely divided into systemic QA and patient-specific QA. Systemic QA engenders periodic QA of target localization, image localization, CT simulation, image registration, treatment planning calculation, basic dosimetry, output, and treatment delivery. These QA measures are performed on a scheduled, routine basis. Output should be assessed and verified daily. For radiosurgery specifically, target localization accuracy is of paramount importance and must be plumbed routinely. Small beam dosimetry is also very important but can be challenging. Systemic QA ensures smooth and proper operation of the day-to-day operations of a department. Patient-specific QA assesses the reliability of the process on an individual patient treatment basis.

A number of commercial packages offering "end-to-end" SRS quality assurance have become available. In addition to our custom devices, two such models (Fig. 44.20) that UAB has familiarity with are STEEV (stereotactic end-to-end verification and treatment), CIRS® and Lucy 3D QA Phantom,

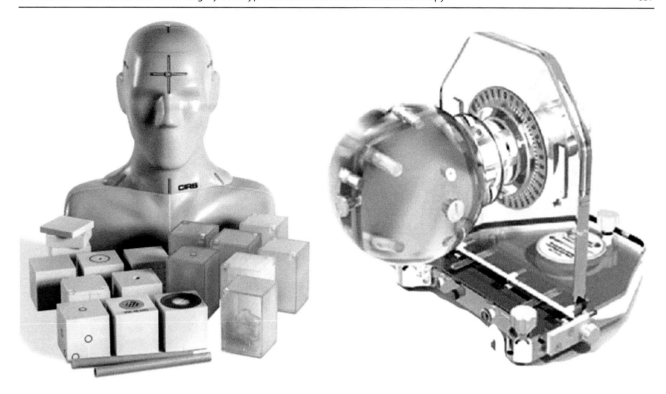

**Fig. 44.20** (left) STEEV (CIRS) and (right) Lucy (standard imaging), two examples of commercially available end-to-end stereotactic QA phantoms

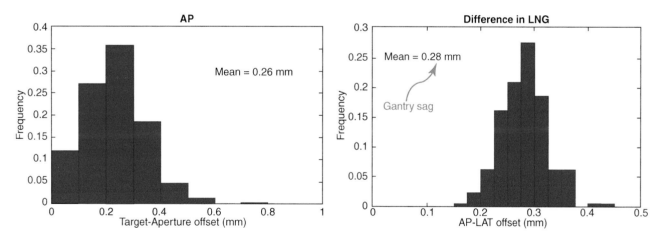

**Fig. 44.21** Mean spatial discrepancy between target and aperture for AP and longitudinal axes for series of University of Alabama SRS cases

and Standard Imaging®. Both have had their efficacy validated in the literature at multiple sites [115–120].

Programs willing to treat small targets in single fractions should be confident that their end-to-end spatial accuracy including all factors from CT-MR registration to isocenter positioning and treatment delivery is less than 1 mm and that they have the imaging capability to verify that level of accuracy. The gamma index corresponding to agreement of calculated and delivered dose distribution should be at or better than 5%/1 mm. At UAB, our end-to-end spatial accuracy is consistently at or within 0.3 mm and our gamma index within 3%/1 mm (Figs. 44.21 and 44.22).

Quality does not just apply to the radiosurgery workflow. Installing systematicity and protocol for all aspects of the patient encounter and treatment process increases efficiency and decreases the likelihood of an accident or misadministration. Examples of known quality-improving measures include implementation of checklists, verification of patient ID at all steps of the treatment process, ease of reporting incidents without fear of reprisal, and routine assessments by the physicians and physicists that therapists, dosimetrist, and nurses are comfortable with all aspects of their job and not afraid to alert a supervisor when they are uncomfortable.

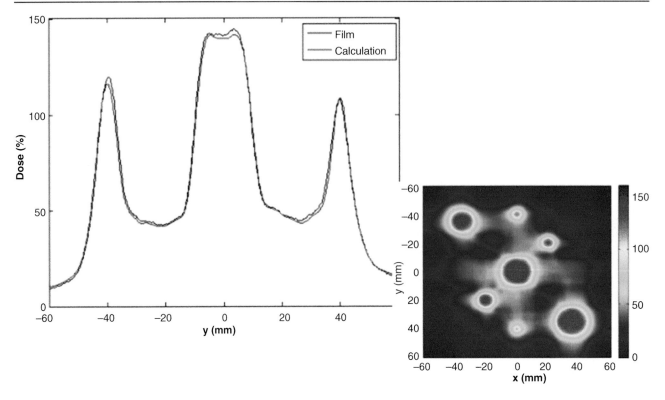

**Fig. 44.22** Planning system calculation accuracy for multiple small targets (Eclipse AAA v13 and EBT2 radiographic film)

## Conclusions

Tremendous advancement has occurred in the technology available to treat intracranial neoplasms with linac-based SRS or hfSRT. Dosimetrically equivalent plan equality between linac-based treatments and Gamma Knife is now possible even for complex multiple brain metastasis plans. Frameless treatments with rigid thermoplastic masks improve the patient experience and facilitate hypofractionation when desired at no compromise to treatment precision. High-resolution image guidance and 6DOF couch alignment allow submillimetre positioning accuracy. Flattening filter-free beam modes allow treatments to be delivered in a fraction of the time, that comparable treatment would have taken on the Gamma Knife (Elekta AB, Stockholm, Sweden).

The use of linac-based SRS and hfSRT will continue to increase both as indications for WBRT continue to wane, and SRS-capable linacs are increasingly deployed not only in academic centers but community centers as well.

The decision to hypofractionate a single radiosurgical treatment into three or five fractions can be made when there is concern for toxicity due to lesion size or critical structure proximity. Most lesions up to 2.5–3 cm can be treated in a single fraction up to 18 Gy with low risk of complication. Larger lesions should like receive a BED-appropriate hypofractionated treatment rather than a reduced prescription dose that would compromise local control.

## Case Study

A 50-year-old African-American female with nine brain metastases from metastatic high-grade carcinoma ex pleomorphic adenocarcinoma, originally of the left parotid. She was initially treated with parotidectomy, bilateral neck dissection, and chemo/RT (cisplatin and 66 Gy/33fx) on protocol but found to be metastatic to inguinal lymph node shortly after completion of adjuvant therapy. Her tumor was sequenced for actionable mutation, but none were found. She underwent first-line salvage with Taxotere/carboplatin and then was ultimately switched to pembrolizumab. Disease progression stable for approximately 9 months, until increase in an inguinal lymph node, prompted re-imaging with PET, which showed equivocal avidity in axilla and inguinal regions, as well as hyperdense avidity lateral to posterior limb of right internal capsule of the brain. MRI showed nine brain metastases, the largest measuring 1.4 × 1.1 cm with associated vasogenic edema. The patient was neurologically intact and otherwise of good performance status, KPS 90 (Fig. 44.23).

Given patient's high performance status and limited extracranial disease burden, the patient was given SRS instead of WBRT. Total gross tumor volume was 3.5 cc. 18 Gy in a single fraction was delivered to each of the metastases, with four noncoplanar arcs and a single metastasis as below.

Plan quality metrics were:
RTOG CI = 1.20 (for entire plan).
V12 Gy = 14.4 cc (for all 9 lesions).

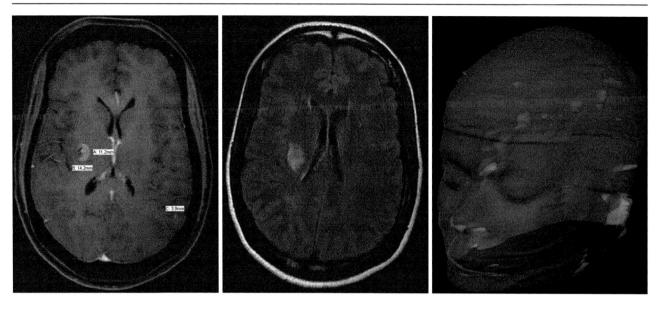

**Fig. 44.23** T1 post-contrast MRI (left, middle) and three-dimensional distribution (right) of intracranial metastases being targeted for treatment

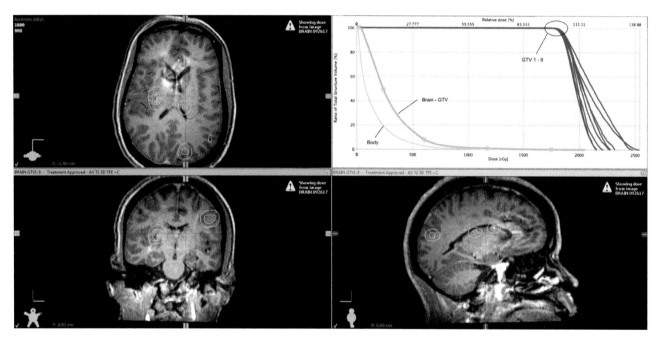

**Fig. 44.24** V100% (yellow) and V50% (green) isodose levels for 9 target single-isocenter, single-fraction linac radiosurgery plan. The DVH for the 9 targets, the body, and the normal brain tissue is displayed in the upper right corner

Mean brain dose = 297 cGy.

The patient was immobilized and simulated using a Qfix Encompass ™ SRS mask. A single-isocenter, 4 noncoplanar VMAT SRS plan was developed according to the methodology referenced earlier in the chapter (isodose curves and DVH above). Patient-specific QA was performed, with radiographic film measurements at site of largest and smallest metastasis, showing agreement between calculated and measured dose within 3%. The patient's initial alignment and positioning within 1 mm were verified using orthogonal kV and CBCT imaging on 6DOF couch. The treatment was delivered on a Varian Edge™ linear accelerator with 2.5 mm HD-MLC in flattening filter-free mode at 2400 MU/min. The treatment time was approximately 17 min including room entry for each table adjustment. The patient was given 10 mg IM dexamethasone after treatment, which the authors' clinical institutional experience has found to reduce the incidence of posttreatment Grade 2 headache. The patient was brought back to clinic with follow-up MR imaging at 1 month posttreatment. Each of the lesions was either stable or decreased in size. No new lesions were identified. The patient remains clinically stable, KPS 90 (Fig. 44.24).

## Summary

- Radiosurgery enjoys a rich history, originating shortly after the value of the practice of stereotaxy was realized and buffeted by important developments such as CT- and MR-based imaging.
- Technological improvements such as VMAT and FFF delivery in recent years have led to substantial improvements in linac SRS plan quality and treatment efficiency.
- Linac-based SRS/hfSRT, when appropriately implemented, can and has been used for virtually every application that Gamma Knife has; clinical outcomes and comparisons between the two modalities have not shown any difference.
- The same metrics used to evaluated Gamma Knife plans can be used to evaluate linac plans
- When treating with a linac, to realize sharp gradients, it is critical to use multiple noncoplanar beam entry points.
- Hypofractionation of a plan can mitigate risk of toxicity associated with treatment of larger target volumes.
- Quality assurance, both systematic and patient-specific, is vital for a linac SRS plan.
- Collaboration between radiation oncologists, neurosurgeons, and medical physicists is paramount in maintenance of a safe and effective linac radiosurgery program.

## Self-Assessment Questions

1. Which invention was most important in facilitating the initial application of CT imaging to the practice of stereotactic irradiation?
   A. Linear accelerator
   B. Relocatable stereotactic frame
   C. Thermoplastic head frame
   D. Six degrees of freedom couch

2. Which of the following treatment planning strategies is most important when considering treatment of a pituitary adenoma with SRS or hfSRT?
   A. 3D isotropic conformality
   B. Organ avoidance

3. All attempts should be made to enforce homogeneity in a linac SRS/hfSRT plan. (True or False)
   A. True
   B. False

4. The purpose of hypofractionated SRT in comparison to single-fraction radiosurgery is:
   A. To decrease the likelihood of toxicity for a large treatment volume
   B. To bill more
   C. To allow the patient more time to become comfortable with their stereotactic frame or thermoplastic mask
   D. To increase the amount of time the treating physician can interact with the patient

5. Which of the following plan quality metric has been commonly associated with radionecrosis in a single fraction?
   A. Maximum dose (dmax)
   B. Mean brain dose
   C. Volume of tissue receiving 12 Gy ($V_{12Gy}$)
   D. Volume of tissue receiving 4 Gy ($V_{4Gy}$)

## Answers

1. B
   *Explanation*: The relocatable stereotactic frame allowed a patient to be treated in the same position and orientation in which they were imaged, facilitating application of a 3D coordinate system to treatment planning. Choice A is incorrect because early CT-based stereotactic irradiations were not performed on linac. Choices C and D are incorrect because these developments entered wide use much later than CT-based stereotaxy.

2. B
   *Explanation*: When treating a pituitary adenoma, given that there are many data supporting the ability to control the adenoma with treatment at an acceptably low risk of visual toxicity, the most important consideration is ensuring that dose associated with toxicity to the nearby optic chiasm is minimized.

3. B
   *Explanation*: Enforcing homogeneity within a target volume worsens the gradient of a plan and increases the spill of moderate isodose. This should only be done for a legitimate clinical reason, such as intended preservation of normal tissue within a target volume. There is no justification for doing so when focally treating a malignant target.

4. A
   *Explanation*: Increasing the number of fractions from 1 to 3 or 5 reduces the likelihood of toxicity to the patient, particularly symptomatic radionecrosis. It may also compensate for the increased volume of treatment if it is necessary to add a CTV or PTV margin to target.

5. C
   *Explanation*: Only Choice C, the V12Gy, has been shown to be a correlative factor with radionecrosis.

## References

1. Leksell L. Stereotactic radiosurgery. J Neurol Neurosurg Psychiatry. 1983;46(9):797–803.

2. Gildenberg PL. Stereotactic surgery: present and past. In: Stereotactic neurosurgery. Baltimore: Williams & Wilkins; 1988. p. 2.
3. Hernaman-Johnson F. On the value of combined treatment, with special reference to surgery, electricity and X rays. Arch Radiol Electrother. 1920;24(10):325–33.
4. Kavanagh BD, Sheehan JP. Stereotactic irradiation: CNS tumors. In: Clinical radiation oncology 4th ed. New York: Elsevier, 2010. p. 419–26. e2.
5. Leksell L. The stereotaxic method and radiosurgery of the brain. Acta Chir Scand. 1951;102:316–9.
6. Brown RA. A stereotactic head frame for use with CT body scanners. Investig Radiol. 1979;14(4):300–4.
7. Gill SS, Thomas DGT, Warrington AP, et al. Relocatable frame for stereotactic external beam radiotherapy. Int J Radiat Oncol Biol Phys. 1991;20(3):599–603.
8. Schulder M, Patil V. The history of stereotactic radiosurgery. In: Principles and practice of stereotactic radiosurgery. New York, NY: Springer; 2008. p. 3–7.
9. Hall EJ, Giaccia AJ. Radiobiology for the radiologist. Philadelphia: Lippincott Williams & Wilkins; 2006.
10. Fahrig A, Ganslandt O, Lambrecht U, et al. Hypofractionated stereotactic radiotherapy for brain metastases. Strahlenther Onkol. 2007;183(11):625–30.
11. Marcrom SR, McDonald AM, Thompson JW, et al. Fractionated stereotactic radiation therapy for intact brain metastases. Adv Radiat Oncol. 2017;2(4):564–71.
12. Stupp R, Hegi ME, Mason WP, et al. Effects of radiotherapy with concomitant and adjuvant temozolomide versus radiotherapy alone on survival in glioblastoma in a randomised phase III study: 5-year analysis of the EORTC-NCIC trial. Lancet Oncol. 2009;10(5):459–66.
13. ASTRO model policies guidelines, "Stereotactic radiosurgery". Retrieved from: https://www.astro.org/uploadedFiles/_MAIN_SITE/Daily_Practice/Reimbursement/Model_Policies/Content_Pieces/ASTROSRSModelPolicy.pdf
14. Leksell L, Herner T, Liden K. Stereotactic radiosurgery of the brain: report of a case. Kungl fysiograf sällsk Lund förh. 1955;25:142.
15. Sheehan J, Pouratian N, Sansur C. Psychiatric and pain disorders. In: Principles and practice of stereotactic radiosurgery. New York, NY: Springer; 2008. p. 563–72.
16. Khan FM. The physics of radiation therapy. Philadelphia: Lippincott Williams & Wilkins; 2010.
17. Betti O, Derechinsky V. Hyperselective encephalic irradiation with linear accelerator. In: Advances in stereotactic and functional neurosurgery. 6th ed. Wien: Springer; 1984. p. 385–90.
18. Winston KR, Lutz W. Linear accelerator as a neurosurgical tool for stereotactic radiosurgery. Neurosurgery. 1988;22(3):454–64.
19. Colombo F, Benedetti A, Pozza F, et al. Stereotactic radiosurgery utilizing a linear accelerator. Stereotact Funct Neurosurg. 1985;48(1–6):133–45.
20. Loeffler JS, Shrieve DC, Wen PY, et al. Radiosurgery for intracranial malignancies. In: Seminars in radiation oncology. New York: Elsevier; 1995.
21. Alexander E 3rd, Loeffler J. Radiosurgery using a modified linear accelerator. Neurosurg Clin N Am. 1992;3(1):167–90.
22. Loeffler JS, Alexander E, Siddon RL, et al. Stereotactic radiosurgery for intracranial arteriovenous malformations using a standard linear accelerator. Int J Radiat Oncol Biol Phys. 1989;17(3):673–7.
23. Loeffler JS, Kooy HM, Wen PY, et al. The treatment of recurrent brain metastases with stereotactic radiosurgery. J Clin Oncol. 1990;8(4):576–82.
24. Podgorsak EB, Olivier A, Pla M, et al. Dynamic stereotactic radiosurgery. Int J Radiat Oncol Biol Phys. 1988;14(1):115–26.
25. Adler JR Jr, Chang SD, Murphy MJ, et al. The Cyberknife: a frameless robotic system for radiosurgery. Stereotact Funct Neurosurg. 1997;69(1–4):124–8.
26. Adler JR. Apparatus for and method of performing stereotaxic surgery. Google Patents; 1993.
27. Nedzi LA, Kooy HM, Alexander E, et al. Dynamic field shaping for stereotactic radiosurgery: a modeling study. Int J Radiat Oncol Biol Phys. 1993;25(5):859–69.
28. Cardinale RM, Benedict SH, Wu Q, et al. A comparison of three stereotactic radiotherapy techniques; ARCS vs noncoplanar fixed fields vs. intensity modulation. Int J Radiat Oncol Biol Phys. 1998;42(2):431–6.
29. Solberg TD, Boedeker KL, Fogg R, et al. Dynamic arc radiosurgery field shaping: a comparison with static field conformal and noncoplanar circular arcs. Int J Radiat Oncol Biol Phys. 2001;49(5):1481–91.
30. Yu CX. Intensity-modulated arc therapy with dynamic multi-leaf collimation: an alternative to tomotherapy. Phys Med Biol. 1995;40(9):1435.
31. Otto K. Volumetric modulated arc therapy: IMRT in a single gantry arc. Med Phys. 2008;35(1):310–7.
32. Brown PD, Jaeckle K, Ballman KV, et al. Effect of radiosurgery alone vs radiosurgery with whole brain radiation therapy on cognitive function in patients with 1 to 3 brain metastases: a randomized clinical trial. JAMA. 2016;316(4):401–9.
33. Ma L, Nichol A, Hossain S, et al. Variable dose interplay effects across radiosurgical apparatus in treating multiple brain metastases. Int J Comput Assist Radiol Surg. 2014;9(6):1079–86.
34. Ma L, Petti P, Wang B, et al. Apparatus dependence of normal brain tissue dose in stereotactic radiosurgery for multiple brain metastases. J Neurosurg. 2011;114(6):1580–4.
35. McDonald D, Schuler J, Takacs I, et al. Comparison of radiation dose spillage from the gamma knife Perfexion with that from volumetric modulated arc radiosurgery during treatment of multiple brain metastases in a single fraction. J Neurosurg. 2014;121(Suppl 2):51–9.
36. Keeling V, Algan O, Ahmad S, et al. SU-D-BRB-04: plan quality comparison of intracranial stereotactic radiosurgery (SRS) for gamma knife and VMAT treatments. Med Phys. 2015;42(6):3211–2.
37. Thomas EM, Popple RA, Wu X, et al. Comparison of plan quality and delivery time between volumetric arc therapy (RapidArc) and gamma knife radiosurgery for multiple cranial metastases. Neurosurgery. 2014;75(4):409–18.
38. Clark GM, Popple RA, Prendergast BM, et al. Plan quality and treatment planning technique for single isocenter cranial radiosurgery with volumetric modulated arc therapy. Practical radiation oncology. 2012;2(4):306–13.
39. Park HS, Wang EH, Rutter CE, et al. Changing practice patterns of gamma knife versus linear accelerator-based stereotactic radiosurgery for brain metastases in the US. J Neurosurg. 2016;124(4):1018–24.
40. Shaw E, Kline R, Gillin M, et al. Radiation therapy oncology group: radiosurgery quality assurance guidelines. Int J Radiat Oncol Biol Phys. 1993;27(5):1231–9.
41. Flickinger JC, Kondziolka D, Kalend AM, et al. Radiosurgery-related imaging changes in surrounding brain: multivariate analysis and model evaluation. Radiosurgery 1995. 1. Basel: Karger Publishers; 1996. p. 229–36.
42. Korytko T, Radivoyevitch T, Colussi V, et al. 12 Gy gamma knife radiosurgical volume is a predictor for radiation necrosis in non-AVM intracranial tumors. Int J Radiat Oncol Biol Phys. 2006;64(2):419–24.
43. Blonigen BJ, Steinmetz RD, Levin L, et al. Irradiated volume as a predictor of brain radionecrosis after linear accelerator stereotactic radiosurgery. Int J Radiat Oncol Biol Phys. 2010;77(4):996–1001.
44. Minniti G, Clarke E, Lanzetta G, et al. Stereotactic radiosurgery for brain metastases: analysis of outcome and risk of brain radionecrosis. Radiat Oncol. 2011;6(1):48.

45. Minniti G, D'Angelillo RM, Scaringi C, et al. Fractionated stereotactic radiosurgery for patients with brain metastases. J Neurooncol. 2014;117(2):295–301.

46. Thomas EMFC-GKDKRJFRPMB, editor Treatment of 27 brain metastases with single-isocenter VMAT Radiosurgery: a case report. 13th International Stereotactic Radiosurgery Society Congress; 2017 May 28, 2017; Montreux, Switzerland.

47. Huang Y, Chin K, Robbins JR, et al. Radiosurgery of multiple brain metastases with single-isocenter dynamic conformal arcs (SIDCA). Radiother Oncol. 2014;112(1):128–32.

48. Kirkpatrick JP, Soltys SG, Lo SS, et al. The radiosurgery fractionation quandary: single fraction or hypofractionation? Neuro Oncol. 2017;19(suppl_2):ii38–49.

49. RadsWiki. In: Vestibular-schwannoma-003, editor. Wikimedia Commons. Retrieved from: https://commons.wikimedia.org/wiki/File:Vestibular-schwannoma-003.jpg

50. Badakhshi H, Graf R, Böhmer D, et al. Results for local control and functional outcome after linac-based image-guided stereotactic radiosurgery in 190 patients with vestibular schwannoma. J Radiat Res. 2013;55(2):288–92.

51. Combs SE, Welzel T, Schulz-Ertner D, et al. Differences in clinical results after LINAC-based single-dose radiosurgery versus fractionated stereotactic radiotherapy for patients with vestibular schwannomas. Int J Radiat Oncol Biol Phys. 2010;76(1):193–200.

52. Friedman WA, Bradshaw P, Myers A, et al. Linear accelerator radiosurgery for vestibular schwannomas. J Neurosurg. 2006;105(5):657–61.

53. Okunaga T, Matsuo T, Hayashi N, et al. Linear accelerator radiosurgery for vestibular schwannoma: measuring tumor volume changes on serial three-dimensional spoiled gradient-echo magnetic resonance images. J Neurosurg. 2005;103(1):53–8.

54. Rutten I, Baumert BG, Seidel L, et al. Long-term follow-up reveals low toxicity of radiosurgery for vestibular schwannoma. Radiother Oncol. 2007;82(1):83–9.

55. Spiegelmann R, Lidar Z, Gofman J, et al. Linear accelerator radiosurgery for vestibular schwannoma. J Neurosurg. 2001;94(1):7–13.

56. Hsu P-W, Chang C-N, Lee S-T, et al. Outcomes of 75 patients over 12 years treated for acoustic neuromas with linear accelerator-based radiosurgery. J Clin Neurosci. 2010;17(5):556–60.

57. Roos DE, Potter AE, Zacest AC. Hearing preservation after low dose linac radiosurgery for acoustic neuroma depends on initial hearing and time. Radiother Oncol. 2011;101(3):420–4.

58. Suh JH, Barnett GH, Sohn JW, et al. Results of linear accelerator-based stereotactic radiosurgery for recurrent and newly diagnosed acoustic neuromas. Int J Cancer. 2000;90(3):145–51.

59. Yomo S, Carron R, Thomassin J-M, et al. Longitudinal analysis of hearing before and after radiosurgery for vestibular schwannoma. J Neurosurg. 2012;117(5):877–85.

60. Kano H, Kondziolka D, Khan A, et al. Predictors of hearing preservation after stereotactic radiosurgery for acoustic neuroma. J Neurosurg. 2009;111(4):863–73.

61. Karam SD, Tai A, Strohl A, et al. Frameless fractionated stereotactic radiosurgery for vestibular schwannomas: a single-institution experience. Front Oncol. 2013;3:121.

62. Meijer O, Vandertop W, Baayen J, et al. Single-fraction vs. fractionated linac-based stereotactic radiosurgery for vestibular schwannoma: a single-institution study. Int J Radiat Oncol Biol Phys. 2003;56(5):1390–6.

63. Morimoto M, Yoshioka Y, Kotsuma T, et al. Hypofractionated stereotactic radiation therapy in three to five fractions for vestibular schwannoma. Jpn J Clin Oncol. 2013;43(8):805–12.

64. Song DY, Williams JA. Fractionated stereotactic radiosurgery for treatment of acoustic neuromas. Stereotact Funct Neurosurg. 1999;73(1–4):45–9.

65. Tsai J-T, Lin J-W, Lin C-M, et al. Clinical evaluation of CyberKnife in the treatment of vestibular schwannomas. Biomed Res Int. 2013;2013:297093.

66. Vivas EX, Wegner R, Conley G, et al. Treatment outcomes in patients treated with CyberKnife radiosurgery for vestibular schwannoma. Otol Neurotol. 2014;35(1):162–70.

67. Simpson D. The recurrence of intracranial meningiomas after surgical treatment. J Neurol Neurosurg Psychiatry. 1957;20(1):22.

68. Hadelsberg U, Nissim U, Cohen ZR, et al. LINAC radiosurgery in the management of parasagittal meningiomas. Stereotact Funct Neurosurg. 2015;93(1):10–6.

69. Correa SFM, Marta GN, Teixeira MJ. Neurosymptomatic carvenous sinus meningioma: a 15-years experience with fractionated stereotactic radiotherapy and radiosurgery. Radiat Oncol. 2014;9(1):27.

70. Spiegelmann R, Cohen ZR, Nissim O, et al. Cavernous sinus meningiomas: a large LINAC radiosurgery series. J Neurooncol. 2010;98(2):195–202.

71. Torres RC, Frighetto L, De Salles AA, et al. Radiosurgery and stereotactic radiotherapy for intracranial meningiomas. Neurosurg Focus. 2003;14(5):1–6.

72. Shafron DH, Friedman WA, Buatti JM, et al. Linac radiosurgery for benign meningiomas. Int J Radiat Oncol Biol Phys. 1999;43(2):321–7.

73. Rodolfo H, Eben A III, Jay SL, et al. Results of linear accelerator-based radiosurgery for intracranial meningiomas. Neurosurgery. 1998;42(3):446–54.

74. Chung LK, Mathur I, Lagman C, et al. Stereotactic radiosurgery versus fractionated stereotactic radiotherapy in benign meningioma. J Clin Neurosci. 2017;36:1–5.

75. Pollock BE, Stafford SL, Utter A, et al. Stereotactic radiosurgery provides equivalent tumor control to Simpson grade 1 resection for patients with small-to medium-size meningiomas. Int J Radiat Oncol Biol Phys. 2003;55(4):1000–5.

76. Tdvorak. Meningioma, MRI T1 with contrast, sagittal. Wikimedia Commons. Retrieved from: https://commons.wikimedia.org/wiki/File:Tumor_Meningioma3.JPG.

77. Adler JR Jr, Gibbs IC, Puataweepong P, et al. Visual field preservation after multisession cyberknife radiosurgery for perioptic lesions. Neurosurgery. 2006;59(2):244–54.

78. Puataweepong P, Dhanachai M, Hansasuta A, et al. The clinical outcome of hypofractionated stereotactic radiotherapy with cyberknife robotic radiosurgery for perioptic pituitary adenoma. Technol Cancer Res Treat. 2016;15(6):NP10–5.

79. Runge MJ, Maarouf M, Hunsche S, et al. LINAC-radiosurgery for nonsecreting pituitary adenomas. Strahlenther Onkol. 2012;188(4):319–27.

80. Wilson PJ, De-Loyde KJ, Williams JR, et al. A single centre's experience of stereotactic radiosurgery and radiotherapy for non-functioning pituitary adenomas with the Linear Accelerator (Linac). J Clin Neurosci. 2012;19(3):370–4.

81. Mitsumori M, Shrieve DC, Alexander E, et al. Initial clinical results of LINAC-based stereotactic radiosurgery and stereotactic radiotherapy for pituitary adenomas. Int J Radiat Oncol Biol Phys. 1998;42(3):573–80.

82. Yoon SC, Suh TS, Jang HS, et al. Clinical results of 24 pituitary macroadenomas with linac-based stereotactic radiosurgery. Int J Radiat Oncol Biol Phys. 1998;41(4):849–53.

83. Iwata H, Sato K, Tatewaki K, et al. Hypofractionated stereotactic radiotherapy with CyberKnife for nonfunctioning pituitary adenoma: high local control with low toxicity. Neuro Oncol. 2011;13(8):916–22.

84. Posner J, Chernik N. Intracranial metastases from systemic cancer. Adv Neurol. 1978;19:579–92.

85. Takakura K. Metastatic tumors of the central nervous system. Tokyo: Igaku-Shoin Medical Publishers; 1982.

86. Nayak L, Lee EQ, Wen PY. Epidemiology of brain metastases. Curr Oncol Rep. 2012;14(1):48–54.

87. Gaspar L, Scott C, Rotman M, et al. Recursive partitioning analysis (RPA) of prognostic factors in three radiation therapy oncol-

ogy group (RTOG) brain metastases trials. Int J Radiat Oncol Biol Phys. 1997;37(4):745–51.

88. Sperduto PW, Yang TJ, Beal K, et al. Estimating survival in patients with lung cancer and brain metastases: an update of the graded prognostic assessment for lung cancer using molecular markers (lung-molGPA). JAMA Oncol. 2017;3(6):827–31.

89. Yamamoto M, Serizawa T, Shuto T, et al. Stereotactic radiosurgery for patients with multiple brain metastases (JLGK0901): a multi-institutional prospective observational study. Lancet Oncol. 2014;15(4):387–95.

90. Scorsetti M, Navarria P, Ascolese A, et al. OS03.4 Gammaknife versus Linac based (EDGE) radiosurgery (SRS) for patients with limited brain metastases (BMS) from different solid tumor: a phase III randomized trial. Neuro Oncol. 2017;19(suppl_3):iii5–6.

91. Souhami L, Seiferheld W, Brachman D, et al. Randomized comparison of stereotactic radiosurgery followed by conventional radiotherapy with carmustine to conventional radiotherapy with carmustine for patients with glioblastoma multiforme: report of radiation therapy oncology group 93-05 protocol. Int J Radiat Oncol Biol Phys. 2004;60(3):853–60.

92. Cardinale R, Won M, Choucair A, et al. A phase II trial of accelerated radiotherapy using weekly stereotactic conformal boost for supratentorial glioblastoma multiforme: RTOG 0023. Int J Radiat Oncol Biol Phys. 2006;65(5):1422–8.

93. Redmond KJ, Mehta M. Stereotactic radiosurgery for Glioblastoma. Cureus. 2015;7(12):e413.

94. Gagliardi F, Bailo M, Spina A, et al. Gamma knife radiosurgery for low-grade Gliomas: clinical results at long-term follow-up of tumor control and Patients' quality of life. World Neurosurg. 2017;101:540–53.

95. Heppner PA, Sheehan JP, Steiner LE. Gamma knife surgery for low-grade gliomas. Neurosurgery. 2005;57(6):1132–9. discussion

96. Barcia JA, Barcia-Salorio JL, Ferrer C, et al. Stereotactic radiosurgery of deeply seated low grade gliomas. Acta Neurochir Suppl. 1994;62:58–61.

97. Simonova G, Novotny J Jr, Liscak R. Low-grade gliomas treated by fractionated gamma knife surgery. J Neurosurg. 2005;102(Suppl):19–24.

98. Krane KS, Halliday D. Introductory nuclear physics. New York: Wiley; 1988.

99. Kramers HA. XCIII. On the theory of X-ray absorption and of the continuous X-ray spectrum. Lond Edinb Dubl Phil Mag Sci. 1923;46(275):836–71.

100. Fu W, Dai J, Hu Y, et al. Delivery time comparison for intensity-modulated radiation therapy with/without flattening filter: a planning study. Phys Med Biol. 2004;49(8):1535.

101. Vassiliev ON, Titt U, Pönisch F, et al. Dosimetric properties of photon beams from a flattening filter free clinical accelerator. Phys Med Biol. 2006;51(7):1907.

102. Prendergast BM, Popple RA, Clark GM, et al. Improved clinical efficiency in CNS stereotactic radiosurgery using a flattening filter free linear accelerator. J Radiosurg SBRT. 2011;1(2):117–22.

103. Thomas EM, Popple RA, Prendergast BM, et al. Effects of flattening filter-free and volumetric-modulated arc therapy delivery on treatment efficiency. J Appl Clin Med Phys. 2013;14(6):155–66.

104. Abacioglu U, Ozen Z, Yilmaz M, et al. Critical appraisal of RapidArc radiosurgery with flattening filter free photon beams for benign brain lesions in comparison to GammaKnife: a treatment planning study. Radiat Oncol. 2014;9(1):119.

105. Gasic D, Ohlhues L, Brodin NP, et al. A treatment planning and delivery comparison of volumetric modulated arc therapy with or without flattening filter for gliomas, brain metastases, prostate, head/neck and early stage lung cancer. Acta Oncol. 2014;53(8):1005–11.

106. Stieler F, Fleckenstein J, Simeonova A, et al. Intensity modulated radiosurgery of brain metastases with flattening filter-free beams. Radiother Oncol. 2013;109(3):448–51.

107. Hoogeman MS, Nuyttens JJ, Levendag PC, et al. Time dependence of intrafraction patient motion assessed by repeat stereoscopic imaging. Int J Radiat Oncol Biol Phys. 2008;70(2):609–18.

108. Kim J, Hsia A, Xu Z, et al. Motion likelihood over spine radiosurgery treatments—an intrafraction motion analysis. Int J Radiat Oncol Biol Phys. 2017;99((2):E678.

109. Sharma SD. Unflattened photon beams from the standard flattening filter free accelerators for radiotherapy: advantages, limitations and challenges. J Med Phys. 2011;36(3):123.

110. Pasquier D, Dubus F, Castelain B, et al. Repositioning accuracy of cerebral fractionated stereotactic radiotherapy using CT scanning. Cancer Radiother. 2009;13(5):446–50.

111. Dhabaan A, Schreibmann E, Siddiqi A, et al. Six degrees of freedom CBCT-based positioning for intracranial targets treated with frameless stereotactic radiosurgery. J Appl Clin Med Phys. 2012;13(6):215–25.

112. World Health Organization (WHO). Quality assurance in radiotherapy. Geneva, Switzerland: WHO; 1988.

113. Kutcher GJ, Coia L, Gillin M, et al. Comprehensive QA for radiation oncology: report of AAPM radiation therapy committee task group 40. Med Phys. 1994;21(4):581–618.

114. Schell M, Bova F, Larson D, et al. Aapm report number 54: Stereotactic radiosurgery, report of task group 42. American Institute of Physics. 1995.

115. Niroomand-Rad A, Blackwell CR, Coursey BM, et al. Radiochromic film dosimetry: recommendations of AAPM radiation therapy committee task group 55. Med Phys. 1998;25(11):2093–115.

116. Lightstone A, Benedict SH, Bova FJ, et al. Intracranial stereotactic positioning systems: report of the american association of physicists in medicine radiation therapy committee task group no. 68. Med Phys. 2005;32(7):2380–98.

117. Klein EE, Hanley J, Bayouth J, et al. Task group 142 report: quality assurance of medical accelerators. Med Phys. 2009;36(9):4197–212.

118. Benedict SH, Yenice KM, Followill D, et al. Stereotactic body radiation therapy: the report of AAPM task group 101. Med Phys. 2010;37(8):4078–101.

119. Solberg TD, Balter JM, Benedict SH, et al. Quality and safety considerations in stereotactic radiosurgery and stereotactic body radiation therapy: executive summary. Pract Radiat Oncol. 2012;2(1):2–9.

120. Liu D, Mutanga T. Poster-44: development and implementation of a comprehensive end-to-end testing methodology for linac-based frameless SRS QA using a modified commercial stereotactic anthropomorphic phantom. Med Phys. 2016;43(8):4946–7.

121. Calusi S, Noferini L, Marrazzo L, et al. γTools: a modular multifunction phantom for quality assurance in GammaKnife treatments. Phys Med. 2017;43:34–42.

122. Cabacés LP, Kolster IS, Olmos CP. Evaluation of positioning uncertainty for frameless radiosurgery for three IGRT methods with a head phantom. Phys Med. 2016;32:302–3.

123. Wen N, Li H, Song K, et al. Characteristics of a novel treatment system for linear accelerator–based stereotactic radiosurgery. J Appl Clin Med Phys. 2015;16(4):125–48.

124. Soisson ET, Hardcastle N, Tomé WA. Quality assurance of an image guided intracranial stereotactic positioning system for radiosurgery treatment with helical tomotherapy. J Neurooncol. 2010;98(2):277–85.

125. Choi D, Gordon I, Ghebremedhin A, et al. SU-E-T-268: proton radiosurgery end-to-end testing using lucy 3D QA phantom. Med Phys. 2014;41(6):285.

# Gamma Knife® Stereotactic Radiosurgery and Hypo-Fractionated Stereotactic Radiotherapy

# 45

Dheerendra Prasad

## Learning Objectives

- Understand the technology and technique of Gamma Knife radiosurgery.
- Develop a framework for planning a radiosurgery case.
- Understand dose prescription guidelines and the key Gamma Knife literature supporting them.

## Description and Evolution of Modality

Swedish neurosurgeon, Lars Leksell, proposed the concept of stereotactic radiosurgery [1] as the use of stereotactically directed ionizing beams to ablate intracranial targets in 1951. Sixteen years later, together with physicist Börje Larsson [2], he completed the design of the Leksell Gamma Knife(LGK) as a dedicated tool to perform brain radiosurgery. The LGK in all its various models consists of a number of independent $Co^{60}$ sources that emit gamma radiation in the 1.1 MeV range that are focused through a series of collimators to one focal point (isocenter). The diameter of the isovolume created by the cross-firing of approximately 200 beams can be varied from 4 to 16 mm (18 mm in the early models). Treatment plans are generated by superimposing multiple such dose clouds creating a multi-isocenter dose plan. The target is then stereotactically aligned with the focal point of the unit, and treatment delivery is one isocenter at a time.

The key features of the LGK and the evolution of the technology over the various models are summarized in Fig. 45.1.

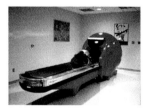
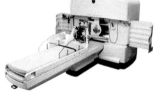
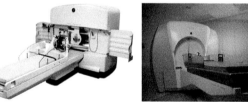
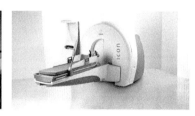

Model U
- Brought the technology to USA
- Totally manual device
- Core idea of fixed target fixed source

Model 4C
- Robotic auto positioning of patient
- Semi-automated
- Core idea of fixed target fixed source
- Allowed increased conformaliity of plans by making it easy to traet multiple isocenters

Prefexion
- Auto positioning plus auto collimation switching
- Fully automated
- Core idea of fixed target fixed source
- Further improvement in conformality and plan quality with use of sectors
- Enhanced radiation safety

Icon
- Integrated imaging and frame and frameless option
- Fully automated
- Core idea of fixed target fixed source
- Permits new workflows
- Onboard imaging and patient motion monitoring with gating

**Fig. 45.1** Key technological highlights for various models of the Leksell Gamma Knife arranged chronologically from left to right

D. Prasad
Department of Radiation Medicine and Neurosurgery, Roswell Park Comprehensive Cancer Center, Buffalo, NY, USA
e-mail: d.prasad@roswellpark.org

© Springer International Publishing AG, part of Springer Nature 2018
E. L. Chang et al. (eds.), *Adult CNS Radiation Oncology*, https://doi.org/10.1007/978-3-319-42878-9_45

## Immobilization Techniques and Image Guidance

Precise delivery of the treatment plan is dependent on the ability of the system to localize the target in stereotactic coordinate space. This requires immobilization of the patient. There are two immobilization techniques that can be used with the LGK: the Leksell stereotactic frame and a thermoplastic mask.

## Leksell Stereotactic Frame

Originally designed for stereotactic neurosurgery, this device is made of high-grade anodized aluminum and uses a Cartesian coordinate system to localize targets in stereotactic space (Fig. 45.2). The coordinates are expressed as a triplet of $x$, $y$, and $z$. The origin of the coordinate system (0,0,0) is on the right—superior—posterior aspect of the skull. The $x$-axis runs from the right to the left; the $y$-axis runs from posterior to anterior and the $z$-axis from superior to inferior. The center of the coordinate system has a value of 100,100,100.

Using the frame provides a very high level of accuracy allowing the device to perform at its calibrated specification which is always better than 0.3 mm. Inaccuracy in imaging and frame displacement as a result of improper application are the major sources of error with this setup.

## Thermoplastic Mask

With the LGK Icon®, it is possible to immobilize the patient using thermoplastic mask and a deformable at cushion (Fig. 45.3). This fixation system permits single as well as hypo-fractionated stereotactic treatments with the Gamma Knife. Stereotactic coordinates are obtained by performing a cone beam computerized tomography (CBCT) using the onboard CBCT system.

## Cone Beam CT

The CBCT in the ICON is integrated into the patient positioning and source unit as one rigid entity. This makes it operate in true Leksell coordinate space—and every voxel in the reconstructed image has known Leksell coordinates, requiring a transformation along only the $z$-axis, while determining true $x$ and $y$ coordinates. This distinguishes it from all other image guidance systems in use. The unit operates at two different computerized tomography dose index (CTDI) settings 2.5 mGy and 6.3 mGy. It is customary to use the higher CTDI setting for the localizing scan when the co-registration is being performed to a pre-planning MRI, allowing more detail for mutual information matching. The lower CTDI setting is used for the daily delivery CBCT which is co-registered to the reference CT.

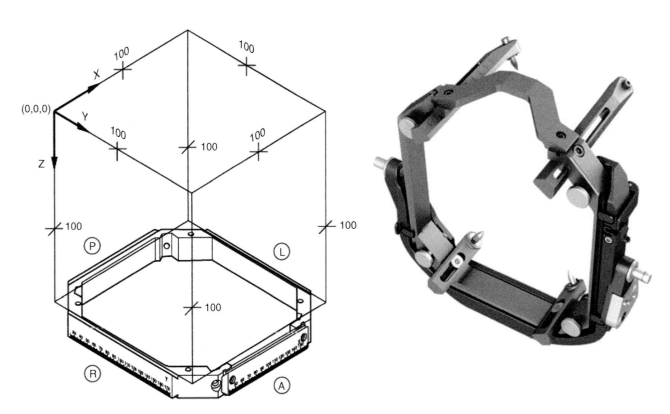

**Fig. 45.2** Leksell coordinate space and the Leksell stereotactic frame model G. [Courtesy of Elekta]

Accuracy of the CBCT system has been verified experimentally (Dalhalwi) and shows excellent concordance with frame-based coordinates in phantom studies. Insert error values here.

## Intra-Fraction Motion Management

In order to ensure "intra-fraction patient position" when a thermoplastic mask is in use, a high-definition motion management system (HDMM) is coupled with the thermoplastic mask (Fig. 45.4). The HDMM uses an infrared reflective marker placed on the nose and tracked by an infrared camera

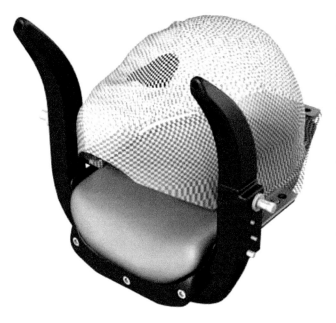

**Fig. 45.3** Thermoplastic mask, moldable cushion, and cradle for hypo-fractionated treatments. [Courtesy of Elekta]

relative to static reflectors located on the patient head cradle. A motion trace for the marker is then displayed on the operator console allowing the operator to set a tolerance level for the maximum deviation of the patient from the initial position. The system automatically suspends (gates) delivery of radiation if the patient exceeds the programmed tolerance. Should the patient return within tolerance in a predefined time interval, treatment delivery will continue; however, if the patient remains out of position for a single or repeated periods exceeding 20 s, then the treatment is interrupted and the patient is ejected from the machine. The operator then decides whether to override the deviation or to perform a new cone beam CT and realign the patient for continued delivery. In practice with a cooperative patient, it is not unusual to have deviations of the nasal marker less than 0.5 mm. Most patients can be delivered to treatment with nose marker deviations under 1.5 mm. It should be pointed out that the marker on the nose is a surrogate for target position, and the relative target deviation depends on target location in the brain. Based on studies conducted on a test system, the corresponding deviation at the target was on average half of that displayed as the nose marker deviation.

## Treatment Planning

Treatment planning for the LGK is performed on a dedicated planning system—Leksell Gamma Plan®—and can be performed manually, semiautomatically as a forward plan with optimization assistance or as a fully automated inverse plan.

At the outset, it is important to understand that the treatment planning with LGK is more akin to brachytherapy rather than a conventional external beam plan. This is due to the fact that the plan is often multi-isocenter and comprised of multiple superimposed dose clouds, each with its own iso-

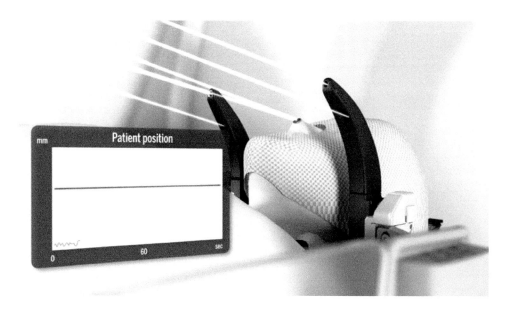

**Fig. 45.4** High-definition motion management for mask-based delivery with the LGK Icon®. [Courtesy of Elekta]

center called a "shot" in LGK parlance. The goal is to create a confluent dose cloud that conformally encloses the target. This fundamental aspect of an LGK plan makes it inherently more conformal but also more prone to heterogeneity. Another key difference from traditional IMRT and SRS plans on a LINAC-based system is the fact that dose is prescribed (or normalized) to isodose lines varying from 90% to 30% (with the mode and median prescription IDL in plans being the 50%). This derives from the fact that the LGK dose profile offers the steepest dose gradient between the 40% and 55% isodose lines based on its physical design characteristics.

## Typical Dose Distribution

At initial loading, LGK houses upward of 6000 curies of radioactivity and a resultant dose rate of 3.3–3.6 Gy/min. Based on the collimator output factors, this dose rate is modified by a factor of 0.8–1.0 for the three collimators 4, 8, and 16 mm. Their numeric designation refers to the diameter in mm of the 80% isovolume of a single shot of a given size. Dose profiles are shown in Figs. 45.5 and 45.6, and typical dose distributions of the three collimators as depicted in Gamma Plan are shown in Fig. 45.7.

In practice the user has to develop a sense for the isovolume generated by each collimator in three dimen-

sions; since visual inspection is dependent on the magnification of the images being viewed, it is best to start by placing a test shot of a given size on the images in question.

When more than one isocenter/shot is present, the superimposed distribution depends on the size of collimators used and the separation between the isocenters. It is common practice to place adjacent shots such that they are overlapping. As shown in Fig. 45.8, the inter-isocenter distance has an effect on both the prescription isodose (yellow) and the appearance of cold and hot spots.

For the Perfexion and Icon models, sources are mounted in groups of 24 on movable conical sections called sectors. Each of the 8 sectors for a given isocenter can be configured to be blocked or open and collimated to the 4, 8, or 16 setting. Since the sectors are arranged along the z-axis, the most intuitive effect of blocking a single sector is in the axial (x–y) plane. The influence on the other planes is not intuitive and is illustrated in Fig. 45.9 since in those planes the skull geometry affects the dose rate from different sectors differently. In addition to choosing the size of the collimation, sector blocks and composite shots (with different collimator settings for different sectors) are other ways to creating shaped dose distributions.

Prescriptions for the LGK were historically normalized to the 50% IDL, but in fact as the more automated models of LGK became available and the number of isocenters used

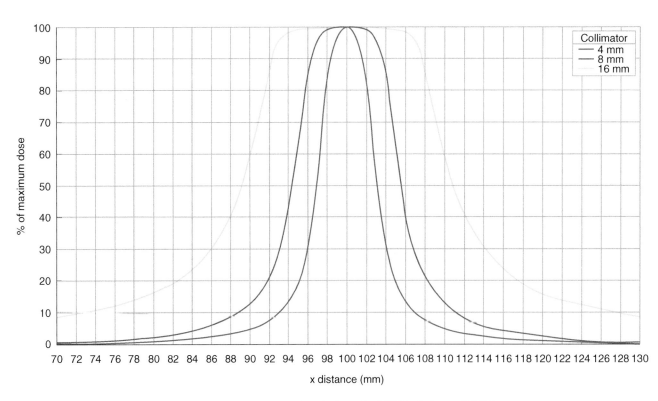

**Fig. 45.5** Dose profiles along x-axis for the three collimators 4, 8, and 16 mm for LGK Perfexion and ICON

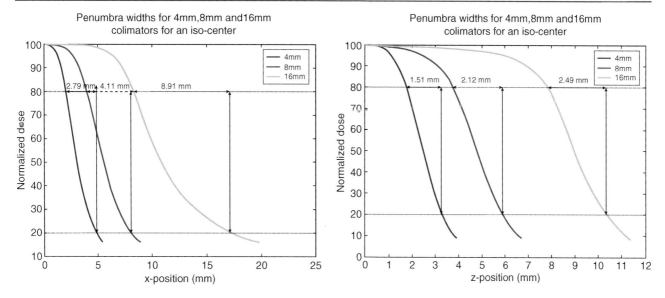

**Fig. 45.6** Penumbra widths for all sources combined for Leksell Gamma Knife Perfexion or ICON

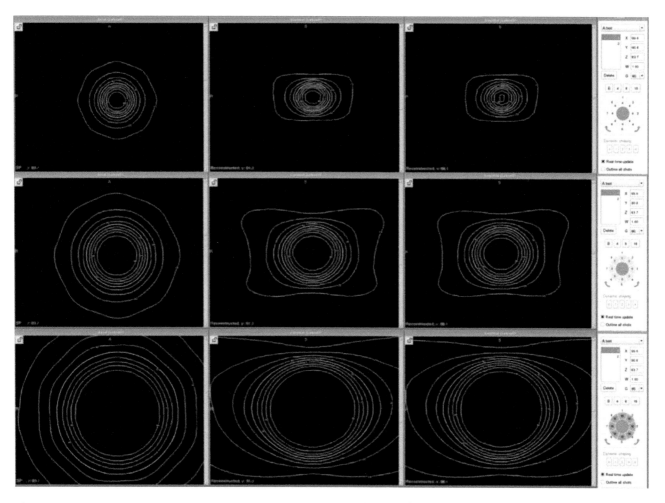

**Fig. 45.7** Typical dose distribution of single 4, 8, and 16 mm collimators. The isodose line in yellow is the 50%. Also represented are 10, 20, 30, 40, 60, 70, 80, and 90% isodose lines in green, axial plan is represented in the left-most column, coronal in the middle column, and sagittal in the right-most column

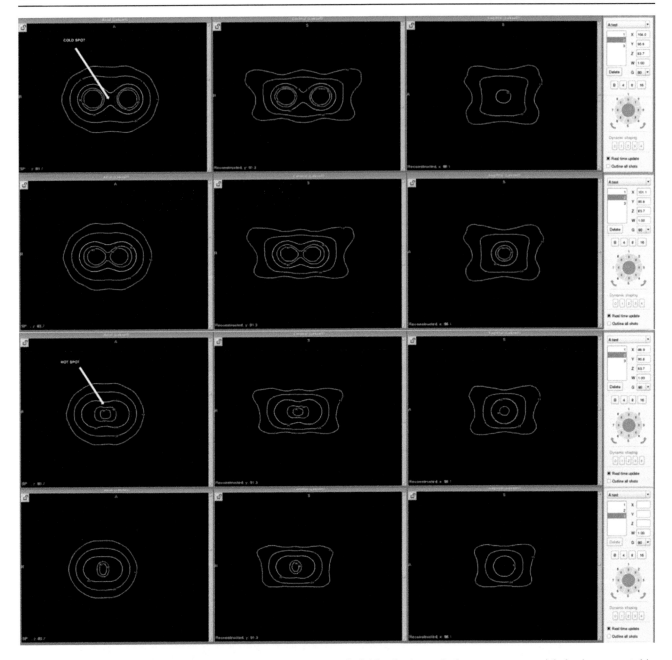

**Fig. 45.8** Two 8 mm collimator shots placed adjacent to each other will yield a resultant dose distribution with a cold spot if they are non-overlapping. As they are moved closer (top to bottom), the cold spot diminishes in size, and a hot spot appears, axial plan is represented in the left-most column, coronal in the middle column, and saggital in the right-most column

increased, this is no longer true. Once multiple isocenter penumbras are combined, the steepest gradient can actually fall anywhere in the 40–55% IDL range. As discussed later this effect will reflect itself in steeper dose gradients and lower values of gradient index with normalization to less than 50% IDL. Care must be exercised in recognizing that the associated peak dose prescription and mean energy delivered by the plan will increase (Fig. 45.10). This can have consequences on the target and its response to the treatment.

## Measures of Plan Quality

Before discussing planning and prescribing techniques with the LGK, it is important to discuss and define the parameters used to assess the quality of a dose plan.

*Coverage*: is defined as the proportion of the target volume (TV) that is covered by the prescription isodose volume (PIV), that is, Volume (PIV∩TV)/Volume (TV).

*Selectivity*: is defined as the proportion of the prescription isodose volume (PIV) that is inside the target volume (TV), that is, Volume (PIV∩TV)/Volume (PIV).

**Fig. 45.9** Influence of sector blocking on the dose distribution from a 4 mm collimator, illustrating the difference between sectors

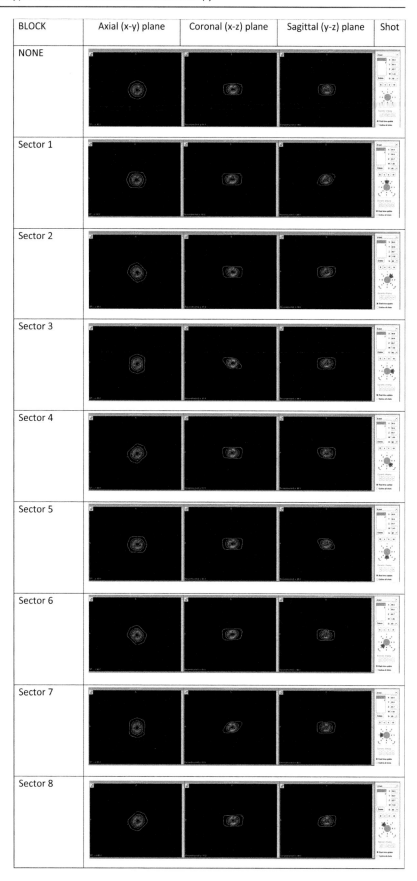

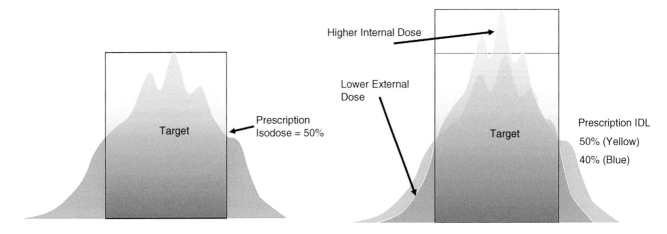

**Fig. 45.10** Dose profile along the long axis of a tumor demonstrating the impact of renormalization of the dose plan from the 50% IDL to the 40% IDL: steeper gradient in normal tissue and elevated hot spot in target. [Courtesy of Ian Paddick]

**Fig. 45.11** Dependence of the gradient index value on the prescription isodose line chosen

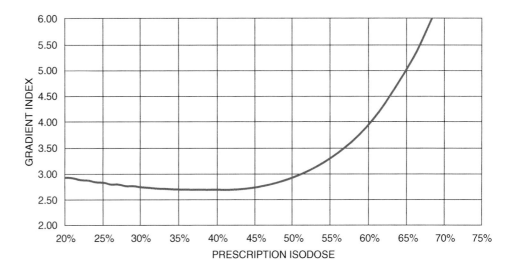

*Gradient Index*: is defined [3] as the quotient between the half-prescription isodose volume size and the prescription isodose volume size, that is, Volume (PIV25%)/Volume (PIV50%) if the planning isodose is 50%. Gradient index is commonly used to quantify the steepness of the dose falloff.

In addition, there are several measures of plan conformality:

*RTOG PITV ratio*: Defined by Shaw et al. [4], this is simply the ratio given by PIV/TV. It has the advantages of being easy to calculate. A value of >1 suggests a treatment volume that exceeds the target and implies irradiation of non-target surrounding tissue.

A value of <1 suggests a that treatment volume is smaller than the target and therefore indicates under-coverage of target. However, this ratio fails to reflect the actual overlap of the two volumes, leaving that determination to the planner.

*Paddick conformity index*: Defined by Paddick [5] this is calculated as the product of the coverage and selectivity. It is therefore $((PIV \cap TV)^2)/(PIV \times TV)$. It has a theoretical maximum value of 1. This index has the advantage of accounting

for the concordance between dose and target as well as being a number that ranges from 0 to 1.

When designing a dose plan, the planner strives to achieve coverage as close to 1 as possible, although in most clinical situations, any value greater than 0.95 is found to be acceptable. Likewise, selectivity should be maximized, and values in 0.75 are easy to achieve and a reasonable target for the plan. Coverage and selectivity are often inversely related to each other, particularly in irreglar targets. Clinical judgment should be exercised to decide the balance netween the two, as long as a minimum of 0.95 in coverage has been achieved.

The achievable gradient index (GI) has a theoretical limit based on the physical characteristics of the LGK around a value of 2.5. The factors that determine the GI include number and size of collimators used as well as the IDL to which the dose is prescribed. For example, in the curve shown in Fig. 45.11 based on one plan shows that the lowest GI would correspond to the 40% IDL. In addition to the global dose gradient, local gradients close to critical structures are also important for treatment plan quality assessment.

## Forward Planning

The process of forward planning begins by delineating a target volume and designating it as such in the planning system. The user then sets a dose grid (called target or matrix) centered on the desired target. There is a separate grid on each target in the dose plan such as in multiple metastases.

The dose plan is then constructed by placing individual shots of varying collimator size and or composite shots in the target. The dose filling strategy varies greatly by operator and both "center out" and "periphery in" filling paradigms are used. In general, while the largest collimator provides the most coverage, it can also provide the sloppiest dose gradient in normal tissue. Thus, an efficient dose plan includes large collimators used away from critical structures and smaller

collimators closer to critical structures. Fig. 45.12 demonstrates the construction of a dose plan for a cavernous sinus meningioma.

## Optimizer-Assisted Forward Planning

The optimizer provided with LGP uses a cost function for optimization. The values of this cost function lie between 0 and 1, and the higher the value, the better the plan quality. The equation for the cost function is:

$$F = \frac{c^{\min(2\alpha,1)} s^{\min((2-2\alpha),1)} + \beta G + \gamma T}{1 + \beta + \gamma}$$

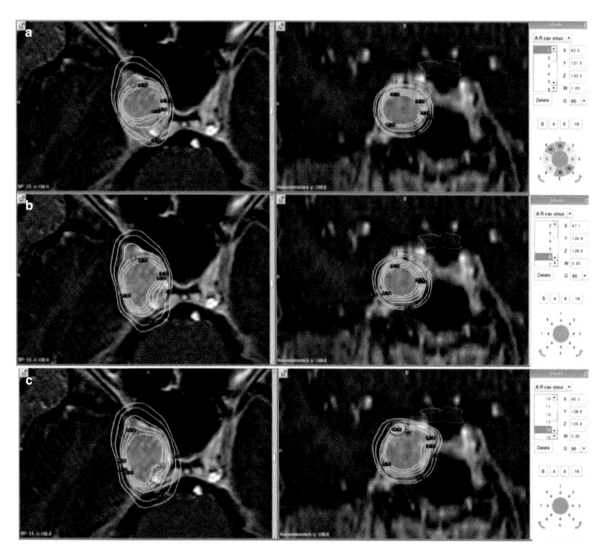

**Fig. 45.12** Development of a forward dose plan for a right cavernous sinus meningioma. The plan begins (**a**) with the a composite 8 and 16 mm shot placed in the center of the tumor (shown are the axial, coronal, and shot configuration representations of the plan), followed by the addition of other shots (**b** and **c**) and the final dose plan in axial and coronal views (**d**) and sagittal and 3D representations (**e**). Note that doses are depicted in Gy. The isodose lines represented in green from outside in are 8, 10, 16, 18, and 20 Gy. The prescription line is 14 Gy shown in yellow. Target volume – red and optic chiasm and pathway (pink)

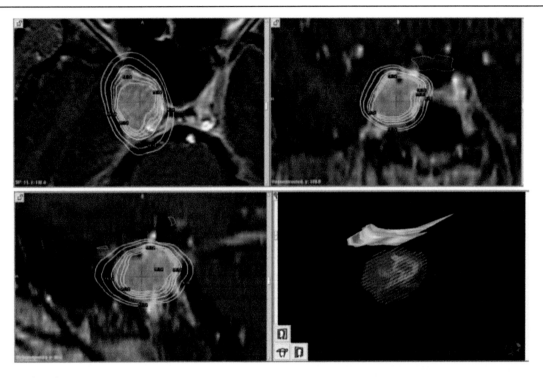

**Fig. 45.12** (continued)

*c* is the target coverage, and *s* is the selectivity (defined previously).

$\alpha$, $\beta$, and $\gamma$ are weights between 0 and 1, set by the user.

*G* and *T* are functions whose values lie between 0 and 1 that describe how "good" the gradient index, *g*, and treatment time, *t*, are. ($G = 1$ if $g < 2.6$, $G = 0$ if $g > 6$ & $T = 1$ if $t < 0.25\ T_0$, $T = 0$ if $T > 1.5\ T_0$, where $T_0$ is the beam-on time at the start of the optimization).

$\alpha$, $\beta$, and $\gamma$ are set by the user with interactive sliders in the inverse planning settings dialog box (Fig. 45.13). The coverage and selectivity sliders are interconnected since they visually reflect the effect of the $\alpha$ parameter which drives the c and s variables in the cost function. The gradient index slider is the $\beta$ parameter and drives the G parameter. Beam-on time represents the $\gamma$ parameter and drives the T function.

Default settings in LGP are $\alpha = 0.5$, $\beta = 0.25$, and $\gamma = 0$. Therefore, if no changes are made, then the cost function ignores the time of plan delivery and concentrates on a good balance of selectivity and coverage with a gradient index which is as low as possible. The algorithm for optimization can change the already placed shots by the user and can even delete shots that are deemed redundant, using simulated annealing to maximize the cost function. The user can restrict the system from changing the manual plan in various ways. It is recommended that optimization be performed on a plan copy. If the lock positions and lock collimator settings boxes are checked (Fig. 45.13), then the only possible changes to the plan that the optimizer can make are shot weights. It is unlikely that this strategy will yield a big improvement in the plan. When only "lock collimator settings" is checked, the planning system will optimize the position and weights of the shots and will weight shots that are not necessary to zero.

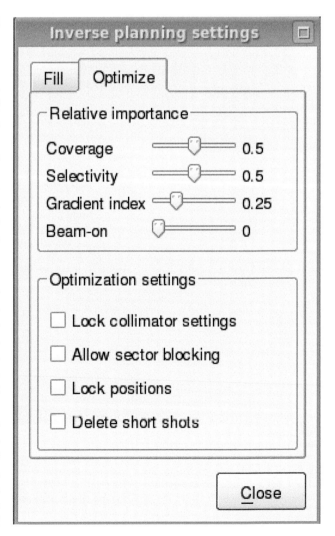

**Fig. 45.13** Options in the inverse planning dialog for Leksell Gamma Plan

This is perhaps the most useful setting for small to mid-size targets where the planner is seeking to optimally place a few shots. It is possible to use this function repeatedly at various stages of the plan as one places for instance different size collimators. When no boxes are checked, the optimizer will introduce composite shots, and while the global dose gradient may improve, the user should evaluate the result with the lower isodose lines displayed so as to prevent locally sloppy gradients in high-risk areas since the optimizer does not take into account avoidance structures. At this stage, no sectors (other than those that were manually blocked by the user) will be blocked by the optimizer. Allowing sector blocking enables that functionality. It is important to reiterate that sector blocking usually negatively impacts gradient – as does normalization to a higher isodose line.

Choosing optimization parameters is often a personal matter and depends on the manner in which the shots are placed by the user and the individualized planning goals for the case in question. Table 45.1 enumerates typical settings for various targets.

## Inverse Planning

Inverse planning requires no a priori placement of shots and uses the fill function of the program before using the optimization techniques described above. The fill dialog (Fig. 45.14) has a few options. The user can choose to use composite collimators or simple collimators. By unchecking the composite box, the dialog changes to display the 3 collimators 16, 8, and 4 and allows the user to decide which collimators are likely to best suit the plan intent.

If composite collimators are allowed, then the software uses the size slider as a guide to choosing composite sectors.

**Table 45.1** Optimizer settings for various targets to obtain the best results with inverse planning with Gamma Plan

| Target | Optimizer settings | | | Optimizer solution | | |
| --- | --- | --- | --- | --- | --- | --- |
| | Coverage /Selectivity | Gradient index | Time | Acceptable coverage | Acceptable selectivity | Acceptable gradient |
| Vestibular schwannoma | 0.5/0.5 | 0.25–0.4 | 0 | > 0.95 | > 0.85 | 2.5–2.8 |
| Cavern. Sinus meningioma | 0.5/0.5 | 0.25–0.4 | 0 | > 0.95 | > 0.85 | 2.5–2.8 |
| Convexity meningioma | 0.6/0.4 | 0.25 | 0.3 | > 0.95 | > 0.7 | 2.5–3.2 |
| Atypical meningioma | 0.8/0.2 | 0.25 | 0.3 | >0.95 | >0.6 | 2.5–4 |
| Large metastasis | 0.7/0.3 | 0.25 | 0.2 | >0.95 | >0.6 | 2.5–4 |
| Small metastasis | 0.6/0.4 | 0.25 | 0 | 1 | >0.6 | 3–7[a] |
| Surgical cavity-metastatic | 0.7/0.3 | 0.25 | 0.2 | >0.95 | >0.6 | 2.5–4 |

[a]Often prescribed to isodose lines higher than 50% and therefore the achievable gradient index is higher

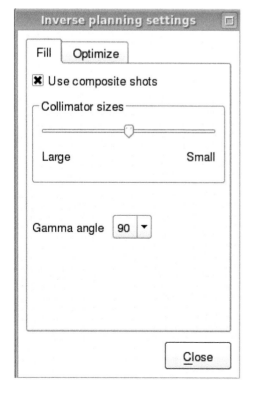
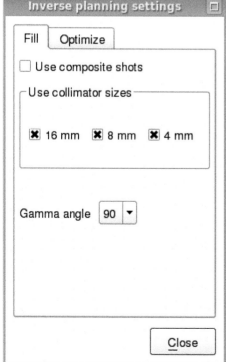

**Fig. 45.14**   The fill dialog

If set to small, then there are unlikely to be size 16 sectors in the placed shots. The program uses a bevy of preconfigured shot templates to fill, starting from the periphery and then populating the center. It initially places the shots without overlap of their 50% isovolume. The final setting is the gamma angle that can be chosen for patient docking based on lesion location and frame placement to avoid collisions (only usable with the stereotactic frame). Once shot filling is completed, the optimizer is used to optimize the dose plan as described in the previous section. Finally, manual placement of shots and or manipulation of the existing shots may be required to complete the process.

## Dose Specification

Traditionally dose prescriptions with the LGK are defined as the minimum dose or dose to the margin of the target along with the percent IDL to which it is normalized. The corresponding maximum and mean doses while recorded are not used in publications when discussing efficacy and side effects. The exception to this pattern are functional targets where it is customary to prescribe the maximum dose to a point (given dose). Care must be taken not to confuse the two approaches to prescription.

## Single Session: SRS

The doses used in single session radiosurgery are well worked out in LGK literature, and representative range is presented in Table 45.2. The outcomes of GKRS for vestibular schwannoma (Table 45.3), meningioma

**Table 45.2** Representative single session dose ranges by pathology

| Diagnosis | Dose in Gy (Modal prescription) | References |
|---|---|---|
| Vestibular schwannoma | 11–13 (12) | [6–18] |
| Meningioma | 10–20 (15) | [19–49] |
| Pituitary adenoma: Nonsecretory | 12–17 (15) | [24, 50–57] |
| Pituitary adenoma: Secretory | 22–28 | [24, 50–57] |
| Craniopharyngioma | 10–15 | [24, 58–61] |
| Low grade astrocytoma | 12–15 | [24, 62–68] |
| High-grade glioma | 17–20 | [68–72] |
| Metastatic tumor | 16–24 | [24, 73–92] |
| Metastatic tumor plus whole brain RT | 16–18 | [24, 73–92] |
| Glomus tumor | 15 | [93–96] |
| Other cranial schwannomas | 12–14 | [97–105] |
| Chordoma/Chondrosarcoma | 17–22 | [106] |

**Table 45.3** Outcomes for vestibular schwannomas treated with single-fraction GKRS

| Study | Number of patients | % with local control | % Facial nerve morbidity | % Loss of hearing |
|---|---|---|---|---|
| Lunsford [6] | 829 | 97 | 1 | 21 |
| Regis [7] | 1000 | 97 | 1.3 | 22 |
| Landy [8] | 34 | 97 | 0 | 0 |
| Rowe [9] | 234 | 92 | 1 | 25 |
| Iwai [10] | 51 | 96 | 0 | 41 |
| Unger [11] | 100 | 96 | 2 | 45 |
| Litvack [12] | 134 | 97 | 0 | 38 |
| Petit [13] | 45 | 96 | 0 | 12 |
| Bertallanfy [14] | 32 | 91 | 12.5 | 21 |
| Prasad [15] | 153 | 92 | 2 | 35 |
| Lisˇcˇák [16] | 122 | 96 | 1.9 | 17 |
| Kwon [17] | 63 | 95 | 5 | 33 |
| Norén [18] | 669 | 95 | 2 | 30 |

**Table 45.4** Tumor control rates for radiosurgery for meningiomas

| Series | Cases | Control % |
|---|---|---|
| Bir et al. [37] | 136 | 98 |
| Bledso e et al. [26] | 116 | 99 |
| Choi et al. [27] | 20 | 73 |
| Chung et al. [28] | 80 | 92 |
| Davidson et al. [29] | 36 | 95 |
| DiBiase et al. [38] | 137 | 86 |
| Feigl et al. [39] | 211 | 86 |
| Franzin et al. [30] | 123 | 91 |
| Hasegawa et al. [31] | 119 | 87 |
| Jo et al. [32] | 69 | 100 |
| Kano et al. [40] | 272 | 96 |
| Kondziolka et al. [33] | 488 | 95 |
| Kreil et al. [41] | 200 | 99 |
| Massager et al. [34] | 120 | 93 |
| Metellus et al. [35] | 36 | 94 |
| Park et al. [42] | 74 | 98 |
| Park et al. [43] | 39 | 92 |
| Pollock et al. [36] | 416 | 96 |
| Sheehan et al. [44] | 575 | 81 |
| Shin et al. [45] | 36 | 91 |
| Starke et al. [46] | 255 | 99 |
| Williams et al. [47] | 138 | 100 |
| Zada et al. [48] | 116 | 100 |
| Zenonos et al. [49] | 23 | 91 |

(Table 45.4), and metastatic tumors (Table 45.5) are provided for reference.

## Multisession SRS (Hypo-Fractionated SRT)

With the introduction of the LGK Icon, it has become more practical to perform multisession SRS (hypo-fractionated SRT), although frame-based hypo-fractionation has been

**Table 45.5**  Outcomes for metastatic tumors treated with single session SRS with GK

| Study | Number of patients | Tumor control rate (%) | Origin |
| --- | --- | --- | --- |
| Gerosa  et al. [73] | 225 | 88 | All |
| Shiau  et al. [74] | 100 | 77 | All |
| Kim  et al. [75] | 77 | 85 | Lung carcinoma |
| Wowra et al. [24, 76] | 126 | 89 | All |
| Mori  et al. [77] | 60 | 88 | Melanoma |
| Mori et al. [78] | 35 | 90 | Renal cell |
| Seung  et al. [79] | 55 | 89 | Melanoma |
| Chen  et al. [80] | 190 | 89 | All |
| Muacevic  et al. [81] | 56 | 83 | All |
| Sneed  et al. [82] | 105 | 71 | All |
| Lavine  et al. [83] | 45 | 97 | Melanoma |
| Sansur  et al. [84] | 173 | 82 | All |
| Amendola  et al. [85] | 68 | 94 | Breast cancer |
| Simonova  et al. [86] | 237 | 91 | All |
| Schöggl  et al. [87] | 67 | 95 | All |
| Firlik  et al. [88] | 30 | 93 | Breast cancer |
| Sheehan  et al. [89] | 273 | 84 | Lung cancer |
| Muacevic  et al. [90] | 151 | 94 | Breast cancer |
| Lippitz  et al. 2004 [91] | 15 | 89 | All |
| Mix et al. [92] | 214 | 87 | Breast |

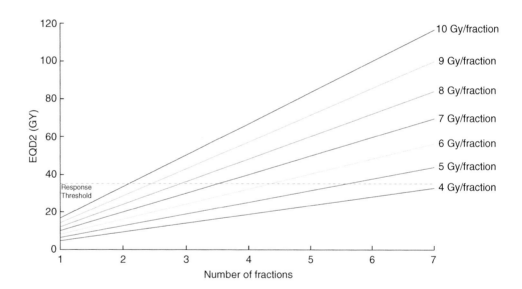

**Fig. 45.15**  Threshold EQD2 based on Martens et al. [108] for local control plotted against different fractionation schemes

performed both with the traditional frame and the Extend® frame.

Using the extend system, McTyre et al. [107] reported 34 cases where they used hypo-fractionation for benign tumors >10 cc in volume or abutting the optic pathway, vestibular schwannoma with the intent of hearing preservation, or a tumor previously irradiated with single-fraction GKRS.

The most challenging aspect of hypo-fractionation is developing an understanding of iso-effective doses with different fractionation schemes in the face of limited literature. One approach is to calculate the equivalent dose in 2 Gy fractions used in standard fractionation the

EQD2. Martens et al. [108] reported a significant difference in median LC 14.9 months for EQD2 > 35 Gy and 3.4 months for EQD2 ≤ 35 Gy($p < 0.004$). In order to allow the reader a quick tool to decide the number and size of fractional doses that will exceed this threshold, Fig. 45.15 is useful.

In single session, the threshold EQD2 dose is exceeded by a dose of 17 Gy, but it takes 2 fractions of 10 Gy, 3 of 8 Gy, and so on to achieve the same EQD2. In more general terms, the most common doses used in treating metastatic tumors can be plotted against the EQD2 for various dose fractionation schemes as shown in Fig. 45.16.

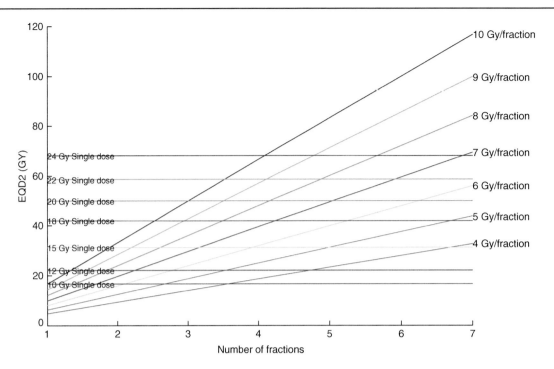

**Fig. 45.16** Single doses commonly used for treating brain metastasis (assume alpha beta ratio of 10) and fractionated schemes using EQD2. This chart is provided as a quick tool and should be used in conjunction with clinical judgment with the understanding that radiobiologic modeling is an imperfect science

**Table 45.6** Outcomes of hypo-fractionated treatment of brain metastases and/or surgical cavities

| Series | Patients (lesions) | Lesion size (median) | Fractionation | EQD2 tumor (Gy) | Local control | Reported toxicity % |
|---|---|---|---|---|---|---|
| Aoyama [109] | 87(159) | 3.3 cc | 8.75 Gy × 4 | 55 | 81% | 7 |
| Lindvall [110] | 47(47) | – | 8 Gy × 5 | 60 | 84% | 6.25 |
| Aoki [111] | 44(65) | – | 5–6 Gy × 3–5 | 19–30 | 72% | 2 |
| Fahrig [112] | 150(228) | 6.1 cc | 6–7 Gy × 5 | 30–50 | – | 22 |
| | | | 5 Gy × 7 | 44 | – | 7 |
| | | | 10 Gy × 4 | 67 | – | 0 |
| Narayana [113] | 20(20) | – | 6 Gy × 5 | 40 | 70% | 15 |
| Giubilei [114] | 30(44) | 2.1 cm/4.8 cc | 6 Gy × 3/ 8 Gy × 4 | 24/48 | 86% | – |
| Kwon [115] | 27(52) | 1.2 cm/0.5 cc | 20–35 Gy in 4–6 | 25–48 | 68% | 5.8 |
| Ogura [116] | 39(46) | 1.8 cm | 7 Gy × 5 or | 50 | 17% | 2.5 |
| | | | WBRT + 4–5 Gy × 5 | 31.2[a] | | |
| Wang [117] | 37(37) | Cavity > 3 cm | 8 Gy × 3 | 36 | 80% | 9 |
| DePotter [118] | 35(58) | 8.6 cc | WBRT + 6 Gy × 5 | 40[a] | 66% | 11 |
| Eaton et al. [119] | 42(42) | 3.9 cm 13.6 cc | 5–8 Gy × 3–5 | 31–36 | 62% | 7 |

[a]*BED of the hypo-fractionated course*

Hypo-fractionated treatment of brain metastasis has been reported by many authors using a wide variety of fractionation schemes and varied success and complication rates. These are summarized in Table 45.6.

## Treatment Delivery

Treatment delivery can follow one of several workflow patterns depending on the fixation used and the fractionation or single session model. It is also dependent on the model of LGK being used. For brevity, we will discuss workflows with the Perfexion and Icon units.

## Frame-Based SRS

The first step in the delivery of frame-based SRS on the day of treatment is the application of the Leksell stereotactic frame to the patients' head. This is performed as a clean or sterile procedure depending on the preference of the surgeon, under anxiolytics, or mild sedation in adults and general anesthesia in children. Local anesthetic is used at the four points on the scalp where the fixation screws penetrate the skin. Fixation is achieved with titanium screws (aluminum if only CT imaging will be used). Following frame application, a collision check cap is placed on the head to ensure that

**Fig. 45.17**   Treatment delivery in a frame-based linear workflow. Red ring indicates image that serves as source of stereotactic coordinates, and green ring is indicative of predelivery verification

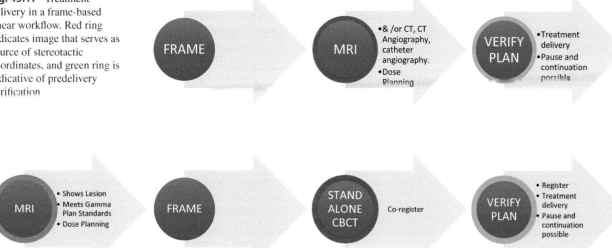

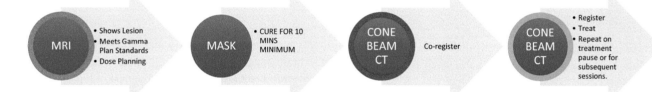

**Fig. 45.18**   Treatment delivery in a pre-imaging/pre-planning frame-based workflow. Orange ring indicates images that are used for getting the anatomical data for dose planning, red ring indicates image that serves as source of stereotactic coordinates, and green ring is indicative of predelivery verification

**Fig. 45.19**   Treatment delivery in a pre-imaging/pre-planning mask-based workflow. Orange ring indicates images that are used for getting the anatomical data for dose planning, red ring indicates image that serves as source of stereotactic coordinates, and green ring is indicative of predelivery verification

there is no risk of collision with the interior of the LGK in any desired target position.

In a linear workflow, this is followed by stereotactic MRI, CT, and catheter angiography as needed (Fig. 45.17). Since the frame limits the size of imaging coils that can be used with the MRI and the sequences that can be performed, sometimes it is preferred to perform the MRI imaging without a frame and co-registration with a frame-based CT (Perfexion), or onboard CBCT (Icon) is used to align the MRI into stereotactic space (Fig. 45.18).

## Mask-Based SRS or Hypo-Fractionated SRT

Planning for mask-based treatments is performed on MRI or diagnostic CT imaging which is obtained with at least one sequence covering the whole head with a slice including air at the top and is designated as the pre-plan reference. More specialized sequences that delineate anatomy relevant to the plan can be used by co-registration with the

pre-plan reference as long as the imaging covers at least a 50 mm thick slab of brain. Thermoplastic mask immobilization can be accomplished on the same day as treatment or prior to treatment. The stereotactic coordinates are obtained from the CBCT obtained at any point after the immobilization has been designed. These images are registered to the pre-plan allowing real Leksell coordinates to be acquired for the treatment plan. Prior to delivery of the actual treatment, several steps are required: (1) the HDMM (IFMM) nose marker has to be placed on the patient, (2) the HDMM camera has to be deployed, (3) the delivery fraction has to brought up on the console, and (4) one Gamma Plan station has to be in treatment mode. At this point a delivery CBCT is obtained and transferred to the Gamma Plan station in treatment mode. A co-registration window opens automatically and permits co-registration and verification of shifts. On accepting the shifts, a treatment evaluation window appears allowing the user to evaluate the influence of the repositioning on the dose plan. This can be viewed both for the current delivery as well as the cumulative delivery of all fractions delivered to that point in time. Since the shifts are applied, the comparison is made between the dynamic re-planned dose and the original plan. This workflow is illustrated in Fig. 45.19.

## Quality Assurance and AAPM Task Group

### Purpose

This section describes a procedure for investigating and verifying the precision of the dose delivery. Various factors may affect the dose distribution, such as the strength of each radiation source, the exact alignment to the collimator system, and the tolerances to which the collimators are manufactured.

### Method

In Leksell Gamma Knife®, with very steep dose gradients and complex geometry, it is recommended to use film dosimetry because of good spatial resolution and low energy dependence. Due to the designs with a large number of sources (201 sources for Leksell Gamma Knife® B, C, 4, and 4C and 192 sources for Leksell Gamma Knife® Perfexion™ and Leksell Gamma Knife® Icon™), it is not possible to measure and investigate the beams from every single source. For Leksell Gamma Knife® B, C, 4, and 4C, the transmission through the collimator helmet would be too high, and more than 50 beams are required to have an excessive transmission of less than 1%. For Leksell Gamma Knife® Perfexion™ and Leksell Gamma Knife® Icon™, it is not possible to use only 1 beam at all, because they are designed with sectors of 24 sources each and individual sources cannot be blocked.

To investigate the precision in dose delivery, it is recommended to test the dose distributions from all beams in a standard geometry at the Leksell coordinate $x,y,z = 100$ mm for the various collimator sizes available on the treatment unit. The standard geometry is a sphere of 8 cm diameter. It is recommended to use the spherical phantom or the Elekta Dosimetry Phantom.

For each collimator size to be investigated:

(a) Prepare two films to the appropriate size for phantom (and collimator size).
(b) In the selected phantom type, mount the film in the center plane of the phantom in the $XY$ plane.
(c) Prepare a test plan with the coordinates $X, Y, Z = 100$ mm, and select an appropriate dose for the film type used (e.g., 5 Gy for Gafchromic EBT type film).
(d) Expose the film to the selected dose.
(e) Repeat **steps 2–4** for the $XZ$ plane.
(f) Prepare eight films to the appropriate size for phantom (and collimator size).
(g) Create a dose-intensity calibration curve.

## Case Study

A 59-year-old female with known metastatic melanoma presents with short onset ataxia and mild headache. MRI of the brain reveals a hemorrhagic metastatic deposit in the R middle cerebellar peduncle. The lesion has a 9 mm solid tumor (0.3 cc) component and a 32 mm hemorrhage (7.9 cc).

Location precluded surgical removal. Given the radioresistant nature of the primary radiosurgery would be a superior method for controlling disease. Since this was a single metastasis, whole brain radiotherapy would not be appropriate. However the volume of the hemorrhage would make single session dose to this area to be restricted to reduce side effects, compromising efficacy.

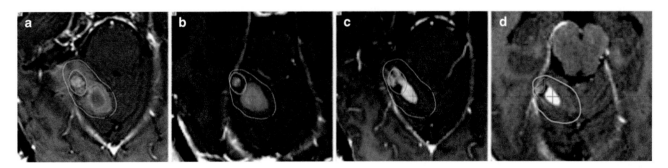

**Fig. 45.20** (**a–d**) Metastatic melanoma with hemorrhage in the cerebellar peduncle treated with hypo-fractionated SRS showing progressive resolution of tumor and hemorrhage

Leveraging the ability to hypo-fractionate with the ICON, the entire hemorrhagic cavity was treated to15 Gy in three fractions and the solid tumor received an additional boost dose of 5 Gy. Figure 45.20 (a) shows the original plan with the hemorrhage covered by the yellow (15 Gy) line and the solid tumor portion in turquoise that received additional 5 Gy. Follow-up imaging at 2 months (b), 4 months (c), and 1 year (d) reveals resolution of hematoma and shrinkage of tumor.

## Summary

Gamma Knife radiosurgery introduced the concept of radiosurgery in the CNS and has become an important tool in the management of CNS tumors in conjunction with or in lieu of microsurgery, fractionated radiotherapy, and chemotherapy. It provides the ability to deliver high doses of radiation with high precision and steep gradients for falloff in normal structures. Long-term results reflect high efficacy and low toxicity rates for the procedure. With the introduction of the ICON®, there are new indications and possibilities for the patients.

## Self-Assessment Questions

1. Tolerance of the optic chiasm to single session SRS is commonly accepted to be:
   A. 12–14 Gy
   B. 2–4 Gy
   C. 5 Gy
   D. 8–10 Gy

2. Tolerance dose to the brain stem in single session SRS is
   A. 50 Gy
   B. 25 Gy
   C. 12 Gy
   D. 10 Gy

3. Gradient index refers to
   A. Homogeneity of dose inside the target
   B. Rapidity of falloff of dose in normal structures
   C. Extent of target covered in adequate dose
   D. Volume of target included in the prescription dose

4. Frame-based radiosurgery with Gamma Knife is capable of achieving a precision of
   A. Less than 2.0 mm
   B. Less than 1.0 mm
   C. Less than 0.5 mm
   D. Less than 0.1 mm

5. Dose normalization with the Gamma Knife is typically in the range of 40–70% because:
   A. It provides more choices for treatment.
   B. Minimizes treatment time.
   C. Allows more coverage.
   D. Permits optimal gradients in normal tissue.

## Answers

1. D
2. C
3. B
4. C
5. D

## References

1. Leksell L. The stereotaxic method and radiosurgery of the brain. Acta Chir Scand. 1951;102(4):316–9.
2. Larsson B. 1931–1998-a multidisciplinary scientist. Acta Oncol. 1999;38:389–90.
3. Paddick I, Lippitz B. A simple dose gradient measurement tool to complement the conformity index. J Neurosurg. 2006;105(Suppl):194–201. https://doi.org/10.3171/sup.2006.105.7.194.
4. Shaw E, Kline R, Gillin M, et al. Radiation therapy oncology group: radiosurgery quality assurance guidelines. Int J Radiat Oncol Biol Phys. 1993;27(5):1231–9.
5. Paddick I. A simple scoring ratio to index the conformity of radiosurgical treatment plans. Technical note. J Neurosurg. 2000;93(Suppl 3):219–22. https://doi.org/10.3171/jns.2000.93.supplement.
6. Lunsford LD, Niranjan A, Flickinger JC, et al. Radiosurgery of vestibular schwannomas: summary of experience in 829 cases. J Neurosurg. 2005;102(Suppl):195–9.
7. Regis J, Delsanti C, Roche PH, et al. Functional outcomes of radiosurgical treatment of vestibular schwannomas: 1000 successive cases and review of the literature. Neurochirurgie. 2004;50(2–3 Pt 2):301–11.
8. Landy HJ, Markoe AM, Wu X, et al. Safety and efficacy of tiered limited-dose gamma knife stereotactic radiosurgery for unilateral acoustic neuroma. Stereotact Funct Neurosurg. 2004;82(4):147–52. https://doi.org/10.1159/000081347.
9. Rowe JG, Radatz MW, Walton L, et al. Clinical experience with gamma knife stereotactic radiosurgery in the management of vestibular schwannomas secondary to type 2 neurofibromatosis. J Neurol Neurosurg Psychiatry. 2003;74(9):1288–93.
10. Iwai Y, Yamanaka K, Shiotani M, et al. Radiosurgery for acoustic neuromas: results of low-dose treatment. Neurosurgery. 2003;53(2):282–7. discussion 287-288
11. Unger F, Walch C, Papaefthymiou G, et al. Long term results of radiosurgery for vestibular schwannomas. Zentralbl Neurochir. 2002;63(2):52–8. https://doi.org/10.1055/s-2002-33975.
12. Litvack ZN, Noren G, Chougule PB, et al. Preservation of functional hearing after gamma knife surgery for vestibular schwannoma. Neurosurg Focus. 2003;14(5):e3.

13. Petit JH, Hudes RS, Chen TT, et al. Reduced-dose radiosurgery for vestibular schwannomas. Neurosurgery. 2001;49(6):1299–306. discussion 1306-1297

14. Bertalanffy A, Dietrich W, Aichholzer M, et al. Gamma knife radiosurgery of acoustic neurinomas. Acta Neurochir. 2001;143(7):689–95.

15. Prasad D, Steiner M, Steiner L. Gamma surgery for vestibular schwannoma. J Neurosurg. 2000;92(5):745–59. https://doi.org/10.3171/jns.2000.92.5.0745.

16. Liscak R, Vladyka V, Urgosik D, et al. Repeated treatment of vestibular schwannomas after gamma knife radiosurgery. Acta Neurochir. 2009;151(4):317–24.; discussion 324. https://doi.org/10.1007/s00701-009-0254-0.

17. Kwon Y, Kim JH, Lee DJ, et al. Gamma knife treatment of acoustic neurinoma. Stereotact Funct Neurosurg. 1998;70(Suppl 1):57–64.

18. Noren G. Long-term complications following gamma knife radiosurgery of vestibular schwannomas. Stereotact Funct Neurosurg. 1998;70(Suppl 1):65–73.

19. Gande A, Kano H, Bowden G, et al. Gamma knife radiosurgery of olfactory groove meningiomas provides a method to preserve subjective olfactory function. J Neuro-Oncol. 2014;116(3):577–83. https://doi.org/10.1007/s11060-013-1335-8.

20. Malik I, Rowe JG, Walton L, et al. The use of stereotactic radiosurgery in the management of meningiomas. Br J Neurosurg. 2005;19(1):13–20. https://doi.org/10.1080/02688690500080885.

21. Pollock BE, Stafford SL, Link MJ. Stereotactic radiosurgery of intracranial meningiomas. Neurosurg Clin N Am. 2013;24(4):499–507. https://doi.org/10.1016/j.nec.2013.05.006.

22. Sheehan JP, Lee CC, Xu Z, et al. Edema following gamma knife radiosurgery for parasagittal and parafalcine meningiomas. J Neurosurg. 2015;123(5):1287–93. https://doi.org/10.3171/2014.12.JNS142159.

23. Starke RM, Przybylowski CJ, Sugoto M, et al. Gamma knife radiosurgery of large skull base meningiomas. J Neurosurg. 2015;122(2):363–72. https://doi.org/10.3171/2014.10.JNS14198.

24. Wowra B, Horstmann GA, Cibis R, et al. Profile of ambulatory radiosurgery with the gamma knife system. 2: report of clinical experiences. Radiologe. 1997;37(12):1003–15.

25. Cohen-Inbar O, Lee CC, Schlesinger D, et al. Long-term results of stereotactic radiosurgery for skull base meningiomas. Neurosurgery. 2016;79(1):58–68. https://doi.org/10.1227/NEU.0000000000001045.

26. Bledsoe JM, Link MJ, Stafford SL, et al. Radiosurgery for large-volume (> 10 cm3) benign meningiomas. J Neurosurg. 2010;112(5):951–6. https://doi.org/10.3171/2009.8.jns09703.

27. Choi CYH, Soltys SG, Gibbs IC, et al. Cyberknife stereotactic radiosurgery for treatment of atypical (who grade II) cranial meningiomas. Neurosurgery. 2010;67(5):1180–8. https://doi.org/10.1227/NEU.0b013e3181f2f427.

28. Chung H-T, Kim DG, Paek SH, et al. Development of dose–volume relation model for gamma knife surgery of non-skull base intracranial meningiomas. Int J Rad Oncol Biol Phys. 2009;74(4):1027–32. https://doi.org/10.1016/j.ijrobp.2008.09.007.

29. Davidson L, Fishback D, Russin JJ, et al. Postoperative gamma knife surgery for benign meningiomas of the cranial base. Neurosurg Focus. 2007;23(4):E6. https://doi.org/10.3171/foc-07/10/e6.

30. Franzin A, Vimercati A, Medone M, et al. Neuroophthalmological evaluation after gamma knife surgery for cavernous sinus meningiomas. Neurosurg Focus. 2007;23(6):E9. https://doi.org/10.3171/foc-07/12/e10.

31. Hasegawa T, Kida Y, Yoshimoto M, et al. Gamma knife surgery for convexity, parasagittal, and falcine meningiomas. J Neurosurg. 2011;114(5):1392–8. https://doi.org/10.3171/2010.11.jns10112.

32. Jo K-W, Kim C-H, Kong D-S, et al. Treatment modalities and outcomes for asymptomatic meningiomas. Acta Neurochir. 2011;153(1):62–7. https://doi.org/10.1007/s00701-010-0841-0.

33. Kondziolka D, Mathieu D, Lunsford LD, et al. Radiosurgery as definitive management of intracranial meningiomas. Neurosurgery. 2008;62(1):53–58; discussion 58-60. https://doi.org/10.1227/01.neu.0000311061.72626.0d.

34. Massager N, De Smedt F, Devriendt D. Long-term tumor control of benign intracranial tumors after gamma knife radiosurgery in 280 patients followed more than 5 years. Acta Neurol Belg. 2013;113(4):463–7. https://doi.org/10.1007/s13760-013-0211-9.

35. Metellus P, Regis J, Muracciole X, et al. Evaluation of fractionated radiotherapy and gamma knife radiosurgery in cavernous sinus meningiomas: treatment strategy. Neurosurgery. 2005;57(5):873–86. https://doi.org/10.1227/01.NEU.0000179924.76551.cd.

36. Pollock BE, Stafford SL, Link MJ, et al. Single-fraction radiosurgery of benign intracranial meningiomas. Neurosurgery. 2012;71(3):604–612; discussion 613. https://doi.org/10.1227/NEU.0b013e31825ea557.

37. Bir SC, Ambekar S, Ward T, et al. Outcomes and complications of gamma knife radiosurgery for skull base meningiomas. J Neurol Surg B. 2014;75(06):397–401. https://doi.org/10.1055/s-0034-1376422.

38. DiBiase SJ, Kwok Y, Yovino S, et al. Factors predicting local tumor control after gamma knife stereotactic radiosurgery for benign intracranial meningiomas. International Journal of Radiation Oncology*Biology*Physics. 2004;60(5):1515–9. https://doi.org/10.1016/j.ijrobp.2004.05.073.

39. Feigl GC, Samii M, Horstmann GA. Volumetric follow-up of meningiomas: a quantitative method to evaluate treatment outcome of gamma knife radiosurgery. Neurosurgery. 2007;61(2):281–286; discussion 286-287. https://doi.org/10.1227/01.neu.0000279999.95953.ea.

40. Kano H, Park K-J, Kondziolka D, et al. Does prior microsurgery improve or worsen the outcomes of stereotactic radiosurgery for cavernous sinus meningiomas? Neurosurgery. 2013;73(3):401–10. https://doi.org/10.1227/01.neu.0000431471.64289.3d.

41. Kreil W, Luggin J, Fuchs I, et al. Long term experience of gamma knife radiosurgery for benign skull base meningiomas. J Neurol Neurosurg Psychiatry. 2005;76(10):1425–30. https://doi.org/10.1136/jnnp.2004.049213.

42. Park S-H, Kano H, Niranjan A, et al. Stereotactic radiosurgery for cerebellopontine angle meningiomas. J Neurosurg. 2014;120(3):708–15. https://doi.org/10.3171/2013.11.jns131607.

43. Park S-H, Kano H, Niranjan A, et al. Gamma knife radiosurgery for meningiomas arising from the tentorium: a 22-year experience. J Neuro-Oncol. 2015;121(1):129–34. https://doi.org/10.1007/s11060-014-1605-0.

44. Sheehan JP, Starke RM, Kano H, et al. Gamma knife radiosurgery for sellar and parasellar meningiomas: a multicenter study. J Neurosurg. 2014;120(6):1268–77. https://doi.org/10.3171/2014.2.jns13139.

45. Shin M, Kurita H, Sasaki T, et al. Analysis of treatment outcome after stereotactic radiosurgery for cavernous sinus meningiomas. J Neurosurg. 2001;95(3):435–9. https://doi.org/10.3171/jns.2001.95.3.0435.

46. Starke RM, Williams BJ, Hiles C, et al. Gamma knife surgery for skull base meningiomas. J Neurosurg. 2012;116(3):588–97. https://doi.org/10.3171/2011.11.jns11530.

47. Williams BJ, Yen CP, Starke RM, et al. Gamma knife surgery for parasellar meningiomas: long-term results including complications, predictive factors, and progression-free survival. J Neurosurg. 2011;114(6):1571–7. https://doi.org/10.3171/2011.1.jns091939.

48. Zada G, Pagnini PG, Yu C, et al. Long-term outcomes and patterns of tumor progression after gamma knife radiosurgery for benign meningiomas. Neurosurgery. 2010;67(2):322–8., discussion 328-329. https://doi.org/10.1227/01.neu.0000371974.88873.15.

49. Zenonos G, Kondziolka D, Flickinger JC, et al. Gamma knife surgery in the treatment paradigm for foramen magnum meningiomas. J Neurosurg. 2012;117(5):864–73. https://doi.org/10.3171/2012.8.jns111554.

50. Chen Y, Li ZF, Zhang FX, et al. Gamma knife surgery for patients with volumetric classification of nonfunctioning pituitary adenomas: a systematic review and meta-analysis. Eur J Endocrinol. 2013;169(4):487–95. https://doi.org/10.1530/EJE-13-0400.

51. Ganz JC. Gamma knife treatment of pituitary adenomas. Stereotact Funct Neurosurg. 1995;64(Suppl 1):3–10.

52. Jackson IM, Noren G. Role of gamma knife therapy in the management of pituitary tumors. Endocrinol Metab Clin N Am. 1999;28(1):133–42.

53. Jagannathan J, Sheehan JP, Pouratian N, et al. Gamma knife radiosurgery for acromegaly: outcomes after failed transsphenoidal surgery. Neurosurgery. 2008;62(6):1262–9.; discussion 1269-1270. https://doi.org/10.1227/01.neu.0000333297.41813.3d.

54. Jagannathan J, Yen CP, Pouratian N, et al. Stereotactic radiosurgery for pituitary adenomas: a comprehensive review of indications, techniques and long-term results using the gamma knife. J Neuro-Oncol. 2009;92(3):345–56. https://doi.org/10.1007/s11060-009-9832-5.

55. Pomeraniec IJ, Dallapiazza RF, Xu Z, et al. Early versus late gamma knife radiosurgery following transsphenoidal resection for nonfunctioning pituitary macroadenomas: a matched cohort study. J Neurosurg. 2016;125(1):202–12. https://doi.org/10.3171/2015.5.JNS15581.

56. Thoren M, Hoybye C, Grenback E, et al. The role of gamma knife radiosurgery in the management of pituitary adenomas. J Neuro-Oncol. 2001;54(2):197–203.

57. Zeiler FA, Bigder M, Kaufmann A, et al. Gamma knife in the treatment of pituitary adenomas: results of a single center. Can J Neurol Sci. 2013;40(4):546–52.

58. Chung WY, Pan DH, Shiau CY, et al. Gamma knife radiosurgery for craniopharyngiomas. J Neurosurg. 2000;93(Suppl 3):47–56. https://doi.org/10.3171/jns.2000.93.supplement.

59. Kobayashi T, Tanaka T, Kida Y. Stereotactic gamma radiosurgery of craniopharyngiomas. Pediatr Neurosurg. 1994;21(Suppl 1):69–74.

60. Prasad D, Steiner M, Steiner L. Gamma knife surgery for craniopharyngioma. Acta Neurochir. 1995;134(3–4):167–76.

61. Ulfarsson E, Lindquist C, Roberts M, et al. Gamma knife radiosurgery for craniopharyngiomas: long-term results in the first Swedish patients. J Neurosurg. 2002;97(5 Suppl):613–22. https://doi.org/10.3171/jns.2002.97.supplement.

62. El-Shehaby AM, Reda WA, Abdel Karim KM, et al. Gamma knife radiosurgery for low-grade tectal gliomas. Acta Neurochir. 2015;157(2):247–56. https://doi.org/10.1007/s00701-014-2299-y.

63. Fuchs I, Kreil W, Sutter B, et al. Gamma knife radiosurgery of brainstem gliomas. Acta Neurochir Suppl. 2002;84:85–90.

64. Gagliardi F, Bailo M, Spina A, et al. Gamma knife radiosurgery for low-grade gliomas: clinical results at long-term follow-up on tumor control and patients' quality of life. World Neurosurg. 2017;101:540–53. https://doi.org/10.1016/j.wneu.2017.02.041.

65. Liao CH, Pan DH, Yang HC, et al. Gamma knife radiosurgery as a treatment modality for low-grade pediatric brainstem gliomas: report of two cases. Childs Nerv Syst. 2012;28(1):175–8. https://doi.org/10.1007/s00381-011-1620-9.

66. Simonova G, Novotny J Jr, Liscak R. Low-grade gliomas treated by fractionated gamma knife surgery. J Neurosurg. 2005;102(Suppl):19–24.

67. Weintraub D, Yen CP, Xu Z, et al. Gamma knife surgery of pediatric gliomas. J Neurosurg Pediatr. 2012;10(6):471–7. https://doi.org/10.3171/2012.9.PEDS12257.

68. Szeifert GT, Prasad D, Kamyrio T, et al. The role of the gamma knife in the management of cerebral astrocytomas. Prog Neurol Surg. 2007;20:150–63. https://doi.org/10.1159/0000100102.

69. Coffey RJ. Boost gamma knife radiosurgery in the treatment of primary glial tumors. Stereotact Funct Neurosurg. 1993;61(Suppl 1):59–64.

70. Elliott RE, Parker EC, Rush SC, et al. Efficacy of gamma knife radiosurgery for small-volume recurrent malignant gliomas after initial radical resection. World Neurosurg. 2011;76(1–2):128–40.; discussion 161-122. https://doi.org/10.1016/j.wneu.2010.12.053.

71. Lowell D, Tatter SB, Bourland JD, et al. Toxicity of gamma knife radiosurgery in the treatment of intracranial tumors in patients with collagen vascular diseases or multiple sclerosis. Int J Radiat Oncol Biol Phys. 2011;81(4):e519–24. https://doi.org/10.1016/j.ijrobp.2011.02.056.

72. Zeiler FA, Kaufmann AM, McDonald PJ, et al. Gamma knife radiosurgery for high grade glial neoplasms: a Canadian experience. Can J Neurol Sci. 2013;40(6):783–9.

73. Gerosa M, Nicolato A, Severi F, et al. Gamma knife radiosurgery for intracranial metastases: from local tumor control to increased survival. Stereotact Funct Neurosurg. 1996;66(Suppl 1):184–92.

74. Shiau CY, Sneed PK, Shu HK, et al. Radiosurgery for brain metastases: relationship of dose and pattern of enhancement to local control. Int J Radiat Oncol Biol Phys. 1997;37(2):375–83.

75. Kim YS, Kondziolka D, Flickinger JC, et al. Stereotactic radiosurgery for patients with nonsmall cell lung carcinoma metastatic to the brain. Cancer. 1997;80(11):2075–83.

76. Wowra B, Czempiel H, Cibis R, et al. Profile of ambulatory radiosurgery with the gamma knife system. 1: method and multicenter irradiation concept. Radiologe. 1997;37(12):995–1002.

77. Mori Y, Kondziolka D, Flickinger JC, et al. Stereotactic radiosurgery for cerebral metastatic melanoma: factors affecting local disease control and survival. Int J Radiat Oncol Biol Phys. 1998;42(3):581–9.

78. Mori Y, Kondziolka D, Flickinger JC, et al. Stereotactic radiosurgery for brain metastasis from renal cell carcinoma. Cancer. 1998;83(2):344–53.

79. Seung SK, Sneed PK, McDermott MW, et al. Gamma knife radiosurgery for malignant melanoma brain metastases. Cancer J Sci Am. 1998;4(2):103–9.

80. Chen JC, O'Day S, Morton D, et al. Stereotactic radiosurgery in the treatment of metastatic disease to the brain. Stereotact Funct Neurosurg. 1999;73(1–4):60–3.

81. Muacevic A, Kreth FW, Horstmann GA, et al. Surgery and radiotherapy compared with gamma knife radiosurgery in the treatment of solitary cerebral metastases of small diameter. J Neurosurg. 1999;91(1):35–43. https://doi.org/10.3171/jns.1999.91.1.0035.

82. Sneed PK, Lamborn KR, Forstner JM, et al. Radiosurgery for brain metastases: is whole brain radiotherapy necessary? Int J Radiat Oncol Biol Phys. 1999;43(3):549–58.

83. Lavine SD, Petrovich Z, Cohen-Gadol AA, et al. Gamma knife radiosurgery for metastatic melanoma: an analysis of survival, outcome, and complications. Neurosurgery. 1999;44(1):59–64. discussion 64-56

84. Sansur CA, Chin LS, Ames JW,et al. Gamma knife radiosurgery for the treatment of brain metastases. Stereotact Funct Neurosurg. 2000;74(1):37–51. doi:56462

85. Amendola BE, Wolf AL, Coy SR, et al. Brain metastases in renal cell carcinoma: management with gamma knife radiosurgery. Cancer J. 2000;6(6):372–6.

86. Simonova G, Liscak R, Novotny J Jr, et al. Solitary brain metastases treated with the Leksell gamma knife: prognostic factors for patients. Radiother Oncol. 2000;57(2):207–13.

87. Schoggl A, Kitz K, Reddy M, et al. Defining the role of stereotactic radiosurgery versus microsurgery in the treatment of single brain metastases. Acta Neurochir. 2000;142(6):621–6.

88. Firlik KS, Kondziolka D, Flickinger JC, et al. Stereotactic radiosurgery for brain metastases from breast cancer. Ann Surg Oncol. 2000;7(5):333–8.

89. Sheehan JP, Sun MH, Kondziolka D, et al. Radiosurgery for non-small cell lung carcinoma metastatic to the brain: long-term outcomes and prognostic factors influencing patient survival time and local tumor control. J Neurosurg. 2002;97(6):1276–81. https://doi.org/10.3171/jns.2002.97.6.1276.

90. Muacevic A, Kreth FW, Tonn JC, et al. Stereotactic radiosurgery for multiple brain metastases from breast carcinoma. Cancer. 2004;100(8):1705–11. https://doi.org/10.1002/cncr.20167.

91. Lippitz BE, Kraepelien T, Hautanen K, et al. Gamma knife radiosurgery for patients with multiple cerebral metastases. Acta Neurochir Suppl. 2004;91:79–87.

92. Mix M, Elmarzouky R, O'Connor T, et al. Clinical outcomes in patients with brain metastases from breast cancer treated with single-session radiosurgery or whole brain radiotherapy. J Neurosurg. 2016;125(Suppl 1):26–30. https://doi.org/10.3171/2016.7.GKS161541.

93. Sheehan JP, Tanaka S, Link MJ, et al. Gamma knife surgery for the management of glomus tumors: a multicenter study. J Neurosurg. 2012;117(2):246–54. https://doi.org/10.3171/2012.4.JNS11214.

94. Liscak R, Vladyka V, Simonova G, et al. Leksell gamma knife radiosurgery of the tumor glomus jugulare and tympanicum. Stereotact Funct Neurosurg. 1998;70(Suppl 1):152–60.

95. Gerosa M, Visca A, Rizzo P, et al. Glomus jugulare tumors: the option of gamma knife radiosurgery. Neurosurgery. 2006;59(3):561–9.; discussion 561-569. https://doi.org/10.1227/01.NEU.0000228682.92552.CA.

96. Chen PG, Nguyen JH, Payne SC, et al. Treatment of glomus jugulare tumors with gamma knife radiosurgery. Laryngoscope. 2010;120(9):1856–62. https://doi.org/10.1002/lary.21073.

97. Madhok R, Kondziolka D, Flickinger JC, et al. Gamma knife radiosurgery for facial schwannomas. Neurosurgery. 2009;64(6):1102–5.; discussion 1105. https://doi.org/10.1227/01.NEU.0000343743.20297.FB.

98. Sun J, Zhang J, Yu X, et al. Stereotactic radiosurgery for trigeminal schwannoma: a clinical retrospective study in 52 cases. Stereotact Funct Neurosurg. 2013;91(4):236–42. https://doi.org/10.1159/000345258.

99. Sheehan J, Yen CP, Arkha Y, et al. Gamma knife surgery for trigeminal schwannoma. J Neurosurg. 2007;106(5):839–45. https://doi.org/10.3171/jns.2007.106.5.839.

100. Phi JH, Paek SH, Chung HT, et al. Gamma knife surgery and trigeminal schwannoma: is it possible to preserve cranial nerve function? J Neurosurg. 2007;107(4):727–32. https://doi.org/10.3171/JNS-07/10/0727.

101. Kato K, Wanifuchi H, Watanabe A. Cyst formation after gamma knife radiosurgery for trigeminal schwannoma: a case report. No Shinkei Geka. 2009;37(6):573–8.

102. Kano H, Niranjan A, Kondziolka D, et al. Stereotactic radiosurgery for trigeminal schwannoma: tumor control and functional preservation. Clinical article. J Neurosurg. 2009;110(3):553–8.

103. Iikubo M, Sakamoto M, Furuuchi T, et al. A case of masticatory disturbance incidental to trigeminal schwannoma: changes in occlusal force and masticatory sensation before and after radiosurgery. Br J Radiol. 2008;81(963):e84–7. https://doi.org/10.1259/bjr/43860468.

104. Muthukumar N, Kondziolka D, Lunsford LD, et al. Stereotactic radiosurgery for jugular foramen schwannomas. Surg Neurol. 1999;52(2):172–9.

105. Pollock BE, Kondziolka D, Flickinger JC, et al. Preservation of cranial nerve function after radiosurgery for nonacoustic schwannomas. Neurosurgery. 1993;33(4):597–601.

106. Kano H, Iqbal FO, Sheehan J, et al. Stereotactic radiosurgery for chordoma: a report from the north American gamma knife consortium. Neurosurgery. 2011;68(2):379–89. https://doi.org/10.1227/NEU.0b013e3181ffa12c.

107. McTyre E, Helis CA, Farris M, et al. Emerging indications for fractionated gamma knife radiosurgery. Neurosurgery. 2017;80(2):210–6. https://doi.org/10.1227/NEU.0000000000001227.

108. Martens B, Janssen S, Werner M, et al. Hypofractionated stereotactic radiotherapy of limited brain metastases: a single-Centre individualized treatment approach. BMC Cancer. 2012;12:497. https://doi.org/10.1186/1471-2407-12-497.

109. Aoyama H, Shirato H, Onimaru R, et al. Hypofractionated stereotactic radiotherapy alone without whole-brain irradiation for patients with solitary and oligo brain metastasis using noninvasive fixation of the skull. Int J Radiat Oncol Biol Phys. 2003;56(3):793–800.

110. Lindvall P, Bergstrom P, Lofroth PO, et al. Hypofractionated conformal stereotactic radiotherapy alone or in combination with whole-brain radiotherapy in patients with cerebral metastases. Int J Radiat Oncol Biol Phys. 2005;61(5):1460–6. https://doi.org/10.1016/j.ijrobp.2004.08.027.

111. Aoki M, Abe Y, Hatayama Y, et al. Clinical outcome of hypofractionated conventional conformation radiotherapy for patients with single and no more than three metastatic brain tumors, with noninvasive fixation of the skull without whole brain irradiation. Int J Radiat Oncol Biol Phys. 2006;64(2):414–8. https://doi.org/10.1016/j.ijrobp.2005.03.017.

112. Fahrig A, Ganslandt O, Lambrecht U, et al. Hypofractionated stereotactic radiotherapy for brain metastases--results from three different dose concepts. Strahlenther Onkol. 2007;183(11):625–30. https://doi.org/10.1007/s00066-007-1714-1.

113. Narayana A, Chang J, Yenice K, et al. Hypofractionated stereotactic radiotherapy using intensity-modulated radiotherapy in patients with one or two brain metastases. Stereotact Funct Neurosurg. 2007;85(2–3):82–7. https://doi.org/10.1159/000097923.

114. Giubilei C, Ingrosso G, D'Andrea M, et al. Hypofractionated stereotactic radiotherapy in combination with whole brain radiotherapy for brain metastases. J Neuro-Oncol. 2009;91(2):207–12. https://doi.org/10.1007/s11060-008-9700-8.

115. Kwon AK, Dibiase SJ, Wang B, et al. Hypofractionated stereotactic radiotherapy for the treatment of brain metastases. Cancer. 2009;115(4):890–8. https://doi.org/10.1002/cncr.24082.

116. Ogura K, Mizowaki T, Ogura M, et al. Outcomes of hypofractionated stereotactic radiotherapy for metastatic brain tumors with high risk factors. J Neuro-Oncol. 2012;109(2):425–32. https://doi.org/10.1007/s11060-012-0912-6.

117. Wang CC, Floyd SR, Chang CH, et al. Cyberknife hypofractionated stereotactic radiosurgery (HSRS) of resection cavity after excision of large cerebral metastasis: efficacy and safety of an 800 cGy x 3 daily fractions regimen. J Neuro-Oncol. 2012;106(3):601–10. https://doi.org/10.1007/s11060-011-0697-z.

118. De Potter B, De Meerleer G, De Neve W, et al. Hypofractionated frameless stereotactic intensity-modulated radiotherapy with whole brain radiotherapy for the treatment of 1-3 brain metastases. Neurol Sci. 2013;34(5):647–53. https://doi.org/10.1007/s10072-012-1091-0.

119. Eaton BR, Gebhardt B, Prabhu R, et al. Hypofractionated radiosurgery for intact or resected brain metastases: defining the optimal dose and fractionation. Radiat Oncol. 2013;8:135. https://doi.org/10.1186/1748-717X-8-135.

# Spinal Stereotactic Body Radiotherapy

# 46

Annie Carbonneau, Arjun Sahgal, and G. Laura Masucci

## Key Terms

- Stereotactic body radiotherapy (SBRT): the precise delivery of highly conformal and image-guided hypofractionated external beam radiotherapy, delivered in a single or few fraction(s), to an extracranial body target with doses at least biologically equivalent to a radical course when given over a conventionally fractionated (1.8–3.0 Gy/fraction) schedule.
- Radiation myelopathy: spinal cord injury secondary to radiotherapy, resulting in an alteration of its function.
- Gross tumor volume (GTV): treatment volume including visible tumor on imaging.
- Clinical tumor volume (CTV): treatment volume including GTV with a margin taking into account microscopic disease.
- Planning tumor volume (PTV): treatment volume including CTV with a margin, usually 2–3 mm, to take into account uncertainties relating to positioning.
- Metastatic epidural spinal cord compression (MESCC): spinal cord compression due to tumor involvement with associated neurological symptoms.

## Learning Objectives

- Understand the delivery of SBRT to spine.
- Discuss appropriate inclusion and exclusion criteria for spine SBRT.
- Learn about pain relief response and local control rates after spine SBRT.
- Identify most common patterns of relapse after spine SBRT.
- Define target volumes specific to spine SBRT.
- Discuss dose limits for organs at risk, including the spinal cord.
- Discuss the optimal dose and fractionation for spine SBRT.
- Consider acute and late toxicities specific to spine SBRT.
- Use appropriate imaging strategy to evaluate response to spine SBRT and recognize challenges with response interpretation due to specific effects of therapy.

## Introduction

It is estimated that nearly 40% of patients diagnosed with cancer will develop spinal metastases at some point during the course of their illness [1]. With improvement in systemic therapies and increasing cancer survivorship, these rates are likely to escalade. Although back pain is the most common initial presenting symptom, patients may also present with mechanical instability and/or neurologic compromise secondary to epidural disease compressing the nerve roots or central neurological structures (spinal cord or thecal sac).

Palliative conventional external beam radiotherapy has had a historical role in the management of spinal metastases with results that are considered suboptimal; partial response

A. Carbonneau
Department of Radiation Oncology, Jewish General Hospital of Montreal, Montreal, QC, Canada

A. Sahgal
Department of Radiation Oncology, Sunnybrook Odette Cancer Centre, Toronto, ON, Canada

G. L. Masucci (✉)
Department of Radiation Oncology, Centre Hospitalier de l'Universite de Montreal (CHUM), Montreal, QC, Canada
e-mail: g.laura.masucci.chum@ssss.gouv.qc.ca

rates are in the order of 60% [2], and complete pain response rates range from 0% to 14% [3, 4].

Stereotactic body radiotherapy (SBRT) is a novel radiation technique that allows delivery of a high radiation dose, potentially ablative, to spinal tumors while minimizing dose to the spinal cord, cauda equina, and other organs at risk (OAR). The Canadian Association of Radiation Oncology (CARO) defined SBRT as "the precise delivery of highly conformal and image-guided hypofractionated external beam radiotherapy, delivered in a single or few fraction(s), to an extracranial body target with doses at least biologically equivalent to a radical course when given over a conventionally fractionated (1.8–3.0 Gy/fraction) schedule." [5]. With the intent to maximize pain relief response and local control rates, spine SBRT is increasingly used.

## Modern Technical Standard for Practice

Spine SBRT demands extreme precision in radiotherapy delivery to within 1–2 mm. It is only with recent technical advances in the entire radiotherapy process, including image guidance (IGRT), that this level of technical excellence is now achievable.

## Technology

### CyberKnife
CyberKnife is a robotic nonisocentric X-band dedicated radiosurgery linear accelerator (LINAC) system. Essentially, it is a compact LINAC that is attached to a robotic arm. Initially, the CyberKnife was put into use by 1990s for treatment of only intracranial lesions. Subsequent developments made it possible to extend the facility to extracranial lesions also, thereby making it a whole-body stereotactic radiotherapy system.

### Technical Innovations to Adapt LINAC
Most commonly used is an isocentric S-band LINAC using multileaf collimators (MLC). It delivers intensity-modulated radiotherapy (IMRT) or volumetric modulated arc therapy (VMAT). It uses onboard image-guidance systems, sophisticated immobilization devices, and treatment couches able to move in all six degrees of freedom (6-DOF) to yield extreme precision.

### Treatment Delivery Unit Considerations
The dose delivery differs significantly between CyberKnife and LINAC technology. The CyberKnife is a nonisocentric X-band LINAC equipped with circular collimators of fixed diameters. It takes advantage of a highly flexible multi-jointed robotic arm to move the compact LINAC with six

degrees of freedom so that beam placement maximizes target coverage while it minimizes directions in which the OAR are directly in the beam's trajectory. It relies on a set of 1–3 beam paths cross-firing from a large number of beam trajectories and angles (approximately 100–200), and the radiation is shaped by a series of circular collimators with apertures ranging from 0.5 to 6 cm. The flexibility of treatment planning is based on the large number of noncoplanar beam angles. The beam intensity is not modulated, and the additive effect of the individual beams results in a conformal dose distribution. The number of beam apertures is relatively few, and therefore treatment planning is not based on IMRT; this results in significant dose heterogeneity within the target volume. This translates to somewhat higher intratumoral maximum doses compared with other technologies. The technology has recently evolved to allow for MLC-based delivery.

The more common technology is an isocentric S-band LINAC using MLC for beam shaping and intensity modulation. It overlaps a large number (approximately 100–300) of shaped apertures (termed beamlets or beam segmentation) from multiple coplanar and/or noncoplanar beam angles (approximately 7–11) to achieve the desired dose distribution. VMAT (volumetric modulated arc therapy) is a new development in MLC-based LINAC radiation delivery technique in which the dose rate, gantry speed, and beam apertures may continuously change while the treatment is being delivered dynamically in a single- or multi-arc treatment. Treatment planning is achieved with an inverse planning algorithm for the optimization of the beam segment shapes and weight, in which the beam opening is maximal for the target while closing areas to block OAR. A more homogeneous dose distribution is created compared with current nonisocentric CyberKnife technology [6].

## Immobilization

Patient immobilization is an important aspect of spine SBRT, in particular for those systems not equipped with near real-time intrafractional image guidance as used in the CyberKnife. Various devices have been used, including a long thermoplastic mask for patients with lesions involving C1 to T3 and near-rigid body immobilization for lesions involving T4 and below. Examples of near-rigid body immobilization devices include the BodyFIX (Medical Intelligence) [7, 8] or in-house, custom-designed device [9, 10]. These immobilization systems serve to minimize potential patient movement, to ensure proper match of the position of the target at time of treatment to that at the time of planning. The aim is to avoid large shift (>2 mm or 2°) as detected with the image-guidance system. Near-rigid body immobilization also reduces the potential for patient motion while the beam is on (intrafractional variation) and increases delivery accuracy, and this is of critical importance for SBRT.

## Image-Guidance System and Online Correction

Image-guided radiotherapy (IGRT) is critical to SBRT. The IGRT system allows 3D imaging of the target just prior to radiation delivery while the patient is immobilized on the treatment couch. It allows the match of the pretreatment position of the tumor to that at the time of simulation and can determine three-dimensionally what corrective actions are required to ensure proper and secure delivery of treatment. Furthermore, because the patient may move while treatment is being delivered, IGRT is used to determine intrafractional positional variations to ensure treatment accuracy. The IGRT systems can be broken down into those based on stereoscopic X-ray- and computed tomography (CT)-based imaging. For spine SBRT, the aim is to ensure precise positioning with an accuracy of 1–2 mm and 1°–2° with either IGRT system [6].

Stereoscopic X-ray imaging, used in the CyberKnife technique, implies simultaneous orthogonal X-ray imaging of the target. The X-rays are processed by software solutions to provide 3D information on the target position indirectly. The position of target is then referenced to that at the time of treatment planning to determine what shifts are required for a match. Bony landmarks are used for spine SBRT. This stereoscopic system allows for fast imaging of the target in near real time and corrects the position of the LINAC to track shifts via the robotic arm while the beam is on.

CT-based imaging results in the direct acquisition of high-quality volumetric images, which provides optimal registration accuracy. Soft tissues and anatomical structures are directly visualized on the transaxial CT images and registered to the corresponding planning CT studies. Necessary shifts for a match are determined. When necessary, shifts are achieved via the robotic couch with up to six degrees of freedom motion. To account for intrafractional variation, interruption of the treatment is necessary to obtain repeat images.

## Planning Imaging

CT-simulation requires fine resolution scans with a slice thickness not exceeding 2.5 mm [5]. Magnetic resonance imaging (MRI) of the target vertebrae, and at least one to two vertebrae above and below, is suggested for accurate delineation of the target, paraspinal soft tissue extension, epidural disease as well as the spinal cord/thecal sac. Axial volumetric T1 and T2 sequences without gadolinium are a standard [11]. The use of gadolinium, however, might be advantageous in delineating paraspinal disease, epidural disease, and in differentiating postoperative surgical fluid from residual disease [12].

Specific to postoperative SBRT, fusion of the preoperative MRI axial images is paramount. In patients with metal artifact from hardware obscuring the critical neural structures, a CT myelogram should be obtained [11, 13].

## Target Volumes

The International Spine Radiosurgery Consortium has published guidelines for target volume definition in spine SBRT [14]. These propose that the gross tumor volume (GTV) should include all gross tumors, including epidural and paraspinal elements. The clinical target volume (CTV) should include the entire vertebral body, particularly including all areas of abnormal bone marrow signal, but should avoid encircling the cord unless there is invasion of the pedicles or extensive epidural tumor. It is recommended that the CTV to planning target volume (PTV) expansion is ≤3 mm and this should be constrained around the spinal cord (Table 46.1).

Recently, a consensus contouring guidelines has been proposed by an international group of experts in the postoperative setting [15]. The GTV is defined as any residual disease visualized on postoperative CT and MRI with attention to residual epidural or paraspinal disease. The CTV should account for the GTV and regions that were

**Table 46.1** Summary of GTV, CTV, and PTV contouring guidelines for spine SBRT

| Target volume | Guidelines |
|---|---|
| GTV | • Contour gross tumor using all available imaging<br>• Include epidural and paraspinal components of tumor |
| CTV | • Include abnormal marrow signal suspicious for microscopic invasion<br>• Include bony CTV expansion to account for subclinical spread<br>• Should contain GTV<br>• Circumferential CTVs encircling the cord should be avoided except in rare instances where the vertebral body, bilateral pedicles/lamina, and spinous process are all involved or when there is extensive metastatic disease along the circumference of the epidural space without spinal cord compression |
| PTV | • Uniform expansion around CTV<br>• CTV to PTV margin ≤3 mm<br>• Modified at dural margin and adjacent critical structures to allow spacing at discretion of the treating physician unless GTV compromised<br>• Never overlaps with cord<br>• Should contain entire GTV and CTV |

Reprinted from Cox BW, Spratt DE, Lovelock M, et al. International Spine Radiosurgery Consortium consensus guidelines for target volume definition in spinal stereotactic radiosurgery. Int J Radiat Oncol Biol Phys. 2012;83(5):e597–605. With permission from Elsevier

involved preoperatively according to CT and MRI. It should include adjacent anatomic compartments at risk of microscopic disease extension based on preoperative bony and epidural involvement using the International Spine Radiosurgery Consortium anatomic classification as a framework. Indeed, a recent pattern of failure analysis found that the location of preoperative epidural disease was more predictive of subsequent failure than the sites of residual disease postoperatively [16]. It is recommended to use judiciously circumferential CTVs limited to cases of preoperative circumferential or near-circumferential osseous and/or epidural involvement. The surgical incision and instrumentation does not need to be included in the treatment volume unless involved. The expansion of a PTV varies between institutions, ranging from no expansion to 2.5 mm uniform expansion. The PTV should be modified so that it does not extend into the cord avoidance structure for treatment planning.

Given the critical nature of the spinal cord and the impact of uncertainties present in the radiotherapy process, a planning risk volume (PRV) is typically applied to the spinal cord [17]. The margin used for the PRV should be based on a robust evaluation of each center's process. Usually, a margin of 1.5–2 mm is added to the spinal cord to generate cord PRV (Table 46.2).

**Table 46.2** Summary of GTV, CTV, and PTV contouring guidelines for postoperative spine SBRT for spinal metastases

| Target volume | Guidelines |
|---|---|
| GTV | • Gross tumor based on postoperative CT MRI with attention to residual epidural or paraspinal disease<br>• Include postoperative residual epidural and paraspinal components of tumor |
| CTV | • Include the postoperative region and entire anatomic compartment corresponding to all preoperative MRI abnormalities suspicious for tumor involvement<br>• Include entire GTV<br>• Surgical instrumentation and incision not included unless involved<br>• Judicious use of circumferential CTVs limited to cases of preoperative circumferential osseous and/or epidural involvement; however, it can be considered for near-circumferential epidural disease involvement<br>• Modified at reconstructed dural space to account for changes in anatomy after surgery at the discretion of treating physician<br>• Consider additional anatomic expansions of up to 5 mm beyond paraspinal extension and cranio-caudally for epidural disease<br>• Uniform CTV to PTV expansion of up to 2.5 mm<br>• Treating physician may modify expansion at the interface with critical organs at risk |
| PTV | • May subtract cord avoidance structure from PTV as a modified PTV for planning and does reporting purposes<br>• Include entire GTV and CTV |

Reprinted from Redmond KJ, Robertson S, Lo SS, et al. Consensus contouring guidelines for postoperative stereotactic body radiation therapy for metastatic solid tumor malignancies to the spine. Int J Radiat Oncol Biol Phys. 2017;97(1):64–74. With permission from Elsevier

## Treatment Planning

Treatment planning can be challenging, particularly in situations where multiple OAR are present such as the bowel, kidneys, and esophagus. The basic strategy is often to determine the spinal cord dose to the maximum allowable safe limit and focus on achieving as steep a dose gradient as possible while maximizing coverage within the epidural space.

Typical techniques include 7- to 11-static-field IMRT or VMAT. Standard characteristics of a spine SBRT treatment plan include hotspots in the target in excess of 20–50% beyond the prescription dose, a steep dose gradient between the cord and the target, and 70–90% target coverage (percent volume receiving the prescribed dose) in order to respect strict OAR tolerances [18].

Treatment planning for SBRT in the postoperative setting is complicated by the presence of surgical hardware leading to electron backscatter and photon attenuation. This may not be accurately captured in standard treatment planning algorithms. Therefore, treatment planning algorithm approved by the RTOG for calculation of dose within a medium with heterogeneities should be used for all postoperative spine SBRT cases [19].

## Patient Selection

A number of factors are taken into account when deciding whether a patient is a good candidate for spine SBRT.

## Epidural Disease Grading

In an effort to standardize the communication of epidural disease extent, a grading system known as the Bilsky grading system has been developed and validated by the Memorial Sloan Kettering Cancer Center group [20]. A schematic representation of the Bilsky grading system is represented in Fig. 46.1. A Bilsky grade 0 implies no extension of the lesion beyond the vertebral body into the epidural space, grade 1A–C refers to epidural disease approaching the spinal cord but not compressing it, grade 2 refers to compression of the spinal cord with cerebrospinal fluid visible in the spinal canal at the level of the compression, and grade 3 refers to complete compression of the spinal cord with no cerebrospinal fluid visible. Spinal metastases graded as a Bilsky 3 should have surgical consultation for consideration of decompression, and if surgery is contraindicated, then conventional EBRT at this time may be most appropriate [21]. For Bilsky 2 tumors, there may be therapeutic benefit to downgrading the epidural disease to a Bilsky 0 or 1 then following with SBRT, as reported by Al-Omair et al.[22]. Otherwise, SBRT for Bilsky 2 disease

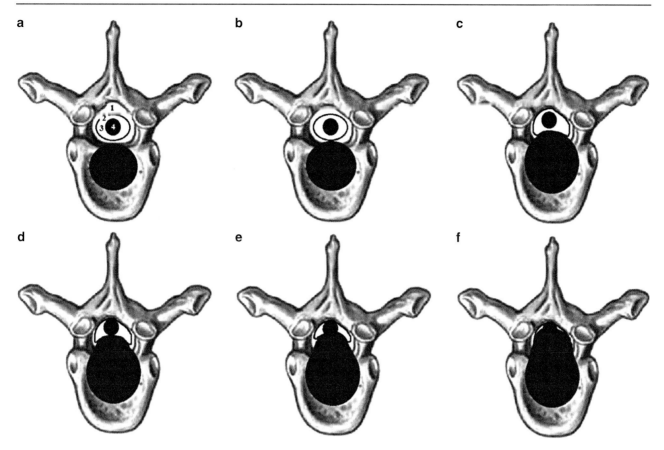

**Fig. 46.1** Schematic of Bilsky six-point grading system applied to the thoracic spine depicting epidural spinal cord compression. (**a**) (1) Epidural space, (2) dural sac, (3) cerebrospinal fluid (CSF), (4) spinal cord. Grade 0, bone involvement only; (**b**) grade 1a, epidural impingement without deformation of the thecal sac; (**c**) grade 1b, deformation of the thecal sac without spinal cord abutment; (**d**) grade 1c, deformation of the thecal sac with spinal cord abutment, but without spinal cord compression; (**e**) grade 2, spinal cord compression with CSF visible around the cord; (**f**) grade 3, spinal cord compression without CSF visible around the cord. [Reprinted from Kumar R, Nater A, Hashmi A. et al. The era of stereotactic body radiotherapy for spinal metastases and the multidisciplinary management of complex cases. Neuro Oncol Pract. 2016;3(1):48–58. With permission from Oxford University Press]

remains appropriate as a relative contraindication. Ideally, there should be at least 2–5 mm between the disease and the spinal cord to maximize CTV coverage [23].

## Mechanical Instability

The Spinal Instability Neoplastic Score (SINS) provides an objective and validated measure of spinal instability [24]. It considers factors including location, pain quality, posterior element involvement, vertebral body collapse, quality of the metastases (e.g., lytic vs. blastic), and vertebral alignment. The key outcome is categorical, with the condition of patients defined as stable (0–6), potentially unstable (7–12), or unstable (13–18). An experienced surgeon should evaluate potentially unstable or unstable deemed patients to determine whether stabilization prior to SBRT is necessary to minimize posttreatment risk of fracture (Table 46.3).

## Neurologic Deficit

Consideration of spine SBRT also requires objective grading of neurologic function. The most accepted score is from the American Spinal Injury Association (ASIA) [25]. An ASIA E rating is normal motor and sensory function, D is incomplete motor impairment with more than half of the key muscles below the affected level having a power of at least 3 out of 5, C is incomplete motor impairment with key muscles below the affected level having a power under 3 out of 5, B is incomplete motor impairment with sensory but no motor function preserved, and A is complete impairment with neither sensory nor motor function preserved. Spinal metastases causing progressive neurologic deficits (ASIA grades A–D), if not definitively responsive to corticosteroids, are considered a strong indication for surgical consultations [13]. ASIA grade A status is usually a contraindication for SBRT [19].

**Table 46.3** Spinal instability neoplastic score

| Element of SINS | Score |
| --- | --- |
| Location | |
| Junctional (occiput–C2, C7–T2, T11–L1, L5–S1) | 3 |
| Mobile spine (C3–C6, L2–L4) | 2 |
| Semirigid (T3–T10) | 1 |
| Rigid (S2–S5) | 0 |
| Pain relief with recumbency and/or pain with movement/loading of the spine | |
| Yes | 3 |
| No (occasional pain but not mechanical) | 1 |
| Pain-free lesion | 0 |
| Bone lesion | |
| Lytic | 2 |
| Mixed (lytic/blastic) | 1 |
| Blastic | 0 |
| Radiographic spinal alignment | |
| Subluxation/translation present | 4 |
| De novo deformity (kyphosis/scoliosis) | 2 |
| Normal alignment | 0 |
| Vertebral body collapse | |
| >50% collapse | 3 |
| <50% collapse | 2 |
| No collapse with >50% body involved | 1 |
| None of the above | 0 |
| Posterolateral involvement of the spinal elements (facet, pedicle, or CV joint fracture or replacement with tumor) | |
| Bilateral | 3 |
| Unilateral | 1 |
| None of the above | 0 |

Reprinted from Fisher CG, DiPaola CP, Ryken TC, et al. A novel classification system for spinal instability in neoplastic disease: an evidence-based approach and expert consensus from Spine Oncology Study Group. Spine (Phila Pa 1976). 2010;35(22):E1221–1229. With permission from Wolters Kluwer Health

## Life Expectancy

One of the most challenging issues in this clinical setting is to identify patients that will long enough to realize the potential benefits of SBRT as compared to palliative conventional EBRT. Typically, a life expectancy of at least 3 months has been identified as inclusion criteria.

Laufer et al. [26] published a decision framework used at the Memorial Sloan Kettering Cancer Center to select the optimal treatment for patients with spinal metastases. This framework, called NOMS, is based on neurologic, oncologic, mechanical, and systemic parameters. It also incorporates the use of conventional EBRT (cEBRT in Fig. 46.2), spine SBRT, and minimally invasive and open surgical procedures. Following the NOMS decision algorithm, SBRT (SRS in Fig. 46.2) should be mainly delivered in patients presenting a low-grade epidural spinal cord compression score and a radioresistant or previously radiated metastases, without signs of vertebral instability [27].

Chao et al. [28] generated a prognostic index based on the recursive partitioning analysis (RPA) for patients undergoing spine SBRT. The authors used a Kaplan-Meier analysis to detect any correlation between survival and several clinical and technical features (Fig. 46.3). Time from primary diagnosis (< or >30 months) and the Karnofsky Performance Status (< or >70) were determined to be significant parameters to identify patients with a better prognosis and, therefore, most likely to benefit from spine SBRT.

Recently, Tang et al. [29] published a scoring system that stratifies patients based on a secondary analysis of overall survival of two mature phase II prospective trials. Two hundred six patients with a minimal follow-up of 3 years were analyzed. They identified four subgroups of patients characterized by different prognoses ranging from excellent to poor. This prognostic index for spinal metastases (PRISM) was based on a multivariate Cox regression model. Five clinical variables (female sex, Karnofsky Performance Status >60, only one bone metastasis, low number of extra-osseous metastatic sites, and an interval from initial diagnosis to detection of spinal metastasis of more than 5 years) and two therapeutic variables (previous surgery at the SBRT site and a previous radiotherapy at the SBRT site) were found to be statistically predictive of good or excellent prognosis after SBRT.

## Indications and Contraindications

Multiple guidelines have been reported detailing appropriate inclusion and exclusion criteria for spine SBRT, including those from the American Society for Therapeutic Radiology and Oncology and the American College of Radiology [11] and from the Canadian Association of Radiation Oncology [5]. In general, patients considered appropriate for spine SBRT have a spinal or paraspinal metastasis from a solid tumor histology in three or less contiguous segments, SINS score revealing a stable or minimally unstable spinal column, low-grade epidural disease, life expectancy of at least 3 months, and a relatively limited systemic disease burden [23]. With respect to the latter, patients with oligometastatic disease are ideal candidates for SBRT given their longer life expectancy and the increasing literature to suggest that a proportion may potentially achieve significant disease-free intervals with aggressive therapy [30]. Furthermore, independent series from various institutions have suggested increased therapeutic benefit in terms of local control and pain relief particularly in tumors stemming from a radioresistant histology such as melanoma, sarcoma, and renal cell carcinoma (RCC) [31–36]. The use of these techniques becomes more critical in a previously irradiated patient in order to deliver a tumoricidal dose and protect critical neural structures simultaneously [23]. A summary of current spine SBRT indications is provided in Table 46.4 and represents an expert opinion considering the data to date and reported consensus.

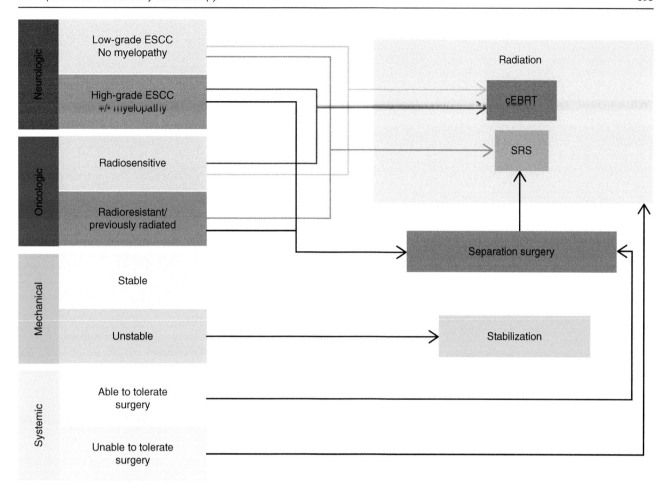

**Fig. 46.2** Schematic depiction of the neurologic, oncologic, mechanical, and systemic (NOMS) decision framework. [Reprinted from Bhattacharya IS, Hoskin PJ. Stereotactic body radiotherapy for spinal and bone metastases. Clin Oncol (R Coll Radiol). 2015;27(5):298–306. With permission from Elsevier]

**Fig. 46.3** RPA tree for overall survival for patients treated with SBRT to the spine. [Reprinted from Chao ST, Koyfman SA, Woody N, et al. Recursive partitioning analysis index is predictive for overall survival in patients undergoing spine stereotactic body radiation therapy for spinal metastases. Int J Radiat Oncol Biol Phys. 2012;82(5):1738–1743. With permission from Elsevier]

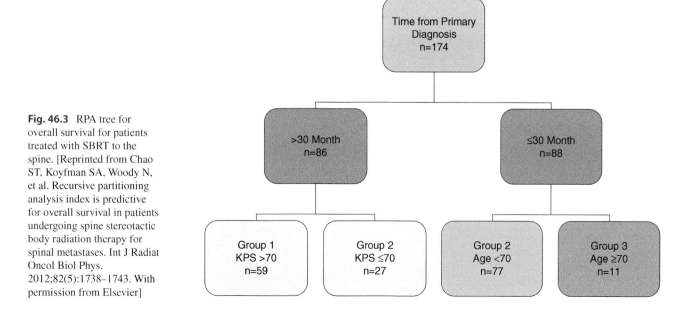

**Table 46.4** Inclusion and relative and major contraindication to spine SBRT

| Optimal inclusion criteria for spine SBRT | Relative contraindication to spine SBRT | Major contraindications to spine SBRT[a] |
|---|---|---|
| • Good to excellent performance status | • Moderate performance status | • Poor performance status (ECOG 3–4; KPS <60) |
| • Oligometastatic disease (≤5 sites extracranial metastases) | • Oligoprogression in patients with widely metastatic and/or rapidly progressive disease | • Widely metastatic and/or rapidly progressive disease with limited life expectancy |
| • Oligoprogression in a patient with oligometastatic disease | | |
| • No more than three spinal levels involved (contiguous or noncontiguous) | • >3 spinal levels involved but nondiffuse spine disease and no more than three contiguous segments | • >3 contiguous spinal levels involved or diffuse spine disease |
| • No or minimal spine instability (SINS 0–6) | • Potential spine instability (SINS 7–12) | • Spine instability (SINS 13–18) |
| • No or minimal epidural disease (Bilsky 0–1) | • Moderate-grade epidural disease (Bilsky 2) | • High-grade epidural disease (Bilsky 3) |
| • "Radioresistant" histology | • "Radiosensitive" history | |
| • No prior cEBRT to affected level or prior cEBRT delivered ≥5 mo of a considered second course of salvage SBRT | • Prior cEBRT delivered 3–5 mo prior to considered course of salvage spine SBRT | • Prior cEBRT <3 mo prior to considered course of salvage spine SBRT |
| • Spine SBRT delivered ≥5 mo of a considered second course of savage SBRT | • Spine SBRT delivered within 3–5 mo of a considered course of salvage SBRT | • Spine SBRT delivered <3 mo prior to a considered second course of salvage SBRT |
| • Robotic LINAC or subcentimeter MLC-based LINAC delivery, CBCT, and/or stereoscopic imaging IGRT; near-rigid body immobilization; fusion of thin-slice MRI sequences for target/CNS contouring; and, in selected postoperative cases, a treatment planning CT myelogram | • If unable to have an MRI, then a treatment planning with CT myelogram for CNS structure contouring provided that the target is identifiable on CT alone with sufficient clinical detail as to paraspinal disease extension/epidural disease extension | • Unable to tolerate near-rigid/supine immobilization<br>• Unable to have a full-spine MRI and/or CT myelogram |

Reprinted from Jabbari S, Gerszten PC, Ruschin M, et al. Stereotactic body radiotherapy for spinal metastasis: practice guidelines, outcomes, and risks. Cancer J. 2016;22(4):280–289. With permission from Wolters Kluwer Health

*CNS* central nervous system (spinal cord, thecal sac), *ECOG* Eastern Cooperative Organization Group, *IGRT* image-guided radiotherapy, *KPS* Karnofsky Performance Status, *MLC* multileaf collimator, *mo* months

[a]Exceptions may exist based on practitioner's experience and clinical scenario

In the postoperative setting, Redmond et al. published a consensus guidelines based on the results of an international survey [19]. Consensus treatment indications included radioresistant primary, 1–2 levels of adjacent disease, and previous radiotherapy. Contraindications included involvement of more than three contiguous vertebral bodies, ASIA grade A status, and postoperative Bilsky grade 3 residual.

## Challenges with Response Interpretation

A clear understanding of response to treatment is crucial in order to make appropriate treatment decisions. As suggested by the recently reported SPIne response assessment in Neuro-Oncology (SPINO) group, MRI is the recommended imaging modality for assessment of tumor response following spine SBRT [12]. However, early morphologic changes are poorly understood, and interpretation of the response can be challenging. Traditional metrics such as bidimensional size measurements and RECIST criteria are not optimal to monitor response, especially when changes in tumor dimensions are subtle. Also, a change in signal

intensity must be interpreted with caution with the knowledge of the clinical context since it may be not be associated with true progression but due to osteoradionecrosis, fibrosis, as well as non-tumor-related vertebral compression fracture.

Pseudoprogression is a specific treatment response to high-dose radiotherapy such as spine SBRT. It is defined as a treatment-related transient tumor growth that mimics true progression. It was first described in gliomas undergoing high-dose radio- and chemotherapy [37] and has been well documented following brain radiosurgery [38], lung SBRT [39, 40], and liver SBRT [41]. The group from MD Anderson Cancer Center (MDACC) [42] and the one from Montreal University Hospital Center (CHUM) [43] reported a pseudoprogression incidence of 14% and 18%, respectively, occurring at 3- to 6-month time intervals after SBRT. Of note, the latter study demonstrated that tumor growth confined to the 80% prescription isodose line and earlier time to tumor enlargement predicted for pseudoprogression.

The SPINO group suggested defining local progression as gross unequivocal increase in tumor volume or linear dimension, any new or progressive tumor within the epidural space, or neurological deterioration attributable to preexisting epidural disease with equivocal increased epidural disease dimension on MRI. Images should be interpreted by a radiation oncologist and radiologist. In circumstances where treatment response is unclear, serial imaging with two to three MRIs, 8–12 weeks apart, is recommended by the group. Although there is increasing use of functional imaging such as PET and perfusion MRI, there are insufficient data to recommend these modalities at this time [12].

## Clinical Outcomes

The two main therapeutic targets of SBRT for spinal metastasis, namely, pain control and local control, have been explored in a number of retrospective series and few phase I and II studies, but data of phase III studies are not available as of yet. Selected series are summarized in Table 46.5. Of note, these reports largely varied in terms of total dose, dose/fraction, and delivery techniques.

**Table 46.5** Results from select series using spine SBRT

| Author (year) | Design | No. of tumors/no. of patients | Prescribed dose (range), Gy/no. of fractions (range) | Median follow-up (range), mo | Local control | Overall survival | Pain response |
|---|---|---|---|---|---|---|---|
| Selected spine SBRT series for spinal metastases with no prior history of radiation (de novo) | | | | | | | |
| Degen (2005) [44] | Retrospective | 72/51 | (10–37.5)/3 (1–5) | 12 (1–22) | N/A | N/A | VAS: 51.5 (baseline) to 17.5 (12 mo) |
| Gerszten (2007) [45] | Prospective | 500/393 | Median, 20 (12.5–25)/1 | 21 (3–53) | 88% | N/A | 86% (overall long-term improvement) |
| Chang (2007) [7] | Phase I/II | 74/63 | (27–30)/(3–5) | 21.3 (0.9–49.6) | 84% (1 y) | 69.8% (1 y) 24.3 mo median | N/A |
| Yamada (2008) [9] | Prospective | 103/93 | Median, 24 (18–24)/1 | 15 (2–45) | 90% (15 mo) | 15 mo median | N/A |
| Gagnon (2009) [46] | Prospective | 274/200 | (21–37.5)/(3–5) | 12 (1–51) | N/A | 17 mo median | VAS: 40.1 (baseline) to 28.6 (12 mo) |
| Nguyen (2010) [36] | Prospective (RCC only) | 55/48 | (24–30)/(1–5) | 13.1 (3.3–54.5) | 82% (1 y) | 72% (1 y) 22 mo median | BPI: no pain 23% (baseline) to 52% (12 mo) |
| Wang (2012) [47] | Phase I/II | 166/149 | (27–30)/3 | 15.9 (1.0–91.6) | 80.5% (1 y) 72.4% (2 y) Tumor progression-free survival | 68.5% (1 y) 46.4% (2 y) 23 mo median | BPI: no pain 26% (baseline) to 54% (6 mo) |
| Garg (2012) [48] | Phase I/II | 63/61 | (18–24)/1 | 19.7 (1.2–52.1) | 88% (18 mo) | 64% (18 mo) 30.4 mo median | BPI: no pain 21% (baseline) to 30% (6 mo) |
| Guckenberger (2014) [49] | Multicentric retrospective | 387/301 | Median, 24 (8–60)/3 (1–20) | 11.8 (0–105) | 89.9% (1 y) 83.9% (2 y) | 64.9% (1 y) 43.7% (2 y) 19.5 mo median | BPI: no pain 18.2% (baseline) to 76.8% (11.5 mo) |
| Selected reirradiation spine SBRT series for spinal metastases | | | | | | | |
| Sahgal (2009) [50] | Retrospective | 37/25 | Median, 24 (8–30)/3 (1–5) | 7 (1–48) | 85% (1 y) 69% (2 y) | 45% (2 y) 21 mo median | N/A |
| Choi (2010) [51] | Retrospective | 51/42 | Median, 20 (10–30)/2 (1–5) | 7 (2–47) | 73% (1 y) | 68% (1 y) | 65% |
| Damast (2011) [52] | Retrospective | 97/94 | 20/5 (42 tumors) 30/5 (55 tumors) | 12.1 (0.2–63.6) | 66% (1 y) | 52–59% (1 y) 13.6 mo median | 85% |

(continued)

**Table 46.5** (continued)

| Author (year) | Design | No. of tumors/no. of patients | Prescribed dose (range), Gy/no. of fractions (range) | Median follow-up (range), mo | Local control | Overall survival | Pain response |
|---|---|---|---|---|---|---|---|
| Garg (2011) [53] | Prospective | 63/59 | (27–30)/3 (3–5) | 17.6 (0.9–67.5) | 76% (1 y) | 76% (1 y) | N/A |
| Mahadevan (2011) [54] | Retrospective | 81/60 | (24–30)/3 (3–5) | 12 (3–39) | 93% (crude) | 11 mo median | 65% |
| Chang (2012) [55] | Retrospective | 54/49 | 27/3 | 17.3 (mean) | 81% (1 y) 79% (2 y) | 11.0 mo median | N/A |
| Selected postoperative spine SBRT series for spinal metastases | | | | | | | |
| Gerszten (2005) [56] | Retrospective | 26/26 | Mean, 18 (16–20)/1 | 16 (11–24) | N/A | N/A | VAS: 92% long-term improvement |
| Moulding (2010) [57] | Retrospective | 21/21 | Median, 24 (18–24)/1 | 10.2 (1.2–54.0) | 90.5% (1 y) | 10.2 mo median | N/A |
| Laufer (2013) [58] | Retrospective | 186/186 | Median, 24/1 or 27 (24–30)/3 or 30 (18–36)/5 | 7.6 (1.0–66.4) | 83.6% (1 y) | 29% (crude) 5.6 mo median | N/A |
| Al-Omair (2013) [22] | Retrospective | 80/80 | Median, 24 (18–40)/2 (1–5) | 8.3 (0.13–39.1) | 84% (1 y) | 64% (1 y) | N/A |
| Tao (2016) [59] | Prospective | 69/66 | 16–24/1 or 27/3 or 30/5 | 30 (1–145) | 85% (1 y) 79% (2 y) 74% (3 y) | 74% (1 y) 60% (2 y) 40% (3 y) 30 mo median | N/A |

*mo* month, *y* year, *VAS* visual analog scale, *N/A* not applicable, *BPI* brief pain inventory

## De Novo Spine SBRT

Several single-institution retrospective series and few prospective studies have reported high rates of both pain control and local tumor control in previously unirradiated spinal metastases treated with SBRT.

In the prospective phase I/II study reported by Wang et al. [47], 149 patients and 166 lesions were treated to a total dose of 27–30 Gy in three fractions. Pain control was assessed using the validated Brief Pain Inventory (BPI) assessment tool. With a median follow-up of 15.9 months, investigators concluded a mean reduction of 3.4 points based on the BPI, and 54% of patients were completely pain-free 6 months post-SBRT. A concomitant statistically significant decrease in opioid use was also reported. Quality of life outcomes demonstrated improvements in disturbed sleep, drowsiness, sadness, fatigue, distress, lack of appetite, nausea, and memory following spine SBRT. This trial also reported a 1-year actuarial tumor progression-free survival rate of 80.5%. No radiation-related spinal cord myelopathy was reported during the study.

Multiple series corroborate the previous data with radiographic and/or clinical local tumor control rates ranging from 80% to 90% in cohort with mixed tumor histology. Furthermore, at least six series have specifically reported on the outcomes in patients with radioresistant histology such

as melanoma, sarcoma, and RCC documenting local tumor control rates of 79–88% [30–35]. More recently, data has been published showing, in patients surviving at least 5 years after treatment, a local recurrence of 9.6% [60].

SBRT is also highly effective at palliation of pain symptoms. In the selected studies summarized in Table 46.5, we observe that complete pain response rates are not often reported but can range up to 86%.

The literature concerning quality of life after SBRT is scarce. However, Degen et al. [44] and Gagnon et al. [46] reported quality of life maintenance after treatment. The 12-item Short Form Health Survey (SF-12) was used to assess quality of life prior to and after treatment. Average SF-12 scores did not vary in either the physical or mental well-being domains throughout follow-up, with assessments at regular intervals from 1 month posttreatment to 18 months posttreatment.

## Spine SBRT Following Previous Conventional External Beam Radiation

It is well known that up to 20% of patients will require retreatment due to the recurrence of pain in the previously radiated area in the short term [21]. One of the major indications for spine SBRT has been failure following palliative conventional EBRT. Equivalent rates of pain and local control in patients with or without prior radiation treated with SBRT are suggested based on a nonrandomized comparison. Selected studies on retreatment with spine SBRT for recurrent spinal metastasis showed 66–93% local control rate over a follow-up period of 7–21 months (Table 46.5). Concerning palliation of pain symptoms, 65–85% of patients experienced a positive response. Another option being studied recently is intraoperative brachytherapy for tumors of the spine involving the dura. It is a useful adjunct to surgical intervention for recurrent spinal metastases, especially in the setting of prior conventional EBRT [61].

## Spine SBRT Following Previous SBRT

As the rate of application of spine SBRT continues to rise, salvage of SBRT failures will become increasingly important. A recent review from the University of Toronto examined outcomes in a group of 40 patients with 56 spinal metastases that were treated using a second course of SBRT after local SBRT failure [62]. Furthermore, 43% had received previous conventional EBRT prior to the first SBRT treatment course. The median prescription dose and number of fractions for the second course of SBRT were 30 Gy and four fractions (range 20–35 Gy in two to five fractions). The 1-year local control rate was 81%, and there were no cases of radiation myelopathy. This series is important as it supports the use of aggressive salvage therapy with SBRT despite initial failure, as opposed to strictly palliative approaches for fear of causing complications with a second course of SBRT.

## Postoperative Spine SBRT

The historical standard adjuvant therapy to surgical decompression and stabilization has been conventional EBRT. The intent is to deliver sufficient dose to be safe to normal tissues while yielding at least short-term local control and pain palliation. Imaging-based local control after palliative conventional EBRT has not been well defined. Based on the few studies that have been reported, these control rates are modest at best and represent an area for improvement [63, 64]. Innovations in radiation technology and surgery have allowed increasing application of SBRT in postoperative patients, and data are emerging to suggest that outcomes with this technique may be superior to those achieved with conventional EBRT.

Few retrospective series and one recently published prospective study looked at postoperative SBRT in particular. Tao et al. [59] reported 66 patients with 69 tumors treated with SBRT after open spinal decompression. They received 16–24 Gy in one fraction, 27 Gy in three fractions, or 30 Gy

in five fractions. After a median follow-up of 30 months, the actuarial 1-year rate of tumor control was 85% and overall survival was 74%. There was no myelopathy reported.

In selected postoperative spine SBRT series, 1-year local control rates range from 83.6% to 90.5%, and pain response rate was reported in one study at 92% (Table 46.5). Posttreatment ambulatory status, although not stated in most series, is 100% in those studies that do report it.

## Pattern of Relapse

Failure in epidural space is the most common pattern reported in the SBRT literature occurring in approximately half of the recurrences. Chang et al. [7] reported specific failures in this area in 8 of 17 failures in their series of 74 tumors treated. Nguyen et al. [36] also reported 6 epidural space failures out of 12 failures in their series of 55 RCC metastases treated.

Sahgal et al. [50] reported local failure in 8 of 60 tumors treated and analyzed the potential for treatment failure as the tumor approached the thecal sac. A trend was found when the minimal distance between the target and the thecal sac was <1 mm, and exploratory analysis showed a significant risk of failure for tumors with extensive epidural disease.

Data illustrates the challenge of treating epidural disease with SBRT, because spinal cord constraints simply limit epidural tumor coverage. Therefore, for tumors abutting the critical neural structures, there may be a therapeutic benefit to epidural disease resection with respect to local control as reported by Al-Omair et al. [22].

Failure at other areas due to intentional avoidance or lack of margin beyond the GTV can occur. Failure in the paravertebral tissue has been reported: 4 out of 17 in Chang et al. [7] and 3 out of 12 in Nguyen et al. [36]. It probably results from the practice of applying no margin to paravertebral disease into the adjacent soft tissues. A small margin of 0.5 cm may be reasonable along the paraspinal muscles when involved, to reduce the risk of marginal failure, given that the muscle is not an anatomical barrier to tumor growth. However, optimal margins are unknown [6]. When the posterior elements were deliberately excluded, failures have been reported: 3 out of 7 in Chang et al. [7] and 5 out of 12 in Nguyen et al. [36]. If disease is located only within the vertebral body based on MR imaging, then it is reasonable to exclude the posterior elements, as suggested in the International Spine Radiosurgery Consortium [14]. Progression in adjacent vertebral bodies is rare and supports SBRT treatment of the involved spinal levels only [65].

As observed for unirradiated patients, failure after retreat SBRT most often occurs within, or close to, the epidural space. Also, after postoperative SBRT, the predominant pattern of failure is within the epidural space. It is the only site of failure in two-thirds of cases [22, 59]. A recent patterns of failure analysis found that the location of preoperative epidural disease was more predictive of subsequent failure than the sites of residual disease postoperatively [16].

## Toxicities and Dose Limits for Organs at Risk

In terms of acute toxicity, the treatment appears to be well tolerated, and most reports indicate limited acute toxicities in relation to the surrounding anatomy. Late toxicities are more of a concern, given that we have little experience with dose-volume limits for high-dose-per-fraction exposure of normal tissues. Furthermore, the risk of harmful permanent tissue damage is greater with higher-dose-per-fraction radiotherapy, and it accumulates with time, often manifesting several months to years postradiation.

## Pain Flare

Pain flare is defined as a temporary increase in pain in the immediate period after radiation. It was specifically studied after spine SBRT in two studies: Chiang et al. [66] and Pan et al. [67] Incidence reported was 23% and 68%, after a median time up to 5 days after SBRT. The prescription of dexamethasone (most commonly 4 mg orally once daily for the time of the treatment and/or for 5 days after SBRT) resulted in a significant decrease in pain scores. As a matter of fact, dexamethasone has been showed to be efficient in the prophylaxis of radiation-induced pain flare after palliative conventional EBRT for bone metastases [68]. It is not yet standard practice to use dexamethasone as a prophylactic intervention following spine SBRT as many reserve it as a rescue intervention should the pain occur. A randomized trial of dexamethasone in patients treated with spine SBRT has been proposed.

## Vertebral Body Compression Fracture (VCF)

VCF after spine SBRT has emerged as the most common adverse effect following SBRT. It includes de novo fracture and fracture progression. The mean time to fracture after SBRT is 3 months. Rates range between 10% and 40% and are more commonly reported after high-dose single-fraction SBRT versus fractionated SBRT. This dose complication relationship is evident. With 24 Gy in a single fraction, the rate of VCF approaches 40%, which was first reported by Rose et al. [69] and later confirmed in a multi-institutional analysis. The risk of VCF is approximately 20% with 20–23 Gy/fraction and 10% with less than 20 Gy/fraction [70]. Other risk factors identified in the literature include spinal misalignment, lytic tumor, baseline fracture, and high

SINS [18]. Less than half of all patients require an intervention and, in those that did, a minimally invasive cement augmentation procedure has been applied as opposed to an open spinal surgery [70].

## Radiation Myelopathy

Radiation myelopathy is generally the most feared complication of spine SBRT. Fortunately, evidence-based dose constraint guidelines have been published to guide spine SBRT both in the setting of no prior irradiation as well as prior conventional EBRT of the spinal cord.

A report published by the American Association of Physicists in Medicine (AAPM) [71] suggests limiting to 7 Gy, 12.3 Gy, and 14.5 Gy the dose delivered to ≤1.2 cc of spinal cord in one, three, and five fractions, respectively. The same report recommends to limit to 10 Gy, 18 Gy, and 23 Gy the dose delivered to ≤0.35 cc of spinal cord in one, three, and five fractions, respectively. These recommendations are however not evidence based.

Spinal cord dose limits have been published by Sahgal et al. based on the updated analysis of nine cases of radiation myelopathy specific to spine SBRT and a dosimetric comparison to a multi-institutional control cohort. It was recommended that the point maximum thecal sac dose (typically equivalent to the true cord plus a 1.5 mm PRV) be constrained to 12.4 Gy in a single fraction, 17 Gy in two fractions, 20.3 Gy in three fractions, 23 Gy in four fractions, and 25.3 Gy in five fractions [72]. Using higher doses is a clinical decision in which tumor control is weighed against toxicity. The Memorial Sloan Kettering Cancer Center practice typically allows a maximum point dose up to 14 Gy within the true spinal cord (typically based on myelogram) in a single fraction. They recently published the largest analysis of single-fraction spinal cord dose limits in patients with no prior radiation, using a prospectively collected cohort of dose-volume histogram data, with the longest follow-up time (14.6 months). For 228 patients treated at 259 sites, the median spinal cord maximum point dose was 13.85 Gy. Radiation myelitis occurred in two patients with maximum point dose to the spinal cord of 13.43 and 13.63 Gy, and the authors conclude based on a model that the risk of radiation myelitis with 14 Gy in a single fraction is <1% [73].

## GI Toxicity

Case reports and at least one retrospective series have reported gastrointestinal tract complications following SBRT. The most serious include perforation of the esophagus and small bowel. Cox et al. [74] reported the risk of esophageal toxicity following single-fraction SBRT in 182 patients and 204 spinal segments. Given a median prescription dose of 24 Gy and median follow-up of 12 months, an incidence of acute and late esophageal toxicities of 15% and 12%, respectively, was reported. More specifically, the overall rate of grade 3 or higher late toxicity was 6.8%. In seven cases of grade 4 or higher toxicity, these were associated with radiation recall reactions with chemotherapy regimens such as gemcitabine or doxorubicin or occurred following procedures involving the esophagus. A volume of esophagus receiving 14 Gy or higher (V14) above 2.5 mL was associated with significantly higher toxicity, and the authors recommended maintaining a V14 of less than 2.5 mL as a planning dose constraint and a maximum point dose of 22 Gy or lower. Few reports of esophageal or bowel toxicity have been reported with more fractionated courses of spine SBRT, as fractionation likely mitigates the risk as compared with single-fraction SBRT.

In practice, the limitations published by the AAPM [71] are often used in order to respect normal tissue tolerance. Dose received by a previous radiation treatment has to be taken in consideration.

## Toxicity Specific to Spine SBRT Following Previous Radiation

The most common acute side effects include grades 1–2 fatigue (up to 40%) and gastrointestinal effects (up to 10–20%; most often nausea, vomiting, diarrhea, and esophagitis). VCFs were reported in approximately 10% of patients. Serious late neurological effects have been observed, with one patient developing radiation myelopathy and one patient developing grade 3 neurological peripheral nerve toxicity. Although limited to grade 1–2 toxicity, 15

patients developed peripheral nerve injury manifesting as paresthesia and pain along the affected dermatome [75].

A multi-institutional international collaboration [76] led to the publication of reirradiation spinal cord dose limits for spine SBRT. The authors recommended limiting the cumulative nBED to <70 Gy 2/2 as determined by the thecal sac point dose maximum. Additional recommendations included a maximum SBRT nBED of 20–25 Gy 2/2 also determined by thecal sac point dose maximum, a minimum interval of 5 months before reirradiation, and a SBRT point maximum nBED to cumulative point maximum nBED ratio not exceeding 0.5. Table 46.6 summarizes reirradiation SBRT dose limits that satisfy the proposed criteria given common initial conventional EBRT practice.

## Toxicity Specific to Postoperative Spine SBRT

The toxicities to adjacent OAR are fundamentally similar to those in patients treated with SBRT for intact metastases. Same spinal cord constraints are applied as de novo SBRT, and no radiation myelopathy has been reported in the limited literature so far. In the recently published consensus guidelines [19], common schemes according to the fractionation schedule and prior radiation doses are provided (Table 46.7).

Toxicities unique to the postoperative setting are wound dehiscence or infection, hardware failure, and VCF. Literature with respect to complications after either postoperative conventional EBRT or SBRT is limited. One series of patients with thyroid cancer managed with surgery with or without conventional EBRT or SBRT noted a 35% rate of postoperative complications [77]. Of 43 patients, 5 (11.6%) required

**Table 46.6** Reasonable reirradiation SBRT doses to the thecal sac $P_{max}$ following common initial conventional radiotherapy regimens

| Conventional radiotherapy (nBED) | Single fraction: SBRT dose to thecal sac $P_{max}$ | Two fractions: SBRT dose to thecal sac $P_{max}$ (Gy) | Three fractions: SBRT dose to thecal sac $P_{max}$ (Gy) | Four fractions: SBRT dose to thecal sac $P_{max}$ (Gy) | Five fractions: SBRT dose to thecal sac $P_{max}$ (Gy) |
|---|---|---|---|---|---|
| 0 | 10 Gy | 14.5 | 17.5 | 20 | 22 |
| 20 Gy in five fractions (30 Gy$_{2/2}$) | 9 Gy | 12.2 | 14.5 | 16.2 | 18 |
| 30 Gy in ten fractions (37.5 Gy$_{2/2}$) | 9 Gy | 12.2 | 14.5 | 16.2 | 18 |
| 37.5 Gy in 15 fractions (42 Gy$_{2/2}$) | 9 Gy | 12.2 | 14.5 | 16.2 | 18 |
| 40 Gy in 20 fractions (40 Gy$_{2/2}$) | N/A | 12.2 | 14.5 | 16.2 | 18 |
| 45 Gy in 25 fractions (43 Gy$_{2/2}$) | N/A | 12.2 | 14.5 | 16.2 | 18 |
| 50 Gy in 25 fractions (50 Gy$_{2/2}$) | N/A | 11 | 12.5 | 14 | 15.5 |

Reprinted from Sahgal A, Ma L, Weinberg V, et al. Reirradiation human spinal cord tolerance for stereotactic body radiotherapy. Int J Radiat Oncol Biol Phys. 2012;82(1):107–116. With permission from Elsevier

$P_{max}$ dose to a point within the thecal sac that receives the maximum dose, *N/A* not applicable, *nBED* normalized biologically effective doses, *SBRT* stereotactic body radiotherapy

**Table 46.7** Common spinal cord constraints that are applied to either true cord or a surrogate of the true cord (cord PRV or thecal sac) according to no prior and common prior radiation dose exposure

| Prior conventional RT dose | Single fraction | Two fractions | Three fractions | Four fractions | Five fractions |
|---|---|---|---|---|---|
| No prior RT but cord compromise | 10–14 Gy $D_{max}$ 10 Gy to <10% cord[a] | 17 Gy $D_{max}$ | 18–21 Gy $D_{max}$ | 23–26 Gy $D_{max}$ | 25–30 Gy $D_{max}$ |
| No prior RT but cord compromise | 8–14 Gy $D_{max}$ 10 Gy to <10% cord[a] | 17 Gy $D_{max}$ | 18–21 Gy $D_{max}$ | 23–26 Gy $D_{max}$ | 25–28 Gy $D_{max}$ |
| 800 cGy in single fraction | 9 Gy $D_{max}$ | 12.2 Gy $D_{max}$ | 14–21 Gy $D_{max}$ | 16.2 Gy $D_{max}$ | 17.5–27.5 $D_{max}$ |
| 2000 cGy in five fractions | 9–12 Gy $D_{max}$ | 12.2 Gy $D_{max}$ | 14–21 Gy $D_{max}$ | 16.2 Gy $D_{max}$ | 15–27.5 Gy $D_{max}$ |
| 3000 cGy in ten fractions | 9–12 Gy $D_{max}$ | 12.2 Gy $D_{max}$ | 14–21 Gy $D_{max}$ | 16.2–24 Gy $D_{max}$ | 17.5–26 Gy $D_{max}$ |
| 4000 cGy in 20 fractions | 9–12 Gy $D_{max}$ | 12.2 Gy $D_{max}$ | 14–21 Gy $D_{max}$ | 16.2 Gy $D_{max}$ | 12–25 Gy $D_{max}$ |
| 4500 cGy in 25 fractions | 9–12 Gy $D_{max}$ | 12.2 Gy $D_{max}$ | 14–21 Gy $D_{max}$ | 16.2 Gy $D_{max}$ | 12–18 Gy $D_{max}$ |

Reprinted from Redmond KJ, Lo SS, Soltys SG, et al. Consensus guidelines for postoperative stereotactic body radiation therapy for spinal metastases: results of an international survey. J Neurosurg Spine. 2017;26(3):299–306. With permission from The Journal of Neurosurgery: Spine

$D_{max}$ maximum point dose

[a]The 10% criterion uses the spinal cord volume 5–6 mm above and below the target volume. Note that these constraints are intended as a summary of practice patterns of experienced spine specialists. However, these constraints are not data driven. They should be utilized with caution and may not be applicable to all clinical scenarios. Evidence-based constraints have been previously published by Sahgal et al. [72, 76]

revision surgery for wound dehiscence or infection. This rate is similar to that recently reported after postoperative conventional EBRT for MESCC (metastatic epidural spinal cord compression), where the overall surgical complication rate was 30% and the rate for risk of wound infection was 10% [78]. Similarly, another recently published article reports the development of wound infections requiring antibiotics postoperatively in 2 of 22 patients (9%) but no new or persistent wound infection after SBRT [79]. It is speculated that SBRT may reduce radiation-related surgical complications as the dose distribution is more conformal, allowing for selective wound sparing. However, it is also important to note that innovations in surgery such as minimally invasive techniques may reduce complications. This was reported in a small series by Massicotte et al. [80], where the time to SBRT after minimally invasive surgery was approximately 1 week. The incision was ≤2 cm, and no wound complications were noted.

It has been hypothesized that SBRT may reduce the rate of hardware failure, limiting the necessity for reoperation. The rationale is that all of the surgical hardware is not exposed to radiotherapy. Only three of the studies reviewed in Table 46.5 specified these data [22, 57, 58]. In aggregate, 6 of 287 patients (2.1%) required revision for hardware failure. This is comparable with the crude cumulative rate of 1.4% reported in the modern study limited to patients receiving conventional EBRT after spine surgery [78].

Similarly, it has been hypothesized that surgical instrumentation may reduce the risk of VCF compared with SBRT for intact vertebral bodies by stabilizing the vertebral column. The risk after SBRT for intact vertebral bodies is well established, ranging from 10% to 40% depending on the dose and fractionation schedule used [69, 70]. One study in Table 46.5 reported cases of VCF specifically in postoperative cases, with 9 of 80 patients (11.3%) having new or progressive loss of vertebral body height [22]. As such, preliminary data suggest that the presence of hardware does

not mitigate this risk, although it remains unclear whether the need for intervention may be reduced because of the presence of hardware.

## Optimal Dose and Fractionation

The total dose, fractionation, and method of prescribing vary significantly among the series in the summarized literature (Table 46.5). There are no dedicated phase I dose escalation studies, nor are there any randomized studies testing various SBRT dose schemes. Therefore, the optimal practice has not been well established and is a source of controversy.

Retrospective and prospective studies have examined single-fraction SBRT for spinal metastases with excellent local control of 88–90% in the selected literature presented in Table 46.5. Yamada et al. [9] from the Memorial Sloan Kettering Cancer Center analyzed their experience in which the SBRT dose was escalated over time and suggest greater rates of local control with a higher single-fraction total dose, up to 24 Gy in a single fraction.

However, Garg et al. [48] from the MD Anderson Cancer Center described significant neurological toxicity in their series of spinal metastases treated with single-fraction SBRT including two cases of grade 3 or greater neurologic sequelae, specifically hemicord syndrome and foot drop from radiculopathy.

Also, VCF is more commonly reported after high-dose single-fraction SBRT versus fractionated SBRT. This dose-complication relationship is evident; with 24 Gy in a single fraction, the rate of VCF approaches 40%, but it is approximately 20% with 20–23 Gy/fraction and 10% with less than 20 Gy/fraction [70].

Pain flare was also reported to be more frequent with single-fraction spine SBRT. As a matter of fact, recent data of prospective spine SBRT studies found that the only significant predictor of the risk of pain flare was the number of fractions. In this study, 34% of patients treated with single-fraction spine SBRT experienced this adverse event compared with 20% of patients receiving three fractions and 8% of patients receiving five fractions [67].

At present, there are no prospective randomized studies comparing outcomes following single-fraction versus multiple-fraction spine SBRT. A single retrospective series compared outcomes in 195 spine lesions treated with single session SBRT and 153 lesions treated with multiple sessions of SBRT. The mean doses were 16.3 Gy in one fraction, 20.6 Gy in three fractions, 23.8 Gy in four fractions, and 24.5 Gy in five fractions. This study found that although pain control was significantly improved in patients receiving a single fraction, local control at up to 2 years following treatment was significantly better in patients treated with multiple fractions (96% vs. 70%) [81]. Similarly, the need for retreatment was significantly lower in patients receiving multiple-fraction therapy than following single-fraction treatment. These preliminary data are inconclusive, and future prospective studies will be necessary to evaluate the proposed hypothesis that single-fraction radiosurgery may improve short-term pain control, while fractionated radiosurgery may lead to more durable control with decreased need for retreatment and decreased risk of toxicities including VCF, pain flare, and radiation-induced spinal cord myelopathy.

Since effective prescription doses include 18–24 Gy in a single fraction, 24 Gy in two fractions, 24–30 Gy in three fractions, and 25–40 Gy in five fractions, individual fractionation regimens need to be prescribed on the basis of previous radiation, proximity of the target to the OAR, and volume of the target. Single-fraction SBRT could be considered in selected patients with radioresistant tumors and life expectancies of less than a year and when the main goal of treatment is pain control. Patients to be treated with single-fraction SBRT should have at least 2–3 mm gap between the spinal metastasis and the cord and no risk factors predisposing the patient to vertebral compression fracture, and the treating center should have the appropriate technical capability, expertise, and experience with planning and delivery of single-fraction SBRT [11]. Fractionated SBRT may hold a particular advantage in cases of large or circumferential tumors, in the postoperative setting, or in cases of reirradiation [82].

For previously irradiated cases, the most common practice after initial conventional EBRT has been to prescribe a total dose in the range of 24–35 Gy delivered in two to five fractions. Of note, no dose-response relationship has been clearly demonstrated [75].

In the postoperative setting, there is data suggesting that higher-dose-per-fraction SBRT may be associated with greater rates of local control as compared with lower doses per fraction. The largest series to date from Laufer et al. [58] recently reported on 168 patients after separation surgery, stabilization, and adjuvant postoperative spine SBRT. SBRT was either delivered as 24 Gy in single fraction, hypofractionated with 24–30 Gy in three fractions (high dose), or hypofractionated with 18–36 Gy in five to six fractions (lower dose). Local control at 1 year was 83.6%, and dose was the only predictor of local control. There was a significant improvement in local control with high-dose single-fraction SBRT and high-dose hypofractionated treatment associated with a 9% and 4.1% risk of local progression, respectively, at 1 year. This is compared with 22.6% in patients receiving lower-dose hypofractionated treatment. The series from Al-Omair et al. [22] also reported that dose per fraction may be a predictive factor, with patients receiving 18–26 Gy in one to two fractions having better control rates than those receiving lower-dose-per-fraction regimens of 18–40 Gy over three to five fractions.

Possible dose and fractionation schemes for postoperative spine SBRT include the following: 16–24 in single fraction, 24 Gy in two fractions, 24–30 Gy in three fractions, 30–32 Gy in four fractions, and 30–40 Gy in five fractions [19].

Some practitioners use an integrated boost to areas of residual tumor. Simultaneous integrated boost doses to the GTV are 16–22 Gy in a single fraction for patients with radiosensitive tumors and 18–25 Gy in a single fraction or 50 Gy in five fractions for patients with radioresistant tumors [19].

The optimal timing of postoperative SBRT is largely unknown, but the commonly used is the 4-week postoperative mark [6, 22, 58].

## Special Circumstance: Concurrent Spine SBRT with Targeted Therapy

Concerning molecular targeted therapy, tyrosine kinase inhibitors have been shown to potentiate the response to radiotherapy in animal and in vitro models [83]. However, little is known about the combination of molecular targeted therapy and SBRT in terms of toxicity and local tumor control in patients with advanced disease. Few clinical data are emerging concerning safety and efficacy of concurrent spine SBRT and molecular targeted therapy. Three retrospective series reporting spinal metastatic lesions from RCC treated with SBRT and targeted molecular treatments showed promising outcome and acceptable toxicity [84–86].

Although data is limited, fatal toxicities have been observed with combination of SBRT and targeted molecular therapy. Especially with anti-angiogenic therapy, ischemic bowel complication including perforation, tracheoesophageal fistula, and surgical complications have been reported [87, 88]. Therefore, caution must be used in combination of these two therapeutic approaches. No clear recommendation exists concerning the timing between this systemic modality and SBRT.

## Cost-Effectiveness

Kim et al. [89] performed a cost-effectiveness analysis to compare single fraction of SBRT and single fraction of conventional EBRT for palliation of vertebral bone metastases. They concluded that selective SBRT used in patients with longer expected survival (11 months and more) might be the most cost-effective approach. Bijlani et al. [90] described and synthesized stereotactic radiosurgery (SRS) and SBRT cost-effectiveness research across several common SRS and SBRT applications including for spinal metastases. He concluded that, from a patient perspective, SRS and SBRT provide patients effective treatment option, while from the payer and provider perspective, SRS and SRT demonstrate cost savings.

## Treatment Surveillance and Follow-Up

Prior to treatment, it is essential that the treatment plan undergo strict quality assurance (QA) testing, in accordance with national and international guidelines [5, 11, 71]. Such QA tests include multidisciplinary peer review, physics QA, and pretreatment patient-specific dose measurements. For treatment delivery, online image guidance is critical to ensure the most accurate patient positioning. Image guidance is often based on cone-beam CT (CBCT) for most systems, but near-continuous stereoscopic imaging is also commonly used. Regardless of imaging technique, the entire target volume must be visualized in the field of view. Strict thresholds for repositioning tolerance are demanded because of the close proximity of the spinal cord to the steep dose gradient. For CBCT-based systems, if the treatment time is protracted over more than 15–20 min, it has also been demonstrated that a mid-treatment CBCT serves to correct for intra-fraction motion [91].

As recommended by the SPINO group, spine MRI should be done every 2–3 months after SBRT for the first 12–18 months and every 3–6 months thereafter [12].

## Ongoing Studies

Prospective randomized trials are few and still underway. RTOG 0631 is a phase III trial comparing conventional EBRT of 8 Gy in single fraction to SBRT of 16–18 Gy in single fraction (https://clinicaltrials.gov/ct2/show/NCT00922974), and the Canadian SC24 is a phase II randomized trial comparing conventional EBRT of 20 Gy in five fractions to 24 Gy in two fractions of SBRT (https://clinicaltrials.gov/ct2/show/NCT02512965). The Canadian SC24 trial has recently been converted to a phase III trial. A prospective randomized phase III trial at MSKCC in New York compares 24 Gy in a single fraction versus three sessions of 9 Gy (total 27 Gy) in effecting durable local control in oligometastatic tumors, including oligometastatic spine disease (MSKCC 10–154).

## Clinical Case Discussion

A 63-year-old patient was referred for an oligometastatic lesion at T8 level. She had a history of breast cancer, stage III, ER/PR+, diagnosed 5 years prior. After being treated with mastectomy and axillary dissection, she underwent chemotherapy and radiotherapy to the breast and lymph nodes and was prescribed hormonotherapy.

She presented with a history of back pain without any neurological symptoms. Bone scan was performed and confirmed the presence of a solitary lesion at T8. A pet scan did not show any evidence of other distant metastases. The presence of the bone lesion in the vertebral body of T8 was confirmed by a MRI (Fig. 46.4) of the spine. Involvement of the right pedicle, lamina, and proximal right transverse process was noted. Epidural disease was present (Bilsky grade 1c); SINS score was evaluated at 5.

In order to maximize local control, the patient was assessed for minimally invasive spinal surgery and underwent resection of the epidural disease. Postoperative MRI did not show any residual disease in the thecal sac (Fig. 46.5).

Patient underwent SBRT treatment after surgery (Fig. 46.6). She received a dose of 24 Gy in two fractions of 12 Gy (Fig. 46.7) using arc therapy. Maximum point dose ($D_{max}$) received by the spine PRV was 17 Gy and by the esophagus 20 Gy.

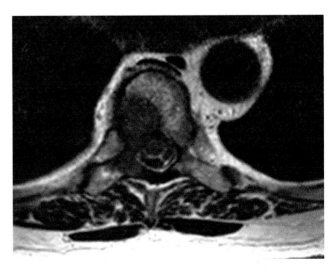

**Fig. 46.4** Preoperative MRI, showing epidural disease, Bilsky grade 1c

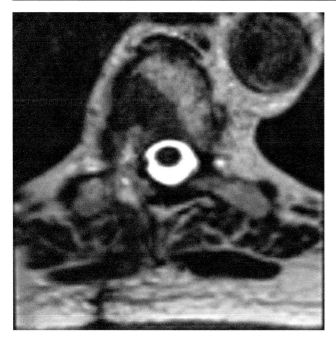

**Fig. 46.5** Postoperative MRI

## Summary

- Recent technical advances in the entire radiotherapy process, including immobilization, planning imaging with MRI, and image-guidance radiotherapy, are critical to achieve the level of precision required for spine SBRT treatment.

- Guidelines have been published for target volume definition in spine SBRT. In the postoperative setting, a consensus contouring guidelines has also been proposed.

- In general, patients considered appropriate for spine SBRT have a spinal or paraspinal metastasis from a solid tumor histology in three or less contiguous segments, SINS score revealing a stable or minimally unstable spinal column, low-grade epidural disease, life expectancy of at least 3 months, and a relatively limited systemic disease burden.

- In the postoperative setting, treatment indications included radioresistant primary, 1–2 levels of adjacent disease, and previous radiotherapy. Contraindications include involve-

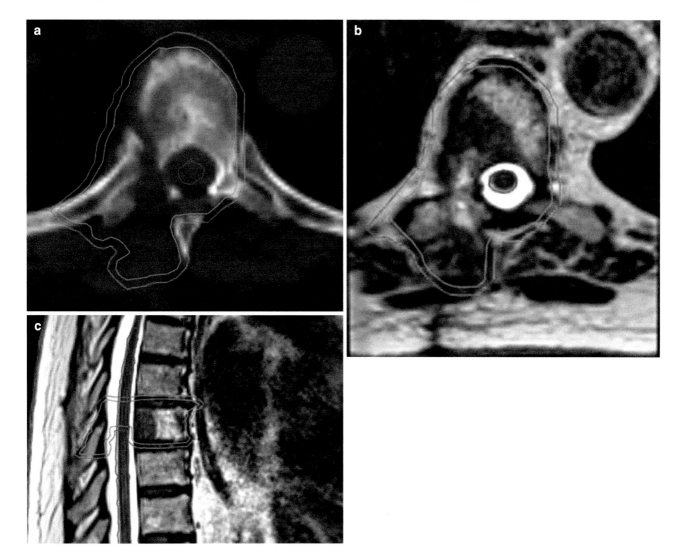

**Fig. 46.6** Axial view of CT scan (**a**), axial view (**b**), and sagittal view of planning MRI (**c**) with CTV, PTV, and spinal cord contoured

**Fig. 46.7** Treatment
administered by arc therapy

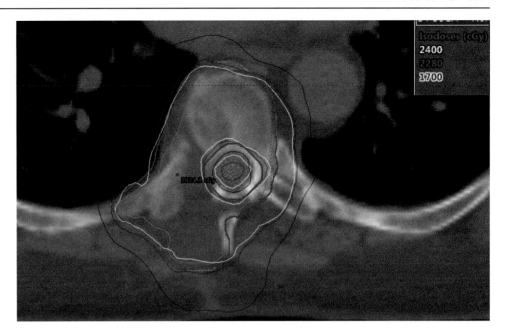

ment of more than three contiguous vertebral bodies, ASIA grade A status, and postoperative Bilsky grade 3 residual.
- Local progression is defined as gross unequivocal increase in tumor volume or linear dimension, any new or progressive tumor within the epidural space, or neurological deterioration attributable to preexisting epidural disease with equivocal increased epidural disease dimension on MRI.
- Several retrospective series and few prospective studies have reported excellent local tumor control rates (ranging from 80% to 90%). Spine SBRT is also associated with good pain control.
- Failure in the epidural space is the most common pattern of recurrence following spine SBRT occurring in more than half of recurrences.
- Vertebral body compression fracture after spine SBRT is a common adverse effect following SBRT with rates of 10–40%.
- Radiation myelopathy is generally the most feared complication of spine SBRT. Evidence-based dose-constraint guidelines have been published to guide spine SBRT in the setting of both no prior irradiation and prior conventional EBRT of the spinal cord.
- Effective prescription doses include 18–24 Gy in a single fraction, 24 Gy in two fractions, 24–30 Gy in three fractions, and 25–40 Gy in five fractions. Individual fractionation regimens need to be prescribed according to the presence of previous radiation, proximity of the target to the organs at risk, and volume of the target.
- For previously irradiated cases, the most common practice after initial conventional EBRT has been to fraction-

ate treatment, with a total dose in the range of 24–35 Gy delivered in three to five fractions.
- Possible dose and fractionation schemes for postoperative spine SBRT include the following: 16–24 Gy in single fraction, 24 Gy in two fractions, 24–30 Gy in three fractions, 30–32 Gy in four fractions, and 30–40 Gy in five fractions.
- MRI is the recommended imaging modality for assessment of tumor response following spine SBRT. Follow-up spine MRI should be done every 2–3 months after SBRT for the first 12–18 months and every 3–6 months thereafter.

## Self-Assessment Questions

1. What is the essential condition for the safe administration of stereotactic body radiotherapy (SBRT) treatment delivery?
   A. Correct volume definition
   B. Image guidance
   C. Correct patient immobilization
   D. All of the above

2. In terms of SBRT doses, higher doses:
   A. Seem to yield better local control results for all patients
   B. Seem to yield better overall survival for all patients
   C. None of the above

3. Recurrence after irradiation occurs most often in:
   A. Paraspinal tissue
   B. Epidural space
   C. Adjacent vertebra

4. Overall survival of patients is influenced by:
   A. Patient Karnofsky Performance Status
   B. Time to reirradiation
   C. Radiosensitive histology
   D. All of the above

5. The risk of vertebral compression fracture depends on:
   A. Dose per fraction
   B. Prior treatment with radiotherapy
   C. Tumor histology

## Answers

1. D
2. C
3. B
4. A
5. A

## References

1. Wong DA, Fornasier VL, MacNab I. Spinal metastases: the obvious, the occult, and the impostors. Spine (Phila Pa 1976). 1990;15(1):1–4.
2. Chow E, Harris K, Fan G, et al. Palliative radiotherapy trials for bone metastases: a systematic review. J Clin Oncol. 2007;25(11):1423–36.
3. Nguyen J, Chow E, Zeng L, et al. Palliative response and functional interference outcomes using the Brief Pain Inventory for spinal bony metastases treated with conventional radiotherapy. Clin Oncol (R Coll Radiol). 2011;23(7):485–91.
4. van der Linden YM, Lok JJ, Steenland E, et al. Single fraction radiotherapy is efficacious: a further analysis of the Dutch Bone Metastasis Study controlling for the influence of retreatment. Int J Radiat Oncol Biol Phys. 2004;59(2):528–37.
5. Sahgal A, Roberge D, Schellenberg D, et al. The Canadian Association of Radiation Oncology scope of practice for lung, liver and spine stereotactic body radiotherapy. Clin Oncol (R Coll Radiol). 2012;24(9):629–39.
6. Sahgal A, Bilsky M, Chang EL, et al. Stereotactic body radiotherapy for spinal metastases: current status, with a focus on its application in the postoperative patient. J Neurosurg Spine. 2011;14(2):151–66.
7. Chang EL, Shiu AS, Mendel E, et al. Phase I/II study of stereotactic body radiotherapy for spinal metastasis and its pattern of failure. J Neurosurg Spine. 2007;7(2):151–60.
8. Shiu AS, Chang EL, Ye JS, et al. Near simultaneous computed tomography image-guided stereotactic spinal radiotherapy: an emerging paradigm for achieving true stereotaxy. Int J Radiat Oncol Biol Phys. 2003;57(3):605–13.
9. Yamada Y, Bilsky MH, Lovelock DM, et al. High-dose, single-fraction image-guided intensity-modulated radiotherapy for metastatic spinal lesions. Int J Radiat Oncol Biol Phys. 2008;71(2):484–90.
10. Yenice KM, Lovelock DM, Hunt MA, et al. CT image-guided intensity-modulated therapy for paraspinal tumors using stereotactic immobilization. Int J Radiat Oncol Biol Phys. 2003;55(3):583–93.
11. Potters L, Kavanagh B, Galvin JM, et al. American Society for Therapeutic Radiology and Oncology (ASTRO) and American College of Radiology (ACR) practice guideline for the performance of stereotactic body radiation therapy. Int J Radiat Oncol Biol Phys. 2010;76(2):326–32.
12. Thibault I, Chang EL, Sheehan J, et al. Response assessment after stereotactic body radiotherapy for spinal metastasis: a report from the SPIne response assessment in Neuro-Oncology (SPINO) group. Lancet Oncol. 2015;16(16):e595–603.
13. Redmond KJ, Lo SS, Fisher C, et al. Postoperative stereotactic body radiation therapy (SBRT) for spine metastases: a critical review to guide practice. Int J Radiat Oncol Biol Phys. 2016;95(5):1414–28.
14. Cox BW, Spratt DE, Lovelock M, et al. International Spine Radiosurgery Consortium consensus guidelines for target volume definition in spinal stereotactic radiosurgery. Int J Radiat Oncol Biol Phys. 2012;83(5):e597–605.
15. Redmond KJ, Robertson S, Lo SS, et al. Consensus contouring guidelines for postoperative stereotactic body radiation therapy for metastatic solid tumor malignancies to the spine. Int J Radiat Oncol Biol Phys. 2017;97(1):64–74.
16. Chan MW, Thibault I, Atenafu EG, et al. Patterns of epidural progression following postoperative spine stereotactic body radiotherapy: implications for clinical target volume delineation. J Neurosurg Spine. 2016;24(4):652–9.
17. Sangha A, Korol R, Sahgal A. Stereotactic body radiotherapy for the treatment of spine metastases: an overview of the University of Toronto, Sunnybrook Health Sciences Odette Cancer Center, technique. J Med Imaging Radiat Sci. 2013;44(3):126–33.
18. Jabbari S, Gerszten PC, Ruschin M, et al. Stereotactic body radiotherapy for spinal metastasis: practice guidelines, outcomes, and risks. Cancer J. 2016;22(4):280–9.
19. Redmond KJ, Lo SS, Soltys SG, et al. Consensus guidelines for postoperative stereotactic body radiation therapy for spinal metastases: results of an international survey. J Neurosurg Spine. 2017;26(3):299–306.
20. Bilsky MH, Laufer I, Fourney DR, et al. Reliability analysis of the epidural spinal cord compression scale. J Neurosurg Spine. 2010;13(3):324–8.
21. Lutz S, Berk L, Chang E, et al. Palliative radiotherapy for bone metastases : an ASTRO evidence-based guideline. Int J Radiat Oncol Biol Phys. 2011;79(4):965–76.
22. Al-Omair A, Masucci L, Masson-Cote L, et al. Surgical resection of epidural disease improves local control following postoperative spine stereotactic body radiotherapy. Neuro Oncol. 2013;15(10):1413–9.
23. Kumar R, Nater A, Hashmi A, et al. The era of stereotactic body radiotherapy for spinal metastases and the multidisciplinary management of complex cases. Neuro Oncol Pract. 2016;3(1): 48–58.
24. Fisher CG, DiPaola CP, Ryken TC, et al. A novel classification system for spinal instability in neoplastic disease: an evidence-based approach and expert consensus from Spine Oncology Study Group. Spine (Phila Pa 1976). 2010;35(22):E1221–9.
25. Kirshblum SC, Burns SP, Biering-Sorensen F, et al. International standards for neurological classification of spinal cord injury. J Spinal Cord Med. 2011;34:535–46.
26. Laufer I, Rubin DG, Lis E, et al. The NOMS framework: approach to the treatment of spinal metastatic tumors. Oncologist. 2013;18(6):744–51.
27. Bhattacharya IS, Hoskin PJ. Stereotactic body radiotherapy for spinal and bone metastases. Clin Oncol (R Coll Radiol). 2015;27(5):298–306.
28. Chao ST, Koyfman SA, Woody N, et al. Recursive partitioning analysis index is predictive for overall survival in patients undergoing spine stereotactic body radiation therapy for spinal metastases. Int J Radiat Oncol Biol Phys. 2012;82(5):1738–43.
29. Tang C, Hess K, Bishop AJ, et al. Creation of a prognostic index for spine metastasis to stratify survival in patients treated with spinal

stereotactic radiosurgery: secondary analysis of mature prospective trials. Int J Radiat Oncol Biol Phys. 2015;93(1):118–25.

30. Salama JK, Milano MT. Radical irradiation of extracranial oligometastases. J Clin Oncol. 2014;32(26):2902–12.

31. Gerszten PC, Burton SA, Quinn AE, et al. Radiosurgery for the treatment of spinal melanoma metastases. Stereotact Funct Neurosurg. 2005;83(5–6):213–21.

32. Leeman JE, Bilsky M, Laufer I, et al. Stereotactic body radiotherapy for metastatic spinal sarcoma: a detailed patterns-of-failure study. J Neurosurg Spine. 2016;25(1):52–8.

33. Folkert MR, Bilsky MH, Tom AK, et al. Outcomes and toxicity for hypofractionated and single-fraction image-guided stereotactic radiosurgery for sarcomas metastasizing to the spine. Int J Radiat Oncol Biol Phys. 2014;88(5):1085–91.

34. Ghia AJ, Chang EL, Bishop AJ, et al. Single-fraction versus multifraction spinal stereotactic radiosurgery for spinal metastases for spinal metastases from renal cell carcinoma: secondary analysis of phase I/II trials. J Neurosurg Spine. 2016;24(5):829–236.

35. Thibault I, Al-Omair A, Masucci GL, et al. Spine stereotactic body radiotherapy for renal cell cancer spinal metastases: analysis of outcomes and risk of vertebral compression fracture. J Neurosurg Spine. 2014;21(5):711–8.

36. Nguyen QN, Shiu AS, Rhines LD, et al. Management of spinal metastases from renal cell carcinoma using stereotactic body radiotherapy. Int J Radiat Oncol Biol Phys. 2010;76(4):1185–92.

37. Brandsma D, van den Bent MJ. Pseudoprogression and pseudoresponse in the treatment of gliomas. Curr Opin Neurol. 2009;22(6):633–8.

38. Walker AJ, Ruzevick J, Malayeri AA, et al. Postradiation imaging changes in the CNS: how can we differentiate between treatment effect and disease progression? Future Oncol. 2014;10(7):1277–97.

39. Frechette KM, Brown LC, Aubry MC, et al. Pseudoprogression after stereotactic body radiotherapy. J Thorac Oncol. 2014;9(4):e29–30.

40. Stauder MC, Rooney JW, Neben-Wittich MA, et al. Late tumor pseudoprogression followed by complete remission after lung stereotactic ablative radiotherapy. Radiat Oncol. 2013;8:167.

41. Jarraya H, Mirabel X, Taieb S, et al. Image-based response assessment of liver metastases following stereotactic body radiotherapy with respiratory tracking. Radiat Oncol. 2013;8:24.

42. Amini B, Beaman CB, Madewell JE, et al. Osseous pseudoprogression in the vertebral bodies treated with stereotactic radiosurgery : a secondary analysis of prospective phase I/II clinical trials. AJNR Am J Neuroradiol. 2016;37(2):387–92.

43. Bahig H, Simard D, Letourneau L, et al. A study of pseudoprogression after spine stereotactic body radiation therapy. Int J Radiat Oncol Biol Phys. 2016;96(4):848–56.

44. Degen JW, Gagnon GJ, Voyadzis JM, et al. CyberKnife stereotactic radiosurgical treatment of spinal tumors for pain control and quality of life. J Neurosurg Spine. 2005;2(5):540–9.

45. Gerszten PC, Burton SA, Ozhasoglu C, et al. Radiosurgery for spinal metastases : clinical experience in 500 cases from a single institution. Spine (Phila Pa 1976). 2007;32(2):193–9.

46. Gagnon GJ, Nasr NM, Liao JJ, et al. Treatment of spinal tumors using CyberKnife fractionated stereotactic radiosurgery: pain and quality-of-life assessment after treatment in 200 patients. Neurosurgery. 2009;64(2):297–306.

47. Wang XS, Rhines LD, Shiu AS, et al. A prospective analysis of the clinical effects of stereotactic body radiation therapy in cancer patients with spinal metastases without spinal cord compression. Lancet Oncol. 2012;13(4):395–402.

48. Garg AK, Shiu AS, Yang J, et al. Phase 1/2 trial of single-session stereotactic body radiotherapy for previously unirradiated spinal metastases. Cancer. 2012;118(20):5069–77.

49. Guckenberger M, Mantel F, Gerszten PC, et al. Safety and efficacity of stereotactic body radiotherapy as primary treatment for vertebral metastases: a multi-institutional analysis. Radiat Oncol. 2014;9:226.

50. Sahgal A, Ames C, Chou D, et al. Stereotectic body radiotherapy is effective salvage therapy for patients with prior radiation of spinal metastases. Int J Radiat Oncol Biol Phys. 2009;74(3):723–31.

51. Choi CY, Adler JR, Gibbs IC, et al. Stereotactic radiosurgery for treatment of spinal metastases recurring in close proximity to previously irradiated spinal cord. Int J Radiat Oncol Biol Phys. 2010;78(2):499–506.

52. Damast S, Wright J, Bilsky M, et al. Impact of dose on local failure rates after image-guided reirradiation of recurrent paraspinal metastases. Int J Radiat Oncol Biol Phys. 2011;81(3):819–26.

53. Garg AK, Wang XS, Shiu AS, et al. Prospective evaluation of spinal reirradiation by using stereotactic body radiation therapy: the University of Texas experience. Cancer. 2011;117(5):3509–16.

54. Mahadevan A, Floyd S, Wong E, et al. Stereotactic body radiotherapy reirradiation for recurrent epidural spinal metastases. Int J Radiat Oncol Biol Phys. 2011;81(5):1500–5.

55. Chang UK, Cho WI, Kim MS, et al. Local tumor control after retreatment of spinal metastasis using stereotactic body radiotherapy: comparison with initial treatment group. Acta Oncol. 2012;51(5):589–95.

56. Gerszten PC, Germanwala A, Burton SA, et al. Combination kyphoplasty and spinal radiosurgery : a new treatment paradigm for pathologic fractures. J Neurosurg Spine. 2005;3(4):296–301.

57. Moulding HD, Elder JB, Lis E, et al. Local disease control after decompressive surgery and adjuvant high-dose single-fraction radiosurgery for spine metastases. J Neurosurg Spine. 2010;13(1):87–93.

58. Laufer I, Iorgulescu JB, Chapman T, et al. Local disease control for spinal metastases following "separation surgery" and adjuvant hypofractionated or high-dose single-fraction stereotactic radiosurgery: outcome analysis in 186 patients. J Neurosurg Spine. 2013;18(3):207–14.

59. Tao R, Bishop AJ, Brownlee Z, et al. Stereotactic body radiation therapy for spinal metastases in the postoperative setting: a secondary analysis of mature phase 1-2 trials. Int J Radiat Oncol Biol Phys. 2016;95(5):1405–13.

60. Moussazadeh N, Lis E, Katsoulakis E, et al. Five Year outcomes of high-dose single-fraction spinal stereotactic radiosurgery. Int J Radiat Oncol Biol Phys. 2015;93(2):361–7.

61. Folkert MR, Bilsky MH, Cohen GN, et al. Local recurrence outcomes using the $^{32}$P intraoperative brachytherapy plaque in the management of malignant lesions of the spine involving the dura. Brachytherapy. 2015;14(2):202–8.

62. Thibault I, Campbell M, Tsen CL, et al. Salvage stereotactic body radiotherapy (SBRT) following in-field failure of initial SBRT for spinal metastases. Int J Radiat Oncol Biol Phys. 2015;93(2):353–60.

63. Klekamp J, Samii H. Surgical results for spinal metastases. Acta Neurochir. 1998;140(9):957–67.

64. Mizumoto M, Harada H, Asakura H, et al. Radiotherapy for patients with metastases to the spinal column: a review of 603 patients at Shizuoka Cancer Center Hospital. Int J Radiat Oncol Biol Phys. 2011;79(1):208–13.

65. Sahgal A, Larson DA, Chang EL. Stereotactic body radiosurgery for spinal metastases: a critical review. Int J Radiat Oncol Biol Phys. 2008;71(3):652–65.

66. Chiang A, Zeng L, Zhang L, et al. Pain flare is a commom adverse event in steroid-naïve patients after spine stereotactic body radiation therapy: a prospective clinical trial. Int J Radiat Oncol Biol Phys. 2013;86(4):638–42.

67. Pan HY, Allen PK, Wang XS, et al. Incidence and predictive factors of pain flare after spine stereotactic body radiation therapy: secondary analysis of phase 1/2 trials. Int J Radiat Oncol Biol Phys. 2014;90(4):870–6.

68. Chow E, Meyer RM, Ding K, et al. Dexamethasone in the prophylaxis of radiation-induced pain flare after palliative radiotherapy for bone metastases: a double-blind, randomised placebo-controlled, phase 3 trial. Lancet Oncol. 2015;16(15):1463–72.

69. Rose PS, Laufer I, Boland PJ, et al. Risk of fracture after single fraction image-guided intensity-modulated radiation therapy to spinal metastases. J Clin Oncol. 2009;27(30):5075–9.

70. Sahgal A, Atenafu EG, Chao S, et al. Vertebral compression fracture after spine stereotactic body radiotherapy: a multi-institutional analysis with a focus on radiation dose and the spinal instability neoplastic score. J Clin Oncol. 2013;31(27):3426–31.

71. Benedict SH, Yenice KM, Followill D, et al. Stereotactic body radiation therapy: the report of AAPM Task Group 101. Med Phys. 2010;37(8):4078–101.

72. Sahgal A, Weinberg V, Ma L, et al. Probabilities of radiation myelopathy specific to stereotactic body radiation therapy to guide safe practice. Int J Radiat Oncol Biol Phys. 2013;85(2):341–7.

73. Katsoulakis E, Jackson A, Cox B, et al. A detailed dosimetric analysis of spinal cord tolerance in high-dose spine radiosurgery. Int J Radiat Oncol Biol Phys. 2017;99(3):598–607.

74. Cox BW, Jackson A, Hunt M, et al. Esophageal toxicity from high-dose, single-fraction paraspinal stereotactic radiosurgery. Int J Radiat Oncol Biol Phys. 2012;83(5):e6661–7.

75. Masucci GL, Eugene Y, Ma L, et al. Stereotactic body radiotherapy is an effective treatment in reirradiating spinal metastases: current status and practical considerations for safe practice. Expert Rev Anticancer Ther. 2011;11(12):1923–33.

76. Sahgal A, Ma L, Weinberg V, et al. Reirradiation human spinal cord tolerance for stereotactic body radiotherapy. Int J Radiat Oncol Biol Phys. 2012;82(1):107–16.

77. Sellin JN, Suki D, Harsh V, et al. Factors affecting survival in 43 consecutive patients after surgery for spinal metastases from thyroid carcinoma. J Neurosurg Spine. 2015;23(4):419–28.

78. Fehlings MG, Nater A, Tetreault L, et al. Survival and clinical outcomes in surgically treated patients with metastatic epidural spinal cord compression: results of the prospective multicenter AOSpine study. J Clin Oncol. 2016;34(3):268–76.

79. Harel R, Emch T, Chao S, et al. Quantitative evaluation of local control and wound healing following surgery and stereotactic spine radiosurgery (SRS) for spine tumors. World Neurosurg. 2016;87:48–54.

80. Massicotte E, Foote M, Reddy R, et al. Minimal access spine surgery (MASS) for decompression and stabilization performed as an out-patient procedure for metastatic spinal tumours followed by spine stereotactic body radiotherapy (SBRT): first report of technique and preliminary outcomes. Technol Cancer Res Treat. 2012;11(1):15–25.

81. Heron DE, Rajagopalan MS, Stone B, et al. Single-session and multisession CyberKnife radiosurgery for spine metastases-University of Pittsburgh and Georgetown University experience. J Neurosurg Spine. 2012;17(1):11–8.

82. Redmond KJ, Sahgal A, Foote M, et al. Single versus multiple session stereotectic body radiotherapy for spinal metastasis: the risk-benefit ratio. Future Oncol. 2015;11(17):2405–15.

83. Schueneman AJ, Himmelfarb E, Geng L, et al. SU11248 maintenance therapy prevents tumor regrowth after fractionated irradiation of murine tumor models. Cancer Res. 2003;63(14):4009–16.

84. Staehler M, Haseke N, Nuhn P, et al. Simultaneous anti-angiogenic therapy and single-fraction radiosurgery in clinically relevant metastases from renal cell carcinoma. BJU Int. 2011;108(5):673–8.

85. Park S, Kim KH, Rhee WJ, et al. Treatment outcome of radiation therapy and concurrent targeted molecular therapy in spinal metastasis from renal cell carcinoma. Radiat Oncol J. 2016;34(2):128–34.

86. Miller JA, Balagamwala EH, Angelov L, et al. Spine stereotactic radiosurgery with concurrent tyrosine kinase inhibitors for metastatic renal cell carcinoma. J Neurosurg Spine. 2016;25(6):766–74.

87. Peters NA, Richel DJ, Verhoeff JJ, et al. Bowel perforation after radiotherapy in a patient receiving sorafenib. J Clin Oncol. 2008;26(14):2405–6.

88. Basille D, Andrejak M, Bentayeb H, et al. Bronchial fistula associated with sunitinib in a patient previously treated with radiation therapy. Ann Pharmacother. 2010;44(2):383–6.

89. Kim H, Rajagopalan MS, Beriwal S, et al. Cost-effectiveness analysis of single fraction of stereotactic body radiation therapy compared with single fraction of external beam radiation therapy for palliation of vertebral bone metastases. Int J Radiat Oncol Biol Phys. 2015;91(3):556–63.

90. Bijlani A, Aguzzi G, Schaal DW, et al. Stereotactic radiosurgery and stereotactic body radiation therapy cost-effectiveness results. Front Oncol. 2013;3:77.

91. Hyde D, Lochray F, Korol R, et al. Spine stereotactic body radiotherapy utilizing cone-beam CT image-guidance with a robotic cough: intrafraction motion analysis accounting for all six degrees of freedom. Int J Radiat Oncol Biol Phys. 2012;82(3):e555–62.

# Proton Beam Therapy (For CNS Tumors)

**47**

Divya Yerramilli, Marc R. Bussière, Jay S. Loeffler, and Helen A. Shih

## Learning Objectives

At the end of this chapter, readers should be able to:

- Understand the physical differences between proton beam therapy and photon beam therapy.
- Identify clinical indications for which proton beam therapy might be appropriate for patients with CNS tumors.
- Evaluate some of the existing data for which proton therapy has been used for patients with intracranial tumors, and understand that research in this field is still ongoing.
- Understand and apply simulation and treatment techniques that are specific to proton beam therapy delivery.
- Apply this knowledge to clinical situations in which patients may be appropriately referred for proton therapy.

## Description and Evolution of Proton Beam Therapy

The use of proton therapy in a clinical setting was first suggested based on the inherent properties of the particle. The mass and the charge of protons confer several physical advantages when applied to radiation therapy. Compared to electrons, protons have approximately 1840 times the mass and therefore scatter at a significantly smaller angle. At certain depths, this results in a sharper lateral distribution than electron or photon beams and allows normal tissue on either side lateral to the target to be better spared [1, 2].

Furthermore, the rate of energy loss of a proton in matter is inversely proportional to its velocity, which results in a characteristic depth-dose distribution. There is a slow increase in dose with depth, followed by a sharp increase near the end of range, and this sharp increase at the end of the particle range is referred to as the Bragg peak. The proton beam can be modified with different techniques to encompass targets of greater thickness than a single Bragg peak. Several beams of various energies are combined and superimposed to result in a spread-out Bragg peak (Fig. 47.1) [3]. This form of passive-scattering delivery results in a beam that is wide enough to cover the target, with the advantage of very little dose distal to the target. Alternatively, the beam can be controlled with magnets and actively scanned across the width of targets with changes in energy to vary the depth.

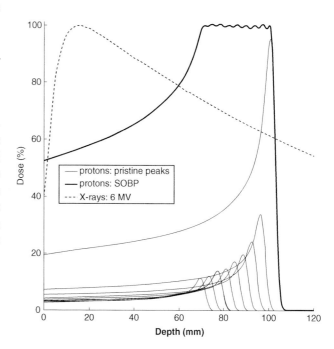

**Fig. 47.1** Depth-dose curve of a proton spread-out Bragg peak (SOBP) with a 10.1 cm range and a 3.5 cm modulation formed by the summation of multiple pristine peaks varying ranges and weights. A 6 MV photon depth dose is plotted for reference

D. Yerramilli
Harvard Radiation Oncology Program, Department of Radiation Oncology, Massachusetts General Hospital, Boston, MA, USA

M. R. Bussière · J. S. Loeffler · H. A. Shih (✉)
Department of Radiation Oncology, Massachusetts General Hospital, Boston, MA, USA
e-mail: hshih@mgh.harvard.edu

© Springer International Publishing AG, part of Springer Nature 2018
E. L. Chang et al. (eds.), *Adult CNS Radiation Oncology*, https://doi.org/10.1007/978-3-319-42878-9_47

This form of delivery is referred to as pencil-beam scanning and achieves higher conformality of radiation therapy than passive-scattering protons and importantly enables intensity-modulated proton therapy (IMPT).

Robert Wilson first anticipated the therapeutic benefits of protons in 1946 and suggested that proton therapy would result in a highly conformal dose distribution with far less collateral dose to adjacent normal tissues [4]. When applied to tumors in the central nervous system, there are several dosimetric advantages, particularly for tumors adjacent to more radiation-sensitive structures [5].

The trend in radiation techniques over time has been toward increasing conformality, to reduce exposure of radiation to normal tissue, whether 3D conformal planning is favored over 2D planning or IMRT is favored over 3D conformal planning [6, 7]. By this logic, the conformality of proton therapy could be considered one technological tool in improving targeted delivery of radiation therapy. In the 1960s, the Harvard Cyclotron Laboratory began preclinical and clinical studies to better characterize the therapeutic applications of proton therapy in partnership with the Massachusetts General Hospital Department of Neurosurgery [8]. In that era, the advantage of conformality from proton therapy was highly promising compared to available radiation techniques, but critics of proton therapy now argue conformality is less expensively achieved with IMRT. Thus, investigations on the potential clinical benefit of lowering nontarget dose radiation with the use of protons as compared to modern photon radiation techniques will be critical to defining the role of each in the future.

While proton therapy offers many physical and anatomic advantages, the energy and charge properties of protons have potential radiobiological advantages as well. Due to the charge of protons, these particles have greater linear energy transfer (LET) in matter, and therefore, they are estimated to have a greater radiobiological effectiveness for cell killing than photons [9]. Since the LET of charged particles increases as the particles slow down near end of range, the relative biological effectiveness (RBE) of the charged particle is greatest in the down slope of the Bragg peak.

There have been many radiobiological studies to determine the RBE of protons in various conditions using various endpoints [10]. Most proton treatment centers commonly apply an RBE of 1.1 for dose calculations and prescriptions, so that clinical workflows can be easily translated across modalities. However, these estimations do not take into account that proton dosimetry has a tendency to be more heterogeneous than the initial calculations estimated, and the true RBE is not fully quantified and remains an active area of study [11, 12]. Taking into account the estimated RBE of protons to photons, for equivalent doses prescribed to the tumor, protons and photons seem to have similar effects on tumor cell killing.

## Clinical Indications

In general, the efficacy of radiation therapy is limited by the dose constraints of normal tissue, which is the primary determinant for unacceptable radiation-related toxicity. For patients with intracranial tumors, there are a variety of pathologies, ranging from incurable malignancies to benign tumors. Malignancies may require high doses for tumor control that far exceed certain normal tissue tolerance, and protons may allow dose escalation where it was previously unachievable with standard photon options. For patients with benign tumors, any additional dose of radiation may expose an otherwise healthy patient to an unnecessary risk of long-term toxicity with lifetime consequences.

For CNS tumors, treatment-related toxicity can have severe implications on a patient's quality of life when considering the treated tumor itself is often not life threatening. Common acute toxicities include alopecia, skin erythema and irritation, fatigue, headaches, nausea, and vomiting, which are managed during treatment with a combination of skin care, over-the-counter pain medications, antiemetics, and steroids. More concerning are the potential long-term consequences of radiation therapy, which include focal neurologic deficits, particularly sensory changes, such as vision, hearing, motor or sensory loss, or vestibular function [13]. In addition, risks of exposure to low doses of radiation, such as a secondary malignancy, are of significance to long-term survivors as seen with diagnoses of lower-grade gliomas, and pituitary adenomas, vestibular schwannomas, among others [14–16].

While these considerations seem to be compelling arguments for treating many brain tumor patients indicated for radiation therapy with proton radiation therapy, protons remain an expensive and limited resource for therapy and must be justly allocated across all patients with appropriate indications [17, 18]. At some institutions, a systematic regular review of patients who may potentially benefit from proton therapy is conducted with a team of physicists, dosimetrists, therapists, and physicians to ensure that candidates for proton therapy are appropriately selected. In general, there are a few consistently agreed upon indications that warrant consideration of proton therapy, including benign tumors or patients with malignant tumors with favorable prognoses, tumors requiring high doses of radiation adjacent to critical structures, patients considered for re-irradiation, and participation in clinical trials. In patients with poor prognoses, more advanced age, or with tumors in locations that are easily treated with little risk to normal tissue, it may be inappropriate to use this costly and limited modality.

## Benign CNS Tumors

The management of patients with benign intracranial tumors is driven heavily by careful considerations of risks versus benefits [19, 20]. While these diseases are benign, intracranial tumors can still significantly impact quality of life, thus necessitating treatment. Because these patients generally have favorable prognoses without significant risk for mortality from their tumors, the guiding principle for treatment of benign conditions is to *Do No Harm*. Therefore, the acute and specifically the late toxicities of radiation therapy must be carefully considered before offering treatment. Proton therapy can offer some advantages, compared to photon-based therapies in this regard. Given the conformality to the target, the volume of normal tissue exposed to low doses of radiation therapy can be reduced (Fig. 47.2). These patients may live decades and have more years at risk for developing treatment-related late normal tissue injury and secondary malignancy.

For patients with arteriovenous malformations (AVMs), photon-based SRS has been used for obliteration, to ultimately reduce a small but real risk of a life-threatening intracranial hemorrhage. However, for patients with larger AVMs, a larger volume of collateral normal tissue is typically irradiated. Proton therapy can provide a way to minimize the integral dose to the surrounding brain and to achieve a superior risk-benefit balance in favor of treatment [21–23].

For patients with vestibular schwannomas (acoustic neuromas) with serviceable hearing, one goal of treatment is to maximize the amount of time with stable hearing. Therefore, patients are often candidates for observation or fractionated radiation treatment. For patients with small tumors and no serviceable hearing, proton radiosurgery can be considered with same dose practice as used with photons, of 12 Gy(RBE), and with both high tumor control and low rates of facial nerve dysfunction [24, 25].

Pituitary adenomas can also be managed with proton therapy with excellent disease control rates [26]. In most series, tumor local control rates are as high as 90–100% regardless of technique or technology, and biochemical control is comparative to photon experiences. In one study, patients with both functional and nonfunctional pituitary adenomas were treated

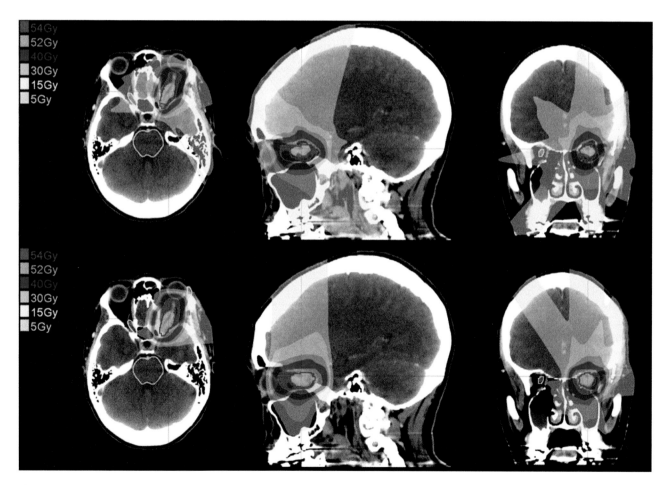

**Fig. 47.2** Treatment plan of an optic nerve sheath meningioma treated with (**a**) photon IMRT versus (**b**) passively scattered proton therapy. Whereas target dose coverage is comparable between the two techniques, there is markedly less collateral irradiation of the normal tissues with proton therapy

with fractionated protons to a median dose of 54 Gy(RBE), with local or hormonal control in all patients assessed in follow-up [27]. Most patients in this series presented in the setting of residual or recurrent disease. In these patients, anticipated benefits of proton radiation are related to reducing exposure of normal brain tissue to low doses of ionizing radiation therapy.

For patients with meningiomas, protons appear to be similarly beneficial with a higher margin of benefit for atypical or malignant meningiomas as compared to benign meningiomas, for which dose and margins are more modest. A study of 31 patients who underwent fractionated proton or photon radiation therapy for either atypical or malignant meningiomas demonstrated significantly improved local control for patients receiving proton radiation versus photon radiation, with target doses of greater than 60 Gy for both [28]. Presumptively, this was related to superior tumor target dose coverage as enabled by the use of protons.

For all of the above tumors, with small target sizes, tumor control outcomes from photon-based and proton-based treatments are likely similar, and doses for benign tumors rarely exceed normal tissue tolerance. However, these patients have excellent prognoses, and the possibility that they may experience late side effects of radiation must be considered. Particularly among long-term survivors of 10–20 years or greater, rare late adverse effects of radiation therapy are not negligible [29, 30].

## Malignant CNS Tumors

The potential role of proton radiation therapy in patients with malignant intracranial tumors must be approached differently. In patients with low-grade gliomas, who have more favorable prognoses, and who are treated to a higher dose that exceed some intracranial normal tissue tolerance parameters, protons may offer real dosimetric advantages. A prospective study single-arm study of patients with grade 2 gliomas treated with 54 Gy(RBE) in 30 fractions demonstrated preservation of excellent quality of life. At a median follow-up of 5.1 years, there was no overall decline in cognitive function, visual ability, attention/working memory, or executive functioning. However, a subset developed predictable neuroendocrine deficiencies when disease involved or abutted the pituitary [31]. While it was a small single-arm study, the results are promising that sparing normal tissue may in fact translate to sustained quality of life outcomes.

For patients with high-grade gliomas, the role of proton radiation therapy is less well established. Late toxicities are less of a concern in this group, given that their competing risk for cancer-specific morbidity and mortality far outweighs the likelihood of developing discernible treatment-related toxicity. However, the potential application of proton therapy in this cohort may allow for safer radiation dose escalation. In a series of 23 patients treated with proton radiation to a dose of 90 Gy(RBE) at 1.8 Gy(RBE) BID, median survival was 18.6 months [32]. Despite the promising median survival outcome, 90 Gy(RBE) was associated with a high rate of tissue necrosis that led to progressive neurological symptoms and need for surgical intervention. The diagnostic skills, treatment planning, and treatment delivery techniques in this study are antiquated by today's standards and such the application of protons in this setting remains under current investigation.

Protons also have a dosimetric advantage with and expectant local control clinical benefit for patients with skull base tumors, such as chordomas or chondrosarcomas. Proton therapy may offer the same anatomic advantages that are anticipated in the treatment of patients with other benign processes of the skull base, such as pituitary adenomas, vestibular schwannomas, or meningiomas. However, the doses to control sarcomas often exceed normal tissue tolerance of adjacent critical intracranial structures, with doses often of 70 Gy(RBE) or higher. One study demonstrated that patients with skull base chordomas who received 3D conformal proton therapy to doses between 77.4 Gy(RBE) and 79.4 Gy(RBE) showed that local control at 2 years was 86% and overall survival was 92%, with grade 2 toxicity of unilateral hearing loss in 18% of the cohort, with no grade 2 or higher toxicities observed for optic structures or brainstem, suggesting that proton therapy allows effective doses of radiation therapy to be delivered without compromising local control or normal tissue function [33]. Pencil-beam scanning may enable even better control and sparing of toxicity. Long-term outcomes of patients with skull base chordoma or low-grade chondrosarcomas treated with pencil-beam scanning proton therapy showed 7-year local control rates of 70.9% for patients with chordoma and 93.6% of patients with chondrosarcoma with mean delivered dose of 72.5 Gy(RBE). However, the gross residual disease was abutting the brainstem or optic apparatus in 32% of patients, and this was ultimately found on multivariate analysis to be independent prognostic factors for poorer local control and overall survival, suggesting there are some patients for whom their target volumes are centered in or around a critical structure which precludes even the most conformal therapy from optimizing control. However, for many of these patients, local control was excellent, and at 7 years, 87.2% of patients survived without evidence of any grade 3 or higher toxicity, including unilateral or bilateral optic neuropathy, temporal lobe necrosis, cerebellum brain necrosis, spinal cord necrosis, and unilateral hearing loss [34].

Where melanomas of the eye have historically been managed with enucleation, proton radiation established the alternative of definitive radiation therapy to manage these small tumors, delivering high radiation doses with no collateral radiation delivered to the brain. Rationale for proton therapy is similar to many intracranial tumors, that of small target size, excellent tumor control to radiation, and the ability to minimize radiation-related toxicity to the structures in the eye. One study of 191 patients treated with either photon-based stereotactic radiosurgery or proton beam therapy demonstrated excellent local control rates, with 98% eye preservation in the SRS group, and 95% in the proton beam therapy group. However, the patients in the SRS group showed poorer visual prognosis with 65% losing significant visual acuity, while only 45% in the proton therapy group had lost the same level of visual acuity. This suggests that while both modalities over excellent local control, proton therapy allows better preservation of function, and less late toxicity [35]. Further attempts to characterize visual acuity outcomes after proton beam therapy in a prospective way have shown that at 60-month follow-up, patients with favorable pretreatment visual acuity retained their visual acuity and will likely retain excellent long-term visual acuity. Multivariate analysis did reveal that the volume of the macula receiving 28 Gy(RBE) and optic nerve were independent dose-volume histogram predictors of post-proton therapy visual acuity loss in patients with good pretreatment vision [36].

## Re-irradiation

For patients with recurrences or progression after initial definitive radiation therapy, proton therapy may facilitate a feasible way to re-irradiate patients and mitigate some risk of exceeding normal tissue tolerances in the setting of prior irradiation (Fig. 47.3) [37].

McDonald et al. reported a retrospective review of 16 patients with a diagnosis of progressive chordoma who under-

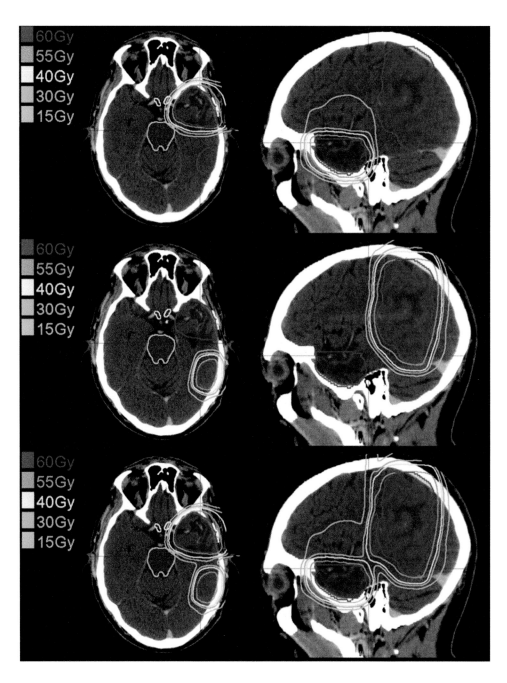

**Fig. 47.3** Re-irradiation treatment plan

went re-irradiation with proton therapy and received a median dose of re-irradiation of 75.6 Gy(RBE) with local control of 85%, overall survival of 80%, and chordoma-specific survival of 88% at 2 years [38]. Late toxicity in this study included bitemporal lobe radionecrosis in one patient, cerebrospinal fluid leak in one patient, and brainstem stroke occurring outside of the radiation field in another. Whereas this study reports on the experience of applying proton therapy as a modality for re-irradiation, it still harbors significant risks and how much less than with photon-based treatments is as yet unclear.

## Participation in Clinical Trials

There continues to be extreme controversy over the role of proton therapy, given the high capital costs of adopting the technology. In this vein, there have been strong calls for greater evidence and randomized clinical trials that study the efficacy and the potential benefits of proton therapy versus photon therapy. In order to answer this call, centers with proton therapy should be supported in their ability to conduct and participate in clinical trials. Furthermore, patients willing to participate in these studies should be allocated proton therapy, in order to justify its continued applications over time. There have been many ongoing clinical trials investigating the application of proton therapy for intracranial tumors. A recently published single-arm study examined overall survival, progression-free survival, and quality of life outcomes of proton therapy for patients with low-grade gliomas and found that patients tolerated proton therapy well with a subset of patients developing neuroendocrine dysfunction, as described above [31]. NRG BN001 is investigating hypofractionated dose-escalated photon IMRT or proton therapy in comparison to standard photon therapy for patients with

glioblastoma with a primary endpoint of overall survival [39]. As previously described, there is also a great interest in proton therapy's ability to mitigate the negative quality of life impact of interest, and there is currently a trial of proton therapy for patients with meningiomas or hemangiopericytomas with primary endpoints of quality of life measures [40]. For this reason, participation in a clinical trial is taken into account in determining allocation for proton therapy [20, 41–43].

## Immobilization Techniques and Image Guidance

Immobilization for proton therapy is of critical importance. Given the benefits of conformality with proton beam radiation therapy, immobilization is paramount to minimizing uncertainty and ensuring that ultimately the entire target is treated to the prescription dose. For intracranial tumors, many types of external frames have been developed for standard fractionated proton radiation treatment using doses ≤3 Gy(RBE) [44]. Because protons are more sensitive than photons to shape and density variations, immobilization equipment must be specifically designed to minimize these factors. Patient compliance and ability to tolerate the immobilization devices is also essential for successful proton treatment, and sedation or anesthesia can be used if patients have considerable difficulty tolerating treatment.

An example of an immobilization frame that has been developed for proton therapy of brain tumors is a modified Gill-Thomas-Cosman (mGTC) frame, comprising a rounded carbon fiber occipital support and low-density cushion in addition to the GTC frame (Fig. 47.4) [45]. This device is used to treat intracranial targets that do not extend to the base

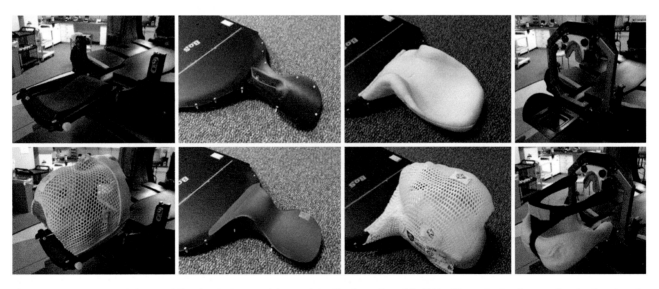

**Fig. 47.4** Proton compatible immobilization devices used for cranial irradiation. Two leftmost images: intracranial mask system with a standard occipital cushion (top) and reinforced thermoplastic mask (top); middle four images: QFix base of skull immobilization system (QFix Products, Avondale, PA) with standard and custom head and neck cushions and mask and the modified Gill-Thomas-Cosman (MGTC) frame with and without a custom occipital cushion

of the skull but requires that the patient have good dentition, as the skull is immobilized using a fixed dental mold to create excellent and reproducible immobilization.

Alternative fixation devices, which do not use dental fixation, make use of thermoplastic masks and custom occipital cushions for a somewhat comfortable yet reproducible immobilization. An example of a proton compatible system is the intracranial (IC) frame assembly, which was originally designed for PET imaging and subsequently adapted for proton therapy (Carbon Head Holder 237HH, Tru-Scan Imaging Inc., Annapolis, MD). The IC frame can be used with a standard head cup or custom occipital cushion and a perforated thermoplastic mask reinforced with a solid sheet polyfoam [46]. The base of the IC device is made of carbon fiber to permit treatment beams to be employed through the frame, enabling lower fields and skull base tumors to be treated, unlike the MGTC frame. It can also be used in patients who have poor or no dentition. A readily available commercial alternative to the IC frame is the Base of Skull (BoS) frame (AccuFix BOS Frame RT-45, Q-Fix WFR-Aquaplast, Avondale, PA) specifically designed for proton therapy. The BoS is similar to the IC frame using a proton friendly designed carbon support in combination with a thermoplastic mask and custom or standard head and neck cushion.

The regular use of cone beam computed tomography (CBCT) and automated corrections is not commonly used with proton beam therapy, yet, and therefore, patients requiring intracranial proton stereotactic radiosurgery can undergo an additional step to improve localization, which may include placement of fiducial markers using minimal anesthetic into the outer table of the skull. This procedure can be performed as an outpatient procedure by a neurosurgeon in approximately 15 min with minimal blood loss. This allows triangulation of the skull for treatment with utmost accuracy [47].

Once these immobilization devices are created, patients undergo CT simulation in a supine position. The use of IV contrast is at the discretion of the treating physician, depending on the ability of the contrast to enhance regions of interest on the CT images and the patient's individual ability to tolerate contrast (with good baseline kidney function and no contrast-related allergies). The use of contrast must be used cautiously, as CT densities are used to estimate stopping power, from which proton ranges are ultimately derived [48]. The discrepancy between the artificial density of IV contrast and the true tissue density may be mitigated by using *pre-contrast* scans. Regardless, in most cases, a recent MRI is often registered to the planning CT scan to give additional anatomic information.

## Treatment Planning

### Target Delineation

Because the potential advantages of proton therapy are related to high-precision conformality, treatment planning demands accurate target and organs at risk (OAR) delineation. For intracranial tumors, MRI fusions are used to assist in delineation of the target volume as well as of critical structures. This fusion must be as accurate as possible to ensure precise tumor volume delineation. A dedicated anatomist can be helpful in delineating critical structures for consistency and highest accuracy for treatment planning.

## Treatment Delivery Systems

Protons employed in therapeutic radiation therapy can be accelerated with either cyclotrons or synchrotrons. Accelerated protons are directed toward the gantry heads using a series of bending magnets, so the energy of each particle can be maintained until it is delivered to the target (Fig. 47.5) Because the beam is delivered as a single beam line, the particle beam must be spread to cover the target, and this can be achieved in a few ways. Protons can be spread from the source by either passive-scattering or by pencil-beam scanning [49]. A single-scattering system may be used for small tumors, while double-scattering allows larger tumors to be treated with a uniform lateral dose. Both forms require custom blocking for lateral conformality, as well as a range compensator, which allows for distal conformality to the target.

There has also been an increasing interest in the use of pencil-beam scanning, in which uniform fields can be produced without loss of range. In pencil-beam scanning, each beam is delivered in a certain array, with a specific spot size and defined energy [50, 51]. The energy for each spot is modulated to deliver dose to a particular depth, and then this is repeated for each position in the array, without the need for a range compensator for distal conformality (Fig. 47.6). Custom blocking with apertures can also be used to sharpen the penumbra but may not be necessary for some applications of pencil-beam scanning. Scanned beams may be delivered with single-field uniform doses (SFUD) where each field covers the target uniformly or using multi-field intensity-modulated proton therapy (IMPT) maps determined from inverse planning optimization. IMPT may be preferred for patients with irregularly shaped tumors, who would similarly benefit from IMRT treatments over forward-planning 3D conformal radiation therapy, with the added advantage of using protons to further spare dose to neighboring critical structures.

Proton therapy can also be used for radiosurgery. At the Massachusetts General Hospital, a fixed stereotactic single-scattering beamline used with a minimal penumbra can deliver highly accurate doses to intracranial tumors, such as brain metastases, arteriovenous malformations, pituitary adenomas, meningiomas, and vestibular schwannomas [52].

In the treatment planning process, there are several ways to account for uncertainty that are unique to proton therapy

**Fig. 47.5** Layout for a shielded single gantry system. Protons are extracted from the cyclotron and degraded to the desired energy before they are transported through a vacuum pipe to the treatment room. Dipole bending magnets (blue; left image insert) deflect the beam by degrees requiring refocusing with the aid of multiple quadrupole magnets (yellow; right image insert). The 35 ton gantry assembly includes two large bending magnets which direct the proton beam to the treatment head which can pivot 360° about isocenter

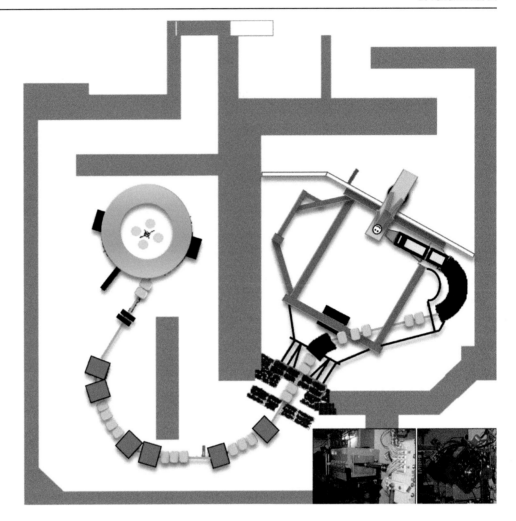

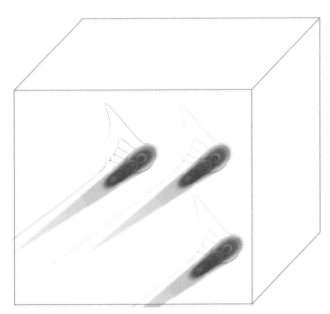

**Fig. 47.6** The pencil-beam treatment head replaces the modulation wheel and scattering elements with fast-responding scanning magnets which are used to deflect un-scattered pristine peaks from the nominal beam-eye-view axis $(x, y)$. A treatment plan provides the map defining the location $(x, y, \text{depth})$ of the individual peaks required to achieve a desired dose distribution. The irradiation sequence is performed one energy layer at a time. Changing the system's energy requires a brief pause in the irradiation

[53]. Variations in patient setup, organ and tumor motion, image guidance, tumor localizations, and uncertainties in dose calculations must be minimized. Adequate margins should be added to the tumor volume, but large margins lose the advantage of sparing normal tissue. In addition to range uncertainty originating from daily setup variations, there is also inherent uncertainty in the conversion of CT Hounsfield numbers to proton stopping power. Some institutions may assess target coverage using a uniform PTV expansion, but corrections should be applied on a per beam basis.

Each proton beam is known to have a degree of uncertainty regarding the range, and dosimetric calculations and distributions must take these uncertainties into account. These uncertainties can be mitigated using a "smearing technique" where the compensator dimensions are adjusted within the range of uncertainty to ensure target volume coverage.

## Typical Dose Distribution

Dose distributions for proton therapy generally are characterized as more conformal as compared to photons with virtually no dose distal to the target per beam, as previously described. This may be varied, depending on the geometry of the tumor, the specifications of the plan, and whether or not the patient is receiving passively scattered proton therapy or pencil-beam scanning. There have been studies that attempt to characterize and model the dose distribution of these various modalities [54–58]. However, special attention must be given to consider neutron dose distribution, which is unique to proton dosimetry and may be underestimated if dose from protons alone is accounted [59].

## Dose Specification

For patients treated with fractionated passive-scattering proton therapy, like 3D photon therapy, prescription doses of radiation therapy are generally prescribed to the center of the spread-out Bragg peak [60]. For patients treated with pencil-beam scanning, the dose is prescribed to the volume because of the complexity of the dose distributions. The same is true for proton radiosurgery, where a GTV/CTV and PTV are delineated, and the dose is prescribed to the PTV, to maintain consistency with photon radiosurgery dose specifications.

## Quality Assurance

Institutions should follow IAEA TRS-398 and ICRU Report 59 for absolute dosimetry characterization and undergo annual independent verification by an accredited laboratory [61, 62]. General quality assurance (QA) recommendations are provided by the ACR and AAPM [63]. However, there are currently no formal AAPM task group report for proton therapy. In absence of comprehensive quality assurance recommendations, references used for photon therapy should be used for guidance. Examples of such references include AAPM reports TG-142 (quality assurance of medical accelerators), TG-54 (stereotactic radiosurgery), TG-100 (application of risk analysis methods to radiation therapy quality management), TG-135 (quality assurance for robotic radiosurgery), TG-101 (stereotactic body radiation therapy), TG-179 (quality assurance for image-guided radiation therapy using CT-based technologies), TG-147 (quality assurance for non-radiographic radiotherapy localization and positioning systems), and TG-53 (quality assurance for clinical radiotherapy treatment planning). Similarly, IAEA 1583 (Commissioning of Radiotherapy Treatment Planning Systems: Testing for Typical External Beam Treatment Techniques) as well as the various AAPM/ACR and ASTRO/ACR practice guidelines should be reviewed [64–70].

As with Linac-based equipment, a comprehensive quality assurance program involves daily, monthly, and annual checks. Daily quality assurance is completed prior to the first patient treatment and may differ depending on the treatment delivery system. For passive scattering, the machines can be tested both in service mode with a range verifier installed in the nozzle that can be used to verify first and second scatterers, timing of modulator wheels, and beam range. Treatment mode can be verified using an ion chamber and Lucite phantom to measure dose outputs for standard fields spanning various equipment settings. More comprehensive dose measurements can be performed using planar ion chamber arrays. Daily QA also incorporates other checks including but not limited to safety interlocks, imaging alignment, and audio/visual monitoring systems. Monthly quality assurance expands on the daily checks, verifying beam range, modulation, field flatness, and symmetry for a fixed set of fields that spans the full set of equipment settings. Proton versus X-ray field coincidence is also measured at regular intervals. Annual QA significantly expands on daily and monthly QA. As with 3D conformal photon plans, individual measurements may not be necessary if an independent verification system is used. However, beam-modifying hardware such as apertures and compensators must be subjected to a QC process.

For individual pencil-beam scanning, patient fields, dose profiles at two to three depths are verified in phantom. A quality assurance program similar to passive scattering, encompassing daily, monthly, and annual checks ensures delivery constancy. In addition to those items described for passive scattering, beam spot position, size, and dose is monitored.

## Case Study

A patient is a 55-year-old woman with no significant past medical history, who initially presents with diplopia and right facial nerve numbness in the V2 and V3 distribution. She undergoes MRI of the brain which demonstrated a complex skull base well-circumscribed and enhancing lesion of the suprasellar, cavernous sinus, sella, Meckel's cave, and petroclival region with spillage into the posterior fossa. The image is consistent with a meningioma. She then undergoes transsphenoidal surgery as well as a right suboccipital craniotomy, with final pathology demonstrating a WHO grade 2 meningioma with prominent nucleoli, architectural sheeting, foci of necrosis, and Ki-67 of 12.4%. Postoperatively, an MRI shows 40% debulking of the tumor beneath the sella in the prepontine cistern and stable component inferior to the right of the chiasm, right of Meckel's cave, and residual tumor in the dorsum of the sella turcica (Fig. 47.7).

She is referred for consultation with radiation oncology, and full history and physical are reviewed. At the treating physician's discretion, several factors are considered, including aggressive pathology, no clinical comorbidities that suggest competing risk, relatively young age, and

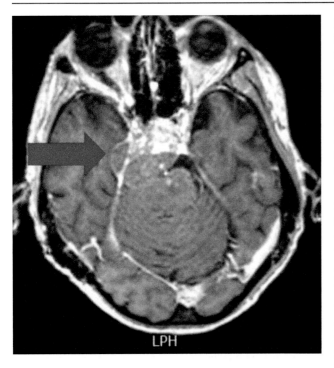

**Fig. 47.7** Preoperative and postoperative MRI of a patient

proximity of the tumor to critical structures that are important for the patient's quality of life. Given these considerations, the treating physician discusses external beam therapy options with the patient, including photon versus proton irradiation, and delineates potential geometric advantages and also discloses that there is no level I evidence that protons are superior to photons but the dosimetric difference is compelling in favor of protons as a safer treatment modality (Fig. 47.8). Furthermore, the patient is eligible for a clinical trial, and she expresses interest in participating.

The patient is then presented to a multidisciplinary team, including other physicians, physicists, and administrative staff, and the case is reviewed for potential benefit of proton therapy. At this meeting, scans are evaluated by physicists to best choose a treatment delivery modality based on size and projected geometry. Physicians examine the clinical history to determine appropriateness of allocation of proton therapy. Schedulers examine wait times for the machines and prioritization of other cases. Enrollment on a clinical trial and contribution to general medical knowledge are also given importance in consideration of allocation of proton therapy. For all of these reasons, the patient is ultimately deemed to

**Fig. 47.8** Comparison of an IMRT (top) and passively scattered proton plan (bottom) for a complex atypical skull base meningioma. The clinical goals included coverage of the target with 59.4 Gy(RBE) with an integrated simultaneous boost to 66 Gy(RBE) to the GTV while limiting the brainstem surface to 66 Gy(RBE), brainstem center to 54 Gy(RBE), optic nerves and chiasm to 60 Gy(RBE), cochlea to 45 Gy(RBE), retina to 45 Gy(RBE), and mean lacrimal glands to 26 Gy(RBE)

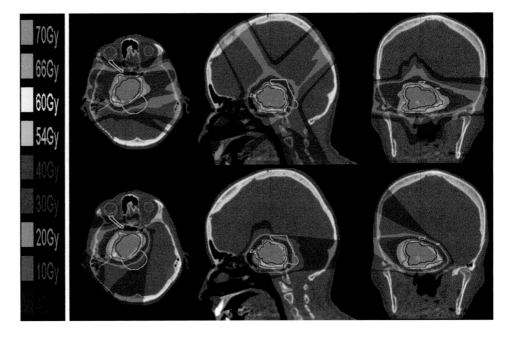

be appropriate for proton therapy and is appropriately scheduled as a medically nonurgent case.

She undergoes placement of three stainless steel fiducials using local topical anesthetic for target localization. She undergoes CT simulation in the supine position. A modified GTC head frame is used for immobilization. Using treatment planning software, recent MRI is fused with the planning CT to aid in target delineation. The treating physician delineates target volumes, and a dedicated anatomist contours neighboring normal tissue critical structures.

Based on these contours, proton-specific planning software is used to generate a proton stereotactic fractionated radiation therapy plan using a single-scattering, passive-scattering, or scanning system. Custom apertures and compensators are fabricated. Treatment planning is executed with prioritization of gross tumor volume coverage, and limiting dose to critical structures under their respective tolerances. A physics peer review is performed before presenting the plan to the physician. Once approved, these plans are then reviewed in chart rounds for broader peer review quality assurance, and the treatment is delivered. Patients are monitored throughout the course of the treatment by nursing staff and undergo weekly treatment management visits with the physician. After the completion of the treatment course, the patient is then closely followed for long-term treatment toxicity and tumor stability.

This case highlights several of the complexities of treating a patient with proton therapy. Clinicians must use stringent clinical criteria to evaluate the appropriateness of resource allocation but allow for some flexibility, given the unique nature of certain cases, and this requires a priori knowledge of the potential benefits of proton therapy. Her enrollment on a clinical trial will also allow the medical community to learn more about the capabilities of proton therapy.

## Special Considerations

There is a great deal of controversy surrounding the use of proton therapy, primarily arising from the high capital cost. Cost ratios per fraction of proton therapy compared to IMRT are the same in 2016 as in 2003: 2.34 times that of IMRT [71].

With the increased number of proton centers being deployed, there have been multiple discussions regarding the utility, the cost-effectiveness, and the appropriate indications for proton therapy. Even in institutions where proton therapy is readily available and used regularly, there is a sense of guardianship over proton therapy as a limited resource, given the high costs. There have been some attempts to study the absolute costs of proton radiation therapy. The subjective arguments range from never using it at all on the basis of cost, using it judiciously and cautiously, and using it more generously with the intent to clarify clinical indications for which the costs are worth it[72–74]. One cost-effectiveness study attempted to model the costs associated with the quality-adjusted life years across four groups of patients: left breast cancer, prostate cancer, head and neck cancer, and childhood medulloblastoma [75]. In this model, they argue that the capital costs may be worth the investment to treat certain patients on the basis of cost alone. As more prospective research comparing proton therapy and standard photon therapy emerge, and toxicity data is quantified, stronger evidenced-based data may emerge that ultimately favor the use of proton therapy for certain indications on the basis of quality of life and cost, while limiting its use when clinically equivalent and wasteful. While rigorous study remains an academic priority, further innovation may make proton therapy less expensive to deliver in the future, obviating much of this controversy.

## Summary

- Proton therapy has been in clinical use for over 50 years, with several clear physical advantages that improve conformality of radiation dose delivery.
- Proton therapy applied for adult CNS indications is most commonly rationed for patients with benign disease or malignant disease adjacent to critical radiation-sensitive structures that can be spared by the use of protons.
- Proton therapy may allow patients to more safely and feasibly undergo re-irradiation.
- There is a need for further level I evidence to characterize the potential clinical benefits of proton therapy compared to photon therapy.

- Patients require special consideration for immobilization for proton intracranial irradiation.
- Proton treatment planning and delivery are complex and can either employ the use of passive-scattering or pencil-beam scattering technology.
- Typical dose distributions of proton therapy depend on the tumor, anatomical site, and plan but generally result in more conformal plans, although the role of neutron scatter must not be ignored.
- There are specific quality assurance guidelines that can be used to ensure maximally safe proton treatment delivery.
- Proton therapy has high capital costs, and cost-effectiveness research is ongoing to identify indications for which it would be financially sustainable.
- Well-selected patients may undergo a complex selection and treatment planning process, resulting in potentially beneficial treatment option with proton therapy and which merits future studies.

## Self-Assessment Questions

1. Proton therapy differs from photon therapy in that:
   A. Protons have a lower RBE.
   B. Protons have increased distal conformality.
   C. Protons are less laterally conformal.
   D. Protons are universally accepted as better treatment for pediatric patients.

2. Which patient might be a suitable candidate for proton therapy?
   A. A 92-year-old gentleman with widely metastatic melanoma with numerous intracranial lesions.
   B. A 51-year-old woman with metastatic breast cancer with diffuse leptomeningeal disease.
   C. A 33-year-old gentleman with NF1 who presents with a low-grade glioma of the cerebellum.
   D. A 63-year-old woman with metastatic lung cancer with a single hemorrhagic brain metastasis in her frontal lobe.

3. Which patient would NOT be a suitable candidate for proton therapy?
   A. A 34-year-old woman with residual functional pituitary adenoma after surgery
   B. A 52-year-old gentleman with an acoustic neuroma with gradual hearing loss
   C. A 21-year-old woman with medulloblastoma
   D. A 75-year-old woman with a completely resected frontal WHO grade I meningioma

4. The following quality assurance guidelines can be used for absolute dosimetry of standard fractionated proton delivery:
   A. No guidelines are available yet, as proton therapy is still a novel technology.
   B. AAPM TG-54.
   C. IAEA TRS-398.
   D. AAPM TG-170.

5. True or false: Full-dose proton therapy can always be used for patients with recurrent disease after prior definitive radiation therapy.

## Answers

1. B
   Protons have higher RBE, increased distal and lateral conformality, and are considered to be potentially beneficial for pediatric patients, although this is not universally accepted.
2. C
   Patients who are younger and may live to see radiation toxicity, including secondary malignancy, should be considered for proton therapy. Older patients with poor prognoses or patients with diffuse disease who have less to benefit from proton radiation dosimetrically are less compelling to be treated with costly and limited technology with unlikely benefit.
3. D
   The patient may be closely observed and can likely be treated with photons without concern for radiation-related toxicity or development of secondary malignancy
4. C
   IAEA TRS-398 can be used. TG-54 is for radiosurgery quality assurance.
5. False
   For patients with in-field recurrences, proton therapy may not necessarily be safely feasible

## References

1. Khan FM, Gibbons JP. Chapter 27: Proton beam therapy. In: Khan's the physics of radiation therapy. Philadelphia, PA: Lippincott Williams & Wilkins; 2014. p. 527–40.
2. Urie MM, Sisterson JM, Koehler AM, et al. Proton beam penumbra: effects of separation between patient and beam modifying devices. Med Phys. 1986;13(5):734–41.
3. Koehler AM, Preston WM. Protons in radiation therapy; comparative dose distributions for protons, photons, and electrons. Radiology. 1972;104(1):191–5.
4. Wilson RR. Radiological use of fast protons. Radiology. 1946;47(5):487–91.

5. Gridley DS, Grover RS, Loredo LN, et al. Proton-beam therapy for tumors of the CNS. Expert Rev Neurother. 2010;10(2):319–30.

6. Teh BS, Woo SY, Butler EB. Intensity modulated radiation therapy (IMRT): a new promising technology in radiation oncology. Oncologist. 1999;4(6):433–42.

7. Shumway DA, Griffith KA, Pierce LJ, et al. Wide variation in the diffusion of a new technology: practice based trends in intensity modulated radiation therapy (IMRT) use in the state of Michigan, with implications for IMRT use nationally. J Oncol Pract. 2015;11(3):e373–9.

8. Suit H, Chu W. History of charged particle radiotherapy. In: De Laney TF, Kooy HM, editors. Proton and charged particle radiotherapy. Philadelphia, PA: Lippincott Williams & Wilkins; 2008. p. 1–8.

9. Urano M, Verhey LJ, Goitein M, et al. Relative biological effectiveness of modulated proton beams in various murine tissues. Int J Radiat Oncol Biol Phys. 1984;10(4):509–14.

10. Paganetti H, Niemierko A, Ancukiewicz M, et al. Relative biological effectiveness (RBE) values for proton beam therapy. Int J Radiat Oncol Biol Phys. 2002;53(2):407–21.

11. Paganetti H. Relative biological effectiveness (RBE) values for proton beam therapy. Variations as a function of biological endpoint, dose, and linear energy transfer. Phys Med Biol. 2014;59(22):R419.

12. Paganetti H, Jiang H, Parodi K, et al. Clinical implementation of full Monte Carlo dose calculation in proton beam therapy. Phys Med Biol. 2008;53(17):4825.

13. Cox JD, Stetz J, Pajak TF. Toxicity criteria of the radiation therapy oncology group (RTOG) and the European organization for research and treatment of cancer (EORTC). Int J Radiat Oncol Biol Phys. 1995;31(5):1341–6.

14. Cardis E, Gilbert ES, Carpenter L, et al. Effects of low doses and low dose rates of external ionizing radiation: cancer mortality among nuclear industry workers in three countries. Radiat Res. 1995;142(2):117–32.

15. Lowe XR, Bhattacharya S, Marchetti F, et al. Early brain response to low-dose radiation exposure involves molecular networks and pathways associated with cognitive functions, advanced aging and Alzheimer's disease. Radiat Res. 2009;171(1):53–65.

16. Lawrence YR, Li XA, El Naqa I, et al. Radiation dose–volume effects in the brain. Int J Radiat Oncol Biol Phys. 2010;76(3):S20–7.

17. Jagsi R, DeLaney TF, Donelan K, et al. Real-time rationing of scarce resources: The Northeast Proton Therapy Center experience. J Clin Oncol. 2004;22(11):2246–50.

18. Bekelman JE, Asch DA, Tochner Z, et al. Principles and reality of proton therapy treatment allocation. Int J Radiat Oncol Biol Phys. 2014;89(3):499–508.

19. Al-Mefty O, Kersh JE, Routh A, et al. The long-term side effects of radiation therapy for benign brain tumors in adults. J Neurosurg. 1990;73(4):502–12.

20. Schulz-Ertner D, Tsujii H. Particle radiation therapy using proton and heavier ion beams. J Clin Oncol. 2007;25(8):953–64.

21. Seifert V, Stolke D, Mehdorn HM, et al. Clinical and radiological evaluation of long-term results of stereotactic proton beam radiosurgery in patients with cerebral arteriovenous malformations. J Neurosurg. 1994;81(5):683–9.

22. Silander H, Pellettieri L, Enblad P, et al. Fractionated, stereotactic proton beam treatment of cerebral arteriovenous malformations. Acta Neurol Scand. 2004;109(2):85–90.

23. Vernimmen FJ, Slabbert JP, Wilson JA, et al. Stereotactic proton beam therapy for intracranial arteriovenous malformations. Int J Radiat Oncol Biol Phys. 2005;62(1): 44–52.

24. Weber DC, Chan AW, Bussiere MR, et al. Proton beam radiosurgery for vestibular schwannoma: tumor control and cranial nerve toxicity. Neurosurgery. 2003;53(3):577–88.

25. Lunsford LD, Niranjan A, Flickinger JC, et al. Radiosurgery of vestibular schwannomas: summary of experience in 829 cases. J Neurosurg. 2005;102(Suppl):195–9.

26. Loeffler JS, Shih HA. Radiation therapy in the management of pituitary adenomas. J Clin Endocrinol Metabol. 2011;96(7): 1992–2003.

27. Ronson BB, Schulte RW, Han KP, et al. Fractionated proton beam irradiation of pituitary adenomas. Int J Radiat Oncol Biol Phys. 2006;64(2):425–34.

28. Hug EB, DeVries A, Thornton AF, et al. Management of atypical and malignant meningiomas: role of high-dose, 3D-conformal radiation therapy. J Neuro-Oncol. 2000;48(2):151–60.

29. Arvold ND, Niemierko A, Broussard GP, et al. Projected second tumor risk and dose to neurocognitive structures after proton versus photon radiotherapy for benign meningioma. Int J Radiat Oncol Biol Phys. 2012;83(4):e495–500.

30. Blomquist E, Bjelkengren G, Glimelius B. The potential of proton beam radiation therapy in intracranial and ocular tumours. Acta Oncol. 2005;44(8):862–70.

31. Shih HA, Sherman JC, Nachtigall LB, et al. Proton therapy for low-grade gliomas: results from a prospective trial. Cancer. 2015;121(10):1712–9.

32. Fitzek MM, Thornton AF, Rabinov JD, et al. Accelerated fractionated proton/photon irradiation to 90 cobalt gray equivalent for glioblastoma multiforme: results of a phase II prospective trial. J Neurosurg. 1999;91(2): 251–60.

33. Deraniyagala RL, Yeung D, Mendenhall WM, et al. Proton therapy for skull base chordomas: an outcome study from the University of Florida Proton Therapy Institute. J Neurol Surg B Skull Base. 2014;75(01):053–7.

34. Weber DC, Malyapa R, Albertini F, et al. Long term outcomes of patients with skull-base low-grade chondrosarcoma and chordoma patients treated with pencil beam scanning proton therapy. Radiother Oncol. 2016;120(1):169–74.

35. Sikuade MJ, Salvi S, Rundle PA, et al. Outcomes of treatment with stereotactic radiosurgery or proton beam therapy for choroidal melanoma. Eye. 2015;29(9): 1194–8.

36. Polishchuk AL, Mishra KK, Weinberg V, et al. Temporal evolution and dose-volume histogram predictors of visual acuity after proton beam radiation therapy of uveal melanoma. Int J Radiat Oncol Biol Phys. 2017;97(1):91–7.

37. Mizumoto M, Okumura T, Ishikawa E, et al. Reirradiation for recurrent malignant brain tumor with radiotherapy or proton beam therapy. Strahlenther Onkol. 2013;189(8):656–63.

38. McDonald MW, Linton OR, Shah MV. Proton therapy for reirradiation of progressive or recurrent chordoma. Int J Radiat Oncol Biol Phys. 2013;87(5):1107–14.

39. Mehta M. Randomized phase II trial of hypofractionated dose-escalated photon IMRT or proton beam therapy versus conventional photon irradiation with concomitant and adjuvant temozolomide in patients with newly diagnosed glioblastoma. In: ClinicalTrials.gov [Internet]. Bethesda (MD): National Library of Medicine (US). 2015. Available from: https://clinicaltrials.gov/ct2/show/NCT02179086?term=bn001&rank=1. NLM Identifier: NCT02179086.

40. Abramson Cancer Center at the University of Pennsylvania. Proton radiation for meningiomas and hemangiopericytomas. In: ClinicalTrials.gov [Internet]. Bethesda (MD): National Library of

Medicine (US). 2015. Available from: https://clinicaltrials.gov/ct2/show/NCT01117844. NLM Identifier: NCT01117844.

41. Olsen DR, Bruland ØS, Frykholm G, et al. Proton therapy–a systematic review of clinical effectiveness. Radiother Oncol. 2007;83(2):123–32.

42. Lodge M, Pijls-Johannesma M, Stirk L, et al. A systematic literature review of the clinical and cost-effectiveness of hadron therapy in cancer. Radiother Oncol. 2007;83(2):110–22.

43. Glimelius B, Montelius A. Proton beam therapy–do we need the randomised trials and can we do them? Radiother Oncol. 2007;83(2):105–9.

44. Winey B, Daartz J, Dankers F, et al. Immobilization precision of a modified GTC frame. J Appl Clin Med Phys. 2012;13(3):12.

45. Bussière MR, Adams JA. Treatment planning for conformal proton radiation therapy. Technol Cancer Res Treat. 2003;2(5):389–99.

46. Engelsman M, Rosenthal SJ, Michaud SL, et al. Intra and interfractional patient motion for a variety of immobilization devices. Med Phys. 2005;32(11):3468–74.

47. Chen CC, Chapman P, Petit J, et al. Proton radiosurgery in neurosurgery. Neurosurg Focus. 2007;23(6):E4.

48. Schneider U, Pedroni E, Lomax A. The calibration of CT Hounsfield units for radiotherapy treatment planning. Phys Med Biol. 1996;41(1):111.

49. Gottschalk B. Passive beam scattering. In: De Laney TF, Kooy HM, editors. Proton and charged particle radiotherapy. Philadelphia, PA: Lippincott Williams & Wilkins; 2008. p. 33–9.

50. Pedroni E. Pencil beam scanning. In: De Laney TF, Kooy HM, editors. Proton and charged particle radiotherapy. Philadelphia, PA: Lippincott Williams & Wilkins; 2008. p. 33–9.

51. Pedroni E, Scheib S, Böhringer T, et al. Experimental characterization and physical modelling of the dose distribution of scanned proton pencil beams. Phys Med Biol. 2005;50(3):541.

52. Bussière M, Loeffler J, Chapman P, et al. Techniques of radiosurgery. Chapter 254. Proton radiosurgery. In: Youmans WH, editor. Neurological surgery. Amsterdam: Elsevier; 2016.

53. De Laney TF, Kooy HM, editors. Proton and charged particle radiotherapy. Philadelphia, PA: Lippincott Williams & Wilkins; 2008.

54. Yock T, Schneider R, Friedmann A, et al. Proton radiotherapy for orbital rhabdomyosarcoma: clinical outcome and a dosimetric comparison with photons. Int J Radiat Oncol Biol Phys. 2005;63(4):1161–8.

55. Boehling NS, Grosshans DR, Bluett JB, et al. Dosimetric comparison of three-dimensional conformal proton radiotherapy, intensity-modulated proton therapy, and intensity-modulated radiotherapy for treatment of pediatric craniopharyngiomas. Int J Radiat Oncol Biol Phys. 2012;82(2):643–52.

56. Verhey LJ, Smith V, Serago CF, et al. Comparison of radiosurgery treatment modalities based on physical dose distributions. Int J Radiat Oncol Biol Phys. 1998;40(2):497–505.

57. Phillips MH, Frankel KA, Lyman JT, et al. Comparison of different radiation types and irradiation geometries in stereotactic radiosurgery. Int J Radiat Oncol Biol Phys. 1990;18(1):211–20.

58. Bolsi A, Fogliata A, Cozzi L, et al. Radiotherapy of small intracranial tumours with different advanced techniques using photon and proton beams: a treatment planning study. Radiother Oncol. 2003;68(1):1–14.

59. Tayama R, Fujita Y, Tadokoro M, et al. Measurement of neutron dose distribution for a passive scattering nozzle at the Proton Medical Research Center (PMRC). Nucl Instrum Methods Phys Res, Sect A. 2006;564(1):532–6.

60. Vynckier S, Bonnett DE, Jones DTL. Supplement to the code of practice for clinical proton dosimetry. Radiother Oncol. 1994;32(2):174–9.

61. Lu HM. Proton therapy: operations and physics QA at MGH. Presented at AAPM, 2013.

62. Sahoo N. Quality assurance implementation in proton therapy centers. Presented at AAPM, 2013.

63. American College of Radiology. ACR-AAPM technical standard for the performance of proton beam radiation therapy. https://www.acr.org/~/media/7BEBF7E77E1141578CB8722F997BDE9B.pdf. Accessed 15 Feb 2017.

64. American College of Radiology. ACR practice parameter for 3D external beam radiation planning and conformal therapy. 2016. https://www.acr.org/~/media/ACR/Documents/PGTS/guidelines/3D_External_Beam.pdf. Accessed 15 Feb 2017.

65. American College of Radiology. ACR technical standard for medical physics performance monitoring of image-guided radiation therapy (IGRT). 2014. https://www.acr.org/~/media/ACR/Documents/PGTS/standards/IGRT.pdf. Accessed 15 Feb 2017.

66. American College of Radiology. ACR–ASTRO practice parameter for image-guided radiation therapy (IGRT) CSC/BOC. 2014. https://www.acr.org/~/media/7B19A9CEF68F4D6D8F0CF25F21155D73.pdf. Accessed 15 Feb 2017.

67. American College of Radiology. ACR practice parameter for intensity modulated radiation therapy (IMRT). 2016. https://www.acr.org/~/media/ACR/Documents/PGTS/guidelines/IMRT.pdf. Accessed 15 Feb 2017.

68. American College of Radiology. ACR practice parameter for the performance of brain stereotactic radiosurgery. 2016. https://www.acr.org/~/media/f80a2737ff0f4753b6ababa73e15d757.pdf. Accessed 15 Feb 2017.

69. American College of Radiology. ACR–ASTRO practice parameter for the performance of stereotactic body radiation therapy. 2014. https://www.acr.org/~/media/A159B3D508C64C918C4C6295BAEC4E2B.pdf. Accessed 15 Feb 2017.

70. American College of Radiology. ACR technical standard for the performance of radiation oncology physics for external beam therapy. http://www.acr.org/~/media/ACR/Documents/PGTS/standards/ROPhysicsExtBeamTherapy.pdf. Accessed 15 Feb 2017.

71. Goitein M, Jermann M. The relative costs of proton and X-ray radiation therapy. Clin Oncol. 2003;15(1):S37–50.

72. Lievens Y, Pijls-Johannesma M. Health economic controversy and cost-effectiveness of proton therapy. Semin Radiat Oncol. 2013;23(2):134–41.

73. Zietman AL. The titanic and the iceberg: prostate proton therapy and health care economics. J Clin Oncol. 2007;25(24):3565–6.

74. Konski A, Speier W, Hanlon A, et al. Is proton beam therapy cost effective in the treatment of adenocarcinoma of the prostate? J Clin Oncol. 2007;25(24):3603–8.

75. Lundkvist J, Ekman M, Ericsson SR, et al. Proton therapy of cancer: potential clinical advantages and cost-effectiveness. Acta Oncol. 2005;44(8):850–61.

# Brachytherapy

# 48

Amandeep Singh Taggar, Antonio L. Damato,
Gil'ad N. Cohen, Laszlo Voros, and Yoshiya Yamada

## Learning Objectives

- To understand the role of brachytherapy in CNS malignancies.
- To develop an understanding of radiobiology of brachytherapy and learn how this can beneficial in CNS malignancies.
- To learn about various isotopes utilized in brachytherapy.
- To provide an overview of various brachytherapy techniques, including low-dose rate and high-dose rate as well as plaque brachytherapy techniques.
- To summarize available data on the use of brachytherapy for various CNS sites and malignancies.

## Evolution of Brachytherapy in CNS

Brachytherapy is one of the oldest forms of radiation therapy as its application for cancer treatment was first described in 1903, shortly after discovery of radium by Marie Curie in 1898 [1]. Hirsch first employed brachytherapy for CNS tumors using radium in 1912 [2], followed by Frazier in 1920 [3] and then by Harvey Cushing, who implanted "radium bomb" into the surgical cavity [4]. However, he was disappointed in the results of brachytherapy and radiation in general due to no improvement in survival of patients with malignant gliomas. Therefore, he abandoned this treatment

A. S. Taggar (✉)
Department of Radiation Oncology, Sunnybrook Odette Cancer Center, Toronto, ON, Canada

Department of Radiation Oncology, University of Toronto, Toronto, ON, Canada
e-mail: aman.taggar@sunnybrook.ca

A. L. Damato · G. N. Cohen · L. Voros
Department of Medical Physics, Memorial Sloan Kettering Cancer Center, New York, NY, USA

Y. Yamada
Department of Radiation Oncology, Memorial Sloan Kettering Cancer Center, New York, NY, USA

approach, and it is seldom mentioned in his writings or teachings [5].

With technological advances in the 1960s and 1970s, especially with development of stereotactic methods and high-energy external beam therapy treatment machines, interest in using radiation for malignant brain tumors reemerged. Over the past four decades, despite significant efforts to improve outcomes for high-grade malignant gliomas using multimodality treatments that include surgery, chemotherapy, and radiation, survival has remained dismal, and nearly all patients will have either rapid tumor progression or recurrence [6, 7]. Patterns of failure studies have shown that >90% of malignant gliomas recur within 2 cm of resection margin. Efforts to escalate radiotherapy dose to decrease local recurrences have gained much interest, especially with development of stereotactic radiosurgery (SRS) as well as advancement of brachytherapy (BT) techniques. Brachytherapy has the advantage of delivering extremely high doses of radiation directly to the tumor site while sparing normal tissue.

## Radiobiology of Brachytherapy

Studies have shown that when radiation is delivered at lower-dose rates, there are significantly lower rates of normal tissue complications, with no impact on tumor control or overall survival [8–10]. Haie-Meder et al. illustrated that by decreasing dose rate from 0.8 to 0.4 cGy/h, there was 15% (45% vs. 30%) reduction in late complications. Similarly, by reducing dose rate from 0.6–1 cGy/h to 0.3–0.6 cGy/h, Mazeron et al. showed a reduction in necrosis from 29% to 12% and observed no significant change in tumor control.

This phenomenon is known as the dose rate effect, i.e., as the dose rate is lowered, the biological effect is reduced and so are the side effects. This is more pronounced in the ranges of 1–100 cGy/h and more so in normal tissue compared to tumors. As dose rates are lowered, the slope of survival curve becomes progressively shallower as a greater proportion of sublethal damage is potentially repaired. Experimental models have shown that reducing dose rate from 1.54 to 0.37 Gy/h results in more cell kill for a given absorbed dose. This is explained by the fact that at a certain dose rate range, cells can move through cell cycle but then are blocked in G2 phase of cell cycle which is relatively more radiosensitive [11]. Furthermore, $\alpha/\beta$ ratio of normal brain tissue is estimated to be between 2 and 3, whereas for malignant gliomas, it ranges from 8 to 10 [12, 13]. This may further explain improved therapeutic effect observed by LDR-based radiotherapy approaches. Using these values of $\alpha/\beta$, Qi et al. predicted that a combination of EBRT and LDR brachytherapy would provide highest BED for malignant gliomas as well as accounts for sparing of normal tissue and an improvement in therapeutic ratio [12]. Furthermore, the late responding tissues (normal brain in this case) generally repair more slowly with a longer half-life (T1/2) than early responding tissues, which generally have shorter T1/2 [14]. Hence the rapid dose falloff and normal tissue sparing that brachytherapy provides make it an attractive option for treatment of CNS tumors.

cern for surrounding critical structures. At the same time, a highly localized dose profile may not be suitable for treatment of deep-seated disease.

Figure 48.1 shows the dose profiles of typically used isotopes in brachytherapy. The dose profiles of high-energy photon-emitting isotopes (e.g., iridium-192 (Ir-192), cobalt-60 (Co-60), ytterbium-169 (Yb-169)) approximate the inverse-square falloff, with small radiation attenuation and scatter corrections. The dose profiles of low-energy photon-emitting isotopes (such as iodine-125 (I-125), palladium-103 (Pd-103), or cesium-131 (Cs-131)) are strongly influenced by the photoelectric attenuation in the tissue and are therefore less penetrating than high-energy sources, but the dose to the target and critical organs is more sensitive to the source placement. Charged particles on the other hand are characterized by even steeper dose profiles. Here the dose cloud is concentrated within a few millimeters of the sources. As such, the treatment for those isotopes is often limited by the dose at the surface of the source (phosphorus-32 (P-32); ytterium-90 (Y-90)).

## Physics of Brachytherapy

### Types of Sources Used for Brachytherapy

Various radioactive sources are used in brachytherapy. They can be high-dose rate (HDR) or low-dose rate (LDR) sources; they can be implanted permanently or placed temporarily to deliver a specific dose of radiation. The selection of a source is based on the dose rate, energy, type of emission, half-value layer, and its half-life. Common sources used in CNS brachytherapy are summarized in Table 48.1.

### Dose Specification

In general the dose delivered is closely related to the isotope used. The more localized the dose profile, the lower the con-

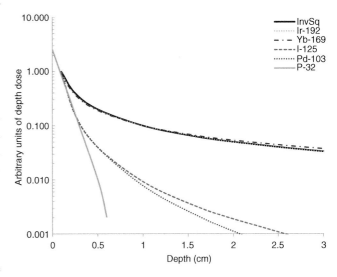

**Fig. 48.1** Depth dose profiles of common brachytherapy sources

**Table 48.1** Brachytherapy sources and their characteristics

| Radioactive isotope | Emission | Mean energy (MeV) | Dose rate (Gy/h) | HVL (in water) | Half-life (days) |
|---|---|---|---|---|---|
| Iridium-192 | Gamma | 0.380 | | 65 mm | 73.83 |
| Iodine-125 | X-ray | 0.028 | Permanent, 0.07 temporary, 0.5–0.6 | 17 mm | 59.4 |
| Cesium-131 | X-ray | 0.030 | Permanent, 0.34 | 18 mm | 9.7 |
| Phosphorus-32 | Beta | 0.695 (Max = 1.7) | 40–802 | Range in water = 7 mm | 14.28 |
| Yttrium-90 | Beta | 0.934 (Max = 2.27) | 40–80 | Range in water = 12 mm | 2.67 |
| Samarium-53 | Beta | 0.225 | | Range in the bone = 1 mm | 1.93 |

## Treatment Delivery Methods

### Permanent Seed Implant

Permanent implantation of low-energy seeds (I-125 or Cs-131), also known as stereotactic brachytherapy, is an effective way to provide dose to the resection cavity while sparing surrounding normal tissue. Seeds are typically provided embedded in sterile suture strands by the manufacturer. Additional, non-sterile seeds from the same seed batch can in some cases be obtained for calibration, and reimbursement of the cost of the additional seeds is in general allowed by insurance. In these cases, the AAPM (American Association of Physicists in Medicine) recommends [15] ordering an additional 5% non-stranded extra seeds or five seeds, whichever is fewer, and calibration can occur before the beginning of the surgical procedure. Alternatively, calibration can be performed in the operating room on 10% or two strands (whichever is larger). Techniques for the batch calibration of stranded seeds while maintaining sterility have been described [16]. In the operating room, the suture strands are cut to the desired length and placed 5 mm to 1 cm apart by the neurosurgeon with the radiation oncologist guidance. Strands can also be sutured into permanent meshes to be used for implantation. Good clinical photography at the time of the implant can simplify the task of seed reconstruction during postoperative dosimetry evaluation. For the evaluation, a CT is acquired 1–7 days after implantation to permit seed reconstruction. An MRI can be fused to the CT to assist with anatomical segmentation. Various reports exist on the clinical use of permanent seed implant to the brain [17–24]. Advantages of this technique include good dose conformity and low dose to the surrounding normal tissues (Fig. 48.2), due to the low-energy spectrum of the seeds. Seed migration is not in general a concern, although an isolated case report exists documenting migration, though a mechanism that has not been understood, within the white matter [25].

### Temporary Seed Implant

Temporary implantation of catheters loaded with I-125 seeds of activity of 3–50 mCi (as opposed to <1 mCi typically used for permanent implant) has been described by numerous authors [26–29] and is more prevalent than permanent seed implantation [30]. Also referred to as stereotactic brachytherapy (SBT), it consists in the placement of a stereotactic frame followed by CT imaging that is used to plan the catheter approach to the treatment site (Fig. 48.3). After implantation, another CT scan is performed for catheter reconstruction in the planning system, often fused with MRI for target definition. A satisfactory dose distribution can typically be achieved with only 1–5 seeds, although up to 28 seeds per plan have been reported [30]. Seeds are encapsulated in the tip of a catheter and manually afterloaded in the implanted catheters (Fig. 48.3). Temporary implants with Ir-192 have also been reported [31]. Treatment usually requires irradiation for 1–50 days [30], depending on the desired dose and dose rate. After irradiation is completed, the sources are retrieved, and the implanted catheters are removed.

### Other Treatment Options

The GliaSite was a device commercialized by IsoRay from 2011 to 2016 for the delivery of temporary radiation to postsurgical cavities in the brain [32]. A balloon applicator is positioned in the resection cavity and inflated with saline

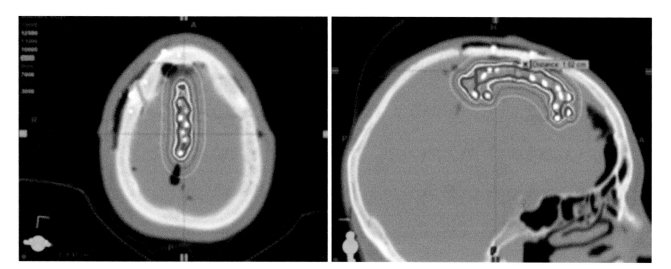

**Fig. 48.2** Post-implantation dosimetry of a permanent brain seed implantation. [Courtesy of Drs. Phillip Devlin and Nils Arvold]

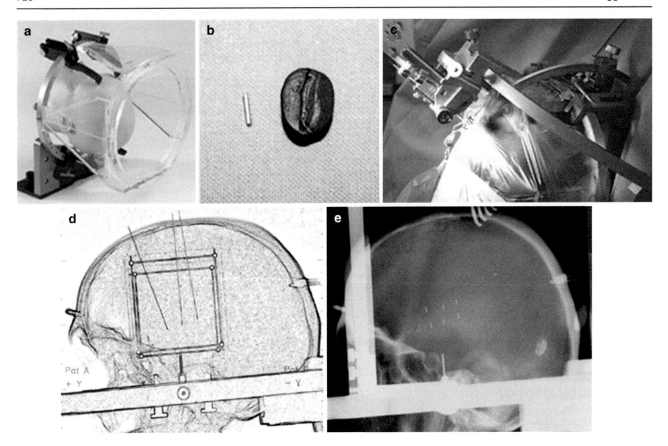

**Fig. 48.3** Steps involved in stereotactic brachytherapy. (**a**) Stereotactic frame with localizer. (**b**) Iodine-125 seed compared to a coffee bean. (**c**) Operative setting with the stereotactic frame, the stereotactic arc, and the inserted seed catheter. (**d**) Positioning of the catheters and seeds, which is then compared with (**e**) the two-plane X-ray images performed after final placement of the seeds' catheters by overlaying. [Courtesy of Dr. Maximilian I. Ruge, MD, PhD, University Hospital of Cologne]

solution to evaluate the desired inflation volume either intra-operatively or with MRI. An access port to the inner lumen of the applicator is secured to the skull and is accessible. Afterward, the saline solution is removed, and an I-125 aqueous source is injected into the balloon. The balloon is then inflated to the planned volume with additional saline solution. Treatment typically lasted 3–7 days, after which the radioactive solution is retrieved and the device may be removed. P-32 use for the treatment of craniopharyngioma has been reported [33]. Other beta-emitting sources have also been used for brain brachytherapy, including Re-186 and Y-90.

## Spinal Plaques

Superficial disease can be treated using electron-emitting sources, achieving even better sparing of underlying structures. A P-32 high-dose rate foil is shown in Fig. 48.4. It is less than 0.35 mm thick and can be placed directly on the surface being treated. With P-32 foils, a treatment of 10 Gy at 1 mm in tissue is delivered. Due to the steep dose profile,

the resulting surface dose is approximately 25 Gy, while typical cord doses are well below 1.0 Gy.

## Spinal HDR Catheters

Vertebral lesions can also be treated with HDR Ir-192 source by inserting catheters directly into vertebral bodies under general anesthesia. As previously described by group from MSKCC [34], catheters can be inserted into the vertebral body:

- Intraoperatively during surgery under direct visualization
- Percutaneously implanted using standard 2D fluoroscopic technique
- Percutaneously implanted using of image-guided surgical navigation systems

Traditional HDR catheter treatments start with placement of the applicators (catheters) into the lesion under fluoroscopic imaging, shown in Fig. 48.5. CT images are then acquired, and a treatment plan is designed based on the

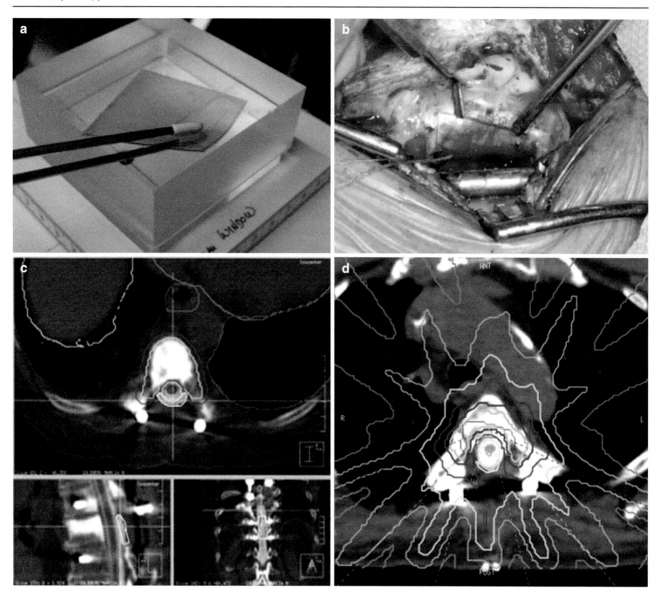

**Fig. 48.4** Spinal P-32 plaque (**a**) and intraoperative application of the plaque (**b**); the plaque is recreated (yellow contour) at the time of external beam treatment (**c**) and made as an avoidance structure. Isodose lines from EBRT plan are shown in (**d**) with spinal dural plaque (in yellow)

given catheters; catheter position is then verified, and treatment is delivered. Multichannel HDR has the advantage to get a more conformal dose to the target tissues. However, it also increases the complexity of the treatment planning. Traditional HDR treatments have been limited by doses to critical structures, such as the cauda, esophagus, and kidneys. Proper source or applicator placement is essential in achieving the separation observed between the dose delivered to the target and structures to be avoided. Oftentimes, the catheter positions have to be optimized prior the insertions (preplanning) in order to get the best possible coverage of the target lesion while minimizing critical structure doses. Preplanned multiple catheter trajectories make the actual catheter placement challenging with the conventional 2D fluoroscopy technique.

The neuro-navigated method described here is one of the most technology intensive techniques in interstitial HDR brachytherapy. A navigation system consists of a CT or CBCT scanner, an infrared or electromagnetic tracking system, special surgical instruments with marking for tracking, and a computer/software for image registration/navigation guidance. Schematic shows setup of an intraoperative 3-dimensional (3D) image (O-arm, Medtronic Navigation, Louisville, CO) system connected with a navigation system (StealthStation Navigation, Medtronic Navigation, Louisville, CO). Prior MRI or CT study can be used to determine the best catheter configuration before the surgery. This optimized configuration (needle trajectories) with the preplanned imaging can be transferred into a navigation system. On the day of the surgery, an optical fiducial (external frame of reference) is

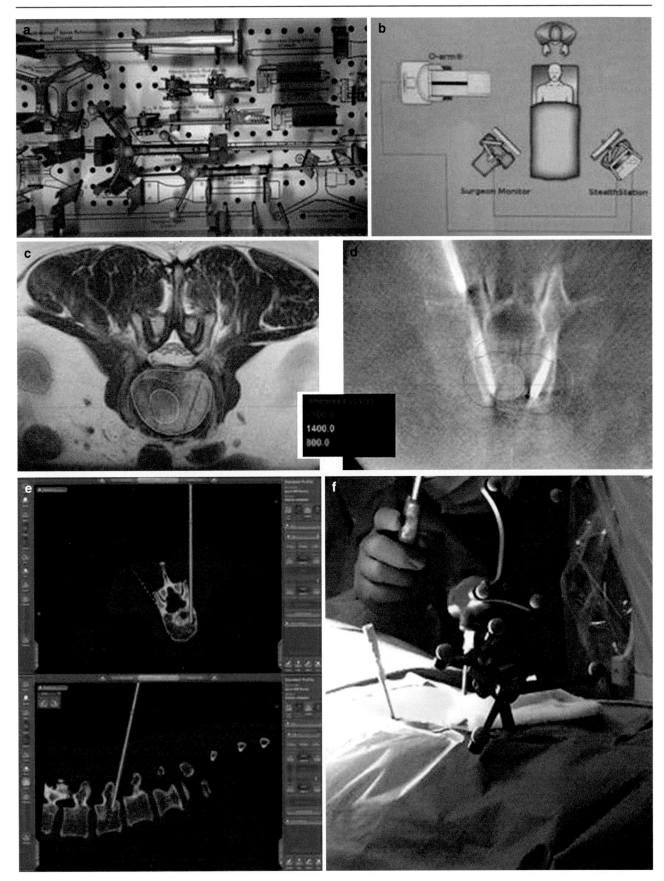

**Fig. 48.5** Neuro-navigated HDR catheter insertion. (**a**) Surgical instruments with passive IR markers, (**b**) navigation system connection setup, (**c**) preplan on diagnostic MRI, (**d**) final catheter insertion, (**e**) axial/sagittal view of navigated PAK needle path (blue line) as progressing over the preplan trajectory (green line) to final position, (**f**) placement of trocars, reference frame, and navigated PAK needle

placed in the patient for registration with the navigation system. An intraoperative (O-arm) CBCT scan is acquired, which is also registered with the navigation system. This scan can be also registered with the previously loaded preplan containing needle positions. Once these two scans are registered to each other, the preplan trajectories and entry points can be transferred into the intraoperative (O-arm) CBCT exam space. This enables the surgeon to pinpoint the entry point on the skin and insert the navigated pedicle access kit (PAK) needle into the vertebral bodies according to the planned trajectory. There are three views (axial, sagittal, coronal) combined with a probe's eye view on the navigation screen to indicate the progress. Final placement and position of the first trocar are shown next to the reference frame and navigated PAK needle. Depth of placement can be checked if needed with fluoroscopic imaging, and a repeated second (O-arm) CBCT scan can be used for verification or final intraoperative planning if an adjustment is necessary. Neuro-navigated HDR catheter insertion can drastically reduce treatment planning time, enabling intraoperative brachytherapy treatment delivery in a shielded OR (operating room) without the necessity of transferring the patient.

## Summary of Clinical Use of Brachytherapy for CNS Lesions

### Brain

#### Introduction

Radiotherapy is essential for treatment of malignant glioma. Impact of radiotherapy dose on survival outcome was established in the 1970s and 1980s and is still maintained [35–37]. However, further attempts to improve survival by increasing radiation dose have shown mixed results [38–40], and higher radiation doses have not been adopted in clinical practice. The primary reason for disappointment in these studies is an increase in toxicity due to higher doses received by normal tissues with external beam techniques. Therefore, alternative approaches for dose escalation, such as interstitial brachytherapy (IBT), were explored. In the proceeding sections of this chapter, we will summarize results of major clinical trials and reports on the use of brachytherapy in primary and recurrent setting for both high-grade and low-grade gliomas as well as metastatic lesions in the brain.

#### High-Grade Glioma

The rationale for brachytherapy in malignant gliomas is based upon following facts:

1. Most malignant gliomas recur locally.
2. In most of the cases, they regrow within 2–3 cm of the original boundary of the primary tumor site.

3. Radiation therapy is one of the most effective tools at our disposal to control their growth.
4. Higher doses of radiation are more effective than lower doses to achieve local control.
5. The radiation emitted by the brachytherapy sources falls off very quickly from the margin, thereby sparing normal brain tissue while delivering very high doses at the center of the tumor.

Early, single-institution reports of brachytherapy in treatment of malignant gliomas indicated encouraging results in selected patients. Typical selection criteria included the Karnofsky performance status (KPS) >70%, well-circumscribed unifocal lesion, supratentorial location, and size <5 (or 6) cm [41–43]. Patients with multifocal or diffuse lesions and those with involvement of the corpus callosum and subependymal region were usually excluded. Table 48.2 summarizes selected publications that used BT in the upfront setting treating malignant gliomas.

Loeffler et al. reported 35 patients implanted with temporary I-125 seeds between 1987 and 1990 at Brigham and Women's Hospital [41]. They compared their results with carefully selected matched cohort (40 patients) from their historical database; these patients were selected based on their eligibility to receive brachytherapy but were never implanted. All 35 patients received maximal safe resection or biopsy followed by external beam radiation (EBRT) to a maximum of 59.4 Gy in 33 daily fractions to the surgical bed plus 3–4 cm margin. Two weeks post-completion of EBRT patients underwent implantation of silicone catheters under stereotactic guidance that were loaded with high-activity I-125 seeds (20–50 mCi, dose rate 30–60 cGy/h). Median BT dose to the residual enhancing tumor was 50.2 Gy (range 37.7–55.4 Gy). Median survival of patients treated with EBRT plus BT was 27 months compared to 11 months for patients treated with EBRT alone. Corresponding 1- and 2-year survival rates were 87% versus 40% ($p < 0.001$) and 57% versus 12.5% ($p < 0.001$), respectively. Forty percent of patients receiving BT required reoperation at median of 6 months post-implantation. Histopathological evaluations revealed radiation necrosis in two patients, while others had microscopic residual disease. There was no perioperative mortality, and procedure-related complications were limited to infection in four patients, an abscess requiring surgery in one patient, and intracranial hemorrhage in one patient at the time of catheter placement. No long-term neurological toxicity was described, but they reported a gradual decline in KPS from 80% at baseline to 70% at 6 months and 60% at 12 months.

The Northern California Oncology Group (NCOG) conducted a single-arm trial of BT boost at the University of California, San Francisco (UCSF), in patients with newly diagnosed glioblastoma multiforme (GBM) and non-

**Table 48.2** Summary of studies using brachytherapy in the initial management of malignant gliomas

| Author | Histology, n | Intervention (isotope, T/P, dose rate cGy/h) | Dose Gy (range) | Follow-up (months) | MS (months) OS | Acute comp | Necrosis | Reoperation |
|---|---|---|---|---|---|---|---|---|
| Loeffler et al. [41] | GBM, 35 | I-125 (T, 30–60) | 50.2 (37.7–55.4) | 15 | 27 1 year = 87% | 17% | 6% | 40% |
| Gutin et al. [42] | GBM, 34 AA, 29 | I-125 (T, 40–60) | 51.2 (42–66.1) 55 (46–75.9) | | 20.5 36.6 | 13% 21% | | 44% 52% |
| Lucas et al. [44] | GBM, 13[a] AA, 7 | Ir-192 (T) | 48 | | 10 22 | 12% | | 9% |
| Prados et al. [43] | GBM, 56 | I-125 (T, 40–60) | 50.1 | | 20.4 3 years = 14% | | | 46% |
| | AA, 32 | | 52.6 | | 37.3 3 years = 32% | | | 56% |
| Scharfen et al. [45] | GBM, 106 NGM, 68 | I-125 (T, 40–60) | 52.9 (40–86.2) 64.4 (37–120) | 33.4 | 20.5 33.1 (HGG) 52.7 (LGG) | 6% G3, 1% G4, <1% G5 | 5% | 40% |
| Malkin et al. [46] | GBM, 20 | I-125 (T, 23–50) | 59.7 (53.2–70.3) | | 22 | 9% G3, 2% G5 | | 40% |
| Wen et al. [47] | GBM, 56 | I-125 (T, 30–60) | 50 | 18 | 18 1 year = 83% | | 17% | 64% |
| Fernandez et al. [48] | GBM, 18 AA, 40 | I-125 (P) | 102 | | 23 >31 | | | 45% |
| Laperriere et al. [49] | AA, 63 | I-125 (T, 21–125) | 60 (57.2–67.7) | | 15.7 | 24%, 6.3% G3 | 17% | 31% |
| Videtic et al. [50] | GBM, 53 | I-125 (P) | 104 | 11 | 16 2 years = 42% | | | |
| Selker et al. [51] | GBM, 123 AA, 10 AO, 3 Mixed, 1 | I-125 (T) | 60 (±10%) | 19.5 | 15.9 | | | |
| Welsh et al. [52] | GBM, 20 | I-125 (T, GliaSite) | 50 (38–70) | 36 | 11.5 | | 10% | |
| Wernicke et al. [53] | GBM, 4 AA, 2 | I-125 (T, GliaSite) | 52 (45–60) | 38 | 17.6 | 0 | 0 | 0 |
| Waters et al. [54] | GBM, 11 | I-125 (n = 9) (T, GliaSite) Ir-192 (n = 2) (T, Mammosite) | 60 | 19 | 15.6 2 years = 42.4% | 9% | 0 | 0 |
| Kickingereder et al. [55] | GBM, 103 | I-125 (T, 4.04) | 60 (30–60) | 9.8 | 11.1 1 year = 45.6% | 7.5% | 1.5% | 0% |

*GBM* glioblastoma multiforme, *AA* anaplastic astrocytoma, *AO* anaplastic oligodendroglioma, *T* temporary, *P* permanent, *MS* median survival, *OS* overall survival, *Acute comp* acute complications (comps include CSF leak, seizure, infection, abscess, meningitis, G3 edema, scalp dehiscence, catheter migration, PE)
[a]Includes six patients with recurrent GBM tumors

glioblastoma anaplastic glioma (NGM) between 1982 and 1990 [42]. A total of 101 patients were enrolled; however, only 63 patients were implanted with temporary I-125 seeds (10–40 mCi, dose rate 40–60 cGy/h). All patients underwent surgical resection, EBRT (up to 60 Gy) and concurrent hydroxyurea followed by BT implant and adjuvant chemotherapy with a combination of lomustine (CCNU), procarbazine, and vincristine (PCV). With median survival of 88 weeks for GBM patients and 157 weeks for NGM patients, this study supported the findings of Loeffler et al., in the setting of newly diagnosed GBM. The reoperation rate in this study was similar at 47.6%, and focal necrosis and edema were the main indications for reoperation. Patients who underwent reoperation had longer median survival

compared to those who did not. Furthermore, patients receiving BT maintained stable or only slightly decreasing KPS (91% at baseline versus 78% at 30 months for NGM patients; 86% at baseline versus 75% at 24 months for GBM patients) and were on either no steroids or stable steroid doses. The authors concluded that while BT boost improved survival in GBM patients, it had no impact on survival of patients with NGM, when compared to their historical data. Two other studies from UCSF with higher number of patients those were not enrolled on the trial, reported similar findings [43, 45]. Prados et al. found that 50% required reoperation, mostly due to symptomatic necrosis, and nonetheless, concluded that BT lengthened survival in select newly diagnosed GBM patients [43]. Reoperation rate in the

Scharfen et al. series was 38% for GBM and 44% high-grade NGM, at median time of 33.1 weeks [45]. The histopathology evaluation showed that 66% of patients undergoing reoperation had both microscopic tumor and radiation necrosis, whereas 5% of patients had necrosis only.

Based on encouraging results of these earlier experiences, two randomized, phase III studies were conducted to compare efficacy of brachytherapy boost in the setting of newly diagnosed malignant glioma. Laperriere et al. at the University of Toronto (UT) enrolled a total of 140 patients with malignant astrocytoma from 1986 to 1996 and randomized them to surgery, EBRT (50 Gy in 25 daily fractions), and oral lomustine with ($n = 71$) or without ($n = 69$) interstitial brachytherapy boost (60 Gy) with temporary I-125 implants [49]. Sixty-three out of 71 patients randomized to BT arm were actually implanted, whereas 8 patients did not receive an implant because of tumor progression (5 cases), death from myocardial infarction (2 cases), and pulmonary embolus (1 case). Intention-to-treat analysis found that median survival of patients in the BT arm was not different from EBRT arm, 13.8 versus 13.2 months, respectively ($p = 0.48$). However, the median survival for the cohort that actually received an implant was slightly higher (15.7 months), and the Cox proportional analysis showed a trend toward improved survival with BT ($p = 0.007$). Ultimately, factors found to be associated with significantly improved survival were age <50, KPS >90, reoperation, and chemotherapy at the time of recurrence. Furthermore, there was 24% rate of acute complications reported in the BT arm and patients required higher doses of steroids, likely due to high rates of necrosis. Interestingly, reoperation rate was same in both arms (31% in implant arm vs. 33% in non-implant arm). The group performed detailed histopathological analysis on all reoperation specimens [56]. Although there was higher amount of necrosis within the tumor samples, the difference in degree of vessel sclerosis, fibrosis, fibrous exudate, calcium deposition, lymphocytic infiltrate, and cystic changes within tumor tissue were not statistically different in implanted patients compared to control group. Nevertheless, these results led the authors to conclude that radiation dose intensification is unlikely to improve survival for most patients with malignant glioma, and hence they abandoned the practice after the conclusion of the trial.

Selker et al. conducted a multi-institutional, phase III trial that compared patients undergoing surgery, EBRT (60.2 Gy in 35 fractions to enhancing tumor plus 3 cm), and Carmustine (BCNU) ($n = 137$) to the same plus interstitial brachytherapy ($n = 133$) using I-125 temporary sources to deliver 60 Gy to enhancing volume with up to 1 cm margin [51]. At median follow-up of 83.4 weeks, there was an approximately 10-week difference in median survival of patients with or without BT at 68.1 versus 58.8 weeks, respectively. This difference, however, was not statistically significant,

$p = 0.101$. Similar to experience by Laperriere et al., among GBM patients, KPS and age were noted to have significant survival differences, hazard ratios 2.67 ($p = 0.0001$), and 1.27 ($p < 0.011$), respectively.

Although, single-institution, retrospective series showed the advantage of radiation dose intensification with BT, two phase III randomized control trials failed to show any survival benefit in newly diagnosed malignant glioma, especially those amenable to surgical resection. Therefore, many neurosurgeons and radiation oncologists have now abandoned the practice in this setting. Nonetheless, some clinicians continue believe that higher dose, when delivered with appropriate means, may lead to improvement in survival. Hence they continue to strive to find new and innovative ways to deliver higher radiation doses to tumor site and surgical bed. Welsh et al. described the use of GliaSite RTS BT in 20 patients accrued in a single-arm prospective protocol opened at 8 different institutions in the USA between 2000 and 2004 [52]. All patients received maximal safe resection and implantation of GliaSite device at the time of surgery followed by 60 Gy of EBRT and adjuvant temozolomide (ten patients). Two to 4 weeks postoperatively, patients returned to the clinic, and the balloon was filled with an aqueous solution of organically bound I-125 (Iotrex [sodium 3-(125I)-iodo-4-hydroxybenzenesulfonate]) with median activity and dose rates of 232 mCi (90–457 mCi) and 53.3 cGy/h (42–64 cGy/h). A reference dose of 50 Gy (38–70 Gy) was prescribed to a depth of 1.0 cm, and the radioisotope solution was left in situ for 78.5 h (67–164 h). Sixteen (80%) of the enrolled patients belonged to recursive partitioning analysis (RPA) class 5 and 6, which generally have median survival of 8.9 months and 4.6 months, respectively. Authors reported a median survival of 11.4 months in these patients with RPA class 5/6 and concluded that additional 3-month survival gain represented a 43% increase in survival which was reported to be significant, $p = 0.03$. They further concluded that GliaSite RTS is safe in delivering brachytherapy boost in the initial management setting, as well as reducing the local recurrences within 2 cm of balloon surface. Others have also confirmed these findings and reported median survival of 15.6–17.6 months for newly diagnosed GBM, treated with surgery, brachytherapy boost using GliaSite RTS, EBRT, and chemotherapy [53, 54]. No grade 3 toxicity was reported in these series. Grade 2 seizures and temporary hemiparesis were observed in 18% of patients. Unfortunately, the company has stopped manufacturing and producing GliaSite RTS, and to our knowledge, there are no ongoing or planned prospective trials evaluating efficacy of brachytherapy with GliaSite in contemporary setting.

Despite disappointing results discussed above in the initial management of GBM, there still may be a role for brachytherapy in situations where the tumor is located in eloquent parts of the brain or is technically challenging to resect. In a study by Kickingereder et al., 201 patients were implanted with low-dose-rate I-125 seeds [55]. One hundred three (51%) patients were with newly diagnosed GBM who were inoperable due to location of tumor. Only patients with tumor diameter <5 cm (before 1997) and <4 cm (after 1997) with KPS >60% were included. A median dose of 60 Gy (30–60 Gy) was prescribed to the gadolinium-enhancing tumor using temporary LDR I-125 seeds (dose rate 4.04 cGy/h). All patients then underwent EBRT to a median dose of 25.2 Gy in 1.8 Gy daily fractions, while temozolomide was given to 31% of patients. At median follow-up of 9.8 months, progression-free and overall survival was 6.2 months and 11.1 months, respectively. Procedure-related transient and permanent complication rates were 7.5% and 2%, respectively, and late grade 3 toxicity (mostly necrosis) was 1.5%. Toxicity was mostly related to the excessive edema associated with larger tumor volumes. The authors concluded that upfront LDR brachytherapy treatment may be an acceptable treatment option for patients with tumors located in eloquent locations that are inoperable.

## Summary

The current standard for treatment of newly diagnosed malignant glioma includes maximal safe resection or biopsy plus external beam radiation plus concurrent and adjuvant temozolomide [57]. Brachytherapy as a part of upfront treatment of malignant glioma has fallen out of favor, especially due to no significant improvement in overall survival seen in two randomized control trials and potential high rates of necrosis. Necrosis, however, can be viewed as the desired effect of radiation, especially within the tumor [46]. Most of the necrotic tissue is absorbed by the circulating macrophages, and the remaining can be removed by craniotomy. Therefore, reoperation after necrosis is part of the management process, rather than a complication. Furthermore, brachytherapy may have an important role in treatment of deep-seated tumors or tumors in eloquent areas of the brain, where adequate dose cannot be delivered with EBRT techniques.

## Low-Grade Glioma

Unlike malignant gliomas, there are no phase III randomized control studies that evaluated efficacy of brachytherapy in low-grade gliomas. Our understanding and recommendations come from single or multi-institutional reports, most of which are summarized in Table 48.3. Theoretically, LDR brachytherapy may have a higher benefit in low-grade gliomas from a radiobiological standpoint. As discussed earlier, due to continuous low-dose irradiation, the therapeutic ratio is increased in part due to ongoing repair of sublethal damage, which has been shown to be more effective in normal tissue compared to neoplastic cells. Furthermore, tumor cells tend to synchronize in the radiosensitive G2 and

M phase as the dose rate is lowered from 154 to 37 cGy/h [11, 70]. Further lowering the dose rate results in less cell kill because of repopulation effect. In low-grade gliomas, however, repopulation is of minor consequence as these are very slow-growing tumors. Therefore, a protracted course of irradiation with very low-dose rates (<10 cGy/h) emerges as a rational treatment strategy [71]. Furthermore, intra-tumoral placement of radiation sources results in highly ablative dose to the middle of the tumor, with steep dose decrease to the periphery. Finally, continuous low-dose radiation also exhibits characteristics of ultra-hyperfractionated radiotherapy particularly at the boundary of the treatment volume [14]. Consequently, unlike malignant glioma, many clinicians that offer brachytherapy implants for low-grade gliomas prefer irradiation sources with much lower-dose rates (<10 cGy/h) as illustrated in discussion in the following paragraphs.

Kreth et al. published one of the first and the largest patient series on the use of brachytherapy in WHO grade I and II gliomas [59]. A total 455 patients were treated between 1979 and 1991, either with permanent I-125 seed implant (1979–1985) or with temporary I-125 sources with dose rate of 10 cGy/h (after 1985), to reference doses of 100 Gy and 60 Gy, respectively. Histological classifications included pilocytic astrocytomas (PA, $n = 97$), grade II astrocytoma ($n = 250$), oligoastrocytoma (OA, $n = 60$), oligodendroglioma (OD, $n = 27$), and gemistocytic astrocytoma (GA, $n = 21$). At median follow-up of 72 months for all surviving patients, corresponding 5- and 10-year OS rates of 85% and 83% for pilocytic astrocytomas and 61% and 51% for grade II astrocytomas were reported. Five-year OS for patients with OA, OD, and GA was 49%, 50%, and 32%, respectively. Authors also reported very low perioperative mortality and morbidity rates of 0.9% and 1.8%, respectively. Radiogenic complications, mostly radionecrosis, were observed in 2.5% patients; this was only noted in patients who received permanent implant. They updated their experience in 2005 on patients with supratentorial grade II astrocytoma ($n = 187$) and oligoastrocytomas ($n = 52$) [61]. They not only confirmed their previous findings but also reported tumor response rates (complete response $n = 18$, partial response $n = 33$, stable disease $n = 146$) as well as malignant transformation rates of 33%, 54%, and 67% at 5, 10, and 15 years, respectively. Updated results showed higher rate of radiogenic complications at 11.3%; eight patients sustained permanent damage (seven required surgery, and one required long-term steroids). Others have also reported similar success rates, morbidity, and long-term complications with the use of temporary I-125 implants for inoperable supratentorial, de novo, or recurrent low-grade gliomas [63, 67].

Although surgery (or microsurgery) is the standard for LGG [72, 73], rates of gross total resection (GTR) in eloquent areas of the brain, especially in pediatric population, range from 0% to 50% [74–76]. Furthermore, surgical

**Table 48.3** Summary of studies using brachytherapy in the initial management of low-grade gliomas

| Author | Histology, n | Intervention (isotope, T/P, dose rate cGy/h) | Dose Gy (range) | Follow-up (months) | 5-year PFS | 5-/10-year OS | Neurological status: improved (1) stable (2) | Necrosis | Perioperative mortality/ morbidity |
|---|---|---|---|---|---|---|---|---|---|
| Mundinger et al. [58] | BSG, 26 | Ir-192 (P, 4.55) | 120 | 40.8 | | 27% | | | 2.4%ᵃ/6.2% |
| | BSG, 29 | I-125 (P, 1.32) | 100 | | | 33% | | | |
| Kreth et al. [59]ᵇ | PA, 97 | I-125 (P, before 1985; T, 1985, 10) | 100 (P) | 72 | MTR₅: 35% | 85%/83% | 1—24.3% | 2.6% | 0.9%/1.8% |
| | GII A, 250 | | 60 (T) | 55 | | 61%/51% | 2—51.7% | | |
| | OA, 60 | | | 52 | | 49% | | | |
| | OD, 27 | | | 76 | | 50% | | | |
| | GA, 21 | | | 52 | | 32% | | | |
| Chuba et al. [60] | BSG, 10ᶜ | I-125 (P, 4) | 82.9 | 7–43 | | MS 8.4 months | | | 0% |
| Kreth et al. [61] | A, 187 | I-125 (P&T) | 100 (P) | 10.3 years | 42% MTR₅: 33% | 56%/37% CR (9%) PR (17%) SD (74%) | | 11.3% | 0.8%/1.2% |
| | OA, 52 | | 60 (T) | | | | | | |
| Peraud et al. [62]ᵇ | Mixed BSG, 11ᵈ | I-125 (T, 10) | 54 | 31.5 | | CR (64%) PR (26%) | 1—45.5% 2—54.5% | 0% | 0% |
| Schnell et al. [63] | Mixed GII, 31ᵈ | I-125 (T, 10) | 54 | 37 | 60% | CR (26%) PR (29%) SD (45%) | | 0% | 0%/27.8% (BT + S) 0%/6.4% (BT) |
| Ruge et al. [64]ᵇ | Mixed GI/II, 147 | I-125 (P, 0.9–30.6 mCi) | 50 (n = 25) 65 (n = 122) | 67.1 | 92% | 93/82% CR (25%) PR (31%) | 1—57.8% 2—23% | 0% | 0%/5.4% |
| Ruge et al. [65]ᵇ | Mixed BSG, 47 | I-125 (P, 3.1) | 65 | 82 | 81% | 97.4%; CR (24%) PR (30%) | 1—50% | 0% | 0%/13% |
| Majdoub et al. [66] | GI/II E, 10ᵉ | I-125 (P&T) | 50–65 (P) | 110 | 100% | 90% CR (17%) PR (58%) SD (25%) 100% CR (11%) PR (56%) SD (33%) | 1—25% | | 0%/4.7% |
| | GIII E, 11ᵉ | | 50 (T) | | | | | | |
| Ruge et al. [67] | Mixed CS GII/III, 60 | I-125 (P) | 50 | 58 | GII 52.5% GIII 34.2% | 94.7% 59.4% | 1/2—83% | 1.7% | 0%/27% 0%/10% |
| Lopez et al. [68] | BSG, 10 | I-125 (T, 9.16) | 60 | 72.5 | 60% | 60% | 1/2—100% | | 0%/0% |
| Kunz et al. [69]ᵇ | GI/II, 58ᶠ | I-125 (T, <12) | 54 | | 87% | 95% CR (17%) PR (48%) SD (34%) | 1—20% 2—14% | 8.6% | 0/6.9% |

*PA* pilocytic astrocytoma, *A* astrocytoma, *OA* oligoastrocytoma, *OD* oligodendroglioma, *GA* gemistocytic astrocytoma, *BSG* brainstem glioma, *E* ependymoma, *CS* central sulcus, *GI* grade 1, *GII* grade 2, *GIII* grade 3, *CR* complete response, *PR* partial response, *SD* stable disease, *MTR₅* malignant transformation rate at 5 years, *BT* brachytherapy, *S* surgery

ᵃIncludes pediatric patients
ᵇIncludes patients without radiation who received biopsy only
ᶜIncludes new and recurrent brainstem gliomas
ᵈDeep-seated and eloquent area gliomas
ᵉTreatment included primary adjuvant and recurrent
ᶠIncludes progressive tumors post-chemotherapy

resection results in high rates of permanent postoperative morbidity, reported to be between 12% and 33% [75, 77–79]. In most instances, where GTR is not achieved, EBRT is generally recommended, and the reported long-term control rates are 50–70% [73]. However, with EBRT large volumes of the brain and normal tissue also receive significant doses that result in severe late effects in children, such as neurocognitive damage, growth arrest, endocrinopathies, as well as secondary cancers. Therefore, stereotactic brachytherapy (SBT) that provides ablative dose to the tumor and very little dose outside the target volume is an attractive alternative for pediatric population. This highly specialized technique, however, is performed only at select centers in the world.

The largest series of SBT in pediatric population includes 155 patients treated at the University of Cologne between 1982 and 2009 [64]. Tumors were located either in eloquent areas or were deep-seated and not amenable to GTR with microsurgery. Inclusion criteria for SBT included KPS >60, radiologically well-circumscribed tumors, and diameter <5 cm (before 1995) and <4 cm (after 1995). All patients were treated with "permanent" I-125 seeds (median activity 5.1 mCi, range 0.9–30.6 mCi) to a surface dose of 50 Gy (first 25 patients) or 65 Gy (all remaining patients). Median follow-up was 67.1 months. Five- and 10-year progression-free survival was 92% and 74%, and corresponding overall survival was 93% and 82%, respectively. 24.6% of patients were deemed to have CR, 31% PR, and 29.6% stable disease. 14.8% of patients presented with tumor recurrence or progression at a median of 36.3 months (6.6–147.6 months). Neurologic status improved in 57.8% of patients and stayed stable in another 23% of patients. There was no periopera-tive mortality and overall rate of morbidity was also low (5.4%). SBT-related late complications manifested as endocrinopathies in 4.7% of patients: thyroid dysfunction in four patients, growth hormone deficiency in two patients, and complete pituitary insufficiency in one patient. Given, excellent tumor control and functional outcomes, authors concluded that SBT is safe and effective treatment for small, well-circumscribed unresectable or incompletely resected LGG located in deep or highly eloquent areas of the brain in pediatric population. Furthermore, because children's brain tissue maybe more vulnerable to harmful effects of ionizing radiation, SBT can be considered as a reasonable alternative to EBRT in other settings as well. Others have also reported similar OS (85–95%), PFS (81–87%), and CR/PR rates as well as improvement in neurological status posttreatment in pediatric LGG [59, 62, 65, 69].

As the LGG patients tend to have long survival, the long-term effect of irradiation on the brain and quality of life must be considered. Sneed et al. reported on long-term impact on quality of life in 28 pediatric patients with primary or recurrent LGG [79]. They did not find significant change in median KPS at 3 or 6–12 years posttreatment: 88% (±9) at baseline compared to 87% (±7) and 87% (±7) at 3 and 6–12 years, respectively.

Brainstem LGG is uncommon in adults; however, available small single-institution series suggest SBT can be safely performed [60, 68]. Despite no perioperative mortality or morbidity associated with the procedure, local control with SBT in these series, however, remains disappointing with essentially all patients recurring within months of procedure.

Experience of using brachytherapy for non-glial tumors is limited. Majdoub et al. treated 21 newly diagnosed or recurrent ependymoma patients (WHO grade 1, 1 patient; grade 2, 9 patients; grade 3, 11 patients) with temporary SBT using LDR I-125 sources [66]. In 5 patients, SBT was employed as the primary treatment modality, whereas in 4 patients it was adjuvant treatment and for other 12 it was used as a salvage maneuver. All patients with grade III disease underwent whole brain RT to a dose of 36 Gy. With a median follow-up of 110 months, authors reported 5-year overall and disease-specific survival to be 100% and CR/PR/ stable disease rates of 16.7%/58.3%/25% for grades 1 and 2 and 11%/56%/33% for grade 3 disease.

## Summary

The use of brachytherapy in the management of low-grade gliomas has resulted in comparable survival outcome to historical controls. The patient population in brachytherapy series, however, includes those with deep-seated tumors or tumors located within eloquent areas of the brain. These patients typically have poorer survival, despite having favorable histology, because high enough dose of radiation cannot be delivered without compromising surrounding normal tissue that results in long-term neurocognitive dysfunction. Therefore, employing brachytherapy to deliver highly ablative dose should be considered. Furthermore, at present molecular subtyping is critical for defining appropriate treatment regimens, especially when targeted therapies can significantly improve survival in select patients. In patients, where current targeted regimens may not achieve desired results, escalating radiation dose with brachytherapy may be beneficial. This, however, needs to be tested in prospective randomized setting.

## Recurrent Gliomas

As it stands now, brachytherapy has limited role in upfront treatment of malignant glioma. It may have a place in the treatment of recurrent gliomas, where prior radiation to the normal tissues limits the delivery of adequate dose to sterilize the recurrent tumor cells. Initial experience in recurrent glioma setting was reported using temporary I-125 sources, as these were commonly used for CNS brachytherapy at the time and are summarized in Table 48.4.

Gutin et al. first described the use of I-125 temporary implants using CT-based stereotaxis at UCSF in recurrent gliomas and metastatic lesions [80]. With typical dose of 3000–12,000 rads with high-activity sources, overall response rate in their cohort was 68%; 11 out of 37 patients had clinical deterioration. With median follow-up of 9 months for recurrent malignant glioma patients only, the overall survival was 48%. Radiation necrosis was identified in five (14.7%) patients; two underwent reoperation, and the other three were treated with steroids. All five patients were

**Table 48.4** Summary of studies using brachytherapy in the initial management of recurrent gliomas

| Author | Histology, n | Intervention (isotope, T/P, dose rate cGy/h) | Dose Gy (range) | Follow-up (months) | PFS (months) | MS (months) | Comps | Necrosis | Reoperation |
|---|---|---|---|---|---|---|---|---|---|
| Gutin et al. [80] | AA, 18 GBM, 13 | I-125 (T, 20–100) | 30–120 | 9 | | 48% at 9 months | 10.8% | 14.7% | |
| Gutin et al. [81] | AA, 23 GBM, 18 | I-125 (T, 25–100) | 57.4–120 | | | 35.7 12.1 | 9.8% | | 47.8% 33.3% |
| Willis et al. [82] | AA, 12 | I-125 (T) | 130 | 6–50 | | 1-year OS 60% | | 41.1% | 47% |
| Scharfen et al. [45] | GBM, 66 NGM, 67 | I-125 (T, 40–60) | 52.9 (40–86.2) 64.4 (37–120) | 33.4 | | 11.4 12.1 HGG 18.9 LGG | | 5% | 40% |
| Malkin et al. [46] | GBM, 24 AA, 12 | I-125 (T, 23–50) | 59.7 (53.2–70.3) | | 10 | | | | 40% |
| Kitchen et al. [83] | GBM/AA (23) | I-125 (T) | 50 | | 5.8 | | | | 8.7% |
| Bernstein et al. [86] | AA, 46 | I-125 (T, 68) | 70 | | | 10.7 | 11% | 26% | 26% |
| Tatter et al. [32] | AA, 6 GBM, 15 | I-125[a] (T, 41–61) | 40–60 | 21.8 patient years | | 17.9 8 | 24% | | |
| Chan et al. [85] | GBM, 24 | I-125[a] (T, 41–70) | 53.1 | 21.8 | | 9.1 | 8.3% | 8.3% | |
| Gabayan et al. [86] | GIII/IV, 94 | I-125[a] (T, 52.3) | 60 | 13.3 | 4.4 | 8.5 1-year OS 31% | 7.4% | 3.2% | |
| Kickingereder et al. [55] | GBM, 98 | I-125 (T, 7.53) | 60 (30–60) | 9.8 | 6.2 | 10.4 | 7.5% | 1.5% | 0% |
| Schwartz et al. [87] | GIII GBM N = 68 | I-125 (T, 4.5–21.6) | 50 | 13.8 | 8.3 | 28.1 9.3 | | 2.9% | |

*GBM* glioblastoma multiforme, *AA* anaplastic astrocytoma, *T* temporary, *P* permanent, *MS* median survival
Comps include CSF leak, seizure, infection, abscess, meningitis, G3 edema, scalp dehiscence, catheter migration, PE
[a]GliaSite radiation therapy system

long-term survivors. The authors updated their experience and reported on a total of 41 patients, all with diagnosis of recurrent malignant glioma [81]. Compared to the historical controls treated with chemotherapy, they found brachytherapy had significant impact on survival, with median survival of 52 weeks for GBM patients and 153 weeks for anaplastic astrocytoma patients. Reoperation rate, unfortunately, was high (40%) in brachytherapy patients, but there was no significant decline in quality of life (QOL) as indicated by median KPS of 80% at the time of successive follow-up compared to 90% prior to implant.

Investigators at the University of Toronto implanted 46 recurrent astrocytoma patients and observed median survival of 46 weeks with a minimum follow-up of 12 months in all patients [84]. KPS of ≥80 vs. <80 at the time of implant was the only prognostic factor that correlated with survival (56 weeks vs. 38 weeks, $p = 0.02$). They noted high rate of necrosis requiring reoperation in 26% of patients. These results, however, were not confirmed by others performing SBT I-125 implants for recurrent gliomas [83].

A plausible explanation for the high rates of radiation necrosis observed in these initial series was dose inhomogeneity with individual seed implantation. Furthermore, I-125

seed implantation involved multiple invasive procedures from installation of stereotactic frame to drilling multiple holes in the skull to place catheters. Therefore, other devices that can deliver high doses more homogenously were sought. GliaSite radiation therapy system (RTS) is one such device, first described by Tatter et al. [32] and discussed in detail in earlier sections. Twenty-one patients with recurrent high-grade astrocytoma were prospectively treated at multiple institutions across the USA. An aqueous solution of organically bound I-125 was instilled in the GliaSite balloon to deliver 40–60 Gy. Authors found that with follow-up of 21.8 patient years, the overall median survival was 12.7 months (8 months for GBM and 17.9 months for AA and OD patients). They did not report any radiation necrosis in their cohort; however, 23.8% patients suffered from procedure-related adverse events that included pseudomeningocele (1), infection (2), and aseptic meningitis (3). At the time, this new device generated enthusiasm among clinicians treating recurrent glioma with radiation and resulted in multiple publications [85, 86, 88, 89]. These reports corroborate initial findings of Tatter et al.'s trial; however, there was no survival or quality of life gain with GliaSite RTS; hence, interest in the use of this product has faded.

Presently there is a renewed interest in using I-125 seeds in combination with temozolomide for newly diagnosed and recurrent malignant gliomas. Two separate reports describe implantation of LDR temporary seeds in recurrent malignant glioma patients [55, 87]. With radiation dose that ranged from 30 to 60 Gy at the tumor margin, median survival was of 10.5 months [55] and 13.4 months [87]. Although survival results are not very impressive in these two series and are comparable to others, the rates of radiation necrosis were extremely low at 1.5% and 2.9%, respectively, especially when compared to historical data [80, 81, 83, 84].

## Summary

Brachytherapy is an effective treatment option for recurrent glioma, especially in the setting when normal brain tissue has seen significant previous radiation. Reported outcomes are encouraging with low rates of perioperative complications and toxicity in long-term survivors.

## Metastatic Lesions

Whole brain radiotherapy (WBRT) and/or supportive care are standard for patients with multiple brain metastases. Surgery, although considered as a standard for solitary metastasis, cannot eliminate microscopic disease at the operative site. Therefore, adjuvant radiation is indicated to improve local control; moreover, surgical plus radiotherapy interventions when combined improve overall survival [90]. Acute and long-term adverse effects associated with WBRT, however, significantly limit its benefit. Other methods of delivering adjuvant radiation include brachytherapy (BT) that employs interstitial implant at the time of resection or stereotactic radiosurgery (SRS) using external beam techniques.

A summary of published literature is provided in Table 48.5. Earlier reports that described interstitial brachytherapy (IBT) for metastatic lesions were mixed with inclusion of other primary CNS lesions [44, 81]. Ostertag et al. published the first largest series of 93 patients with new and recurrent solitary brain metastatic lesions treated with resection followed by I-125 BT alone ($n = 34$) or BT plus EBRT ($n = 38$) for newly diagnosed solitary brain metastasis or BT alone for recurrent lesions ($n = 21$) [92]. BT dose was 60 Gy, and patients with BT + EBRT arm received additional 40 Gy with EBRT. Median survival for patients with recurrent tumors was 6 months post-interstitial implant. Survival was not different for BT alone or BT + EBRT arms, 15 months vs. 17 months, respectively. Importantly, unlike earlier series [44, 81], Ostertag et al. did not report any radiation necrosis or patients requiring reoperation. Bogart et al. from the University of Syracuse reported on 15 patients with solitary brain metastases from non-small cell lung cancer, treated with resection and permanent I-125 seeds to a much higher dose (range 80–160 Gy) [93]. With a median follow-up of 14 months, they reported overall survival of 14 months and relapse in only 3 patients. None of the patients, however, recurred within 2.5 cm of implant. These findings were confirmed by three separate series using permanent I-125 implants post-resection, and that delivered even higher doses of radiation [17, 18, 96]. The local control rates were 88–96%, and median survival ranged from 11.8 to 17.8 months. Rate of symptomatic radiation necrosis was 7.5–23% and was generally associated with larger tumor size. An important feature of Petr et al.'s report was that 67 out of 72 (93%) patients never required WBRT [17]. Recently Shi et al. from the University of Sun Yat-sen and Raleigh et al. from the UCSF reported on permanent I-125 seed implantation

**Table 48.5** Summary of studies using brachytherapy in the initial management of brain metastasis

| Author | n | Isotope (T/P) | Dose, Gy (range) | Median FU (months) | LC | Survival (months) | Comps | Necrosis |
|---|---|---|---|---|---|---|---|---|
| Ostertag et al. [90] | A—38 B—34 C—34 Total = 93 | | 60 | | | A—17 B—15 C—6 | | |
| Bogart et al. [92] | 15 | I-125 (P) | 80–160 | 14 | 80% | 14 | 6.7% | |
| Dagnew et al. [21] | 27 | I-125 (P) | 120–200 at 0.5 cm | 12 | 96% | 17.8 | | 7.4% |
| Huang et al. [18] | 40 | I-125 (P) | 200 (100–300) at 1 cm | 6.1 years | 88% | 11.3 | 13% | 23% |
| Petr et al. [17] | 72 | I-125 (P) | 150 | 16 | 93% | 14 | 1.4% | 5.6% |
| Ruge et al. [26] | 90 | I-125 (T) | 50 | 8.8 | 94.6% | 8.5 | 3.3% | |
| Ruge et al. [27] | 27 | I-125 (T) | 50 | | 96% | 14.8 CR 22.2% PR 50% SD 22.2% | 6.6% | |
| Wernicke et al. [93] | 24 | Cs-131 (P) | 80 at 0.5 cm | 19.3 | 100% | 9.9 | 12.5 | 0% |
| Shi et al. [94] | 24 | I-125 (P) | 130 (90–160) | 19.6 | 62.1% | 2-year OS 83.3% | 4.2% | |
| Raleigh et al. [24] | 95 | I-125 (P) | 135 at 1 cm | 14.4 | 90% | 12 | | 15% |

*A* brachytherapy + external beam RT, *B* brachytherapy only, *C* brachytherapy in recurrent setting, *T* temporary, *P* permanent, *LC* local control
Comps include CSF leak, seizure, infection, abscess, meningitis, G3 edema, scalp dehiscence, catheter migration, PE

of solitary brain metastasis [24, 94]. Shi et al. noted 2-year LC and OS rates of 55% and 83%, respectively, after median follow-up of 19.6 months in patients with metastatic melanoma. Procedure-related complications were minimal and limited to one patient who suffered post-procedural hemorrhage. Raleigh et al. updated a previous experience from their group and reported on 95 new and recurrent (53%) patients of various histologies. LC, OS, complication rates, and late morbidity were similar to what they had previously reported [18, 80, 95].

Wernicke et al. published their experience of 21 patients with newly diagnosed and 3 recurrent patients (previously treated with SRS) that underwent permanent implantation of Cs-131 seeds within the surgical cavity after resection [93]. Cs-131 was selected due to its shorter half-life and with expectation of less radiation necrosis as compared to I-125 seeds reported in other series. At median follow-up of 19.3 months, local freedom from progression (FFP) was 100%; however, distant FFP was 48%, and OS at 1 year was 50%. None of the patients suffered radiation necrosis, but procedure-related complication rate was 12.5% (CSF leak, 1 patient; infection, 1 patient; seizure, 1 patient).

While most groups performing brachytherapy for brain metastasis do permanent implants, a group from the University of Cologne has done temporary LDR I-125 implants [26]. All newly diagnosed and previously irradiated (either with WBRT or SRS) patients were included; with median follow-up of 8.8 (±18.8) months, they reported median survival of 8.5 months. While 1 year local relapse rate was only 5.4% and distant brain failure rate was 46.4%, many patients died of systemic relapse and/or distant brain failure. Importantly there was no grade 3 of higher toxicity or necrosis related to brachytherapy, and the transient morbidity rate was 3.3%, which included CSF leak and infection. The authors then separately reported on patients that received brachytherapy for recurrent tumors post-WBRT or post-SRS [27]. With median survival of 14.8 months, complete response rate as assessed on MRI 3 months post-implant was 22.2%. In both publications, authors observed an average KPS improvement in 94–96% of surviving patients at 3 months following brachytherapy implant.

## Summary

Although SRS has become the mainstay of treatment for limited brain metastasis, brachytherapy with permanent or temporary sources is an attractive alternative for patients with solitary metastasis undergoing resection. Implantation of seeds at the time of resection eliminates protracted postoperative treatment schedules.

## Spine

### Introduction

Radiation myelitis of the spinal cord is one of the most feared complications of the radiation therapy. The spinal cord tolerance to radiation has traditionally been quoted to be between 45 and 50 Gy, in standard fractionation [96, 97]. This limit severely restricts the dose of radiation that can be given safely when using conventional radiotherapy techniques, as many tumors need significantly higher doses of radiation for a reasonable chance of tumor control. The advantages of brachytherapy make it a natural consideration for the treatment of paraspinal tumors. Although the literature is limited, brachytherapy in the spine is an attractive method of improving the therapeutic ratio in the radiotherapy of spine tumors by increasing the total dose delivered to a tumor without significantly increasing the dose delivered to the spinal cord or other nearby dose-sensitive structures. Seminal series of spine brachytherapy are summarized in Table 48.6.

### LDR Brachytherapy in Management of Spinal Lesions

I-125 sources have been the most widely reported isotope used in spinal brachytherapy. Gutin et al. reported the use of I-125 in 13 patients with recurrent primary axial paraspinal and base-of-skull tumors [98]. All patients had undergone prior radiation therapy and multiple surgical interventions. These seeds were placed either as loose seeds via a Mick applicator or as seeds embedded in polyglactin suture and glued with biologic adhesive. Seeds were placed into circular or linear arrays using stereotactic localization. Prescribed doses ranged from 70 to 150 Gy. Chordomas ($N = 5$) and

**Table 48.6** Summary of studies using brachytherapy in the management of spinal lesions

| Author | Isotope | N | Dose, Gy | Notes |
|---|---|---|---|---|
| Gutin et al. [98] | I-125 | 13 | 70–150 | Platinum foil cord shield |
| Kumar et al. [99] | I-125 | 2 | | 1 patient NED 19 months |
| Armstrong et al. [100] | I-125 / Ir-192 | 14 / 21 | 125 / 30 | 50% LC / 50% LC |
| Hamilton et al. [101] | I-125 | 1 | 120 | Gold foil cord shield |
| Rogers et al. [102] | I-125 | 30 | 50–160 | Post-EBRT, no myelitis 73% 2 years OS |
| Delaney et al. [103] | Ir-192 / YT-90 | 3 / 5 | 10 / 10 | 1/3 NED / 1/5 NED |
| Folkert et al. [104] | P-32 | 68 | 10 | LR 18.5% with plaque vs. 34% without ($p = 0.04$) |
| Folkert et al. [34] | Ir-192 (HDR) | 5 | 14 (12–18) | 100% control |

malignant meningioma ($N = 3$) were the most common histologies. Of the nine patients with at least 6-month follow-up, six patients had experienced tumor progression. These results underscore the technical difficulty of implanting sources in these tumors. Even though I-125 emits a relatively low-energy photon, because of the proximity of the spinal cord, extreme care must be taken not to implant too closely to the cord, because the dose given by any one seed in very close proximity to the source is extremely high. Platinum foil was used in one case to shield the spinal cord. The use of gold foil to protect the spinal cord for brachytherapy has also been reported by Hamilton et al. [101]. In a 28-year-old patient with multiply recurrent chondrosarcoma at T2–4 causing epidural cord compression, two layers of gold foil, 0.025 mm thick, were laid in place over the thecal sac after resection of the recurrent tumor. Sixty I-125 seeds were sutured into place in the resection cavity to give 120 Gy at 5 mm. The cord dose with shielding was less than 5%. The patient was reported to be well without evidence of recurrence 18 months after the procedure. Although the use of a foil is an excellent protection against radiation dose from I-125, it has the disadvantage of shielding the dural surface, which in many tumors with epidural extension is at risk for tumor contamination. Kumar et al. have reported the use of I-125 in the management of previously irradiated clival and sacral chordomas [99]. The sacral chordoma showed excellent initial response, but the patient died 3 years post-implant after developing meningeal carcinomatosis with chordoma cell contamination. A previously irradiated clival chordoma was implanted via transnasal approach. This patient was reported to be well 19 months after the procedure.

At the Memorial Sloan Kettering Cancer Center, 35 patients with paraspinal tumors underwent brachytherapy using low-dose Ir-192 temporarily ($n = 21$) or permanent I-125 implantation ($n = 14$) [101]. The median dose for patients receiving Ir-192 was 30 Gy and the 125 Gy with I-125. The spinal cord dose was a median of 20 Gy for Ir-192. Both metastatic disease and primary tumors were treated. All cases were incompletely resected at the time of treatment. Survival was limited in this cohort. Only 23 patients survived longer than 6 months, 16 lived more than 1 year, and 7 survived past 18 months. Dural tumor involvement was a poor prognostic sign. Overall, approximately 50% of patients were locally controlled, but only 22% of these patients were alive beyond the median time to local failure.

The Barrow Neurological Institute reported the use of I-125 brachytherapy in 30 consecutive patients, of which 25 brachytherapy procedures had adequate follow-up for reporting purposes [102]. I-125 seeds in vicryl suture were placed in the resection site. Gelfoam was placed around the dura, and seeds were placed over the Gelfoam to provide approxi-

mately 4 mm distance between the seed and the dural surface. The mean prescribed dose was 101 Gy (50–160 Gy). Most patients also had external beam radiation (mean dose 37.9, range 12–50.4 Gy). With a mean follow-up of nearly 20 months, 87% and 73% actuarial survival was reported at 2 and 3 years, respectively. The mean calculated central spinal cord dose was found to be 33 Gy, giving a composite central spinal cord dose of 70 Gy when external beam radiation was factored in. In those patients who had prior external beam and brachytherapy was the sole form of salvage, the mean central spinal cord dose was 67 Gy (22–167 Gy). No adverse sequelae, including no cases of myelitis were noted.

## Dural Plaque Brachytherapy of Spinal Lesions

Recent advances in image-guided technology have significantly improved the accuracy of delivery of very high-dose radiation therapy to spinal tumors, making it safe to give very high doses of radiation within very close proximity of the spinal cord. However, even with stereotactic body radiotherapy or proton beam radiation techniques, the treatment of contaminated dura is problematic. Delaney et al. have reported the use of a yttrium-90 (Y-90) dural plaque to boost the dura with 10–20 Gy intraoperatively [103]. Y-90 is a short-range beta-particle-emitting isotope, which makes it particularly well suited for dural application. The dose falloff is very steep. The plaque is placed directly on the region of interest (Fig. 48.4). While dura receives 100% of the prescribed dose, the surface of the spinal cord typically receives less than 10% of the dural surface dose. Because of its very low-energy radiation, Y-90 has the added advantage of posing little radiation safety risks to operating room staff. With the use of intensity-modulated radiotherapy, a dose constraint on the dural surface can be applied at the time of postoperative radiation treatment planning to account for the radiation given intraoperatively with the plaque. This allows the inverse treatment planning algorithm to deliver a higher and more homogenous dose to the rest of the tumor resection cavity. With this technique, they report local control of disease in six out of eight patients with no acute or long-term neurological complications [103].

The group at MSKCC has reported the use of phosphorus-32 (P-32) embedded in a thin flexible plastic film to sterilize the dura after decompression of epidural disease [104, 105]. P-32 has a similar shallow depth dose curve to Y-90 but has a longer shelf life and when embedded in a thin plastic film, can be cut to the appropriate shape intraoperatively. Thus, P-32 is easily shielded and can also be used in standard operating theaters with minimal radiation safety concerns. This approach allows for more intraoperative flexibility and avoids the need for preoperative fabrication of a dural plaque required for Y-90. At median follow-up of 10 months in 68 patients treated with P-32 plaque therapy, they report local relapse of 25.5%. In the subgroup of patients who were able to undergo EBRT (single-fraction, hypofractionated, or standard fractionation RT) after surgery and dural plaque therapy, local relapse was significantly lower, 18.5% vs. 34% for those who did not ($p = 0.04$).

## HDR Brachytherapy in Management of Painful Vertebral Lesions

Spine metastasis will develop in 10–40% of cancer patients, resulting in bony pain and vertebral instability. External beam (fractionated or single fraction) is the primary treatment and resolution of pain is variable with <50% to >90% of patients reporting some improvement. Failure rates are high, and repeat irradiation is challenging due to normal tissue tolerance and risk of severe permanent toxicity. Brachytherapy is particularly advantageous in these situations, where a sharp dose drop-off is necessary to protect normal tissues. Folkert et al. described their experience at MSKCC where they used high-dose rate Ir-192 for previously irradiated, painful, and progressive spinal metastasis [34]. Radiation was delivered using intraoperatively or percutaneously placed catheters (Fig. 48.5). At median follow-up of 9 months, they reported 100% control of the disease, and four out of five patients had complete (two) or partial (two) reduction of symptoms.

Stability of spinal column is an important consideration in management of vertebral lesions, and interventions, such as kyphoplasty or vertebroplasty, are often necessary to stabilize the spine. Adjuvant treatment with radiation, however, is still needed for symptom management and tumor control, which is two-step process. Ways to develop one-step treatment for unstable vertebral lesions led to the development of radionuclides being directly injected into the bone at the time kyphoplasty. For example, samarium-153 (Sm-153) has been mixed in with polymethyl methacrylate (PMMA) during kyphoplasty [106]. Sm-153 is a bone-seeking radiopharmaceutical that is often used as an injectable radionuclide to treat bone metastases. It is also mainly a beta-emitting radioisotope with ranges of 0.5 and 3.0 mm in water. Hence it is also a very short range radiation source and can only treat a limited distance from the source, which will limit the amount of tumor that this approach an effectively treat to within a few millimeters of the PMMA.

## Summary

Brachytherapy is an attractive treatment alternative for spinal lesions especially where dural contamination is expected. Spinal plaques can sterilize the dura, while single fraction or fractionated EBRT can be delivered effectively without compromising coverage. In certain scenarios where a patient has received multiple prior radiation courses, HDR brachytherapy can be effective for palliation.

## Case Studies

### Case 1

A 63-year-old woman was diagnosed with breast cancer in 1998 and underwent surgery, adjuvant radiation, and hormone therapy. In 2011, she presented with metastatic disease to the brain, liver, and lung. She underwent stereotactic radiosurgery to the right parietal lobe and right tentorium with CyberKnife. In 2012, she developed three separate spinal recurrences. She underwent surgery for two of the recurrences and palliative radiation (30 Gy in 10 fractions) to the third recurrence. She now presented with re-recurrence at the previously irradiated spinal lesion.

The workup, which included MRI of the brain and spine as well as PET/CT scan, did not show evidence of any other disease, except for the known lesion in spine. Given the absence of any other disease as the indolent nature of the cancer, a multidisciplinary team decision to aggressively treat this lesion was reached. She underwent resection of the recurrence as well as intraoperative P-32 plaque therapy (15 Gy, single placement) to sterilize the dura around the spinal cord. The size of the plaque was determined intraoperatively based on the length of the treatment. Figure 48.4 shows an example of placement of the P-32 dural plaque over the posterior spine after the resection of the tumor. The patient underwent stereotactic body radiotherapy (SBRT) to the rest of the surgical cavity. The area treated by the P-32 plaque was meticulously documented and created as an avoidance structure during SBRT to avoid overdosing spinal cord.

### Case 2

A 44-year-old man with thyroid cancer presented with metastatic disease at T11 causing cord compression with posterior T10, T11, and T12 laminectomy and T9-L1 stabilization and thyroidectomy showing poorly differentiated thyroid cancer in 2014. He developed recurrent spinal cord compression and received palliative radiation to T9-L1 at the end of 2016. Short-interval repeated MRI unfortunately showed persistent cord compression at T11. After discussion at the multidisciplinary case conference, he underwent repeat decompression at T11. To maximize treatment benefit, he was treated with intraoperative P-32 plaque therapy (15 Gy in single placement) with hopes to sterilize microscopic disease over the dura. Refer to Fig. 48.4 for an example of P-32 plaque preparation and placement over the dura post-resection.

## Summary

- Brachytherapy is the placement of radiation sources directly into the tumor and provides highly ablative doses of radiation to the tumor while sparing surrounding normal tissue.
- Low-dose rates of radiation emitted by brachytherapy sources provide radiobiological advantage of decreased normal tissue toxicity compared to higher dose rates of radiation delivered by external beam techniques.
- I-125 is the most common isotope used for brain and spinal brachytherapy.
- Technological advances have allowed placement of brachytherapy sources in deep-seated tumors and tumors at the eloquent areas of the brain that has resulted in excellent clinical outcomes.
- In the setting of recurrent and metastatic brain tumors, placement of brachytherapy sources at the time of surgical resection eliminates protracted external beam radiation courses.
- Dural plaque therapy results in adequate sterilization of tumor cells at the dural surface. This is turn helps in delivery of high doses of EBRT to the rest of the lesion while sparing the spinal cord and dura where plaque therapy was applied.

## Self-Assessment Questions

1. Which of the follow is true regarding brachytherapy of malignant brain gliomas?
   A. The use of brachytherapy has improved overall survival.
   B. Both HDR and LDR brachytherapy have not demonstrated an improvement in overall survival for malignant gliomas.
   C. Brachytherapy can be given without significant toxicity.
   D. Brachytherapy for malignant brain tumors should be done with only beta-emitting isotopes.
   E. None of the above are true.

2. Which of the following are true regarding brachytherapy for malignant gliomas of the brain?
   A. There may be a role for brachytherapy in treating tumors in eloquent areas of the brain that are inoperable.
   B. LDR brachytherapy has not demonstrated a survival advantage for malignant gliomas.
   C. Radionecrosis after LDR brachytherapy is rare.
   D. Stereotactic brachytherapy appears to have a negative impact upon quality of life.

   E. There is no role for LDR brachytherapy in the treatment of malignant gliomas.

3. Regarding the treatment of recurrent brain gliomas:
   A. There is no clear survival advantage with brachytherapy.
   B. Radionecrosis may be associated with dose inhomogeneity.
   C. I-125 is the most commonly used isotope for recurrent brain gliomas.
   D. A typical dose used for recurrent gliomas is 60 Gy.
   E. All of the above are true.

4. Which of the following are true regarding brachytherapy for brain metastases?
   A. With technologies such as stereotactic radiosurgery, brachytherapy has no role in the management of brain metastases.
   B. Cs-131 implantation results in rates of radionecrosis greater than 20%.
   C. The use of I-125 sources for brain metastases results in local failures in excess of 10%.
   D. Brachytherapy has an added advantage over stereotactic radiosurgery in that implanting seeds at the time of resection eliminates protracted treatment with external beam radiation.
   E. None of the above.

5. Regarding spine brachytherapy:
   A. Brachytherapy of the dura should be performed with I-125 plaques.
   B. HDR brachytherapy of the painful spine metatases results in minimal palliation of pain.
   C. P-32 brachytherapy of the dura is best done in a specially shielded operating room.
   D. P-32 dural brachytherapy of the dura is best suited for microscopic residual disease after maximal surgical debulking.
   E. None of the above are true.

6. Which of the following is true regarding spine brachytherapy?
   A. HDR brachytherapy should not be used because it is a high-energy source.
   B. LDR brachytherapy of spine tumors includes the treatment of chordomas.
   C. LDR brachytherapy should not be used in skull base tumors because of the risk of radionecrosis.
   D. When using brachytherapy for spine tumors, supplemental external beam radiotherapy is contraindicated.
   E. None of the above are true.

## Answers

1. B

   Two randomized trials of brachytherapy boosts in the setting of newly diagnosed malignant gliomas have failed to demonstrate an overall survival advantage [42, 49].

2. A

   A large series from Kickingereder et al. [55] and Ruge et al. [66] have described the use of brachytherapy in eloquent and deep-seated areas of the brain.

3. E

   All of the above are true.

4. D

   Brachytherapy at the time of surgical resection provides immediate postoperative radiation and eliminates the need for patients to return for simulation and treatment with external beam radiation [92–96].

5. D

   P-32 has a rapid dose falloff that only penetrates a few millimeters with a therapeutic dose of radiation and best used with minimal residual disease [105, 106].

6. B

   Gutin et al. and Kumar et al. have reported on the use of I-125 for chordomas [99, 100].

## References

1. Goldberg SW, London ES. Zur frage der beziehungen zwischen Becquerel-strahlen und hautaffectionen. Dermatol Zeitschr. 1903;10:457.
2. Hirsch O. Die operative Behandlung von Hypophysentumoren nach endonasalen Methoden. Arch Laryngol Rhinol. 1912;26:529–686.
3. Frazier CH. The effects of radium emanations upon brain tumors. Surg Gynecol Obstet. 1920;31:236–9.
4. Cushing H. Intracranial tumors. Springfield, IL: Charles C Thomas; 1932.
5. Schulder M, Loeffler JS, Howes AE, et al. The radium bomb: Harvey Cushing and the interstitial irradiation of gliomas. J Neurosurg. 1996;84(3):530–2.
6. Sneed PK, Suh JH, Goetsch SJ, et al. A multi-institutional review of radiosurgery alone vs. radiosurgery with whole brain radiotherapy as the initial management of brain metastases. Int J Radiat Oncol Biol Phys. 2002;53(3):519–26.
7. Wallner KE, Galicich JH, Krol G, et al. Patterns of failure following treatment for glioblastoma multiforme and anaplastic astrocytoma. Int J Radiat Oncol Biol Phys. 1989;16(6):1405–9.
8. Haie-Meder C, Kramar A, Lambin P, et al. Analysis of complications in a prospective randomized trial comparing two brachytherapy low dose rates in cervical carcinoma. Int J Radiat Oncol Biol Phys. 1994;29(5):953–60.
9. Lambin P, Gerbaulet A, Kramar A, et al. Phase III trial comparing two low dose rates in brachytherapy of cervix carcinoma: report at two years. Int J Radiat Oncol Biol Phys. 1993;25(3):405–12.
10. Mazeron JJ, Crook JM. Effect of dose rate on local control and necrosis in the reirradiation of faucial arch squamous cell carcinomas with interstitial iridium 192. Int J Radiat Oncol Biol Phys. 1990;18(5):1275.
11. Hall EJ, Brenner DJ. The dose-rate effect revisited: radiobiological considerations of importance in radiotherapy. Int J Radiat Oncol Biol Phys. 1991;21(6):1403–14.
12. Qi XS, Schultz CJ, Li XA. An estimation of radiobiologic parameters from clinical outcomes for radiation treatment planning of brain tumor. Int J Radiat Oncol Biol Phys. 2006;64(05):1570–80.
13. Jones B, Sanghera P. Estimation of radiobiologic parameters and equivalent radiation dose of cytotoxic chemotherapy in malignant glioma. Int J Radiat Oncol Biol Phys. 2007;68(2):441–8.
14. Brenner D, Armour E, Corry P, et al. Sublethal damage repair times for a late-responding tissue relevant to brachytherapy (and external-beam radiotherapy): implications for new brachytherapy protocols. Int J Radiat Oncol Biol Phys. 1998;41(1):135–8.
15. Butler WM, Bice WS, DeWerd LA, et al. Third-party brachytherapy source calibrations and physicist responsibilities: report of the AAPM Low Energy Brachytherapy Source Calibration Working Group. Med Phys. 2008;35(9):3860–5.
16. Butler WM, Dorsey AT, Nelson KR, et al. Quality assurance calibration of 125I rapid strand in a sterile environment. Int J Radiat Oncol Biol Phys. 1998;41(1):217–22.
17. Petr MJ, McPherson CM, Breneman JC, et al. Management of newly diagnosed single brain metastasis with surgical resection and permanent I-125 seeds without upfront whole brain radiotherapy. J Neurooncol. 2009;92(3):393–400.
18. Huang K, Sneed PK, Kunwar S, et al. Surgical resection and permanent iodine-125 brachytherapy for brain metastases. J Neurooncol. 2009;91(1):83–93.
19. Darakchiev BJ, Albright RE, Breneman JC, et al. Safety and efficacy of permanent iodine-125 seed implants and carmustine wafers in patients with recurrent glioblastoma multiforme. J Neurosurg. 2008;108(2):236–42.
20. Chen AM, Chang S, Pouliot J, et al. Phase I trial of gross total resection, permanent iodine-125 brachytherapy, and hyperfractionated radiotherapy for newly diagnosed glioblastoma multiforme. Int J Radiat Oncol Biol Phys. 2007;69(3):825–30.
21. Dagnew E, Kanski J, McDermott MW, et al. Management of newly diagnosed single brain metastasis using resection and permanent iodine-125 seeds without initial whole-brain radiotherapy: a two institution experience. Neurosurg Focus. 2007;22(3):E3.
22. Larson DA, Suplica JM, Chang SM, et al. Permanent iodine 125 brachytherapy in patients with progressive or recurrent glioblastoma multiforme. Neuro Oncol. 2004;6(2):119–26.
23. Wernicke AG, Smith AW, Taube S, et al. Cesium-131 brachytherapy for recurrent brain metastases: durable salvage treatment for previously irradiated metastatic disease. J Neurosurg. 2017;126:1212–9.
24. Raleigh DR, Seymour ZA, Tomlin B, et al. Resection and brain brachytherapy with permanent iodine-125 sources for brain metastasis. J Neurosurg. 2017;126:1749–55.
25. Brahimaj B, Lamba M, Breneman JC, et al. Iodine-125 seed migration within brain parenchyma after brachytherapy for brain metastasis: case report. J Neurosurg. 2016;125(5):1167–70.
26. Ruge MI, Suchorska B, Maarouf M, et al. Stereotactic 125Iodine brachytherapy for the treatment of singular brain metastases: closing a gap? Neurosurgery. 2011;68(5):1209–19.
27. Ruge MI, Kickingereder P, Grau S, et al. Stereotactic biopsy combined with stereotactic (125)iodine brachytherapy for diagnosis and treatment of locally recurrent single brain metastases. J Neurooncol. 2011;105(1):109–18.
28. Suchorska B, Ruge M, Treuer H, et al. Stereotactic brachytherapy of low-grade cerebral glioma after tumor resection. Neuro Oncol. 2011;13(10):1133–42.
29. Korinthenberg R, Neuburger D, Trippel M, et al. Long-term results of brachytherapy with temporary iodine-125 seeds in children with low-grade gliomas. Int J Radiat Oncol Biol Phys. 2011;79(4):1131–8.

30. Schwarz SB, Thon N, Nikolajek K, et al. Iodine-125 brachytherapy for brain tumours--a review. Radiat Oncol. 2012;7:30.

31. Koot RW, Maarouf M, Hulshof MC, et al. Brachytherapy: results of two different therapy strategies for patients with primary glioblastoma multiforme. Cancer. 2000;88(12):2796–802.

32. Tatter SB, Shaw EG, Rosenblum ML, et al. An inflatable balloon catheter and liquid 125I radiation source (GliaSite Radiation Therapy System) for treatment of recurrent malignant glioma: multicenter safety and feasibility trial. J Neurosurg. 2003;99(2):297–303.

33. Ansari SF, Moore RJ, Boaz JC, et al. Efficacy of phosphorus-32 brachytherapy without external-beam radiation for long-term tumor control in patients with craniopharyngioma. J Neurosurg Pediatr. 2016;17(4):439–45.

34. Folkert MR, Bilsky MH, Cohen GN, et al. Intraoperative and percutaneous iridium-192 high-dose-rate brachytherapy for previously irradiated lesions of the spine. Brachytherapy. 2013;12(5):449–56.

35. Salazar OM, Rubin P, Feldstein ML, et al. High dose radiation therapy in the treatment of malignant gliomas: final report. Int J Radiat Oncol Biol Phys. 1979;5(10):1733–40.

36. Bleehen NM, Stenning SP. A Medical Research Council trial of two radiotherapy doses in the treatment of grades 3 and 4 astrocytoma. The Medical Research Council Brain Tumour Working Party. Br J Cancer. 1991;64(4):769–74.

37. Walker MD, Strike TA, Sheline GE. An analysis of dose-effect relationship in the radiotherapy of malignant gliomas. Int J Radiat Oncol Biol Phys. 1979;5(10):1725–31.

38. Werner-Wasik M, Scott CB, Nelson DF, et al. Final report of a phase I/II trial of hyperfractionated and accelerated hyperfractionated radiation therapy with carmustine for adults with supratentorial malignant gliomas. Radiation Therapy Oncology Group Study 83-02. Cancer. 1996;77(8):1535–43.

39. Coughlin C, Scott C, Langer C, et al. Phase II, two-arm RTOG trial (94-11) of bischloroethyl-nitrosourea plus accelerated hyperfractionated radiotherapy (64.0 or 70.4 Gy) based on tumor volume (> 20 or < or = 20 cm(2), respectively) in the treatment of newly-diagnosed radiosurgery-ineligible glioblastoma multiforme patients. Int J Radiat Oncol Biol Phys. 2000;48(5):1351–8.

40. Piroth MD, Pinkawa M, Holy R, et al. Integrated boost IMRT with FET-PET-adapted local dose escalation in glioblastomas. Results of a prospective phase II study. Strahlenther Onkol. 2012;188(4):334–9.

41. Loeffler JS, Alexander E, Wen PY, et al. Results of stereotactic brachytherapy used in the initial management of patients with glioblastoma. J Natl Cancer Inst. 1990;82(24):1918–21.

42. Gutin PH, Prados MD, Phillips TL, et al. External irradiation followed by an interstitial high activity iodine-125 implant "boost" in the initial treatment of malignant gliomas: NCOG study 6G-82-2 gliomas: NCOG study 6H-82-2. Int J Radiat Oncol Biol Phys. 1991;21(3):601–6.

43. Prados MD, Gutin PH, Phillips TL, et al. Interstitial brachytherapy for newly diagnosed patients with malignant gliomas: the UCSF experience. Int J Radiat Oncol Biol Phys. 1992;24(4):593–7.

44. Lucas GL, Luxton G, Cohen D, et al. Treatment results of stereotactic interstitial brachytherapy for primary and metastatic brain tumors. Int J Radiat Oncol Biol Phys. 1991;21(3):715–21.

45. Scharfen CO, Sneed PK, Wara WM, et al. High activity iodine-125 interstitial implant for gliomas. Int J Radiat Oncol Biol Phys. 1992;24(4):583–91.

46. Malkin MG. Interstitial implant radiosurgery of brain tumors: radiobiology, indications, and results. In: Wiestler OD, Schlegel U, Schramm J, editors. Molecular neuro-oncology and its impact on the clinical management of brain tumors, Recent results in cancer research, vol. vol 135. Berlin: Springer; 1994.

47. Wen PY, Alexander E, Black PM, et al. Long term results of stereotactic brachytherapy used in the initial treatment of patients with glioblastomas. Cancer. 1994;73(12):3029–36.

48. Fernandez PM, Zamorano L, Yakar D, et al. Permanent iodine-125 implants in the up-front treatment of malignant gliomas. Neurosurgery. 1995;36(3):467–73.

49. Laperriere NJ, Leung PM, McKenzie S, et al. Randomized study of brachytherapy in the initial management of patients with malignant astrocytoma. Int J Radiat Oncol Biol Phys. 1998;41(5):1005–11.

50. Videtic GM, Gaspar LE, Zamorano L, et al. Implant volume as a prognostic variable in brachytherapy decision-making for malignant gliomas stratified by the RTOG recursive partitioning analysis. Int J Radiat Oncol Biol Phys. 2001;51(4):963–8.

51. Selker RG, Shapiro WR, Burger P, et al. The Brain Tumor Cooperative Group NIH Trial 87-01: a randomized comparison of surgery, external radiotherapy, and carmustine versus surgery, interstitial radiotherapy boost, external radiation therapy, and carmustine. Neurosurgery. 2002;51(2):343.

52. Welsh J, Sanan A, Gabayan AJ, et al. GliaSite brachytherapy boost as part of initial treatment of glioblastoma multiforme: a retrospective multi-institutional pilot study. Int J Radiat Oncol Biol Phys. 2007;68(1):159–65.

53. Wernicke AG, Sherr DL, Schwartz TH, et al. Feasibility and safety of GliaSite brachytherapy in treatment of CNS tumors following neurosurgical resection. J Cancer Res Ther. 2010;6(1):65–74.

54. Waters JD, Rose B, Gonda DD, et al. Immediate post-operative brachytherapy prior to irradiation and temozolomide for newly diagnosed glioblastoma. J Neurooncol. 2013;113(3):467–77.

55. Kickingereder P, Hamisch C, Suchorska B, et al. Low-dose rate stereotactic iodine-125 brachytherapy for the treatment of inoperable primary and recurrent glioblastoma: single-center experience with 201 cases. J Neurooncol. 2014;120(3):615–23.

56. Siddiqi SN, Provias J, Laperriere N, et al. Effects of iodine-125 brachytherapy on the proliferative capacity and histopathological features of glioblastoma recurring after initial therapy. Neurosurgery. 1997;40(5):910.

57. Stupp R, Mason WP, van den Bent MJ, et al. Radiotherapy plus concomitant and adjuvant temozolomide for glioblastoma. N Engl J Med. 2005;352(10):987–96.

58. Mundinger F, Braus DF, Krauss JK, et al. Long-term outcome of 89 low-grade brain-stem gliomas after interstitial radiation therapy. J Neurosurg. 1991;75(5):740–6.

59. Kreth FW, Faist M, Warnke PC, et al. Interstitial radiosurgery of low-grade gliomas. J Neurosurg. 1995;82(3):418–29.

60. Chuba PJ, Zamarano L, Hamre M, et al. Permanent I-125 brain stem implants in children. Childs Nerv Syst. 1998;14(10):570–7.

61. Kreth FW, Faist M, Grau S, et al. Interstitial 125I radiosurgery of supratentorial de novo WHO Grade 2 astrocytoma and oligoastrocytoma in adults: long-term results and prognostic factors. Cancer. 2006;106(6):1372–81.

62. Peraud A, Goetz C, Siefert A, et al. Interstitial iodine-125 radiosurgery alone or in combination with microsurgery for pediatric patients with eloquently located low-grade glioma: a pilot study. Childs Nerv Syst. 2007;23(1):39–46.

63. Schnell O, Schöller K, Ruge M, et al. Surgical resection plus stereotactic 125I brachytherapy in adult patients with eloquently located supratentorial WHO grade II glioma - feasibility and outcome of a combined local treatment concept. J Neurol. 2008;255(10):1495–502.

64. Ruge MI, Simon T, Suchorska B, et al. Stereotactic brachytherapy with iodine-125 seeds for the treatment of inoperable low-grade gliomas in children: long-term outcome. J Clin Oncol. 2011;29(31):4151–9.

65. Ruge MI, Kickingereder P, Simon T, et al. Stereotactic iodine-125 brachytherapy for treatment of inoperable focal brainstem gliomas of WHO grades I and II: feasibility and long-term outcome. J Neurooncol. 2012;109(2):273–83.

66. El Majdoub F, Elawady M, Blau T, et al. Intracranial ependymoma: long-term results in a series of 21 patients treated with stereotactic (125)iodine brachytherapy. PLoS One. 2012;7(11):e47206.

67. Ruge MI, Kickingereder P, Grau S, et al. Stereotactic iodine-125 brachytherapy for the treatment of WHO grades II and III gliomas located in the central sulcus region. Neuro Oncol. 2013;15(12):1721–31.

68. Lopez WO, Trippel M, Doostkam S, et al. Interstitial brachytherapy with iodine-125 seeds for low grade brain stem gliomas in adults: diagnostic and therapeutic intervention in a one-step procedure. Clin Neurol Neurosurg. 2013;115(8):1451–6.

69. Kunz M, Nachbichler SB, Ertl L, et al. Early treatment of complex located pediatric low-grade gliomas using iodine-125 brachytherapy alone or in combination with microsurgery. Cancer Med. 2016;5(3):442–53.

70. Hall EJ, Giaccia AJ. Radiobiology for the radiologist. 7th ed. Philadelphia, PA: Wolters Kluwer; 2011.

71. Kreth FW, Thon N, Siefert A, et al. The place of interstitial brachytherapy and radiosurgery for low-grade gliomas. Adv Tech Stand Neurosurg. 2010;35:183–212.

72. Freeman CR, Farmer JP, Montes J. Low-grade astrocytomas in children: evolving management strategies. Int J Radiat Oncol Biol Phys. 1998;41(5):979–87.

73. Recinos PF, Sciubba DM, Jallo GI. Brainstem tumors: where are we today? Pediatr Neurosurg. 2007;43(3):192–201.

74. Sandri A, Sardi N, Genitori L, et al. Diffuse and focal brain stem tumors in childhood: prognostic factors and surgical outcome. Experience in a single institution. Childs Nerv Syst. 2006;22(9):1127–35.

75. Farmer JP, Montes JL, Freeman CR, et al. Brainstem gliomas. A 10-year institutional review. Pediatr Neurosurg. 2001;34(4):206–14.

76. Lesniak MS, Klem JM, Weingart J, et al. Surgical outcome following resection of contrast-enhanced pediatric brainstem gliomas. Pediatr Neurosurg. 2003;39(6):314–22.

77. Teo C, Siu TL. Radical resection of focal brainstem gliomas: is it worth doing? Childs Nerv Syst. 2008;24(11):1307–14.

78. Pollack IF, Gerszten PC, Martinez AJ, et al. Intracranial ependymomas of childhood: long-term outcome and prognostic factors. Neurosurgery. 1995;37(4):655.

79. Sneed PK, Russo C, Scharfen CO, et al. Long-term follow-up after high-activity 125I brachytherapy for pediatric brain tumors. Pediatr Neurosurg. 1996;24(6):314–22.

80. Gutin PH, Phillips TL, Wara WM, et al. Brachytherapy of recurrent malignant brain tumors with removable high-activity iodine-125 sources. J Neurosurg. 1984;60:61–8.

81. Gutin PH, Leibel SA, Wara WM, et al. Recurrent malignant gliomas: survival following interstitial brachytherapy with high-activity iodine-125 sources. J Neurosurg. 1987;67(6):864–73.

82. Willis BK, Heilbrun MP, Sapozink MD, et al. Stereotactic interstitial brachytherapy of malignant astrocytomas with remarks on postimplantation computed tomographic appearance. Neurosurgery. 1988;23(3):348–54.

83. Kitchen ND, Hughes SW, Taub NA, et al. Survival following interstitial brachytherapy for recurrent malignant glioma. J Neurooncol. 1994;18(1):33–9.

84. Bernstein M, Laperriere N, Glen J, et al. Brachytherapy for recurrent malignant astrocytoma. Int J Radiat Oncol Biol Phys. 1994;30(5):1213–7.

85. Chan TA, Weingart JD, Parisi M, et al. Treatment of recurrent glioblastoma multiforme with GliaSite brachytherapy. Int J Radiat Oncol Biol Phys. 2005;62(4):1133–9.

86. Gabayan AJ, Green SB, Sanan A, et al. GliaSite brachytherapy for treatment of recurrent malignant gliomas: a retrospective multi-institutional analysis. Neurosurgery. 2006;58(4):701.

87. Schwartz C, Romagna A, Thon N, et al. Outcome and toxicity profile of salvage low-dose-rate iodine-125 stereotactic brachytherapy in recurrent high-grade gliomas. Acta Neurochir. 2015;157(10):1757.

88. Payne JT, St Clair WH, Given CA, et al. Double balloon GliaSite in the management of recurrent glioblastoma multiforme. South Med J. 2005;98(9):957–8.

89. Gobitti C, Borsatti E, Arcicasa M, et al. Treatment of recurrent high-grade gliomas with GliaSite brachytherapy: a prospective mono-institutional Italian experience. Tumori. 2011;97(5):614–9.

90. Patchell RA, Tibbs PA, Walsh JW, et al. A randomized trial of surgery in the treatment of single metastases to the brain. N Engl J Med. 1990;322(8):494–500.

91. Ostertag CB, Kreth FW. Interstitial iodine-125 radiosurgery for cerebral metastases. Br J Neurosurg. 1995;9(5):593–603.

92. Bogart JA, Ungureanu C, Shihadeh E, et al. Resection and permanent I-125 brachytherapy without whole brain irradiation for solitary brain metastasis from non-small cell lung carcinoma. J Neurooncol. 1999;44(1):53–7.

93. Wernicke AG, Yondorf MZ, Peng L, et al. Phase I/II study of resection and intraoperative cesium-131 radioisotope brachytherapy in patients with newly diagnosed brain metastases. J Neurosurg. 2014;121(2):338–48.

94. Shi F, Zhang X, Wu K, et al. Metastatic malignant melanoma: computed tomography-guided 125I seed implantation treatment. Melanoma Res. 2014;24(2):137–43.

95. Dagnew E, Kanski J, McDermott MW, et al. Management of newly diagnosed single brain metastasis using resection and permanent iodine-125 seeds without initial whole-brain radiotherapy: a two-institution experience. Neurosurg Focus. 2007;22(3):1–3.

96. Emami B, Lyman J, Brown A, et al. Tolerance of normal tissue to therapeutic irradiation. Int J Radiat Oncol Biol Phys. 1991;21(1):109–22.

97. Kirkpatrick JP, van der Kogel AJ, Schultheiss TE. Radiation dose-volume effects in the spinal cord. Int J Radiat Oncol Biol Phys. 2010;76(3 Suppl):S42–9.

98. Gutin PH, Leibel SA, Hosobuchi Y, et al. Brachytherapy of recurrent tumors of the skull base and spine with iodine-125 sources. Neurosurgery. 1987;20(6):938–45.

99. Kumar PP, Good RR, Skultety FM, et al. Local control of recurrent clival and sacral chordoma after interstitial irradiation with iodine-125: new techniques for treatment of recurrent or unresectable chordomas. Neurosurgery. 1988;22(3):479–83.

100. Armstrong JG, Fass DE, Bains M, et al. Paraspinal tumors: techniques and results of brachytherapy. Int J Radiat Oncol Biol Phys. 1991;20(4):787–90.

101. Hamilton AJ, Lulu B, Stea B, et al. The use of gold foil wrapping for radiation protection of the spinal cord for recurrent tumor therapy. Int J Radiat Oncol Biol Phys. 1995;32(2):507–11.

102. Rogers CL, Theodore N, Dickman CA, et al. Surgery and permanent 125I seed paraspinal brachytherapy for malignant tumors with spinal cord compression. Int J Radiat Oncol Biol Phys. 2002;54(2):505–13.

103. DeLaney TF, Chen GT, Mauceri TC, et al. Intraoperative dural irradiation by customized 192iridium and 90yttrium brachytherapy plaques. Int J Radiat Oncol Biol Phys. 2003;57(1):239–45.

104. Folkert MR, Bilsky MH, Cohen GN, et al. Local recurrence outcomes using the $^{32}$P intraoperative brachytherapy plaque in the management of malignant lesions of the spine involving the dura. Brachytherapy. 2015;14(2):202–8.

105. Folkert MR, Bilsky MH, Cohen GN, et al. Intraoperative 32P high-dose rate brachytherapy of the dura for recurrent primary and metastatic intracranial and spinal tumors. Neurosurgery. 2012;71(5):1003–10.

106. Ashamalla H, Cardoso E, Macedon M, et al. Phase I trial of vertebral intracavitary cement and samarium (VICS): novel technique for treatment of painful vertebral metastasis. Int J Radiat Oncol Biol Phys. 2009;75(3):836–42.

# Index

Printed by Printforce, the Netherlands